K.J. Lee's Essential Otolaryngology

K.J. Lee's Essential Otolaryngology
Head & Neck Surgery
Eleventh Edition

Edited by

YVONNE CHAN, MD, FRCSC, MSc, HBSc
Continuing Education & Professional Development Director,
Department of Otolaryngology—Head & Neck Surgery
Assistant Professor, University of Toronto
Toronto, Ontario, Canada

JOHN C. GODDARD, MD
Otology, Neurotology, and Skull Base Surgery
Department of Otolaryngology—Head & Neck Surgery
Northwest Permanente, PC
Portland, Oregon

New York Chicago San Francisco Athens London Madrid
Mexico City Milan New Delhi Singapore Sydney Toronto

K.J. Lee's Essential Otolaryngology, Eleventh Edition

1 2 3 4 5 6 7 8 9 0   DOC/DOC   20 19 18 17 16 15

ISBN 978-0-07-184992-0
MHID 0-07-184992-0

This book was set in Minion pro by Cenveo® Publisher Services.
The editors were Brian Belval and Christie Naglieri.
The production supervisor was Catherine Saggese.
Project management was provided by Tanya Punj, Cenveo Publisher Services.
RR Donnelley was printer and binder.
This book is printed on acid-free paper.

Library of Congress Cataloging-in-Publication Data

K.J. Lee's Essential otolaryngology : head & neck surgery/edited by Yvonne Chan, John C. Goddard.—Eleventh edition.
     p. ; cm.
    Includes bibliographical references and index.
    ISBN 978-0-07-184992-0 (paperback : alk. paper)-ISBN 0-07-184992-0 (paperback : alk. paper)
I. Chan, Yvonne, 1973-, editor.   II. Goddard, John C. (John Christopher), editor.
    [DNLM: 1. Otorhinolaryngologic Diseases-surgery-Outlines. 2. Otorhinolaryngologic Surgical Procedures-Outlines.   WV 18.2]
  RF58
  617.5'1-dc23
                                                 2015009153

Contents

Part 1   General Otolaryngology   1

Contributors

Peter A. Adamson, MD, FRCSC, FACS [48]
Professor and Head
Division of Facial Plastic and Reconstructive Surgery
Department of Otolaryngology—Head & Neck Surgery
Staff Surgeon
Toronto General Hospital
University Health Network
Ontario, Canada

Vijay K. Anand, MD, FACS [29]
Clinical Professor
Department of Otolaryngology—Head & Neck Surgery
Weill Cornell Medical College
Attending Surgeon
New York Presbyterian Hospital Weill Cornell
    Medical Center
Consultant Surgeon
Department of Surgery
Memorial Sloan Kettering Cancer Center
New York, New York

Oneida Arosarena, MD [49]
Associate Professor
Head and Neck Institute
Temple University
Philadelphia, Pennsylvania

Jamil Asaria, MD, FRCSC [48]
Director
FACE Cosmetic Surgery
Clinical Lecturer
Division of Facial Plastic and Reconstructive Surgery
Department of Otolaryngology—Head & Neck Surgery
University of Toronto
Ontario, Canada

Seilesh Babu, MD [17]
Neurotologist/Skull Base Surgeon
Chief Financial Officer
Michigan Ear Institute
Farmington Hills, Michigan
Clinical Assistant Professor
Department of Otolaryngology
Wayne State University School of Medicine
Detroit, Michigan
Clinical Assistant Professor
Department of Surgery
William Beaumont Oakland University School of
    Medicine
Rochester, Michigan

Victoria Banuchi, MD, MPH [43]
Assistant Professor
Division of Otolaryngology
Weill Cornell Medical Center
New York, New York

Craig Berzofsky, MD [44]
Assistant Professor Otolaryngology
New York Medical College Laryngologist
ENT Faculty Practice
New York, New York

Kathleen C. M. Campbell, PhD [14]
Distinguished Scholar and Professor
Southern Illinois University School of Medicine
Springfield, Illinois

Yvonne Chan, MD, FRCSC, MSc, HBSc [11, 12, 27, 54]
Continuing Education & Professional Development
    Director
Department of Otolaryngology—Head & Neck
    Surgery
Assistant Professor
University of Toronto
Ontario, Canada

Janet Chung, BSc, MD, FRCSC [12]
Lecturer
Department of Otolaryngology—Head & Neck
    Surgery
University of Toronto
Ontario, Canada

Robin T. Cotton, MD [47]
Director, Aerodigestive and Esophageal Center
Cincinnati Children's Hospital
Professor
University of Cincinnati College of Medicine
Cincinnati, Ohio

Marion Couch, MD, PhD, MBA, FACS [8]
Professor and Chair
Department of Otolaryngology—Head & Neck
    Surgery
Physician Executive
IU School of Medicine
Indianapolis, Indiana

David J. Crockett, MD [46]
Pediatric Otolaryngology—Head & Neck Surgery
Arizona Otolaryngology Consultants Section
Vice Chief of Otolaryngology
Phoenix Children's Hospital
Phoenix, Arizona

Subinoy Das, MD, FACS [9, 54]
Medical Director
US Institute for Advanced Sinus Care and Research
Columbus, Ohio

Christopher M. DeBacker, MD, FACS [51]
Assistant Clinical Professor
Department of Ophthalmology
University of Texas Health Science Center at San
    Antonio
San Antonio, Texas

Angela M. Donaldson, MD [29]
Department of Otolaryngology—Head &Neck
    Surgery
Atlanta Institute for ENT
Atlanta, Georgia

Carlos S. Ebert, Jr. MD, MPH [10]
Associate Professor
Department of Otolaryngology—Head &Neck Surgery
University of North Carolina
Chapel Hill, North Carolina

David Eibling, MD, FACS [31]
Professor of Otolaryngology
Department of Otolaryngology—Head & Neck Surgery
University of Pittsburgh School of Medicine
Pittsburgh, Pennsylvania

David W. Eisele, MD, FACS [30]
Andelot Professor and Director
Department of Otolaryngology—Head & Neck
    Surgery
Johns Hopkins University School of Medicine
    Baltimore, Maryland

Carolyn Falls, MClSc, Reg. CASLPO [16]
Manager, Centre for Advanced Hearing and Balance
Manager, Munk Hearing Centre
Lecturer, University of Toronto, Faculty of Medicine
Toronto General Hospital, University Health Network
Ontario, Canada

Jessica Feinleib MD, PhD [4]
Assistant Professor
Department of Anesthesiology
Yale School of Medicine
West Haven, Connecticut

Bruce J. Gantz, MD [22, 24]
Professor and Head
University of Iowa
Department of Otolaryngology—Head & Neck Surgery
University of Iowa Hospitals and Clinics
Iowa City, Iowa

Marion Boyd Gillespie, MD, Msc [32]
Professor
Department of Otolaryngology—Head & Neck
  Surgery
Medical University of South Carolina
Charleston, South Carolina

John C. Goddard, MD [13, 18, 23, 45]
Otology, Neurotology, and Skull Base Surgery
Department of Otolaryngology—Head & Neck Surgery
Northwest Permanente, PC
Portland, Oregon

John E. Godwin, MD, MS [5]
Physician Program Leader, Hematologic Malignancies
Providence Cancer Center Oncology & Hematology
  Care Clinic - Eastside
Robert W. Franz Cancer Research Center in the Earle
  A Chiles Research Institute
Portland, Oregon

Debra Gonzalez, MD [39]
Assistant Professor
Department of Otolaryngology
Washington University School of Medicine
St. Louis, Missouri

Steven Goudy, MD [46]
Director of Pediatric Otolaryngology
Emory University School of Medicine
Atlanta, Georgia

Amandeep S. Grewal, MD, FRCSC [12]
Lecturer
Department of Otolaryngology—Head & Neck Surgery
University of Toronto
Ontario, Canada

Patrick Ha, MD, FACS [30]
Associate Professor
Johns Hopkins Department of Otolaryngology
Johns Hopkins Head and Neck Surgery
Baltimore, Maryland

Heather Herrington, MD [8]
Assistant Professor of Otolaryngology
Head & Neck Surgery
University of Vermont
Burlington, Vermont

Benjamin L. Hodnett [38]
Fellow in Head and Neck Oncology & Microvascular
  Reconstruction
Department of Otorhinolaryngology—Head & Neck
  Surgery
University of Pennsylvania
Philadelphia, Pennsylvania

David E. E. Holck, MD, FACS [51]
EyePlasTX
Associate Clinical Professor
Department of Surgery
The University of Texas at San Antonio, Health
  Sciences Center
San Antonio, Texas

Zain Husain, MD [41]
Assistant Professor
Department of Therapeutic Radiology
Yale University School of Medicine
West Haven, Connecticut

Natalia Issaeva, PhD [42]
Department of Surgery, Otolaryngology
Yale School of Medicine
Yale Cancer Center
New Haven, Connecticut

Ali O. Jamshidi, MD [6]
Department of Neurological Surgery
The Ohio State University Wexner
Columbus, Ohio

Courtney A. Jatana, DDS [34]
Assistant Professor
Division of Oral and Maxillofacial Surgery and
    Anesthesiology
The Ohio State University College of Dentistry
Columbus, Ohio

Kris R. Jatana, MD, FAAP, FACS [34]
Associate Professor-Clinical
Department of Otolaryngology—Head & Neck
    Surgery
The Ohio State University and Nationwide
    Children's Hospital
Columbus, Ohio

Pardis Javadi, MD [54]
Assistant Professor of Otolaryngology,
Head & Neck Surgery
Southern Illinois University
Springfield, Illinois

Jonas T. Johnson, MD, FACS [38]
Distinguished Service Professor of Otolaryngology
The Dr. Eugene N. Myers Professor and Chairman
    of Otolaryngology
University of Pittsburgh School of Medicine
Pittsburgh, Pennsylvania

Robert M. Kellman, MD [50]
Professor and Chair
Department of Otolaryngology and Communication
    Sciences
SUNY Upstate Medical University
Syracuse, New York

David W. Kennedy, MD [26]
Rhinology Professor
Perelman School of Medicine
University of Pennsylvania
Philadelphia, Pennsylvania

Dennis H. Kraus, MD, FACS [43]
Director, New York Head & Neck Institute
Center for Head & Neck Oncology
NS-LIJ Cancer Institute
Professor of Otolaryngology
Hofstra North Shore-LIJ School of Medicine
Hempstead, New York

Jack H. Krouse, MD, PhD, MBA [53]
Professor and Chairman
Department of Otolaryngology—Head & Neck Surgery
Director, Temple Head and Neck Institute
Associate Dean for Graduate Medical Education
Temple University School of Medicine
Philadelphia, Pennsylvania

Andrew P. Lane, MD [25]
Professor
Department of Otolaryngology—Head & Neck Surgery
Director
Division of Rhinology and Sinus Surgery
Johns Hopkins School of Medicine
Baltimore, Maryland

John M. Lee, MD, FRCSC, MSc [26]
Assistant Professor
Department of Otolaryngology—Head & Neck
    Surgery
University of Toronto
St. Michael's Hospital
Ontario, Canada

K. J. Lee, MD, FACS [1, 4, 7, 13, 17, 21, 45, 52, 54]
Associate Clinical Professor
Yale University School of Medicine
Adjunct Associate Clinical Professor
Hofstra University School of Medicine
Emeritus Chief of Otolaryngology
Hospital of St. Raphael
Chief Medical and Experience Officer
IQ-EQ Systems
Intelligent Cloud and Advisory Group
New Haven, Connecticut

Flora Levin, MD, FACS [52]
Clinical Assistant Professor
Yale School of Medicine
New Haven, Connecticut

Jill Mazza, MD [25]
Instructor
Department of Otolaryngology—Head & Neck Surgery
Johns Hopkins University School of Medicine
Baltimore, Maryland

Theodore R. McRackan, MD [18, 23]
Assistant Professor
Otolaryngology Head & Neck Surgery
Division of Neurotology
Medical University of South Carolina
Charleston, South Carolina

Richard T. Miyamoto, MD, FACS, FAAP [20]
Arilla Spence DeVault Professor Emeritus
Department of Otolaryngology—Head & Neck Surgery
Indiana University School of Medicine
Indianapolis, Indiana

Wojciech Mydlarz, MD [30]
Assistant Professor
Department of Otolaryngology—Head & Neck Surgery
Johns Hopkins University School of Medicine
Baltimore, Maryland

James Netterville, MD [35]
Mark C. Smith Professor
Director of Head and Neck Oncologic Services
Executive Vice Chair
Department of Otolaryngology
Vanderbilt University Medical Center
Nashville, Tennessee

Thomas J. Ow, MD, FACS [37]
Assistant Professor
Department of Otorhinolaryngology—Head & Neck Surgery
Department of Pathology
Montefiore Medical Center
Albert Einstein College of Medicine
Bronx, New York

Paige M. Pastalove, AuD, CCC-A, FAAA [15]
Director
Division of Audiology
Assistant Director
Temple Head and Neck Institute
Instructor
Temple University School of Medicine
Philadelphia, Pennsylvania

James E. Peck, PhD [14]
Associate Professor Emeritus
Division of Audiology
Department of Otolaryngology and Communicative Sciences
University of Mississippi Medical Center
Jackson, Mississippi

Natasha Pollak, MD [19]
Associate Professor
Department of Otolaryngology—Head & Neck Surgery
Temple University School of Medicine
Associate Director
Temple Head & Neck Institute
Philadelphia, Pennsylvania

Dr. David Pothier, MSc, MBChB, FRCS (ORL-HNS) [16]
Staff Neurotologist Assistant Professor
Department of Otolaryngology
University of Toronto
Head and Neck Surgery Toronto General Hospital
University Health Network
Ontario, Canada

Daniel Prevedello, MD [6]
Associate Professor of Neurological Surgery
Department of Neurological Surgery
The Ohio State University, Wexner Medical Center
Columbus, Ohio

Evan J. Propst, MD, MSc, FRCSC [47]
Assistant Professor
Department of Otolaryngology—Head & Neck
  Surgery
Hospital for Sick Children
University of Toronto
Ontario, Canada

Gregory W. Randolph, MD, FACS, FACE [33]
Director of the General and Thyroid-Parathyroid
  Endocrine Surgical Divisions
Mass Eye and Ear Infirmary
Member Endocrine Surgery Service
Mass General Hospital
Boston, Massachusetts

Krishna A. Rao, MD, PhD [40]
Associate Professor
Division of Hematology/Medical Oncology
Departments of Internal Medicine, Medical
  Microbiology, and Simmons Cancer Institute
Southern Illinois University School of Medicine
Springfield, Illinois

Shilpa Renukuntla, MD [38]
Assistant Professor
General Otolaryngology
University of South Florida
Tampa, Florida

K. Thomas Robbins, MD, FRCSC, FACS [39]
Professor and Executive Director Emeritus
Simmons Cancer Institute at SIU
Southern Illinois University School of Medicine
Springfield, Illinois

Joseph P. Roche, MD [10]
Neurotology Fellow
Otology, Neurotology & Lateral Skull Base Surgery
Department of Otolaryngology—Head & Neck
  Surgery
The University of Iowa Hospitals and Clinics
Iowa City, Iowa

Allan Rodrigues, MD [7]
Attending Physician
Pulmonary and Critical Care Medicine
Hospital of Saint Raphael
New Haven, Connecticut

Dr. Brian W. Rotenberg, MD, MPH, FRCSC [2]
Associate Professor
Director of Sleep Surgery Program
Sinonasal & Skull Base Surgery
Dept of Otolaryngology—Head & Neck Surgery
Western University, London
Ontario, Canada

John Rutka, MD, FRCSC [16]
Professor of Otolaryngology—Head & Neck Surgery
University of Toronto
Staff Otologist/Neurotologist
University Health Network
Toronto General Hospital
Ontario, Canada

Ryan Scannell, MD [54]
New England ENT & Facial Plastic Surgery
North Andover, Massachusetts

Joseph Scharpf, MD [33]
Staff, Head and Neck Institute
Cleveland Clinic Foundation
Associate Professor of Surgery CCLCM
Cleveland, Ohio

Dimitrios Sismanis, MD [51]
Private Practice
Oculoplastic and Reconstructive Surgery
Richmond, Virginia

Susan L. Tan, BSc(Hon), MD, FRCSC [48]
Facial Plastic and Reconstructive Surgery Fellow
Art of Facial Surgery
University of Toronto
Ontario, Canada

Thomas G. Takoudes, MD [36]
Clinical Instructor in Surgery
Department of Surgery
Division of Otolaryngology—Head & Neck Surgery
Yale University School of Medicine
New Haven, Connecticut

Elizabeth H. Toh, MD, FACS [21]
Director, Balance and Hearing Implant Center
Lahey Hospital & Medical Center
Burlington, Massachusetts

Randal S. Weber, MD [37]
Professor and Chairman Department of Head &
  Neck Surgery
John Brooks Williams and Elizabeth Williams
Distinguished University Chair in Cancer Medicine
Professor of Radiation Oncology
University of Texas MD Anderson Cancer Center
Houston, Texas

Gayle E. Woodson, MD, FACS [44]
Professor Emeritus
Southern Illinois University School of Medicine
Springfield, Illinois

Wendell Yarbrough, MD, FACS, MMHC [42]
Professor & Chief, Otolaryngology Yale
Co-Director, Molecular Virology Program Yale
  Cancer Center
Director, Head and Neck Disease Center, Smilow
  Cancer Hospital
New Haven, Connecticut

Jeff Yeung, MD [11]
Department of Otolaryngology—Head & Neck
  Surgery
University of Ottawa
Ottawa, Ontario

Adam Zanation, MD [28]
Associate Professor
Director of Practice Development
Department of Otolaryngology—Head & Neck
  Surgery
Director of the Skull Base Surgery Fellowship
Co-Director of the Advanced Rhinology and Skull
  Base Surgery Fellowship
Division of Head & Neck Oncology
Division of Rhinology/Sinus Surgery
Skull Base Surgery
Chapel Hill, North Carolina

Preface

It is a privilege and great pleasure for me to introduce two excellent editors for the 11th edition of K. J. Lee's Essential Otolaryngology—Head and Neck Surgery, Dr. Yvonne Chan and Dr. John Goddard.

The first edition of *Essential Otolaryngology*, published in 1973, was based predominantly on my own notes that had helped me through my Board examination. Because of the enthusiastic reception among practicing clinicians and the universal acceptance of this book among residents in the United States and abroad, I have found keeping this book current a most satisfying endeavor. Dr. Anthony Maniglia arranged for the 6th edition to be translated into Spanish by Drs. Blanco, Cabezas, Cobo, Duque, Reyes, and Santamaria. The 7th edition was also translated into Spanish by Drs. Rendón, Araiza, Pastrana, Enriquez, and González. The 8th edition was translated into Turkish by Professor Metin Onerci and Dr. Hakan Korkmaz and translated into Chinese by Professor Chen and her colleagues. A previous edition was also translated into Turkish by Professor Vecdet Kayhan, Doc. Dr. Tayfun Sunay, and Uz. Dr. Cetin Kaleli. It has also been translated into other languages without our knowledge.

Although the original material still forms a significant portion of the book, Dr. Chan and Dr. Goddard have assembled a broad panel of authorities in several subspecialities to present additional information, which is considered the most current in their areas of expertise.

Neither a complete review of otolaryngology nor a comprehensive textbook on the subject, *K.J. Lee's Essential Otolaryngology,* 11th edition, remains true to its original intent—to serve as a guide for Board preparation as well as a practical and concise reference text reflecting contemporary concepts in clinical otolaryngology. Senior medical students, residents, and fellows; Board-eligible, Board-certified otolaryngologists; primary care physicians; and specialists in other fields will all find this edition to be an even more useful and indispensable resource.

I thank Dr. Chan and Dr. Goddard.

K. J. Lee

Acknowledgments

For this 11th edition, I want to thank our two editors, Dr. Yvonne Chan and Dr. John Goddard, who have done a tremendous job. Particularly, I would like to thank the one person who has been by my side even before the appearance of the very 1st edition of this book in 1973, my lovely and devoted wife of 49 years, Linda. Our three sons, Ken, Lloyd, and Mark, used to help with editorial assistance, but are now busy with their respective professions, law, private equity, and movie production; Jeannie Grenier, my nurse for over 31 years and editorial associate, worked hard on previous editions. I thank the McGraw-Hill staff for their diligence, great work, and congeniality.

I thank my parents for the gene and nurturing environment that allowed me to develop a passion for hard work, a sense for organization, and an ability to distill complex materials into simple facts. These are the three cornerstones that have shaped this book from the 1st edition. I am thrilled to see these traits are also inherent in Yvonne and John.

And to those newcomers at the frontiers of medical science who have contributed to this edition, I also extend my thanks for taking the time to share their own expertise and, by doing so, helping to keep this book up-to-date.

K. J. Lee

Part 1
General Otolaryngology

Chapter 1
Syndromes and Eponyms

Syndromes and Diseases

Adult Respiratory Distress Syndrome

Adult respiratory distress syndrome (ARDS) is characterized by a delay in onset (12-24 hours) following injury, shock, and/or successful resuscitative effort. Septic shock, extrathoracic trauma, central nervous system (CNS) pathology, fat embolism, oxygen toxicity, head and facial injuries, and massive blood transfusions can lead to ARDS. It is characterized by hypoxia and pulmonary infiltrates secondary to increased pulmonary vascular permeability, microvascular hemorrhage, or both.

Aide Syndrome

Aide syndrome is characterized by decreased pupillary reaction and deep tendon reflex. The etiology is unknown.

Alagille Syndrome

Alagille syndrome is marked by cardiovascular abnormalities, characteristic facial appearance, chronic cholestasis, growth retardation, hypogonadism, mental retardation, vertebral arch defect, temporal bone anomalies in the cochlear aqueduct, ossicles, semicircular canals (SCCs), and subarcuate fossa. Liver transplantation is a possible treatment.

Albers-Schönberg Disease

A genetic disorder also known as osteopetrosis, Albers-Schönberg disease results in progressive increase in the density (but also increase in weakness) of the bones in the skeletal system. Vascular nutrition to affected bones is also decreased by this disease. Broken down into three categories, there is osteopetrosis with precocious manifestations, osteopetrosis with delayed manifestations, and pyknodysostosis. In the mandible long-term antibiotic therapy, multiple debridements, sequestrectomies, or even resection are possible treatments.

Albright Syndrome

Polyostotic fibrous dysplasia usually manifests early in life as multicentric lesions involving the long bones and bones of the face and skull with scattered skin lesions similar to melanotic café au lait spots and precocious puberty in female patients. Frequently, there is an elevation of serum alkaline phosphatase as well as endocrine abnormalities.

Aldrich Syndrome

Thrombocytopenia, eczema, and recurrent infections occur during the first year of life. It is inherited through a sex-linked recessive gene. The bleeding time is prolonged, the platelet count is decreased, and the bone marrow megakaryocytes are normal in number.

Amalric Syndrome

Granular macular pigment epitheliopathy (foveal dystrophy) is associated with sensorineural hearing loss. Visual acuity is usually normal. Amalric syndrome may be a genetic disorder, or it may be the result of an intrauterine rubella infection.

Aortic Arch Syndrome

See Takayasu Disease.

Apert Syndrome

Apert syndrome is not to be confused with Pfeiffer syndrome, which has different types of hand malformations.

Ascher Syndrome

Ascher syndrome is a combination of blepharochalasis, double lip, and goiter.

Auriculotemporal Syndrome (Frey Syndrome)

Auriculotemporal syndrome is characterized by localized flushing and sweating of the ear and cheek region in response to eating. It usually occurs after parotidectomy. It is assumed that the parasympathetic fibers of the ninth nerve innervate the sweat glands after parotidectomy. It has been estimated that 20% of the parotidectomies in children result in this disorder.

Avellis Syndrome

Unilateral paralysis of the larynx and velum palati, with contralateral loss of pain and temperature sensitivity in the parts below the larynx characterize Avellis syndrome. The syndrome is caused by involvement of the nucleus ambiguus or the vagus nerve along with the cranial portion of the ninth nerve.

Babinski-Nageotte Syndrome

Babinski-Nageotte syndrome is caused by multiple or scattered lesions, chiefly in the distribution of the vertebral artery. Ipsilateral paralysis of the soft palate, larynx, pharynx, and sometimes tongue occurs. There is also ipsilateral loss of taste on the posterior third of the tongue, loss of pain and temperature sensation around the face, and cerebellar asynergia. Horner syndrome with contralateral spastic hemiplegia and loss of proprioceptive and tactile sensation may also be present.

Baelz Syndrome

Painless papules at the openings of the ducts of the mucous glands of the lips with free exudation of mucus are characteristic. Congenital and familial forms are precancerous. Acquired forms are benign and caused by irritating substances.

Bannwarth Syndrome (Facial Palsy in Lymphocytic Meningoradiculitis)

A relatively benign form of acute unilateral or bilateral facial palsy that is associated with lymphocytic reactions and an increased protein level in the cerebrospinal fluid (CSF) with minimal, if any, meningeal symptoms is known as Bannwarth syndrome. Neuralgic or radicular pain without facial palsy and unilateral or bilateral facial palsy of acute onset are symptoms of this syndrome. A virus has been suggested as a possible etiology. Males are more often affected than females, with the greatest number of cases occurring in the months of August and September.

Barany Syndrome

Barany syndrome is a combination of unilateral headache in the back of the head, periodic ipsilateral deafness (alternating with periods of unaffected hearing), vertigo, and tinnitus. The syndrome complex may be corrected by induced nystagmus.

Barclay-Baron Disease

Vallecular dysphagia is present.

Barre-Lieou Syndrome

Occipital headache, vertigo, tinnitus, vasomotor disorders, and facial spasm due to irritation of the sympathetic plexus around the vertebral artery in rheumatic disorders of the cervical spine are characteristic. It is also known as cervical migraine.

Barrett Syndrome

Barrett syndrome is characterized by esophagitis due to change in the epithelium of the esophagus.

Barsony-Polgar Syndrome

A diffuse esophageal spasm, caused by disruption of the peristaltic waves by an irregular contraction resulting in dysphagia and regurgitation, is evidence of this syndrome. It most commonly affects excitable elderly persons.

Basal Cell Nevoid Syndrome

This familial syndrome, non–sex-linked and autosomal dominant with high penetrance and variable expressivity, manifests early in life. It appears as multiple nevoid basal cell epitheliomas of the skin, cysts of the jaw, abnormal ribs and metacarpal bones, frontal bossing, and dorsal scoliosis. Endocrine abnormalities have been reported and it has been associated with medulloblastoma. The cysts in the jaw, present only in the maxilla and mandible, are destructive to the bone. The basal cell epitheliomas are excised as necessary, and the cysts in the jaw rarely recur after complete enucleation.

Bayford-Autenrieth Dysphagia (Arkin Disease)

Dysphagia lusoria is said to be secondary to esophageal compression from an aberrant right subclavian artery.

Beckwith Syndrome

This is a congenital disorder characterized by macroglossia, omphalocele, hypoglycemia, pancreatic hyperplasia, noncystic renal hyperplasia, and cytomegaly of the fetal adrenal cortex.

Behçet Syndrome

Of unknown etiology, this disease runs a protracted course with periods of relapse and remission. It manifests as indolent ulcers of the mucous membrane and skin, stomatitis, as well as anogenital ulceration, iritis, and conjunctivitis. No definitive cure is known, though steroids help.

Besnier-Boeck-Schaumann Syndrome

Sarcoidosis is present.

Bloom Syndrome

An autosomal recessive growth disorder, Bloom syndrome is associated with chromosomal breaks and rearrangements. It is also associated with an unusually high rate of cancer at an early age. Associated with facial erythema, growth retardation, immunodeficiency, infertility, and sun sensitivity, diagnosis is confirmed by chromosome analysis. Anomalous numbers of digits or teeth, asymmetric legs, heart malformation, hypopigmented spots in blacks, protruding ears, sacral dimple, simian line, and urethral or meatal narrowing are less common characteristics. For head and neck tumor patients, there is an increased chance of secondary and primary tumors.

Bogorad Syndrome

Bogorad syndrome is also known as the syndrome of crocodile tears, characterized by residual facial paralysis with profuse lacrimation during eating. It is caused by a misdirection of regenerating autonomic fibers to the lacrimal gland instead of to the salivary gland.

Bonnet Syndrome

Sudden trigeminal neuralgia accompanied by Horner syndrome and vasomotor disorders in the area supplied by the trigeminal nerve are manifestations of this syndrome.

Bonnier Syndrome

Bonnier syndrome is caused by a lesion of Deiters nucleus and its connection. Its symptoms include ocular disturbances (eg, paralysis of accommodation, nystagmus, diplopia), deafness, nausea, thirst, and anorexia, as well as other symptoms referable to involvement of the vagal centers, cranial nerves VIII, IX, X, and XI, and the lateral vestibular nucleus. It can simulate Ménière disease.

Bourneville Syndrome

Bourneville syndrome is a familial disorder whose symptoms include polyps of the skin, harelip, moles, spina bifida, and microcephaly.

Bowen Disease

Bowen disease is a precancerous dermatosis characterized by the development of pinkish or brownish papules covered with a thickened horny layer. Histologically, it shows hyperchromatic acanthotic cells with multinucleated giant cells. Mitoses are frequently observed.

Branchio-Oto-Renal Syndrome

Branchio-Oto-Renal syndrome is an autosomal dominant disorder characterized by anomalies of the external, middle, and inner ear in association with preauricular tissues, branchial cleft anomalies, and varying degrees of renal dysplasia, including aplasia. Many of the following symptoms (but not necessarily all) are present:

A. Conductive or mixed hearing loss
B. Cup-shaped, anteverted pinnae with bilateral preauricular sinuses
C. Bilateral branchial cleft fistulas or sinuses
D. Renal dysplasia

This syndrome is among a group of syndromes characterized by deformities associated with the first and second branchial complexes. The precise incidence of the disorder is unknown.

Briquet Syndrome

Briquet syndrome is characterized by a shortness of breath and aphonia due to hysteric paralysis of the diaphragm.

Brissaud-Marie Syndrome

Unilateral spasm of the tongue and lips of a hysteric nature are characteristic.

Brown Syndrome

Brown syndrome is a congenital or acquired abnormality of the superior oblique muscle tendon characterized by vertical diplopia and the inability to elevate the eye above midline or medial gaze. This syndrome is of two types: true and simulated. True Brown syndrome is always congenital. Simulated Brown syndrome is either congenital or acquired. The congenital simulated type may be caused by thickening of an area in the posterior tendon or by the firm attachment of the posterior sheath to the superior oblique tendon. The acquired simulated type may be caused by inflammation extending from the adjacent ethmoid cells to the posterior sheath and tendon, an orbital floor fracture, frontal ethmoidal fracture, crush fracture of nasal bones, sinusitis, frontal sinus surgery, or surgical tucking of the superior oblique tendon.

Brun Syndrome

Vertigo, headache, vomiting, and visual disturbances due to an obstruction of CSF flow during positional changes of the head are seen. The main causes of this syndrome include cysts and cysticercosis of the fourth ventricle as well as tumors of the midline cerebellum and third ventricle.

Burckhardt Dermatitis

Burckhardt dermatitis appears as an eruption of the external ear. It consists of red papules and vesicles that appear after exposure to sunlight. The rash usually resolves spontaneously.

Caffey Disease (Infantile Cortical Hyperostosis)

Of familial tendency, its onset is usually during the first year of life. It is characterized by hyperirritability, fever, and hard nonpitting edema that overlie the cortical hyperostosis. Pathologically, it involves the loss of periosteum with acute inflammatory involvement of the intratrabecular bone and the overlying soft tissue. Treatment is supportive, consisting of steroids and antibiotics. The prognosis is good. The mandible is the most frequently involved site.

Caisson Disease

This symptom complex occurs in men and women who work in high air pressures and are returned too suddenly to normal atmospheric pressure. Similar symptoms may occur in fliers when they suddenly ascend to high altitudes unprotected by counterpressure. It results from the escape from solution in the body fluids of bubbles (mainly nitrogen) originally absorbed at higher pressure. Symptoms include headache; pain in the epigastrium, sinuses, and tooth sockets; itchy skin; vertigo; dyspnea; coughing; nausea; vomiting; and sometimes paralysis. Peripheral circulatory collapse may be present. Nitrogen bubbles have been found in the white matter of the spinal cord. It also can injure the inner ear through necrosis of the organ of Corti. There is a question of rupture of the round window membrane; hemotympanum and eustachian tube obstruction may occur.

Camptomelic Syndrome

The name is derived from a Greek word meaning *curvature of extremities*. The syndrome is characterized by dwarfism, craniofacial anomalies, and bowing of the tibia and femur, with malformation of other bones. The patient has cutaneous dimpling overlying the tibial bend. Respiratory distress is common, and the patient has an early demise in the first few months of life. In the otolaryngologic area, the patient exhibits a prominent forehead, flat facies with a broad nasal bridge and low-set ears, cleft palate, mandibular hypoplasia, and tracheobronchial malacia that contributes to the respiratory distress and neonatal death. Histologically, two temporal bone observations showed defective endochondral ossification with no cartilage cells in the endochondral layer of the otic capsule. The cochlea was shortened and flattened, presenting a scalar communis. The vestibule and the SCC were deformed by bone invasion.

This syndrome is often of unknown etiology, although some believe it is autosomal recessive. Others believe it may be due to an exogenous cause.

This syndrome is not to be confused with Pierre Robin syndrome, which presents with very similar clinical features.

Cannon Nevus

This is an autosomal dominant disorder characterized by spongy white lesions of the oral and nasal mucosa. The lesions are asymptomatic and may be found from the newborn period with increasing severity until adolescence. The histologic picture is that of keratosis, acanthosis, and parakeratosis.

Carcinoid Syndrome

The symptoms include episodic flushing, diarrhea, and ascites. The tumor secretes serotonin. Treatment is wide excision. The tumor may give a positive dopa reaction.

Carotid Sinus Syndrome (Charcot-Weiss-Barber Syndrome)

When the carotid sinus is abnormally sensitive, slight pressure on it causes a marked fall in blood pressure due to vasodilation and cardiac slowing. Symptoms include syncope, convulsions, and heart block.

Castleman Disease

Castleman disease was first described by Castelman et al in 1954. It is a benign lymphoepithelial disease that is most often mistaken for lymphoma. It is also known as localized nodal hyperplasia, angiomatous lymph node hyperplasia, lymphoid hamartoma, and giant lymph nodal hyperplasia. Symptoms include tracheobronchial compression, such as cough, dyspnea, hemoptysis, or dysphagia. Masses in the neck are also not uncommon. There are two histologic types: the hyaline vascular type and the plasma cell type. Follicles in the hyaline vascular type are traversed by radially oriented capillaries with plump endothelial cells and collagenous hyalinization surrounding the vessels. The follicles in the plasma cell type are normal in size without capillary proliferation or hyalinization. Intermediate forms exist but are rare. Treatment entails complete excision of the mass. Etiology is unknown.

Cavernous Sinus Syndrome

The cavernous sinus receives drainage from the upper lip, nose, sinuses, nasopharynx, pharynx, and orbits. It drains into the inferior petrosal sinus, which in turn drains into the internal jugular vein. The cavernous sinus syndrome is caused by thrombosis of the cavernous intracranial sinus, 80% of which is fatal. The symptoms include orbital pain (V_1) with venous congestion of the retina, lids, and conjunctiva. The eyes are proptosed with exophthalmos. The patient has photophobia and involvement of nerves II, III, IV, and V_1. The treatment of choice is anticoagulation and antibiotics. The most common cause of cavernous sinus thrombosis is ethmoiditis. The ophthalmic vein and artery are involved as well. (The nerves and veins are lateral to the cavernous sinus, and the internal carotid artery is medial to it.)

Cestan-Chenais Syndrome

Cestan-Chenais syndrome is caused by occlusion of the vertebral artery below the point of origin of the posteroinferior cerebellar artery. There is paralysis of the soft palate, pharynx, and larynx. Ipsilateral cerebellar asynergia and Horner syndrome are also present. There is contralateral hemiplegia and diminished proprioception and tactile sensation.

Champion-Cregah-Klein Syndrome

This is a familial syndrome consisting of popliteal webbing, cleft lip, cleft palate, lower lip fistula, syndactyly, onychodysplasia, and pes equinovarus.

Chapple Syndrome

This disorder is seen in the newborn with unilateral facial weakness or paralysis in conjunction with comparable weakness or paralysis of the contralateral vocal cord, the muscles of deglutition, or both. The disorder is secondary to lateral flexion of the head in utero, which compresses the thyroid cartilage against the hyoid or cricoid cartilages or both, thereby injuring the recurrent or superior laryngeal nerve, or both.

Charcot-Marie-Tooth Disease

This is a hereditary and degenerative disease that includes the olivopontocerebellar, cerebelloparenchymal, and spinocerebellar disorders and the neuropathies. This disease is characterized by chronic degeneration of the peripheral nerves and roots; and distal muscle atrophy in feet, legs, and hands. Deep tendon reflexes are usually nil. It is also associated with hereditary cerebellar ataxia features, optic atrophy, and other cranial involvement. Some suggest that this disease is linked to auditory dysfunction and that it is also linked to other CNS dysfunctions. This disease can be progressive, and it can also spontaneously arrest.

CHARGE Syndrome

CHARGE syndrome (Coloboma of the eye, Heart defects, Atresia of the choanae, Retardation of growth and development, Genital and/or urinary abnormalities and Ear abnormalities and deafness) is a genetic pattern of birth defects which occur one in 10,000 births worldwide, without any family history. It involves heart defects, breathing and swallowing difficulties, hearing loss, vision loss, and balance problems.

Major Features of CHARGE Syndrome (Very Common in CHARGE and Relatively Rare in Other Conditions)

Feature	Includes	Frequency (%)
Coloboma of the eye	Coloboma (sort of like a cleft) of the iris, retina, choroid, macula, or disc (not the eyelid); microphthalmos (small eye) or anophthalmos (missing eye): *Causes vision loss*	80-90
Choanal atresia or stenosis	They can be stenosed or atretic. It can be unilateral or bilateral, bony, or membranous.	50-60
Cranial nerve abnormality	I—Missing or decreased sense of smell	90-100
	IX/X—Swallowing difficulties, aspiration	70-90
	VII—Facial palsy (one side or both)	40
CHARGE outer ear	Short, wide ear with little or no lobe, "snipped off" helix, prominent antihelix which is discontinuous with tragus, triangular concha, decreased cartilage (floppy), often stick out, usually asymmetric	> 50
CHARGE middle ear	Malformed bones of the ossicles: *Conductive hearing loss*	Common
CHARGE inner ear	Mondini defect; small or absent semicircular canals: *Balance problems and sensorineural loss*	90

Minor Characteristics of CHARGE: Significant, But More Difficult to Diagnose or Less Specific to CHARGE

Feature	Includes	Frequency (%)
Heart defects	Can be any type, but many are complex, such as tetralogy of Fallot	75
Cleft lip ± cleft palate	Cleft lip with or without cleft palate, cleft palate, submucous cleft palate	20
TE fistula	Esophageal atresia, tracheoesophageal fistula (TEF), H-shaped TEF	15-20
Kidney abnormalities	Small kidney, missing kidney, misplaced kidney, reflux	40
Genital abnormalities	Males: small penis, undescended testes	50
	Females: small labia, small or missing uterus	25
	Both: lack of puberty without hormone intervention	90
Growth deficiency	Growth hormone deficiency	15
	Other short stature	70
Typical CHARGE face	Square face with broad prominent forehead, arched eyebrows, large eyes, occasional ptosis, prominent nasal bridge with square root, thick nostrils, prominent nasal columella, flat midface, small mouth, occasional small chin, larger chin with age. Facial asymmetry even without facial palsy	
Palm crease	Hockey-stick palmar crease	50
CHARGE behavior	Perseverative behavior in younger individuals, obsessive compulsive behavior (OCD) in older individuals	> 50

Chédiak-Higashi Syndrome

Chédiak-Higashi syndrome is the result of an autosomal recessive trait. It is characterized by albinism, photophobia, nystagmus, hepatosplenomegaly, anomalous cellular granules, and development of lymphoma. These patients usually die during childhood of fulminant infections.

Cleft Lip Palate and Congenital Lip Fistulas

This syndrome is transmitted in an autosomal dominant manner with 80% penetrance; it occurs in 1 per 100,000 live births. Usually bilateral, symmetrically located depressions are noted on the vermilion portion of the lower lip and communicate with the underlying minor salivary glands. The lip pits may be an isolated finding (33%) or be found with cleft lip palate (67% of cases). Associated anomalies of the extremities may include talipes equinovarus, syndactyly, and popliteal pterygia. Congenital lip pits have also been seen in association with the oral-facial-digital syndrome.

Cockayne Syndrome

Cockayne syndrome is autosomal recessive, progressive bilateral sensorineural hearing loss, associated with dwarfism, facial disharmony, microcephaly, mental deficiency, retinitis pigmentosa, optic atrophy, intracranial calcification, and multiple dental caries. Patients succumb to respiratory or genitourinary infection in the teens or twenties.

Cogan Syndrome

Nonsyphilitic interstitial keratitis and vestibuloauditory symptoms are characteristics of Cogan syndrome. Interstitial keratitis gives rise to rapid visual loss. Symptoms include episodic severe vertigo accompanied by tinnitus, spontaneous nystagmus, ataxia, and progressive sensorineural hearing loss. There are remissions and exacerbations. It is believed to be related to periarteritis nodosa. Eosinophilia has been reported in this entity. Pathologically, it is a degeneration of the vestibular and spiral ganglia with edema of the membranous cochlea, SCCs, and inflammation of the spiral ligament. Treatment with steroids has been advocated.

Cyclophosphamide and azathioprine have been used in addition to prednisone (40 mg daily). This syndrome is not to be confused with Ménière disease despite vertiginous symptoms and fluctuating hearing loss. Vogt-Koyanagi-Harada syndrome is also similar but involves alopecia, poliosis, and exudative uveitis. Syphilis is also confused with this syndrome, but in syphilis, the interstitial keratitis is old and usually does not demonstrate active inflammatory changes. Syphilitic involvement of the cornea is often centrally located. Follow-up treatment of patients must be thorough in order to detect more extensive involvement, such as systemic vasculitis or aortitis.

Collet-Sicard Syndrome

The 9th, 10th, and 11th nerves are involved with normal sympathetic nerves. The etiology is usually a meningioma or other lesion involving the nerves in the posterior cranial fossa.

Conradi-Hünermann Syndrome

The most common variant of chondrodysplasia punctata; this syndrome is characterized by punctate epiphyseal calcifications. Clinical features include saddle nose deformity, micromelia, rhizomelia, short stature, flexion contractures, and dermatoses. This syndrome is also known as chondrodystrophia epiphysialis punctata, stippled epiphysis disease, dysplasia epiphysialis punctata, chondroangiopathia calcarea punctata, and Conradi disease. Some cases point to sporadic mutations and others to autosomal dominant patterns of inheritance. The clinical features of this syndrome are so varied from case to case that only a complete workup can exclude other versions of this syndrome.

Costen Syndrome

Costen syndrome is a temporomandibular joint (TMJ) abnormality, usually due to impaired bite and characterized by tinnitus, vertigo, and pain in the frontal, parietal, and occipital areas with a blocked feeling and pain in the ear. After a careful workup to rule out other abnormalities, the patient is treated with aspirin, heat, and slow exercise of the joint. An orthodontist may help the patient. The TMJ differs from other joints by the presence of avascular fibrous tissue covering the articulating surfaces with an interposed meniscus dividing the joint into upper and lower compartments. The right and left TMJs act as one functional unit. The condyle is made up of spongy bone with marrow and a growth center. The condyle articulates with the glenoid fossa of the temporal bone (squamosa). The squamotympanic fissure separates the fossa from the tympanic bone. The joint is a ginglymoarthrodial joint with hinge and transverse movements. The key supporting ligament of the TMJ is the temporomandibular ligament. The boundaries of the glenoid fossa are as follows:

Anterior:	Margins of the articular eminence
Posterior:	Squamosotympanic fissure
Lateral:	Zygomatic process of the temporal bone
Medial:	Temporal spine

The TMJ derives its nourishment from the synovial membrane, which is richly vascularized and produces a mucinous-like substance. The joint has a gliding motion between the meniscus and the temporal bone (upper compartment). It has a hinge motion between the disk and the condyle (lower compartment). It is innervated by the auriculotemporal nerve, masseter nerve, lateral pterygoid nerve, and temporal nerve. It is supplied by the superficial temporal artery and the anterior tympanic branch of the internal maxillary artery. The lateral pterygoid muscle protracts the jaw, and the masseter, medial pterygoid, and temporalis muscles act as elevators. All these muscles are innervated by V_3. The sphenomandibular and stylomandibular ligaments have no function in TMJ articulation.

Cowden Syndrome

This is a familial syndrome characterized by adenoid facies, hypoplasia of the mandible and maxilla, high-arched palate, hypoplasia of the soft palate and uvula, microstomia, papillomatosis of the lips and pharynx, scrotal tongue, multiple thyroid adenomas, bilateral breast hypertrophy, pectus excavatum, and liver and CNS abnormalities.

Creutzfeldt-Jakob Disease

Creutzfeldt-Jakob disease is a rare spongiform encephalopathy. Constitutional symptoms lead to mental retardation and movement disorder.

Cri du Chat Syndrome

Cri du Chat syndrome is a condition caused by a B group chromosome with a short arm; its symptoms are mental retardation, respiratory stridor, microcephaly, hypertelorism, midline oral clefts, and laryngomalacia with poor approximation of the posterior vocal cords.

Crouzon Disease

See Chapter 17.

Curtius Syndrome

Curtius syndrome is a form of hypertrophy that may involve a single small part of the body or an entire system (ie, muscular, nervous, or skeletal systems). It is also known as congenital hemifacial hypertrophy.

Dandy Syndrome

Oscillopsia or jumbling of the panorama common in patients after bilateral labyrinthectomy is characteristic of this syndrome. These patients are unable to focus while walking or moving.

Darier Disease (Keratosis Follicularis)

Autosomal dominant, this skin disorder of the external auditory canal is characterized by keratotic debris in the canal. Some investigators have advocated the use of vitamin A or steroids.

De'Jean Syndrome

Exophthalmos, diplopia, superior maxillary pain, and numbness along the route of the trigeminal nerve are found with lesions of the orbital floor in this syndrome.

Déjérine Anterior Bulbar Syndrome

This syndrome is evidenced by thrombosis of the anterior spinal artery, resulting in either an alternating hypoglossal hemiplegia or an alternating hypoglossal hemianesthetic hemiplegia.

Demarquay-Richter Syndrome

Demarquay-Richter syndrome is a congenital orofacial disorder characterized by cleft lip, cleft palate, lower lip fistulas, and progeria facies. Defective dentition, heart defects, dwarfism, and finger abnormalities may be seen.

DIDMOAD Syndrome

DIDMOAD syndrome is an autosomal recessive disorder associating **d**iabetes **i**nsipidus, **d**iabetes **m**ellitus, **o**ptic **a**trophy, and **d**eafness. Diabetes mellitus is usually juvenile in onset and insulin dependent. The diabetes insipidus has a varied time of onset and is vasopressin sensitive, indicative of degeneration of the hypothalamic cells or of the supraopticohypophyseal tract. The hearing loss is sensorineural and progressive, and primarily affects the higher tones. Urinary tract abnormalities ranging from atonic bladder to hydronephrosis and hydroureter have been reported with this disorder.

DiGeorge Syndrome

Lischaneri reported three categories of this syndrome:

A. Third and fourth pharyngeal pouch syndrome, characterized by cardiovascular and craniofacial anomalies as well as abdominal visceral abnormalities
B. DiGeorge syndrome (thymus agenesis)
C. Partial DiGeorge syndrome (thymic hypoplasia in which the thymus gland weighs less than 2 g)

The patients have small malformed pinnae with narrow external auditory canals and abnormal ossicles. The patients also have shortened cochlea of the Mondini type as well as an absence of hair cells in the hook region, hypertelorism with nasal cleft, shortened philtrum, and micrognathia. Other middle ear anomalies include an absence of stapedial muscle, hypoplastic facial nerve, and absent oval window. Most of the findings are symmetrical.

Down Syndrome

See section on trisomy in Chapter 17.

Dysphagia Lusoria

Dysphagia lusoria is secondary to an abnormal right subclavian artery. The right subclavian arises abnormally from the thoracic aorta by passing behind or in front of the esophagus, thus compressing it.

Eagle Syndrome

The patient has elongation of the styloid process or ossification of the stylohyoid ligament causing irritation of the trigeminal, facial, glossopharyngeal, and vagus nerves. Symptoms include recurrent nonspecific throat discomfort, foreign body sensation, dysphagia, facial pain, and increased salivation. Carotidynia may result from impingement of the styloid process on the carotid artery, producing regional tenderness or headaches. The only effective treatment for Eagle syndrome is surgical shortening of the styloid process.

Ectodermal Dysplasia, Hidrotic

See Chapter 17.

Ectodermal Dysplasia, Hypohidrotic

This syndrome consists of hypodontia, hypotrichosis, and hypohidrosis. Principally, the structures involved are of ectodermal origin. Eyelashes and especially eyebrows are entirely missing. Eczema and asthma are common. Aplasia of the eccrine sweat glands may lead to severe hyperpyrexia. The inheritance is X-linked recessive.

18q Syndrome

This syndrome consists of psychomotor retardation, hypotonia, short stature, microcephaly, hypoplastic midface, epicanthus, ophthalmologic abnormalities, cleft palate, congenital heart disease, abnormalities of the genitalia, tapered fingers, aural atresia, and conductive hearing loss.

Eisenlohr Syndrome

Numbness and weakness in the extremities; paralysis of the lips, tongue, and palate; and dysarthria are evidenced.

Elschnig Syndrome

Extension of the palpebral fissure laterally, displacement of the lateral canthus, ectropion of the lower lid, and lateral canthus are observed. Hypertelorism, cleft palate, and cleft lip are frequently seen.

Empty Sella Syndrome

The patient has an enlarged sella, giving the appearance of a pituitary tumor. An air encephalogram shows an empty sella. The syndrome consists of the abnormal extension into the sella turcica of an arachnoid diverticulum filled with CSF, displacing and compressing the pituitary gland. Four causal theories of this syndrome exist: (1) rupture of an intrasellar or parasellar cyst; (2) infarction of a pituitary adenoma; (3) pituitary hypertrophy and subsequent involution; and (4) the most common theory, the syndrome is due to CSF pressure through a congenitally deficient sella diaphragm leading to the formation of an intrasellar arachnoidocele. A trans-septal or trans-sphenoidal route to the sella is a treatment to consider.

The primary empty sella syndrome is due to congenital absence of the diaphragm sella, with gradual enlargement of the sella secondary to pulsations of the brain. Secondary empty sella syndrome may be due to necrosis of an existing pituitary tumor after surgery, postirradiation directed at the pituitary, or pseudotumor cerebri.

Face-Hand Syndrome

Face-hand syndrome is a reflex sympathetic dystrophy that is seen after a stroke or myocardial infarction. There may be edema and erythema of the involved parts along with persistent burning.

Fanconi Anemia Syndrome

Patients have aplastic anemia with skin pigmentation, skeletal deformities, renal anomalies, and mental retardation. Death due to leukemia usually ensues within 2 years. The disorder rarely occurs in adults. (A variant is congenital hypoplastic thrombocytopenia, which is inherited as an autosomal recessive trait.) It is characterized by spontaneous bleeding and other congenital anomalies. The bleeding time is prolonged, the platelet count is decreased, and the bone marrow megakaryocytes vary from decreased to absent.

It is associated with unrepaired chromosome breakage. Congenital anomalies of the inner, middle, and external ear could be causes of the deafness that accompanies this syndrome.

Felty Syndrome

Felty syndrome is a combination of leukopenia, arthritis, and enlarged lymph nodes and spleen.

First and Second Branchial Arch Syndromes (Hemifacial Microsomia, Lateral Facial Dysplasia)

This disorder consists of a spectrum of craniofacial malformations characterized by asymmetric facies with unilateral abnormalities. The mandible is small with hypoplastic or absent ramus and condyle. Aural atresia, hearing impairment, tissue tags from the tragus to the oral commissure, coloboma of the upper eyelid, malar hypoplasia, and cleft palate also may be present. Cardiovascular, renal, and nervous system abnormalities have been noted in association with this disorder.

Fish Odor Syndrome

Clinical symptoms of this peculiar syndrome consist of a fish odor emanating from the mucus, particularly in the morning. A challenge test with either choline bitartrate or trimethylamine is diagnostic of this disease. Eating non–choline-containing foods usually helps. No long-term effects are known.

Fordyce Disease

Fordyce disease is characterized by pseudocolloid of the lips, a condition marked by the presence of numerous, small yellowish-white granules on the inner surface and vermilion border of the lips. Histologically, the lesions appear as ectopic sebaceous glands.

Foster Kennedy Syndrome

Patients with this disorder show ipsilateral optic atrophy and scotomas and contralateral papilledema occurring with tumors or other lesions of the frontal lobe or sphenoidal meningioma. Anosmia may be seen.

Fothergill Disease

The combination of tic douloureux and anginose scarlatina is characteristic of this disease.

Foville Syndrome

Facial paralysis with ipsilateral paralysis of conjugate gaze and contralateral pyramidal hemiplegia are diagnostic. Tinnitus, deafness, and vertigo may occur with infranuclear involvement. Loss of taste of the anterior two-thirds of the tongue with decreased salivary and lacrimal secretions is seen with involvement of the nervus intermedius.

Frey Syndrome

In the normal person, the sweat glands are innervated by sympathetic nerve fibers. After parotidectomy, the auriculotemporal nerve sends its parasympathetic fibers to innervate the sweat glands instead. The incidence of Frey syndrome after parotidectomy in children has been estimated to be about 20%.

Also called preauricular gustatory sweating, parotidectomy is considered the most common etiology.

Friedreich Disease

The disease consists of facial hemihypertrophy involving the eyelids, cheeks, lips, facial bones, tongue, ears, and tonsils. It may be seen alone or in association with generalized hemihypertrophy.

Garcin Syndrome

Paralysis of cranial nerves III through X, usually unilateral or occasionally bilateral, is observed. It may be the result of invasion by neoplasm, granulomas, or infections in the retropharyngeal space.

Gard-Gignoux Syndrome

Gard-Gignoux syndrome involves paralysis of the eleventh nerve and the tenth nerve below the nodose ganglion. The cricothyroid function and sensation are normal. The symptoms include vocal cord paralysis and weakness of the trapezius and sternocleidomastoid muscles.

Gardner Syndrome

Gardner syndrome is an autosomal dominant disease whose symptoms include fibroma, osteoma of the skull, mandible, maxilla, and long bones, with epidermoid inclusion cysts in the skin and polyps in the colon. These colonic polyps have a marked tendency toward malignant degeneration.

Gargoylism (Hurler Syndrome)

See Chapter 17.

Gaucher Disease

As an autosomally recessive inherited disorder of lipid metabolism, this syndrome results in a decrease in activity of the glucocerebrosidase. This leads to an increased accumulation of glucocerebrosides, particularly in the retroendothelial system. There are three classifications of the disease: (1) the chronic non-neuronopathic form, characterized by joint pain, aseptic necrosis, pathologic fractures, hepatosplenomegaly, thrombocytopenia, anemia, and leukopenia; (2) the acute neuronopathic Gaucher disease (infantile form), causing increased neurologic complications that often end in death before the first 2 years of life; and (3) the juvenile and less severe forms than the infantile form.

Gerlier Disease

With the presence of vertigo and kubisagari, it is observed among cowherds. It is marked by pain in the head and neck with visual disturbances, ptosis, and generalized weakness of the muscles.

Giant Apical Air Cell Syndrome

Giant apical air cell syndrome, first described in 1982, consists of giant apical air cells, spontaneous CSF rhinorrhea, and recurrent meningitis. It is caused by the constant pounding of the brain against the dura overlying the giant apical air cell, which leads to dural rupture and CSF leak.

Gilles de la Tourette Syndrome

Characterized by chorea, coprolalia, and tics of the face and extremities, it affects children (usually boys 5-10 years old). Repetitive facial grimacing, blepharospasms, and arm and leg contractions may be present. Compulsive grunting noises or hiccupping subsequently become expressions of frank obscenities.

Goldenhar Syndrome

A rare, nonhereditary congenital variant of hemifacial microsomia, Goldenhar syndrome is a congenital syndrome of the first and second arch. It is characterized by underdevelopment of craniofacial structures, vertebral malformations, and cardiac dysfunction. Clinical features of this syndrome are malar and maxillary hypoplasia, poor formation of external auditory canal, supernumerary ear tags and antetragal pits, orbit, enlarged mouths, renal anomalies, and missing growth centers in the condyle, causing delayed eruption of teeth and teeth crowding. Intelligence is usually normal or mildly retarded. Maxillofacial reconstruction in young patients demands consideration of future growth and development. It is also recommended for psychologic reasons as well as reasons involving the proper expansion of the skin that will later aid in further reconstruction. This syndrome is not to be confused with Treacher Collins, Berry, or Franceschetti-Zwahlen-Klein syndromes. These tend to show well-defined genetic patterns (irregular but dominant), whereas Goldenhar syndrome does not.

Goodwin Tumor (Benign Lymphoepithelial Lesion)

This syndrome is characterized by inflammatory cells, lymphocytes, plasma cells, and reticular cells.

Gradenigo Syndrome

Gradenigo syndrome is due to an extradural abscess involving the petrous bone. The symptoms are suppurative otitis, pain in the eye and temporal area, abducens paralysis, and diplopia.

Grisel Syndrome

Grisel syndrome, also known as nasopharyngeal torticollis, is the subluxation of the atlantoaxial joint and is usually associated with children. It is associated with pharyngitis, nasopharyngitis, adenotonsillitis, tonsillar abscess, parotitis, cervical abscess, and otitis media. This syndrome has been known to occur after nasal cavity inflammation, tonsillectomy, adenoidectomy, mastoidectomy, choanal atresia repair, and excisions of a parapharyngeal rhabdomyosarcoma. Proposals for etiology include overdistention of the atlantoaxial joint ligaments by effusion, rupture of the transverse ligament, excessive passive rotation during general anesthesia, uncoordinated reflex action of the deep cervical muscles, spasm of the prevertebral muscles, ligamentous relaxation from decalcification of the vertebrae, and weak lateral ligaments. Clinical features include spontaneous torticollis in a child, a flexed and rotated head with limited range of motion, flat face, and Sudeck sign (displacement of the spine of the axis to the same side as the head is turned). Treatment includes skeletal skull traction under fluoroscopic control to realign the odontoid process within the transverse ligament sling, followed by 6 to 12 weeks of immobilization. Timely treatment is usually successful.

Guillain-Barré Syndrome

Guillain-Barré syndrome is infectious polyneuritis of unknown etiology ("perhaps" viral) causing marked paresthesias of the limbs, muscular weakness, or a flaccid paralysis. CSF protein is increased without an increase in cell count.

Hallermann-Streiff Syndrome

Hallermann-Streiff syndrome consists of dyscephaly, parrot nose, mandibular hypoplasia, proportionate nanism; hypotrichosis of scalp, brows, and cilia; and bilateral congenital cataracts. Most patients exhibit nystagmus or strabismus. There is no demonstrable genetic basis.

Hanhart Syndrome

A form of facial dysmorphia, Hanhart syndrome is characterized by (1) bird-like profile of face caused by micrognathia, (2) opisthodontia, (3) peromelia, (4) small growth, (5) normal intelligence, (6) branchial arch deformity resulting in conductive hearing loss, (7) tongue deformities and often a small jaw, and (8) possibly some limb defects as well. Ear surgery should be carefully considered because of the abnormal course of the facial nerve due to this syndrome.

Heerfordt Syndrome or Disease

In Heerfordt syndrome, the patient develops uveoparotid fever. Heerfordt syndrome is a form of sarcoidosis (see Chapter 12).

Hick Syndrome

Hick syndrome is a rare condition characterized by a sensory disorder of the lower extremities, resulting in perforating feet and by ulcers that are associated with progressive deafness due to atrophy of the cochlear and vestibular ganglia.

Hippel-Lindau Disease

Hippel-Lindau disease consists of angioma of the cerebellum, usually cystic, associated with angioma of the retina and polycystic kidneys.

Hollander Syndrome

With Hollander syndrome, there is appearance of a goiter during the third decade of life related to a partial defect in the coupling mechanism in thyroxine biosynthesis. Deafness due to cochlear abnormalities is usually related to this.

Homocystinuria

Homocystinuria is a recessive hereditary syndrome secondary to a defect in methionine metabolism with resultant homocystinemia, mental retardation, and sensorineural hearing loss.

Horner Syndrome

The presenting symptoms of Horner syndrome are ptosis, miosis, anhidrosis, and enophthalmos due to paralysis of the cervical sympathetic nerves.

Horton Neuralgia

Patients have unilateral headaches centered behind or close to the eye accompanied or preceded by ipsilateral nasal congestion, suffusion of the eye, increased lacrimation and facial redness, and swelling.

Hunt Syndrome

A. Cerebellar tumor, an intention tremor that begins in one extremity gradually increasing in intensity and subsequently involving other parts of the body
B. Facial paralysis, otalgia, and aural herpes due to disease of both motor and sensory fibers of the seventh nerve
C. A form of juvenile paralysis agitans associated with primary atrophy of the pallidal system

Hunter Syndrome

A hereditary and sex-linked disorder, this incurable syndrome involves multiple organ systems through mucopolysaccharide infiltration. Death, usually by the second decade of life, is often caused by an infiltrative cardiomyopathy and valvular disease leading to heart failure. Physical characteristics include prominent supraorbital ridges, large flattened nose with flared nares, low-set ears, progressive corneal opacities, generous jowls, patulous lips and prognathism, short neck, abdominal protuberance, hirsutism, short stature, extensive osteoarthritis (especially in the hips, shoulders, elbows, and hands), TMJ arthritis, pseudopapilledema, and low-pressure hydrocephalus. Chondroitin sulfate B and heparitin in urine, mental retardation, beta-galactoside deficiency, and hepatosplenomegaly are also features of this syndrome. There is cerebral storage of three gangliosides: GM_1, GM_2, and GM_3. Compressive myelopathy may result from vertebral dislocation. High spinal cord injury is a great complication in surgery. Neurologic development is often slowed or never acquired. Abdominal abnormalities, respiratory infections, and cardiovascular troubles plague the patient.

Immotile Cilia Syndrome

This syndrome appears to be a congenital defect in the ultrastructure of cilia that renders them incapable of movement. Both respiratory tract cilia and sperm are involved. The clinical picture includes bronchiectasis, sinusitis, male sterility, situs inversus, and otitis media. Histologically, there is a complete or partial absence of dynein arms, which are believed to be essential for cilia movement and sperm tail movement. Also no cilia movements were observed in the mucosa of the middle ear and the nasopharynx.

Inversed Jaw-Winking Syndrome

When there are supranuclear lesions of the fifth nerve, touching the cornea may produce a brisk movement of the mandible to the opposite side.

Jackson Syndrome

Cranial nerves X, XI, and XII are affected by nuclear or radicular lesion. There is ipsilateral flaccid paralysis of the soft palate, pharynx, and larynx with weakness and atrophy of the sternocleidomastoid and trapezius muscles and muscles of the tongue.

Jacod Syndrome

Jacod syndrome consists of total ophthalmoplegia, optic tract lesions with unilateral amaurosis, and trigeminal neuralgia. It is caused by a middle cranial fossa tumor involving the second through sixth cranial nerves.

Job Syndrome

Job syndrome is one of the groups of hyperimmunoglobulin E (hyper-IgE) syndromes that are associated with defective chemotaxis. The clinical picture includes fair skin, red hair, recurrent staphylococcal skin abscesses with concurrent other bacterial infections and skin lesions, as well as chronic purulent pulmonary infections and infected eczematoid skin lesions. This syndrome obtained its name from the Biblical passage referring to Job being smitten with boils. It is of interest to the otolaryngologist because of head and neck infections.

Jugular Foramen Syndrome (Vernet Syndrome)

Cranial nerves IX, X, and XI are paralyzed, whereas XII is spared because of its separate hypoglossal canal. Horner syndrome is not present because the sympathetic chain is below the foramen. This syndrome is most often caused by lymphadenopathy of the nodes of Krause in the foramen. Thrombophlebitis, tumors of the jugular bulb, and basal skull fracture can cause the syndrome. The glomus jugulare usually gives a hazy margin of involvement, whereas neurinoma gives a smooth, sclerotic margin of enlargement. The jugular foramen is bound medially by the occipital bone and laterally by the temporal bone. The foramen is divided into anteromedial (pars nervosa) and posterolateral (pars vascularis) areas by a fibrous or bony septum. The medial area transmits nerves IX, X, and XI as well as the inferior petrosal sinus. The posterior compartment transmits the internal jugular vein and the posterior meningeal artery. The right foramen is usually slightly larger than the left foramen.

Kallmann Syndrome

Kallmann syndrome consists of congenital hypogonadotropic eunuchoidism with anosmia. It is transmitted via a dominant gene with variable penetrance.

Kaposi Sarcoma

Patients have multiple idiopathic, hemorrhagic sarcomatosis particularly of the skin and viscera. Radiotherapy is the treatment of choice.

Kartagener Syndrome

The symptoms are complete situs inversus associated with chronic sinusitis and bronchiectasis. It is also called the Kartagener triad.

Cilia and flagella of a patient lack normal dynein side arms of ciliary A-tubes. Deficient mucociliary transport causes sterility in both sexes.

Keratosis Palmaris et Solaris

This disorder is an unusual inherited malformation. If these people live to 65 years of age, 50% to 75% of them develop carcinoma of the esophagus.

Kimura Disease

Kimura disease was first described by Kimura et al in 1949 as a chronic inflammatory condition occurring in subcutaneous tissues, salivary glands, and lymph nodes. Etiology is unknown. Histologically, there is dense fibrosis, lymphoid infiltration, vascular proliferation, and eosinophils. This is different from angiolymphoid hyperplasia with eosinophilia (ALHE). It is much more prevalent in people of Oriental descent. Laboratory studies show eosinophilia and elevated IgE. Differential diagnosis includes ALHE, eosinophilic granuloma, benign lymphoepithelial lesion, lymphocytoma, pyogenic granuloma, Kaposi sarcoma, hamartoma, and lymphoma. Treatment includes corticosteroids, cryotherapy, radiation, and surgery.

The differences between Kimura disease and ALHE are as follows:

Kimura	Age:	30-60 (ALHE age 20-50)
	Sex:	Male (ALHE female)
	Larger lesions	(ALHE < 1 cm)
	Deep	(ALHE superficial)
	More lymphoid follicles than ALHE	
	Fewer mast cells than ALHE	
	Less vascular hyperplasia than ALHE	
	More fibrosis than ALHE	
	More eosinophilia than ALHE	
	More IgE than ALHE	

Kleinschmidt Syndrome

Symptoms include influenzal infections, resulting in laryngeal stenosis, suppurative pericarditis, pleuropneumonia, and occasionally meningitis.

Klinefelter Syndrome

Klinefelter syndrome is a sex chromosome defect characterized by eunuchoidism, azoospermia, gynecomastia, mental deficiency, small testes with atrophy, and hyalinization of seminiferous tubules. The karyotype is usually XXY.

Klinkert Syndrome

Paralysis of the recurrent and phrenic nerves due to a neoplastic process in the root of the neck or upper mediastinum is evidenced. The sympathetics may be involved. (Left-side involvement is more common than right-side involvement.) It can be a part of Pancoast syndrome.

Lacrimoauriculodentodigital Syndrome

Autosomal dominant, occasional middle ear ossicular anomaly with cup-shaped ears, abnormal or absent thumbs, skeletal forearm deformities, sensorineural hearing loss, and nasolacrimal duct obstruction are the characteristics of lacrimoauriculodentodigital syndrome.

Large Vestibular Aqueduct Syndrome

The large vestibular aqueduct as an isolated anomaly of the temporal bone is associated with sensorineural hearing loss. It is more common in childhood than in adulthood. In this syndrome, the rugose portion of the endolymphatic sac is also enlarged. Endolymphatic sac procedures to improve hearing are not often successful. A vestibular aqueduct is considered enlarged if its anteroposterior diameter on computed tomography (CT) scan is greater than 1.5 mm.

Larsen Syndrome

Larsen syndrome is characterized by widely spaced eyes, prominent forehead, flat nasal bridge, midline cleft of the secondary palate, bilateral dislocation of the knees and elbows, deformities of the hands and feet, and spatula-type thumbs; sometimes tracheomalacia, stridor, laryngomalacia, and respiratory difficulty are present. Therapy includes maintaining adequate ventilation.

Lemierre Syndrome

First discussed by André LeMierre in 1936, usually caused by anaerobic, nonmotile gram-negative rod, *Fusobacterium necrophorum*, Lemierre syndrome can be found in normal flora of oropharynx, gastrointestinal (GI), female genital tract; sensitive to clindamycin and metronidazole, penicillin, and chloramphenicol. Usually in young adults first presenting with oropharynx infection, progress to neck and parapharyngeal abscess, leading to internal jugular and sigmoid sinus thrombosis leading to septic embolism causing septic arthritis, liver and splenic abscess, sigmoid sinus thrombosis findings include headache, otalgia, vertigo, vomiting, otorrhea and rigors, proptosis retrobulbar pain, papilledema, and ophthalmoplegia.

Lermoyez Syndrome

Lermoyez syndrome is a variant of Ménière disease. It was first described by Lermoyez in 1921 as deafness and tinnitus followed by a vertiginous attack that relieved the tinnitus and improved the hearing.

Lethal Midline Granuloma Syndrome

Destroying cartilage, soft tissue, and bone, this disease manifests itself by a number of entities, including idiopathic midline destructive disease, Wegener granulomatosis, polymorphic reticulosis, nasal lymphoma, and non-Hodgkin lymphoma (NHL). High-dose local radiation totaling 5000 rad is the treatment of choice for localized cases. Chemotherapy involving an alkylating agent (cyclophosphamide) is recommended for disseminated cases.

Löffler Syndrome

Löffler syndrome consists in pneumonitis characterized by eosinophils in the tissues. It is possibly of parasitic etiology.

Loose Wire Syndrome

Loose wire syndrome occurs in patients with stapedectomy and insertion of a prosthesis that attaches to the long process of the incus by means of a crimped wire. It is a late complication, occurring on an average 15 years after surgery. A triad of symptoms is present that improves temporarily with middle ear inflation: auditory acuity, distortion of sound, and speech discrimination. Treatment in revision surgery involves finding the loose wire attachment at the incus and tightening that wire to allow the incus and prosthesis to move as one.

Louis-Bar Syndrome

This autosomal recessive disease presents as ataxia, oculocutaneous telangiectasia, and sinopulmonary infection. It involves progressive truncal ataxia, slurred speech, fixation nystagmus, mental deficiency, cerebellar atrophy, deficient immunoglobulin, and marked frequency of lymphoreticular malignancies. The patient rarely lives past age 20.

Maffucci Syndrome

Maffucci syndrome is characterized by multiple cutaneous hemangiomas with dyschondroplasia and often enchondroma. The origin is unknown, and it is not hereditary. Signs and symptoms of this syndrome usually appear during infancy. It equally affects both sexes and has no racial preference. The dyschondroplasia may cause sharp bowing or an uneven growth of the extremities as well as give rise to frequent fractures. Five to 10% of Maffucci syndrome patients have head and neck involvement giving rise to cranial nerve dysfunction and hemangiomas in the head and neck area. The hemangiomas in the nasopharynx and larynx could cause airway compromise as well as deglutition problems. Fifteen to 20% of these patients later undergo sarcomatous degeneration in one or more of the enchondromas. The percentage of malignant changes is greater in older patients, with the percentage of malignant degeneration approaching 44% in patients older than 40.

This syndrome is not to be confused with Klippel-Trenaunay syndrome, which causes no underdeveloped extremities, Sturge-Weber syndrome, or von Hippel-Lindau syndrome. No treatment is known for this syndrome, although surgical procedures to treat the actual deformities are sometimes necessary.

Mal de Debarquement Syndrome

Mal de Debarquement syndrome (or MDDS) is an imbalance or rocking sensation that occurs after prolonged exposure to motion (most commonly after a sea cruise or a long airplane flight). Travelers often experience this sensation temporarily after disembarking, but in the case of MDDS sufferers, it can persist for 6 to 12 months or even many years in some cases.

The imbalance is generally not associated with any nausea, nor is it alleviated by typical motion sickness drugs such as scopolamine or meclizine. Symptoms are usually most pronounced when the patient is sitting still; in fact, the sensations are usually minimized by actual motion such as walking or driving.

The functional cause of MDDS is unknown. (Vestibular and CNS tests for MDDS patients invariably turn out normal results.)

Speculation about the cause of MDDS includes the following:

- Psychiatric condition (particularly linked to depression)
- A hormonal-related condition (may occur more often in females)
- Otolith organ or CNS abnormalities
- Some link to a variant of migraine

Diagnosis of MDDS is generally a process of exclusion.

The medical literature describes MDDS as *self-limiting* condition.

Valium and other derivatives (particularly *Klonopin*) have been known to help alleviate some of the severe symptoms in MDDS patients, but there is always a worry that these are habit forming and may prolong the eventual disappearance of the condition.

In general, physical activity is recommended for vestibular rehabilitation.

Marcus Gunn Syndrome (Jaw-Winking Syndrome)

Marcus Gunn syndrome results in an increase in the width of the eyelids during chewing. Sometimes the patient experiences rhythmic elevation of the upper eyelid when the mouth is open and ptosis when the mouth is closed.

Marie-Strümpell Disease

Marie-Strümpell disease is rheumatoid arthritis of the spine.

Masson Tumor

Masson tumor is intravascular papillary endothelial hyperplasia caused by excessive proliferation of endothelial cells. It is a benign condition. Differential diagnosis includes angiosarcoma, Kaposi sarcoma, and pyogenic granuloma.

Melkersson-Rosenthal Syndrome

(Triad: Recurrent orofacial swelling, one or more episodes of facial paralysis, and lingua plicata.)
Melkersson-Rosenthal syndrome is a congenital disease of unknown etiology, and it manifests

as recurring attacks of unilateral or bilateral facial paralysis (see Chapter 21), swelling of the lips, and furrowing of the tongue. It is associated with high serum levels of angiotensin-converting enzyme during affliction, and also known as orofacial granulomatosis, cheilitis granulomatosis, Scheuermann glossitis granulomatosis, and Miescher cheilitis.

Treatment should focus on facial paralysis and edema. Steroids and facial nerve decompression have had limited success.

Meyenburg Syndrome (Familial Myositis Fibrosa Progressiva)

Meyenburg syndrome is a disease in which the striated muscles are replaced by fibrosis. Fibrosarcoma rarely originates from this disease.

Middle Lobe Syndrome

Middle lobe syndrome is a chronic atelectatic process with fibrosis in one or both segments of the middle lobe. It is usually secondary to obstruction of the middle lobe bronchus by hilar adenopathy. The hilar adenopathy may be transient, but the bronchiectasis that resulted persists. Treatment is surgical resection.

Mikulicz Disease

The symptoms characteristic of Mikulicz disease (swelling of the lacrimal and salivary glands) occur as complications of some other disease, such as lymphocytosis, leukemia, or uveoparotid fever.

Millard-Gubler Syndrome

Patients present with ipsilateral paralysis of the abducens and facial nerves with contralateral hemiplegia of the extremities due to obstruction of the vascular supply to the pons.

Möbius Syndrome

Möbius syndrome is a nonprogressive congenital facial diplegia (usually bilateral) with unilateral or bilateral loss of the abductors of the eye, anomalies of the extremities, and aplasia of the brachial and thoracic muscles. It frequently involves other cranial nerves. Saito showed evidence that the site of nerve lesions is in the peripheral nerve. The etiology could be CNS hypoplasia, primary peripheral muscle defect with secondary nerve degeneration, or lower motor neuron involvement.

Morgagni-Stewart-Morel Syndrome

Morgagni-Stewart-Morel syndrome occurs in menopausal women and is characterized by obesity, dizziness, psychologic disturbances, inverted sleep rhythm, and hyperostosis frontalis interna. Treatment is supportive.

Multiple Endocrine Adenomatosis

Multiple Endocrine Adenomatosis Type IIA (Sipple Syndrome) Sipple syndrome is a familial syndrome consisting of medullary carcinoma of the thyroid, hyperparathyroidism, and pheochromocytoma.

Multiple Endocrine Adenomatosis Type IIB This multiple endocrine adenomatosis (MEA) variant consists of multiple mucosal neuromas, pheochromocytoma, medullary carcinoma of the thyroid, and hyperparathyroidism. This syndrome is inherited in an autosomal dominant pattern. Mucosal neuromas principally involve the lips and anterior tongue. Numerous white medullated nerve fibers traverse the cornea to anastomose in the pupillary area.

Munchausen Syndrome

Munchausen syndrome was named after Baron Hieronymus Karl Freidrich von Münchausen (1720-1791) by Asher in 1951. The integral features of this syndrome include the following:

A. A real organic lesion from the past that has left some genuine signs but is causing no organic symptoms.
B. Exorbitant lying with dramatic presentation of nonexistent symptoms.
C. Traveling widely with multiple hospitalizations.
D. Criminal tendencies.
E. Willingness to undergo painful and dangerous treatment.
F. Presenting challenging illnesses for treatment.
G. Unruly behavior during hospital stays and early self-discharge without prior approval.
H. Patients often inflict pain on their own children and forcibly create symptoms to indirectly receive hospital treatment.

The patients usually go from one medical center to another to be admitted with dramatic presentations of nonorganic symptoms related to a real organic lesion on the past medical history.

Nager Syndrome (Acrofacial Dysostosis)

Acrofacial dysostosis patients have facies similar to those seen with Treacher Collins syndrome. They also present with preaxial upper limb defects, microtia, atresia of the external auditory canals, and malformation of the ossicles. Conductive and mixed hearing losses may occur.

Nager de Reynier Syndrome

Hypoplasia of the mandible with abnormal implantation of teeth associated with aural atresia characterizes this syndrome.

Neurofibromatosis (von Recklinghausen Disease)

Salient Features
A. Autosomal dominant.
B. Mental retardation common in families with neurofibromatosis.
C. Arises from neurilemmal cells or sheath of Schwann and fibroblasts of peripheral nerves.
D. Café au lait spots—giant melanosomes (presence of six or more spots > 1.5 cm is diagnostic of neurofibromatosis even if the family history is negative).
E. Of all neurofibromatoses, 4% to 5% undergo malignant degeneration with a sudden increase in growth of formerly static nodules. These nodules may become neurofibrosarcomas, and they may metastasize widely.

External Features
A. Café au lait spots
B. Fibromas

Internal Features
A. Pheochromocytoma.
B. Meningioma.
C. Acoustic neuroma: bilateral in type 2 neurofibromatosis.
D. GI bleeding.
E. Intussusception bowel.
F. Hypoglycemia (intraperitoneal fibromas).

G. Fibrous dysplasia.
H. Subperiosteal bone cysts.
I. Optic nerve may be involved, causing blindness and proptosis.
J. May present with macroglossia.
K. May involve the parotid or submaxillary gland.
L. The nodules may be painful.
M. Nodules may enlarge suddenly if bleeding of the tumor occurs or if there is malignant degeneration.

The treatment is only to relieve pressure from expanding masses. It usually does not recur if the tumor is completely removed locally.

Nothnagel Syndrome

The symptoms include dizziness, a staggering and rolling gait with irregular forms of oculomotor paralysis, and nystagmus often is present. This syndrome is seen with tumors of the midbrain.

Oculopharyngeal Syndrome

Oculopharyngeal syndrome is characterized by hereditary ptosis and dysphagia, and is an autosomal dominant disease having equal incidence in both sexes. It is related to a high incidence of esophageal carcinoma. Age of onset is between 40 and 50 years, and it is particularly common among French Canadians. Marked weakness of the upper esophagus is observed together with an increase in serum creatinine phosphokinase. It is a myopathy and not a neuropathy. Treatment includes dilatation and cricopharyngomyotomy.

Ollier Disease

Ollier disease consists of multiple chondromatosis, 10% of which is associated with chondrosarcoma.

Ondine Curse

Failure of respiratory center automaticity with apnea, especially evident during sleep, is symptomatic. Also known as the alveolar hypoventilation syndrome, it may be associated with increased appetite and transient central diabetes insipidus. Hypothalamic lesions are thought to be the cause of this disorder.

Oral-Facial-Digital Syndrome I

See Chapter 17 for oral-facial-digital syndrome I.

A lethal trait in men, it is inherited as an X-linked dominant trait limited to women. Symptoms include multiple hyperplastic frenula, cleft tongue, dystopia canthorum, hypoplasia of the nasal alar cartilages, median cleft of the upper lip, asymmetrical cleft palate, digital malformation, and mild mental retardation. About 50% of the patients have hamartoma between the lobes of the divided tongue. This mass consists of fibrous connective tissue, salivary gland tissue, few striated muscle fibers, and rarely cartilage. One-third of the patients present with ankyloglossia.

Orbital Apex Syndrome

Orbital apex syndrome involves the nerves and vessels passing through the superior sphenoid fissure and the optic foramen with paresis of cranial nerves III, IV, and VI. External ophthalmoplegia is associated with internal ophthalmoplegia with a dilated pupil that does not react to either light or convergence. Ptosis as well as periorbital edema are due to fourth nerve paresis. Sensory changes are secondary to the lacrimal frontal nasal ciliary nerves as well as the three branches of the ophthalmic nerve. The optic nerve usually is involved.

Ortner Syndrome

Cardiomegaly associated with laryngeal paralysis secondary to compression of the recurrent laryngeal nerve is observed with this syndrome.

Osler-Weber-Rendu Disease (Hereditary Hemorrhagic Telangiectasia)

Osler-Weber-Rendu disease is an autosomal dominant disease in which the heterozygote lives to adult life, whereas the homozygous state is lethal at an early age. The patient has punctate hemangiomas (elevated, dilated capillaries and venules) in the mucous membrane of the lips, tongue, mouth, GI tract, and so on. Pathologically, they are vascular sinuses of irregular size and shape lined by a thin layer of endothelium. The muscular and elastic coats are absent. Because of their thin walls these vascular sinuses bleed easily, and because of the lack of muscular coating the bleeding is difficult to control. The patient has normal blood elements and no coagulation defect. The other blood vessels are normal. If a person with this disease marries a normal person, what are the chances that the offspring will have this condition? Because the patient with this disease is an adult, we can assume that he is heterozygous, as the homozygote dies early in life. Therefore, the child will have a 50% chance of having this hereditary disease.

Otopalatodigital Syndrome

Otopalatodigital syndrome is characterized by skeletal dysplasia, conductive hearing loss, and cleft palate. Middle ear anomalies are also associated with this syndrome. Although the mode of inheritance is not known, some suggest that X-linked recessive inheritance is possible. Symptoms tend to be less severe in females than in males. The diagnosis of otopalatodigital (OPD) syndrome is sometimes based on characteristic facies and deformities of hands and feet. Physical features include mild dwarfism, mental retardation, broad nasal root, frontal and occipital bossing, hypertelorism, small mandible, stubby, clubbed digits, low-set and small ears, winged scapulae, malar flattening, downward obliquity of the eye, and down-turned mouth. The inner ear has been known to display deformities likened to a mild type of Mondini dysplasia. Surgical attempts to improve hearing loss are not always recommended since certain deformities, such as a missing round window, make such attempts unsuccessful.

Paget Disease (Osteitis Deformans)

See Chapter 17.

This term also is used to characterize a disease of elderly women who have an infiltrated, eczematous lesion surrounding the nipple and areola associated with subjacent intraductal carcinoma of the breast.

Paget Osteitis

This disorder is related to sarcomas.

Pancoast Syndrome

See Chapter 7.

Pelizaeus-Merzbacher Disease

Pelizaeus-Merzbacher disease is an X-linked recessive sudanophilic leukodystrophy. The CNS myelin forms improperly and never matures, sometimes ending in death by the age of 2 or 3 years.

Nystagmoid eye movements are characteristic at age 4 to 6 months, followed by a delay in motor development. Prenatal amniocentesis is not useful in detecting this disease. Neonatal stridor, a specific genealogy combined with a characteristic auditory brain stem response (ABR) wave can lead to early diagnosis. Characteristic waves have been known to be missing rostral waves and normal wave I latency. Males are afflicted, whereas females are unknowing carriers.

Pena-Shokeir Syndrome

Rare autosomal recessive, affects newborn camptodactyly, multiple ankylosis, pulmonary hypoplasia, and facial anomaly. Generally poor prognosis and die shortly after birth.

Peutz-Jeghers Syndrome

The patient has pigmentation of the lips and oral mucosa and benign polyps of the GI tract. Granulosa theca cell tumors have been reported in female patients with this syndrome.

Pheochromocytoma

Pheochromocytoma is associated with neurofibromatosis, cerebellar hemangioblastoma, ependymoma, astrocytoma, meningioma, spongioblastoma, multiple endocrine adenoma, or medullary carcinoma of the thyroid. Pheochromocytoma with or without the tumors may be inherited as an autosomal dominant trait. Some patients have megacolon, others suffer neurofibromatosis of Auerbach and Meissner plexuses.

Pierre Robin Syndrome

Pierre Robin syndrome consists of glossoptosis, micrognathia, and cleft palate. There is no sex predilection. The etiology is believed to be intrauterine insult at the fourth month of gestation, or it may be hereditary. Two-thirds of the cases are associated with ophthalmologic difficulties (eg, detached retina or glaucoma), and one-third are associated with otologic problems (eg, chronic otitis media and low-set ears). Mental retardation is present occasionally. If the patient lives past 5 years, he or she can lead a fairly normal life (see Chapter 17). The symptoms are choking and aspiration as a result of negative pressure created by excessive inspiratory effort. Passing a nasogastric (NG) tube may alleviate the negative pressure. Aerophagia has to be treated to prevent vomiting, airway compromise, and aspiration. Tracheotomy may not be the answer.

A modification of the Douglas lip–tongue adhesion has helped prevent early separation of the adhesion. One theory explains that the cause may be that the fetus's head is flexed, preventing forward growth of the mandible, forcing the tongue up and backward between the palatal shelves, and producing the triad of micrognathia, glossoptosis, and cleft palate.

Plummer-Vinson Syndrome (Paterson-Kelly Syndrome)

Symptoms include dysphagia due to degeneration of the esophageal muscle, atrophy of the papillae of the tongue, as well as microcytic hypochromic anemia. Achlorhydria, glossitis, pharyngitis, esophagitis, and fissures at the corner of the mouth also are observed. The prevalence of this disease is higher in women than in men, and usually presents in patients who are in their fourth decade. Treatment consists of iron administration, with esophagoscopy for dilatation and to rule out carcinoma of the esophagus, particularly at the postcricoid region. Pharyngoesophageal webs or stenosing may be noted.

This disease is to be contrasted with pernicious anemia, which is a megaloblastic anemia with diarrhea, nausea and vomiting, neurologic symptoms, enlarged spleen, and achlorhydria. Pernicious anemia is secondary to failure of the gastric fundus to secrete intrinsic factors necessary for vitamin B12 absorption. Treatment consists of intramuscular vitamin B12 (riboflavin).

Folic acid deficiency also gives rise to megaloblastic anemia, cheilosis, glossitis, ulcerative stomatitis, pharyngitis, esophagitis, dysphagia, and diarrhea. Neurologic symptoms and achlorhydria are not present. Treatment is the administration of folic acid.

Potter Syndrome

One of every 3000 infants is born with Potter syndrome. Most of them die during delivery and the rest die shortly after birth. Potter syndrome is characterized by severely malformed, low-set ears bilaterally, a small lower jaw, and extensive deformities of the external and middle ear (eg, an absence of auditory ossicles, atresia of the oval window, and abnormal course of the facial nerve). The cochlear membranous labyrinth is normal in its upper turn but contains severe hypoplasia in its basal turn, a rare cochlear anomaly.

One cause for this syndrome that has been proposed is fetal compression caused by oligoamnios.

Pseudotumor Cerebri Syndrome

Also known as benign intracranial hypertension, pseudotumor cerebri syndrome is characterized by increased intracranial pressure without focal signs of neurologic dysfunction. Obstructive hydrocephalus, mass lesions, chronic meningitis, and hypertensive and pulmonary encephalopathy should be ruled out and not confused with this syndrome. The patient is typically a young, obese female with a history of headaches, blurring of vision, or both. Facial pain and diplopia caused by unilateral or bilateral abducens nerve paralysis are less common symptoms. The CSF opening pressure on a patient lies between 250 and 600 mm of water. CSF composition, electroencephalogram (EEG), and CT scans of the head are typically normal. X-rays of the skull may reveal enlargement of the sella turcica or thinning of the dorsum sellae. This simulates a pituitary tumor, but pituitary function is normal. This syndrome is self-limited and spontaneous recovery usually will occur within a few months. Auscultation of ear canal, neck, orbits, and periauricular regions should be performed for diagnosis, as well as funduscopic examination to identify papilloma. Complete audiologic evaluations, electronystagmography (ENG), and radiographic examinations should also be made. Occlusion of the ipsilateral jugular vein by light digital pressure should make the hum disappear by cessation of blood flow in this structure.

Purpura-Like Syndrome

Purpura-like syndrome is autoimmune thrombocytopenic purpura, which can be accompanied by systemic lupus erythematosus (LE), chronic lymphocytic leukemia, or lymphoma. There seems to be a strong association between syndromes resembling autoimmune thrombocytopenia and nonhematologic malignancies.

Pyknodysostosis

Pyknodysostosis is a syndrome consisting of dwarfism, osteopetrosis, partial agenesis of the terminal phalanges of the hands and feet, cranial anomalies (persistent fontanelles), frontal and occipital bossing, and hypoplasia of the angle of the mandible. The facial bones are usually underdeveloped with pseudoprognathism. The frontal sinuses are consistently absent, and the other paranasal sinuses are hypoplastic. The mastoid air cells often are pneumatized. Toulouse-Lautrec probably had this disease.

Raeder Syndrome

This relatively benign, self-limiting syndrome consists of ipsilateral ptosis, miosis, and facial pain with intact facial sweating. Pain exists in the distribution of the ophthalmic division of the fifth cranial nerve. It results from postganglionic sympathetic involvement in the area of the internal carotid artery or from a lesion in the anterior portion of the middle cranial fossa.

Reichert Syndrome

Neuralgia of the glossopharyngeal nerve, usually precipitated by movements of the tongue or throat, is present.

Reiter Syndrome

Arthritis, urethritis, and conjunctivitis are evident.

Reye Syndrome

Reye syndrome is an often fatal disease primarily afflicting young children during winter and spring months. Its cardinal pathologic features are marked encephalopathy and fatty metamorphosis of the liver. Though its etiology is unclear, Reye syndrome has been known to occur after apparent recovery from a viral infection, primarily varicella or an upper respiratory tract infection. In some patients, there is also structural damage in cochlear and vestibular tissues of the membranous labyrinth.

Intracranial pressure monitoring and respiratory support may limit brain edema. Tracheal diversion and pulmonary care may be necessary.

Riedel Struma

This disorder is a form of thyroiditis seen most frequently in middle-aged women manifested by compression of surrounding structures (ie, trachea). There is loss of the normal thyroid lobular architecture and replacement with collagen and lymphocyte infiltration.

Rivalta Disease

Rivalta disease is an actinomycotic infection characterized by multiple indurated abscesses of the face, neck, chest, and abdomen that discharge through numerous sinus tracts.

Rollet Syndrome (Orbital Apex-Sphenoidal Syndrome)

Caused by lesions of the orbital apex that cause paralysis of cranial nerves III, IV, and VI, Rollet syndrome is characterized by ptosis, diplopia, ophthalmoplegia, optic atrophy, hyperesthesia or anesthesia of the forehead, upper eyelid and cornea, and retrobulbar neuralgia. Exophthalmos and papilledema may occur.

Romberg Syndrome

Romberg syndrome is characterized by progressive atrophy of tissues on one side of the face, occasionally extending to other parts of the body that may involve the tongue, gums, soft palate, and cartilages of the ear, nose, and larynx. Pigmentation disorders, trigeminal neuralgia, and ocular complications may be seen.

Rosai-Dorfman Disease

Rosai-Dorfman disease is benign, self-limiting lymphadenopathy, and has no detectable nodal involvement. Histiocytosis, plasma cell proliferation, and lymphophagocytosis may all be present.

Rutherford Syndrome

A familial oculodental syndrome characterized by corneal dystrophy, gingival hyperplasia, and failure of tooth eruption.

Samter Syndrome

Samter syndrome consists of three symptoms in combination:

    A. Allergy to aspirin
    B. Nasal polyposis
    C. Asthma

Scalenus Anticus Syndrome

The symptoms for scalenus anticus syndrome are identical to those for cervical rib syndrome. In scalenus anticus syndrome, the symptoms are caused by compression of the brachial plexus and subclavian artery against the first thoracic rib, probably as the result of spasms of the scalenus anticus muscle bringing pressure on the brachial plexus and the subclavian artery. Any pressure on the sympathetic nerves may cause vascular spasm resembling Raynaud disease.

Schafer Syndrome

Hereditary mental retardation, sensorineural hearing loss, prolinemia, hematuria, and photogenic epilepsy are characteristics. Schafer syndrome is due to a deficiency of proline oxidase with a resultant buildup of the amino acid proline.

Schaumann Syndrome

Schaumann syndrome is generalized sarcoidosis.

Schmidt Syndrome

Unilateral paralysis of a vocal cord, the velum palati, the trapezius, and the sternocleidomastoid muscles are found. The lesion is located in the caudal portion of the medulla and is usually of vascular origin.

Scimitar Syndrome

This congenital anomaly of the venous system of the right lung gets its name from the typical shadow formed on a thoracic roentgenogram of patients afflicted with it. (The scimitar is a curved Turkish sword that increases in diameter toward its distal end.) The most common clinical features are dyspnea and recurrent infections. The cause of scimitar syndrome is abnormal development of the right lung bed. The syndrome may be the result of vascular anomalies of the venous and arterial system of the right lung, hypoplasia of the right lung, or drainage of part of the right pulmonary venous system into the inferior vena cava, causing the scimitar sign on the thoracic roentgenogram.

This syndrome occurs between the fourth and sixth weeks of fetal life. Clinical features include displacement of heart sounds as well as heart percussion shadow toward the right. When dextroposition of the heart is marked, tomography can also help in diagnosis. Bronchography and angiography also aid in diagnosis and in providing exact information for surgical correction.

Seckel Syndrome

Seckel syndrome is a disorder that consists of dwarfism associated with a bird-like facies, beaked nose, micrognathia, palate abnormalities, low-set lobeless ears, antimongoloid slant of the palpebral fissures, clinodactyly, mental retardation, and bone disorders.

Secretion of Antidiuretic Hormone Syndrome

Secretion of antidiuretic hormone syndrome is also referred to as the syndrome of inappropriate secretion of antidiuretic hormone (SIADH). Antidiuretic hormone helps maintain constant serum osmolality by conserving water and concentrating urine. This syndrome involves low serum osmolality, elevated urinary osmolality less than maximally dilute urine, and hyponatremia. This can lead to lethargy, anorexia, headache, convulsions, coma, or cardiac arrhythmias. Increased CSF and intracranial pressure are possible etiologies. Fluid restriction can help prevent this condition.

Sheehan Syndrome

Ischemic necrosis of the anterior pituitary associated with postpartum hypotension characterizes Sheehan syndrome. It is seen in menopausal women and is associated with rheumatoid arthritis, Raynaud phenomenon, and dental caries. Changes in the lacrimal and salivary glands resemble those of Mikulicz disease. Some physicians attribute this syndrome to vitamin A deficiency. A positive LE preparation, rheumatoid factor, and an abnormal protein can be identified in this disorder.

Shy-Drager Syndrome

Usually presented in late middle age, Shy-Drager syndrome (SDS) is a form of neurogenic orthostatic hypotension that results in failure of the autonomic nervous system and signs of multiple systems atrophy affecting corticospinal and cerebellar pathways and basal ganglia. Symptoms include postural hypotension, impotence, sphincter dysfunction, and anhidrosis with later progression to panautonomic failure. Such autonomic symptoms are usually followed by atypical parkinsonism, cerebellar dysfunction with debilitation, or both, and then death. SDS should always be considered when the patient displays orthostatic hypotension, laryngeal stridor, restriction in range of vocal cord abduction (unilaterally or bilaterally), vocal hoarseness, intermittent diplophonia, and slow speech rate. This syndrome is often compared with Parkinson disease. However, SDS involves the nigrostriatal, olivopontocerebellar, brain stem, and intermediolateral column of the spinal cord. It is a multiple system disorder, whereas Parkinson disease involves only the nigrostriatal neuronal system. The symptoms, such as autonomic failure, pyramidal disease, and cerebellar dysfunction, have been associated with pathology of the pigmented nuclei and the dorsal motor nucleus of the vagus.

Sjögren Syndrome (Sicca Syndrome)

Sjögren syndrome is often manifested as keratoconjunctivitis sicca, dryness of the mucous membranes, telangiectasias or purpuric spots on the face, and bilateral parotid enlargement. It is a chronic inflammatory process involving mainly the salivary and lacrimal glands and is associated with hyperactivity of the B lymphocytes and with autoantibody and immune complex production. One of the complications of this syndrome is the development of malignant lymphoma. CT aids in the diagnosis.

Sleep Apnea Syndrome

The definition of apnea is a cessation of airflow of more than 10 seconds in duration. The conditions for sleep apnea syndrome are said to be met when at least 30 episodes of apnea occur within a 7-hour period or when 1% of a patient's sleeping time is spent in apnea. The cause of sleep apnea is unclear. Some people believe it is of central origin; others think that it may be aggravated by hypertrophied and occluding tonsils and adenoids. Some investigators classify sleep apnea into central apnea, upper airway apnea, and mixed apnea. Monitoring of the EEG and other brain stem-evoked response measurements may help identify central apnea.

Sluder Neuralgia

The symptoms are neuralgia of the lower half of the face, nasal congestion, and rhinorrhea associated with lesions of the sphenopalatine ganglion. Ocular hyperemia and increased lacrimation may be seen.

Stevens-Johnson Syndrome

Stevens-Johnson syndrome is a skin disease (erythema multiforme) with involvement of the oral cavity (stomatitis) and the eye (conjunctivitis). Stomatitis may appear as the first symptom. It is most common during the third decade of life. Treatment consists largely of steroids and supportive therapy. It is a self-limiting disease but has a 25% recurrence rate. The differential diagnosis includes herpes simplex, pemphigus, acute fusospirochetal stomatitis, chicken pox, monilial infection, and secondary syphilis.

Still Disease

Rheumatoid arthritis in children is sometimes called Still disease (see a pediatric textbook for more details).

Sturge-Weber Syndrome

Sturge-Weber syndrome is a congenital disorder that affects both sexes equally and is of unknown etiology. It is characterized by venous angioma of the leptomeninges over the cerebral cortex, ipsilateral port wine nevi, and frequent angiomatous involvement of the globe, mouth, and nasal mucosa. The patient may have convulsions, hemiparesis, glaucoma, and intracranial calcifications. There is no specific treatment.

Subclavian Steal Syndrome

Stenosis or occlusion of the subclavian or innominate artery proximal to the origin of the vertebral artery causes the pressure in the vertebral artery to be less than that of the basilar artery, particularly when the upper extremity is in action. Hence the brain receives less blood and may be ischemic. The symptoms consist of intermittent vertigo, occipital headache, blurred vision, diplopia, dysarthria, and pain in the upper extremity. The diagnosis, made through the patient's medical history, can be confirmed by the difference in blood pressure in the two upper extremities, by a bruit over the supraclavicular fossa, and by angiography.

Superior Semicircular Canal Dehiscence Syndrome

Vertigo, oscillopsia induced by loud noise, changes in middle ear, or intracranial pressure, positive Hennebert sign, and Tullio phenomenon. Dehiscence of bone overlying the superior SCC can lead to vestibular as well as auditory symptoms and signs. The vestibular abnormalities include vertigo (an illusion of motion) and an oscillopsia (the apparent motion of objects that are known to be stationary) induced by loud noises and/or by maneuvers that change middle ear or intracranial pressure. Patients with this syndrome can have eye movements in the plane of the superior canal in response to loud noises in the affected ear (Tullio phenomenon). Insufflation of air into the external auditory canal or pressure on the tragus can, in some patients, result in similar abnormalities (Hennebert sign).

The auditory abnormalities include autophony, hypersensitivity for bone-conducted sounds, and pulsatile tinnitus. Patients may complain of seemingly bizarre symptoms as hearing their eye movements in the affected ear. They may also experience an uncomfortable sensation of fullness or pressure in the ear brought about by activities that lead to vibration or motion in the long bones such as running. The Weber tuning fork test (512 Hz) often localizes to the affected ear. The audiogram will frequently show an air–bone gap in the low frequencies, and bone conduction thresholds may be better than 0-dB NHL. The findings on audiometry can resemble those in otosclerosis. Some patients with superior canal dehiscence have undergone stapedectomy, which does not lead to closure of the air–bone gap. Acoustic reflex testing can be beneficial in distinguishing an air–bone gap due to superior canal dehiscence from one due to otosclerosis. Acoustic reflexes will be absent in the affected ear of a patient with otosclerosis whereas these responses will be present in superior canal dehiscence. Patients with intact acoustic reflex responses and an air–bone gap on audiometry should undergo further investigation for superior canal dehiscence such as a high-resolution CT scan of the temporal bones before proceeding with surgical exploration of the middle ear.

Some patients have exclusively vestibular manifestations, others have exclusively auditory manifestations, and still others have both auditory and vestibular abnormalities from superior canal dehiscence. The reasons for these differences are not known. The mechanism underlying both the vestibular and auditory manifestations of this syndrome can be understood based upon the effects of the dehiscence in creation of a "third mobile window" into the inner ear.

Vestibular-evoked myogenic potential (VEMP) responses are short-latency relaxation potentials measured from tonically contracting sternocleidomastoid muscles that relax in response to ipsilateral presentation of loud sounds delivered as either clicks or tone bursts. The VEMP response is typically recorded from the sternocleidomastoid muscle that is ipsilateral to the side of sound presentation. Patients with superior canal dehiscence have a lowered threshold for eliciting a VEMP response in the ear(s) affected by the disorder. The VEMP response can also have a larger than normal amplitude in superior canal dehiscence.

High-resolution temporal bone CT scans have been used to identify dehiscence of bone overlying the superior canal. The parameters used for these CT scans are important for maximizing the specificity of the scans. Conventional temporal bone CT scans are performed with 1-mm collimation, and images are displayed in the axial and coronal planes. These scans have a relatively low specificity (high number of false positives) in the identification of superior canal dehiscence because of the effects of partial volume averaging.

The surgery is typically performed through the middle cranial fossa approach. A recent comparison of surgical outcomes in patients who underwent either canal plugging or resurfacing (without plugging of the canal lumen) revealed that complete resolution of vestibular symptoms and signs is more commonly obtained with canal plugging than with resurfacing alone.

Superior Orbital Fissure Syndrome (Orbital Apex Syndrome, Optic Foramen Syndrome, Sphenoid Fissure Syndrome)

There is involvement of cranial nerves III, IV, V1, and VI, the ophthalmic veins, and the sympathetics of the cavernous sinus. The syndrome can be caused by sphenoid sinusitis or any neoplasia in that region. Symptoms include paralysis of the upper eyelid, orbital pain, photophobia, and paralysis of the above nerves. The optic nerve may be damaged as well.

Superior Vena Cava Syndrome

This syndrome is characterized by obstruction of the superior vena cava or its main tributaries by bronchogenic carcinoma, mediastinal neoplasm, or lymphoma. Rarely, the presence of a substernal goiter causes edema and engorgement of the vessels of the face, neck, and arms, as well as a nonproductive cough and dyspnea.

Takayasu Disease

Also called "pulseless disease" and aortic arch syndrome, this disease involves narrowing of the aortic arch and its branches. Possibly an autoimmune disorder, the etiology is unknown. Symptoms often originate in the head and neck area. Sensorineural hearing loss is often an associated symptom. An association has also been found with B-cell alloantigens DR4 and MB3. Steroid treatment and cyclophosphamide have been known to help, as does surgery, although operating during a relatively inactive phase of the disease is recommended.

Tapia Syndrome

Unilateral paralysis of the larynx and tongue is coupled with atrophy of the tongue; the soft palate and cricothyroid muscle are intact. Tapia syndrome is usually caused by a lesion at the point where the 12th and 10th nerves, together with the internal carotid artery, cross one another.

Trauma is the most common cause of this syndrome. Pressure neuropathy due to inflation of the cuff of an endotracheal tube within the larynx, rather than within the trachea, is associated with the palsy of the laryngeal nerve.

Tay-Sachs Disease

An infantile form of amaurotic familial idiocy with strong familial tendencies, it is of questionably recessive inheritance. It is more commonly found among those of Semitic extraction. Histologically, the nerve cells are distorted and filled with a lipid material. The juvenile form is called Spielmeyer-Vogt disease, and the patient is normal until after 5 to 7 years of age. The juvenile form is seen in children of non-Semitic extraction as well.

Tietze Syndrome

Tietze syndrome is a costal chondritis chondropathia tuberosa of unknown etiology. Its symptoms include pain, tenderness, and swelling of one or more of the upper costal cartilages (usually the second rib). Treatment is symptomatic.

Tolosa-Hunt Syndrome

Tolosa-Hunt syndrome is a cranial polyneuropathy usually presenting as recurrent unilateral painful ophthalmoplegia. Cranial nerves II, III, IV, V1, and VI may be involved. The etiology is unknown, and there is a tendency for spontaneous resolution and for recurrence. An orbital venogram may show occlusion of the superior ophthalmic vein and at least partial obliteration of the cavernous sinus. The clinical course often responds well to systemic steroids.

Erroneous diagnoses include inflammation, tumor, vascular aneurysm, thrombus involving the orbit, superior orbital fissure, anterior cavernous sinus, parasellar area, or posterior fossa. An extension of nasopharyngeal carcinoma, mucocele, or contiguous sinusitis must also be ruled out. Sources of infection in the head and neck region, such as the tonsils, can be treated, relieving the pain of ophthalmoplegia.

Tourette Syndrome

Tourette syndrome is a disorder of the CNS, characterized by the appearance of involuntary tic movements, such as rapid eye blinking, facial twitches, head jerking, or shoulder shrugging. Involuntary sounds, such as repeated throat clearing, "nervous" coughing, or inappropriate use of words, sometimes occur simultaneously. Tourette syndrome in many cases responds to medication. It has a higher rate of absorption, or binding at D_2 dopamine receptors on cells in the caudate nucleus. The etiology of this syndrome is unknown.

Toxic Shock Syndrome

Cases of toxic shock syndrome have been found related to nasal packing and to staphylococcal infection of surgical wounds. Although the pathogenesis of the disease is incompletely understood, it is believed that packing left too long can cause bacterial overgrowth, leading to toxic shock syndrome. Symptoms include fever, rash, hypotension, mucosal hyperemia, vomiting, diarrhea, laboratory evidence of multiorgan dysfunction, and desquamation during recovery. It has been found that although antibiotic impregnation into the packing material may reduce bacterial overgrowth, it does not provide absolute protection against toxic shock syndrome.

Single-dose antimicrobial prophylaxis has proven highly effective as a treatment. Additionally, screening for toxic shock syndrome toxin (TSST)-1–producing *Staphylococcus aureus* is helpful in pointing out high-risk patients for this syndrome.

Treacher Collins Syndrome

See Chapter 17.

Trigeminal Trophic Syndrome

Trigeminal trophic syndrome, also called trigeminal neurotrophic ulceration or trigeminal neuropathy with nasal ulceration, involves ulceration of the face, particularly ala nasi, and histologic features, such as chronic, nonspecific ulceration and crusting, erythema, tendency to bleed easily, and predominant granulation tissue. Whether caused by self-induced trauma, surgery, or any process involved with the trigeminal nerve or its connections, the etiologies of nasal ulceration to be excluded with this syndrome are basal cell carcinoma, blastomycosis, leishmaniasis, leprous trigeminal neuritis, lethal midline granuloma, paracoccidioidomycosis, postsurgical herpetic reactivation, pyoderma gangrenosum, and Wegener granulomatosis. Treatment should focus on prevention of trauma to lesion and prevention of secondary infection.

Trotter Syndrome (Sinus of Morgagni Syndrome)

Neuralgia of the inferior maxillary nerve, conductive hearing loss secondary to eustachian tube blockage, preauricular edema caused by neoplastic invasion of the sinus of Morgagni, ipsilateral akinesia of the soft palate, and trismus are observed in Trotter syndrome.

Tube Feeding Syndrome

See Chapter 53.

Turner Syndrome

See Chapter 17.

Turpin Syndrome

Patients have congenital bronchiectasis, megaesophagus, tracheoesophageal fistula, vertebral deformities, rib malformations, and a heterotopic thoracic duct.

Vail Syndrome

Vail syndrome consists of unilateral, usually nocturnal, vidian neuralgia that may be associated with sinusitis.

VATER Syndrome (VACTERL Syndrome)

VATER syndrome is a nonrandom association of vertebral defects, anal atresia, tracheoesophageal fistula with esophageal atresia, renal defects, and radial limb dysplasia. Vascular anomalies, such as ventricular septal defect and single umbilical artery, have also been associated with this syndrome. Vertebral anomalies consist of hypoplasia of either the vertebral bodies or the pedicles, leading to secondary scoliosis in children. Anal and perineal anomalies consist of hypospadias, persistent urachus, female pseudohermaphroditism, imperforate anus, and genitourinary fistulas. GI anomalies include duodenal atresia, esophageal atresia, and tracheoesophageal fistula. Radial anomalies include supernumerary digiti, hypoplastic radial rays, and preaxial lower extremity anomalies. Renal anomalies include aplasia or hypoplasia of the kidneys with ectopia or fusion as well as congenital hydronephrosis and hydroureter. Hold-Oram syndrome is often confused with this syndrome, but VATER syndrome is random whereas Hold-Oram is inherited. This syndrome is suggested to be formed prior to the fifth week of fetal life during organogenesis.

Vernet Syndrome

See Jugular Foramen Syndrome (Vernet Syndrome).

Villaret Syndrome

Villaret syndrome is the same as the jugular foramen syndrome except that Horner syndrome is present here, suggesting more extensive involvement in the region of the jugular foramen, the retroparotid area, and the lateral pharyngeal space.

Vogt-Koyanagi-Harada Syndrome

Spastic diplegia with athetosis and pseudobulbar paralysis associated with a lesion of the caudate nucleus and putamen, bilateral uveitis, vitiligo, deafness, alopecia, increased CSF pressure, and retinal detachment are evidenced.

von Hippel-Lindau Disease

von Hippel-Lindau disease is associated with cerebellar, medullary, and spinal hemangioblastoma, retinal angiomata, pheochromocytoma, and renal cell carcinoma. Sometimes this fatal disease is predisposed to papillary adenoma of the temporal bone. The etiology is unknown.

Wallenberg Syndrome

Also called syndrome of the posterior–inferior cerebellar artery thrombosis or lateral medullary syndrome, Wallenberg syndrome is due to thrombosis of the posteroinferior cerebellar artery giving rise to ischemia of the brain stem (lateral medullary region). Symptoms include vertigo, nystagmus, nausea, vomiting, Horner syndrome, dysphagia, dysphonia, hypotonia, asthenia, ataxia, falling to the side of the lesion, and loss of pain and temperature sense on the ipsilateral face and contralateral side below the neck.

Weber Syndrome

Weber syndrome is characterized by paralysis of the oculomotor nerve on the side of the lesion and paralysis of the extremities, face, and tongue on the contralateral side. It indicates a lesion in the ventral and internal part of the cerebral peduncle.

Whistling Face Syndrome

Also known as craniocarpotarsal dysplasia, whistling face syndrome is mostly transmitted through autosomal dominant genes (although heterogenic transmission is not unknown). The main physical features are antimongoloid slant of the palpebral fissures, blepharophimosis, broad nasal bridge, convergent strabismus, enophthalmos, equinovarus with contracted toes, flat midface, H-shaped cutaneous dimpling on the chin, kyphosis–scoliosis, long philtrum, mask-like rigid face, microglossia, microstomia, protruding lips, small nose and nostrils, steeply inclined anterior cranial fossa on roentgenogram, thick skin over flexor surfaces of proximal phalanges, ulnar deviation, and flexion contractures of fingers.

Wildervanck (Cervico-Oculo-Acoustic) Syndrome

Wildervanck syndrome consists of mixed hearing loss, Klippel-Feil anomalad (fused cervical vertebrae), and bilateral abducens palsy with retracted bulb (Duane syndrome). Occurring in more female than male subjects, in almost a 75:1 ratio, it has sex-linked dominance with lethality in the homozygous male subject.

Wilson Disease (Hepatolenticular Degeneration)

There are two chief types of Wilson disease: one rapidly progressive that occurs during late childhood and the other slowly progressive occurring in the third or fourth decades. Familial, its symptoms are cirrhosis with progressive damage to the nervous system and brown pigmentation of the outer margin of the cornea, called Kayser-Fleischer ring. It can present with hearing loss as well.

Winkler Disease (Chondrodermatitis Nodularis Chronica Helicis)

Arteriovenous anastomosis and nerve ending accumulation at the helical portion of the ear are evident. It presents with pain and is characterized by hard, round nodules involving the skin and cartilage of the helix. Ninety percent of all cases occur in men. The treatment is to excise the nodules or administer steroids.

Xeroderma Pigmentosum (Autosomal Recessive)

This disorder presents as photosensitive skin with multiple basal cell epitheliomas. Squamous cell carcinoma or malignant melanoma can result from it. The condition occurs mainly in children. These children should be kept away from the sun.

Eponyms

Abrikossoff Tumor (Granular Cell Myoblastoma)

Causes pseudoepithelial hyperplasia in the larynx, the site most favored in the larynx being the posterior half of the vocal cord. Three percent of granular cell myoblastoma progress to malignancy. In order of decreasing frequency of involvement, the granular cell myoblastoma occurs in tongue, skin, breast, subcutaneous tissue, and respiratory tract.

Adenoid Facies

Adenoid facies is characterized by crowded teeth, high-arched palate, and underdeveloped nostrils.

Adler Bodies

Deposits of mucopolysaccharide are found in neutrophils of patients with Hurler syndrome.

Antoni Types A and B

See Chapter 53.

Arnold-Chiari Malformation

Type I:	Downward protrusion of the long, thin cerebellar tonsils through the foramen magnum
Type II:	Protrusion of the inferior cerebellar vermis through the foramen
Type III:	Bony occipital defect with descent of the entire cerebellum
Type IV:	Cerebellar hypoplasia

Arnold Ganglion

Otic ganglion.

Aschoff Body

Rheumatic nodule is found in rheumatic disease.

Ballet Sign

Ballet sign is characterized by paralysis of voluntary movements of the eyeball with preservation of the automatic movements, and is sometimes present with exophthalmic goiter and hysteria.

Bechterew Syndrome

Bechterew syndrome is characterized by paralysis of facial muscles limited to automatic movements. The power of voluntary movement is retained.

Bednar Aphthae

Bednar aphthae is characterized by symmetrical excoriations of the hard palate in the region of the pterygoid plates due to sucking of the thumb, foreign objects, or scalding.

Bezold Abscess

Bezold abscess is abscess in the sternocleidomastoid muscle secondary to perforation of the tip of the mastoid by infection.

Gland of Blandin

Gland of Blandin is a minor salivary gland situated in the anterior portion of the tongue.

Brooke Tumor (Epithelioma Adenoides Cysticum)

Brooke tumor originates from the hair follicles in the external auditory canal and auricle and of basal cell origin. Treatment is local resection.

Broyle Ligament

Broyle ligament is anterior commissure ligament of the larynx.

Brudzinski Sign

With meningitis, passive flexion of the leg on one side causes a similar movement to occur in the opposite leg. Passive flexion of the neck brings about flexion of the legs as well.

Brunner Abscess

Brunner abscess is abscess of the posterior floor of the mouth.

Bruns Sign

Bruns sign is characterized by intermittent headache, vertigo, and vomiting, especially with sudden movements of the head. It occurs in cases of tumor of the fourth ventricle of the brain.

Bryce Sign

A gurgling is heard in a neck mass. It suggests a laryngocele.

Carhart Notch

Maximum dip at 2000 kHz (bone conduction) is seen in patients with otosclerosis.

Charcot-Leyden crystals

Crystals are in the shape of elongated double pyramids, composed of spermine phosphates, and present in the sputum of asthmatic patients. Synonyms are Charcot-Newman crystals and Charcot-Robin crystals. Also found in fungal infection.

Charcot Triad

The nystagmus, scanning speech, and intention tremor are seen in multiple sclerosis.

Cherubism

Cherubism is familial, with the age of predilection between 2 and 5 years. It is characterized by giant cell reparative granuloma causing cystic lesions in the posterior rami of the mandible. The lesions are usually symmetrical. It is a self-limiting disease with remissions after puberty. The maxilla also may be involved.

Chvostek Sign

Chvostek sign is the facial twitch obtained by tapping the distribution of the facial nerve. It is indicative of hypocalcemia and is the most reliable test for hypocalcemia.

Curschmann Spirals

Curschmann spirals are spirally twisted masses of the mucus present in the sputum of bronchial asthmatic patients.

Dalrymple Sign

Upper lid retraction with upper scleral showing is a clinical manifestation of Graves orbitopathy (exophthalmos).

Demarquay Sign

Demarquay sign is characterized by absence of elevation of the larynx during deglutition. It is said to indicate syphilitic induration of the trachea.

Di Sant'Agnese Test

Di Sant'Agnese test measures the elevated sodium and chloride in the sweat of cystic fibrotic children.

Dupre Sign

Meningism.

Gustatory Glands of Ebner

These glands are the minor salivary glands near the circumvallate papillae.

Escherich Sign

In hypoparathyroidism, tapping of the skin at the angle of the mouth causes protrusion of the lips.

Flexner-Wintersteiner Rosettes

True neural rosettes of grades III and IV esthesioneuroblastoma.

Galen Anastomosis

An anastomosis between the superior laryngeal nerve and the recurrent laryngeal nerve.

Goodwin Tumor

Benign lymphoepithelioma.

Griesinger Sign

Edema of the tip of the mastoid in thrombosis of the sigmoid sinus.

Guttman Test

In the normal subject, frontal pressure on the thyroid cartilage lowers the tone of voice produced, whereas lateral pressure produces a higher tone of voice. The opposite is true with paralysis of the cricothyroid muscle.

Guyon Sign

The 12th nerve lies directly upon the external carotid artery, whereby this vessel may be distinguished from the internal carotid artery. (The safer way prior to ligation of the external carotid artery is to identify the first few branches of the external carotid artery.)

Glands of Henle

They are the small glands situated in the areolar tissue between the buccopharyngeal fascia anteriorly and the prevertebral fascia posteriorly. Infection of these glands can lead to retropharyngeal abscess. Because these glands atrophy after age 5, retropharyngeal abscess is less likely to occur after that age.

Hennebert Sign

See Chapter 17. The presence of a positive fistula test in the absence of an obvious fistula is called Hennebert sign. The patient has a normal-appearing tympanic membrane and external auditory canal. The nystagmus is more marked upon application of negative pressure. This sign is present with congenital syphilis and is believed to be due to an excessively mobile footplate or caused by motion of the saccule mediated by fibrosis between the footplate and the saccule.

Hering-Breuer Reflex

A respiratory reflex from pulmonary stretch receptors. Inflation of the lungs sends an inhibitory impulse to the CNS via the vagus nerve to stop inspiration. Similarly, deflation of the lungs sends an impulse to stop expiration. This action is the Hering-Breuer reflex.

Homer-Wright Rosettes

Pseudorosette pattern seen in grade I esthesioneuroblastoma.

Kernig Sign

When the subject lies on the back with the thigh at a right angle to the trunk, straightening of the leg (extending the leg) elicits pain, supposedly owing to the pull on the inflamed lumbosacral nerve roots. This sign is present with meningitis.

Kiesselbach Plexus

This area is in the anterior septum where the capillaries merge. It is often the site of anterior epistaxis and has also been referred to as Little's area.

Koplik Spot

Pale round spots on the oral mucosa, conjunctiva, and lacrimal caruncle that are seen in the beginning stages of measles.

Krause Nodes

Nodes in the jugular foramen.

Lhermitte Sign

A rare complication of radiation to the head and neck region causing damage to the cervical spinal cord, symptoms of Lhermitte sign consist of lightning-like electrical sensation spreading to both arms, down the dorsal spine, and to both legs upon neck flexion.

Lillie-Crowe Test

Lillie-Crowe test is used in the diagnosis of unilateral sinus thrombophlebitis. Digital compression of the opposite internal jugular vein causes the retinal veins to dilate.

Little Area

See Kiesselbach Plexus.

Luschka Pouch

See Thornwaldt Cyst.

Marcus Gunn Phenomenon

Unilateral ptosis of the eyelid with exaggerated opening of the eye during movements of the mandible.

Marjolin Ulcer

Marjolin ulcer is a carcinoma that arises at the site of an old burn scar. It is a well-differentiated squamous cell carcinoma that is aggressive and metastasizes rapidly.

Meckel Ganglion

Sphenopalatine ganglion.

Mikulicz Cells

These cells are macrophages in rhinoscleroma. (Russell bodies, which are eosinophilic, round structures associated with plasma cells, are also found with rhinoscleroma.)

Mollaret-Debre Test

Mollaret-Debre test is performed for cat scratch fever.

Sinus of Morgagni

A dehiscence of the superior constrictor muscle and the buccopharyngeal fascia where the eustachian tube opens.

Ventricle of Morgagni

Ventricle of Morgagni separates the quadrangular membrane from the conus elasticus in the larynx.

Nikolsky Sign

Detachment of the sheets of superficial epithelial layers when any traction is applied over the surface of the epithelial involvement in pemphigus is characteristic of Nikolsky sign. Pemphigus involves the intraepithelial layer, whereas pemphigoid involves the subepithelial layer. The former is a lethal disease in many instances.

Oliver-Cardarelli Sign

Recession of the larynx and trachea is synchronous with cardiac systole in cases of aneurysm of the arch of the aorta or in cases of a tumor in that region.

Parinaud Sign

Extraocular muscle impairment with decreased upward gaze and ptosis seen in association with pinealomas and other lesions of the tectum.

Paul-Bunnell Test

Paul-Bunnell test measures the elevated heterophile titer of infectious mononucleosis.

Physaliferous Cells

"Soap bubble" cells of chordoma.

Psammoma Bodies

Found with papillary carcinoma of the thyroid.

Rathke Pouch

See Thornwaldt Cyst.

Reinke Tumor

A "soft" tumor variant of lymphoepithelioma in which the lymphocytes predominate. (With the hard tumor the epithelial cells predominate; it is called Schmincke tumor.)

Romberg Sign

If a patient standing with the feet together "falls" when closing the eyes, the Romberg test is positive. It is indicative of either abnormal proprioception or abnormal vestibular function. It does not necessarily distinguish central from peripheral lesions. Cerebellar function is not evaluated by this test.

Rosenbach Sign

Fine tremor of the closed eyelids seen in hyperthyroidism and hysteria.

Rouvier Node

Lateral retropharyngeal node, Rouvier node is a common target of metastases in nasopharyngeal carcinoma.

Russell Bodies

Eosinophilic, round structures; associated with plasma cells found in rhinoscleroma.

Santorini Cartilage

Corniculate cartilage of the larynx, composed of fibroelastic cartilage.

Santorini Fissures

Fissures in the anterior cartilaginous external auditory canal leading to the parotid region.

Schaumann Bodies

Together with asteroids, they are found in sarcoid granuloma.

Schmincke Tumor

The "hard" variant of lymphoepithelioma in which the epithelial cells predominate (see Reinke Tumor).

Schneiderian Mucosa

Pseudostratified ciliated columnar mucosa of the nose.

Seeligmüller Sign

Contraction of the pupil on the affected side in facial neuralgia.

Semon Law

Semon law is a law stating that injury to the recurrent laryngeal nerve results in paralysis of the abductor muscle of the larynx (cricoarytenoid posticus) before paralysis of the adductor muscles. During recovery, the adductor recovers before the abductor.

Straus Sign

With facial paralysis, the lesion is peripheral if injection of pilocarpine is followed by sweating on the affected side later than on the normal side.

Sudeck Sign

Sudeck sign is sometimes associated with Grisel syndrome and is recognized by the displacement of the spine of the axis to the same side as the head is turned.

Sulkowitch Test

Sulkowitch test determines an increase in calciuria.

Thornwaldt Cyst

A depression exists in the nasopharyngeal vault that is a remnant of the pouch of Luschka. When this depression becomes infected, Thornwaldt cyst results. In the early embryo, this area has a connection between the notochord and entoderm. Thornwaldt cyst is lined with respiratory epithelium with some squamous metaplasia. Anterior to this pit, the path taken by Rathke pouch sometimes persists as the craniopharyngeal canal, running from the sella turcica through the body of the sphenoid to an opening on the undersurface of the skull.

Tobey-Ayer-Queckenstedt Test

Tobey-Ayer-Queckenstedt test is used in the diagnosis of unilateral and bilateral sinus thrombophlebitis. In cases where the lateral sinus is obstructed on one side, compression of the jugular vein on the intact side causes a rise in CSF pressure, whereas compression of the obstructed side does not raise the CSF pressure.

Toynbee Law

When CNS complications arise in chronic otitis media, the lateral sinus and cerebellum are involved in mastoiditis, whereas the cerebrum alone is involved in instances of cholesteatoma of the attic.

Trousseau Sign

With hypocalcemia a tourniquet placed around the arm causes tetany.

Tullio Phenomenon

See Chapter 17. This phenomenon is said to be present when a loud noise precipitates vertigo. It can be present in congenital syphilis, with a SCC fistula, or in a postfenestration patient if the footplate is mobile. The tympanic membrane and ossicular chain must be intact with a mobile footplate.

Wartenberg Sign

Intense pruritus of the tip of the nose and nostril indicates cerebral tumor.

Warthin-Finkeldey Giant Cells

Warthin-Finkeldey giant cells are found in the lymphoid with measles.

Warthin-Starry Stain

Warthin-Starry stain is used to identify cat scratch bacillus.

Weber Glands

Weber glands are minor salivary glands in the superior pole of the tonsil.

Wrisberg Cartilage

Wrisberg cartilage is the cuneiform cartilage of the larynx, composed of fibroelastic cartilage.

Xeroderma Pigmentosa

Xeroderma pigmentosa is hereditary precancerous condition that begins during early childhood. These patients die at puberty.

Zaufal Sign

Saddle nose.

Zellballen

Nest of cells surrounded by sustentacular cells seen in paragangliomas.

Clinical Entities Presenting With Dysequilibrium

The clinical entities presenting with vertigo or dysequilibrium have been named by their mode of presentation. As more information becomes available about clinical entities, the emphasis is shifting toward finding an etiology for the symptoms. When evaluating a patient with vertigo, one should try to differentiate between vertigo of peripheral origin and that of central origin. The following list of differential diagnoses constitutes the more common etiologies of the dizzy patient:

Acoustic Neuroma (Vestibular Schwannoma)

Acoustic neuroma, a benign, slow-growing tumor, has its origin most commonly in the vestibular division of the eighth cranial nerve. Most patients with acoustic neuromas complain of unsteadiness rather than episodic vertigo. As the enlarging tumor spills over into the cochlear division of the eighth nerve or compromises the artery to the inner ear, hearing symptoms become manifest. These symptoms include unilateral tinnitus, hearing loss, or both. Initially the findings may be indistinguishable from Ménière syndrome. With time, there is a progressive hearing loss, with a disproportionate loss of speech discrimination occurring long before a total hearing loss occurs. Acoustic neuroma accounts for 80% of cerebellar–pontine (CP) angle tumors.

Even though the facial nerve is in close proximity, visible signs of facial nerve (VII) palsy occur only rarely in advanced cases. More commonly, the first modality affected by the pressure on the fifth (trigeminal) nerve is demonstrated by altered corneal sensation. Later, there may be symptoms of numbness in any or all divisions of the trigeminal nerve. On rare occasions, trigeminal neuralgia has been a presenting symptom.

The audiologic evaluation may vary from normal pure tone hearing with poor speech discrimination to a pure tone sensorineural hearing loss and poor or absent speech discrimination. A search for the acoustic stapedial reflexes with the impedance bridge may show reflexes present at normal levels without evidence of decay in about 18% of the tumors. The reflexes are helpful when they are absent or show evidence of decay when the behavioral pure tones are in the normal range. ABR is the most sensitive test in detecting acoustic neuromas, abnormal in 82% of small intracanalicular tumors.

When there is an absent caloric response in the suspect ear with no history of dysequilibrium, the vestibular evaluation heightens one's suspicion.

Magnetic resonance imaging (MRI) with intravenous contrast (gadolinium-DPTA) is a reliable and cost-effective method of identifying tumors and may be selected as the first or only imaging technique. Tumors as small as 2 mm may be enhanced and identified.

Presbystasis (Dysequilibrium of Aging) and Cardiovascular Causes

Age-related decline in peripheral vestibular function, visual acuity, proprioception, and motor control has a cumulative effect upon balance and is the most common cause of dysequilibrium.

Arrhythmias usually produce dysequilibrium. They rarely present to the otologist but are seen in consultation with the cardiologist. However, consideration must be given when seeing a new patient with dysequilibrium.

Benign Paroxysmal Positional Vertigo

The symptoms include sudden attacks of vertigo precipitated by sitting up, lying down, or turning in bed. These attacks have been reported to be prompted by sudden movement of the head to the right or left or by extension of the neck when looking upward. The sensation of vertigo is always of short duration even when the provocative position is maintained. Diagnosis can be confirmed by positional testing (Dix-Hallpike test), which indicates positional nystagmus with latency and fatigability.

Etiologies include degenerative changes, otitis media, labyrinthine concussion, previous ear surgery, and occlusion of the anterior vestibular artery. The cause is thought to involve abnormal sensitivity of the SCC ampulla, specially the posterior, to gravitational forces stimulated by free-floating abnormally dense particles (canaliths). These particles can be repositioned and the symptoms resolved in a high percentage of cases, by canalith repositioning procedure.

To effectively carry out the procedure, one should be able to envision the ongoing orientation of the SCCs while carrying out the head maneuvers.

Internuclear Ophthalmoplegia

Internuclear ophthalmoplegia is a disturbance of the lateral movements of the eyes characterized by a paralysis of the internal rectus on one side and weakness of the external rectus on the other. In testing, the examiner has the patient follow his or her finger, first to one side and then to the other, as when testing for horizontal nystagmus. Internuclear ophthalmoplegia is recognized when the adductive eye (third nerve) is weak and the abducting eye (sixth nerve) moves normally and displays a coarse nystagmus ("perhaps" vestibular nuclei involvement). The pathology is in the medial longitudinal fasciculus (MLF). When the disorder is bilateral, it is pathognomonic of multiple sclerosis. When it is unilateral, one should consider a tumor or vascular process.

Intracranial Tumors

There are a small but definite number of patients that present with dysequilibrium associated with primary or secondary intracranial tumors. The use of CT and MRI scanning, without and with intravenous contrast, in selected patients helps identify these otherwise silent lesions.

Ménière Disease

The symptoms, when complete and classically present, include fluctuating sensorineural hearing loss, fluctuating tinnitus, and fluctuating fullness in the affected ear. In addition, as the tinnitus, fullness, and hearing loss intensify, an attack of episodic vertigo follows, lasting 30 minutes to 2 hours. The process may spontaneously remit, never occur again, and leave no residual or perhaps a mild hearing loss and tinnitus. In 85% of the patients, the disease affects only one ear. However, should the second ear become involved, it usually happens within 36 months. The natural history is final remission occurs in about 60% of the patients.

Cochlear hydrops, vestibular hydrops, or Lermoyez syndrome have aural fullness as the common denominator. *Cochlear hydrops* is characterized by the fluctuating sensorineural hearing loss and tinnitus. *Vestibular hydrops* has episodic vertigo as well as the aural fullness. *Lermoyez syndrome* is characterized by increasing tinnitus, hearing loss, and aural fullness that is relieved after an episodic attack of vertigo. Recurrence of this phenomenon can be expected. *Crisis of Tumarkin or drop attack* is another variant of Ménière syndrome in which the patient loses extensor powers and falls to the ground suddenly and severely. There is no loss of consciousness and complete recovery occurs almost immediately. This occurs late in the disease process with no warning.

Audiometric tests show a fluctuating low-tone sensorineural hearing loss, and little to no tone decay. The ENG findings commonly show very little between the initial episodes. During the attack, there may be active spontaneous nystagmus with direction changing components even in the midst of caloric testing.

Because the stage at which a spontaneous remission occurs cannot be predicted, several medical and surgical therapies have evolved to alter the natural history. The medical therapies are aimed at the symptoms and include vestibular suppressants, vasodilators, and diuretics. The surgical therapies are either destructive, or preservative of residual hearing. The first includes labyrinthectomy or translabyrinthine eighth nerve section when there is no useful hearing. Procedures when there is useful hearing include selective (middle cranial fossa, retrolabyrinthine, or retrosigmoid) vestibular nerve section, gentamicin or streptomycin application to the inner ear. Conservative procedures include those performed on the endolymphatic sac. They range from sac decompression to endolymphatic–mastoid shunts. The latter appears directed at correcting the resultant mechanical or production–reabsorption changes seen in the histopathology of endolymphatic hydrops in the temporal bone. Cochleosacculotomy is indicated in elderly patients, with disabling vertigo, poor hearing, and residual vestibular function under local anesthesia.

Glycerol Test It is speculated that the administration of glycerol in an oral dose of 1.2 mL/kg of body weight with the addition of an equal amount of physiologic saline to a patient with Ménière syndrome may have diagnostic value in clinical management. Within 1 hour of administration, the patient may sense an improvement in the hearing loss, tinnitus, and sensation of fullness in the ear with maximum effects occurring within 2 to 3 hours. After 3 hours, the symptoms slowly return.

Metabolic Vertigo

There are no clinical symptoms that separate the metabolic form from other forms of vertigo. A prerequisite may be an abnormally functioning vestibular system. In this instance, the metabolic factor exaggerates or interferes with the compensatory mechanisms and brings about the symptoms. Dietary modification often results in a striking improvement in symptoms.

Hypothyroidism is an extremely rare but definite cause. Many times the patients are not otherwise clinically hypothyroid.

Allergic causes are very elusive in the management of the dizzy patient, but the screening IgE assay may give a clue. Radioallergosorbent test (RAST) or skin testing may provide more precise findings about an allergic cause and its treatment. When there is no clear-cut history and in the absence of any other clearly defined cause, an allergic management should be undertaken.

Multiple Sclerosis

Multiple sclerosis is one of the more common neurologic diseases encountered in a clinical practice. Vertigo is the presenting symptom of multiple sclerosis in 7% to 10% of the patients or eventually appears during the course of disease in as many as one-third of the cases. The patient usually complains of unsteadiness along with vertigo. Vertical nystagmus, bilateral internuclear ophthalmoplegia, and ataxic eye movements are other clues to this disease. *Charcot triad* (nystagmus, scanning speech, and intention tremor) may be present. Electronystagmography may show anything from normal findings to peripheral findings to central findings. Auditory brain stem-evoked potentials may show delay of central conduction. More likely, there is a significant delay of the visually evoked potentials. Research into an etiology for this disorder is pointing to an autoimmune disorder of the myelin.

Oscillopsia (Jumbling of the Panorama) Dandy Syndrome

Since our heads bob up and down while walking, the otolithic system controls eye movement to maintain a constant horizon when walking. When there is bilateral absent vestibular function as seen with ototoxic drug use, *the loss of otolithic function results in oscillopsia,* which is the inability to maintain the horizon while walking.

Otitis Media

Suppurative or serous otitis media may have associated vestibular symptoms. In serous otitis media, the presence of fluid in the middle ear restricting the round window membrane, serous labyrinthitis, may be responsible for the vestibular symptoms. Removing the serous fluid either medically or surgically gives rise to remission of the dizziness.

In the presence of suppuration there may be reversible serous labyrinthitis or irreversible suppurative labyrinthitis, and the more extensive sequestrum with a dead ear and facial nerve palsy. In this instance, judgment about the disease and its effects determines the proper treatment.

Otosclerosis (Otospongiosis)

There appears to be three areas where otosclerosis may bear relation to dysequilibrium. The first occurs in relation to the fixed footplate. There may be a change in the fluid dynamics of the inner ear, giving rise to vestibular symptoms. In a large number of patients, the symptoms are cleared by stapedectomy.

Sometimes vertigo begins after stapedectomy. It may occur with a perilymph fistula that requires revision and repair. A total, irreversible loss of hearing with vertigo may also occur. A destructive surgical procedure of labyrinthectomy with or without eighth nerve section is indicated if the vestibular suppressants fail to control the dysequilibrium.

The coexistence of otosclerotic foci around the vestibular labyrinth with elevated blood fats or blood glucose abnormalities may give rise to vestibular symptoms. Effective treatment requires fluoride therapy.

There is also evidence that an otosclerotic focus may literally grow through the vestibular nerve. In this instance, a reduced vestibular response (RVR) is found on ENG testing. This clinical presentation may look like vestibular neuronitis in the absence of a hearing loss.

Ototoxic Drugs

Ototoxic drugs, predominantly aminoglycoside antibiotics, are usually used in lifesaving situations where no other antibiotics are judged to be as effective. The main symptom is oscillopsia and results from lack of otolithic input to allow the eyes to maintain a level horizon. This is found while the head is bobbing up and down as the individual walks.

The use of rotational testing, especially at the higher frequencies, may reveal function that is not evident on caloric testing. The presence of this rotational function indicates intact responses in other areas of vestibular sensitivity. This intact function may separate the patient who will benefit from vestibular rehabilitation from the patient who will not. This may also explain the difference in the degree of disability between patients.

Sometimes the usual vestibular suppressants aid the patient. In other instances, one is frustrated by an inability to adequately treat this condition.

Perilymph Fistula

In the absence of hearing loss, perilymph fistula is a cause of vertigo. The history should be straightforward for impulsive trauma or barotrauma, and the resultant symptoms clearly follow. However, this is not always the case, as a sneeze or vigorous blowing of the nose may be the inciting event. The resultant vertigo may not occur for some time. The clue in the history is one of an episodic nature usually related to exertion. Many patients are asymptomatic on awakening in the morning only to have symptoms appear once they are up and around. A positive fistula sign with or without ENG results is helpful, although a negative sign does not rule out a fistula.

Associated symptoms of ear fullness, tinnitus, and mild or fluctuating hearing loss help localize the problem to the ear. Many patients demonstrate nystagmus with the affected ear down; however, this finding alone is not a reliable sign to determine the pathologic ear. The definitive diagnosis occurs at surgery, but there are instances where there are equivocal findings at surgery.

Posttraumatic Vertigo

Posttraumatic vertigo comprises a history of head trauma followed by a number of possible symptoms, such as dysequilibrium. If there is a total loss of balance and hearing function, the use of vestibular suppressants may result in a cure that is sustained after cessation of the suppressants. In some instances when there is no cure, a labyrinthectomy or eighth nerve section ameliorates the symptoms. Occasionally, there is a progressive hearing loss.

After trauma, delayed Ménière syndrome may develop. This may be resistant to medical therapy and requires surgery. In this instance, endolymphatic sac surgery can improve the symptoms if there is no fracture displacement through the endolymphatic duct.

The statoconia of the otolithic system may have become dislodged by the trauma. With head movement, they roll toward the ampullated end of the posterior SCC. Their weight deflects the ampullary contents producing a gravity stimulus that stimulates a positional vertigo of a post-traumatic type. The nystagmus is said to occur with the affected ear down. The most effective treatment is with habituation exercises. Vestibular neurectomy is also a recommended therapy.

Syphilis: Congenital and Acquired

The neurotologic findings associated with syphilis usually present with bilateral Ménière syndrome. There is a significant hearing loss and usually bilateral absent caloric function. Another common clinical manifestation is the presence of interstitial keratitis. The patients, as a rule, are in their midforties; however, when the onset occurs during childhood, the hearing loss is abrupt, bilaterally symmetrical, and more severe.

These patients usually have a positive Hennebert sign (ie, positive fistula test without any demonstrable fistula along with a normal external auditory canal and tympanic membrane). The positive fistula test indicates an abnormally mobile footplate or an absence or softening of the bony plate covering the lateral SCC. The patient also may demonstrate Tullio phenomenon.

Histopathologically, the soft tissue of the labyrinth may demonstrate mononuclear leukocyte infiltration with obliterative endarteritis, inflammatory fibrosis, and endolymphatic hydrops. Osteolytic lesions are often seen in the otic capsule.

The treatment consists of an intensive course of penicillin therapy for an adequate interval. Patients allergic to penicillin should be desensitized to this drug in the hospital and given 20 million units of penicillin intravenously daily for 10 days. The use of steroids may result in a dramatic improvement in hearing and a reduction of vestibular symptoms. Usually, the steroids must be maintained indefinitely to retain the clinical improvement.

Temporal Bone Fracture and Labyrinthine Concussion

Transverse Fracture Because a transverse fracture destroys the auditory and vestibular function, the patient has no hearing or vestibular response in that ear. Initially, the patient is severely vertiginous and demonstrates a spontaneous nystagmus whose fast component is away from the injured side. The severe vertigo subsides after a week, and the patient may remain mildly unsteady for 3 to 6 months. The patient may also have labyrinthine concussion of the contralateral side, and facial nerve palsy is not uncommon.

Longitudinal Fracture Longitudinal fractures constitute 80% of the temporal bone fracture. With this type of fracture, there is usually bleeding into the middle ear with perforation of the tympanic membrane and disruption of the tympanic ring. Thus, there may be a conductive hearing loss from the middle ear pathology and a sensorineural high-frequency hearing loss from a concomitant labyrinthine concussion. There may also be evidence of peripheral facial nerve palsy. Dizziness may be mild or absent except during positional testing.

Labyrinthine Concussion Labyrinthine concussion is secondary to head injury. The patient complains of mild unsteadiness or light-headedness, particularly with a change of head position. Audiometric testing may reveal a high-frequency hearing loss. The ENG may show a spontaneous or positional nystagmus, an RVR, or both. As the effects of the concussion reverse, the symptoms and objective findings also move toward normal.

Vascular Insufficiency and Its Syndromes

Vascular insufficiency can be a common cause of vertigo among people over the age of 50 as well as patients with diabetes, hypertension, or hyperlipidemia. The following syndromes have been recognized among patients with vascular insufficiency.

Labyrinthine Apoplexy Labyrinthine apoplexy is due to thrombosis of the internal auditory artery or one of its branches. The symptoms include acute vertigo with nausea and vomiting. Hearing loss and tinnitus may also occur.

Wallenberg Syndrome Wallenberg syndrome is also known as the lateral medullary syndrome secondary to infarction of the medulla, which is supplied by the posterior inferior cerebellar artery. This syndrome is believed to be the most common brain stem vascular disorder. The symptoms include the following:

A. Vertigo, nausea, vomiting, nystagmus
B. Ataxia, falling toward the side of the brain
C. Loss of the sense of pain and temperature sensations on the ipsilateral and contralateral body
D. Dysphagia with ipsilateral palate and vocal cord paralysis
E. Ipsilateral Horner syndrome

Subclavian Steal Syndrome

Subclavian steal syndrome is characterized by intermittent vertigo, occipital headache, blurred vision, diplopia, dysarthria, pain in the upper extremity, loud bruit or palpable thrill over the supraclavicular fossa, a difference of 20 mm Hg in systolic blood pressure between the two arms, and a delayed or weakened radial pulse. The blockage can be surgically corrected.

Anterior Vestibular Artery Occlusion This symptom complex includes:

A. A sudden onset of vertigo without deafness
B. A slow recovery followed by months of positional vertigo of the benign paroxysmal type
C. Signs of histologic degeneration of the utricular macula, cristae of the lateral and superior SCCs, and the superior vestibular nerve

Vertebrobasilar Insufficiency

The symptoms of vertebrobasilar insufficiency include vertigo, hemiparesis, visual disturbances, dysarthria, headache, and vomiting. These symptoms are a result of a drop in blood flow to the vestibular nuclei and surrounding structures. The posterior and anterior inferior cerebellar arteries are involved. Tinnitus and deafness are unusual symptoms.

Drop attacks without loss of consciousness and precipitated by neck motion are characteristic of vertebrobasilar insufficiency.

Cervical Vertigo

Cervical vertigo can be caused by cervical spondylosis as well as by other etiologies. Cervical spondylosis can be brought about by degeneration of the intervertebral disk. As the disk space narrows, approximation of the vertebral bodies takes place. With mobility, the bulging of the annulus is increased, causing increased traction on the periosteum to which the annulus is attached and stimulating proliferation of bone along the margins of the vertebral bodies to produce osteophytes.

Barre believed that the symptoms of cervical spondylosis (including vertigo) are due to irritation of the vertebral sympathetic plexus, which is in close proximity to the vertebral artery. It is claimed that spondylosis irritates the periarterial neural plexus in the wall of the vertebral and basilar arteries leading to contraction of the vessels. Temporary ischemia then gives rise to vertigo. Others claimed that the loss of proprioception in the neck can give rise to cervical vertigo. Emotional tension, rotation of the head, and extension of the head can cause the neck muscle (including the scalenus anticus) to be drawn tightly over the thyrocervical trunk and subclavian artery, compressing these vessels against the proximal vertebral artery. In elderly individuals, a change from the supine to the upright position may give rise to postural hypotension, which in turn may cause vertebrobasilar insufficiency. The aortic arch syndrome and subclavian steal syndrome may also cause cervical vertigo.

Symptoms include the following:

A. Headache, vertigo
B. Syncope
C. Tinnitus and loss of hearing (usually low frequencies)
D. Nausea and vomiting (vagal response)
E. Visual symptoms, such as flashing lights (not uncommon), due to ischemia of the occipital lobe, supplied by the posterior cerebral artery, a branch of the basilar artery
F. Supraclavicular bruit seen by physical examination in one-third of the patients

Each of these symptoms usually appears when the head or neck assumes a certain position or change of position.

Proper posture, neck exercises, cervical traction, heat massage, anesthetic infiltration, and immobilization of the neck with a collar temporarily are all good therapeutic measures. If traction is required, it can be given as a few pounds horizontally for several hours at a time. For cervical spondylosis without acute root symptoms, heavy traction (100 lb) for 1 to 2 minutes continuously or 5 to 10 minutes intermittently is considered by some to be more effective.

Vertiginous Epilepsy

Dysequilibrium as a symptom of epilepsy is seen in two forms. The first is an aura of a major Jacksonian seizure. The second is the momentary, almost petit mal seizure whose entire brief moment is experienced as dysequilibrium. The diagnosis of the latter form may require a sleep EEG. These patients respond to usual seizure control therapy.

Cortical vertigo either can be as severe and episodic as Ménière disease or it may manifest itself as a mild unsteadiness. It is usually associated with hallucinations of music or sound. The patient may exhibit daydreaming and purposeful or purposeless repetitive movements. Motor abnormalities such as chewing, lip smacking, and facial grimacing are not uncommon. The patient may experience an unusual sense of familiarity (déjà vu) or a sense of strangeness (*jamais vu*). Should the seizure discharge spread beyond the temporal lobe, grand mal seizures may ensue.

Vertigo due to Whiplash Injury

Patients often complain of dizziness following a whiplash injury. In some cases, there is no physiologic evidence for this complaint. In others, ENG has documented objective findings, such as spontaneous nystagmus. The onset of dizziness often occurs 7 to 10 days following the accident, particularly with head movements toward the side of the neck most involved in the whiplash. The symptoms may last months or years after the accident.

Otologic examination is usually normal. Audiometric studies are normal unless there is associated labyrinthine concussion. Vestibular examination can reveal spontaneous nystagmus or positional nystagmus with the head turned in the direction of the whiplash. The use of ENG is essential for evaluation of these patients.

Vertigo With Migraine

Vertebrobasilar migraine is due to impairment of circulation of the brain stem. The symptoms include vertigo, dysarthria, ataxia, paresthesia, diplopia, diffuse scintillating scotomas, or homonymous hemianopsia. The initial vasoconstriction is followed by vasodilatation giving rise to an intense throbbing headache, usually unilateral. A positive family history is obtained in more than 50% of these patients. Treatment of migraine includes butalbital (Fiorinal), ergot derivatives, and methysergide (Sansert). The latter has the tendency to cause retroperitoneal fibrosis.

Vestibular Neuronitis

Occasionally referred to as viral labyrinthitis, vestibular neuronitis begins with a nonspecific viral illness followed in a variable period of up to 6 weeks by a sudden onset of vertigo with nausea, vomiting, and the sensation of blacking out accompanied by severe unsteadiness. The patient, however, does not lose consciousness. The severe attack can last days to weeks. Cochlear symptoms are absent and without associated neurologic deficits. When seen initially, the patient has spontaneous nystagmus to the contralateral side, and ENG demonstrates a unilaterally reduced caloric response. The remainder of the evaluation is negative for a cause. In most patients, vestibular compensation clears the symptoms in time. The remission may be hastened by the effective use of vestibular suppressant medication for a period of up to 6 weeks. After the acute episode has subsided, which may take weeks, the patient continues to experience a slight sensation of light-headedness for some time, particularly in connection with sudden movements. The acute episode may also be followed by a period of positional vertigo of the benign paroxysmal type.

A small percentage of afflicted patients do not respond to vestibular suppression or to vestibular compensation. In these patients, an evaluation for metabolic, otosclerotic, or autoimmune factors is indicated. If these other factors are identified and the appropriate treatment initiated, the symptoms may disappear. If after an appropriate treatment and observation period, and if incapacitating symptoms persist, a retrolabyrinthine vestibular nerve section is indicated. Abnormal myelination has been found in some of these nerve specimens.

Bibliography

Hennekam R, Krantz I, Allanson J, eds. Gorlin's Syndromes of the Head and Neck. 5th ed. New York, NY: Oxford University Press; 2010.

Questions

1. Which of the following is characterized by hypoplastic malar eminences, down-slanting palpebral fissures, normal IQ, and aural atresia?
   A. Waardenburg syndrome
   B. Goldenhar syndrome
   C. Treacher-Collins syndrome
   D. Apert syndrome

2. Zellballen is best described as
   A. Whorled cellular pattern with psammoma bodies
   B. Cellular nests and sustentacular cells
   C. Keratin pearls
   D. Palisading cells and Verocay bodies

3. Sipple syndrome is a familial syndrome consisting of
   A. Medullary carcinoma of the thyroid
   B. Hyperparathyroidism
   C. Pheochromocytoma
   D. All of the above

4. Nonsyphilitic interstitial keratitis and progressive hearing loss with vestibular symptoms is characteristic of
   A. Meniere disease
   B. Alport syndrome
   C. Cogan syndrome
   D. Behçet disease

5. Which of the following syndromes is characterized by cerebellar, medullary, and spinal hemangioblastoma, pheochromocytoma, and bilateral papillary adenocarcinoma of the temporal bone?
   A. Chediak Higashi syndrome
   B. von Hippel-Lindau syndrome
   C. Takayasu disease
   D. Costen syndrome

Chapter 2
Obstructive Sleep Apnea

Obstructive sleep apnea (OSA) is a highly prevalent disorder typified by repeated episodes of complete or partial pharyngeal collapse and airway obstruction occurring during sleep. It is estimated by the seminal Wisconsin Sleep Cohort that OSA affects 3% of middle-aged women and 9% of middle-aged men, with incidence increasing in parallel with society's worsening obesity rates. This disorder is among the most common problems presenting to Otolaryngology—Head and Neck surgeons, and a recent NEJM (The New England Journal of Medicine) editorial has described OSA as a "perioperative epidemic."

Sleep Disordered Breathing

The term *sleep disordered breathing* (SDB) refers to a large number of sleep-related breathing problems, of which OSA is just one, the others being beyond the scope of this chapter. In regard to obstructive diseases specifically, the severity can range from simple snoring to life-threatening obstruction. The more commonly employed terms are stated below.

Primary Snoring

This is defined as snoring without concomitant arousals or sleep fragmentation. All patients with OSA will snore, but not all snorers have OSA. Although not pathological in and of itself, snoring can be associated with altered sleep habits (because of bed partner dissatisfaction). Additionally there is emerging evidence that the physical trauma of the snoring vibrations on neck structures can be independently associated with carotid artery stenosis and stroke.

Upper Airway Resistance

This syndrome remains poorly defined in the literature. It is generally accepted to consist of respiratory events during sleep that are not severe enough to qualify as apneas or hypopneas, but still lead to sleep fragmentation and daytime symptoms.

Obstructive Sleep Apnea

Obstructive sleep apnea is formally defined as repetitive episodes of airway obstruction consisting of either hypopneas (partial obstruction associated with hypoxia and brief sleep arousal) or apneas (complete obstruction for minimum of 10 seconds associated with hypoxia and brief arousal). In OSA, evidence must also exist of respiratory effort being made in association with the decreased or absent airflow, in order to differentiate this from central sleep apnea (in which no respiratory efforts are made). Respiratory events in OSA are more common during Stage 2 or rapid-eye-movement (REM) sleep, which in the adult is the largest proportional sleep stage.

Impact of OSA on Personal Health

- Snoring
- Witnessed choking or gasping
- Frequent body moments
- Disproportionate fatigue
- Daytime somnolence
- Morning headaches
- Sensation of unrefreshing sleep
- Memory loss
- Sexual dysfunction
- Personality changes

Impact of OSA on Society

- Increased odds-ratio of motor vehicle accidents (MVAs).
- Loss of economic productivity.
- Workplace accidents.
- Patients with OSA are known to use more health-care resources.

Medical Consequences of Untreated OSA

Hypertension

OSA is an independent risk factor for hypertension (HTN) development as shown by the Sleep Heart Health Study. This is thought to be associated with increased sympathetic tone from chronic hypoxia and the frequent cortical arousals. Once an apnea occurs the cardiac output decreases, triggering increased firing of the sympathetic nervous system and associated increased systemic vascular resistance. This cycle happens repeatedly throughout the apneic sleep time and eventually persists throughout the day too. Successful treatment of OSA is known to decrease HTN severity even in patients resistant to pharmacotherapy.

Cardiovascular Disease

OSA is well known to be associated with increased risk of heart attack, stroke, and death. This has been prominently demonstrated in the Busselton Health Study, showing that untreated OSA was an independent mortality risk factor. OSA can also worsen preexisting congestive heart failure by decreasing cardiac output as well as altering catecholamine levels. Cardiac arrhythmias can also be seen in patients with OSA, with the most common being brady- or tachyarrhythmias.

Cerebrovascular Disease

Like the heart, the brain is also under hypoxic stress during OSA. In the midst of apneic events there can be increases in the intracranial pressure leading to decreased cerebral perfusion, which correspondingly increases stroke risk. Additionally the snoring associated with OSA can lead to atherosclerotic changes in the carotid arteries, worsening the chance of an embolic event in the brain.

Making the Diagnosis

History

Diagnosis begins with a thorough history. Patients should be questioned about sleep habits and hygiene, typical sleep initiation and wake-up times, and shift work, in addition to asking about the standard symptoms and signs of sleep apnea. History can also be used to distinguish fatigue from OSA versus other type of sleep disorders such as insomnia or simple lack of sleep. Comorbidities of OSA should be pursued. It is very important to question patients about their sleepiness at work or while driving, as in some jurisdictions or for certain occupations the physician is required by law to notify the transportation authorities or company about excessively drowsy patients who are at risk of driving or operating equipment. If possible a history should be taken from the bed partner, who can both corroborate and expand on the patient's complaints. It is not surprising to find patients who claim to either be asymptomatic, or downplay their symptoms, as over years of untreated disease a process of normalization occurs. Screening tools can be also used to help quantify disease severity. The most commonly employed is the Epworth sleepiness scale (Figure 2-1), which is a validated measure of daytime somnolence (although not specific

EPWORTH SLEEPINESS SCALE

Please answer the following questions based on this scale:

0. Would never fall asleep
1. Slight chance of dozing
2. Moderate chance of dozing
3. High chance of dozing

Situation	Chance of Dozing
Reading	_____
Watching TV	_____
Sitting in a public place (eg, theater or meeting place)	_____
Driving a car, stopped at a traffic light	_____
As a passenger in a car for an hour without a break	_____
During quite time after lunch without alcohol	_____
Lying down to rest when circumstances permit	_____
Total Score:	_____

Epworth Score < 8 = Normal

Figure 2-1 The Epworth sleepiness scale.

to OSA). A score over 10 is considered problematic. The Berlin scale is useful as a screening test for OSA as it is more specific, but is also more complex to employ. Quality of life scoring is valuable to assess the impact of disease on personal health. Performance vigilance testing is important as a direct measure of the impact of OSA on wakefulness—these tests are widely available on the Internet.

Physical Findings

All patients suspected of having OSA should undergo a complete head and neck examination to assess for areas of obstruction. The body mass index (BMI) should be calculated as well. Specific areas to examine include the following:

Nose
- Deviated septum
- Turbinate hypertrophy
- Nasal polyposis
- Concha bullosa

The nasal cavity should be examined both with a speculum and endoscope. If the nose is blocked, this can lead to downstream increases in airflow resistance both directly (by nasal obstruction) and secondarily (by forcing mouth opening which in turn drops the tongue and pushes the hyoid backward).

Nasopharynx
- Adenoid tissue

Oral Cavity
- Size and position of tongue
- Scalloping of tongue edges
- Mandibular or palatine tori
- Assess occlusive status and jaw position

Scalloping of the tongue can indicate relative macroglossia. Jaw occlusion and position (Angle Classification II in particular) should be noted as a retrognathic jaw, which means the tongue will be relatively posteriorly positioned. Tori of large size can also decrease room inside the oral cavity, which can in turn malposition the malleable tongue.

Oropharynx
- Tonsil size and position
- Soft palate thickness and position
- Uvular size, wrinkles, thickness, and position
- Medialized lateral pharyngeal walls

One of the most important physical assessments in OSA is the relationship between the tonsils, tongue, and palate. This can be graded using the Friedman staging system. The tonsils are Friedman graded from 0 to 4: 0 = no tonsil (prior tonsillectomy); 1 = small, lateral to the pillars; 2 = extend to edge of tonsil pillars; 3 = extend beyond tonsil pillars; 4 = hypertrophic and midline contact. The Friedman palate position grading differs from the anesthesiology Mallampati classification. In the Friedman system the tongue is not protruded and remains in a neutral position with mouth open, whereas the Mallampati classification involves having the patient open their mouth wide and protrude the tongue. The Friedman palate grades are: I = posterior pharyngeal wall visible; II = uvula visible; III = soft palate visible; IV = hard palate visible (Figure 2-2). The Mallampati system is not correct to use when assessing OSA, as it is not an accurate reflection of the patient's oropharyngeal anatomical relationships during sleep.

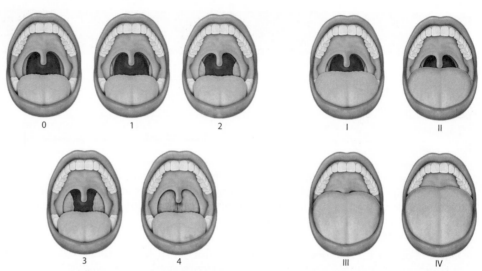

Figure 2-2 *Friedman tonsil and palate grading scales. (Reproduced with permission from Friedman M, Ibrahim H, Bass L: Clinical staging for sleep-disordered breathing,* Otolaryngol Head Neck Surg. *2002 Jul;127(1):13-21.)*

Hypopharynx
- Size and position of tongue base relative to epiglottis
- Lingual tonsil hypertrophy

The hypopharynx should be examined with a flexible fiberoptic endoscope to study both the retropalatal and retrolingual areas. The Mueller maneuver (MM) is a commonly employed examination test during which the patient's mouth is closed and nose pinched after which they are asked to inhale and the examiner can see which areas of the pharynx collapse. This is done with the patient both sitting and lying down. MM is simple to perform and inexpensive but is hampered by poor inter- and intra-rater reliability. Additionally there is a low correlation with intraoperative findings and a low positive-predictive value for success at pharyngeal sleep surgery. Another valuable method of endoscopic assessment is to identify areas of obstruction seen in the pharynx at end-expiration (which is thought to be the time of the respiration cycle most prone to collapse). This is a more reproducible maneuver and also more valid than the MM.

Supraglottis
- Epiglottis shape
- Epiglottis position relative to posterior pharyngeal wall
- Size and position of tongue base relative to epiglottis

An increasing body of evidence has shown that the larynx may play a more prominent role in OSA than previously thought, especially in cases resistant to standard therapies.

Drug-Induced Sleep Endoscopy

Office-based assessments of the patient are hampered by the fact that anatomical and physiological findings while aware are known to be different from those during sleep. Drug-induced sleep endoscopy (DISE) is a method of examination performed while the patient is asleep and in recent years has gained considerable traction in the sleep community. Under appropriate anesthetic supervision, sleep is induced via either midazolam or propofol after which the endoscope is inserted and the relevant anatomical subsites examined in a structured fashion. Various

Structure	Degree of Obstruction[a]	Configuration[c]		
		A–P	Lateral	Concentric
Velum				
Oropharynx lateral walls[b]				
Tongue Base				
Epiglottis				

For each structure, there should be a classification as to the degree of obstruction and configuration of obstruction. *Open boxes* reflect the potential configuration that can be visualized related to a specific structure. *Shaded boxes* reflect the fact that a specific structure-configuration cannot be seen (eg, oropharynx lateral walls in an anteroposterior direction).

A-P Anteroposterior.

[a]Degree of obstruction has one number for each structure: 0, No obstruction (no vibration); 1, Partial obstruction (vibration); 2, Complete obstruction (collapse); X, Not visualized.

[b]Oropharynx obstruction can be distinguished as related solely to the tonsils or including the lateral walls, with or without a tonsillar component.

[c]Configuration noted for structures with degree of obstruction greater than 0.

Figure 2-3 The VOTE scoring system used during DISE.

protocols, most commonly the VOTE system, allow for valid and reproducible examinations to be performed (Figure 2-3). Patients who have very severe OSA or are morbidly obese represent relative contraindications to DISE. There remain open questions regarding the cost-effectiveness of DISE and its predictive value to surgical outcomes. Since it is resource intensive DISE is not indicated for all patients with OSA; it is rather suggested for use in the following situations:

- Where clinical findings do not match sleep study outcomes
- Failure of primary surgery
- Prior to major surgical intervention

Polysomnography

Sleep studies are currently considered the gold standard in making the diagnosis of OSA as well as tracking responses to therapy. The American Academy of Sleep Medicine (AASM) has defined four levels of sleep studies.

Level 1 Polysomnography (PSG) This is the prototypical attended hospital-based overnight study, requiring 6 hours of recording sleep at an efficiency of 70% or better to make an accurate recording. A technician is preset to hook up all recording leads and remains present overnight to adjust or correct as necessary as well as to observe the patients' sleep behaviors. Specific recordings made include: Electroencephalogram (EEG), ECG (Electrocardiogram), Electro-oculogram (EOG), nasal airflow, oxygen saturation (Sao_2), thoracic and abdominal movements, leg movements, body position, and snoring sound. From the Level 1 PSG is derived the fundamental diagnostic measure of OSA, that being the apnea-hypopnea index (AHI). Disease severity can be subdivided into mild (AHI < 15), moderate (AHI 15-30), and severe (AHI > 30). Typically blood pressure is at risk when the AHI is greater than 30, but the other cut-offs are less objectively defined. The level 1 PSG is also able to distinguish central from obstructive sleep apnea. Performing this as a split-night study with the addition of continuous positive airway pressure (CPAP) for the second half of the night allows for immediate therapy and titration.

Although considered the gold-standard test for OSA, level 1 PSG is also highly resource intensive and expensive and considered by many practitioners to be overly detailed beyond what is required to initiate and maintain therapy. There are also questions as to validity of the study in that patients frequently report that their sleep in the lab was different than that which they do at home.

Level 2 PSG This is performed in the patient's home without a technician present, but is otherwise identical in recording channels to a level 1 PSG. This test is rarely performed due to a higher incidence of lost data from misplaced leads.

Level 3 PSG (Ambulatory Sleep Study) This is performed in the patient's home as well but records fewer outcomes, most typically Sao_2, body motion, snoring, and chest movement. Modern devices are far more sensitive than those from the past, and mobile software has also improved accuracy tremendously. In many jurisdictions, ambulatory studies are rapidly overtaking level 1 PSG as the primary test for OSA due to their convenience, decreased cost, and improved accuracy. Patients tend to believe the diagnosis more if the test takes place in their own bed, and this in turn increases therapeutic adherence. As demand increases for sleep diagnostics and technology continues to improve, level 3 ambulatory sleep studies are likely to grow in importance. Practice standards for ambulatory sleep studies have been developed based on American and Canadian Thoracic Society guidelines, and practitioners in sleep medicine and surgery should familiarize themselves with these documents. In general, it is necessary that ambulatory sleep studies when used are part of a comprehensive sleep program, that quality assurance checks exists, and that the result is interpreted by a qualified or experienced sleep expert.

Level 4 PSG This is essentially home oximetry. Although simple to perform, the test is insufficiently detailed for therapeutic planning and can lead to false positives (in patients with mild chronic obstructive pulmonary disease) and false negatives (in a subgroup of patients with problematic OSA but only mild desaturations). This test is rarely performed.

Nonsurgical Therapy of OSA

Behavioral Modifications

Various conservative measures have been shown to improve both the fundamental indices of OSA as well as symptoms. Patients should be warned against excessive alcohol or sedative consumption as these can disturb respiratory drive. Patients who are feeling sleepy also commonly feel the need to take stimulants (eg, excess caffeine) that can further alter sleep hygiene. Weight reduction is the key in treatment of OSA, but despite the physician's well-meaning intentions and suggestions, weight loss of the degree needed to alter OSA is frequently unattainable by the patient, and therefore consideration should be given to refer the morbidly obese patient to bariatric surgery. Positional therapy (by retraining the body not to sleep supine) can also be attempted either by commercially available devices or homemade products.

CPAP

CPAP has been considered the gold standard of OSA therapy. It functions as a pneumatic splint to prevent airway collapse. In the past the air pumps were cumbersome and loud, but modern devices are both stylish and far quieter. CPAP may be delivered in three main ways: via nasal mask, nasal cannula, or full-face mask. When patients are able to tolerate CPAP and wear it frequently, their disease will be effectively treated. Newer machines have built-in compliance monitors as well as self-diagnostics to check for air leak as well as auto-titration of the air pressure. Bilevel positive airway pressure (BiPAP) devices can help deliver higher air pressure than CPAP can by altering the pressure during inspiration versus expiration to more comfortable levels.

The AASM defines adequate therapy as 4 hours per night, 5 nights per week. However, numerous studies indicate that generally only approximately 50% of patients are still able to use the device at this rate. Although the AHI improvement while on CPAP is almost always robust, generally only the lab-based PSG results are reported, as opposed to long-term results when considered over total sleep time at home, which are likely to be less impressive. It is not sufficient to simply prescribe CPAP as one would a medication, but rather extensive coaching and long-term support should be offered to help maximize therapeutic adherence. Reasons for CPAP nonadherence include the following:

- Comfort
- Cost
- Claustrophobia
- Convenience
- Side effects (skin rashes, nasal irritation, eye irrigation, and nasal congestion)

Oral Appliance Therapy

Oral-mandibular splints can be utilized to prevent oropharyngeal or hypopharyngeal collapse during sleep. There are numerous marketed devices, but the common theme is to hold the mandible relatively protruded compared to the maxilla, in turn bringing the soft pharyngeal structures forward thereby opening the airway. Some newer devices can be titrated to patient comfort and also record adherence. Most devices are very effective for snoring, and in some cases these can also be used as a therapy bridge if CPAP cannot be consistently used. The most common complications of mandibular repositioning devices are temporomandibular joint discomfort, malocclusion, and an overly dry mouth.

Surgical Treatment of OSA

Surgery for OSA is intended to expand the pharyngeal airway, thus restoring patency and improving both AHI and symptomatic outcomes. The modern concept of multilevel surgery suggests that operations should take place at more than one level of the pharynx, the goal being to address the multiple collapsing segments and obtain cure. Multilevel surgery can either be staged or performed simultaneously based on clinician's discretion and patient characteristics. Indications for surgery for OSA include the following:

- CPAP nonadherence
- Favorable anatomy
- Cardiovascular dysfunction
- Patient preference

Nasal Surgery

Whenever nasal obstruction exists in the setting of OSA, corrective measures should be offered. Options for nasal surgery include the following:

- Septoplasty (open vs endoscopic)
- Nasal valve surgery (functional septorhinoplasty)
- Turbinate surgery
- Polypectomy
- Endoscopic adenoidectomy
- Removal obstructive concha bullosa

Does Nasal Surgery Affect OSA or Snoring? Nasal surgery is not intended to affect either snoring or the AHI. The nose is not a collapsing segment, and thus altering airflow therein is unlikely to change the patient's OSA. Many patients need to be educated in that regard. Correction of nasal obstruction can, however, improve the perception of sleep quality as well as decrease daytime fatigue.

Does Nasal Surgery Facilitate CPAP Use? Correction of nasal obstruction has been shown to both improve CPAP adherence and potentially decrease the machine's pressure (if nasal CPAP is prescribed). The literature is as yet unable to provide guidance as to the optimal time to resume nasal CPAP use after surgery, so clinicians should use their individual judgement in terms of optimal early resumption versus the effect the mask may have on the healing nose.

Oropharyngeal Surgery

The oropharynx holds some of the most compliant tissues in the upper airway and is frequently cited as the main area of collapse. Numerous surgical options exist, and it is important that the clinicians not have a one-size-fits-all approach, but rather tailor the choice of which procedure to use with the right anatomical characteristics of the patient. The modern options for oropharyngeal surgery include the following:

- Isolated tonsillectomy
- Uvulopalatopharyngoplasty (UPPP)
- Uvulopalatal flap (UPF)
- Expansion sphincteroplasty (ES)
- Transpalatal advancement pharyngoplasty (TPA)
- Cautery-assisted palate stiffening operation (CAPSO)
- Soft palate implants (SPI)

Isolated Tonsillectomy Extremely hypertrophic tonsils are rare in adults. Both Friedman's original publications and subsequent data suggest that grade 3 or 4 tonsils only occur in 10% to 12% of the population. However, these patients represent optimal candidates for tonsillectomy and both AHI and symptomatic improvement can be high in this group.

Uvulopalatopharyngoplasty This procedure has long been synonymous with OSA surgery. Introduced by Fujita in 1981, it consists of tonsillectomy simultaneous to trimming of redundant tissue from the soft palate, uvula, and palatoglossus muscles. The posterior pillars are then sutured anteriorly, as is the back of the palate to the front, in order to expand the whole oropharyngeal airway anteriorly. When considering all patients, UPPP has a suboptimal historical success rate of approximately 50%. However, using the Friedman staging system in a thoughtful manner to perform this procedure on more anatomically favorable patients (ie, those with Friedman tonsil grade 2-4 and palate position I-II), long-term success rates of over 85% can be reliably obtained; this stands in contradistinction to the long-term problematic adherence to CPAP. UPPP is not appropriate as an isolated procedure when tongue base contributions to OSA are strongly suspected. Complications of UPPP include the following:

- Pain
- Infection
- Bleeding
- Velopharyngeal insufficiency (due to malfunction of levator palatini)
- Nasopharyngeal stenosis (due to over-resection of the levator palatini)

Uvulopalatal Flap UPF is a variant of UPPP introduced by Powell and Riley in which the posterior palate is denuded of mucosa and the resulting defect is closed via a rotation flap from the uvula (Figure 2-4). This procedure is advantageous to UPPP because the muscle is left intact,

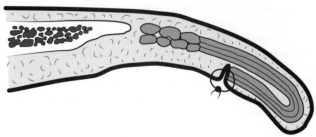

Figure 2-4 Saggital depiction of a completed UPF.

which both decreases pain and minimizes levator dysfunction. Outcomes from surgery are similar to UPPP. UPF is contraindicated if the palate is overly thick as otherwise patients can feel the resulting flap that can lead to problematic gagging.

Expansion Sphincteroplasty Some patients with OSA have narrowing in the lateral dimension more than that in the anteroposterior, often caused by excessively thick palatopharyngeus muscles. Pang introduced ES as means of treating this subgroup. The palatopharyngeus muscle is divided two-thirds of the way down its length and then dissected off the underlying superior constrictor. Two channels are created in the lateral soft palate, and the palatopharngeal stumps are rotated superolaterally and inset into the palate with a tendon stitch. This has the effect of widely opening the pharynx in the lateral dimension. Randomized level evidence has shown that this procedure is more effective than UPPP for appropriately chosen patients.

Transpalatal Advancement Patients with excessively lengthy hard palates are candidates for this procedure. The posterior edge of the hard palate is trimmed and the now free-floating soft palate is advanced anteriorly and sutured to the new hard palate edge. This opens the pharyngeal airway without the need for soft tissue resection. Although this procedure carries good success, it is hampered by problematic oronasal fistula rates.

CAPSO This is an office-based surgery in which needle-tip electrocautery is used to remove a diamond-shaped strip of mucosa off the soft palate. This induces scar tissue to form, which stiffens the palate. Although this carries good success for snoring improvement, this procedure is unlikely to be of benefit for OSA.

Soft Palate Implants Palatal implants made of polyethylene terephthalate have been developed for insertion using a preloaded hand-piece (Medtronic). The implants are inserted in the midline and laterally, just distal to the hard/soft palate junction. The implants themselves are relatively stiff, and the resulting scar tissue from insertion further stiffens the palate. Snoring outcomes are typically very good for the first year after insertion, but then deteriorate in subsequent years (although remaining improved compared to baseline). However, the procedure is relatively painless in comparison to CAPSO. Implant rejection rates have consistently hovered at 1% over the years since introduction.

Hypopharyngeal and Supraglottic Surgery

The hypopharynx and supraglottis are increasingly being identified as major components of the pathological OSA airway. Surgery on these areas should be contemplated if they are identified as collapsing segments. The options to treat the hypopharynx and supraglottis include the following:

- Radiofrequency ablation of the tongue base
- Lingual tonsillectomy

- Hyoid suspension
- Tongue suspension
- Midline glossectomy
- Supraglottoplasty

Radiofrequency Ablation of the Tongue Base Radiofrequency (RF) energy is a temperature-controlled method of delivering relatively high-power current over a longer period of time, inducing scar tissue via plasma formation but at a lower temperature than seen for typical mono-/bipolar cautery. This has significant advantages in terms of reducing pain and swelling after surgery. Numerous published protocols exist, but most involve creating 4 to 6 paired lesions at the base of the tongue within the muscle tissue. The resulting scar stiffens the tongue and also over time reabsorbs, thus volumetrically reducing the tongue size. Potential complications include ulceration, taste change, foreign body sensation, and infection. Tongue base ablation has been shown in several studies to tremendously augment UPPP success rates in higher Friedman stage patients.

Lingual Tonsillectomy The lingual tonsils form part of Waldeyer lymphatic ring of tissue and in many patients with OSA they can be markedly hypertrophic. Multiple methods for reduction exist, most commonly using RF or Coblation technology to shrink them down or ablate at a low temperature (Figure 2-5). Adequate visualization can be achieved via use of a transoral 70-degree endoscope. Potential complications are similar to that of RF ablation of tongue muscle.

Hyoid Suspension In some patients with OSA the hyoid bone is thought to be posteriorly positioned, thus dragging the tongue backward too. Suspending the hyoid anteriorly by transecting the strap muscles and affixing it to the thyroid cartilage may open the airway anteriorly. This procedure is not commonly done and is most useful as augmentative as opposed to stand-alone.

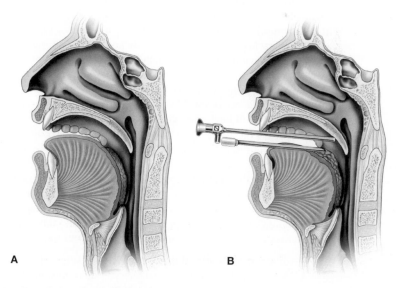

A   **B**

Figure 2-5 (A and B) Before and after views of lingual tonsillectomy.

Tongue Suspension The tongue can be suspended from the genial tubercle using a commercially available low-torque screw and suture system (Medtronic). Suspending the tongue is thought to help prevent posterior collapse. Some patients notice the feeling of an altered swallow or foreign body sensation after this surgery.

Midline Glossectomy Resecting tissue from the base of the tongue in the midline may be done transorally using RF or Coblation technology as well as using the endoscopic microdebrider. Exposure can be improved with the use of endoscopes. The end result is volume reduction at the base of the tongue with an increase in the hypopharyngeal airway. Complications include bleeding from the lingual artery, hypoglossal nerve injury, hematoma, abscess, dysphagia, and taste disturbance.

Supraglottoplasty During DISE or office examination, certain patients are observed to have significant epiglottic collapse either due to configuration of the cartilage or from redundant arytenoid soft tissue. These cases may also be resistant to CPAP, because the pneumatic splint can actually augment the epiglottic collapse. Laser or microdebrider trimming of this tissue can markedly open the airway and improve OSA. All standard laryngeal surgery considerations should apply when this type of surgery is contemplated.

Osseous Surgery for OSA

In addition to soft tissue operations, the other way to consider OSA surgery is that of enlarging the bony confines of the pharynx. Options for osseous surgery include the following:

- Genioglossus advancement
- Maxillomandibular advancement (MMA)

Genioglossus Advancement A rectangular geniotubercle osteotomy is made, the resulting block pulled forward and then rotated and affixed to the anterior mandible with a screw (after removing the anterior table to prevent cosmetic deformity). This advances the tongue forward, thus opening the posterior airway. Potential complications include dental injury, mental nerve injury, mandible fracture, and hematoma. This procedure, like hyoid suspension, is considered augmentative as opposed to stand-alone.

Maxillomandibular Advancement Of all surgeries for OSA, this is the single most effective aside from tracheostomy (Figure 2-6). By performing a series of osteotomies (LeFort 1 for the maxilla and saggital split for the mandible), the boney confines of the airway can be moved anteriorly, taking with them the soft tissue collapsing segments. The moved bone is affixed with plates. Typically orthodontic work may often be required both before and after surgery to optimize healing and occlusion. MMA is most commonly indicated in significantly retrognathic patients who would likely not benefit from traditional soft-tissue surgery, although it also has a role as salvage procedure when primary OSA surgery has failed.

Tracheostomy for OSA

Tracheostomy is the only surgery that definitively cures OSA. Via bypass of the obstructive segments, full airway patency is restored. Tracheostomy in this patient population is often challenging due to morbid obesity and perioperative anesthetic and respiratory concerns. This procedure carries significant personal and social implications, and thus it is rarely performed. The indications for tracheostomy for OSA include the following:

- Failure of conventional therapy (CPAP +/− surgery)
- Not a candidate for traditional pharyngeal expansion procedures
- Significant cardiovascular comorbidities
- Life-threatening OSA

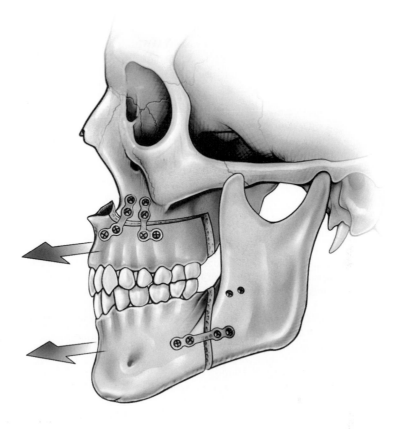

Figure 2-6 Maxillomandibular advancement.

Monitoring After Surgery for Sleep Apnea

A debate has emerged regarding the need for, and the extent of, postoperative Sao_2 monitoring after surgery for OSA. Patients with OSA are theoretically at risk for postoperative respiratory complications because of altered oxygenation physiology, and therefore many hospitals would routinely admit patients for overnight monitoring in high-intensity units. This philosophy has been challenged in recent years because of more modern evidence suggesting that this level of observation is excessive for many patients, the actual rate of respiratory complications is very low, and the admitted patients do not benefit from observation. Current OSA-specific indications for admission and Sao_2 monitoring after surgery include the following:

- Severe symptomatic OSA with highly elevated AHI
- Cardiovascular comorbidities
- Major tongue base surgery

Defining Successful Treatment of OSA

Unlike many other disorders of the head and neck, there is a significant disconnect between the symptoms of OSA and the results of PSG testing. Some patients with elevated AHI are relatively asymptomatic, whereas various patients with lower AHI describe disproportionate symptoms. When treating patients with OSA it is not simply sufficient to aim for a goal of a lowered AHI on postoperative PSG, but also to identify improvement in both symptoms and comorbidities. Broadly speaking, success at surgical therapy can be defined as:

- Decrease in AHI to less than 50% of baseline
- Decrease in AHI to less than 20
- Improvement in witnessed apneas (as noted by bed partner)
- Improvement in daytime symptoms
- Improvement in comorbidities (eg, HTN)
- Improvement in ancillary measures of OSA (quality of life, performance tests)

Bibliography

Aurora RN, Casey KR, Kristo D, et al. Practice parameters for the surgical modifications of the upper airway for obstructive sleep apnea in adults. *Sleep*. 2010;33(10):1408-1413.

Friedman M, Ibraham H, Bass L. Clinical staging for sleep-disordered breathing. *Otolaryngol Head Neck Surg*. 2002;127(1):13-21.

George CF. Reduction in motor vehicle collisions following treatment of sleep apnoea with nasal CPAP. *Thorax*. 2001;56(7):508-512.

Rotenberg BW, Theriault J, Gottesman S. Redefining the timing of surgery for obstructive sleep apnea in anatomically favorable patients. *Laryngoscope*. 2014. Doi: 101002/lary.24720.

Young T, Peppard PE, Gottlieb DJ. Epidemiology of obstructive sleep apnea: a population health perspective. *Am J Respir Crit Care Med*. 2002;165(9):1217-1239.

Questions

1. The definition of an apnea includes
   A. cessation of airflow for 10 seconds
   B. cessation of airflow for 10 seconds with an arousal
   C. hypoxia after decreased airflow for 10 seconds
   D. cessation of airflow for 20 seconds with an arousal

2. All of the following are indications for surgery for OSA except
   A. nonadherence to CPAP
   B. patient preference
   C. favorable anatomy
   D. small tonsils

3. When performing Friedman staging of a patient's oropharynx, which of the following is true?
   A. The tongue is protruded.
   B. The patient is instructed to say "ahh".

    C. The patient is asked to swallow.

    D. The patient is asked to open mouth without any other action.

4. The only curative surgery for OSA is
   A. UPPP
   B. tracheostomy
   C. MMA
   D. lingual tonsillectomy

5. Indications for drug-induced sleep endoscopy include all of the following except
   A. mandatory before any surgery takes place
   B. where clinical findings do not match sleep study outcomes
   C. failure of primary surgery
   D. prior to major surgical intervention

Chapter 3
Laser and Radiofrequency Surgery

Lasers in Otolaryngology

History

- *Laser* is an acronym for "light amplification by stimulated emission of radiation."
- In 1917, Albert Einstein described the theoretical basis of lasers in his paper *Zur Quantentheorie der Strahlung*. The first functional laser was constructed in 1957 by Theodore Maiman, a physicist at Hughes Research Laboratories in Malibu, California.

Physics of Lasers

A laser is a resonant cavity flanked by two mirrors and filled with an active medium that can be gas, liquid, or solid. One of the mirrors is 100% reflective and the other is partially reflective (leaky). A laser also has a pump or external energy source. Pumping the laser can be accomplished by passing current through the active medium or by using a flash lamp. When a laser is pumped, energy is absorbed by the atoms of the active medium, raising electrons to higher energy levels. The high-energy electrons then spontaneously decay to their lower-energy "ground state," emitting a photon in a random direction. This process is called *spontaneous emission*. Most of these spontaneously emitted photons are absorbed and decay; however, the photons emitted in the direction of the long axis of the resonant cavity are retained as they bounce between the two mirrors of the laser. When these photons encounter an atom in the excited state, they stimulate an excited electron to decay to its ground state and emit another photon of the same wavelength in the same direction. This process is called *stimulated emission*. When more than half of the atoms in the active medium reach the high-energy state, *population inversion* occurs. This is a necessary condition for a laser to start working. As light is amplified in the active medium through the process of stimulated emission, the partially reflective mirror begins emanating light that is uniform in wavelength, direction, phase, and polarization. This creates the familiar laser beam (Figure 3-1).

Properties of Laser Light

- Laser light is monochromatic, unidirectional, and uniform in phase and polarization.
- Laser beam spreads over distances, and can be focused with lenses.
- Once laser light exits the main resonance chamber, it has to be delivered to tissue via one of two major delivery mechanisms. The preferred delivery medium is the optical fiber. Light in the visible spectrum easily travels through an optical fiber and can be

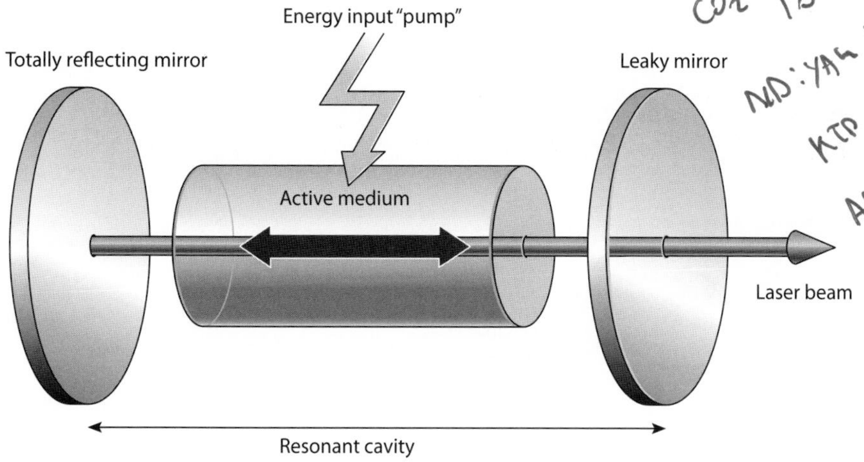

[handwritten: CO₂ 10600 (IR)]
[handwritten: ND:YAG 1080 nm (near-IR)]
[handwritten: KTP 532 nm]
[handwritten: Argon 516nm]

Figure 3-1 Components of a laser include an active medium flanked by two mirrors and a pumping mechanism that delivers energy to the active medium.

delivered directly to target tissues through a handpiece without significant energy loss. Even the near-infrared light of the Nd:YAG laser (1.06 μm) can be delivered through a fiber; however, infrared (IR) light of the CO_2 laser (10.6 μm) cannot be delivered via optical fiber, a major shortcoming of this highly popular laser. CO_2 laser light is delivered through waveguides that are essentially a series of articulated hollow tubes and mirrors. OmniGuide (Cambridge, MA) developed a flexible delivery system for the CO_2 laser, resembling the flexibility of an optical fiber, which allows the surgeon to deliver CO_2 laser light through a handpiece directly to target tissues.

Laser–Tissue Interaction

[handwritten: · In visible light longer = deeper]
[handwritten: · Not for IR BR near-IR easily absorbed by water]

- Tissue interacts only with laser light that is absorbed, not reflected, transmitted, or scattered.
- In general, lasers with longer wavelengths have deeper tissue penetration. This rule holds for lasers in the visible spectrum, but not for IR lasers such as CO_2 and Er:YAG. These lasers in the IR range (3-10 μm) are easily absorbed by water and have shallow tissue penetration.
- Ultraviolet lasers (UV), currently used in ophthalmology, work by tissue heating and photodissociation of bonds. Visible and IR lasers, commonly used in otolaryngology, work by heating tissue only. Laser energy is absorbed and converted to heat.
- *Thermal relaxation time*—time needed for tissue to dissipate half of its heat.
- A laser characteristically produces a wound with the following layers: tissue vaporization, necrosis, and thermal conductivity and repair (reversible damage) (Figure 3-2).
- High laser energy delivered in short pulses minimizes thermal injury by allowing time for heat to diffuse between pulses.
- Laser parameters under surgeon's control are power, spot size, and exposure time.
- Tissue effect depends on the amount of energy deposited into tissue (J/cm^2).
- The surgeon can change the spot size and energy delivered per unit area by changing the lens strength or simply working in and out of focus.
- *Chromophore*—the target molecule that absorbs laser light. For example, in laser skin resurfacing, the chromophore is water contained in the skin. When ablating a vascular

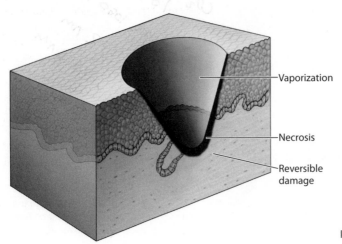

Figure 3-2 Layers of a laser wound.

lesion, the chromophore is hemoglobin. When removing a tattoo, the chromophore is the dye contained within the skin. When removing a pigmented skin lesion or dark hair, the chromophore is melanin.

- Spectral analysis of hemoglobin shows the highest absorption peak at 405 to 420 nm (*blue*) and two secondary peaks at 538 nm (*green*) and 578 nm (*yellow*). Absorption drops off abruptly at wavelengths longer than 600 nm. Because of shallow tissue penetration of blue light and competitive absorption of blue light by melanin, medical lasers targeting vascular lesions exploit the secondary absorption peaks (530-600 nm). The melanin absorption curve is smoother. Melanin absorption is best at blue wavelengths in the 400-nm range and slowly decreases as wavelength increases. Melanin absorption drops off rapidly at wavelengths longer than 700 nm. The third major chromophore for medical applications is water. Water absorbs IR light. Water absorption starts in the 800- to 900-nm range and increases as the wavelength increases, peaking at 2.94 μm that corresponds to the Er:YAG laser output. At 2.94 mm, water-containing tissue is easily ablated.

Commonly Used Medical Lasers

- *Argon (514 nm—blue green)*: transmits easily through clear tissues. Light is absorbed by hemoglobin and pigmented tissue. Used for photocoagulation of pigmented lesions, port-wine stains, hemangiomas, and telangiectasias.
- *Copper vapor (511 nm—green, 578 nm—yellow)*: The green 511-nm laser is best absorbed by melanin and is used to treat superficial pigmented lesions, café au lait spots, nevi, and freckles. The yellow 578-nm variety is better absorbed by hemoglobin and is used for vascular lesions.
- *KTP (potassium titanyl phosphate, 532 nm—green)*: absorbed by hemoglobin better than the argon laser. Used for pigmented dermal lesions and port-wine stains. Light can easily be delivered through a flexible fiberoptic bronchoscope for management of tracheobronchial lesions. KTP laser has been used in endoscopic sinus surgery and management of sinonasal polyps. Major advantage of the KTP laser in sinonasal surgery is excellent hemostasis.

- *Tunable dye laser (585 nm—yellow)*: Dye is chosen for best absorption by hemoglobin. Used for treatment of vascular lesions such as hemangiomas and port-wine stains.
- *Ruby (694 nm—red)*: absorbed by melanin. This laser was used for hair and tattoo removal, works best in patients with light skin complexion.
- *Alexandrite (755 nm—red)*: absorbed by melanin. Alexandrite laser is frequently used for hair and tattoo removal in patients with a range of Fitzpatrick skin types.
- *Nd:YAG (neodymium yttrium aluminum garnet, 1.06 μm—near IR)*: It produces a layer of tissue coagulation and necrosis 4 mm deep, and precise control is not possible. This laser allows good control of hemorrhage. It is used for palliation of obstructive esophageal and tracheobronchial lesions, photocoagulation of vascular lesions, and lymphatic malformations. Nd:YAG laser wavelength can be transmitted through optical fibers, allowing easy delivery via flexible endoscopes.
- *Er:YAG (erbium yttrium aluminum garnet, 2.94 μm—near IR)*: This laser wavelength is near the peak of water absorption, resulting in very shallow tissue penetration. It produces a clean incision with minimal thermal damage to adjacent tissue. Because of shallow penetration, hemostasis is difficult. Used for facial skin resurfacing and epidermal lesions.
- CO_2 *(10.6 μm—IR)*: This wavelength is invisible and needs a coaxial helium-neon (He-Ne) red laser as an aiming beam. CO_2 laser light is strongly absorbed by tissue with high water content. Tissue penetration is shallow. Precision and good hemostasis of small vessels are major advantages. This wavelength cannot be delivered via optical fiber; however, specialized flexible waveguides (eg, OmniGuide) have been developed that allow delivery of this IR wavelength directly to the tissues through a handpiece. The CO_2 laser is the most widely used laser in otolaryngology with a wide range of applications in otology, laryngology, sinonasal surgery, and facial skin resurfacing.
- *Semiconductor (diode) lasers*: These lasers are available in multiple wavelengths. New semiconductor lasers are being developed for medical applications. Advantage is their *compact size* and decreased cost as these technologies mature. Laser properties, depth of tissue penetration, delivery methods, and applications are wavelength dependent. Semiconductor lasers have been used in a variety of otolaryngologic procedures including otology, laryngology, and facial cosmetic procedures.

Laser Applications in Otolaryngology

- Lasers targeting hemoglobin and vascular lesions generally have short wavelengths, 530 to 600 nm.
- Lasers used for hair and tattoo removal operate in the 694- to 755-nm range (Ruby and alexandrite). A semiconductor (diode) laser operating at 800 nm has been marketed for hair removal as well.
- Lasers used in middle ear and stapes surgery are argon, KTP, and CO_2. Recently CO_2 and semiconductor lasers have gained popularity.

Laser Skin Rejuvenation

- Lasers used for facial skin resurfacing operate in the IR range (Er:YAG 2.94 μm, CO_2 10.6 μm), are well absorbed by water, and have shallow tissue penetration.
- Unlike dermabrasion, CO_2 laser allows precise control of depth of tissue penetration. CO_2 laser removes approximately 50 to 100 μm of surface tissue in one pass. CO_2 laser allows for "bloodless" skin resurfacing because small blood vessels in target skin are coagulated. Facial skin reepithelializes within 2 weeks.

- Er:YAG laser's major chromophore is water. This mid-IR laser is superbly absorbed by water, resulting in very shallow tissue penetration depth when used for skin resurfacing. Energy is absorbed in the epithelium; therefore this laser is used for skin with mild to moderate signs of aging, predominantly contained within the epidermis. Er:YAG laser removes only about 25 to 30 μm of the skin surface. Some bleeding is encountered as the Er:YAG light is unable to coagulate the small vessels within the target skin. Skin reepithelializes in 5 to 7 days.
- Nd:YAG laser can also be designed to lase at 1.32 μm (eg, CoolTouch Corp, Roseville, CA) and is used for nonablative skin rejuvenation. Water absorbs the 1.32-μm IR wavelength well but not great. Enough heat is generated to produce a fibroblast reaction but skin is not ablated. Posttreatment pain is an issue. The wavelength range for nonablative skin rejuvenation lasers is approximately 1.30 to 1.45 μm. Longer wavelengths will ablate the epidermis.
- *Perioperative considerations*: For herpes prophylaxis, valacyclovir 500 mg bid is started 24 hours before the procedure and continued until the 10th postoperative day. Some surgeons also use ciprofloxacin for *Pseudomonas* coverage. Lidocaine with epinephrine skin injections are used for analgesia before CO_2 laser skin resurfacing. Er:YAG laser is less painful and application of topical eutectic mixture of local anesthetics (EMLA) provides sufficient analgesia. After the procedure, an occlusive dressing or mupirocin 2% (Bactroban) is applied. After day 2, the postoperative care regimen involves washing the face with an antibacterial cleansing soap (Cetaphil), soaking the face in dilute acetic acid solution and applying a Vaseline-based ointment until reepithelialization occurs.
- *Complications of laser skin resurfacing*: prolonged erythema, scarring, and hyperpigmentation may occur. Patients with Fitzpatrick skin types III or higher are at increased risk of pigmentary changes.
- *Contraindications to laser skin resurfacing*: use of isotretinoin (Accutane) in the past 1 to 2 years as this could impair reepithelialization, scleroderma, active acne, history of facial burns, or head and neck radiation therapy. Please refer to Chapter 48 for a discussion of additional facial rejuvenation techniques.

Laser Safety

- Most hospitals have laser committees and laser safety officers who develop guidelines for laser use, certify physicians in laser use, and ensure that safety protocols are implemented.
- Eye safety—Visible laser light is transmitted easily through the clear portions of the eye and can cause retinal burns. IR laser light is absorbed by water and can cause injury to the anterior chamber, that is, cornea and lens. The patient's eyes must be protected from laser light. Saline-soaked eyepads are acceptable. All operating room personnel must use wavelength-specific protective eyewear.
- Good suctioning is necessary to remove the laser plume.
- Anesthesia and airway safety considerations:
- Partial pressure of oxygen in the inhaled gas mixture is reduced to a minimum when lasing in the airway. Airway fires are possible with laser use in the upper aerodigestive system.
- Wavelength-specific endotracheal tubes are available from various manufacturers. If these are not available, flexible metallic or insulated silicone endotracheal tubes should be used. PVC endotracheal tubes can ignite and cause an airway fire.
- Nitrous oxide should be avoided during laser surgery. The common inhalational agents such as halothane, enflurane, and isoflurane are generally considered nonflammable.

Radiofrequency Surgery

Background and Physics

- Radiofrequency energy is delivered to tissue where particles are ionized and a layer of plasma develops. The high-energy plasma particles are capable of causing bond dissociation in tissue at relatively low temperatures (40°-70°C). This allows tissue removal, tissue shrinkage, or vessel coagulation without significant thermal damage.

Radiofrequency Ablation (Coblation) Tonsillectomy

- Introduced in 2001 as an alternative technology for tonsillectomy. Since then, use of Coblation (ArthroCare Corp, Sunnyvale, CA) for tonsillectomy has become widespread. Multiple studies comparing Coblation tonsillectomy outcomes to other common techniques have found Coblation to be comparable, or possibly superior to electrocautery when considering postoperative pain and hemorrhage rates.

Radiofrequency Ablation of the Tongue Base

- Radiofrequency ablation of the tongue base is a relatively new approach to the treatment of obstructive sleep apnea. An instrument is inserted in the tongue base near the foramen cecum and radiofrequency energy is delivered to the tissue. A controlled area of thermal damage is created, which reduces the volume of bulky tongue base tissue as it heals.
- A 2008 meta-analysis found that radiofrequency surgery of the tongue base and palate in obstructive sleep apnea patients results in 45% reduction in long-term (> 24 months) respiratory distress index (RDI).
- When operating on the tongue base, care should be taken to avoid injury to the neurovascular bundle which is located 2.7 cm deep and 1.6 cm lateral to the foramen cecum.

Bibliography

Burton MJ, Doree C. Coblation versus other surgical techniques for tonsillectomy. *Cochrane Database Syst Rev.* 2007;18(3):CD004619.

Einstein A. *Zur Quantentheorie der Strahlung.* Physikalische Zeitschrift, Band 18, Seite 1917:121-128.

Farrar J, Ryan J, Oliver E, Gillespie MB. Radiofrequency ablation for the treatment of obstructive sleep apnea: a meta-analysis. *Laryngoscope.* 2008;118(10):1878-1883.

Lauretano AM, Li KK, Caradonna DS, Khosta RK, Fried MP. Anatomic location of the tongue base neurovascular bundle. *Laryngoscope.* 1997;107(8):1057-1059.

Wilson YL, Merer DM, Moscatello AL. Comparison of three common tonsillectomy techniques: a prospective randomized, double-blinded clinical study. *Laryngoscope.* 2009;119(1):162-170.

Questions

1. In general, lasers with longer wavelength have deeper tissue penetration. Which of the following lasers is an exception to this rule?

   A. Alexandrite, 755 nm

   B. CO_2, 10.6 μm

    C. Argon, 514 nm

    D. KTP, 532 nm

    E. Tunable dye, 585 nm

2. During an operative procedure utilizing a laser, the following safety precautions should be observed:

    A. Patient's eyes must be protected with moist eye pads.

    B. All operating room personnel must wear wavelength-specific protective glasses.

    C. While the laser is not in use, it should be in "stand by" mode.

    D. In laser aerodigestive tract surgery, partial pressure of oxygen in the gas mixture should be reduced to a minimum.

    E. All of the above.

3. Which of the following lasers would be appropriate for treatment of superficial vascular lesions?

    A. CO_2, 10.6 μm

    B. Er:YAG, 2.94 μm

    C. Alexandrite, 755 nm

    D. Copper vapor, 578 nm

    E. Holmium:YAG, 2.1 μm

4. All of the following are contraindications to laser skin resurfacing, except

    A. Use of isotretinoin (Accutane) within the past 1 to 2 years

    B. Scleroderma

    C. Active smoking

    D. Active acne

    E. History of a facial burn

5. Which of the following statements regarding laser surgery is true?

    A. Alexandrite laser (755 nm) is frequently used for tattoo and hair removal.

    B. CO_2 laser is often used for treatment of superficial vascular lesions.

    C. CO_2 laser light (10.6 μm) can be transmitted through an optical fiber.

    D. Postoperative pigmentary changes after laser skin resurfacing are more pronounced in patients with low Fitzpatrick classes (I and II).

    E. CO_2 laser light is visible.

Chapter 4
Anesthesia for Head and Neck Surgery

Overview

Superlative surgical outcomes rarely occur by chance but are the product of a complex process that starts long before the day of surgery and lasts for at least 30 days after. This process is based on two factors: (1) active perioperative optimization of the patient's medical comorbidities and (2) consistent surgical and anesthetic approaches to procedures. To achieve this goal, active collaboration and communication with anesthesiologists, internists, and other consultants is necessary throughout the perioperative period. Anesthesiologists are uniquely situated in the health care system to implement the "perioperative surgical home" model of care. Therefore, anesthesia for head and neck surgery includes an understanding of pharmacology, fluid, airway, and medial comorbidity management to act as a framework for these collaborations.

Anesthetic agents are classified by their primary actions; sedative hypnotics, amnestic, analgesics, and muscle relaxants. Most agents provide a combination of these effects and can be utilized solely or in combination with one another to provide surgical conditions and minimize patient risk.

Continuum of Depth of Sedation

- Minimal sedation anxiolysis
  (a) Normal response to verbal stimuli
- Moderate sedation/analgesia ("conscious sedation")
  (a) Active response to verbal or tactile stimuli
- Deep sedation/analgesia
  (a) Active response to painful stimuli only
- General anesthesia
  (a) Unarousable to any stimuli

It is critical to understand that only the patient's response to stimuli defines the level of sedation. Therefore, the level of sedation is never defined by a particular anesthetic agent, its dose, or the airway management technique or device utilized. For example, it is possible, in a very rare patient, to achieve the level of general anesthesia with propofol and a nasal cannula or conversely an intubated patient with minimal sedation anxiolysis. Additionally, any level of sedation may be combined with local anesthetics, nerve blocks, or nonsedating systemic analgesics to improve surgical conditions and decrease patient risk. Monitored anesthesia care (MAC) is not synonymous with moderate sedation or any particular pharmacological agents. MAC is defined by the anesthesiologist's ability to assess the patient, anticipate physiological derangements, and medical sequelae of the procedure as well as the anesthesiologist's ability to intervene to rescue a patient's airway and convert to general anesthesia if required.

A majority of patients have some degree of apprehension concerning an upcoming surgical procedure, and more often than not, the "anesthesia" figures prominently in this anxiety. It is therefore crucial that the anesthesiologist devotes the necessary time to explain the sequence of events comprising the anesthetic and to thoroughly answer any questions that patients or their family may have.

Anesthetic Agents

Sedative Hypnotics and Amnestics In general, it is thought that anesthetics act by reversibly inhibiting neurosynaptic function of various regions or components of the cell membrane, either through action on membrane proteins or lipids or through modulation of the inhibitory neurotransmitter gamma-amino butyric acid (GABA). Because these compounds are involved in a number of multisynaptic pathways, they have repercussions far beyond their local sites of action. By altering sympathetic tone, these agents affect almost all organ systems, especially the cardiovascular system.

Each of these drugs has advantages and disadvantages in its clinical profile, so that no one drug can be considered the "ideal" agent in all circumstances.

Combinations of various drugs, such as benzodiazepines and opioids along with propofol, ketamine, and etomidate, can be titrated to the desired level of consciousness. These, in turn, can also be combined with volatile anesthetics and gases. The permutations of these mixtures are endless and can be thoughtfully tailored to the comorbidities of the patient and the surgical necessities.

Intravenous Anesthetics Thiopental's (ultra-short-acting barbiturate) widespread use has come to a close and is not available in the United States currently, but it is encountered in other countries. It is associated with cardiac and respiratory depression and may accumulate after repeated doses, thereby prolonging emergence. It is a highly effective treatment of last resort for status epilepticus. The usual induction dose is 3 to 5 mg/kg IV. Once popular in the United States, secobarbital and pentobarbital are now only encountered when on foreign medical missions. Methohexital is the last remaining available agent in this class. It can be used for procedural sedation but is generally reserved for electroconvulsive therapy due to its unusual ability to lower the seizure threshold.

Propofol is an IV sedative hypnotic agent that rapidly produces hypnosis, usually within about 40 seconds, and is quickly eliminated with minimal accumulation after repeated doses, allowing for a rapid return to consciousness. Propofol has also been associated with a lesser incidence of nausea and vomiting. Therefore, it is the most common agent of choice for induction of general anesthesia (1.5-2.5 mg/kg) and for deep procedural sedation (given as boluses of 10-20 mg or as an infusion of 25-75 μg/kg/min). Its advantages make it particularly suited to outpatient surgery. It is also associated with several important side effects: arterial hypotension (about 20%-30% decrease), apnea, airway obstruction, and subsequent oxygen desaturation. The therapeutic window between sedation, deep sedation, and general anesthesia is very narrow. These facts have earned it a *Food and Drug Administration* (FDA) black box warning, stating that "the agent should be administered only by those trained in the administration of general anesthesia and not involved in the procedure."

Intimidate, a **GABA$_A$ receptor modulator**, rapidly induces general anesthesia while preserving ventilatory drive, cardiovascular stability, and decreasing intracranial pressure.

However, etomidate also causes suppression of corticosteroid synthesis and can lead to primary adrenal suppression. As always, all of its effects must be considered with patient selection.

Ketamine, a phencyclidine derivative that acts as an **NMDA (*N*-Methyl-D-Aspartate) receptor antagonist**, induces dissociative anesthesia in which patients are unresponsive to noxious stimuli but may appear to be awake. Pharyngeal and laryngeal reflexes and respiratory drive also remain intact until very deep levels of anesthesia are attained. Additionally, ketamine has potent analgesic properties (through action on the NMDA receptor) and is therefore useful as a low-dose infusion (0.1-0.2 mg/kg/h) and is commonly used for repeated dressing changes. Ketamine produces increased intracranial pressure (ICP), tachycardia, and a dysphoric reaction, all of which should be considered in patient selection and subsequent monitoring. Of note, recent data suggest that prolonged low-dose infusions (8-72 hours) are therapeutic in the treatment of depression and chronic pain syndromes. Additionally, ketamine is an effective bronchodilator.

Dexmedetomidine, an **alpha-2 adrenergic agonist**, is a relatively new sedative hypnotic with minimal analgesic properties. It maintains ventilatory drive and is, therefore, useful during airway examinations or intubations. However, this medication must be administered as a continuous infusion (0.2-1 µg/kg/h) that must be preceded by a 10-minute loading dose (1 µg/kg/10 min). This is due to its ability to cause hypotension, bradycardia, and even asystole when titrated too rapidly.

Benzodiazepines have enjoyed widespread popularity because of their ability to reliably provide amnesia, reduce anxiety, and increase the seizure threshold without undue respiratory or cardiovascular depression. The three most commonly used benzodiazepines are diazepam (Valium), lorazepam (Ativan), and midazolam (Versed). Midazolam has several advantages: it is water soluble, which reduces the pain of injection associated with diazepam; it is approximately twice as potent as diazepam, with a more rapid peak onset (30-60 minutes) and an elimination half-time of 1 to 4 hours. It is, therefore, well suited to shorter procedures where extubation is anticipated or for sedation during local anesthesia (1-2 mg IV in adults). Recent papers have suggested that use of midazolam produces a higher rate of postoperative delirium in the elderly and other at risk populations (posttraumatic stress disorder patients).

The specific benzodiazepine antagonist is flumazenil (Romazicon), which is supplied in solutions containing 0.1 mg/mL. The recommended dose is 0.2 mg IV over 15 seconds, which can be repeated every 60 seconds for four doses (1 mg total) with more than 3 mg over 1 hour is advised. It is important to note that flumazenil's half-life ($t_{1/2}$) is 7 to 15 minutes and that repeated dose may be required over an extended period when it is used to treat overdosing of long-acting benzodiazepines (lorazepam's $t_{1/2}$ is 9-16 hours).

Droperidol, a **butyrophenone,** has been used extensively in the past as a sedating agent. However, in 2001 the FDA included a black box warning for this medication, citing data of QT prolongation and torsade de pointes when given at higher doses of 2.5 to 7.5 mg. Subsequently, 0.625 to 1.25 mg of droperidol is occasionally used for its antiemetic properties. This is done with active ECG monitoring only and is contraindicated in patients with QT intervals that are lengthy at baseline.

Haloperidol (Haldol), a **butyrophenone,** is a long-acting antipsychotic medication that may be useful in treating acute delirium in the postoperative period. However, due to the QT prolongation that it produces its routine use is not recommended.

Diphenhydramine (Benadryl), an **antihistamine**, has sedative and anticholinergic as well as antiemetic properties. The usual dose is 25 to 50 mg pod, IM, or IV. Because it blocks histamine release, it can be used in conjunction with steroids and H_2 blockers as prophylaxis for potential allergic reactions.

Inhalation Agents

The inhalation anesthetics are those volatile agents and gases that are administered via the lungs. They are administered by mask or through an endotracheal tube, attain a certain concentration in the alveoli, diffuse across the alveolar-capillary membrane, and are transported by the blood to their sites of action in the central nervous-system (CNS). Many factors affect the uptake and distribution of the volatile agents, including agent concentration, minute ventilation, diffusion capacity across the alveolar membrane, blood-gas partition coefficient (solubility), cardiac output, alveolar-arterial gradient, and the blood-brain partition coefficient.

The potency of the inhalation anesthetics is usually described in terms of minimal alveolar concentration (MAC). This is defined as the concentration of anesthetic at one atmosphere that will prevent movement in response to a surgical stimulus (surgical incision) in 50% of individuals. This allows for a somewhat quantitative assessment of the amount of anesthetic delivered. MAC decreases by 6% per decade of age increase, producing a 25% decrease in MAC for a 70-year-old patient versus a 30-year-old patient. It should be noted that MAC is additive; for example, if one-half MAC of two agents is delivered simultaneously, this is equivalent to one MAC of a single agent. Therefore, fractions of MAC of several anesthetic agents, inhalational and intravenous, can be combined to provide adequate anesthesia with reduced side effects from large doses of any one agent.

Nitrous Oxide (N_2O)

- MAC: 104% (therefore, one MAC of N_2O cannot be delivered)
- Blood-gas partition coefficient: 0.47

N_2O is a sedative hypnotic that has profound analgesic properties, but importantly no amnestic effects. It is mainly used as a short-term adjunct to general anesthesia at 30% to 70%. This is due to four properties: (1) rapid onset and offset, (2) potentiation of volatile anesthetics via the second gas effect, (3) improved cardiac stability, and (4) analgesia. These advantages are offset by N_2O role in postoperative nausea and vomiting and its expansion of air-filled spaces. Because N_2O is 34 times more soluble than nitrogen, N_2O can double the volume of a compliant air-filled space in 10 minutes and triple it in 30 minutes. Of clinical importance, N_2O may cause a significant expansion of the closed middle ear space and potential disruption of a tympanic graft. For this reason, N_2O is not used during procedures involving air-filled closed spaces or when a patient is at risk of a pneumothorax. Additionally, air-filled cuffs are also subject to this effect and cuff pressure should be carefully monitored when nitrous oxide is in use.

Isoflurane

- Type: Halogenated methyl ethyl ether
- MAC: 1.15%
- Blood-gas partition coefficient: 1.4
- Uses: Isoflurane is rarely used in modern anesthetic practice, but found in developing nations. It is the most soluble of the volatile agents, therefore it is eliminated most slowly and produces the prolonged emergence.
- Notes: Recently isoflurane has been linked to a possible increase in postoperative cognitive dysfunction in the elderly and increased risk of neurodegeneration in pediatric patients. The FDA and the anesthetic community are actively investigating these concerning issues.

Sevoflurane

- Type: Fluorinated methyl isopropyl ether
- MAC: 2.2%
- Blood-gas partition coefficient: 0.6
- Uses: Suitable for inhalational inductions

- Notes: When used with heated desiccated and exhausted soda lime, it has been shown to produce the nephrotoxin compound A. Frequent changes to fresh soda lime and fresh gas flows above 2 L/min have eliminated this risk. It also decreases airway irritability and can be used to treat status asthmaticus.

Desflurane
- Type: Fluorinated methyl ethyl ether
- MAC: 6%
- Blood-gas partition coefficient: 0.42
- Uses: It is the least soluble of the volatile agents, therefore it is eliminated most rapidly. This produces a shortened emergence and is suitable for use in obese patients, as it does not readily accumulate in adipose tissue.
- Notes: Requires a heated vaporizer because of its lower partial pressure.
- At concentrations above 10%, desflurane produces clinically significant tachycardia and airway irritability. This combined with its pungent odor make it unsuitable for inhalation inductions.

Muscle Relaxants

All volatile anesthetics and sedative hypnotics will provide varying degrees of muscle relaxation when given at the appropriate dose. There are, however, surgical procedures when patient movement is extremely detrimental to their outcome and these procedures warrant the use of other agents to ensure muscle relaxation.

Neuromuscular Blocking Drugs Neuromuscular blocking drugs are capable of interrupting nerve impulse conduction at the neuromuscular junction. This allows for muscle relaxation, which is used to facilitate intubation of the trachea and to provide for optimum surgical working conditions. They can be classified as either depolarizing muscle relaxants, of which succinylcholine is the only clinically available example, or nondepolarizing muscle relaxants. There are many nondepolarizing muscle relaxants, but currently only vecuronium, atracurium, rocuronium, and cisatracurium are readily available. Pancuronium and mivacurium are unavailable in the United States due to marketing and manufacturing issues.

The nondepolarizing agents can be further subdivided into short-, intermediate-, and long-acting drugs.

Succinylcholine	Onset: 30-60 sec	Duration: 5-10 min
Rocuronium	Onset: 60-90 sec	Duration: 45-70 min
Vecuronium	Onset: 90-180 sec	Duration: 30-40 min
Atracurium	Onset: 60-120 sec	Duration: > 30 min
Cisatracurium	Onset: 90-120 sec	Duration: 60-80 min

Monitoring of neuromuscular blockade is accomplished by a supramaximal electric stimulation delivered to a muscle via a neuromuscular stimulator. Decreased twitch height (depolarizing relaxants) or fade (nondepolarizing relaxants) to either train-of-four (four 2-Hz impulses in 2 seconds) or tetanus (50-100 Hz for 5 seconds) is proportional to the percentage of neuromuscular blockade. In this way, with at least one twitch of a train-of-four present, reversal of the blockade can be reliably achieved. Reversal is primarily accomplished with neostigmine 40 to 75 µg/kg and as second choices edrophonium 1 mg/kg or pyridostigmine 0.2 mg/kg. These acetylcholinesterase inhibitors cause accumulation of acetylcholine at the neuromuscular junction, thereby facilitating impulse transmission and reversal of the blockade. Of importance, anticholinergic drugs (glycopyrrolate or atropine) must accompany administration of the reversal agents to avoid the undesirable muscarinic effects (only the nicotinic, cholinergic effects are necessary). Occasionally, prolonged neuromuscular blockade is required postoperatively. In these cases, it is of the utmost importance to monitor the patient's depth of sedation using a spectral index (BIS) monitor, which is a form of electroencephalograph (EEG), while the patient is rendered incapable of voluntary and involuntary movement.

Sugammadex, the first selective relaxant binding agent, binds to and rapidly reverses the effects of rocuronium and vecuronium. This drug has been approved in Europe since 2008 and is still being investigated by the FDA prior to its approval for use in the United States.

Analgesics

Before pain is treated, it is of the utmost importance to diagnosis its character, acute or chronic, and its etiology. Only then can the correct therapeutic modality be selected. It is dangerous to ever assume the cause of a patient's pain before examining or conferring with them. To not do so is to risk missing critical clinical events and to put your patient in harm's way.

Local Anesthesia

Local anesthesia is the blockade of sensation in a circumscribed area. Local anesthetics interfere with the functioning of the sodium channels, thereby decreasing the sodium current. When a critical number of channels are blocked, propagation of a nerve impulse (action potential) is prevented, as in the refractory period following depolarization. All of the clinically useful agents belong to either the aminoester or aminoamide groups. In addition, they are all diffusible, reversible, predictable, water soluble, and clinically stable and they do not produce local tissue irritation.

Chemistry

Local anesthetics consist of three parts: tertiary amine, intermediate bond, and an aromatic group. The intermediate bond can be either of two types: ester (R-COO-R) or amide (R-NHCO-R); local anesthetics are therefore classified as aminoesters or aminoamides.

In general, there are three basic properties that will influence their activity:

A. *Lipid solubility:* This will affect the potency and duration of effect.

B. *Degree of ionization*: According to the Henderson-Hasselbalch equation, the local hydrogen ion concentration will determine where chemical equilibrium lies. The greater the pKa, the smaller the proportion of nonionized form at any pH. The ester pKa values are higher than the amide, accounting for their poor penetrance. The nonionized form is essential for passage through the lipoprotein diffusion barrier to the site of action. Therefore, decreasing the ionization by alkalinization will increase the initial concentration gradient of diffusible drug, thereby increasing the drug transfer across the membrane. Importantly, infected tissues have a decreased pH and causes less nonionized drug to be present (or more ionized drug), and therefore a lesser concentration of drug at the site of action, resulting in a poor or nonexistent local block. Blocking the relevant nerves proximally to the CNS in healthy uninfected tissue can circumvent this effect.

C. *Protein binding*: A higher degree is seen with the longer-acting local anesthetics.

Uptake, Metabolism, and Excretion

Most local anesthetic agents diffuse away from the site of action in the mucous membranes and subcutaneous tissues and are rapidly absorbed into the bloodstream. Factors that affect this process are the physicochemical and vasoactive properties of the agent: the site of injection, dosage, presence of additives such as vasoconstrictors in the injected solution, factors related to the nerve block, and pathophysiologic features of the patient. Certain sites of particular interest to the otolaryngologist (eg, laryngeal and tracheal mucous membranes) are associated with such a rapid uptake of local anesthetics that the blood levels approach those achieved with an intravenous injection.

Amide local anesthetics are metabolized by the liver in a complex series of steps beginning with N-dealkylation. Ester drugs are hydrolyzed by cholinesterases in the liver and plasma. Both degradation processes depend on enzymes synthesized in the liver; therefore, both processes are compromised in a patient with parenchymal liver disease. Many of the end products of catabolism of both esters and amides are excreted to a large extent by the kidneys. Catabolic by-products may retain some activity of the parent compound and may, therefore, contribute to toxicity.

Toxicity

A toxic blood level of local anesthetic can be achieved by rapid absorption, excessive dose, or inadvertent intravascular injection.

Significant symptoms of local anesthetic systemic toxicity are predominantly confined to the central nervous system (CNS) and cardiovascular system. The CNS responses to local anesthetic toxicity begin with an excitatory phase, followed by depression. The extents of these symptoms are dose dependent and include circumoral paresthesias, tinnitus, and mental status changes. They can progress to tonic-clonic seizures and eventual coma, producing respiratory depression and respiratory arrest. Initial symptoms can be treated with benzodiazepines such as diazepam or less effectively midazolam, always remembering that they too can exacerbate respiratory depression. Should seizures ensue, symptomatic therapy should continue with the above-mentioned drugs and an adequate airway and oxygenation must be ensured.

Local anesthetics exert direct dose-related depressive effects on the cardiovascular system. Increasing levels of local anesthetic agents diminishes both myocardial contractility and peripheral vascular tone. Toxic doses of local anesthetics can produce rapid and profound cardiovascular collapse. If local anesthetic systemic toxicity occurs, ACLS (advanced cardiac life support) protocols should be instituted immediately. During ACLS an initial dose of 1.5 mL/kg 20% lipid emulsion (Intralipid) should be administered. If needed, this dose can be followed by additional doses and an infusion of 0.5 mL/kg/min, up to a 30-minute maximal dose of 10 mL/kg. In cases where this protocol has been followed, a full recovery of the patient has resulted. Intralipid therapy may also be instituted to treat CNS local anesthetic toxicity. Please refer to http://www.lipidrescue.org/ for additional information.

Epinephrine is often added to local anesthetic mixtures to increase the duration of the nerve block, to decrease systemic absorption of the local anesthetic, and to decrease operative blood loss. In commercially prepared solutions of local anesthetics, epinephrine is usually found in a 1:100,000 (1 mg/100 mL) or 1:200,000 (1 mg/200 mL) concentration. Tachycardia and hypertension are the most common side effects of this medication and can be treated with short-acting beta-adrenergic blocking drugs (esmolol). Hypertensive crisis can be precipitated by epinephrine in patients taking tricyclic antidepressants and monoamine oxidase inhibitors. Epinephrine toxicity can produce restlessness, nervousness, a sense of impending doom, headache, palpitations, and respiratory distress. These symptoms may progress to ventricular irritability and seizures.

True allergic reactions to local anesthetics account for < 1% of all adverse reactions and most commonly are attributed to the methylparaben or metabisulfite preservative. True allergy to local anesthetics is more common among ester derivatives; it is extremely rare among the amide local anesthetics.

Choosing the anesthetic technique for a patient with a history of local anesthetic allergy is a not-infrequent clinical problem. A careful history with documentation, if possible, should help sort out those with toxic reactions from those with true allergy. Some authorities have advocated provocative intradermal testing, but this should only be undertaken when prepared to treat anaphylaxis and can still be unreliable. Alternatively, some authors suggest using a preservative free local anesthetic from the opposite class of the one suspected. If doubt still exists, one must consider alternative techniques, such as general anesthesia.

Both prilocaine and benzocaine can reduce hemoglobin to methemoglobin, which has a diminished ability to transport oxygen to the peripheral tissues. (*Note:* A pulse oximeter cannot measure methemoglobin. If significant quantities of methemoglobin are present, the oxygen saturation will read 85% regardless of what the actual saturation is and therefore may be grossly in error and unreliable.) Patients with glucose-6-phosphate deficiencies are more susceptible to methemoglobinemia. The treatment of methemoglobinemia is intravenous administration of a 1% methylene blue solution to a total dose of 1 to 2 mg/kg.

Local Anesthetic Agents

Aminoester Agents

Cocaine

- Type: Benzoic acid ester.
- Activity: Extremely potent as a topical anesthetic.
- Onset time: 5 to 10 minutes.
- Duration: 30 to 60 minutes.
- Maximum dose: 2 to 3 mg/kg.
- Formulation: 4% solution.
- Metabolism: Hydrolyzed by plasma cholinesterase.
- Uses: Topical application to mucosal surfaces. (Rarely used clinically.)
- Notable issues: Cocaine is unique in producing vasoconstriction.
- Additionally it blocks reuptake of norepinephrine and dobutamine at adrenergic nerve endings, thereby causing tachycardia, hypertension, mydriasis, cortical stimulation, addiction, and sensitization of the myocardium to catecholamines.
- Elective surgery in acutely intoxicated patients should be aborted.
- It may precipitate hypertensive crisis by reducing catecholamine catabolism.

Procaine Hydrochloride

- Type: Weak ester-type
- Activity: Ineffective as topical
- Onset time: 2 to 5 minutes
- Duration: 30 to 90 minutes
- Maximum dose: 1000 mg
- Percent protein binding: 6%
- Formulation: 2%
- Metabolism: Rapidly hydrolyzed by plasma cholinesterase (may prolong succinylcholine effects)
- Uses: Field and nerve blocks

Chloroprocaine

- Type: A halogenated derivative of procaine, a weak ester
- Activity: Ineffective as topical
- Onset time: 2 to 5 minutes
- Duration: 30 to 60 minutes
- Maximum dose: 800 mg plain and 1000 mg with epinephrine

- Percent protein binding: Not applicable
- Formulation: 2% solution
- Metabolism: Hydrolyzed more rapidly than procaine by plasma cholinesterase (may prolong succinylcholine effects)
- Uses: Field, nerve blocks and epidural
- Notable issues: Low systemic toxicity

Tetracaine
- Type: Potent ester
- Activity: Excellent topical anesthetic
- Onset time: 5 to 10 minutes
- Duration: 30 minutes
- Maximum dose: 20 mg single dose
- Percent protein binding: 94%
- Formulation: 0.25%, 0.5%, 1%, and 2% solutions
- Metabolism: Hydrolyzed by plasma cholinesterase
- Uses: As an aerosol for topical anesthesia of the upper respiratory tract; also used for ophthalmic anesthesia and spinal anesthesia
- Notable issues: 1 mL of 2% solution with maximal dose

Benzocaine
- Type: Ester of para-amino benzoic acid similar to procaine.
- Activity: Excellent topical anesthetic.
- Onset time: 5 to 10 minutes.
- Duration: 30 to 60 minutes.
- Maximum dose: 200 mg.
- Formulation: Ointments and 20% solution.
- Metabolism: Hydrolyzed by plasma cholinesterase.
- Uses: Topical airway anesthetic or as an ointment for wound dressings.
- Notable issues: Can cause methemoglobinemia. Hurricaine solution contains 20% benzocaine in a flavored, water-soluble polyethylene glycol base. It provides rapid topical anesthesia to mucous membranes, but when used improperly toxicity is common and should be used with caution. Since 2006, the VA has banned its use. The FDA has stated that it should not be used in teething infants.

Aminoamide Agents
Lidocaine
- Type: Aminoamide.
- Activity: Excellent topical anesthetic.
- Onset time: 5 to 10 minutes.
- Duration: 1 to 3 hours.
- Maximum dose: 5 mg/kg plain and 7 mg/kg with epinephrine.
- Percent protein binding: 64%.
- Formulation: 0.5% to 2% solution for injection and a 4% solution for direct topical application. Also comes in viscous liquid at 4% and at 5% in an ointment.
- Metabolism: Transformed by hepatic carboxylesterases and cytochrome P450 enzymes.
- Uses: Topical anesthesia for mucosal membranes. Also used field blocks, nerve blocks, epidural and spinal anesthesia.
- Notable issues: 0.5% to 2% solutions are intended for injection into tissue. 4% can be used for trans-tracheal anesthesia, atomized or nebulized for airway anesthesia. IV lidocaine (1.5 mg/kg) can be given during intubation and extubation to blunt the response to tracheal stimulation. The practice of using lidocaine to suppress automaticity in ectopic myocardial foci has been supplanted by the use of amiodarone.

Mepivacaine

- Type: Aminoamide.
- Activity: Moderate to poor topical anesthetic.
- Onset time: 30 seconds to 4 minutes.
- Duration: 1 to 4 hours (depending on location).
- Maximum dose: 6 mg/kg and in some texts 400 mg maximum adult dose.
- Percent protein binding: 77%.
- Formulation: 3% and 2% solutions.
  (a) Produces less vasodilation than lidocaine, therefore used without epinephrine
- Metabolism: Transformed by hepatic carboxylesterases and cytochrome P450 enzymes.
- Uses: Effective for infiltration and peripheral nerve blockade, producing a dense block. Commonly used for dental anesthesia.
- Notable issues: 2% solution contains levonordefrin 1:20,000 (a sulfite), which can cause anaphylactic symptoms.

Prilocaine (Citanest)

- Type: Aminoamide.
- Activity: Excellent topical anesthetic.
- Onset time: 2 to 4 minutes.
- Duration: 1 to 2 hours.
- Maximum dose: 8 mg/kg but 600 mg maximum adult dose.
- Percent protein binding: 55%.
- Formulation: 4% solutions.
  (a) Produces less vasodilation than lidocaine, therefore used without epinephrine
- Metabolism: Transformed by hepatic carboxylesterases and cytochrome P450 enzymes.
- Uses: Similar to lidocaine produces a dense block.
- Notable Issues: A known side effect of prilocaine is methemoglobinemia with dose equal to and greater than 600 mg.
- EMLA cream, a mixture of lidocaine 2.5% and prilocaine 2.5% in an emulsion is effective in lessening the pain associated with venipuncture, catheter placement, and has been successfully employed in the harvesting of split-thickness skin grafts. Satisfactory anesthesia is achieved by placing the cream under an occlusive dressing at least 1 hour prior to the procedure and persists for 2 hours after removal. Weight-based dosing is extremely important as there have been many reports of toxicity in pediatric patients.

Bupivacaine

- Type: Aminoamide.
- Activity: Poor topical anesthetic.
- Onset time: 5 to 10 minutes.
- Duration: 3 to 10 hours.
- Maximum dose: 2 to 3 mg/kg.
- Percent protein binding: 95%.
- Formulation: 0.125% to 0.75%.
- Metabolism: Transformed by hepatic carboxylesterases and cytochrome P450 enzymes.
- Uses: Infiltration, peripheral nerve blockade, spinal and epidural anesthesia. At lower concentrations, it produces a purely sensory block and at higher concentrations it produces a sensory and motor block.
- Notable issues: Bupivacaine is tightly bound to tissue and plasma protein and does not produce high blood levels when appropriately administered. However, toxic doses do not produce classic symptoms prior to cardiovascular collapse, so patients should be closely monitored during administration. Bupivacaine produces cardiac toxicity prior to CNS toxicity.

Of note, the FDA recently approved a liposomal formulation of bupivacaine (Exparel) that has duration of 72 to 96 hours. (FDA labeled only for bunionectomy and hemorrhoidectomy.)

Ropivacaine

- Type: Aminoamide (single isomer of bupivacaine).
- Activity: Poor topical anesthetic.
- Onset time: 5 to 10 minutes.
- Duration: 4 to 12 hours.
- Maximum dose: 1 to 3 mg/kg.
- Percent protein binding: 94%.
- Formulation: 0.2% to 1.0% solutions.
- Metabolism: Transformed by hepatic carboxylesterases and cytochrome P450 enzymes.
- Uses: Infiltration, peripheral nerve blockade, and epidural anesthesia. Produces less motor blockade than bupivacaine.
- Notable issues: Ropivacaine is tightly bound to tissue and plasma protein and does not produce high blood levels when appropriately administered. It is less cardiotoxic than bupivacaine at lower doses. Therefore, it is often used for continuous infusions catheters (1-4 days). Use with epinephrine has no advantages in block prolongation.

Etidocaine

- Type: Aminoamide (chemically similar to lidocaine).
- Activity: Poor topical anesthetic.
- Onset time: 3 to 8 minutes.
- Duration: 2 to 12 hours.
- Maximum dose: 300 (without epinephrine) to 400 mg (with epinephrine).
- Percent protein binding: 94%.
- Formulation: 0.5% to 1.0% solutions.
- Metabolism: Transformed by hepatic carboxylesterases and cytochrome P450 enzymes.
- Uses: Local infiltration. Produces less motor blockade than bupivacaine.
- Notable issues: Induces both a sensory and intense motor blockade.

Miscellaneous Agents

CYCLONITE

- Type: A 4,-butoxy-3-piperindinopropiophonone (neither an ester nor an amide).
- Activity: Excellent topical anesthetic.
- Onset time: 2 to 10 minutes.
- Duration: 30 minutes.
- Maximum dose: 300 mg single dose.
- Formulation: 0.5%.
- Uses: Topical anesthesia (irritating when injected).
- Notable issues: Because it is neither an ester nor an amide, it may be used if allergy to both these classes has been documented.

CETACAINE

- Combination: Benzocaine, butyl aminobenzoate, and tetracaine hydrochloride
- Use: Anesthetize mucous membranes
- Onset: 30 seconds
- Maximum dose: 400 mg or 2 doses of 1-second sprays

Opioids

The opioid narcotics, especially fentanyl, morphine, and hydromorphone, are the most frequently used of this class in the operative setting. They have classically been employed to relieve pain, but may also be administered prior to painful stimuli; this is known as pre-emptive analgesia.

The opioids provide analgesia and sedation with relative cardiovascular stability. One must keep in mind, though, that side effects of these drugs include CNS and respiratory depression and also nausea and vomiting. The elderly may be more sensitive to their effects, and caution should be used in this group of patients as they are at high risk for postoperative cognitive dysfunction. Opioids are often given in conjunction with induction of general anesthesia, but are not necessary for induction and are rarely if ever used anymore as an induction agent.

Morphine is the oldest of these agents, but is by no means the most ideal. Its effect is best titrated in incremental doses. It should not be used in patients with reactive airway disease because of its ability to cause histamine release along with increased central vagal tone. Other patients suffer from pruritus due to morphine-induced histamine release; this can be more troublesome than their pain. Additionally, active morphine metabolites (morphine-glucuronides) are excreted via the kidney and will accumulate in patients with renal failure. Therefore, doses subsequent to initial administration should be based solely on clinical need not a dosing regimen.

Hydromorphone (Dilaudid) is five times more potent than morphine, therefore 0.2 mg of dilaudid is as effective as 1 mg of morphine. When compared to morphine, hydromorphone causes less pruritus and nausea and vomiting. Therefore, it is an excellent drug of choice for PCA dosing.

Fentanyl (Sublimaze), **sufentanil** (Sufenta), and **alfentanil** (Alfenta), the synthetic opioids, can be given as pre-medications, although in general they are given intravenously in small amounts at the induction of general anesthesia, titrated for conscious sedation or postoperative pain relief. All these agents all exhibit context sensitive half-lives and how much drug has been given over a period of time will determine their elimination time.

Remifentanil is an ultra-short-acting selective micro-opioid receptor agonist. It is about 15- to 30-fold more potent than alfentanil. Remifentanil is rapidly hydrolyzed by nonspecific plasma and tissue esterases, making onset and recovery rapid, with no cumulative effects and its metabolism is unaffected by impaired renal clearance or hepatic function. Because of this a remifentanil infusion (0.1-0.5 µg/kg/min) is often used during total intravenous anesthesia to maintain the general anesthetic state. In cases where significant postoperative pain is anticipated longer acting opiates should be titrated while remifentanil is discontinued.

Combined agonist/antagonist drugs also exist, such as pentazocine, butorphanol, and nalbuphine. They do, however, exhibit a ceiling effect with regard to analgesia, and therefore may be less useful. The specific opioid antagonist is **naloxone** (Narcan). It is provided in ampules of 0.4 mg/mL (400 µg/mL) but, unless an emergency situation exists, can be titrated in doses of 20- to 40-µg increments to achieve the desired level of arousal. Naloxone has been associated with flash pulmonary edema when administered rapidly in larger doses.

Meperidine (Demerol) is rarely used now to treat pain due to the risk of serotonin syndrome when combined with MAOIs, as well as other antidepressants, muscle relaxants, and benzodiazepines. Is now only used at low doses (12.5-25 mg) in the treatment of postoperative shivering.

Codeine (a methylated morphine) and **hydrocodone** (a codeine derivative) can be given PO as a single agent or in combination with acetaminophen or ibuprofen and are commonly prescribed for postoperative relief. When given as a combined medication it is important to educate patients about avoiding toxic doses of acetaminophen of ibuprofen by escalating consumption of the combination tablet or be adding additional NSAIDs. It is important to note that codeines effect relies on its metabolism by the CYP2D6 enzyme and that significant genetic variability occurs in the number of this gene. Therefore, patients can vary from ultra-fast metabolizers (1%-2% of patients) all the way to nonmetabolizers (5%-10% of patients) and will experience ultra-high active metabolite concentrations or no active metabolite, respectively.

A patient history of their experience with this medication will often uncover this difference. Alternatively, a patient's first dose of this medication can be given in the recovery room and its effect assessed.

Nonsteroidal Anti-inflammatory Drugs (NSAIDs)

Nonsteroidal anti-inflammatory drugs (NSAIDs) that can be administered either PO or IV are useful first-line agents, as per the WHO pain ladder. The only medications in this class discussed here are those currently available in the operative setting.

- Acetaminophen
  - (a) Dose: 650 mg PO or 1 g IV Q6h   Maximal: 4 g/24 h
  - (b) Contraindications: Hepatic failure.
  - (c) Notes: Stable nondrinking cirrhotics have been shown to take this medication safely.
- Ketorolac
  - (a) Dose: 30 mg IV Q8h   Maximal: 2 days of dosing
  - (b) Contraindications: Renal failure, reactive airway disease, Samter triad, and active bleeding or high risk for hematoma formation.

Belladonna Derivatives

- **Atropine sulfate** 0.4 to 0.8 mg IM or IV
  - (a) Antimuscarinics act centrally to produce either sedation or excitation, most potent vagolytic.
- **Scopolamine** 0.2 to 0.4 mg IM
  - (a) Antimuscarinics and antisialogogues act centrally to produce either sedation or excitation.
- **Glycopyrrolate** 0.2 to 0.4 mg
  - (a) Antimuscarinics and antisialogogues

Antiemesis

Nausea and vomiting usually are a protective physiological function against ingested toxins, but in the case of postoperative nausea and vomiting (PONV) it is deleterious. Occurring in about a third of untreated surgical patients, PONV may result in surgical wound dehiscence, delayed hospital stay, unanticipated hospital admissions, and increased aspiration rates. PONV prevention improves patient safety, medical outcomes, enhances patient satisfaction, and contains medical costs. Risk factors predicting the incidence of PONV include female sex, history of PONV, procedure, nonsmoker, and age less than 40. A combination of these factors can produce a PONV risk reaching 75%. This process may be triggered directly via the medullary chemoreceptor trigger zone and indirectly through gastric enterochromaffin cells and the vestibular system both of which are transmitted via efferent cranial nerves. These signals all culminate in activation of the vomiting center.

The most common cause of nausea in the PACU (postanaesthetic care unit) is PONV, however other serious causes should always be part of the differential diagnosis, including gastric irritants, hypoxia, hypotension, hypoglycemia, increased ICP, and myocardial infarction.

There is a current array of pharmacologic therapies targeting the multifactorial triggers of PONV with an incidence reduction of 20% to 25% per therapeutic modality. Optimal risk reduction will not be achieved by a reactive therapeutic approach relying on rescue. In contrast, optimal PONV risk reduction requires strategic anticipatory planning and employment of a multi-tiered patient specific approach. This includes a reduction of emetogenic agents, gastric suctioning of blood, and a multimodal approach to prevention of PONV.

To that end the reduction of patient's opiate requirement with the use of NSAIDS (ketorolac and IV acetaminophen) alone or even better in combination, can substantially attenuate their risk of PONV.

Pharmacological Antiemetics

The **cholinergic antagonist,** scopolamine, historically used as an anesthesia pre-induction agent, is now being revived in the form of a prophylactic antiemetic. With patients or procedures that are deemed high risk for PONV, a scopolamine transdermal patch placed 8 to 12 hours before surgery.

The **glucocorticoid** dexamethasone has long been used during otolaryngological procedures to prevent PONV and airway edema. However, these benefits should be weighed against the risks of poor glucose control, possible deficiencies in wound healing as well as the other well described side effects of steroidal therapy.

Droperidol, a **butyrophenone** and potent anti-dopaminergic, once a ubiquitously employed therapy, is now only used in low doses (0.625-1.25 mg) as a rescue antiemetic. This is because of QT prolongation incurred at higher doses and the FDAs black box warning of this effect. That being said with proper monitoring it can be invaluable in the treatment of PONV.

Pre-emergence administration of **5-HT3 (serotonin) receptor antagonists** (ondansetron, palonosetron, granisetron, and dolasetron) has become the standard of care in the prevention of PONV. Ironically, they were initially touted as alternatives to droperidol, and avoiding QT prolongation, however they are now known to induce the same effect.

Neurokinin-1 receptor antagonists are a new and promising class of antiemetics that are effective in preventing delayed PONV (POD #1-3). These include the PO formulation aprepitant (Emend) and the newer IV version fosaprepitant (Ivemend).

Histamine-2 receptor antagonists, Ranitidine (Zantac) 150 mg PO or 50 mg IV and famotidine (Pepcid) 40 mg PO or 20 mg IV, can be administered as part of the pre-medication regimen. They are used to raise the pH of subsequently secreted gastric acid above the critical level of 2.5, thereby reducing the pulmonary sequelae should aspiration occur.

The **phenothiazines** have excellent antiemetic and anticholinergic properties, but can also be sedating. Therefore, promethazine (Phenergan) 25 to 50 mg and prochlorperazine (Compazine) 5 to 10 mg are commonly used as rescue antiemetics only.

Nonpharmacological Antiemetics

Recently multiple studies have demonstrated the effectiveness of nonpharmacological and nontraditional techniques to avoid PONV. These include the use of acupressure and acupuncture of the P6 point. However, options that are more readily available include the use of glucose containing IV fluids and aromatherapy. D5LR given during the perioperative period has been shown to reduce the use of PONV rescue medications in the PACU. Additionally, recovery room use of a commercially available aromatic inhaler containing peppermint, ginger and spearmint (QueaseEase) reduces nausea. The physiologic mechanism by which these therapies work is still unknown, but as they present a very low-risk profile any benefit derived is worth attempting.

Postoperative Pain Management

NSAIDs that can be administered either PO or IV are useful first-line agents (ketorolac and acetaminophen). In addition, single shot nerve blocks used for surgical procedures may provide relief in the immediate postoperative period. This pain relief can be extended with the use of local anesthetic infusions either directed to a specific nerve bundle or as a field block.

Patient-controlled analgesia (PCA) has become a well-established method of delivering opiates to postoperative surgical patients. Morphine was the original agent, but dilaudid has become the preferred agent as it produces less nausea and pruritus. PCA is generally well accepted by patients because it provides them with some degree of control over their situation and is adaptable to pediatric and geriatric patients. Additionally, in some circumstances low-dose ketamine infusions have proved highly effective in opiate tolerant patients. As with all analgesics, a multimodal approach is the most effective.

Airway Management

More than any other surgical specialty, otolaryngology presents four major airway management challenges to the anesthesiologist: intubation, airway devices, estuation, and airway security.

Intubation: The otolaryngologist's nasal fiber optic examination provides extremely useful preoperative data to the anesthesiologist and provides excellent data for a discussion on the best approach to patients with anomalous airway anatomy. As always this discussion must be tempered with the acknowledgment that the original plan may fail and that multiple backup plans should also be put in motion. Including a surgical approach to the airway in the planning phase is essential. An airway tragedy has occurred with both anesthesiologist and otolaryngologist in attendance, but lacking communication and foresight. Additionally, all airway management equipment should be readily available; the use of a "difficult airway cart" provides the most reliable solution.

Airway devices: Often, otolaryngological procedures require specialized endotracheal tubes. These too should be included in preoperative consultation with the anesthesiologist to ensure their availability and any change in the anesthetic plan that they introduce. Neural integrity monitoring electromyogram tracheal (NIMS) tubes use is predicated on the lack of neuromuscular junction blockade (NMJB) at the time of monitoring. NIMS tubes do not preclude the use of NMJB at the other times during the procedure, but require a dynamic collaboration between the anesthesia and surgical teams.

With the advent of electrocautery and lasers in surgery, the potential for airway fires has increased. The oxygen-enriched and/or nitrous oxide-enriched atmosphere created in the oropharynx will readily support combustion of flammable materials such as an endotracheal tube. The laser type and object material will determine how much time is necessary to ignite an object. First, the lowest possible concentration of oxygen should be used (21%-40% FIO_2) that will maintain adequate patient oxygen saturation. Next, the placement of an endotracheal tube wrapped with reflective material to reduce the amount of energy absorbed, is advantageous. Placement in the area surrounding the surgical field of saline-soaked pads and a methylene-blue-colored saline filled cuff will also help dissipate excess heat energy. Limiting the bursts to a short duration will help to reduce the risk of an airway fire. Should an airway fire occur, fresh gas flow should be stopped, the endotracheal tube removed, any additional burning material extinguished, removed, and the patient re-intubated immediately. A protocol should be devised and readily available to deal with such emergencies.

Extubation: Over the recent years, there has been a substantial reduction in airway loss events during anesthetic induction. This has not occurred by chance but by active efforts on the part of the anesthesia community. Data collected for the fourth National Audit Project (NAP4) in the United Kingdom identified a surprising number lost airways after failed estuation. The cause they identified was the "failure to plan for failure." Therefore, the same planning and collaboration that now exists surrounding the induction phase of the anesthetic should also be applied to the emergence and estuation phase. Continuous end-tidal CO_2 monitoring is now available for all intubated patients outside of the operating room setting and is now becoming routine for monitoring patients who maintain their own airway are deemed at risk.

Airway security: Any patient with a demonstrated or suspected difficult airway (can't intubate or can't ventilate) should be notified of their condition in writing. Importantly, their critical airway data should be transmitted to future providers to avoid unnecessary tragedies. The written notification that the patient receives is a first step in this process, but is best followed with a flag in the patient's record, written or electronic. The Medic Alert foundation currently maintains an international difficult airway/intubation registry that has been endorsed by the Society for Airway Management. All providers can access this airway data log and patients may opt into the bracelet identification system.

Surgical patients who are extubated and transferred out of the postanaesthetic care unit (PACU) are still at risk of losing their airway. Additionally, patients with acute airway events often present to the hospital and patients with known difficult airways are often admitted by other services for treatment of other comorbid conditions. The existence of these classes of patients has engendered the establishment of difficult airway rescue teams (DART). These teams include anesthesiologists, otolaryngologists, nursing, and technical staff. In institutions supporting these predetermined teams supplied with specifically designated equipment carts many of these patients have been rescued in a timely manner.

Fluid and Transfusion Management

Data from other surgical specialties have demonstrated improved outcomes through goal-directed fluid management and tailored blood transfusion criteria. Invasive monitors are no longer a favorite option because of their lackluster risk-benefit profile in noncritical patients. The application of goal-directed fluid management, using recently developed noninvasive and minimally invasive volume status monitors (Delta CardioQ) has improved clinical outcomes in a large variety of cases.

Less-favorable long-term outcomes for oncological surgical patients have been linked to blood product transfusions, likely due to immunosuppression. This has led to attempts to remediate anemia in the perioperative period and to transfuse only those patients with demonstrated requirements for increased oxygen carrying capacity, such as cardiovascular disease. This is an evolving area of research in the field of otolaryngology.

Complications

This discussion of complications of general anesthesia is confined to those that are of relevance to otolaryngologists. However, one should not lose sight of the fact that anesthesia affects all organ systems, which may be a source of potential complications.

Aspiration pneumonitis (Mendelson syndrome) may occur either during intubation or extubation of the trachea or with sedation and a loss of airway reflexes. Gastric contents of greater than 200 mL with a pH less than 2.5 are associated with a high risk of aspiration syndrome. Postaspiration respiratory tree lavage has not been demonstrated to reduce this syndrome. This syndrome is treated supportively and may require postoperative intubation and can progress to acute respiratory distress syndrome. Of particular concern is that aspiration can also occur with a properly positioned, cuffed endotracheal tube and may be as high as 5%. Foreign matter (blood, secretions, or gastric contents) that is permitted to accumulate may gain access to the respiratory tree. Sodium citrate (Bicitra) 15 to 30 mL administered just prior to induction of anesthesia is effective in raising the pH of gastric contents already present in the stomach and reduce the risk of aspiration pneumonitis.

Many of the inhalation anesthetics are associated with sensitization of the myocardium to catecholamines. In the presence of excess endogenous or exogenous catecholamines, patients may develop cardiac arrhythmias (ventricular ectopy or fibrillation). It is therefore recommended that the dose of epinephrine administered not exceed 10 mL of a 1:100,000 solution (ie, 100 μg) in any 10-minute period when these anesthetics are in use.

Malignant hyperthermia (MH) is a rare (incidence of 1:10,000-1:50,000 anesthetics) and potentially lethal entity. It is triggered by the potent inhalation agents and succinylcholine and is associated with a genetic predisposition. Once triggered, MH causes a massive increase in intracellular calcium and uncoupling of metabolic pathways, resulting in an extreme elevation of temperature, increase in CO_2 production, metabolic acidosis, cardiac arrhythmias, and, if untreated, eventual cardiovascular collapse. Dantrolene is the only directed therapeutic agent; it acts by blocking intracellular calcium release. If a patient has a known history of MH or MH susceptibility—associated with masseter muscle rigidity (MMR), positive family history—a "nontriggering technique" in a "clean anesthesia machine" should be used.

Block Techniques

Specific nerve blocks or field blocks reduce patient's pain, thereby reducing the need for systemic analgesics and in some cases obviate the need for general anesthesia. Therefore, these techniques improve patient safety and experience of the procedure. The majority of nerve blocks are currently preformed utilizing landmarks and increasingly under ultrasound guidance. Eliciting a paresthesia, once used as a technique to locate nerves, is to be avoided as this incurs a high risk of nerve injury. The specific goals of concomitant IV sedation must be kept clearly in mind when utilizing a block technique. Importantly, sedation should never substitute for an adequate local anesthetic block.

Laryngoscopy, Tracheostomy

The larynx and trachea receive their sensory nerve supply from the superior and inferior laryngeal nerves, which are branches of the vagus nerve.

Anesthesia may be provided to the larynx by the topical application of local anesthesia (using a laryngeal syringe) to the mucous membrane of the pyriform fossa (deep into which runs the superior laryngeal nerve) and to the laryngeal surface of the epiglottis and the vocal folds (Figure 4-1). Local anesthesia of the larynx and trachea also may be accomplished by the percutaneous infiltration of local anesthetic solution around the superior laryngeal nerve and the transtracheal application of local anesthetic to the tracheal mucosa. For percutaneous infiltration, the superior laryngeal nerve is located as it pierces the thyrohyoid membrane (Figure 4-2). The transtracheal application of local anesthesia requires insertion of a 25-gauge needle through the cricothyroid membrane in the midline (Figure 4-3).

Reduction of Dislocated Temporomandibular Joint

In the common presentation of temporomandibular dislocation, the condyle rests on the anterior slope of the articular eminence (Figure 4-4). There is intense pain and severe spasm of the surrounding mandibular musculature. Reduction of this dislocation may frequently be accomplished by unilateral intracapsular injection of local anesthesia.

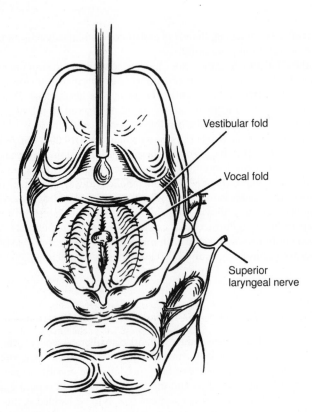

Vestibular fold

Vocal fold

Superior
laryngeal nerve

Figure 4-1 Topical anesthesia to
the larynx.

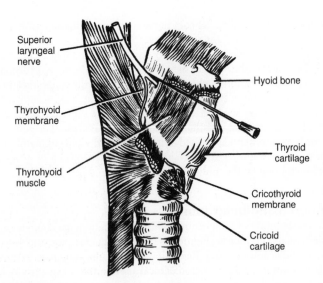

Superior
laryngeal
nerve

Thyrohyoid
membrane

Thyrohyoid
muscle

Hyoid bone

Thyroid
cartilage

Cricothyroid
membrane

Cricoid
cartilage

Figure 4-2 (1) Palpate the greater
cornu of the hyoid bone. (2) Insert
a 25-gauge needle approximately
1 cm caudal to this landmark.
(3) The needle is inserted to a depth
of approximately 1 cm until the
firm consistency of the thyrohyoid
membrane is identified. (4) Inject
3 mL of local anesthetic solution.

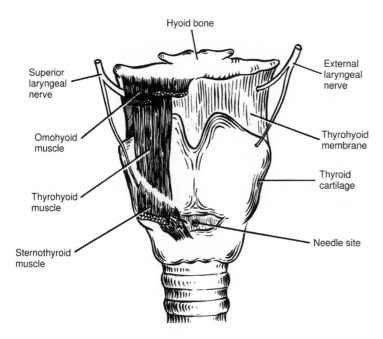

Hyoid bone

Superior laryngeal nerve

Omohyoid muscle

Thyrohyoid muscle

Sternothyroid muscle

External laryngeal nerve

Thyrohyoid membrane

Thyroid cartilage

Needle site

Figure 4-3 (1) Introduce the 25-gauge needle in the midline between the thyroid and cricoid cartilages. (2) Puncture the cricothyroid membrane. It is readily felt as a "pop." Free aspiration of air with the attached syringe verifies the intratracheal position of the needle tip. (3) Instill 4 mL of local anesthetic solution. In addition to anesthesia of the larynx and trachea (steps 1 and 2), the topical application of local anesthesia to the oropharynx is required for adequate visualization for laryngoscopy and tracheoscopy.

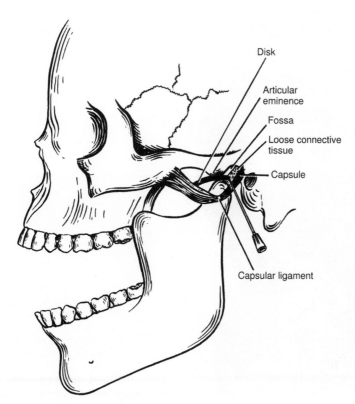

Disk

Articular eminence

Fossa

Loose connective tissue

Capsule

Capsular ligament

Figure 4-4 (1) With the head of the condyloid process locked anteriorly, the depression of the glenoid fossa is easily palpated. (2) The needle is inserted into the depression of the glenoid fossa and directed anteriorly toward the head of the condyloid process. (3) When the condyloid process is contracted, the needle is slightly withdrawn. (4) Instill 2 mL of local anesthetic solution into the capsule.

Reduction and Fixation of Mandibular Fracture

Complete anesthesia for reduction and fixation of a mandibular fracture requires adequate anesthesia of the maxillary and mandibular branches of the trigeminal nerve and superficial branches of the cervical plexus (Figure 4-5).

The mandibular branch of the trigeminal nerve is readily anesthetized near its exit from the skull through the foramen ovale (Figure 4-6). Anesthesia of the maxillary division of the trigeminal nerve may be accomplished in the pterygopalatine fossa near the foramen rotundum, where the nerve exits from the skull (Figure 4-7). The most frequent complication of mandibular and maxillary nerve block is hemorrhage into the cheek, which usually is managed conservatively. Subarachnoid injections and facial nerve blocks are two other rarely reported complications.

The superficial branches of the cervical plexus are easily blocked as they emerge along the posterior margin of the sternocleidomastoid muscle; infiltration is accomplished along the posterior margin of this muscle using 10 to 15 mL of anesthetic solution.

Otology

The sensory innervation of the external ear is illustrated in Figure 4-8. The middle ear receives its sensory innervation through the tympanic plexus (cranial nerves V3, IX, and X).

- V3—auriculotemporal nerve
- IX—Jacobson nerve
- X—auricular nerve

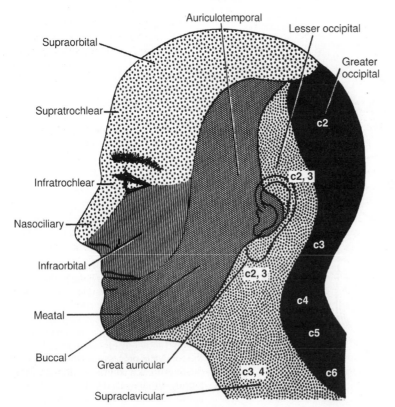

Figure 4-5 Cutaneous innervation of the head and neck.

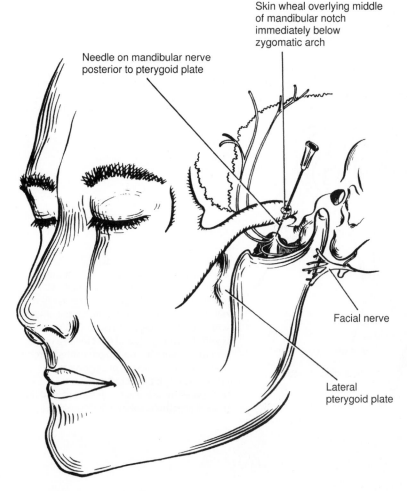

Skin wheal overlying middle
of mandibular notch
immediately below
zygomatic arch

Needle on mandibular nerve
posterior to pterygoid plate

Facial nerve

Lateral
pterygoid plate

Figure 4-6 (1) A skin wheal is raised at the midpoint between the condyle and coronoid process of the mandible and just below the zygoma. (2) An 8-cm needle is introduced perpendicular to the skin until contact with the pterygoid plate occurs, usually at a depth of 4 cm. (3) The needle is withdrawn and then reinserted slightly posterior to a depth of approximately 6 cm. (4) When paresthesia in the mandibular division is elicited, the needle is fixed, and approximately 5 mL of anesthetic solution is administered.

Myringotomy

For myringotomy, inject the cartilaginous and bony junction of the external auditory canal. Instead of introducing local anesthetic through the classic 12, 3, 6, and 9 o'clock infiltration, infiltrate at 12, 2, 4, 6, 8, and 10 o'clock. After the first injection, the subsequent injection sites are already anesthetized before the needle prick. For myringotomy alone, it is not necessary to infiltrate the skin of the bony canal wall and no local anesthetic agent should infiltrate into the middle ear cavity. (See "Complications" later in text.)

Stapedectomy

In addition to the technique described for myringotomy, with stapedectomy it is necessary to infiltrate the tympanomeatal flap. This technique ensures adequate anesthesia while providing vasoconstriction (1% lidocaine with epinephrine 1:100,000) for hemostasis.

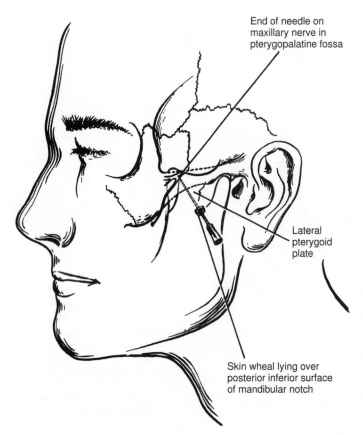

End of needle on
maxillary nerve in
pterygopalatine fossa

Lateral
pterygoid
plate

Skin wheal lying over
posterior inferior surface
of mandibular notch

Figure 4-7 (1) A skin wheal is raised just over the posterior-inferior surface of the mandibular notch. (2) An 8-cm needle is inserted transversely and slightly anterior to a depth of 4-5 cm, where it comes into contact with the lateral pterygoid plate. (3) The needle is withdrawn slightly and directed in a more anterosuperior direction to pass anterior to the pterygoid plate into the pterygopalatine fossa. (4) The needle is advanced another 0.5-1.5 cm until paresthesia is elicited. A total of 5-10 mL of local anesthetic solution is deposited.

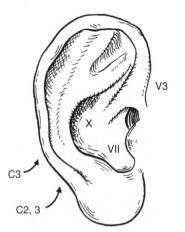
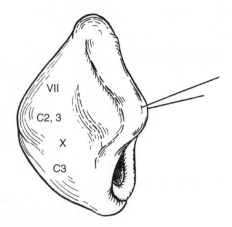

Figure 4-8 Sensory innervation of the external ear.

Complications

Two transient complications have been reported from local anesthetic infiltration for stapedectomy. These result from diffusion of the local anesthetic from the tympanomeatal flap to the middle ear cavity.

A. Temporary facial nerve paralysis results from the local anesthetic coming into contact with the dehiscent facial nerve. Patience and reassurance for a few hours resolve the problem.

B. Violent vertigo with nystagmus (similar to Ménière attack) can occur 45 minutes after infiltration. Provided no damage has been done to the vestibular labyrinth, this problem is secondary to the effect of lidocaine on the membranous labyrinth through the oval or round windows.

These complications are particularly distressing if they occur after an office myringotomy. Therefore, we recommend that there be no infiltration of local anesthetic into the skin of the bony canal wall. Local anesthetic applied at the junction of the bony and cartilaginous canal is adequate and does not risk migrating into the middle ear cavity.

Tympanoplasty and Mastoidectomy (Canalplasty, Meatoplasty)

Tympanoplasty and mastoidectomy are usually performed under general anesthesia, although they may be done under local anesthesia. In addition to the stapedectomy infiltration, postauricular and conchal infiltration are necessary (see Figure 4-8) for sensory innervation. The skin of the anterior canal wall needs to be anesthetized if surgery is to include that anatomic site.

Nasal Surgery

Nasal Polypectomy

Cocaine pledgets along the mucosal surfaces, as well as those in contact with the sphenopalatine ganglion, supply adequate anesthesia for polypectomy. Occasionally, it is necessary to supplement this anesthesia with infiltration, as for rhinoplasty.

Septoplasty and Rhinoplasty

The sensory innervation of the septum and external nose is illustrated in Figures 4-9 to 4-13 and in Tables 4-1 to 4-3. In addition to local infiltration, as shown in Figure 4-13, cocaine pledgets along the mucosal surfaces and sphenopalatine ganglion are used for septoplasty and rhinoplasty. For the best hemostasis and anesthesia result, it is wise to wait at least 20 minutes before performing the surgery.

Sinus Surgery

Caldwell-Luc Operation To achieve good anesthesia for sinus surgery, one needs to block the infraorbital nerve, the sphenopalatine ganglion, and the posterior superior dental nerve. The posterior-superior dental nerve exists from the maxillary nerve adjacent to the sphenopalatine ganglion. To block the sphenopalatine ganglion and posterior-superior dental nerve, introduce local anesthesia through the greater palatine foramen via a curved needle.

Further topical anesthesia is with cocaine pledgets applied intranasally against the sphenopalatine ganglion. Local infiltration of the mucosa in the canine fossa supplies the hemostasis needed over the line of incision.

Ethmoid Sinuses The sensory innervation of the ethmoid sinuses is intertwined with that of the nose and septum. In addition, they are innervated by the anterior ethmoid nerve (branch of the nasociliary, V_1) and the posterior ethmoid nerve (branch of the infratrochlear, V_1).

Sphenoid Sinuses The sensory innervation of the sphenoid sinuses is from the pharyngeal branch of the maxillary nerve as well as the posterior ethmoid nerve.

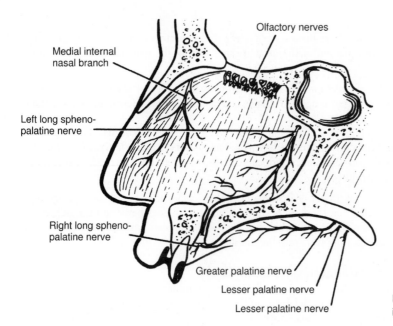

Olfactory nerves

Medial internal
nasal branch

Left long spheno-
palatine nerve

Right long spheno-
palatine nerve

Greater palatine nerve

Lesser palatine nerve

Lesser palatine nerve

Figure 4-9 Sensory innervation of the internal nose.

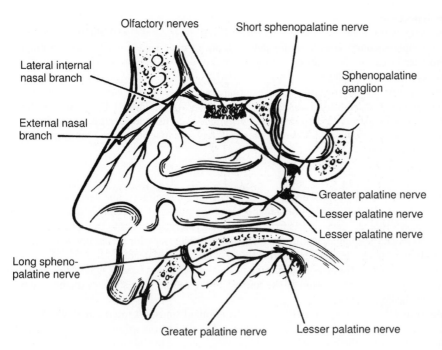

Olfactory nerves

Short sphenopalatine nerve

Lateral internal
nasal branch

Sphenopalatine
ganglion

External nasal
branch

Greater palatine nerve

Lesser palatine nerve

Lesser palatine nerve

Long spheno-
palatine nerve

Greater palatine nerve

Lesser palatine nerve

Figure 4-10 Sensory innervation of the nose.

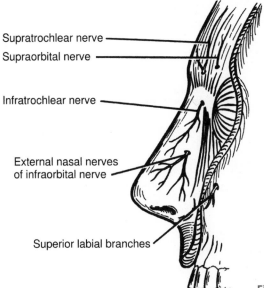

Supratrochlear nerve

Supraorbital nerve

Infratrochlear nerve

External nasal nerves
of infraorbital nerve

Superior labial branches

Figure 4-11 Sensory innervation of the nose.

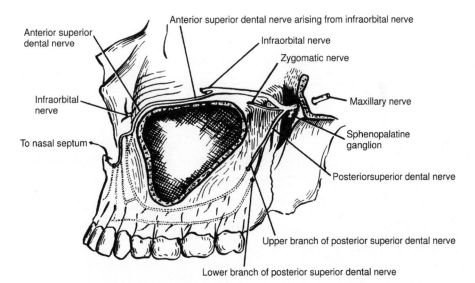

Anterior superior dental nerve arising from infraorbital nerve

Anterior superior
dental nerve

Infraorbital nerve

Zygomatic nerve

Infraorbital
nerve

Maxillary nerve

To nasal septum

Sphenopalatine
ganglion

Posteriorsuperior dental nerve

Upper branch of posterior superior dental nerve

Lower branch of posterior superior dental nerve

Figure 4-12 Sensory innervation of the nose.

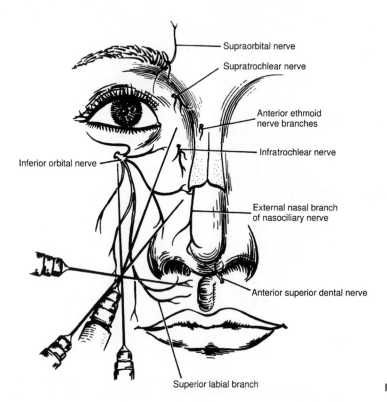

Figure 4-13 Infiltration for rhinoplasty.

Labels in figure:
- Supraorbital nerve
- Supratrochlear nerve
- Anterior ethmoid nerve branches
- Infratrochlear nerve
- Inferior orbital nerve
- External nasal branch of nasociliary nerve
- Anterior superior dental nerve
- Superior labial branch

Table 4-1 **Nasal Sensory Innervation**

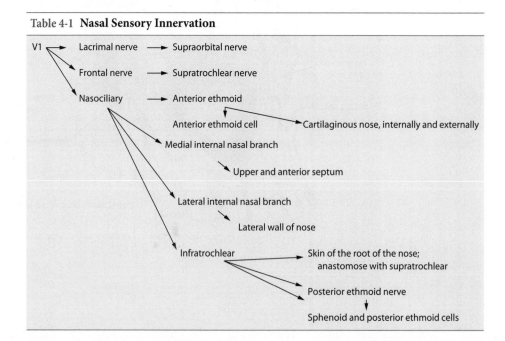

V1 → Lacrimal nerve ⟶ Supraorbital nerve
→ Frontal nerve ⟶ Supratrochlear nerve
→ Nasociliary ⟶ Anterior ethmoid
Anterior ethmoid cell ⟶ Cartilaginous nose, internally and externally
Medial internal nasal branch
Upper and anterior septum
Lateral internal nasal branch
Lateral wall of nose
Infratrochlear → Skin of the root of the nose; anastomose with supratrochlear
Posterior ethmoid nerve
Sphenoid and posterior ethmoid cells

Table 4-2 **Nasal Sensory Innervation**

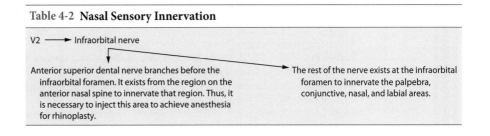

Table 4-3 **Nasal Sensory Innervation**

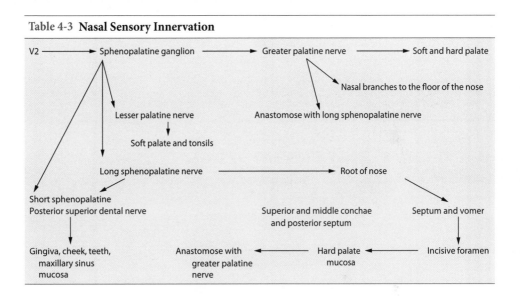

Conclusion

Anesthesia for head and neck surgery may provide some of the most challenging and stressful moments in the operating room. Although many of the procedures may be considered "minor" because they do not involve the major organs or cavities of the body, the access required and manipulation of the airway constantly test the limits of an anesthesiologist's ability to foresee and prevent potentially serious complications. It is, therefore, of supreme importance that the anesthesiologist and otolaryngologist work in tandem to ensure a successful outcome.

Bibliography

ASA perioperative surgical home. http://www.asahq.org/psh.

Barash PG, Cullen BF, Stoelting RK, Cahalan M, Stock MC, Ortega R. *Clinical Anesthesia.* 7th ed. Philadelphia, PA: Wolters Kluwer Health; 2013.

4th National Audit Project (NAP4): Major complications of airway management in the United Kingdom Report and Findings–March 2011.

MedicAlert Foundation difficult airway registry. http://www.medicalert.org/everybody/difficult-airwayintubation-registry.

Richard AJ, Stanley IS, Clifford AS, Brenda G. *Anesthesiologist's Manual of Surgical Procedures.* 4th ed. Philadelphia, PA: Wolters Kluwer Health/Lippincott Williams & Wilkins; 2009.

Chapter 5
Surgical Hemostasis and Clotting Mechanisms

Introduction

The most important considerations for maintaining surgical hemostasis begin before the operation starts. This chapter provides practical tools to approach patients before, during, and after the surgical procedure. Below is a summary explanation of normal hemostasis, and how it can be conceptualized into four basic components. Explanations are provided to illustrate the uses and limitations of the routine coagulation tests. Common coagulation disorders are briefly discussed. Preoperative management of anticoagulants is discussed. The routine clinical application of these basic concepts of blood coagulation can enhance practice and benefit patients.

Basic Concepts of Hemostasis

- *Hemostasis* is a term describing the complex processes that keep blood in its fluid state within the vasculature while allowing it to clot to stop hemorrhage.

The Four Conceptual Components of Hemostasis

- The process of normal hemostasis can be divided conceptually into four basic components of the blood: (1) blood vessel, (2) platelets, (3) coagulation system, and (4) fibrinolytic system (Table 5-1).
- These four components undergo a series of regulated events that lead to clot formation.

Primary Hemostasis

- Blood vessel and platelet interactions
  - (a) Initial reaction with the blood vessel itself triggering vasoconstriction.
  - (b) Platelet adhesion.
    - ○ The initial contact interaction between platelets and *any nonplatelet surface*
    - ○ Mediated by a platelet surface glycoprotein receptor termed GPIb complex and the plasma protein, von Willebrand factor (vWF)
  - (c) Platelet aggregation.
- Results in the formation of a platelet membrane surface receptor, "the aggregation receptor," which is not present on unstimulated platelets.
- The platelet aggregation receptor is made up of two platelet surface proteins, termed *GPIIb/GPIIIa*.

Table 5-1 **Four Conceptual Hemostasis Components**

Component	Composition/Reactions
Blood vessel	Vessel wall; vasoconstriction extravascular proteins, eg, collagen; and tissue factor
Platelet	Adhesion, release, aggregation
Coagulation system	All coagulation factors, vWF, and natural anticoagulant proteins, eg, protein C, AT3
Fibrinolytic system	Clot lysis, split products

      (d) Platelet release.
        ◦ Starts the next process of blood coagulation, termed *secondary hemostasis*
      (e) This whole sequence, from vasoconstriction to the formation of a platelet plug and finally a platelet aggregate and release, constitutes the process of primary hemostasis.
      (f) This process is independent of blood coagulation and occurs even in patients with hemophilia.
      (g) This process is, however, insufficient to completely stop hemorrhage—you need adequate secondary hemostasis.

Secondary Hemostasis

- After primary hemostasis, a series of interdependent enzyme-mediated reactions initiate the formation of a stable fibrin clot, which replaces the unstable platelet plug.
- The key player = tissue factor (TF)—the changing faces of tissue factor biology. A personal tribute to the understanding of the "extrinsic coagulation activation."
      (a) Probably the most important discovery over the last 25 years has been that TF combined with activated factor FVII (FVIIa) *initiates* the clotting cascade.
      (b) TF constitutive expression by fibroblasts outside all blood vessels is termed the "hemostatic barrier."
- The end result of these activation events is the generation of a large amount of thrombin to form hemostatic clot. Knowing these parts of hemostasis helps one understand bleeding risks and drug actions.

Preoperative Screening: Use of Tests of Coagulation

- Preoperative clinical history and examination are the most important components of a preoperative evaluation of the patient's hemostatic ability.

History and Physical

- A careful bleeding history is better than coagulation laboratory tests.
      (a) Several retrospective reviews have repeatedly proven that routine coagulation screening tests do not predict bleeding risks in surgical patients, and specifically in patients undergoing tonsillectomy.
      (b) However, considerable variation occurs in the adequacy of a preoperative screening history and examination.
- A careful bleeding history.

There are three simple questions to remember in taking a bleeding history.
- A. "Have you ever had any surgery?"
    - i. Do not forget to ask about dental surgery.
    - ii. A positive response to this question, that is prior surgery without bleeding problems, serves as a "hemostatic stress test."
    - iii. If the patient has had recent major surgery (within 1-2 years) without bleeding, and no active signs or symptoms of bleeding, one can feel confident that the chances of a hemostatic defect are exceedingly small.
- B. "What do you take for pain?"
    - i. This is the simplest way to elicit information regarding the patient's use of nonsteroidal anti-inflammatory drugs (NSAIDs) and aspirin (ASA).
    - ii. Additional uncommon drugs with some hemorrhagic tendency are "garlic," vitamin E, and fish oil supplements.
- C. "Is there a family history of bleeding or clotting?"
    - i. This question obviously attempts to elicit a familial hemostatic defect that has not yet become clinically apparent, or may only emerge in the postoperative setting.

How to Use Screening Tests of Coagulation

- *If* coagulation tests are used, you will still need a careful bleeding history.
- The following are the common screening tests of coagulation:
    - (a) Prothrombin time (PT), activated partial thromboplastin time (aPTT), complete blood count (CBC) (platelet number)
- The hemostasis components that coagulation tests measure are listed in Table 5-2.
- These coagulation tests are functional global assays.
- Brief study of Table 5-2 shows that it is apparent why these tests are insufficient measures to assess bleeding risk or ensure hemostatic integrity.
    - (a) The bleeding time is insensitive to many hereditary disorders, such as von Willebrand disease.
    - (b) The PT and aPTT are artificial reflections of normal hemostasis, often insensitive. Table 5-2 points out that there is no routinely available screening tool to assess the fibrinolytic system.

Table 5-2 **Testing the Four Hemostatic Components**

Conceptual Hemostatic Component	*Coagulation Screening Tests*
Blood vessel	Bleeding time
Platelet	Bleeding time; CBC
Coagulation system	PT, aPTT, TT
Fibrinolytic system	Not measured

PTT, activated partial thromboplastin time; CBC, complete blood count; PT, prothrombin time; TT, thrombin time.

Anticoagulants in Surgical Patients

Understanding anticoagulation in surgical patients is extremely important in preventing and treating postoperative complications, such as thromboembolism. Moreover, this knowledge is critical in patients undergoing surgery who are already on anticoagulants for various reasons.

Understanding Heparins

Standard or Unfractionated Heparin

- Heparin is a heterogeneous molecule with molecular weight ranging from 3000 to 30,000 Da.
- Heparin is not absorbed orally and must be given intravenously (IV) or subcutaneously (SQ).
- Only one-third of heparin molecules administered have anticoagulant function.
- These heparin molecules act by binding to antithrombin (AT).
- Unfractionated heparin (UFH) also nonspecifically binds to a number of plasma proteins and platelets.
- SQ dosing is higher than IV due to bioavailability.
- Nonspecific UFH binding results in variability in anticoagulant response in different patients.
- The anticoagulant response to UFH is nonlinear—intensity and duration rise disproportionately with increasing dose.
- Four hours is usually sufficient to clear IV heparin (4×60 minutes half-life at 100 U/kg).
- Dosage of UFH varies based on the indication—treatment or prophylaxis.
- Treatment.
  - (a) Weight-based dosing of UFH is preferred over fixed dosing.
  - (b) For deep vein thrombosis (DVT), IV dosing is 80 to 100 U/kg bolus (max 10,000)—followed by 18 U/kg/h continuous infusion.
  - (c) DVT SQ dosing (not used in the United States) is 333 U/kg bolus SQ—followed by 250 U/kg q12h SQ.
  - (d) Dosing for coronary syndromes is lower than that for DVT.
    - ○ IV dose 70 U/kg (max 5000)—followed by 12 to 15 U/kg continuous infusion.
  - (e) UFH monitoring.
    - ○ Therapeutic range—an aPTT ratio 1.5 to 2.5 (upper limit control) is commonly used for DVT therapy based on retrospective data from the 1970s.
    - ○ This range can result in excess heparin exposure and bleeding due to instrument variation.
    - ○ Preferred method—hospital established therapeutic aPTT heparin range.
    - ○ This is done with hospital reagent and instruments, corresponding to an anti-Xa assay of 0.3 to 0.7 IU/mL.
  - (f) Prophylaxis.
    - ○ Prophylaxis dose is generally administered SQ at a dose of 5000 units every 8 or 12 hours.
    - ○ Prophylaxis dose is not monitored by aPTT, and it should not prolong aPTT.

Low-Molecular-Weight Heparin

- Low-molecular-weight heparins (LMWHs) are obtained by depolymerization of UFH yielding fragments between 4000 and 5000 Da.
- Since the depolymerization yields smaller fragments, the extent of nonspecific binding to plasma proteins and platelets is much less for LMWH than UFH.
- This small size changes the pharmacology of LMWH.

- LMWHs give reproducible anticoagulant effects—fixed dosing without monitoring.
- LMWHs do not prolong the aPTT.
  (a) LMWHs act via AT and potentiate the inhibition of coagulation factors Xa and IIa.
  (b) The ratio of anti-Xa/anti-IIa activity is greater than 4 with LMWH and equal to 1 with UFH.
  (c) Anti-Xa assay *can be used* to monitor LMWH activity and is recommended:
    ○ In patients who weigh more than 150 kg
    ○ In patients with renal insufficiency
    ○ In patients who are pregnant
  (d) The anti-Xa activity should be measured 4 hours after the subcutaneous administration with a therapeutic target of 0.6 to 1.0 IU/mL for enoxaparin.
  (e) The mean target anti-Xa activity for tinzaparin, nadroparin, and dalteparin is 0.85, 1.3, and 1.03 IU/mL, respectively.
- There are several LMWHs, including the following:
  (a) Enoxaparin
  (b) Dalteparin
  (c) Nadroparin
  (d) Tinzaparin
  (e) Danaparoid sodium
- The most commonly used LMWHs in the United States are enoxaparin and dalteparin.
- Danaparoid is not available in the United States.

Other Anticoagulants

- Fondaparinux is a new synthetic and selective inhibitor of factor Xa.
- This is distinctly different from UFH and LMWHs.
- It is modeled after the pentasaccharide sequence in heparin that is responsible for binding to AT.
- It does not affect the aPTT, PT, or clotting time.
- Drug levels can only be monitored by special anti-Xa assays, although not widely available.
  (a) Although no oral anti-Xa inhibitors are Food and Drug Administration (FDA) approved in the United States, these are approved in Europe.
    ○ Rivaroxaban is a novel oral *direct* anti-Xa inhibitor approved in more than 100 countries worldwide.
    ○ Apixaban.
    ○ Edoxaban.
    ○ Dabigatran is a specific reversible thrombin inhibitor.
  (b) All these drugs have issues with lack of an antidote or reversibility for surgical procedures.
  (c) Consult hematologist or cardiologist if you encounter a patient on any of these drugs.

Warfarin

- The anticoagulant effect of warfarin results from the inhibition of the vitamin K–dependent clotting factors II, VII, IX, and X.
- The half-life of warfarin ranges from 20 to 60 hours with a mean of 40 hours. The duration of effect is up to 5 days with a maximum effect seen at 48 hours.
- The anticoagulant effect of warfarin is measured by international normalized ratio (INR).

- The antithrombotic effect of warfarin to prevent clot expansion is not present until approximately the fifth day of therapy.
- This effect depends on the clearance of functional factor II (prothrombin), which has a half-life of approximately 50 hours in patients with normal hepatic function.
- Do not use loading doses of warfarin (ie, ≥10 mg/d) as these are of limited value and may increase the patient's risk of bleeding.
- In acute thrombosis (DVT/pulmonary embolism [PE], etc), a full 5-day overlap of warfarin with either UFH or LMWH until the target INR is achieved.

New Oral Anticoagulants

- The anticoagulant effects of the new US-approved oral anticoagulants (dabigatran, rivaroxaban, apixaban) are due to direct, reversible inhibition of thrombin or factor Xa.
- These target-specific oral anticoagulants (rivaroxaban, dabigatran, apixaban) are currently used in clinical practice at fixed doses without the need for routine coagulation monitoring.
- Dabigatran extilate (Pradaxa) is a small molecule prodrug that upon oral administration is converted by nonspecific esterases in the gut, plasma, and liver, into a competitive reversible inhibitor of the active site of thrombin (factor IIa).
- Dabigatran prolongs the PTT, and thrombin time (TT), and PT/INR. However, the INR is relatively insensitive to dabigatran and cannot be used for monitoring.
- Rivaroxaban (Xarelto) is a small molecule competitive, reversible inhibitor of factor Xa (activated factor X clotting factor).
- Rivaroxaban prolongs the PT/INR, PTT, and anti-Xa assays. Special requirements are necessary to use anti-Xa assays to measure levels of rivaroxaban.
- Apixaban (Eliquis) is a small molecule competitive, reversible inhibitor of factor Xa.
- Apixaban prolongs the PT/INR and PTT, but it is not useful for monitoring the drug. Modified anti-Xa assays can be used to measure levels of apixaban.

Reversal of Anticoagulation and Perioperative Anticoagulation Management

UFH

- There is an antidote for UFH—protamine.
- Protamine is a protein derived from fish sperm that binds to heparin to form a stable salt and neutralize the UFH.
- A milligram of protamine will neutralize approximately 100 units of UFH.
- Therefore, an appropriate intravenous dosage should be calculated—based on the estimated heparin in the patient.
  (a) For example, a patient on 1000 U/h of UFH would require 10 mg of protamine.
- Administer intravenously over 1 to 3 minutes to avoid bradycardia and hypotension.
- The aPTT can be used to assess the effectiveness of protamine.

LMWH

- Unlike UFH, the LMWHs have no proven reversing agent.
- In vitro and animal studies demonstrate up to 60% anti-Xa neutralization by protamine sulphate.

- However, its translation into clinical benefit is unclear, and complete reversal is not achieved.
    - (a) The current American College of Chest Physician (ACCP) guidelines recommend using 1 mg of protamine per 100 antifactor Xa units.
        - ○ If the last LMWH dose is less than 8 hours and 0.5 mg of protamine per 100 antifactor Xa units if the last dose is greater than 8 hours.
        - ○ For example, 1 mg enoxaparin equals approximately 100 antifactor Xa units.

Warfarin

- Supratherapeutic INR with warfarin therapy is extremely common in clinical practice.
- Management should be based on the level of the supratherapeutic INR if associated with bleeding.
- No bleeding.
    - (a) For elevation of INR up to 8, in a patient with no other bleeding risk factors:
        - ○ Hold warfarin and following INRs closely until it decreases to less than 4.
    - (b) In patients with INR greater than 8 or with other risk factors for bleeding:
        - ○ Hold warfarin and following INRs closely until it decreases to less than 4.
        - ○ Orally administer phytomenadione (vitamin K_1) at a dose of up to 2.5 mg.
- Bleeding major or minor.
    - (a) *Minor*: for any elevation of INR (> 4)
        - ○ Warfarin should be stopped.
        - ○ Five milligrams of phytomenadione can be given either orally, intravenously, or subcutaneously.
    - (b) *Major*: for any elevation of INR (> 4)
        - ○ Warfarin should be stopped.
        - ○ Five milligrams of phytomenadione can be given either orally, intravenously, or subcutaneously.
        - ○ Two to four units of fresh frozen plasma (FFP) should be given along with vitamin K_1.
        - ○ An INR should be measured 4 to 6 hours after the vitamin K_1 therapy as it may take up to 6 hours to see an effect.
        - ○ Hemodynamic support and transfusion, as needed.
        - ○ Consider prothrombin complex concentrates and recombinant factor VIIa (rFVIIa) with intracranial bleeding.
        - ○ rFVIIa is indicated for treatment of bleeding in patients with congenital and acquired hemophilia.
        - ○ It has been used off label for warfarin bleeding, liver transplant or trauma bleeding, heparin overdose, platelet, and von Willebrand disease bleeding.

New Oral Anticoagulants

Unlike warfarin, the new target-specific oral anticoagulants have no proven reversal agent (Table 5-3).

Use of procoagulant reversal agents such as prothrombin complex concentrate, or recombinant FVIIa, may be considered, but no clear dosing guidelines are available, and clinical experience is limited.

There are new agents in development, including an imitation factor Xa without biological properties, which reverses the anticoagulant action of the factor Xa inhibitors (including

Table 5-3 New Oral Anticoagulants

	Dabigatran IIa	*Rivaroxaban* Xa	*Apixaban* Xa
Tmax	1.5-3 h	2-4 h	1-3 h
Half-life	12-14 h	9-13 h	8-15h
Dose	150 mg bid	15 mg bid × 3 wk/20 mg daily	5 mg bid
FDA approval	A. fib VTE Rx	A. fib VTE prevention VTE Rx	A. fib VTE prevention

rivaroxaban and apixaban), and a fragment of an antibody (Fab), under development, which is a specific antidote to dabigatran.

At least 24 hours off drug are recommended before invasive procedures, for the target-specific new oral anticoagulants.

Perioperative Anticoagulation Management

Warfarin Bridging

Assess the risk of thrombosis for holding warfarin.

- *Low risk:* atrial fibrillation, PE/DVT over 3 months ago, cardiomyopathy, DVT prophylaxis, coronary artery disease, venous access device prophylaxis
- *Intermediate risk:* multiple low-risk factors, or less than 1 month on anticoagulation
- *High risk:* PE/DVT less than 3 months ago, transient ischemia/stroke of cardiac origin, mechanical heart valve hypercoagulable disorders, vascular access occlusion
  - (a) Low-risk patients
    - Consider no heparin bridging; or use prophylactic LMWH or UFH dosing.
    - Prophylactic LMWH dosing—Lovenox 40 mg SQ; UFH 5000 q12h.
    - Day 5—hold warfarin 5 days prior to surgery.
    - Day 1—24 hours before surgery—no LMWH.
    - Day 0—surgery.
    - Day 0—night postoperation no bleeding; start warfarin (double the patient's normal dose) and continue prophylactic LMWH dosing.
    - Day 2—draw INR, continue LMWH and warfarin until therapeutic INR × 2.
  - (b) Intermediate- and high-risk patients
    - Bridging with LMWH or UFH is required.
    - Day 5—hold warfarin 5 days prior to surgery.
    - Day 4—24 hours after stopping warfarin start LMWH (or UFH) at full dose.
    - Continue LMWH days 4 through 2.
    - Day 1—24 hours before surgery—no LMWH.
    - Day 0—surgery.
    - Day 0—night postoperation no bleeding; start warfarin (double the patient's normal dose).
    - Day 1 postoperation—start LMWH, continue warfarin at normal dose.
    - Day 2—draw INR, continue LMWH and warfarin until therapeutic INR × 2.

Full-Dose UFH and LMWH Dosing for Bridging

- Admit for full-dose IV heparin per nomogram.
- Enoxaparin 1 mg/kg SQ bid.
- Enoxaparin 1.5 mg/kg SQ qd.
- Home SQ heparin 215 U/kg SQ q12h (target PTT 45-60, 6 hours after shot).
- If the surgery is urgent, the anticoagulant reversal should follow:
    - (a) INR reversal bleeding major or minor
    - (b) Heparin reversal protamine
    - (c) LMWH reversal protamine and consider rFVIIa

Antiplatelet Drug Therapy: Considerations and Discontinuation Before Operation

- Elective and emergent surgeries may often involve consideration for the risk of bleeding and thrombosis in patients on antiplatelet drug therapy.
- *Antiplatelet agents*: aspirin, NSAIDs, thienopyridines (ie, clopidogrel and ticlopidine).
- Before the procedure, one should consider the risks of (1) bleeding and (2) thrombo-embolic event related to interruption of antithrombotic therapy.
    - (a) The risks of bleeding due solely to endoscopic procedure are outlined in Table 5-4.
    - (b) The thrombotic risks are outlined in Table 5-5.
- Do not stop ASA/clopidogrel for low-risk bleeding procedures.
    - (a) We recommend that aspirin and/or NSAIDs may be continued for all endoscopy when biopsy is not anticipated, and with skin biopsy or other minor dermatologic procedures, ophthalmic surgery excluding major lid or orbital surgery, or dental procedures associated with continuing the antiplatelet.

Coronary Stents

- Do not stop ASA/clopidogrel in first 12 months post stent.
    - (a) We recommend that elective procedures be deferred in patients with a recently placed vascular stent or acute coronary syndrome (ACS) until the patient has received antithrombotic therapy for the minimum recommended duration per current guidelines.
    - (b) Once this minimum period has elapsed, we suggest that clopidogrel or ticlopidine be withheld for approximately 7 to 10 days before endoscopy and aspirin should be continued.

In Emergencies

- For patients who have had placement of a bare metal coronary stent in the 4 weeks or a drug-eluting coronary stent in the 12 months preceding the anticipated procedure, continuing aspirin and clopidogrel (Plavix) through the perioperative period is recommended independent of the bleeding risk of the procedure.

Table 5-4 Common and Uncommon Blood Vessel Bleeding Disorders

Blood Vessel Bleeding Disorders	
Hereditary	Ehlers-Danlos syndrome
	Williams-Beuren syndrome
	Osteogenesis imperfecta
Acquired	Scurvy
	Amyloidosis

Table 5-5 **Common and Uncommon Platelet Bleeding Disorders**

Functional Platelet Bleeding Disorders	
Hereditary	Bernard-Soulier syndrome
	Glanzmann thrombasthenia
	Storage pool disorders
	Chediak-Higashi
	Hermansky-Pudlak
	Wiskott-Aldrich syndrome
	Scott syndrome
	Gray platelet syndrome
	Platelet-type von Willebrand disease
	ADP receptor P2 defects
	Platelet thromboxane A2 (TXA2) receptor deficiency
	Platelet thromboxane synthase deficiency
	Platelet cyclo-oxygenase deficiency
Acquired	Essential thrombocythemia
	Polycythemia vera
	Pseudo-Bernard Soulier syndrome
	Type I Gaucher disease
	Acute megakaryoblastic leukemia
	Postcardiac bypass pump

When to Worry About Preoperative Coagulation Test Results

Approach to a Patient With Elevated aPTT or PT/INR

- Routine preoperative anesthesia evaluation or laboratory evaluation may reveal prolonged aPTT or PT or both.
- Elective surgeries should be postponed for further evaluation.
    (a) Isolated prolongation of PT is usually seen in factor VII deficiency, due to vitamin K or liver disease.
    (b) Prolongation of aPTT or both aPTT/PT reflects multiple factor deficiencies or if there is an acquired inhibitor.
    (c) Extremely important to know whether the patient has a factor deficiency or an acquired inhibitor.
    (d) This is accomplished by ordering *mixing study* laboratory test.
    (e) If the mixing study corrects the PT or aPTT, it is suggestive of a factor deficiency.
    (f) Mixing study will not be corrected if an inhibitor antibody is present.
    (g) Diagnosis of some inhibitors may need incubation of the plasma mixture for several hours.

(h) Factor VIII inhibitors and circulating lupus anticoagulants are the most frequently encountered inhibitors.
- ○ Acquired factor VIII inhibitor is dangerous and may cause large, rapidly expanding hematomas that may impinge on the trachea or on other vital structures resulting in death.
- ○ Lupus anticoagulants are antiphospholipid immunoglobulin G or M antibodies that prolong phospholipid-dependent coagulation in vitro and generally are not dangerous.
- ○ Lupus anticoagulants do not cause bleeding.
- ○ Lupus anticoagulants in some patients may cause thrombosis.
- ○ These were first recognized in a patient with systemic lupus erythematosus, as such called lupus anticoagulant (LA), although it is more frequently encountered in patients without lupus.

Tables of Common and Uncommon Clinical Bleeding Disorders

Tables 5-6 through 5-9 list common and uncommon bleeding disorders by the conceptual component of hemostasis that is affected.

Multifaceted Disorders
Dissemination Intravascular Coagulation and Heparin-Induced Thrombocytopenia
Disseminated Intravascular Coagulation

- Disseminated intravascular coagulation (DIC) is characterized by systemic intravascular activation of coagulation, leading to widespread fibrin deposition and multiorgan failure.

Table 5-6 Common and Uncommon Coagulation Bleeding Disorders

Coagulation Bleeding Disorders	
Hereditary	Hemophilia FVIII, FIX, FXI
	All other clotting factor deficiencies
	von Willebrand disease
	Factor XIII deficiency
	Hypofibrinogenemia
	Dysfibrinogenemia
Acquired	Acquired specific factor inhibitors
	Acquired von Willebrand disease
	DIC
	Lupus anticoagulant, factor II deficiency
	Amyloidosis
	Acquired heparin-like anticoagulant

Table 5-7 **Common and Uncommon Fibrinolytic Bleeding Disorders**

Fibrinolytic Bleeding Disorders	
Hereditary	Deficiency of plasminogen activator inhibitor-1
Acquired	DIC
	Liver disease
	Postcardiac bypass pump

Table 5-8 **Procedure Bleeding Risks**

High Risk	*Low Risk*
Major operations including cancer surgery, reconstruction, surgical removal of the adenoids (adenoidectomy) or tonsils (tonsillectomy), nasal surgeries, sinus surgeries, microsurgical procedures, and complex facial repair	Skin procedures—face and pinna Endoscopy without biopsy Lip laceration repair
PEG placement, pneumatic or other dilation	Dental procedures

Data from ASGE Standards of Practice Committee. Management of antithrombotic agents for endoscopic procedures. *Gastrointest Endosc.* 2009;70(6):1061-1070.

Table 5-9 **Thrombotic Risks for Discontinuation of Antiplatelet Therapy**

High Risk	*Low Risk*
Atrial fibrillation associated with valvular heart disease, prosthetic valves, left ventricular ejection fraction < 35%, a history of a thromboembolic event	Uncomplicated or paroxysmal nonvalvular atrial fibrillation
Recently (≤ 1 year) placed coronary stent	Bioprosthetic valve
Deep vein thrombosis	Mechanical valve in the aortic position
Acute coronary syndrome	
Nonstented percutaneous coronary intervention after myocardial infarction	

Adapted with permission from ASGE Standards of Practice Committee. Management of antithrombotic agents for endoscopic procedures, *Gastrointest Endosc.* 2009 Dec;70(6):1060-1070.

- Most common underlying causes of DIC include the following:
  - (a) Severe infection
  - (b) Inflammation
  - (c) Trauma
  - (d) Cancer
  - (e) Obstetrical calamities such as amniotic fluid embolism or abruptio placentae

- A diagnosis of DIC can be made by the clinical history presentation along with a combination of laboratory abnormalities. See Table 5-2.
- Chronic low-grade DIC is generally seen in patients with history of malignancies.

Management of DIC

Heparin-Induced Thrombocytopenia

- Heparin-induced thrombocytopenia (HIT) is a potentially devastating, common iatrogenic complication occurring from patient exposure to UFH or LMWH.
- HIT is defined as a platelet drop of less than 150,000/µL *or* 50% reduction from the baseline count, 5 to 14 days after the initial exposure to these drugs.
- It may also occur more rapidly if the patient has had a recent prior exposure to these anticoagulants (generally, within 100 days).
- It may also be manifested as *delayed-onset HIT* occurring 9 to 30 days after the discontinuation of UFH/LMWH therapy.
- The incidence of HIT in patients exposed to UFH is 3% to 5% and it is up to 1% in patients exposed to LMWH with up to 600,000 cases and resulting in up to 90,000 deaths yearly.
- HIT is a highly prothrombotic state.
- Most of the thromboses are venous in nature, but arterial thrombosis is seen as well.
- HIT is a clinical diagnosis supported by laboratory testing.
- Identifying the typical platelet drop after exposure to UFH is crucial in the diagnosis of HIT.
- Clinical diagnosis may be challenging as other causes of thrombocytopenia including dilutional, drug-induced, postoperative bleeding, DIC, and sepsis need to be excluded, and HIT may occur in conjunction with the other disorders.
- Laboratory tests include functional activation assays and an antigen assay.
  - (a) The functional assays include heparin-induced platelet aggregation assay (HIPA) and serotonin release assay (SRA).
    - ○ These are less sensitive and more specific.
  - (b) The Heparin-PF4 antibody assay is highly sensitive but less specific.
  - (c) Both types of assays should be performed if the diagnosis is under question.
- Treatment of HIT includes prompt cessation of all heparin products.
  - (d) Including infusions, injections, flushes, heparin-coated intravenous central catheters, heparin in total parenteral nutrition, and during hemodialysis.
- LMWH is contraindicated in patients with HIT due to cross-reactivity to the antibodies.
- The two FDA-approved drugs for the treatment of HIT:
  - (a) Argatroban and lepirudin.
  - (b) These are direct thrombin inhibitors (DTI) that bind and inhibit free and clot-bound thrombin.
  - (c) Argatroban is metabolized in the liver and should be used with caution in mild hepatic insufficiency.
  - (d) Lepirudin is renally metabolized and should be avoided in patients with renal insufficiency.
  - (e) Both of these require aPTT monitoring, and interfere and prolong the PT/INR levels.
- It is extremely important to remember that warfarin *should not* be used alone to treat HIT.
- Warfarin initiation must be postponed until the patient's platelet count has recovered to near-normal levels (< 150,000/µL).

- Warfarin should be started at a low dose (2.5-5 mg) overlapping with argatroban or lepirudin.
- Warfarin should be continued for 3 months if HIT is not associated with thrombosis.

Bibliography

Bartholomew JR, Hursting MJ. Transitioning from argatroban to warfarin in heparin-induced thrombocytopenia: an analysis of outcomes in patients with elevated international normalized ratio (INR). *J Thromb Thrombolysis*. 2005;19:183-188.

Carmeliet P, Mackman N, Moons L, et al. Role of tissue factor in embryonic blood vessel development. *Nature*. 1996;383:73-75.

Hirsh J, Raschke R. Heparin and low-molecular-weight heparin: the Seventh ACCP Conference on Antithrombotic and Thrombolytic Therapy. *Chest*. 2004;126:188S-203S.

Howells RC, Wax MK, Ramadan HH. Value of preoperative prothrombin time/partial thromboplastin time as a predictor of postoperative hemorrhage in pediatric patients undergoing tonsillectomy. *Otolaryngol Head Neck Surg*. 1997;117:628-632.

Ruff, CT, Guigliano RP. Comparison of the efficacy and safety of new oral anticoagulants with warfarin in patients with atrial fibrillation: a meta-analysis of randomised trials. *Lancet*. 2014:383:955-962.

QUESTIONS

1. Why is a bleeding history more likely to reveal a bleeding disorder, than screening tests of coagulation?
   A. The PT/PTT tests do not measure fibrinolytic bleeding.
   B. The bleeding time often misses mild von Willebrand disease.
   C. Antiplatelet drugs such as Plavix may not affect the PT/PTT or bleeding time.
   D. A bleeding history is likely to uncover hemostatic stress such as dental extractions.
   E. All of the above.

2. Which of the following are true statements regarding the differences or similarities between standard UFH and LMWH?
   A. Both UFH and LMWH prolong the PTT.
   B. Only LMWH requires monitoring using the PTT or anti-Xa.
   C. Only LMWH requires dose adjustment in renal failure.
   D. A weight-based nomogram for UFH avoids the need for PTT monitoring.
   E. Only UFH is a polysaccharide with a specific binding site for antithrombin three.

3. Which of the following statements are true regarding typical HIT?
   A. The platelet drop in HIT is less than 100,000.
   B. The platelet drop in HIT is 50% or more from baseline.
   C. The drop in platelets is typically 24 hours after heparin exposure.
   D. The drop in platelets never occurs days after heparin is stopped.
   E. HIT is more common with the use of LMWH.

4. Which of the following statements are true regarding DIC?

   A. DIC is diagnosed by specific laboratory findings.

   B. DIC is only a clinical diagnosis.

   C. DIC can manifest clinically in overt and occult syndromes.

   D. DIC is always treated by heparin therapy to stop thrombosis.

   E. The D-dimer test is diagnostic of DIC.

5. A 35-year-old woman presents to emergency room (ER) with history of bruising easily over the past 1½ weeks. She also reports a large bruise over the right thigh associated with pain and difficulty in walking and also another bruise on her left forearm, which was spontaneous. She did not have history of a fall or trauma prior to this. She did have an upper respiratory tract infection (URI) and was prescribed Augmentin 2 weeks prior. She denies bleeding from anywhere. She also denies history of bleeding excessively after a dental extraction or since childhood or menorrhagia. There is no family history of bleeding in her family. On laboratory evaluation her PT is 12.7 and aPTT is 58. CBC has a white blood cell (WBC)—6.7, Hgb—9.0, platelet (PLT)—145. On physical examination she has a large hematoma over her right thigh. Before surgical management to the hematoma, you would:

   A. Call the laboratory to perform a bleeding time.

   B. Obtain a 50:50 mixing study to evaluate presence of factor deficiency or inhibitor.

   C. Check for lupus anticoagulant.

   D. Order a DIC panel.

Chapter 6
Related Neurology and Neurosurgery

Neurology

A. Headache syndromes
  i. Migraine
    a. Trigeminovascular syndrome
    b. Paroxysmal headache (HA) associated with multiple signs and symptoms that can overlap with sinus symptoms
      1. Unilateral
      2. Throbbing pulsatile headache in the frontotemporal or orbital area
      3. Aura
        • Can arise before or during the HA
        • Usually visual but can be sensory or motor
      4. Pain builds over 1 to 2 hours and progresses posteriorly
      5. Headache lasts 4 to 72 hours
      6. Photophobia, phonophobia
      7. Nausea—80%, vomiting—50%, anorexia and food intolerance and light-headedness
      8. Signs
        • Cranial/cervical tenderness
        • Horner syndrome
        • Conjunctival injection
        • Tachycardia or bradycardia
        • Hypertension or hypotension
        • Hemisensory changes or hemiparesis
        • Adie's-like pupil (light-near dissociation)
    c. Diagnosis
      1. Two of the following characteristics:
        • Unilateral location
        • Pulsating quality
        • Moderate to severe pain
        • Aggravated or caused by physical activity
      2. During the HA patient must have one of the following:
        • Nausea and/or vomiting
        • Photophobia and phonophobia

d. Imaging
   1. Diagnostic imaging is not necessary in patients with stable history of migraine headaches and a normal neurologic examination.
e. Management recommendations
   1. Computed tomography (CT) is not recommended for headache evaluation when magnetic resonance imaging (MRI) is available, unless in an emergency situation.
   2. Persistent over-the-counter (OTC) pain medication for the treatment of headache is not advised as this symptom may indicate underlying brain pathology.
   3. First-line treatment for migraine should not include opioid or butalbital-containing medications as first-line treatment for recurrent headache.
   4. Lifestyle modifications
      - Avoidance of carrying heavy purses or bags over one shoulder
      - Avoidance of certain foods
      - Maintaining hydration status
      - Sleep hygiene
      - Limit stress
   5. Integrative medicine
      - Magnesium
      - Riboflavin
      - Coenzyme Q10
   6. Abortive medications
      - These medications aim to reverse or at least stop the progression of a headache.
      - Most effective when given within 15 minutes of symptom onset when the pain is mild.
      - Types:
        (a) Triptans: selective serotonin receptor agonists
        (b) Ergot alkaloids: ergotamine, dihydroergotamine
        (c) Analgesics and nonsteroidal anti-inflammatory drugs (NSAIDs)
        (d) Combination medications
           ○ Acetaminophen, aspirin, and caffeine (Excedrin)
           ○ Butalbital, aspirin, and caffeine (Fiorinal)
           ○ Isometheptene, dichloralphenazone, acetaminophen (Midrin, Duradrin, and others)
        (e) Antiemetics
   7. Prophylactic medications
      - Indication
        (a) More than two headaches per month
        (b) Duration of headache is more than 24 hours
        (c) Significant disability for 3 or more days
        (d) Abortive therapy fails or is overused
        (e) Abortive medications used more than twice a week
      - Types
        (a) Antiepileptic drugs
        (b) Beta-blockers
        (c) Tricyclic antidepressants

          (d) Ca^{2+} channel blockers

          (e) Botulinum toxin: up to nine treatment cycles for progressive improvement in symptoms

ii. Tension headache

   a. Most common type of recurring headache thought to be related to muscular factors and psychogenic forces (stressful event).

   b. Throbbing quality with onset more gradual than migraines; usually tension headaches are more constant and less severe.

   c. Headaches can last up to 7 days, not associated with nausea or vomiting, photophobia and/or phonophobia.

   d. Diagnostic criteria.

      1. Two of the following must be present:
- Tightening in frontal-occipital locations
      (a) Occipitonuchal
      (b) Bifrontal
- Bilateral
- Mild to moderate intensity
- Not aggravated by physical activity

   e. Management.

      1. Imaging is only required if headache pattern has changed and is not a common primary headache disorder, such as migraine, cluster, or tension headache.

   f. Treatment.

      1. Massage, relaxation techniques

      2. Lifestyle modification: regular exercise, balanced meals, adequate sleep

      3. Trigger points injection/occipital nerve block

      4. NSAIDs

      5. Tricyclic antidepressants, muscle relaxers

iii. Cluster headache

   a. Group of headaches (known as histamine headaches) with multiple characteristics

      1. Severe unilateral pain that is orbital, supraorbital, or temporal.

      2. Each headache lasts 15 to 180 minutes and can occur 8 times a day or every other day.

      3. The HA may occur one to eight times a day for as long as 4 months.

      4. HAs are often nocturnal, during sleep or early morning hours.

      5. Associated with one or more of the following ipsilateral signs:
- Conjunctival injection
- Lacrimation
- Nasal congestion
- Rhinorrhea
- Facial hydrosis
- Miosis
- Ptosis

      6. Two main forms of cluster headaches:
- Episodic: at least two cluster headache phases that last 7 days to 1 year are separated by a cluster-free interval of 1 month or longer
- Chronic: cluster occurs more than once a year without remission or the cluster-free interval is less than 1 month

b. Management
  1. Pharmacologic approach
     - Abortive treatment
       (a) Oxygen
           ○ 8 L/min for 10 minutes or 100% by mask
       (b) Triptans
           ○ Stimulation of 5-HT 1 receptors produces vasoconstrictive effect and may abort attack.
           ○ Sumatriptan has been studied the most in the setting of cluster headache.
           ○ Intranasal administration effective.
       (c) Ergot alkaloids
           ○ Stimulation of alpha receptors to cause vasoconstriction.
           ○ Most effective when given early in a cluster headache attack.
           ○ Intranasal administration is effective.
     - Preventive/prophylactic treatment
       (a) Calcium channel blockers
           ○ Verapamil considered most effective.
           ○ Can be combined with ergotamine and lithium.
     - Anticonvulsant
       (a) Topiramate and divalproex found to be most effective for prophylaxis.
       (b) Mechanism of action is unclear.
  2. Surgical approach
     - Percutaneous radiofrequency ablation of the gasserian ganglion
       (a) 50% success rate.
       (b) 20% have fair-to-good results.
       (c) 30% failure rate.
     - Gamma knife radiosurgery
       (a) Increased risk for disturbance in facial sensation
     - Occipital nerve block
       (a) Abortive procedure for cluster headache
     - Deep brain stimulation (DBS)
       (a) Electrodes placed in ipsilateral posterior inferior hypothalamus.
       (b) Candidates for DBS are the patients who have chronic cluster headaches refractory to pharmacologic therapy.
     - Stimulation of the pterygopalatine ganglion
       (a) Candidate for stimulation are select patients with chronic cluster headaches.

B. Facial pain
  i. Trigeminal neuralgia
    a. Characteristics
      1. Distinct, sudden, lancinating pain following the sensory distribution of the trigeminal nerve.
      2. Pain is most similar to an "electric shock" that worsens in less than 20 seconds and begins to fade to burning.
         - Pain shoots from the corner of the mouth to the angle of the jaw in 60%.
         - Pain shoots from the upper lip or teeth to the eyebrow or area around the eye in 30%.
         - V1 involved in less than 5% of cases.

- V2 and V3 distribution affected in 35% of patients.
        3. Triggers: chewing, talking, smiling, drinking hot or cold fluids, touching, shaving, teeth cleaning, encountering cold air on the face.
        4. Common causes include vascular compression at the root entry zone or demyelination due to diseases such as multiple sclerosis (MS).
    b. Diagnosis
        1. No laboratory, radiographic, or electrophysiologic studies are routinely needed for patients with characteristic history and normal neurologic examination.
        2. Criteria established by the International Headache Society
            - Paroxysmal attacks of pain that lasts up to 2 minutes and involves a distribution of the trigeminal nerve (V1-V3).
            - Pain has at least one of the following characteristics: intense, sharp, superficial, or stabbing, or pain starts from specific trigger areas or by triggering factors.
            - Attacks are stereotyped in the patient.
            - No neurologic deficit based on clinical examination.
            - Pain is not attributed to another disorder.
    c. Management
        1. Multiple treatment options
            - Pharmacologic therapy
                (a) 75% of patients have substantial relief and adequate control with medical therapy.
                (b) Carbamazepine best studied and only indicated drug by the Food and Drug Administration (FDA).
                    ○ Initial response to carbamazepine is diagnostic.
                    ○ Side effects: ataxia (15%), dizziness (44%), drowsiness (32%), nausea (29%), vomiting (18%).
                (c) Lamotrigine and baclofen are second-line options; gabapentin has been shown effective particularly with MS patients.
            - Percutaneous glycerol or thermal rhizotomy of the gasserian ganglion
            - Balloon compression
            - Open cranial procedures (ie, microvascular decompression)
                (a) Most durable treatment option
            - Radiation therapy (ie, gamma knife radiosurgery)
    ii. Cranial neuropathy syndromes
        a. Tolosa-Hunt syndrome
            1. Episodic unilateral orbital or retro-orbital pain with ophthalmoplegia.
            2. Involvement of cranial nerves (CN) III to VI.
            3. Thought to be due to a nonspecific granulomatous inflammation involving the posterior superior orbital fissure, orbital apex, and cavernous sinus.
            4. Diagnosis of exclusion (MRI needed to rule out other pathologies).
            5. Symptoms last for average of 8 weeks if untreated.
            6. Treatment: steroids.
        b. Raeder syndrome
            1. First division of trigeminal nerve involved causing neuropathic pain or sensory loss; other divisions of trigeminal nerve can also be involved.
            2. Sympathetic dysfunction also (miosis, ptosis) without anhidrosis.
            3. Neuroimaging necessary to exclude other diagnoses.

        4. Syndrome not specific to any underlying pathologic process.

   c. Gradenigo syndrome
      1. Apical petrositis: infection of petrous temporal bone
      2. Due to infection extending from middle ear and mastoid air cells into the pneumatized petrous apex via the perilabyrinthine air tract
      3. Involvement of Dorello's canal and possibly the trigeminal nerve → Abducens nerve palsy with possible orbital or retro-orbital pain

   d. Vernet syndrome
      1. Lesion (tumor, infection, fracture, thrombosis) of the jugular foramen
      2. CN IX-XI affected: ipsilateral trapezius and sternocleidomastoid weakness, dysphonia, dysphagia, loss of taste over posterior one-third of the tongue, depressed pharyngeal sensation

   e. Collet-Sicard syndrome
      1. Unilateral palsy of CN IX-XI
      2. Lack of sympathetic dysfunction

  iii. Stroke syndromes
   a. **Rule of thumb:** acute neurologic deterioration with ipsilateral CN deficit(s) and contralateral sensory or motor dysfunction localizes the stroke to the brainstem (midbrain, pons, medulla)

   b. Dejerine-Roussy syndrome
      1. Stroke of the thalamus involving the (PCA)
      2. Contralateral sensory loss, contralateral dysesthesia (thalamic pain), ballistic or choreoathetoid movements, transient hemiparesis

   c. Weber syndrome
      1. Stroke of the caudal midbrain involving the posterior cerebral artery (PCA)
      2. Ipsilateral gaze weakness (oculomotor nerve palsy), contralateral weakness

   d. Benedikt syndrome
      1. Stroke of the tegmentum (midbrain floor) involving the PCA
      2. Oculomotor nerve palsy, contralateral hemichorea, hemiathetosis (red nucleus damage)

   e. Raymond syndrome
      1. Stroke of the pons involving the paramedian branches of the basilar artery
      2. Ipsilateral lateral gaze weakness, contralateral weakness

   f. Foville syndrome
      1. Stroke of inferior medial pons involving the basilar artery
      2. Contralateral hemiparesis, ipsilateral facial palsy (CN VII), lateral gaze palsy (CN VI), reduced touch and position sense (medial lemniscus)

   g. Millard Gubler syndrome
      1. Stroke of the basis pontis (caudal pons) involving the basilar artery
      2. Contralateral weakness, ipsilateral lateral gaze weakness, ipsilateral facial weakness

   h. Palatopharyngeal paralysis of Avellis
      1. Stroke of cephalad portion of nucleus ambiguous
      2. Paralysis of the palatal, pharyngeal muscles with sparing of laryngeal muscles
      3. Somatotopic organization of motor nucleus places laryngeal muscles caudal

   i. Dejerine anterior bulbar syndrome

1. Stroke of paramedian medulla involving the basilar artery
2. Sudden onset of reduced touch and position sense (dorsal column/medial lemniscus) of the contralateral side of body with contralateral hemiplegia, preservation of pain and temperature, with ipsilateral tongue weakness (CN XII) and upbeat nystagmus, without facial droop

j. Wallenberg syndrome
1. Stroke of lateral medulla involving the vertebral artery
2. Ipsilateral loss of facial sensation, ataxia, nystagmus/vertigo/nausea (vestibular nucleus involvement), dysphagia (nucleus ambiguous), Horner syndrome, contralateral hemisensory loss (spinothalamic tract)

iv. Seizure disorders
a. Infantile spasms (West syndrome)
1. Sudden flexor or extensor spasms of the head, trunk, or limbs
2. Associated with tuberous sclerosis (neurocutaneous syndrome)
3. On electroencephalogram (EEG), see hypsarrhythmia

b. Juvenile myoclonic epilepsy
1. Myoclonic jerks that arise usually in the morning.
2. Patients have normal intelligence.
3. On EEG, see 4- to 6-Hz spike waves and polyspike discharges.

c. Benign focal epilepsy of childhood
1. Generalized seizures at night, focal seizures during the day
2. On EEG see di- or triphasic sharp waves

d. Petit mal
1. Frequent, blank staring spells
2. On EEG, see generalized, symmetric 3-Hz spike-wave discharge

e. Gelastic seizures
1. Involuntary laughter with alternating crying or sobbing spells; with precocious puberty when associated with hypothalamic hamartoma
2. 25% associated with hypothalamic hamartoma
3. 21% of patients with hypothalamic hamartoma have gelastic seizures
4. Hypothalamic hamartoma associated with other midline deformities (ie, callosal agenesis)

f. Temporal lobe seizures
1. Most common in adults.
2. Involves mesial temporal structures.
3. Associated with **auras** (hallucinations, sensory illusions, viscerosensory symptoms, eg, sensation over the abdomen or chest wall) and **automatisms** (stereotyped repetitive movement of the mouth, tongue, lips or jaw → lip smacking).
4. Anterior temporal lobe resection is 80% effective.
5. On EEG, see focal temporal slowing or epileptiform sharp waves or spikes in the anterior temporal lobe region.

v. Inflammatory disorders of the nervous system
a. Multiple sclerosis
1. Acquired relapsing demyelinating disease that is disseminated throughout the central nervous system in time and space.
2. Female predilection with peak presentation at age 35 years.
3. Optic neuritis and trigeminal neuralgia are common symptoms.

4. Multiple patterns of presentation
   - Relapsing-remitting: most common; occasional symptoms that resolve on their own.
   - Secondary progressive: begin as relapsing-remitting but then become progressively worse.
   - Primary progressive: symptoms do not relapse and become progressive.
   - Progressive with relapses: symptoms that resolve but when they return are worse than the prior symptom.
   - Benign MS: patient with symptoms but remain functionally active for over 15 years.
5. Radiographic signs
   - Dawson's fingers: hyperintense lesions seen on MRI FLAIR (fluid-attenuated inversion recovery) sequence that are perpendicular to the ventricles.
   - Open ring sing: enhancement is often incomplete on contrasted MRI studies.
   - Lesions are often hyperintense on T2 MRI.
6. Laboratory evaluation
   - IgG and albumin values from the serum and CSF should be measured to obtain the IgG index (a value > 0.7 is elevated).
   - Oligoclonal bands are often seen in cerebrospinal fluid (CSF).
b. Amyotrophic lateral sclerosis
   1. Disease of the upper and lower motor neurons.
   2. Signs of anterior horn cell disease without sensory neuropathy.
   3. Associated with Parkinson-like dementia complex.
   4. Most patients die within 5 years of symptom onset.
c. Progressive multifocal leukoencephalopathy
   1. Due to activation of JC virus (papovavirus) in immunocompromised patients.
   2. Reactivated virus attacks oligodendrocytes of subcortical white matter.
   3. Usually affects the parietal-occipital lobes.
   4. Seen in 4% of AIDS patients and in patients with leukemia and lymphoma.
   5. MRI findings: hyperintense on T2 and FLAIR sequences, nonenhancing.
   6. Dx confirmed by polymerase chain reaction (PCR) analysis of JC virus RNA in CSF.
d. Neuroborreliosis
   1. Neurologic symptoms that arise after tick bite from *Borrelia burgdorferi*
   2. Most common symptom → painful sensory radiculitis
   3. Other symptoms: Bell palsy, limb paresis, oculomotor weakness, arthralgias, cardiomyopathy
   4. Tx: penicillin or ceftriaxone
e. Meningitis
   1. Bacterial meningitis
      - Most common in the winter months
      - Glucose decreased, protein elevated, CSF leukocytosis, and elevated opening pressure
   2. Tuberculous meningitis
      - Secondary to infection elsewhere, usually the lungs.
      - Mortality rate higher than in bacterial meningitis.
      - Early treatment prevents poor outcome.

- Involves skull base (basal meningitis).
- Tx: isoniazid (INH), rifampin, pyrazinamide, ethambutol.
  (a) Tx given for 18 to 24 months.
  (b) INH depletes B6; therefore its use mandates replacement.
- CSF profile: slight increase in intracranial pressure (ICP), pleocytosis with lymphocytic predominance, increased protein, decreased glucose.
- CSF glucose should be normally 60% of serum glucose, usually 45 mg/dL or greater.
3. Viral meningitis/encephalitis
- CSF profile: lymphocytic pleocytosis, mild elevation in protein, normal glucose.
- Peaks in the summer and fall seasons.
- RNA viruses: enteroviruses, arboviruses, rhabdoviruses, arenaviruses.
- DNA viruses: herpes simplex virus type 1 (HSV-1), HSV-2, varicella zoster virus (VZV), Cytomegalovirus (CMV), human herpesvirus-6 (HHV-6).
- Enteroviruses are the most common cause of viral meningitis.

vi. Gerstmann syndrome
  a. Syndrome due to lesion of the dominant parietal lobe (inferior parietal lobule).
  b. Acalculia, agraphia without alexia, right and left confusion, finger agnosia (inability to distinguish fingers of the hand).
  c. Anosognosia (unawareness of the contralateral side of the body) involves the nondominant parietal lobe.

vii. Central pontine myelinolysis
  a. Due to aggressive correction of chronic hyponatremia.
  b. Sx: seizures, dysarthria, pseudobulbar palsy, dysphagia, hyperreflexia, quadriplegia, coma.
     1. Can also occur without symptoms
  c. Dx: confirm with MRI; CSF studies can show elevated myelin basic protein.
  d. To avoid this condition, correct sodium by 12 mmol/L in 24 hours.

viii. Vitamin deficiency
  a. Thiamine (B$_1$) deficiency
     1. Wernicke encephalopathy:
        - Ophthalmoplegia, nystagmus, anisocoria, gait ataxia, confusion, coma, death
     2. Korsakoff psychosis:
        - Confabulation, psychosis, amnesia
        - Mammillary bodies effected
     3. With treatment, symptoms of Wernicke encephalopathy involving the eyes improve; confusion improves to a varying degree; Korsakoff's amnesia is left in about 80% of patients.
  b. B$_{12}$ deficiency
     1. Subacute combined degeneration of the spinal cord
        - Degeneration of posterior and lateral columns of the spinal cord
        - Decreased pressure, vibration, and touch sense
        - Weakness of the extremities, especially legs
        - Ataxia

ix. Neurodegenerative diseases
  a. Huntington disease

1. Trinucleotide repeat (CAG) localized on chromosome 4.
2. Autosomal dominant disease with complete penetrance.
3. More common in males with symptoms beginning at age 35 to 40.
4. Abnormal gene products cause damage to inhibitory pathway between the motor cortex and subcortical structures causing hyperkinesia and choreoathetosis.
5. Disease progresses to death within 20 years of symptom onset.

  b. Friedreich ataxia
1. Trinucleotide repeat (GAA) located on chromosome 9.
2. Frataxin gene not expressed in this disease; frataxin is an iron storage protein that is not expressed.
3. Symptoms related to degeneration of spinal cord tracts, medulla, and deep nuclei → ataxia, dysarthria, areflexia.
4. Sx begin between 10 and 15 years and disorder is deadly by middle age (40-50).

  c. Alzheimer disease
1. A type of dementia associated with language dysfunction, intellectual loss, and memory loss.
2. Can be a rare cause of new-onset auditory hallucinations.
3. Diagnosis based on history, physical examination, and brain imaging so as to exclude reversible causes of dementia.
4. Several genes associated with AD → the E4 allele of the apolipoprotein E (chromosome 19) is associated with 25% to 40% of all cases.
5. Degeneration of the nucleus basalis of Meynert causes decreased cholinergic input to the frontal cortex.
6. Tx: Tacrine (central acting acetylcholinesterase inhibitor) and donepezil (reversible acetylcholinesterase inhibitor) may slow cognitive decline.

x. Brainstem auditory evoked response (BAER)
  a. Can be measured from several important components of the auditory pathway.
  b. Seven peaks in BAER:
1. Wave 1: auditory nerve
2. Wave 2: cochlear nucleus
3. Wave 3: superior olive
4. Wave 4: lateral lemniscus
5. Wave 5: inferior colliculus
6. Wave 6: medial geniculate body
7. Wave 7: auditory radiations/cortex

  c. BAER shows prolonged latency with structural lesion of the brainstem or auditory nerve.
  d. BAER is abnormal in 90% of patient with acoustic schwannoma and usually consists of delayed conduction from the auditory nerve to the caudal pons (wave 1-3).
  e. BAER is abnormal in 33% of MS patients and usually involves increased latency between waves 3 and 5.

Neurosurgery

A. Subarachnoid hemorrhage (SAH)
  i. Patients present with acute-onset, "thunder clap" headache.

  ii. Most devastating complication related to vasospasm and delayed cerebral ischemia.

   a. "Triple H" therapy used to treat vasospasm: hypertension, hypervolemia, hemodilution; risks of treatment associated with hyponatremia, pulmonary edema, cerebral edema, and myocardial infarction.

   b. Balloon angioplasty and spasmolysis with verapamil via and endovascular route are also treatments for vasospasm.

  iii. Hunt and Hess grade is a prognostic scale based on presentation.

   a. Grade 1: asymptomatic or mild headache with slight nuchal rigidity; 11% mortality

   b. Grade 2: moderate to severe headache with nuchal rigidity with no neurologic deficit other than CN palsy; 26% mortality

   c. Grade 3: drowsiness, confusion, mild focal deficit; 37% mortality

   d. Grade 4: stupor, moderate to severe hemiparesis; 71% mortality

   e. Grade 5: deep coma, decerebrate rigidity, moribund appearance; 100% mortality

  iv. Modified Fisher scale is a radiographic score that predicts risk for vasospasm.

   a. Grade 0: no SAH or intraventricular hemorrhage (IVH)

   b. Grade 1: focal or diffuse thin (< 1 mm) SAH, no IVH; positive predictive value (PPV) of 10%

   c. Grade 2: focal or diffuse thin (< 1 mm) SAH with IVH; PPV of 20%

   d. Grade 3: focal or diffuse thick (> 1 mm) SAH, no IVH; PPV of 30%

   e. Grade 4: focal or diffuse think (> 1 mm) SAH, with IVH; PPV of 40%

B. Carotid-cavernous fistula

  i. These fistulas are divided into traumatic or spontaneous.

  ii. Both traumatic and spontaneous fistulas present with retro-orbital pain, chemosis, pulsatile proptosis, ocular or cranial bruit, decreased visual acuity, diplopia, and rarely epistaxis and SAH.

  iii. Symptoms depend on the direction of venous flow and volume of blood flow through the fistula.

  iv. Four types of fistula:

   a. Type A: direct, high-flow shunt between the internal carotid artery (ICA) and CS

   b. Type B: low-flow shunt between dural branches of intracavernous ICA and CS

   c. Type C: low-flow shunt; supply from the meningeal branches of external carotid artery (ECA) and CS

   d. Type D: low-flow shunt between the dural branches of the ICA and ECA with the CS

  v. Treatment

   a. Half of all low-flow fistulas spontaneously resolve.

   b. Mainstay of treatment is transarterial balloon occlusion for type A fistulas.

   c. Transvenous balloon occlusion via the inferior petrosal sinus for Type B-D fistulas.

C. Dural arteriovenous fistulas

  i. Arteriovenous shunts involving dural vessels that usually arise because of thrombosis of a dural venous sinus (transverse sinus most common).

  ii. Presentation: includes pulsatile tinnitus, exophthalmus (due to increased drainage into venous system, ie, venous hypertension), visual symptoms, papilledema, hydrocephalus, and intracranial hemorrhage.

        iii. The presence of retrograde cortical venous drainage indicates the potential for intracranial hemorrhage and mandates urgent treatment because of the higher bleeding risk.

        iv. Hemorrhage in the setting of a DAVF has a high morbidity with about 30% mortality.

        v. Borden classification:

           a. Venous drainage directly into dural venous sinus or meningeal vein; 2% have aggressive behavior (hemorrhage or neurologic deficit).

           b. Venous drainage directly into dural venous sinus or meningeal vein with venous reflux to normal subarachnoid veins; 39% have aggressive behavior.

           c. Venous drainage directly into subarachnoid veins; 79% with aggressive behavior.

D. Arteriovenous malformation (AVM)

    i. Lack intervening capillary network.

    ii. Composed of feeding arteries, a nidus (shunting arterioles and interconnected venous loops), draining veins.

    iii. Increased flow through feeding arteries can cause the formation of aneurysms in the nidus.

    iv. Most AVMs are solitary (98%); 2% are multiple and can be associated with Osler-Weber-Rendu syndrome or Mason-Wyburn syndrome.

    v. Spetzler-Martin AVM grading system.

        a. Composite score to assess surgical risk of resection, maximum score of 5 points associated with the highest morbidity

        b. Size of nidus

           1. < 3 cm = 1 point

           2. 3-6 cm = 2 points

           3. > 6 cm = 3 points

        c. Eloquence of surrounding brain

           1. Noneloquent = 0

             • Fontal lobe, nondominant temporal lobe, cerebellar hemispheres

           2. Eloquent = 1

             • Sensorimotor cortex, language cortex, visual cortex, internal capsule, thalamus, hypothalamus, brainstem, cerebellar nuclei, regions adjacent to these structures

        d. Venous draining

           1. Superficial = 0

           2. Deep = 1

    vi. Treatment includes embolization, microsurgical resection or radiosurgery.

E. Head trauma

    i. Herniation syndromes related to Monro-Kellie doctrine, which states that that cranial vault holds a constant volume that is the sum of brain parenchyma, CSF, and blood.

    ii. An increase in the volume of any one of these components will increase ICP.

    iii. Herniation syndromes

        a. Uncal herniation

           1. Herniation of the uncus through the tentorial incisura

           2. Pupil dilation with down and out appearance of the globe due to compression of the oculomotor nerve (CN III)

        3. Kernohan's notch: mass effect on to the contralateral cerebral peduncle causing ipsilateral hemiparesis; a "false-localizing" sign

   b. Central herniation

        1. Diencephalon and parts of the temporal lobes are squashed inferiorly under the tentorium cerebelli.

        2. Branches of the basilar artery can stretch and cause fatal bleeding if they rupture (Duret hemorrhage).

   c. Cingulate (subfalcine) herniation

        1. The medial frontal lobe is pushed under the falx cerebri.

        2. Pressure can be placed on the anterior cerebral arteries.

   d. Transcalvarial/external herniation

        1. Herniating brain contents outside the confines of the calvarium

        2. Usually due to skull fracture or as a therapeutic surgical procedure for raised ICP (craniectomy)

   e. Upward cerebellar herniation

        1. Increased pressure in the posterior fossa can push the cerebellum rostrally.

   f. Tonsillar/downward cerebellar herniation

        1. Movement of the cerebellar tonsils through the foramen magnum.

        2. Coning of the tonsils can cause compression of the lower brainstem and upper spinal cord leading to respiratory and cardiac dysfunction.

        3. Fatal.

   g. Medical treatment for elevations in ICP

        1. Raising the head of bed, reducing jugular venous pressure, hypertonic saline, mannitol, acute hyperventilation, chemically induced coma.

        2. Mannitol and hyperventilation should be used with caution due to the risk for aggravating ischemia.

           • Mannitol can deplete intravascular volume and hyperventilation can cause vasoconstriction.

           • Hypertonic saline (3%) can be used as a resuscitative fluid that can also reduce ICP acutely.

           • Nevertheless, once primary survey is complete, mannitol and hyperventilation are recommended to acutely reduce elevations in ICP, which may last up to 6 hours.

           • Other risks of mannitol: opens blood-brain barrier and can worsen vasogenic edema; can cause nonketotic hyperosmolar state with high associated mortality; overuse can cause hypertension and increased CBF if autoregulation is defective; high doses can cause acute renal failure (especially when there is sepsis or if serum osm > 320, underlying kidney disease, co-use of nephrotoxic drug).

  iv. Dissection or thrombosis of vertebral artery

   a. Injury due to transverse foramen fracture or blunt injury to the vessel.

   b. Dissection or thrombosis can lead to infarction of the posterior fossa contents.

   c. An occluded vessel has the potential for recanalization and subsequent distal embolization.

        1. The precise incidence of recanalization is unknown, but many favor sacrificing the involved artery via an endovascular approach if there is enough collateral circulation.

   d. Other options include observation and beginning antiplatelet therapy.

      e. Patient with dissection or pseudoaneurysm formation of the vertebral arteries or extracranial carotid arteries may pose a difficult treatment dilemma because optimal treatment has not been defined.

         1. Many authors agree to start heparin drip for 1 to 2 weeks followed by bridge to warfarin for additional 4 to 12 weeks.

         2. Most injuries heal within 6 weeks.

      f. For patients with high hemorrhage risk, aspirin and/or Plavix can be used as an alternative to anticoagulation because it is thought that there could be less risk for bleeding although further studies need to clarify this point.

      g. New stenting techniques with flow diversion technology can also be considered; stent placement would mandate the use of antiplatelet therapy as well.

F. Trigeminal neuralgia

    i. Electric shock-like pain that typically radiates in a V2 and/or V3 distribution; rarely have pain in a V1 distribution.

    ii. Primary treatment includes carbamazepine and/or oxcarbazepine.

    iii. Other treatments include peripheral alcohol injection, glycerol rhizolysis, radio-frequency thermocoagulation, and microvascular decompression.

    iv. Typically the superior cerebellar artery compresses the trigeminal nerve at the root entry zone.

    v. Decompression of the nerve using telfa pledgets can cure this disease.

    vi. Microvascular decompression (MVD) is not an appropriate treatment for MS patients.

G. Craniovertebral junction abnormalities

    i. Chiari 1 malformation associated with tonsillar herniation 6 mm below the foramen magnum and crowding of the foramen magnum causing obstruction of CSF flow into the cervical cistern.

    ii. Occipitocervical instability seen in Down syndrome (trisomy 21) and Klippel-Feil syndrome (complex genetic syndrome causing faulty segmentation with subsequent autofusion of the segments of the vertebral column; commonly effects the cervical spine).

    iii. Platybasia is the abnormal flattening of the clivus with an associated skull base angle of over 143 degrees.

    iv. Basilar invagination is the rostral migration of the odontoid process through the foramen magnum; associated with platybasia.

    v. Rheumatoid arthritis (RA) associated with a number of abnormalities: patients are at risk for developing atlanto-occipital instability/atlantoaxial instability (AAI), superior migration of the odontoid process/cranial settling, and subaxial subluxation (SAS); any form of long-term instability can be associated with the formation of a reactive pannus that can compress the spinal cord.

    vi. These conditions can cause myelopathy, obstructive hydrocephalus, and cranial neuropathies; therefore decompression and stabilization are the mainstays of treatment.

      a. For irreducible lesions (nothing gained by cervical traction) → decompression at the site of encroachment (ventral or posterior) as well as stabilization are often required.

      b. For reducible lesions, immobilization alone with posterior spinal or craniospinal fusion without decompression is the mainstay of treatment.

    vii. Late neurologic deterioration in patients with RA or Chiari is concerning for syrinx formation, but this is very rare.

H. Spontaneous intracranial hypotension
  i. Usually occurs from leakage of CSF outside the cranial cavity.
  ii. Headaches resemble postspinal tap headaches and are positional; caffeine and hydration can help treat these postural headaches.
  iii. Diagnosis can be made with lumbar tap: dry tap or very low opening pressure.
  iv. CSF profile does show elevated protein and pleocytosis.
  v. B2 transferrin can also be sent to confirm whether any collected fluid from the nares is suspicious for CSF.
  vi. MR cisternography can localize the leak, but standard MRI protocols are usually sufficient to localize the skull base defect.
  vii. Contrasted MRI of the brain reveals dural enhancement over the cerebral and cerebellar convexities, tentorium, and falx; this finding is reversible with the resolution of symptoms.
  viii. Surgical closure of the fistula is needed for those patients with persistent CSF rhinorrhea or otorrhea.
    a. Clinical suspicion for pseudotumor cerebri should be high for patients presenting with spontaneous CSF leak.
I. Craniopharyngioma
  i. World Health Organization (WHO) grade 1 tumor that can be found any where between the infundibulum and the pituitary gland.
  ii. Arises from Rathke's cleft.
  iii. Bimodal distribution with peaks during childhood from age 10 to 14 and again during middle age.
    a. Children most often present with adamantinomatous subtype and adults usually present with papillary subtype.
  iv. Imaging.
    a. MRI findings reveal a sellar mass usually associated with suprasellar extension, contrast enhancement, calcification, T1 hyperintensity with tumors containing more protein, blood, or cholesterol (adamantinomatous subtype).
  v. If papillary, the tumor will be isointense to T1.
  vi. After surgery most will have predictable endocrine deficiency; these findings are most often seen in children.
    a. Most serious is obesity which develops in about 50% of patients.
      1. Patients are unable to control their appetite secondary to damage to hypothalamic satiety center.
    b. 50% of patients will require GH replacement.
    c. Diabetes insipidus (DI) occurs in 90% of patients and is usually permanent.
    d. 90% of patients will require hydrocortisone and thyroid replacement therapy after surgery.
J. Pituitary adenoma
  i. Benign WHO grade 1 tumors that can be functional or nonfunctional.
  ii. Microadenomas are less than 10 mm and macroadenomas are greater than 10 mm in size.
  iii. 65% are functional and 35% are nonsecretory.
    a. Prolactin secreting: 48%
    b. Growth hormone secreting: 10%
    c. Adrenocorticotropic hormone (ACTH) secreting: 6%
    d. Thyrotropin (TSH) secreting: 1%

      iv. Prolactinomas should most often be initially treated with bromocriptine or caber-goline whereas patients with other functional adenomas should be offered surgery as their initial treatment strategy.

      v. Nonfunctional pituitary adenomas can be associated with endocrinopathies.
- a. Elevated prolactin can be due to stalk effect that occurs due to the tonic inhibition of dopamine (inhibits prolactin secretion).
- b. Prolactin levels are usually less than 200 ng/mL in setting of stalk effect.
- c. Secondary hypothyroidism can also occur due to the presence of the pituitary adenoma and its mass effect on the adenohypophysis.

      vi. Unless symptomatic, benign nonfunctional tumors can be managed with serial imaging surveillance.

      vii. Pituitary apoplexy.
- a. Hemorrhage of the pituitary gland and adenoma due to venous infarction.
- b. Patients usually present with symptoms of SAH, panhypopituitarism, and cranial neuropathies and visual changes caused by mass effect on to the neural elements of the cavernous sinus as well as the optic apparatus.

      viii. Imaging.
- a. The morphology of adenomas is best appreciated on sagittal and coronal reconstruction views of axial MRIs.
- b. Microadenomas.
  1. Adenomas are hypointense areas within the more hyperintense normal pituitary on T1-weighted images.
  2. Normal gland enhances, which accentuates the hypointense signal of the tumor.
- c. Macroadenomas.
  1. Isointense to slightly hypointense on T1-weighted images.
  2. Hyperintense on T2-weighted images.
  3. Blood within the pituitary usually has a high signal on T1-weighted images.

      ix. Tumors that cause neurologic decline and nonprolactinomas should be treated with surgical excision; the authors endorse endoscopic assisted transsphenoidal surgery as the modality of choice for their resection.
- a. Postoperatively patients should be closely monitored every 6 hours for DI (urine specific gravity < 1.003; rising serum sodium > 145; and normal postoperative pituitary function).

K. Meningioma
    i. Dura-based extra-axial tumors that are predominantly WHO grade 1 and comprise up to 34.7% of all primary brain tumors.
- a. Grades 2 and 3 tumors are less common and make up 7% and 2.4% of all meningiomas, respectively.

    ii. Can be found in multiple locations in the skull base: olfactory groove, planum sphenoidale, tuberculum sellae, sphenoid wing, cavernous sinus, tentorial, diaphragma sellae, petroclival, foramen magnum, etc.

    iii. Presentation usually related to the location of the meningioma.

    iv. Imaging.
- a. Usually isointense on T1 and hyperintense on T2 MRI.
- b. Homogeneous contrast enhancement.
- c. Dural tail: reactive process in the dura adjacent to a meningioma that causes contrast enhancement.

      d. CSF cleft sign: represents the tumor-brain interface between extra-axial lesions and parenchyma; usually hyperintense rim on T2.

      e. Mother-in-law sign: because of the highly vascular nature of meningiomas, angiography can show the stasis of contrast within the tumor during the venous phase.

      f. Hyperostosis of surrounding bone.

    v. These tumors can encase critical neurovascular structures and cause compression of these elements.

    vi. Decompression is critical → surgical management is the mainstay of treatment.

    vii. Simpson grading: meningioma recurrence rate is dependent on extent of resection.

      a. Grade I
        1. Complete removal including resection of underlying bone and associated dura
        2. 9% symptomatic recurrence at 10 years

      b. Grade II
        1. Complete removal and coagulation of dural attachment
        2. 19% symptomatic recurrence at 10 years

      c. Grade III
        1. Complete removal without resection or coagulation of dura
        2. 29% symptomatic recurrence at 10 years

      d. Grade IV
        1. Subtotal resection
        2. 44% symptomatic recurrence at 10 years

      e. Grade V
        1. Decompression with or without biopsy
        2. 100% symptomatic recurrence at 10 years (small sample in original paper)

    viii. The authors reserve radiation therapy for patients who have a tissue diagnosis and decompression of the CNs has been achieved.

Bibliography

Brain Trauma F, American Association of Neurological S, Congress of Neurological S, et al. Guidelines for the management of severe traumatic brain injury. XV. Steroids. *J neurotrauma.* 2007;24(suppl 1):S91-95.

Lal D, Rounds A, Dodick DW. Comprehensive management of patients presenting to the otolaryngologist for sinus pressure, pain, or headache. *Laryngoscope.* Sep 12 2014.

Maarbjerg S, Gozalov A, Olesen J, Bendtsen L. Trigeminal neuralgia—a prospective systematic study of clinical characteristics in 158 patients. *Headache.* Sep 18 2014.

Russin J, Cohen-Gadol AA. Editorial: what did we learn from the ARUBA trial? *Neurosurg Focus.* Sep 2014;37(3):E9.

van Gijn J, Kerr RS, Rinkel GJ. Subarachnoid haemorrhage. *Lancet.* Jan 27 2007;369(9558):306-318.

Questions

1. A 35 year-old woman presents with the primary complaint of "sinus pain." She states that she has had severe pain around her eye that is associated with tearing, nasal congestion, and

rhinorrhea; all of her symptoms are on the right side. Upon further questioning, she reveals that she has had these symptoms throughout most of her adult life and says that these symptoms are quite persistent for 2 to 3 weeks and then relapse; she is symptom free for 1 to 2 months before the symptoms return. She believes most of her symptoms occur with changes in the weather and she does not complain of associated nausea, vomiting, or photophobia. What is her diagnosis?

A. Migraine headache

B. Chronic sinusitis

C. Allergic rhinitis

D. Cluster headache

E. Tension headache

2. A 45-year-old man presents to your clinic with left eye pain. Upon examination he has no extraocular movement from his left eye. Other than a frozen eye and a slightly dilated pupil that does not normally constrict to light, he has a normal neurologic examination. An MRI shows abnormal enhancement of the anterior cavernous sinus, superior orbital fissure, and orbital apex without signs of mass effect or of a dural tail extending posteriorly or laterally. What is the diagnosis?

A. Raeder syndrome

B. Tolosa-Hunt syndrome

C. Gradenigo syndrome

D. Vernet syndrome

3. A 55-year-old man presents to clinic with a 1-year history of facial pain. He states that he has sharp, lancinating pain radiating down his mandible that is exacerbating by shaving, brushing his teeth, and by cool air touching his face. You correctly diagnose him with trigeminal neuralgia. What is the first-line treatment for trigeminal neuralgia?

A. Microvascular decompression

B. Thermal rhizotomy

C. Lamotrigine

D. Carbamazepine

4. A 29-year-old man presents with a history of a seizure disorder. He states that his seizures are associated with lip smacking and odd sensations over his chest wall that lead to unconsciousness and generalized tonic-clonic activity. What is the seizure disorder that affects this patient?

A. Gelastic seizures

B. West syndrome

C. Temporal lobe seizures

D. Petit-mal seizures

5. A 65-year-old woman presents with headache, personality changes, anosmia, central scotoma of the right eye, optic nerve atrophy of the right eye, and papilledema of left eye. She is diagnosed with Foster-Kennedy syndrome, and an MRI of her brain is ordered, which reveals a large mass of the anterior cranial fossa most consistent with an olfactory groove meningioma. She undergoes an endoscopic, endonasal approach for the resection of the

mass, which involves coagulation of the ethmoidal arteries, removal of the crista galli, and cribriform plate of the ethmoid bone, resection of the involved dura underlying the meningioma, and extirpation of the mass. What is the Simpson grade for the degree of resection of the meningioma?

A. Grade 1
B. Grade 2
C. Grade 3
D. Grade 4
E. Grade 5

Chapter 7
The Chest for ENT

A simple overview of lung function is the intention of this chapter. It is meant to outline basic aspects of respiratory physiology and function, but as with any organ system it is but the tip of the iceberg. The following information is meant as a basic introduction as well as a stimulus for the curious to dig deeper.

Definitions

Lung volumes can be divided into primary volumes and capacities.

A. Primary volumes
   i. *Tidal volume (TV)*: The volume of gas that is either inspired or expired during each normal respiratory cycle.
   ii. *Residual volume:* The amount of gas that remains in the lungs at the end of a maximal expiratory effort
B. Capacities
   i. *Total lung capacity*: The amount of gas contained in the lung at the end of a maximal inspiratory effort
   ii. *Vital capacity*: The maximum volume of gas exhaled when a patient makes a forceful exhalation after inspiring to the total lung capacity
   iii. *Functional residual capacity*: The volume of gas that remains in the lung at the end of quiet exhalation

Dynamic lung volumes are as follows:

A. *Forced expiratory volume in 1 second (FEV$_1$)*: The volume of gas exhaled from the lung after initiation of a forceful exhalation following a maximal inspiration
B. *Forced expiratory volume in 1 second/forced vital capacity (FEV$_1$/FVC) ratio*: The ratio of the volume of gas exhaled from the lungs during the first second after forceful exhalation divided by the total volume of gas exhaled after forceful exhalation

Basic Tests of Pulmonary Function

Lung Volumes and Capacities

Despite being simple, Figure 7-1 is an excellent way to understand the various lung volumes and capacities.

There are three points of reference: (1) total lung capacity which is at the point of maximal inspiratory effort; (2) the total volume at maximal voluntary expiration, or residual volume; and (3) the volume at the end of passive expiration, or functional residual capacity.

This appears to be best reinforced and understood if one performs the maneuvers that are involved in achieving the volumes and capacities.

The lung volumes should be viewed in the context of two opposing forces that are seeking to expand or retract the lung.

Spirometry

The spirometer is widely used in pulmonary function laboratories because it has a nitrogen or helium analyzer, which allows the physician to obtain data concerning lung volumes, capacities, and dynamic lung volumes. By analyzing data obtained with a spirometer, the physician is able to determine whether a patient has normal or abnormal lung function. In addition, the spirometer enables the physician to assess the abnormalities of function and place the individual into one of two major pulmonary disease categories: chronic airflow limitation (diseases such as asthma, chronic bronchitis, and pulmonary emphysema) or restrictive lung disease (diseases such as pulmonary fibrosis).

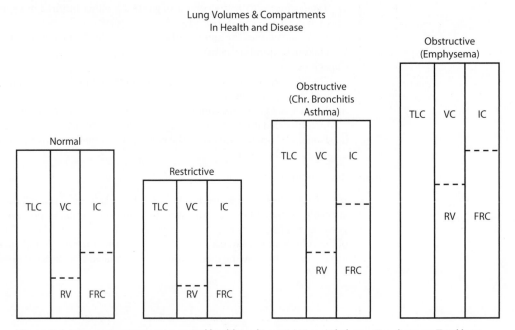

Figure 7-1 Lung compartments in normal health and in restrictive and obstructive diseases. Total lung capacity and residual volumes are generally largest in emphysema.

Flow Volume Loops

The maximal expiratory flow volume curve has been widely used by pulmonary laboratories for the past several years. In a spirometer tracing, volume is plotted against time (FEV_1 is the volume of gas exhaled during the first second after exhalation from a maximal inspiration). If the volume-time relation is normal, the flow rate is presumed to be normal; flow is never actually measured. In the flow volume loop, however, instantaneous flow is measured by means of a pneumotachograph, and flow is plotted against lung volume. Conditions that produce airflow limitation cause a reduction in measured flow rates throughout the patient's FVC maneuver.

Figure 7-2 illustrates a normal flow volume loop and a flow volume loop from a patient with chronic airflow limitation (such as chronic obstructive pulmonary disease [COPD]). Note that the shape of the curve is concave in the normal patient but convex in the patient with limited flow. Note also that the flow volume loop characterizes the relations between flow and volume during the inspiratory portion of the respiratory cycle. The uses of this portion of the curve are discussed in a subsequent section of this chapter.

As with patients whose spirometry tracings indicate airflow limitation, bronchodilator medication is administered to patients with abnormal flow volume loops compatible with airflow limitation. Patients with reversible disease demonstrate a 15% to 20% improvement in the flow volume loop after bronchodilator administration. Patients with restrictive lung diseases have abnormal flow volume loops, but because they do not have an abnormality of the airways,

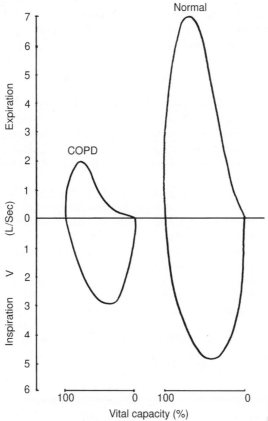

Figure 7-2 Flow volume loop. Note the reduction in flow.

their FEV$_1$/FVC ratio is usually normal. The slope of the expiratory loop in these patients is normal, in keeping with their normal airways.

Additional Uses of the Flow Volume Curve As noted, the flow volume curve can be used to evaluate inspiration as well as exhalation. This feature enables the pulmonary physiologist to evaluate the upper airway and assess the presence or absence of upper airway obstruction; this can also be a useful test for an otolaryngologist.

The ability of the flow volume loop to detect upper airway obstruction is based on the following physiologic principle: on inspiration, pleural pressure becomes more negative than the intraluminal pressure in the intrathoracic airways.

Consequently, on inspiration the caliber of the airways located within the chest increases. In the extrathoracic airways, such as the trachea, however, inspiration leads to a reduction in the intraluminal pressure, making atmospheric pressure greater than the pressure within the tracheal lumen. As a result, during inspiration the caliber of the tracheal lumen tends to diminish because atmospheric pressure exceeds intratracheal pressure.

In patients with variable extrathoracic (upper airway) obstruction, the obstruction tends to narrow the tracheal lumen. On inspiration, this narrowing becomes more pronounced by the effect of inspiration, which also causes a reduction in the size of the tracheal lumen. Hence, on inspiration, patients with variably obstructing lesions of the upper airway show a reduction in inspiratory flow, so that the inspiratory curve often appears flattened. On exhalation, intratracheal pressure becomes greater than atmospheric pressure, which causes the tracheal lumen to expand. This expansion tends to negate the effect of a variably obstructing tracheal lesion, and the expiratory portion of the flow volume curve appears normal even if there is a variably obstructing lesion present. Thus, in a patient with a variably obstructing lesion of the upper airway, the inspiratory curve is flattened whereas the expiratory curve appears normal. Figure 7-3 illustrates the curve produced by variably obstructing extrathoracic (upper airway) lesions.

Lung Compliance

The compliance of the lung refers to the elastic properties of that organ. Compliance is a measure of the distensibility, or elasticity, of the lung parenchyma. Many physicians are confused by the term elasticity. Elasticity refers to the ability of a structure to resist deformation. A rubber band is often referred to as an "elastic band"; it is an elastic structure not because it can be stretched but because it reverts to its original length when released. Hence, elasticity is the property whereby the original shape is preserved.

Distensibility, on the other hand, is the ease with which shape can be altered. An elastic structure is not distensible, whereas a distensible structure does not possess elastic qualities. In the lung, distensibility refers to the ease with which changes in distending pressure change lung volume. A lung in which small distending pressures produce large changes in volume is a highly distensible (or highly compliant) lung. A lung in which high distending pressures are required to produce even small changes in lung volume is poorly distensible and poorly compliant. It is also a highly elastic (or "stiff") lung. Clinical examples are (1) the emphysematous lung, which is highly distensible, highly compliant, and poorly elastic secondary to the destruction of the elastic structures of the lung, and (2) the fibrotic lung, which is poorly compliant, poorly distensible, and very elastic or stiff owing to the increased deposition of collagen. Figure 7-4 illustrates compliance curves in patients with normal, highly compliant (emphysematous), or "stiff" (fibrotic) lungs.

Diffusing Capacity

The diffusing capacity refers to the quantity of a specific gas that diffuses across the alveolar-capillary membrane per unit of time. The diffusing capacity is often used to assess the size of the

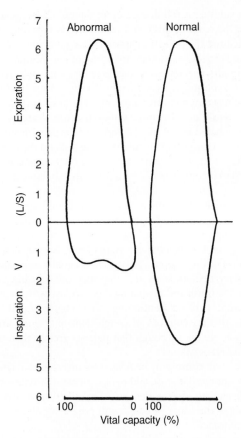

Figure 7-3 Extrathoracic obstruction.

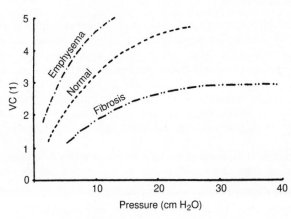

Figure 7-4 Compliance curve: pressure-volume relation.

pulmonary capillary blood volume. A full discussion of the methods employed to measure the diffusing capacity is beyond the scope of this text. In most pulmonary function laboratories, carbon monoxide is used to measure the diffusing capacity. This gas avidly binds to hemoglobin. In clinical practice, the diffusing capacity is thought to represent the volume of capillary blood into which carbon monoxide can dissolve. Diseases such as emphysema, which are characterized by a reduction in capillary blood volume, are associated with a low diffusing capacity.

Six-Minute Walk A simple test that measures a patient's exercise capacity and essentially measures the distance walked in 6 minutes. The more elaborate test is a cardiopulmonary stress test, which involves measure of exhaled gases and measures of oxygen consumption. It should be noted that there is a good correlation between the 6-minute test and the cardiopulmonary stress test and in patients with COPD has better correlation than the conventionally measured FEV_1. It again emphasizes the need to incorporate the muscle pump or bellows into our understanding of the respiratory system.

Immune Function The appreciation of the lungs as an integral part of our immune mechanisms has been recognized since the late 18th century, but suffice it to say we have made some progress in the understanding. The alveolar macrophage is the effector cell in controlling response to pathogens, but given the ongoing exposure of the alveolar membrane to these triggers the mechanism of control of the response to triggers is equally important.

Drug-induced pulmonary toxicity is an area that may offer an insight into mechanisms that balance the processing of stimuli and mediating the response which could be as damaging.

Cough/Sinusitis and Asthma It bears mentioning in the chapter titled Chest that the most interwoven problems relate to the symptom of cough. Not only does sinonasal disease and asthma commonly serve as etiology of a cough that persists greater than an 8-week duration, but there are numerous other associations.

Difficult-to-treat asthma will commonly be related to unrecognized sinonasal disease.

The chronicity of both sinonasal disease and persistent asthma syndromes sometimes may lead to a cough that may develop an independent self-perpetuating process.

Vocal cord dysfunction as the cause of cough will pose a significant clinical challenge to both ENT and pulmonary physicians.

Postulates about the association of sinusitis and asthma include the following:

A. Bacterial seeding
B. Enhanced beta-blockade
C. Nasobronchial reflex
D. Eosinophil activation
E. Simple nasal obstruction

If one works through the algorithm of cough management and difficult-to-treat asthma, it is easy to appreciate the interactions between asthma, sinonasal disease, and gastroesophageal reflux disease. The three disease states and the use of angiotensin-converting enzyme inhibitors will be the causative etiology of a cough that persists for greater than 8 weeks in the setting of a normal chest x-ray. A third of the time more than one etiology will be responsible.

Work of Breathing The concept or understanding of the factors that alter a patient's work of breathing and also the sensation of dyspnea is one aspect of respiratory physiology that continues to be better understood. However, one should approach it with the knowledge that we are still learning.

Consider the example of the test used to assess a patient's ability to be weaned from mechanical ventilation to outline some of the mechanisms. When a patient has been on ventilator support, the assessment for potential exhaustibility is assessed with a spontaneous breathing trial.

If the patient has a "rapid shallow breathing index" (RSBI) of less than 105 over a 30-minute period, he or she has an 85% chance of successful extubation. The *RSBI* is the frequency of breathing divided by the tidal volume measured in liters. The tachypnea as an indication of failure appears to be intuitive, but the reason for the tachypnea is not. The tachypnea is related to the assessment of the load per breath as a ratio of the maximal sustainable load, and the respiratory center adopts rapid shallow breathing as a protective mode to prevent respiratory muscle fatigue.

A real-life analogy would be to think of a distance runner who works his pace up to a point and then reduces it to "cruising" at which time there is tolerance of respiratory effort that will not cause immediate fatigue. This phenomenon is a contributing factor to what is referred to as a second wind.

This becomes a clinical issue in the elderly patient with common comorbidities of pulmonary disease, cardiac disease, and obesity, where there is commonly an attendant component of deconditioning. This reduces the denominator, that is, maximum work load, and hence increases dyspnea.

The mechanism of dyspnea in various disease states is beyond the scope of this review.

Blood Gases

Alveolar ventilation refers to the volume of gas in each breath that participates in gas exchange multiplied by the respiratory rate. Alveolar ventilation determines the level of arterial carbon dioxide; in the clinical setting, the adequacy of alveolar ventilation is assessed by measuring the arterial partial pressure of carbon dioxide (Pco_2).

In clinical practice, the most common causes of hypoxemia are simple hypoventilation and ventilation-perfusion inequality. Other causes of hypoxemia include anatomic shunts and abnormalities of diffusion, but these problems are rarely found in clinical hypoxemia.

The otolaryngologist is often confronted with a patient whose blood gas measurements reveal hypoxemia, and it is important that the attending physician be able to distinguish patients who have intrinsic pulmonary disease from those with simple hypoventilation (such as may be produced by anesthetic administration) and normal lungs. One useful technique for evaluating the presence or absence of intrinsic lung disease is the determination of the alveolar-arterial (A-a) gradient. A simple way to calculate the A-a gradient is to assume that the alveolar oxygen tension is 148-arterial $Pco_2 \times 1.2$. If the alveolar oxygen tension is calculated and the arterial Po_2 measured, the A-a gradient can be estimated. If there is less than a 20 mm Hg gradient between alveolar and arterial oxygen tensions, it is likely that the lungs are normal and that alveolar hypoventilation is the sole abnormality producing the hypoxemia. Patients with normal lungs who have primary alveolar hypoventilation exhibit normal oxygen tensions when the cause of the alveolar hypoventilation is removed. A patient with a sedative overdose has normal oxygenation when the effects of the sedative on respiratory drive wear off.

Diseases that produce widened A-a gradients produce hypoxemia that cannot be corrected by simply increasing the level of alveolar ventilation. As stated, the most common cause of hypoxemia in these patients is maldistribution of alveolar ventilation and pulmonary blood flow. Diseases such as asthma, bronchitis, and emphysema impair ventilation because of abnormal airway flow. The reduction in flow produces abnormal ventilation-blood flow relations, which creates the observed hypoxemia.

The rationale for the treatment of hypoxemia produced by ventilation-perfusion abnormalities is illustrated in Figure 7-5. If alveolus 1 has a reduction in ventilation due to airway narrowing, the alveolar oxygen tension in alveolus 1 decreases. The saturation of red blood cells (RBCs)

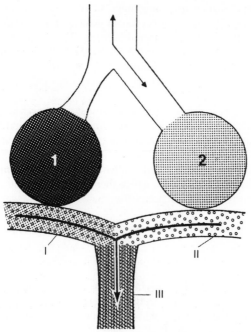

Figure 7-5 Ventilation perfusion mismatch. 1, 2, alveoli; I, II, III, blood vessels.

in blood vessel I supplying alveolus 1 also decreases. Alveolus 2, which receives normal ventilation, has a normal alveolar oxygen tension. RBCs in blood vessel II supplying alveolus 2 are normally saturated. Blood vessel III, which receives blood from vessels I and II, thus holds partially and fully saturated RBCs, so that the saturation of RBCs in III is reduced. Ventilation-perfusion abnormalities cannot be corrected by simple hyperventilation because hyperventilation does not increase the alveolar oxygen tension in alveolus 1 enough to increase the saturation of RBCs in vessel I. Hyperventilation may slightly increase the alveolar oxygen tension in alveolus 2, but the RBCs in blood vessel II are already fully saturated, and, therefore, the increase in alveolar oxygen tension cannot improve the saturation in the blood vessels supplying the alveolus. Thus vessel III, supplied by vessels I and II, remains with less than optimal RBC saturation. On the other hand, if the inspired oxygen tension delivered to the patient is increased, the alveolar oxygen tension in alveolus 1 can be improved and the saturation of RBCs will increase. Samples of blood from vessel III will show an increase in saturation as well.

As shown in Figure 7-6, the shape of the oxyhemoglobin dissociation curve is such that small increments in oxygen tension may be associated with significant improvement in oxygen saturation if the increments occur on the steep slope of the dissociation curve. A higher inspired oxygen tension creates a situation in which the alveolar oxygen tension in alveolus 1 rises, thus raising the RBC saturation in vessel I. As already noted, RBCs in vessel II are fully saturated, but now vessel III has improved RBC saturation in RBCs emanating from vessel I plus normally saturated blood from vessel II. It is evident that if the inspired oxygen tension delivered to the patient is increased, the alveolar oxygen tension in alveolus 1 can be improved and the saturation of RBCs will increase. Samples of blood drawn from vessel III will demonstrate an increase in saturation as well.

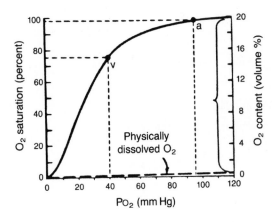

Figure 7-6 Oxyhemoglobin dissociation curve. O_2 saturation is given by the vertical axis on the left and O_2 content by the vertical axis on the right. Note the S shape of the curve and the location of the arterial point on the flat part of the dissociation curve and the venous point on the steep portion of the curve. The hemoglobin content of this blood is 15 g/dL, and the amount of O_2 carried in physical solution is much less than that bound to hemoglobin, as indicated by the bracket on the O_2 content axis.

It is for these reasons that diseases characterized by ventilation-perfusion mismatching show improvement in hypoxemia when treated with higher inspired oxygen tensions. However, if there is a true anatomic shunt present in alveolus 1, so that blood vessel I does not come into contact with the alveolus, raising the inspired oxygen tension will have no effect on the hypoxemia because the RBC saturation in vessel I cannot be increased. True anatomic shunts do not respond to increases in inspired oxygen tension.

Pulmonary Volumes and Capacities

A. *TV*: Depth of breathing, volume of gas inspired or expired during each normal respiratory cycle, 0.5 L (average).
B. *Inspired reserve volume (IRV)*: Maximum that can be inspired from end-inspiratory position, 3.3 L (average).
C. *Expired reserve volume (ERV)*: Maximum volume that can be expired from end-respiratory level, 0.7-1.0 L (average).
D. *RV*: Volume left in lungs after maximum expiration, 1.1 L (average).
E. *FEV_1*: Should be 80% or more of predicted value from a normative chart.
F. *FVC*: Should be 80% or more of predicted value from a normative chart. The FEV_1/FVC ratio should be more than 0.75 for younger patients and 0.70 for older individuals.
G. *Total lung capacity (6 L for men, 4.2 L for women)*: IRV + TV + ERV + RV (total volume contained in the lungs after maximum inspiration).
H. *Vital capacity (4.8 L for men, 3.1 L for women)*: IRV + TV + ERV (maximum volume that can be expelled from the lungs for effort following maximum inspiration).
I. *Functional residual capacity (2.2 L for men, 1.8 L for women)*: RV + ERV (volume in the lungs at resting expiratory level).
J. *Physiologic dead space (dead space of upper airway bypassed by tracheotomy, 70-100 mL)*: Anatomic dead space + the volume of gas that ventilates the alveoli that have no capillary blood flow + the volume of gas that ventilates the alveoli in excess of that required to arteriolize the capillary blood.

Mean Normal Blood Gas and Acid-Base Values

	Arterial blood	Mixed venous blood
pH	7.40	7.37
P_{CO_2}	41 mm Hg	46.5 mm Hg
P_{O_2}	95 mm Hg	40 mm Hg
O_2 saturation	97.1%	75.0%
HCO_3	4.0 mEq/L	25.0 mEq/L

Miscellaneous Information

A. Silo-filler disease (bronchiolitis obliterans) is a pathologic entity consisting of a collection of exudate in the bronchioles obliterating the lumen. This complication often follows inhalation of nitrogen dioxide, exposure to open bottles of nitric acid, and exposure to silos. The diagnosis is based on a history of exposure, dyspnea, cough, and x-ray findings similar to those of miliary tuberculosis. Treatment is symptomatic. Prognosis is poor; most patients eventually succumb to this disease.

B. Bronchogenic cysts are congenital, arise from the bronchi, and are lined with epithelial cells. Furthermore, their walls may contain glands, smooth muscles, and cartilage. In the absence of infection, they may remain asymptomatic; otherwise, they give a productive cough, hemoptysis, and fever. The recommended treatment is surgical excision.

C. Blebs or bullae are air-containing structures resembling cysts, but their walls are not epithelium lined.

D. Anthracosilicosis is also called coal miner's pneumoconiosis.

E. Berylliosis is characterized by an infiltration of the lungs by beryllium. It often is found in workers at fluorescent lamp factories.

F. Bagassosis is characterized by an infiltration of the lungs by sugarcane fibers.

G. Byssinosis is characterized by an infiltration of the lungs by cotton dust.

H. Adenocarcinoma of the bronchus is the leading primary pulmonary carcinoma in women, and bronchogenic (squamous cell) carcinoma is most common in men.

I. Pancoast syndrome (superior sulcus tumor) is caused by any process of the apex of the lung that can invade the pleural layers and infiltrate between the lower cords of the brachial plexus, and may involve the cervical sympathetic nerve chain, phrenic, and recurrent laryngeal nerves. It is usually secondary to a benign or malignant tumor; however, a large inflammatory process may cause this syndrome as well. The symptoms are as follows:

  i. Pain in shoulder and arm, particularly in the axilla and inner arm

  ii. Intrinsic hand muscle atrophy

  iii. Horner syndrome (enophthalmos, ptosis of the upper lid, constriction of the pupil with narrowing of the palpebral fissure, and decreased sweating homolaterally)

J. Congenital agenesis of the lung has been classified by Schneider as follows:

  i. *Class I*: Total agenesis.

  ii. *Class II*: Only the trachea is present.

  iii. *Class III*: Trachea and bronchi are present without any pulmonary tissue.

K. Apnea after tracheotomy is due to carbon dioxide narcosis causing the medulla to be depressed. Prior to the tracheotomy, the patient was breathing secondary to the lack of oxygen. After the tracheotomy this oxygen drive is removed, and hence the patient remains apneic. Treatment is to ventilate the patient until the excess carbon dioxide level is reduced. Mediastinal emphysema and pneumothorax are the most common complications of tracheotomy.

L. Hypoxemia is defined as less than 75% oxygen saturation or less than 40 mm Hg Po_2. A methemoglobin level of more than 5 mg/dL produces cyanosis.

M. Bronchogenic cyst is a defect at the fourth week of gestation. It constitutes less than 5% of all mediastinal cysts and tumors.

N. The bronchial tree ring is cartilaginous until it reaches 1 mm in diameter. These small bronchioles without cartilaginous rings are held patent by the elastic property of the lung. The bronchial tree is lined by pseudostratified columnar ciliated epithelium as well as nonciliated cuboidal epithelium.

O. The adult trachea measures 10 to 12 cm and has 16 to 20 rings. The diameter is approximately 20 mm × 15 mm.

P. The larynx descends on inspiration and ascends on expiration. It also ascends in the process of swallowing and in the production of a high-pitched note.

Q. The esophageal lumen widens on inspiration.

R. The total lung surface measures 70 m². The lung contains 300 million alveoli. It secretes 200 mL of fluid per day.

S. During inspiration, the nose constitutes 79% of the total respiratory resistance, the larynx, 6%, and the bronchial tree, 15%. During expiration, the nose constitutes 75% of the resistance; the larynx, 3%, and the bronchial tree, 23%.

T. Tracheopathia osteoplastica is a rare disease characterized by growths of cartilage and bone within the walls of the trachea and bronchi that produce sessile plaques that project into the lumen. There is no specific treatment other than supportive. It is of unknown etiology. The serum calcium is normal, and there are no other calcium deposits.

U. Calcification found in a pulmonary nodule implies that it is a benign nodule.

V. Middle lobe syndrome may be present.

W. The right upper lobe and its bronchus is the lobe that is most susceptible to congenital anomaly.

X. Cystic fibrosis (mucoviscidosis) is familial and may be autosomal recessive. The patient presents with multiple polyps, pulmonary infiltration with abscesses, and rectal prolapse. The pancreas is afflicted with a fibrocystic process and produces no enzymes. Trypsin is lacking in the gastric secretion. Ten to fifteen percent of the patients pass trypsin in the stool. There is general malabsorption of liposoluble vitamins. Treatment consists of a high-protein, low-fat diet with water-soluble vitamins and pancreatic extracts. Many patients die of pulmonary abscesses.

Y. A person ventilated with pure oxygen for 7 minutes is cleared of 90% of the nitrogen and can withstand 5 to 8 minutes without further oxygenation.

Mediastinum

A. Suprasternal fossa has these characteristics:
   i. It is the region in which the sternocleidomastoid muscles converge toward their sternal attachments. Bound inferiorly by the suprasternal notch, they have no superior boundary.
   ii. The deep cervical fascia splits into an anterior and a posterior portion. These portions are attached to the anterior and posterior margins of the manubrium, respectively.

  iii. The space between these fascial layers is the small suprasternal space containing (1) anterior jugular veins and (2) fatty connective tissues.

  iv. Behind this space lies the pretracheal fascia.

  v. Laterally on each side are the medial borders of the sternohyoid and sternothyroid muscles.

B. In the adult the innominate artery crosses in front of the trachea, behind the upper half of the manubrium. In the child it crosses over the level of the superior border of the sternum.

C. The trachea enters the mediastinum on the right side.

D. The trachea bifurcates at T4-T5 or about 6 cm from the suprasternal notch. As a person approaches 65 years of age or more, it is possible that the trachea bifurcates at T6.

E. To the left of the trachea are the aorta, left recurrent laryngeal nerve, and left subclavian artery. To the right of the trachea are the superior vena cava, azygos vein, right vagus, and right lung pleura.

F. The innominate and left carotid arteries lie anterior to the trachea near their origin. As they ascend, the innominate artery lies to the right of the trachea.

G. The pulmonary artery passes anterior to the bronchi and assumes a position superior to the bronchi at the hilus, with the exception that the right upper lobe bronchus is superior to the right pulmonary artery.

H. The left main bronchus crosses in front of the esophagus. It presses on the esophagus and together with the aorta forms the bronchoaortic constriction. The first part of the aorta is to the left of the esophagus. As it descends it assumes a left posterolateral position to the esophagus.

I. The course of the esophagus is as shown in Figure 7-7. The esophagus has four constricting points:

  i. Cricopharyngeus muscle.

  ii. Aorta crossing.

  iii. Left main stem bronchus crossing.

  iv. Diaphragm ($a < b = c < d$). At the level of c the esophagus passes from the superior mediastinum to the posterior mediastinum.

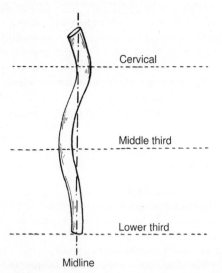

Cervical

Middle third

Lower third

Midline

Figure 7-7 Course of the esophagus.

    J. The following structures are found within the concavity of the aorta:
      i. Left main stem bronchus
      ii. Left recurrent laryngeal nerve
      iii. Tracheobronchial nodes
      iv. Superficial part of the cardiac plexus
    K. The right main stem bronchus is wider, shorter, and follows a more vertical course than the left one.
    L. The interior thyroid vein is immediately in front of the trachea in its infraisthmic portion.
    M. Ten percent of the population has a thyroidea ima artery. It arises from either the innominate artery or the aorta and passes upward along the anterior aspect of the trachea.

Course of the Vagus
Left Side
    A. It passes inferiorly between the left subclavian and the left carotid.
    B. It follows the subclavian to its origin.
    C. It passes to the left of the arch of the aorta.
    D. It gives off the recurrent laryngeal nerve, which passes superiorly along the left border of the tracheoesophageal groove (between the esophagus and trachea).
    E. The main vagus continues to descend behind the left main stem bronchus.
Right Side
    A. It descends anterior to the subclavian where it gives off the recurrent laryngeal nerve that loops around the subclavian artery and ascends posteromedial to the right common carotid artery to reach the tracheoesophageal groove (between the esophagus and the trachea).
    B. The main trunk descends posteriorly along the right side of the trachea, between the trachea and right pleura.
    C. It descends posterior to the right bronchus.

Fascia of the Mediastinum
The space between the various mediastinal organs is occupied by loose areolar tissues. The fascial layers of the mediastinum are a direct continuation of the cervical fascia. A portion of the cervical fascia, the perivisceral fascia, encloses the larynx, pharynx, trachea, esophagus, thyroid, thymus, and carotid sheath contents. This space enclosed by this perivisceral fascia extends to the bifurcation of the trachea. Anteriorly it is bound by the pretracheal fascia. The pretracheal fascia is an important landmark in mediastinoscopy in that dissection should be done only beneath this layer.

Boundaries of the Mediastinum
See Figure 7-8.

    A. *Lateral*: Parietal pleura
    B. *Anterior*: Sternum
    C. *Posterior*: Vertebrae
    D. *Inferior*: Diaphragm
    E. *Superior*: Superior aperture of the thorax
Superior Mediastinum
The boundaries are as follows:
    A. *Superior*: Superior aperture of the throat
    B. *Anterior*: Manubrium with sternothyroid and sternohyoid muscles

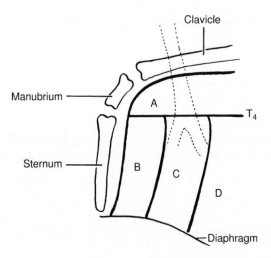

Figure 7-8 Various chambers of the mediastinum. A. superior mediastinum; B. anterior
mediastinum; C. middle mediastinum; D,
posterior mediastinum.

   C. *Posterior*: Upper thoracic vertebrae
   D. *Inferior*: Manubrium to fourth vertebra

Structures of the superior mediastinum are the thymus, innominate veins, aorta, vagus, recurrent laryngeal nerve, phrenic nerve, azygos vein, esophagus, and thoracic duct.

Anterior Mediastinum It lies between the body of the sternum and the pericardium and contains the following:

   A. Loose areolar tissues
   B. Lymphatics
   C. Lymph nodes
   D. Thymus gland

Middle Mediastinum It contains the heart, ascending aorta, superior vena cava, azygos vein, bifurcation of the main bronchus, pulmonary artery trunk, right and left pulmonary veins, phrenic nerves, and the tracheobronchial lymph nodes.

Posterior Mediastinum Anteriorly lie the bifurcation of the trachea, the pulmonary vein, the pericardium, and the posterior part of the upper surface of the diaphragm. Posteriorly lies the vertebral column from T4 to T12. Laterally lies the mediastinal pleura.

The posterior mediastinum contains the thoracic aorta, azygos vein, hemizygous vein, cranial nerve X, splanchnic nerve, esophagus, thoracic duct, posterior mediastinal lymph nodes, and the intercostal arteries.

Lymph Nodes of the Thorax

See Figure 7-9.
   A. Parietal nodes are inconsequential clinically. They are grouped into intercostal, sternal, and phrenic nodes.
   B. Visceral nodes are of greater clinical importance. They are grouped as follows:
      i. Peritracheobronchial
         a. Paratracheal
         b. Pretracheal

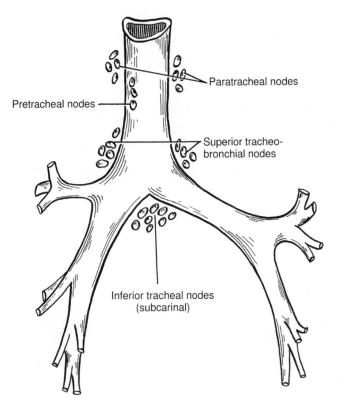

Pretracheal nodes

Paratracheal nodes

Superior tracheo-
bronchial nodes

Inferior tracheal nodes
(subcarinal)

Figure 7-9 Thoracic lymph nodes.

    c. Superior tracheobronchial
    d. Inferior tracheobronchial
  ii. Bronchopulmonary (hilar nodes)
 iii. Anterior mediastinal or prevascular
  iv. Pulmonary
   v. Posterior mediastinal

Lymphatic Drainage of the Lung
Right Side
  A. *Superior area (anteromedial area of the right upper lobe)*: Right paratracheal nodes
  B. *Middle area (posterolateral area of right upper lobe, right middle lobe, and superior right lower lobe)*: Right paratracheal nodes and inferior tracheobronchial nodes
  C. *Inferior area (lower half of right lower lobe)*: Inferior tracheobronchial nodes and posterior mediastinal nodes
Left Side
  A. *Superior area (upper left upper lobe)*: Left paratracheal, anterior mediastinal, and sub-aortic nodes
  B. *Middle area (lower left upper lobe and upper left lower lobe)*: Left paratracheal, inferior tracheobronchial, and anterior mediastinal nodes

    C. *Inferior area (inferior part of the left lower lobe)*: Inferior tracheobronchial nodes. (Inferior tracheobronchial nodes drain into the right paratracheal nodes.)
  i. *Right upper lung*: Right neck
  ii. *Right lower lung*: Right neck
  iii. *Left lower lung*: Right neck
  iv. *Left upper lung*: Left neck
  v. *Lingular lobe*: Both sides of the neck

Purposes of Mediastinoscopy

Barium swallow and tracheogram are usually obtained before mediastinoscopy if indicated.

    A. Histologic diagnosis
    B. To determine which nodes are involved
    C. To make the diagnosis of sarcoidosis

Mediastinal Tumors

One-third of all mediastinal tumors are malignant. Among the malignant ones, lymphoma is most commonly encountered.

    A. *Superior mediastinum*: Thyroid, neurinoma, thymoma, parathyroid
    B. *Anterior mediastinum*: Dermoid, teratoma, thyroid, thymoma
    C. *Low anterior mediastinum*: Pericardial cyst
    D. *Middle mediastinum*: Pericardial cyst, bronchial cyst, lymphoma, carcinoma
    E. *Posterior mediastinum*: Neurinoma, enterogenous cyst

Superior Vena Cava Syndrome

    A. *Etiology*: Malignant metastasis, mediastinal tumors, mediastinal fibrosis, vena cava thrombosis
    B. *Signs and symptoms*: Edema and cyanosis of the face, neck, and upper extremities; venous hypertension with dilated veins; normal venous pressure of lower extremities; visible venous circulation of the anterior chest wall

Endoscopy

Size of Tracheotomy Tubes and Bronchoscopes

Age	Tracheotomy tubes	Bronchoscope (mm)
Premature	No. 000 × 26 mm to No. 00 × 33 mm	3
6 months	No. 0 × 33 mm to No. 0 × 40 mm	3.5
18 months	No. 1 × 46 mm	4
5 years	No. 2 × 50 mm	5
10 years	No. 3 × 50 mm to No. 4 × 68 mm	6
Adult		7

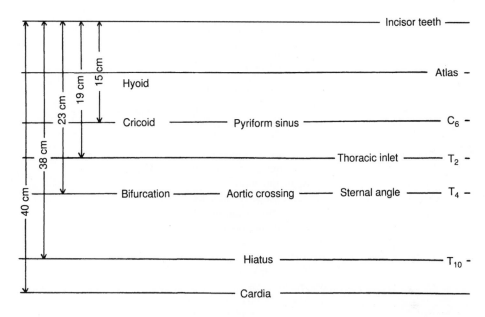

Figure 7-10 Relative landmarks for esophagoscopy.

Esophagoscopy

A. Size of esophagoscope.
B. *Child*: 5 mm × 35 mm or 6 mm × 35 mm.
C. *Adult*: 9 mm × 50 mm.
D. Average distance from incisor teeth to other areas during esophagoscopy (Figure 7-10).
E. *Left lung*: Lobes and segments.
  i. Upper division of upper lobe
    a. Apical posterior
    b. Anterior
  ii. Lower division of upper lobe
    a. Superior
    b. Inferior
  iii. Lower lobe
    a. Superior
    b. Anteromedial basal
    c. Lateral basal (4)
    d. Posterior basal
F. *Right lung*: lobes and segments
  i. Upper lobe
    a. Apical
    b. Posterior
    c. Anterior
  ii. Middle lobe
    a. Lateral
    b. Medial

        iii. Lower lobe
- a. Superior
- b. Medial basal
- c. Anterior basal
- d. Lateral basal
- e. Posterior basal

G. Relative contraindications for esophagoscopy
- i. Aneurysm of the aorta
- ii. Spinal deformities, osteophytes
- iii. Esophageal burns and steroid treatment

H. Relative contraindications for bronchography
- i. Acute infection
- ii. Acute asthmatic attacks
- iii. Acute cardiac failure

I. Causes of hemoptysis (in order of decreasing frequency):
- i. Bronchiectasis
- ii. Adenoma
- iii. Tracheobronchitis
- iv. Tuberculosis
- v. Mitral stenosis
   - a. Foreign bodies
      1. *Right upper lobe bronchus*: Most common site
      2. *Left upper lobe bronchus*: Second most common site
      3. *Trachea*: Least likely site
      4. *Cervical esophagus*: Most common site for esophageal foreign bodies
      5. *Most common foreign bodies in children*: Peanuts, safety pins, coins
      6. *Most common foreign bodies in adults*: Meat and bone

Vascular Anomalies

See Chapter 45. The normal great vessels are shown in Figure 7-11.

A. *Double aortic arch*: This anomaly is a true vascular ring. It is due to the persistence of the right fourth branchial arch vessel. The symptoms include stridor, intermittent dysphagia, and aspiration pneumonitis. The right posterior arch is usually the larger of the two arches.

B. *Right aortic arch with ligamentum arteriosus*: It is due to the persistence of the right fourth branchial arch vessel becoming the aorta instead of the left fourth arch vessel. This vessel crosses the trachea, causing an anterior compression.

C. *Anomalous right subclavian artery*: It is due to the right subclavian artery arising from the dorsal aorta, causing posterior compression of the esophagus. There is no constriction over the trachea.

D. *Anomalous innominate and/or left common carotid*: The innominate arises too far left from the aorta. It crosses the trachea anteriorly, causing anterior compression. The left common carotid arises from the aorta on the right or from the innominate artery. It also causes anterior compression of the trachea. In a variant of this anomaly, the innominate and the right common carotid arise from the same trunk, and when they divide they encircle the trachea and esophagus, causing airway obstruction as well as dysphagia.

E. Patent ductus arteriosus.

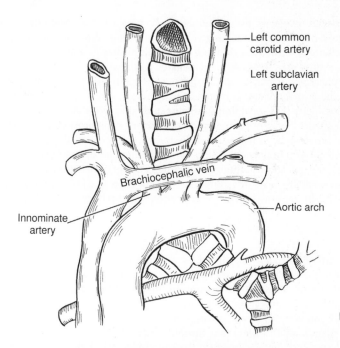

Figure 7-11 Normal great vessels.

F. Coarctation of the aorta.
G. *Enlarged heart*: An enlarged heart, especially with mitral insufficiency, can compress the left bronchus.
H. *Dysphagia lusoria*: This term is used to include dysphagia caused by any aberrant great vessel. The common cause is an abnormal subclavian artery arising from the descending aorta.
I. *Anomalous innominate arteries*: They have been estimated to be the most common vascular anomaly. They cause anterior compression of the trachea. During bronchoscopy, if the pulsation is obliterated with the bronchoscope, the radial pulse on the right arm and the temporal pulse are reduced. In the case of a subclavian anomaly, the bronchoscope compressing the abnormal subclavian produces a decrease of the radial pulse, although the temporal pulse remains normal. A bronchoscope compressing a double aortic arch pulsation produces no pulse changes in either the radial or the temporal pulse.

Diseases Producing Limitation of Airflow

Pulmonary diseases that produce a reduction in the flow of air through airways more than 2 mm in diameter produce spirometric evidence for this limited airflow. Airflow limitation is reflected on the spirometer tracings as a reduction in FVC and FEV_1. In addition, the FEV_1/FVC ratio falls below the predicted normal value. Functional residual capacity is elevated, as is the RV. In more advanced cases, the total lung capacity is also increased.

An abnormal spirogram does not indicate the cause of disease, as asthma, chronic bronchitis, and emphysema all show evidence of airflow limitation. When a spirometric tracing reveals evidence of airflow limitation, the patient is normally given a bronchodilator (eg, metaproterenol) and the test is repeated.

Patients with reversible airflow limitation, such as asthma, most often demonstrate 15% to 20% improvement in dynamic lung volumes following administration of a bronchodilator. These patients are described as exhibiting "reversible airflow limitation."

Patients whose pre- and postbronchodilator tracings do not vary may have chronic bronchitis or emphysema, or may be in the throes of an asthmatic attack that is so severe that the response to the bronchodilator is muted. It is, therefore, not possible to eliminate asthma as a diagnostic possibility if the postbronchodilator study does not show reversibility.

Because the incidence of postoperative pulmonary complications increases with the severity of airflow limitation, it is important to perform spirometry on all patients who, on the basis of history and physical findings, are likely to have pulmonary diseases characterized by obstruction of flow. If the spirogram is abnormal and indicative of obstruction, a bronchodilator should be given. If reversibility is demonstrated, the patient is given a bronchodilator prior to surgery to maximize his or her lung function preoperatively and reduce the incidence of postoperative complications.

Restrictive Lung Disease

The spirometric abnormality produced by patients with restrictive lung disease differs significantly from the curves produced by patients with chronic airflow limitation. Patients with restrictive lung disease exhibit a reduction in their total lung capacity. Diseases that produce restriction include diseases in which a functioning lung is replaced by granulomas or fibrosis (eg, sarcoid or interstitial fibrosis), diseases that lead to restricted expansion of the lungs as seen in primary neurologic disorders (amyotrophic lateral sclerosis) or primary muscle disorders (muscular dystrophy), diseases in which there is a reduction in the amount of functioning lung (pneumonectomy), and diseases in which there is a reduction in lung expansion (scoliosis and fibrothorax).

The spirometric tracing of a patient with restrictive lung disease demonstrates a reduction in FVC and FEV_1, but the FEV_1/FVC ratio is preserved. Whereas with chronic airflow limitation the values for functional residual capacity, RV, and total lung capacity are elevated, in restrictive lung diseases these values are reduced.

Patients with restrictive lung diseases do not demonstrate improvement after the administration of bronchodilators, as the defect in restrictive lung diseases does not lie in the airways per se.

Bibliography

Bates D. *Respiratory Function in Disease.* 3rd ed. Philadelphia, PA: W.B. Saunders; 1989.

Bickerman HA. Lung volumes, capacities, and thoracic volumes. In: Chusid EL, ed. *The Selective and Comprehensive Testing of Adult Pulmonary Function.* United Kingdom, UK: Futura Publishing Company; 1983:5.

Bone RC, Dantzker DR, George RB, et al. *Pulmonary and Critical Care Medicine.* Vol 1 and 2. St. Louis, MO: Mosby Year Book; 1993.

Cherniack N. *Chronic Obstructive Pulmonary Disease.* Philadelphia, PA: W.B. Saunders; 1991.

Comroe JH Jr. *Physiology of Respiration.* 2nd ed. Chicago, IL: Mosby Year Book; 1974.

Questions

1. Spirometric evidence of obstructive airways disease is based on
   A. Reduced FEV_1
   B. Reduced FEV_1/FEV ratio
   C. Both

2. Increased work of breathing could be due to
   A. Decreased pulmonary function
   B. Airway obstruction
   C. Decreased muscle function
   D. All of the above

3. A 6-minute walk distance is a good indicator of cardiopulmonary performance.
   A. True
   B. False

4. Amiodarone lung toxicity may provide a good model for understanding immune function of the lung.
   A. True
   B. False

5. Flow volume loops can help distinguish between intra- and extrathoracic sites of airway obstruction.
   A. True
   B. False

Chapter 8
Nutrition, Fluid, and Electrolytes

Malnutrition is common in patients with head and neck cancer due to dysphagia, pain, poor appetite, and poor dietary intake. This is defined as weight loss greater than 10% of ideal body weight, with preferential loss of adipose tissue over muscle. The resting energy expenditure is reduced. Improved caloric intake of nutritious food or nutritional supplements will often reverse malnutrition and starvation.

However, this is very different from the unintentional weight loss associated with cancer cachexia. This wasting syndrome, commonly seen in patients with advanced head and neck cancer, is metabolically distinct from malnutrition and even from starvation. These patients do not have reduced caloric intake; in fact, they often report increased food intake although they may have early satiety. It is not reversed by improved caloric intake or nutritional supplements alone. Cancer cachexia syndrome is defined as a loss of lean body mass, with or without adipose mass, often associated with inflammation, anorexia, and insulin resistance. Muscle atrophy occurs due to a decrease in protein synthesis and an increase in degradation. Cytokines such as interleukin-6, tumor necrosis factor, and interleukin-1β are elevated. Resting energy expenditure inappropriately increases in many cases. There is an exuberant inflammatory response and amino acids from the breakdown of muscle are shunted into acute phase response proteins in the liver. This results in liver hypertrophy. Clinically, patients exhibit unintentional weight loss of 5% of their pre-morbid body weight. There is loss of the "vanity muscles" such as the biceps and quadriceps. This syndrome manifests itself in weakness, increased fatigue, and a decrease in quality of life. Approximately 30% of all cancer patients will die from cancer cachexia, which ultimately results in such severe muscle wasting that respiratory distress ensues.

The importance of diagnosing and treating both malnutrition and cancer cachexia is evident in the increased perioperative morbidity when untreated. Poor wound healing, increased rates of sepsis, and increased rates of wound infections are seen with malnutrition. Increased complications from surgery, radiation, and chemotherapy are seen in patients with cancer cachexia. There is mounting evidence that cancer cachexia profoundly affects cardiac structure and function, causing significant impairment in patients who previously had no history of cardiac dysfunction. The implications of this for patients who undergo major surgical ablation may be profound, especially in the perioperative period. During therapy, weight loss is an independent poor prognostic sign. Morbidly obese patients can still be profoundly malnourished and weight loss during treatment is not necessarily healthy for them. This form of sarcopenic obesity may be difficult to diagnose and treat.

The use of feeding tubes often helps bypass areas of severe mucositis in patients undergoing radiation or chemoradiation therapy. The ability of feeding tubes to maintain weight during therapy should be considered in selected patients undergoing chemoradiation. Even young, healthy patients such as those being treated for human papillomavirus (HPV)-related oropharyngeal carcinoma may require a temporary feeding tube to avoid weight loss during therapy but this is controversial. Nutritional assessment and counseling by a certified nutritionist is a critical part of the evaluation of patients with head and neck cancer. Early intervention with speech pathologists is an integral part of many multidisciplinary oncology pathways for head and neck cancer.

Patient Evaluation

History

- Document weight loss in the past 3 to 6 months
  (a) Intentional
  (b) Unintentional—consider cancer cachexia
- Alcohol abuse
- Note dysphagia or pain when swallowing
- Document anorexia

Physical Examination

- Loss of muscle mass, especially Type II fast twitch muscles such as biceps or quadriceps
- Evidence of vitamin deficiencies such as dry scaling skin, cheilosis, or stomatitis

Anthropometric

- Body mass index (BMI) = weight (kg)/height (cm) × 100.
- Midarm circumference can be used to estimate skeletal muscle mass.
- Magnetic resonance imaging (MRI) scans or CT scans can be used to measure diaphragm or other muscle groups.

Laboratory Measures

- Albumin levels less than 3.0 g/dL are associated with perioperative morbidity.
- Prealbumin has a short half-life and can be used to assess nutritional status and the need for supplementation.
- Transferrin, an acute phase protein with a short 7-day half-life, more accurately reflects short-term changes in nutritional status. Transferrin less than 150 mg/dL indicates malnutrition. It may be calculated from the total iron-binding capacity (TIBC). Transferrin = (0.68 × TIBC) + 21.
- Anemia is associated with cancer cachexia.
- Elevated C-reactive protein (CRP) is also seen in patients with cancer cachexia.
- Serum glucose levels may help detect insulin resistance, seen in patients with cancer cachexia.
- A total lymphocyte count (TLC) of less than 1700/μL is a gross measurement of humoral immunity and is associated with a fivefold increase in the risk of wound infection. Cell-mediated immunity can be measured by the intradermal placement of antigens such as tetanus, *Candida*, or purified protein derivative (PPD).
- The prognostic nutritional index (PNI) is predictive of complications and morbidity.

    PNI = 158 − 16.6 (albumin) − 0.78 (triceps skinfold) − 0.20 (transferrin)
    − 0.58 (delayed hypersensitivity)

Summary

Unintentional weight loss may be due to a paraneoplastic syndrome, cancer cachexia. Anemia, hypoglycemia, and elevated CRP are hallmarks of this wasting syndrome. It is not treatable with nutritional supplementation alone, although this is an integral part of the therapy. There are no FDA-approved remedies for cancer cachexia, but current management strategies include corticosteroids and megesterol acetate (Megace). Future strategies may include nutraceuticals, omega-3 fatty acids in nutritional supplements, and targeted treatments using Ghrelin analogs. There is preliminary data that nonsteroidal anti-inflammatory drugs may be useful in dampening the inflammatory response that is associated with this. A nutritional consult is a critical part of evaluating patients. If patients are malnourished, nutritional supplements should be considered part of the treatment plan.

Refeeding Syndrome

Patients who have had negligible nutrient intake for 5 days may be at risk for refeeding syndrome, which occurs within 4 days of starting to feed them. Profound electrolyte imbalances may occur, such as hypophosphatemia, which may be accompanied by cardiac arrhythmias, coma, confusion, and convulsions. The underlying mechanisms causing this potentially fatal syndrome is the switching from ketone bodies derived from fatty acids (as the main source of energy) and suppression of insulin secretion to increased secretion of insulin during refeeding. The increased glycogen, fat, and protein synthesis that occur during refeeding require phosphates, potassium, and magnesium, which are already dangerously low. Any residual stores are used up. The basal metabolic rate is increased, further depleting electrolytes. Glucose and thiamine level often drop. The shifting of electrolytes and fluid balance increases cardiac workload. Increased oxygen consumption strains the respiratory system. These patients merit close monitoring. Replenishing vital electrolytes (potassium, phosphate, and magnesium) in a controlled setting is essential.

Nutritional Requirements

For the malnourished patient, the physician must determine the nutrient and caloric requirements needed.

- The average adult needs 30 to 35 kcal/kg/d.
- To avoid protein-calorie malnutrition, provide 6.25 g of protein per 125 to 150 kcal.
- Nitrogen balance should be assessed through serial laboratory and body weight assessments.

Nutritional Delivery Techniques

Always use oral nutritional supplements and enteral feedings when possible.

Enteral Feedings

The route of feeding may be via a nasogastric (NG) tube, gastrostomy (G) tube, or jejunostomy (J) tube. The main advantage of a NG tube is the ease of placement but the disadvantages include short-term use only, esophageal reflux, and tissue inflammation from contact in the nose and posterior pharynx.

G-tubes are well tolerated for long-term use but need a surgical procedure for placement. Another disadvantage is that the G-tube site may become infected and necrotizing fasciitis is possible. Buried bumper syndrome occurs when the G-tube bumper erodes through the stomach wall causing an abdominal catastrophe, so abdominal pain must be thoroughly evaluated.

J-tubes reduce the incidence of reflux which is critical for patients with laryngeal and/or oropharyngeal reconstruction but must also be placed during a surgical procedure. J-tube feedings do not allow for bolus feeds, so the infusion of tube feeds is steadily given throughout the day, which may be inconvenient for patients.

Parenteral Nutrition

This route of nutritional delivery provides for rapid nutritional replacement without being dependent on a functioning alimentary tract. Peripheral parenteral nutrition (PPN) is administered via a peripheral IV and is not adequate for complete nutritional supplementation. It is often given as a supplement consisting of 5% to 10% dextrose, 3.5% amino acids, and lipids to provide 1000 to 2000 cc/d.

Total parenteral nutrition (TPN) must be given via a dedicated central venous catheter. The indications are as follows:

- Nonfunctioning gastrointestinal (GI) tract
- Severe protein malnutrition with loss of normal GI function
- Chyle leak after neck dissection

It allows for rapid replacement of nutritional deficits (1-2 weeks) and does not depend on the GI tract function.

Fluid, Electrolytes, and Acid-Base Balance

Trauma, operative procedures, and multiple medical diseases can produce alterations in the composition, distribution, and volume of the body fluids. Critical disturbances in the fluid, electrolyte, or acid-base balance of the body may have no outward signs or symptoms and may only be diagnosed by laboratory testing. Surgical patients are particularly prone to such disturbances due to the effects of anesthesia, parenteral feedings, underlying medical diseases, and postoperative fluid shifts.

The average 70-kg male is composed of 60% (42 L) water. Of this 42 L approximately two-thirds (28 L) is intracellular and one-third (14 L) is extracellular. The extracellular compartment can be further divided into the interstitial fluid (10 L) and the plasma (4 L). Various electrolytes are distributed among the different fluid compartments of the body (Table 8-1).

Fluid Exchange

Routes		*Average daily volume (mL)*
Water Gains:	Oral fluids	800-1500
	Solid foods	500-700
	Water oxidation	250
Water Loss:	Urine output	800-1500
	Intestinal	250
	Insensible	500-700

Table 8-1 **Body Fluid Electrolyte Composition**

Substance	Extracellular fluid (mEq/L)	Intracellular fluid (mEq/L)
Sodium	140	10
Potassium	4	150
Magnesium	1.7	40
Chloride	105	10
Bicarbonate	28	10
Phosphate/sulfate	3.5	150
Protein anions	15	40

Fluid Requirements

Adults:		35 cc/kg/24 h
Children:	First 10 kg:	100 cc/kg/24 h or 4 cc/kg/h
	Second 10 kg:	50 cc/kg/24 h or 2 cc/kg/h
	Second > 20 kg:	25 cc/kg/24 h or 1 cc/kg/h
Fever		500 cc/24 h/C above 38.3°C (101°F)

Fluid Disturbances

- Overhydration (volume excess)
  (a) Polyuria
  (b) Urine Na greater than 30 mEq/L
  (c) Pulmonary edema
  (d) Distended neck veins
  (e) Ascites
  (f) Peripheral edema
  (g) Systolic hypertension
  (h) Elevated wedge pressure
- Dehydration (volume depletion)
  (a) Oliguria
  (b) Urine Na less than 10 mEq/L
  (c) Hypotension
  (d) Poor skin turgor
  (e) Sunken eyeballs
  (f) Thirst
  (g) Tachycardia
  (h) Hemoconcentration
  (i) Low wedge pressure

Sodium

- Normal serum Na levels: 135 to 145 mEq/L
- Normal intake Na 1 mEq/kg/24 h

- Hypernatremia (Na >150 mEq/L)
  - (a) Etiology
    - ○ *Lost free water*: Diabetes insipidus, sweating, burns, diarrhea, vomiting, osmotic, insensible losses
    - ○ *Solute loading*: Tube feeding, brainstem injury, inappropriate IV, Cushing syndrome
  - (b) *Therapy*: Depends on the fluid status but basic principle is to treat the underlying disorder and slowly rehydrate with hypotonic fluid. Rapid rehydration can lead to cerebral edema or congestive heart failure (CHF).
- Hyponatremia (Na <130 mEq/L)
  - (a) *Etiology*: Iatrogenic, water intoxification, sepsis, renal failure, cirrhosis, syndrome of inappropriate antidiuretic hormone (SIADH), CHF, myxedema, hyperglycemic osmotic effect (correct 2 mEq for every 100 mg of excess glucose to give a serum sodium that correctly reflects the sodium/fluid status).
  - (b) *Therapy*: Depends on the fluid status of the patient. If fluid is overloaded (CHF, renal failure), then restrict fluid and use diuretics. If volume is depleted, then rehydrate with normal saline. In case of severe symptoms (central nervous system [CNS]), replace one-half deficit over 4 to 6 hours with 3% hypertonic saline. Replace the remainder over the next 24 to 48 hours.

Potassium

- Normal serum K^+ levels: 3.5 to 5.0 mEq/L
- Normal intake
  - (a) *Adults*: 40 to 60 mEq/24 h
  - (b) *Children*: 2 mEq/kg/24 h
- Hyperkalemia (K^+ > 5.5)
  - (a) *Etiology*: Excess intake, renal failure, rhabdomyolysis, crush injury, acidosis, angiotensin-converting enzyme (ACE) inhibitors, K^+-sparing diuretics.
  - (b) *Diagnosis*: Weakness, loss deep tendon reflexes (DTRs), confusion, irritable, electrocardiogram (ECG) changes (peaked T waves, prolong QRS, sinus arrest, asystole).
  - (c) *Therapy*: Remove exogenous sources, Kayexalate, emergency situation with K^+ greater than 7.5 or ECG changes combination of D50/insulin/$NaHCO_3$/Ca. Consider dialysis.
- Hypokalemia (K^+ < 3.0 mEq/L)
  - (a) *Etiology*: Decreased intake, GI loss especially NG suction, vomiting, diarrhea, laxative abuse, diuretics, steroid therapy
  - (b) *Diagnosis*: Anorexia, nausea, vomiting, ileus, weakness, ECG changes (prolonged QT, ST depression, premature ventricular contractions)
  - (c) *Therapy*: Replete maximum rate of 40 mEq/h (monitoring)
    - ○ Peripheral 20 mEq in 50 to 100 cc D_5W
    - ○ Central 20 to 40 mEq in 50 to 100 cc D_5W

Remember serum pH will affect serum K^+ (acidosis will produce an increase in serum K^+, while alkalosis produces a decrease).

Calcium

- Normal serum Ca^{2+} levels: 8.5 to 10.6 mg/dL
- Normal intake
  - (a) 1 to 3 g/24 h.

(b) Total body stores 1 to 2 g.

(c) Serum Ca^{2+} 50% ionized, 50% nonionized.

(d) Serum total Ca^{2+} decreases with decreasing serum protein; however, ionized Ca^{2+} remains constant. Check ionized Ca^{2+} or correct serum Ca^{2+} while decreased 0.8 mg/dL Ca^{2+} is seen with each 1.0 g/dL decrease in serum albumin below 4.0 g/dL.

- Hypocalcemia (Ca^{2+} < 8 mg/dL)

  (a) *Etiology*: Hypoparathyroidism (iatrogenic most common), decreased albumin, pancreatitis, renal failure, hypomagnesemia, vitamin D deficiency, malabsorption, pseudohypoparathyroidism

  (b) *Diagnosis*: Usually symptomatic below 7.5 mg/dL, numbness, tingling, headaches, cramps, Chvostek sign (facial nerve irritability), Trousseau sign (carpopedal spasm)

  (c) *Therapy*: Emergent Ca gluconate or chloride 1 g (10 cc of 10% solution = 1 ampule) intravenous pyelogram (IVP) over 10 to 15 minutes with cardiac monitor
    ○ Remember to check Mg.
    ○ Chronic hypocalcemia replaces with Os-cal 1.5 to 3.0 g/d with vitamin D (calcitriol 0.25-2.0 μg/d); start 0.25 μg/d then may increase by 0.25 μg/d q2-4 weeks as needed.
    ○ Transient hypocalcemia (7-8) after thyroid surgery may not require treatment (Rx).
    ○ New rapid parathyroid hormone (PTH) assays may guide surgeon postthyroid-ectomy with immediate post-thyroid PTH greater than 10 to 12 pg/mL at very low risk of postthyroidectomy hypocalcemia.

- Hypercalcemia (Ca^{2+} > 10.6)

  (a) *Etiology*: Hyperparathyroidism, ectopic PTH production, malignancy, bony metastases, milk-alkali syndrome, vitamin D toxicity, sarcoid, tuberculosis (TB), Paget disease, thiazides, parathyroid malignancy

  (b) *Diagnosis*: Mild elevations (< 11.5) often asymptomatic and may require no Rx, nocturia, polydipsia, anorexia, nausea, vomiting, abdominal pain, confusion

  (c) Greater than 14 to 16 emergency levels

  (d) Therapy
    ○ Treat the underlying disorder.
    ○ Hydration (normal saline 1-2 L q2h).
    ○ Diuretics.
    ○ Phosphates, steroids, calcitonin, mithramycin.

Magnesium

- Normal serum Mg levels: 1.6 to 2.5 mg/dL
- Normal intake 20 mEq/d
- Hypomagnesemia Mg^{2+} less than 1.5 mg/dL

  (a) *Etiology*: Laxative abuse, diuretics, SIADH, parathyroidectomy, burns, decreased intake (ethyl alcohol [EtOH] abuse, TPN, malnutrition), decreased GI absorption

  (b) *Diagnosis*: Muscle weakness, cardiac arrhythmia, myoclonus

  (c) Therapy
    ○ Urgent, 1 to 2 g $MgSO_4$ (8-16 mEq) over 15 to 30 minutes then 1 g IM q 4 to 6 h or Mg oxide (Uro-Mag) 2 tabs bid
    ○ Important to correct low Mg if patient hypocalcemic

- Hypermagnesemia Mg^{2+} greater than 3 mg/dL

  (a) *Etiology*: Renal failure, excess intake

      (b) *Diagnosis*: Hypertension, nausea, vomiting, lethargy, weakness, ECG changes (aortic valve [AV] block, prolong QT)

      (c) *Therapy*: Urgent Ca gluconate 20 cc 10% solution IVP, eliminate exogenous sources, dialysis

Acid-Base Disorders

The acid-base system is designed to maintain the pH at a level of 7.4 for optimal cellular function. A number of mechanisms including the respiratory system, renal system, extracellular buffers (primarily HCO_3^-), and intracellular buffers (proteins, phosphates, and hemoglobin) exist to control the pH within this narrow range (Table 8-2).

Excess hydrogen ion (acid) is eliminated by the lungs based on the reaction:

$$H^+ + HCO_3 = H_2CO_3 = CO_2 + H_2O$$

Most of the excess hydrogen is eliminated by this route, with a relatively small amount (~70 mEq) eliminated by the renal system. Both the pulmonary and renal systems make adjustments to compensate for the alterations in the acid-base balance (Table 8-2). There are four general categories of acid-base disorders: respiratory acidosis and alkalosis, and metabolic acidosis and alkalosis.

Respiratory Acidosis

Primary respiratory acidosis is characterized by an increase in the partial pressure of arterial CO_2 (P_{CO_2}) secondary to disorders that limit pulmonary function. This is most commonly seen in diseases that limit the body's ability to eliminate CO_2 such as chronic obstructive pulmonary disease, impairment of central respiration (head injuries or drugs), or chest wall trauma that prevents adequate ventilation. The diagnosis is confirmed by an arterial blood gas that demonstrates a low pH and an elevated P_{CO_2}. The lowered pH reflects the body's attempt to compensate for the rising P_{CO_2} as depicted in the above-mentioned formula. In chronic situations, the renal system may contribute to the compensation by retaining HCO_3^-. Treatment is centered around addressing the chronic hypoventilation and may include steroids, antibiotics, inhalers, reversal of respiratory suppression, and consideration of intubation/mechanical ventilation.

Table 8-2 Acid-Base Disturbances

Disturbance	pH	H⁺	Compensation	Examples
Metabolic acidosis	Decrease	Increase	P_{aCO_2} decreases by 1.3 mm Hg for each mEq/L decrease in HCO_3	Lactic acidosis, ketoacidosis
Metabolic alkalosis	Increase	Decrease	P_{aCO_2} increases by 5-7 mm Hg for each mEq/L increase in HCO_3	Vomiting, NG tube suction, Cushing syndrome
Respiratory acidosis	Decrease	Increase	HCO_3 increases by 1 mEq/L for each 10 mm Hg increase in P_{aCO_2}	Hypoventilation, CNS lesion
Respiratory alkalosis	Increase	Decrease	HCO_3 decreases by 2 mEq/L for each 10 mm Hg decrease in P_{aCO_2}	Hypervent, fever/sepsis, hypoxemia

Respiratory Alkalosis

Primary respiratory alkalosis is characterized by hyperventilation that leads to a reduction in Pco_2. The two primary etiologies are direct stimulation of the central respiratory centers (aspirin, CNS tumors/trauma/cerebral vascular accident [CVA]) or indirect stimulation through hypoxia. It may also be seen in psychogenic hyperventilation, sepsis, errors in mechanical ventilation, and fevers. The diagnosis is confirmed by an arterial blood gas that demonstrates an elevated pH (> 7.45) with a low Pco_2 (< 35). Treatment is directed to the correction of the underlying disorder.

Metabolic Acidosis

Metabolic acidosis results from a variety of disorders that result in an excess acid load, decreased acid secretion, or excess bicarbonate loss. It is characterized by a low arterial pH (< 7.36) and a low HCO_3 (< 22). The reduction in arterial pH leads to a compensatory hyperventilation that decreases the Pco_2 and minimizes the change in arterial pH. Important in distinguishing among the many causes of a metabolic acidosis is the anion gap. The anion gap allows the clinician to classify the causes of metabolic acidosis into a high anion gap versus a normal anion gap (Table 8-3). The anion gap is calculated by subtracting the sum of the chloride and the bicarbonate from the sodium concentration. The usual value is 10 mEq/L.

Diagnosis is confirmed by an arterial blood gas that reflects a low pH and a lowering of the HCO_3^-. The anion gap should be calculated to help guide the determination of an etiology. Treatment is directed toward the underlying disorder. In many cases of mild metabolic acidosis (pH > 7.25), no treatment is necessary. The use of bicarbonate to treat metabolic acidosis is controversial and in some patients with lactic acidosis and ketoacidosis it may cause more harm than benefit. In selected situations (pH < 7.20, HCO_3^- < 10 mEq/L), some clinicians would use bicarbonate while addressing the underlying cause of the acidosis.

Metabolic Alkalosis

A metabolic alkalosis is caused by a primary elevation in plasma HCO_3^- above 27 mEq/L leading to an increased pH greater than 7.44. The increased pH stimulates a decrease in pulmonary ventilation. The drop in ventilation leads to an increase in the Pco_2 thereby attempting to minimize the alterations in the blood pH. The underlying causes of metabolic alkalosis are due

---

Table 8-3 Etiology of Metabolic Acidosis

- Normal anion gap

- Excess acid intake (HCl, NH_4Cl)

- Bicarbonate loss
   (a) GI tract (diarrhea, fistulas, NG tube)
   (b) Proximal renal tubular acidosis
   (c) Distal renal tubular acidosis
- Increased anion gap

- Ketoacidosis (diabetes mellitus, alcohol)

- Lactic acidosis

- Poisons (aspirin, ethylene glycol)

- Renal failure

Table 8-4 **Etiology of Metabolic Alkalosis**
• Acid loss (generally HCl)
• GI (vomiting, NG tube)
• Increased urine acidification
(a) Diuretics
(b) Aldosterone excess
(c) Bartter syndrome
• Excess alkali
(a) Alkali abuse
(b) Overtreatment of metabolic acidosis (ie, HCO_3^-)
• Severe potassium depletion

to a loss of acid or excess alkali intake. Table 8-4 lists the most common causes of metabolic alkalosis. By far the most common cause is related to the loss of acids (HCl). In general, there is no classic clinical picture of metabolic alkalosis. Most commonly the laboratory values will indicate an elevated serum bicarbonate (> 30 mEq/L). An arterial blood gas will then need to be obtained to assess the acid-base status and rule out a metabolic alkalosis or the elevated bicarbonate may reflect a true respiratory acidosis with the elevated bicarbonate representing a compensatory response.

Once the metabolic workup confirms an elevated HCO_3^- with an alkalotic pH, the next step is to assess the patient's volume status. Most commonly, GI losses (vomiting, NG tube) will account for the metabolic alkalosis and treatment can be focused on restoring an adequate volume, chloride, and potassium intake which will allow the body to self-correct the acid-base equilibrium. Obviously, the underlying disorder must be addressed while at the same time providing the necessary fluids and electrolytes that allow the renal system to excrete the excess bicarbonate. The amount of fluid and electrolytes will be guided by the patient's clinical response but often several liters of normal saline and several hundred milliequivalents of potassium will be needed over several days.

Bibliography

Couch M, Lai V, Cannon T, et al. Cancer cachexia syndrome in head and neck cancer patients: part I. Diagnosis, impact on quality of life and survival, and treatment. *Head Neck*. 2007; 29(4):401-411.

Der-Torossian H, Gourin CG, Couch ME. Translational implications of novel findings in cancer cachexia: the use of metabolomics and the potential of cardiac malfunction. *Curr Opin Support Palliat Care*. 2012;6(4):446-450.

Gann DS, Amaral JF. Fluid and electrolyte management. In: Sabiston DC, ed. *Essentials of Surgery*. Philadelphia, PA: W.B. Saunders; 1987:29-61.

Hall JC. Nutritional assessment of surgery patients. *J Am Coll Surg*. 2006;202:837-843.

Richey LM, George JR, Couch ME, et al. Defining cancer cachexia in head and neck squamous cell carcinoma. *Clin Cancer Res*. 2007;13(22 Pt 1): 6561-6567.

Questions

1. Most excess hydrogen ion in the body is eliminated via the
   A. Kidneys
   B. Liver
   C. Lungs
   D. GI tract

2. Which of the following is NOT a common cause of hyperkalemia?
   A. Renal failure
   B. Rhabdomyolysis
   C. Beta-blocker use
   D. Acidosis

3. What are the indications for TPN?
   A. Nonfunctioning of GI tract
   B. Severe protein malnutrition with loss of normal gastrointestinal (GI) function
   C. Chyle leak after neck dissection
   D. All of the above

4. Which of the following symptoms can be seen in hypocalcemia?
   A. Extremity tingling
   B. Headaches
   C. Cramps
   D. Positive Chvostek sign
   E. All of the above

5. Following a period of nutrient deprivation, profound electrolyte imbalances occurring with nutrient intake is called
   A. Cancer cachexia
   B. Gastroenteritis
   C. Refeeding syndrome
   D. Metabolic acidosis

Chapter 9
Antimicrobial Therapy in Otolaryngology—Head and Neck Surgery

Name	Common uses	Mechanism of action	Side effects
AMINOGLYCOSIDES			
Amikacin Gentamycin Neomycin Tobramycin	*Pseudomonas*, other gram negatives (*Escherichia coli*, *Klebsiella*). Not for anaerobes or Methicillin-resistant *Staphylococcus* aureus (MRSA)	Binds 30S ribosomal subunit, bacteriocidal causing misreading of mRNA	Cochleotoxic (2%-10%), vestibulotoxic, nephrotoxic
Cochleotoxicity and vestibulotoxicity: neomycin > amikacin > gentamycin = tobramycin			
CARBAPENEMS			
Ertapenem Imipenem/cilastatin Meropenem	Broad spectrum Not MRSA, not beta-lactamase strains	Beta-lactam cell wall-synthesis inhibitor, antibiotic of last resort	Seizures in high doses New Delhi metallo-beta-lactamase (NDM-1) coliforms resistant
CEPHALOSPORINS (FIRST GENERATION)			
Cefazolin (Ancef, Kefzol) Cephalexin (Keflex)	Gram positives, skin flora	Beta-lactam cell wall-synthesis inhibitor	Nausea with alcohol
Preferred antibiotic for surgical prophylaxis in Medicare Physician Quality Reporting Initiative (PQRI), to be given within 1 h prior to incision.			
CEPHALOSPORINS (SECOND GENERATION)			
Cefoxitin Cefprozil (Cefzil) Cefuroxime (Ceftin)	Less gram positive More gram negative Not *Pseudomonas* or penicillin-resistant *Streptococcus pneumoniae* (PRSP)	Beta-lactam cell wall-synthesis inhibitor	More diarrhea than first generation

CEPHALOSPORINS (THIRD GENERATION)			
Cefdinir (Omnicef) Cefixime (Suprax) Ceftazidime (Fortaz) Ceftriaxone (Rocephin)	Gram negative except *Pseudomonas*, has cerebrospinal fluid (CSF) penetration	Beta-lactam cell wall-synthesis inhibitor	Omnicef binds iron-causing red stools, need to distinguish any diarrhea between this and pseudomembranous colitis from *Clostridium difficile*
CEPHALOSPORINS (FOURTH GENERATION)			
Cefepime (Maxipime)	Antipseudomonal (also third-generation Fortaz)	Beta-lactam cell wall-synthesis inhibitor	increased mortality compared to other antibiotic (abx) in 2007 meta-analysis
GLYCOPEPTIDES			
Vancomycin	MRSA, *C difficile*, not active against gram negatives	Inhibits incorporation of *N*-acetylmuramic acid (NAM) and *N*-acetylglucosamine (NAG) into peptidoglycan	Red man syndrome (flushing of head/neck due to non-specific mast cell degranulation from too fast of an infusion), nephrotoxic, ototoxic
LINCOSAMIDES			
Clindamycin	Anaerobes, some MRSA, some gram positives, (most aerobic gram negatives (GNs) are resistant, eg, *Pseudomonas*, *Haemophilus*, *Moraxella*)	Binds 50S ribosomal subunit, reduces toxin formation (abx of choice for toxic shock)	Most frequent cause of *Pseudomembranous colitis* (*C difficile*)
Treat *P colitis* with metronidazole or oral vancomycin.			
LIPOPEPTIDES			
Daptomycin (Cubicin)	Gram positives only, MRSA	Novel mechanism of action, binds to cell membrane causing depolarization to cell dysfunction	Eosinophilic pneumonia, myalgias

MACROLIDES		
Erythromycin Clarithromycin Azithromycin	Broad spectrum, many gram positives and gram negatives, many atypical infections, effective against *Haemophilus, Moraxella, Helicobacter;* not effective against MRSA	Binds 50S ribosomal subunit, concentrates in phagocytes, also with strong anti-inflammatory effects, likely poor in clearing mucosal biofilming organisms	Motilin agonist (cramping and diarrhea), inhibits P450, cause drug-drug interactions Prolonged QT False-positive cocaine test; myalgia with statins Less than 1% experience side effects, reduces birth control effectiveness
MONOBACTAMS		
Aztreonam	Strong activity against *Pseudomonas*	Inhibits mucopeptide synthesis of cell wall	Rarely toxic epidermal necrolysis, eosinophilia
NITROFURANS		
Nitrofurantoin (Macrobid)	Safe in pregnant women (up to 38 weeks) for gram negatives (*E coli*)	Damages bacterial DNA Concentrates in urine	Hypersensitivity pneumonitis, hemolytic anemia in newborns
PENICILLINS		
Amoxicillin Ampicillin Dicloxacillin Methicillin Oxacillin Penicillin VK	Broad spectrum, much resistance from beta-lactamases; alteration of penicillin-binding protein; active efflux out of the cell	Beta-lactam (functional moiety of penicillin) inhibits D-alanyl-D-alanine carboxypeptidase that crosslinks peptidoglycan	Rash, ampicillin causes rash with mononucleosis, 50% of rashes do not recur; true anaphylaxis rare (1/10,000), IV antibiotics greater risk of life-threatening anaphylaxis
PENICILLIN COMBINATIONS		
Amoxicillin/clavulanate Ampicillin/sulbactam Piperacillin/tazobactam Ticarcillin/clavulanate	Beta-lactamase inhibitor restores sensitivity to many species	Beta-lactamase has no intrinsic antibiotic activity on its own	Increased diarrhea, requires refrigeration

POLYPEPTIDES			
Bacitracin	Gram positives	Inhibits peptidoglycan transport, topical	Contact dermatitis
Polymyxin	Gram negatives (except *Proteus*)	Destabilizes membrane, topical	Severe systemic toxicities, contact dermatitis
QUINOLONES			
Ciprofloxacin (Ciprodex)	Gram negative aerobes, poor gram positive	Inhibits DNA gyrase	Irreversible peripheral neuropathy, tendon rupture (ischemic noninflammatory damage), QT prolongation, toxic epidermal necrolysis, vision damage, concomitant steroid use, and advanced age may increase tendon rupture risk
Levofloxacin (Levaquin)	Increased gram positive, some anaerobes		
Moxifloxacin (Avelox)	Broad spectrum with anaerobic coverage		
Ofloxacin (Floxin)			
SULFONAMIDES			
Trimethoprim-sulfamethoxazole (Bactrim, Septra)	Broad spectrum including some MRSA, significant resistance	Competitive antagonist of para-aminobenzoic acid (PABA) needed for bacterial folic acid	Rash, increases warfarin levels; bone marrow suppression
TETRACYCLINES			
Doxycycline	Broad spectrum with significant resistance	Impairs 30S ribosomal subunit and transfer RNA binding	Stains developing teeth (even during pregnancy)
Tetracycline			
OTHER ANTIBACTERIAL			
Linezolid	Vancomycin-resistant enterococcus (VRE), MRSA, vancomycin-resistant *S aureus* (VRSA)	Protein synthesis inhibitor, disrupts formation of initiation complex	Relatively safe but expensive and antibiotic of last resort, altered taste, tongue discoloration
	No gram negatives		
Metronidazole	Anaerobes only, preferred for *C difficile*	Destabilizes anaerobic DNA	Metallic taste, bone marrow suppression, peripheral neuropathy
Mupirocin (Bactroban)	*S aureus* including MRSA (topical)	Inhibits *S aureus* RNA synthesis	Contact dermatitis
Rifampin	Broad spectrum, only for dual therapy second to quick resistance	RNA polymerase inhibitor	Red-colored tears
Raxibacumab (Abthrax)	Neutralizes anthrax toxin	Monoclonal antibody	Rash, itching

ANTIFUNGALS			
Amphotericin B	All including *Mucor,* some *Candida albicans* resistance	Binds ergosterol	Severe side effects include infusion reactions, nephrotoxicity, cardiac, neuro, and hepatic
Nystatin	All	Similar to amphotericin B, topical only	Rash, itching
Azoles	Skin infections	Inhibits lanosterol conversion to ergosterol	Variable and less compared to amphotericin but with similar side effects including severe and lethal systemic effects
Ketoconazole (Nizoral)	Skin infections		
Clotrimazole (Lotrimin)	Not *Mucor*		
Fluconazole (Diflucan)	*Candida, Aspergillus*		
Itraconazole (Sporanox)	*Fusarium*, not *Mucor*		
Voriconazole (VFend)	Possibly against *Mucor*		
Posaconazole (Posanol)			
Caspofungin	*Candida, Aspergillus*	Inhibits fungal cell wall	Hepatotoxicity
ANTIVIRALS			
Valacyclovir (Valtrex)	Herpes virus family	Inhibits viral polymerase	Bone marrow suppression, Stevens-Johnson syndrome
Oseltamivir (Tamiflu)	Influenza A and B	Neuraminidase inhibitor	Rare neuropsychiatric issues

Antibiotic Pearls

Bacteriocidal versus bacteriostatic refers to strict in vitro conditions and have little clinical relevance. For example, bacteriostatic agents (clindamycin, linezolid, etc) have been effectively used in meningitis and osteomyelitis. The ultimate guide to treatment of any infection should be clinical outcome.

Penicillin allergy is reported by 10% of patients. Only 1% have a true IgE-mediated allergy; only 0.01% will suffer anaphylaxis. Penicillin skin testing is the best test to identify true allergy. Allergic patients may benefit from desensitization. Cephalosporins generally are safe even in patients with true penicillin allergy, though Keflex may have greater risk than other cephalosporins.

Signs of IV cephalosporin anaphylaxis: Occurs within minutes, pain at site of injection, itching/swelling of throat, labored respirations, weak pulses, hypovolemic shock

Treatment: Immediate IV/IM epinephrine, volume expansion with normal saline, 100% oxygen, hydrocortisone 200 mg, cardiac support

Treatment Options and Recommendations

Acute Otitis Media

Bacteriology: Nontypeable *Haemophilus influenzae* (50% penicillin resistant), *S pneumoniae* (40% penicillin resistant), *Moraxella catarrhalis* (nearly 100% penicillin resistant).

Treatment: When antibiotics are chosen over observation, first choice (mild infections) is amoxicillin 80 to 90 mg/kg; first choice (moderate to severe infections) is Augmentin;

Omnicef for penicillin-allergic patients; antibiotics may help relieve pain and speed recovery; antibiotic use in polymicrobial mucosal biofilm infections does not follow classic culture and sensitivity testing.

Chronic Suppurative Otitis Media

Bacteriology: Mixed and includes *S aureus, Pseudomonas aeruginosa*, anaerobic bacteria, and others in addition to those commonly found in acute otitis media.

Treatment: Antimicrobial/antiseptic topical therapy combined with aural toilet is better than aural toilet alone. Adding oral antibiotics and the choice of topical antibiotic is controversial. Vinegar/alcohol, quinolone topical antibiotics, and neomycin-polymyxin-steroid otic drops are safe and effective. Aminoglycoside topical antibiotics may be ototoxic.

Acute Otitis Externa

Bacteriology: *P aeruginosa, S aureus*; (less than 2% of acute otitis externa are fungal infections, viral infections, or eczema)

Treatment: Antiseptic topical therapy (acetic acid/alcohol, topical antimicrobials) and debris removal/wicking

Acute Bacterial Rhinosinusitis

Bacteriology: *H influenzae, S pneumoniae, M catarrhalis*, rarely *Streptococcus pyogenes, S aureus, P aeruginosa* (often in cystic fibrosis), anaerobic (odontogenic sinusitis).

Treatment: Many resolve without antibiotics. Amoxicillin for 10 to 14 days is a reasonable first-line agent. Bactrim or doxycycline is reasonable in true penicillin-allergic patients. Amoxicillin/clavulanate, currently a second-line antibiotic, is currently more effective than cephalosporins. The benefit of culture-directed antibiotics is limited in polymicrobial mucosal biofilm infections.

Chronic Rhinosinusitis

Bacteriology: Chronic bacterial rhinosinusitis, a subset of chronic rhinosinusitis (CRS), is multi-factorial and poorly understood. Healthy sinuses have diverse commensal microbiota located on the surface of sinus epithelium. This diversity is reduced in CRS. Innate immune dysfunction and anatomic obstruction are often contributors if not the cause. Bacteria detected in sinuses with CRS are mixed and include *S aureus, P aeruginosa*, and a large mix of aerobic and anaerobic bacteria.

Treatment: Multiple oral/topical antibiotics have been used. Generally, longer-term antibiotic use leads to longer symptom relief; however, it has been difficult to cure CRS with antibiotic use alone. Polymicrobial biofilms share resistance genes through extensive horizontal gene transfer, decreasing the effectiveness of oral antibiotics. Cell wall-synthesis inhibiting antibiotics may be less effective than non–cell wall synthesis-inhibiting antibiotics. Combined use of quinolones and steroids may lead to more tendonopathy.

Acute Bacterial Tonsillitis/Pharyngitis

Bacteriology: *S pneumoniae*, group A beta-hemolytic *Streptococcus* (*S pyogenes*), *H influenza*.

Treatment: Antibiotics may be held for up to 9 days without increasing the risk for acute rheumatic fever, poststreptococcal glomerulonephritis. Penicillin is currently effective for *S pyogenes*, penicillin-resistant *S pneumoniae* becoming highly prevalent. Amoxicillin will cause rash in patients with Epstein-Barr virus (EBV) pharyngitis.

Deep Neck Infections

Bacteriology: Mixed, often with both aerobic (*Streptococcus, Staphylococcus*) and anaerobic bacteria (foul smelling, poorly detected in culture)

Treatment: Broad-spectrum IV antibiotics followed by blood and/or abscess culture-directed antibiotics

Antibiotic Surgical Prophylaxis

Antibiotic surgical prophylaxis is used to reduce the risk of nosocomial postsurgical wound infections. It has been a focus of the Surgical Care Improvement Project sponsored by the Centers for Medicare and Medicaid Services; hospital reimbursements are tied to reporting of the proper use of antibiotics in surgical cases.

As per the current guidelines, antibiotics should be administered no more than 1 hour prior to incision, infusions should be completed prior to surgical incision, and antibiotics should be discontinued within 24 hours of surgical closure.

For skin incisions, cefazolin is recommended to cover against *S aureus*.

For mucosal incisions, clindamycin or ampicillin/sulbactam may be used to cover a broad spectrum of aerobic and anaerobic bacteria.

For dirty/infected wounds, antibiotic use should not be discontinued until clinically appropriate.

Bibliography

US Food and Drug Administration Information for Healthcare Professionals (Drugs): http://www.fda.gov/Drugs/ResourcesForYou/HealthProfessionals/default.htm.

Questions

1. Which of the following drugs has the least ototoxicity?
   A. Amikacin
   B. Tobramycin
   C. Vancomycin
   D. Clindamycin

2. Which of the following fluoroquinolones has the least anaerobic coverage?
   A. Ofloxacin
   B. Levofloxacin
   C. Ciprofloxacin
   D. Moxifloxacin

3. Which of the following antibiotics is not a cell wall-synthesis inhibitor?
   A. Aztreonam
   B. Cefepime
   C. Doxycycline
   D. Meropenem

4. Which of the following antibiotics is not appropriate for MRSA?
   A. Cubicin
   B. Mupirocin
   C. Linezolid
   D. Cefepime

5. Which of the following antifungals is most appropriate for rhinocerebral mucormycosis in a patient with immunosuppression from chemotherapy?
   A. Amphotericin B
   B. Voriconazole
   C. Caspofungin
   D. Fluconazole

Chapter 10
Pharmacology and Therapeutics

Antimicrobials

- The reader is directed to Chapter 9 for review of antibiotics, antivirals, and antifungal medicinal therapies.

Chemotherapy

- The reader is directed to Chapter 40: Chemotherapy for Head and Neck Cancer for review of chemotherapeutic drugs and their applications and indications.

Perioperative Drugs

- The reader is directed to Chapter 4: Anesthesia for Head and Neck Surgery for review of local anesthetics, narcotics, sedatives, and the various other perioperative drugs.

Allergy Medications

- The reader is directed to Chapter 52: Allergy for review of antihistamines, decongestants, corticosteroid, mast cell stabilizers, leukotriene antagonists, and the treatment of anaphylaxis conditions.

Corticosteroids

- Utilized in the treatment of a variety of inflammatory and immune-mediated disorders (eg, sarcoidosis). Can be administered topically or systemically.
- Common systemic corticosteroids include prednisone and dexamethasone.
- Unless systemic use is brief (3-5 days), a taper is needed to prevent adrenal insufficiency from hypothalamic-pituitary-adrenal (HPA) suppression.
- Common topical corticosteroids include fluticasone and mometasone; no taper is needed with prolonged use, as there is little impact on the HPA axis.

- The available corticosteroids have differing potencies. The list below provides the equi-efficacious dose for several commonly utilized corticosteroids:

Hydrocortisone	1
Prednisone	4
Prednisolone	4
Methylprednisolone	5
Triamcinolone	5
Dexamethasone	25

- Adverse effects of prolonged systemic corticosteroid use include hypertension, increased glucose tolerance and difficulty controlling diabetes, mental status changes (anxiety, insomnia), increased intraocular pressures, cataract (posterior subcapsular) formation, reduction of overall bone mineral density, avascular necrosis of the hip, and peptic ulcer formation.
- Topically administered corticosteroids typically have few or no systemic adverse effects.
- Local adverse effects include epistaxis and rarely nasal septum perforation with intra-nasal administration.
- The most common indication for topical corticosteroids is the treatment of inflammatory conditions of the nose and paranasal sinuses including allergic and nonallergic rhinitis, vasomotor rhinitis, and inflammatory chronic rhinosinusitis (CRS).
- Other indications include as combination therapy in the treatment of infectious otitis externa or as single modality therapy for eczematous otitis externa.
- Several antibiotic and corticosteroid otic drops formulations are available and commonly utilized.
- The table below lists and compares several commonly employed topical nasal corticosteroids:

Drug	Youngest approved age	Possible growth suppression in children	Nasal polyposis indication	Pregnancy approved	Scented
Beclomethasone propionate	6	Yes	No	No	Yes
Budesonide	6	N/A	Yes	Yes	No
Ciclesonide	6	N/A	No	No	No
Flunisolide	6	N/A	No	No	Yes
Fluticasone propionate	6	No	No	No	Yes
Fluticasone furoate	2	No	No	No	No
Mometasone	2	No	Yes	No	No

- Multiple studies have demonstrated the efficacy of nasal corticosteroid sprays in the treatment nasal polyposis, though only two carry formal indications.
- Pre- and postoperative systemic steroid use has been shown to decrease intraoperative bleeding during sinus surgery (prednisone 30 mg PO daily for 5 days before and after surgery). This regimen has no long-term symptom benefit.

Anticholinergics

- Muscarinic acetylcholine receptor antagonists (parasympatholytics) are the most commonly employed anticholinergics in the head and neck conditions.
- Available in both topical and systemic formulations.

Nasal Preparations

- Ipratropium bromide is the only available nasal spray, available in 0.03% and 0.06% preparations. Decreases parasympathetic mediated nasal secretions.
- Rapid onset and low systemic absorption.
- Indications include conditions with elevated nasal secretions including virally mediated rhinitis, allergic and nonallergic rhinitis, and especially vasomotor rhinitis.

Systemic Preparations

- Utilized for motion sickness, systemic secretions reduction, and treatment of vagal reactions and as part of advanced cardiac support during code events.
- Scopolamine is commonly employed in the treatment of motion sickness by blocking vestibular input to the central vestibular system that is responsible for the vegetative symptoms. See below in the section Antiemetics.
- Both systemic and transdermal formulations have demonstrated efficacy with prophylaxis; neither has literature support for active symptom management.
- Glycopyrrolate is a quaternary amine (does not cross the blood-brain barrier) and is commonly used to reduce oral, pharyngeal, and respiratory secretions prior to endoscopy without significant central effects.
- Atropine is typically used in the treatment of bradycardia or cardiac arrest events.
- Adverse effects are mediated by the blockage of normal parasympathetic activity resulting in tachycardia, flushing, blurred vision, urinary retention, decreased gastrointestinal motility and constipation, mental status changes (decreased arousal), and xerostomia.
- "Blind as a bat, mad as a hatter, hot as a hare, dry as a bone" is one mnemonic to remember these adverse effects.

Vasocontrictors

- Employed to decrease the size of mucous membranes and/or decrease bleeding by decreasing arterial inflow via arteriolar vasoconstriction.

Epinephrine (Adrenaline)

- Potent agonist of alpha-1, alpha-2, beta-1, and beta-2 receptors; normal synthesis occurs in the adrenal medulla.
- Vasoconstriction is mediated by alpha-1 receptors.
- Beta-1 receptors agonism results in positive effects on cardiac inotropy, chronotropy, and dromotropy, while beta-2 agonism induces smooth muscle relaxation (coronary vasodilation and bronchodilation).
- Can be administered topically (mucus membranes, aerosolized).

- Topical use on the nasal mucosa produces pallor and shrinkage due to vasoconstriction, which can be useful in sinus surgery. Typically 1:1000 or 1:2000 dilutions are used.
- Commonly used with local anesthetics to increase duration of activity by preventing interstitial drug washout and to decrease bleeding by inducing vasoconstriction.

Ephedrine

- Induces the release of preformed stores of catecholamines and is therefore an indirect, nonselective sympathomimetic drug.
- Can be administered topically or systemically.
- *Pseudoephedrine* is a commonly used analog employed as a systemic decongestant.
  (a) There are now regulations on the over-the-counter (OTC) availability due to its use in the manufacture of methamphetamine.

Phenylephrine

- Alpha-1 agonist, sympathomimetic.
- Commonly employed as a topical nasal decongestant; it can be used as a vasopressor in critical care situations.

Cocaine

- Local anesthetic (LA) with vasoconstrictive properties; most LAs cause vasodilation.
- Works by blocking the reuptake of catecholamines at synapses.
- Most commonly used in nasal endoscopy when debridement is performed after sinus surgery.
- Both serum (3 hours) and urinary (6 hours) levels can be detected after topical use in the nose.
- Maximum dose is about 2 to 3 mg/kg; most prevalent preparation is a 4% solution.
- Oxymetazoline is a common alpha-1 agonist used topically for nasal decongestion.
- Both phenylephrine and oxymetazoline use for longer than 3 to 5 days can result in tachyphylaxis (blunted response to the same dose of drug) and rebound nasal congestion (rhinitis medicamentosa) with cessation of use.

Treatment of Gastric Acidity

- Laryngopharyngeal reflux (LPR) and gastroesophageal reflux disease are important to the otolaryngologist.
- Symptoms include vocal changes (hoarseness), dry cough, globus sensation, and repeated throat clearing.
- Gastric acid can also have significant deleterious effects on airway inflammation and healing after airway surgery.
- Treatment typically starts with lifestyle modifications and moves to medicinal therapy if these are not satisfactory.
- The goals of pharmacotherapy are to reduce gastric acid production (antihistamines and proton pump inhibitors) and neutralize gastric acid (antacids) or clearance of gastric contents distally (promotility agents).

Acid Neutralization

- Antacids neutralize gastric acid by providing hydroxide ions or congregate bases to bind with hydrogen ions.
- Examples include aluminum hydroxide, magnesium hydroxide, sodium bicarbonate, and calcium carbonate.
- Typically taken at or shortly after a meal once acid production has commenced.
- Generally very safe if taken in moderation (per manufacturer's instructions), though caution should be exercised in patients with sodium sensitivity (eg, congestive heart failure).

Protective Barriers

- Alginic acid is a polysaccharide derived from brown algae. It is used to form a protective barrier to gastric acid.
- Gaviscon is an example of alginic acid containing medication.

Antihistamines

- The H_2 histamine receptor promotes acid production from gastric parietal cells.
- Ranitidine, famotidine, nizatidine, and cimetidine are OTC H_2-receptorspecific antihistamines available for acid suppressive therapy.
- Should be taken before meals to block acid production stimulation.
- Cimetidine is a cytochrome P450 inhibitor; drug interactions should be investigated prior to recommendation of this drug.

Proton Pump Inhibitors

- Proton pump inhibitors (PPIs) block the production of gastric acid by inhibiting the production of hydrogen ions by the H^+/K^+ ATPase enzyme on the luminal surface of parietal cells.
- Available drugs include omeprazole, pantoprazole, lansoprazole, rabeprazole as well as specific enantiomers of several of these medications.
  (a) Examples include esomeprazole and dexlansoprazole.
- These medications should be taken 1 hour before a meal to allow for maximal antagonism.
- Long-term use can lead to several adverse effects including negative Ca^{2+} homeostasis (possible risk of fractures) and B_{12} deficiency (megaloblastic anemia).
- Supplemental calcium intake is reasonable recommendation if long-term treatment is to be considered.

Promotility Agents

- Metoclopramide is a dopaminergic antagonist promotility agent. It also increases the tone of the lower esophageal sphincter, decreases the tone of the pyloric sphincter, and increases the motility of the gastric antrum.
- Must be aware of possible extrapyramidal symptoms (dystonias) and need to be aware of other dopamine antagonists (typical and atypical antipsychotics) the patient is taking.

Hemostatic Agents

- Desmopression acetate (ddAVP/arginine vasopression) works by increasing the secretion of von Willebrand factor (vWF) from endothelial cells.
- This can be useful in patients with hemophillia A (Factor-8 deficiency), Type-I von Willebrand disease or prolonged bleeding times (platelet dysfunction) from conditions such as renal insufficiency.

- ddAVP can also stimulate the release of tissue-type plasminogen activator (fibrinolysis).
- Aminocaproic acid can be given to counter this effect.
  (a) Analog of lysine, which interferes with enzymes that bind to lysine residues
- Fibrin sealants–bovine and human thrombin combined with fibrin; examples include Tisseel, Hemaseel, and Crosseal.
- Gelatin hemostatic agents–purified gelatin; serves as a mechanical plug.
- Combination products–examples include FloSeal, which is a combination of gelatin matrix and thrombin.
- Oxidized regenerated cellulose – examples include Surgicel and Surgicel Fibrillar. Made from oxidized plant cellulose that helps as a matrix for clot formation.
- Microfibrillar collegen–Avitene is an example. Purified bovine collagen that stimulates hemostasis via the intrinsic pathway.
- Cyanoacrylate–Dermabond is an example. Polymerizes when it contacts water-containing tissues, which stimulates the polymerization reaction. Typically used in skin closures.

Ototoxicity

- Ototoxicity encompasses both cochlear and vestibular effects. Common classes of medications/substances include aminoglycosides antibiotics, loop diuretics, platinum-based chemotherapeutics, quinine-containing substances and salicylates.
- The following table summarizes the main ototoxic mediation classes:

Drug class	Duration	Primary target	Site of damage
Aminoglycosides	Permanent	Drug specific	1. Inner row of outer hair cells (OHCs) at cochlear basal turn 2. Stria vascularis
Platinum-based chemotheraputics	Permanent	Cochlea	1. Inner row of OHCs at cochlear basal turn 2. Stria vascularis
Loop diuretics	Transient	Cochlea	Stria vascularis
Quinine	Transient	Cochlea	1. Stria vascularis 2. Organ of Corti
Salicylates	Transient	Cochlea	None

Aminoglycosides (AGs)

- Typically with systemic administration and results in bilateral, permanent high-frequency sensorineural hearing loss (SNHL).
- Toxicity is associated with serum levels above therapeutic target levels.
- Renally cleared making renal dosing and kidney function monitoring essential.
- Drug levels concentrate and persist in the inner ear fluids (endolymph).
- AGs bind to a phospholipid (phosphatidylinositol) on the cell membrane.

- AGs chelate iron, which participates in free radical formation and subsequent cell damage starting with the inner row of OHCs and progressing to the remaining two rows over time.
- Proceeds in a base to apex direction explaining the high-frequency SNHL seen early.
- Histopathologic findings include intermittent OHC loss and stria vascularis damage.
- A1555G mutation in the mitochondrial 12S ribosomal RNA imparts exquisite AG sensitivity. Seen in certain Chinese populations.
- While all AGs will damage both the cochlear and vestibular hair cells, many affect one or the other primarily.
- Vestibulotoxic AGs include stretomycin, gentamicin, and tobramycin (**T**errible **G**ait **S**tability).
- Cochleotoxic AGs include amikacin, neomycin, and kanamycin.
- Otic preparations of AGs carry *significant* risk of inner ear toxicity if the tympanic membrane is **not** intact (must be able to visualize the entire TM prior to administration).
  (a) Middle ear AG administration is the access route used in medical vestibular ablation for vestibular hyperfunction.

Platinum-based Chemotherapeutics

- Cisplatin and carboplatin are commonly used in the treatment of upper aerodigestive squamous cell cancers.
- There is a dose-dependent ototoxicity, typically SNHL between 4 and 8 kHz but this can progress to lower hertz over time.
- Histopathology is similar to AG damage outlined above.
- SNHL is seen in more than 50% of patients and tinnitus is seen in 7%. A few of these patients progress to have speech understanding deficits.

Quinine and Chloroquine

- Examples include quinine and chloroquine, which are antimalarial treatments.
- Primarily cochleotoxic due to reversible vasculitis and ischemia of the inner ear with degenerative changes being found in the organ of Corti and stria vascularis.
- Neonates born to mother taking these medications can exhibit bilateral SNHL even if the mother's hearing is normal.

Loop Diuretics

- Main examples are ethacrynic acid (1% of usage) and furosemide (~6% of usage), which work to block the action of the Na^+-K^+-$2Cl^-$ symporter in the ascending loop of Henle.
- Ototoxic effects from loop diuretics are typically transient.
- Impact is through electrolyte imbalances in the endolymph by blocking the H^+/K^+ ATPase enzyme.
- Toxicities can be minimized if parenteral administration is given over time versus a bolus.

Salicylates

- Aspirin (acetylsalicylic acid/ASA) and other salicylates produce reversible hearing loss and tinnitus.
- Doses greater than 2.7 g of ASA are needed to produce the toxicities.
- Renally cleared; once systemically cleared, cochlear effects subside.

Dermatologic Agents

Minoxidil

- Direct vasodilator when given systemically. Topical preparations are used to treat male pattern baldness (FDA [Food and Drug Administration] indication).
- Mechanism of action is speculated to be through the stimulation of increased scalp blood flow and epidermal DNA synthesis.
- Adverse effects include local pruritus, irritation, and hypertrichosis.
- Available in 2% and 5% OTC preparations with the 5% formulation being more efficacious.

Finasteride

- Finasteride is an orally available 5-alpha reductase inhibitor (testosterone to dihydrotestoserone [DHT] conversion).
- DHT is responsible for androgeneic alopecia.
- Hair regrow is seen in 90% of patients.
- Few short-term adverse effects, long-term effects unknown.

Vitamin A Analogs

- Tretinoin is a form of Vitamin A used to improve the appearance of aging skin, particularly photoaged skin.
- Improves collagen synthesis in the papillary dermis, which can improve the appearance of rhytids.
- Used to help prepare skin prior to chemical peels (chemexfoliation).
- Can be a potent teratogen, so strong counseling to avoid pregnancy is warranted. Can consider pharmacologic contraceptives if prolonged use in females of child-bearing age is being planned.

Sunscreens

- Ultraviolent (UV) radiation skin exposure is associated with photoaging and skin cancer.
- UV radiation is separated into UVA (320-400 nm) and UVB (290-320 nm). The shorter the wavelength, the higher the energy available to cause damage.
- UVB can directly damage cells; UVA causes indirect damage by the creation of reactive oxygen species (ROS).
- Historically, most sunscreen available primarily blocked UVB, though this is changing.
- Sunscreen use has been shown to decrease the risk of skin photodamage, actinic keratosis, and squamous cell cancer. Data regarding basal cell carcinoma and melanoma are less clear.
- Sunscreen should be applied 30 minutes before sun exposure and every 2 hours during UV exposure.
- The effectiveness of sunscreen can be estimated by the sun protection factor (SPF), an imperfect measure.

- 10-minute exposure for a burn x SPF 30 = 300-minute exposure for a burn with sunscreen.
- Active ingredients are either radiopaque inorganic compounds (zinc and titanium oxides) that block UV radiation or organic compounds (para-aminobenzoic acid) that absorb the UV radiation.
- Organic compounds tend to become less effective as UV exposure increases.
- Inorganic compounds have typically been available as thick pastes with a white appearance. New formulations with nanoparticles are available with less cosmetic concerns.
- Inorganic compounds provide superior protection in general, though consistent, persistent use of any sunscreen is superior to intermittent or inadequate use.

Botulinum Toxin

- Extremely potent neurotoxin produced by the bacterium *Clostridium botulinum*.
- Secreted exotoxin composed of 1 heavy and 1 light chain; taken into the presynaptic terminals through endocytosis.
- The light chain is an enzyme that selectively cleaves presynaptic SNARE proteins involved with vesicular fusion (acetylcholine-containing vesicles mainly).
- Results in flaccid paralysis of affected neuromuscular junctions.
- Reinnervation occurs through growth of collaterals within 3 months.
- Clinical indications have grown in recent years and include: effacement of rhytids, treatment of facial dystonias, adductor spastic dysphonia, bruxism, strabismus, achalasia, hyperhidrosis, and sialorrhea.
- Seven different serotypes exist (A-G), each targeting unique locations in vesicular and target SNARE proteins.
- Serotypes A (BOTOX) and B (MYOBLOC) are commercially available; only serotype A is indicated for cosmetic use.

Antiemetics

- Most agents target receptors in the chemoreceptor trigger zone (CTZ) found in the floor of the ventricle or the emetic center in the lateral reticular formation in the medulla.
- Histamine and acetylcholine receptors are found in the lateral reticular formation and dopamine receptors in the CTZ.
- Dopamine antagonists include prochloperazine and metoclopramide.
- Metoclopromide is a promotility agent used to increase gastric emptying, often used with diabetic gastroparesis.
- Care must be taken in patients taking antidopaminergic agents to prevent extrapyramidal symptoms. Special attention should be paid to patients taking typical or atypical antipsychotics.
- Antihistamines include scopolamine and promethazine, which can be taken systemically or transdermally.
- Anticholinergics include diphenhydramine.
- Most antihistamines and all anticholinergics can have adverse effects outside the central nervous system (see above).
- Selective serotonin agonists for the 5-HT$_3$ receptors are commonly used due to their very favorable side effect profile, though they are only FDA approved for chemotherapy-induced nausea. Ondansetron is the most commonly used.

- The most common adverse effect is headache (5%-27%).
- Use with caution in patients with prolonged QTc interval; 5-HT3 agonists can prolong the QT interval, which can lead to Torsade de Pointe. Be sure to correct any significant electrolyte abnormalities prior to use systemically.

Mucolytics and Expectorants

- Mucolytic agents work by depolymerizing mucopolysaccharides and increasing their solubility.
- *N*-Acetylcysteine (NAC) is an example; uses include thinning of secretions in asthma, paracetamol (acetaminophen) overdose, and renal protectant with the use of IV radiocontrast.
- Guaifenesin is an example of an expectorant. The mechanism of action is poorly understood.
- Other agents include ammonium and iodide salts.

Selected Therapeutic Regimens

Xerostomia

- Seen commonly in patients with autoimmune salivary gland conditions (Sjögren syndrome) or postradiation sequelae.
- Conservative treatments include drinking small, frequent sips of water, use of sugar-free sialogogues and use of cellulose-based salivary substitutes.
- Cholinergic agonists (parasympathomimetic) stimulate the saliva production when functioning parenchyma is present. Pilocarpine and cevimeline are examples.
- Due to cholinergic systemic effects (diarrhea, hyperhidrosis, increased airway secretions), use is typically limited.

Treatment of Aphthous Stomatitis

- Recurrent aphthous ulcers (aka canker sores) are common, affecting between 20% and 50% of the population. Etiology is unclear and no definitive treatments exist.
- *Topical corticosteroids*: 0.05% clobetaol and 0.05% fluocinonide are more potent and effective than triamcinolone.
- *Antimicrobial*: Tetracycline antibiotic solutions reduces ulcer size, duration, and pain.
- *Anti-inflammatory*: Amlexanox paste 5% facilitates healing but does not reduce frequency of outbreaks.
- *Anesthetic*: Viscous lidocaine at various concentrations can be used to help control pain.

Smoking-Cessation Therapy

- Multiple medications are FDA approved as part of a comprehensive approach to tobacco use cessation therapy.
- Nicotine replacement therapies include transdermal patches and gums.
- Bupropion and varenicline are medicinal options.

- Bupropion's mechanism of action is unknown.
- Varenicline is a partial agonist at central nicotinic acetylcholine receptors; nicotine binds poorly in this state.
- Both nicotine cravings and withdrawal symptoms are reduced when taking varenicline.

Tinnitus

- No medicinal treatments have demonstrated long-term benefit in symptom reduction.
- Agents showing benefit in placebo-controlled trials include benzodiazepines (alprazolam, clonazepam) and tricyclic antidepressants (amitriptyline).
- Anticonvulsants, selective serotonin reuptake inhibitors, gabapentin, and anti-NMDA (*N*-methyl-D-aspartate) glutamate receptor agents (memantine) have failed to show a benefit over placebo in clinical trials.

Chronic Cough

- No strong medication options for the persistent chronic cough exist at the present time.
- Opiates are the mainstay of the refractory, chronic cough; extended-release morphine demonstrates highest efficacy (5 mg dose).
- Other centrally acting medications include amitriptyline, paroxetine, gabapentin, and carbamazepine and locally acting agents such as benzonatate; none have demonstrated effectiveness in clinical trials.

Bibliography

Bailey BJ, Johnson JT, Newlands SD. *Head & Neck Surgery—Otolaryngology*. 4th ed. Philadelphia, PA: Lippincott Williams & Wilkins; 2006.

Flint PW, Cummings CW. Otolaryngology Head & Neck Surgery. 5th ed. Philadelphia, PA: Mosby/Elsevier; 2010.

Lee KJ. *Essential Otolaryngology: Head & Neck Surgery*. 10th ed. New York, NY: McGraw Hill, Medical Publishing Division; 2012.

Questions

1. The mechanism of action of glycopyrrolate is
   A. Sympathomimetic
   B. Blockade of norepinephrine reuptake
   C. Competitive inhibition of cholinergic receptors
   D. Blockade of acetylcholine release
   E. Inhibition of acetylcholinesterase

2. The antihistamine most likely to have significant drug interactions is
   A. Famotidine
   B. Cimetidine

   C. Ranitidine

   D. Nizatidine

3. Genetic predisposition to aminoglycoside toxicity occurs via which of the following inheritance patterns?

   A. X-linked recessive

   B. Autosomal recessive

   C. Autosomal dominant

   D. Mitochondrial

   E. X-linked dominant

4. The wavelength spectrum of UVB is

   A. 200 to 240 nm

   B. 290 to 320 nm

   C. 320 to 400 nm

   D. 430 to 470 nm

   E. 490 to 540 nm

5. The mechanism of action of botulinum toxin is

   A. Cholinergic receptor antagonist

   B. Acetylcholinesterase activity

   C. Presynaptic intracellular cleavage of vesicle fusion proteins

   D. Cellular excitotoxicity

   E. Cholinergic agonist

Chapter 11
HIV

Overview

- Human immunodeficiency virus (HIV) is a blood-borne and sexually transmitted infection that leads to acquired immunodeficiency syndrome (AIDS).
- HIV belongs to the *Lentivirus* genus of the retroviridae family.
- An enveloped, single-stranded RNA virus that primarily infects CD4+ T lymphocytes (though it can infect other cell that express CD4, such as macrophages).
- Viral life cycle
  - (a) Infection of the host cell via binding to CD4 and fusion of the viral envelope and cell membrane.
  - (b) The viral RNA is reverse transcribed in DNA and integrated into the host genome.
  - (c) There is a period of latency, followed by an active viral replication phase.
  - (d) New viral particles "bud off" of the cell membrane of the infected cell.
  - (e) This eventually results in cellular destruction and consequently impairment of the host's immune system.

Clinical Presentation

- HIV can spread via blood, semen, vaginal fluid, or breast milk.
- Primary HIV infection can be asymptomatic or present as a viral prodrome occurring 2 to 4 weeks after exposure.
- Symptoms include fever, reactive cervical lymphadenopathy, pharyngitis, maculopapular rash, orogenital ulcers, and meningoencephalitis.
- Leukopenia and decreased CD4 count can also occur with associated opportunistic infections.

Diagnosis

- HIV is diagnosed via anti-HIV antibodies detected in serum. These are persistently present 3 months following exposure.

Table 11-1 **1993 CDC Classification System for Adults and Adolescents**			
CD4 count	A. Asymptomatic	B. Symptomatic, not A or C	C. AIDS-defining illness
≥500 cells/mm³	HIV	HIV	AIDS
200-499 cells/mm³	HIV	HIV	AIDS
<200 cells/mm³	AIDS	AIDS	AIDS

World Health Organization (WHO) Clinical Staging System

- Takes into account the myriad of clinical manifestations associated with HIV infection (Appendices A and B).
- Useful for establishing baseline, assessing the effect of therapy, monitoring long-term follow-up, and prognosticating.
- Immune status (as measured by CD4 count) is useful in clinical decision-making.
- The likelihood of developing clinical manifestations of immunodeficiency has been shown to correlate with decreasing CD4 count.
- Normal absolute CD4 count in adults is 500 to1500 cells per mm³ of blood (normal values require age-adjustment, as children generally have higher CD4 counts than adults). Opportunistic infections and other manifestations of HIV become more likely when CD4 counts drop below 200 cells/mm³.

Center for Disease Control (CDC) Classification System

- Incorporates both clinical manifestations and CD4 count. It was initially designed for surveillance purposes, though it provides an adequate overview of a patient's clinical picture (Table 11-1).
- The three clinical categories are as follows:
  (a) Asymptomatic HIV infection or persistent generalized lymphadenopathy.
  (b) Clinical manifestations that are not HIV-specific (ie, opportunistic infections) that are not included in A or C.
  (c) AIDS-defining illness (ie, Kaposi sarcoma, *Pneumocystis jiroveci infection*, etc). The CD4 count is stratified into three levels: >500, 200-500, and <200 cells/mm³.

Management

- Consists primarily of medications that target specific viral enzymes and comprises a treatment regimen known as highly active antiretroviral therapy (HAART).
- Initiated when CD4 count drops below 350 cells/mm³ or there is presence of an AIDS-defining illness.
- Five classes of drugs and treatment consist of a cocktail of three or four agents.
  (a) Nucleoside/nucleotide reverse transcriptase inhibitors (NRTIs)
  (b) Nonnucleoside reverse transcriptase inhibitors (NNRTIs)
  (c) Protease inhibitors (PI)
  (d) Entry inhibitors (EIs)
  (e) Integrase inhibitors

Epidemiology

- Approximately 33 million individuals worldwide have HIV, with over one million of those living in the United States.
- Up to 50% of immunosuppressed patients present with head and neck complaints. HIV and immunodeficiency may present in the salivary gland, aerodigestive tract, sinonasal cavity, temporal bone, or cervical lymph nodes.
- The head and neck manifestations of HIV present in four general categories of diseases:
  - (a) Infectious/inflammatory conditions as a result of immunodeficiency
  - (b) Complicated infection as a result of immunodeficiency
  - (c) Malignancy related to immunodeficiency
  - (d) AIDS-related illness

Infectious/Inflammatory Conditions Associated With HIV

Salivary Gland

- HIV may affect any of the salivary glands, but the parotid gland is the most common due to the presence of intraparotid lymph nodes.
- Salivary gland lesions are particularly prevalent in the pediatric population, representing up to 18% of the primary complaints that yield a diagnosis of HIV.
- The initial evaluation of the parotid gland should include a thorough history and head and neck physical examination.
- Parotid lesions are generally infectious, inflammatory, or neoplastic in nature.
- Parotid neoplasms can be further grouped as follows:
  - (a) Primary lesions of the salivary gland itself (benign or malignant)
  - (b) Primary tumors arising from the parotid lymph nodes
  - (c) Metastatic tumors to the parotid lymph nodes
- Specific differential diagnoses need consideration in the evaluation of the HIV positive patient. Benign lymphoepithelial cysts and diffuse infiltrative lymphocytosis are common benign etiologies of the salivary gland. When malignancy is suspected, the common malignancies seen in HIV-positive patients must be considered, particularly Kaposi sarcoma, lymphoma, and metastatic cutaneous malignancies.
- Diagnosis can be confirmed via fine needle aspiration in the majority of cases.
- Diagnostic imaging with U/S, CT, or MRI is useful when clinically indicated.
- Approximately 75% of parotid lesions are benign lymphoepithelial cysts. About 6% represent neoplasms and the remainder consists of infectious/inflammatory processes.

Benign Lymphoepithelial Cyst

- The most common parotid gland lesions seen in HIV-positive patients.
- Etiology is related to viral inflammation.
- May present as unilateral lesions but imaging often reveals subclinical disease bilaterally. Benign lymphoepithelial cyst (BLECs) are bilateral in up to 80% of cases.
- Typically present asymptomatically, though compression of the parotid ducts from the cysts can cause pain and sialadenitis.
- Cervical lymphadenopathy is present in up to 90% of cases.
- BLEC may be confused for papillary cystadenoma lymphomatosum (Warthin tumor)– both are cystic and bilateral.

Management
- No definitive surgical excision is required for BLEC.
- Treatment goals consist of decreasing the viral load with use of HAART, which causes regression of the cysts.
- Options include the following:
  - (a) Serial aspiration for cosmesis.
  - (b) Sclerotherapy with doxycycline injections has also been described.
  - (c) Parotidectomy is typically reserved for large, disfiguring lesions or if malignancy is suspected.

Diffuse Infiltrative Lymphocytosis Syndrome
- Clinically similar to Sjogren syndrome seen in HIV-positive patients.
- Incidence is approximately 1% of HIV patients.
- *Clinical presentation*: Diffuse parotid enlargement and sicca symptoms (ie, xerostomia and xerophthalmia).
- Associated with interstitial lymphocytic pneumonitis in 50% of cases.
- Histologically, diffuse infiltrative lymphocytosis syndrome is characterized by lymphocytic infiltration with CD8 lymphocytes (vs CD4 in Sjogren syndrome).

Management
- Primarily symptom control with salivary substitutes and sialogogues.
- As with other causes of xerostomia, dental caries are a potential complication and referral to dentistry is warranted.

Oral Cavity

- Common amongst patients with HIV.
- The immunodeficiency caused by HIV results in opportunistic infections and inflammatory conditions. Many of these have a strong association with HIV.
- The incidence of oral cavity lesions has decreased in the HAART era, with reductions of 10% to 50% reported. However, HIV patients presenting with oral cavity lesions continue to exist, especially in patients who have had longstanding HIV infection. Moreover, this population is expected to grow as HIV-related mortality decreases.
- Due to the increased risk of malignancy in these patients, index of suspicion must remain high and nonresolving or suspicious lesions should be biopsied.

Oral Candidiasis
- Oral candidiasis is the most common oral cavity lesion seen in HIV/AIDS, though incidence has decreased since the introduction of HAART.
- The most common causative organism is *Candida albicans*.
- There are four types of oral candida:
  - (a) *Pseudomembranous (aka oral thrush)*: Most common type, presents as white curd-like plaques that can be scraped off with a tongue depressor. The underlying mucosa is erythematous and occasionally raw.
  - (b) *Atrophic (aka erythematous candidiasis)*: The mucosa is erythematous, with loss of tongue papillations.
  - (c) *Angular chelitis*: Involvement of the oral commissure, with cracking, ulceration, and pseudomembranous formation.
  - (d) *Hyperplastic*: The rarest type, often involving the buccal mucosa, presents as thick white plaque that cannot be scraped off.
- The diagnosis is confirmed by potassium hydroxide preparation or by periodic acid-Schiff stain.

Management

- CD4 count >200 cells/mm^3, topical antifungals such as nystatin mouthwash can be used.
- CD4 count <200 cells/mm^3, systemic antifungals such as fluconazole are recommended.
- HIV patients are at risk of developing fluconazole-resistant candidiasis following repeated courses of treatment.

Oral Histoplasmosis

- Histoplasmosis is a fungal infection caused by *Histoplasma capsulatum* and is an AIDS-defining illness.
- Histoplasmosis classically affects the lungs and in the United States is endemic to areas surrounding the Ohio River valley.
- Presence of oral histoplasmosis in a previously healthy individual should prompt HIV testing.
- *Clinical presentation*: Painful, erythematous mucosa, which progresses to granulomatous lesions with or without pseudomembrane formation. Enlarged cervical lymph nodes may also be present.
- Diagnosis is confirmed through biopsy of the lesion for fungal culture.

Management

- Management is based on severity of illness and degree of systemic involvement.
- Treatment consists of a course of systemic antifungals, such as amphotericin B or itraconazole.

Oral Hairy Leukoplakia

- As the name suggests, oral hairy leukoplakia (OHL) is a white, corrugated, hyperkeratotic lesion, which most commonly affects the lateral tongue.
- The lesions are asymptomatic.
- Ebstein-Barr virus (EBV) is the causative agent and presence of EBV in the biopsy sample confirms the diagnosis.
- OHL has a strong association with HIV infection and its presence in a previously healthy individual should warrant workup for HIV.

Management

- OHL does not require any specific management, as it does not harbor malignant transformation potential.
- However, one must be mindful that the differential diagnosis for OHL includes lichen planus, idiopathic leukoplakia, and carcinoma in situ and thus observation is required for evolution.

Gingival and Periodontal Disease

- The pathogenesis is hypothesized to be related to a combination of altered/decreased immune response and bacterial/fungal overgrowth.
- Gingival disease, especially when necrotizing or ulcerative, is highly suggestive of HIV infection.
- Presentation in a previously healthy patient should warrant serologic testing for HIV.
- Periodontal disease in HIV is staged as follows:
    (a) *Linear gingival erythema*: Fiery red band of marginal gingiva that is out of proportion with the degree of dental plaque. These areas are prone to hemorrhage and persist despite removal of dental plaque.
    (b) *Necrotizing ulcerative gingivitis/periodontitis/stomatitis*: Spectrum of the same pathology. Characterized by progressive recession of the gingiva and associated bleeding, tissue sloughing, pain, malodor, and loss of the interdental papillae.

- Investigations should include dental roentographs and/or CT to assess the extent of alveolar resorption.
- When the degree of bony destruction is out of proportion with the amount of mucosal injury, malignant neoplasms and bacillary angiomatosis must be considered. Biopsy should be taken for histopathologic and microbiologic analysis.

Management

- Initial management consists of topical therapy to cover bacterial and fungal etiologies, such as chlorhexidine and nystatin mouthwash.
- Dentistry referral should be made to manage the periodontal disease.
- Frankly necrotic tissue requires debridement.
- Failure of topical management may necessitate the use of oral or parenteral antimicrobial therapy.

Complicated Infections as a Result of HIV

- Like immunocompetent individuals, patients with HIV also have a high incidence of sinonasal and otologic infections.
- The microbiology of these infections is similar to immunocompetent patients, with the most common organisms represented by *Streptococcus pneumoniae, Haemophilus influenzae, and Moraxella catarrhalis*.
- For patients with relatively normal CD4 counts (> 200 cells/mm^3), the management of these infections is no different from that of an immunocompetent patient.
- AIDS patients are at risk of developing complicated infections of the middle ear, temporal bone, and paranasal sinuses from opportunistic organisms. Furthermore, infections in the immunosuppressed patient have a propensity for perineural and perivascular spread.
- Must maintain a high clinical suspicion for severe head and neck infections such as malignant otitis externa and invasive fungal sinusitis.

HIV-associated Malignancies

- HIV-associated malignancies are categorized into AIDS-defining and non-AIDS defining.
- In the era of HAART, the incidence of AIDS-defining malignancies has been declining. However, several other malignancies, including cancers of the lung, liver, kidney, anus, and head and neck have been on the rise.

Kaposi Sarcoma

- Kaposi sarcoma (KS) is an angioproliferative tumor commonly associated with HIV infection.
- Caused by human herpes virus 8 (HHV8).
- The incidence of KS in HIV patients is approximately 5%.
- There are four epidemiologically distinct clinical variants of KS.
  (a) AIDS-associated KS
  (b) Classic KS (seen in Mediterranean and Easter European populations)

        (c) Endemic KS (common in Africa)

        (d) Transplant-related KS

Clinical Presentation

- AIDS-associated KS frequently presents in the head and neck in as many as 70% of cases.
- Presentation can be variable based on the site of the lesion.
- The lesions can also range from being relatively indolent to aggressive.
- KS in AIDS patients commonly presents in the oral cavity, with the most frequent subsites consisting of the hard palate, gingiva, and tongue. These mucosal lesions may be associated with pain, ulceration, bleeding, and loose teeth. Gingival lesions resemble and may be misdiagnosed for cyclosporine-associated gingival hyperplasia.
- Cutaneous KS presents as a maculopapular violaceous lesion that does not blanche.

Workup

- Diagnosis is confirmed with biopsy and histopathologic analysis, which demonstrates slit-like vascular channels, extravasated erythrocytes, and spindle cell proliferation.
- Initial evaluation should aim to identify other mucosal, cutaneous, or visceral lesions. Visceral KS has been shown to be present in up to 25% of AIDS patients, and commonly present in the GI tract, liver, spleen, and lungs.
- Immune status and CD4 count should be investigated.

Management

- There is currently no curative treatment for KS. While the natural history of KS is quite variable, patients inevitably succumb to complications and conditions related to their immunosuppression.
- The primary management goal in KS is to successfully treat the underlying cause. This can cause regression of the lesions.
- The role for surgery in KS is palliative.
- Other options for controlling lesions include external beam radiation, cryotherapy, laser excision, intralesional chemotherapy, and systemic chemotherapy.

Lymphoma

- Both non-Hodgkin lymphoma (NHL) and Hodgkin lymphoma (HL) occur at an increased frequency in HIV patients.
- Lymphomas are the second most common malignancy seen in HIV patients, with an incidence of up to 19%.
- Lymphoma in immunocompromised patients is commonly associated with Ebstein-Barr Virus (EBV, also known as human herpes virus 5) and the same is true of HIV-associated lymphomas.
- EBV is detected in up to 50% of HIV-associated lymphoma cases.

Clinical Presentation

- Symptoms are consistent with lymphoma of other etiologies and include B symptoms (fever, night sweats, unexplained weight loss of greater than 10% body mass) as well as enlarging lymph nodes. Depending on the location of the mass, compressive symptoms may also be a presenting complaint.
- HIV-associated lymphoma also presents frequently in the head and neck, as with lymphoma seen in immunocompetent patients.
- HIV-associated lymphoma tends to present at a later stage.
- Furthermore, many AIDS-related illnesses are directly related to decreasing CD4 count; this is, however, *not* the case with lymphoma (particularly Burkitt lymphoma).

Workup

- Fine needle aspiration biopsy may be used to confirm the diagnosis, but open biopsy is preferable, as it is typically required to identify the specific type of lymphoma.
- Cross-sectional imaging of the body is required for staging. Positron emission tomography has also been used for staging.

WHO Classification for AIDS-Related Lymphoma

A. Occurring in immunocompetent patients (Burkitt, diffuse large B cell, immunoblastic, anaplastic)

B. Occurring specifically in HIV-positive patients (primary effusion lymphoma and plasmablastic lymphoma)

C. Also occur in other immunodeficiency states (posttransplantation lymphoproliferative disorder-like B cell lymphoma associated with HIV)

Management

- The fundamentals of managing HIV-associated lymphoma are eradication of the malignant cells while minimizing further immunosuppression.
- The standard treatment consists primarily of chemotherapy with concurrent HAART.
- External beam radiotherapy is also used for locoregional control and palliation.
- Targeted therapies such as rituximab (an anti-CD20 monoclonal antibody) are currently being investigated for their role in treatment of HIV-associated lymphoma.
- Poor prognosis is associated with age (> 60 years), advanced stage, elevated serum lactate dehydrogenase, poor performance status, and more than one extranodal metastasis.
- The outcomes have improved in the HAART era, with 3-year overall survival approaching 50% for all comers.

Burkitt Lymphoma

- Burkitt lymphoma is a type of B-cell lymphoma that was originally described in Ugandan children in the 1950s. This disease commonly presented as a tumor.
- It is the fastest growing tumor in humans, with a doubling time of 24 to 48 hours.
- WHO Classification of Burkitt lymphoma:
  (a) Endemic
  (b) Sporadic (in areas where malaria is not present)
  (c) Immunodeficiency related
- HIV comprises the majority of immunodeficiency-related Burkitt lymphoma. EBV is isolated in about 40% of cases.
- The incidence of Burkitt lymphoma in HIV does not appear to correlate with low CD4 counts.
- The clinical presentation differs from that of the endemic form. It rarely presents as a jaw lesion and more commonly presents as a mass elsewhere in the head and neck or in the abdomen.

Management

- HIV-associated Burkitt lymphoma is treated with a combination of high-dose chemotherapy and HAART.
- The prognosis is dependent on the age of the patient. A series of adult HIV patients treated in this manner achieved a remission rate of 70% and a 2-year overall survival of 47%.

Plasmablastic Lymphoma

- Plasmablastic lymphoma (PBL) is a rare variant of diffuse large B-cell lymphoma.
- It is only a relatively newly recognized entity, being first described in 1997. Because of this, it has been described almost exclusively in case reports and series.
- Classically, it is associated with HIV and immunodeficiency states.
- It is not associated with EBV or HHV8 infection.
- The diagnosis of plasmablastic lymphoma should warrant subsequent investigation of HIV status.

Clinical Presentation

- The majority of cases, particularly in HIV positive patients, presents as lesions in the oral cavity, although other sites have also been involved.
- Extra-oral PBL is seen more frequently in HIV-negative patients and is more likely to be advanced stage at presentation.
- The prognosis is poor, as patients tend to recur despite aggressive chemotherapy. No 5-year survival data has been reported but analysis case reports suggest 50% to 60% disease-related mortality within the first 12 months of diagnosis.

Hodgkin Lymphoma

- Hodgkin lymphoma is the most common non-AIDS defining malignancy seen in HIV-positive patients and presents distinctively in comparison to immunocompetent/HIV-negative individuals.
- Diagnosis is confirmed histopathologically by the presence of Reed-Sternberg cells.
- Four types
  (a) Nodular sclerosing
  (b) Mixed cellularity
  (c) Lymphocyte rich
  (d) Lymphocyte depleted
- Tends to present at a more advanced stage and with a less favorable histopathologic type, specifically mixed cellularity and lymphocyte-depleted types. (In contrast, the nodular sclerosing type is the most common in HIV-negative patients).
- Incidence has risen in the HAART era in contrast to other manifestations of HIV and low CD4 counts.
- The 5-year overall survival is 41%, which is considerably worse than HL seen in HIV-negative patients.

Nonmelanotic Skin Cancer

- Nonmelanotic cutaneous malignancies are more common in immunosuppressed patients and this is true of HIV patients as well.
- Additional risk factors for nonmelanotic skin cancer (NMSC) are the same as in immunocompetent patients (history of sun exposure, Fitzpatrick score, and family history of skin cancer).
- The most common NMSC in HIV patients is basal cell carcinoma.

Management

- The management of NMSC in HIV-positive patients is consistent with standard management for these malignancies and includes wide local excision, removal of the draining lymph node basins, and adjuvant therapy based on the presenting tumor and stage.
- HIV-positive patients have a worse prognosis in comparison to immunocompetent patients. Thus, vigilant screening for new lesions is required.

AIDS-defining Illness

- In the early 1990s, the CDC devised a list of illnesses that, in the presence of HIV infection, confirms the diagnosis of AIDS.
- These illnesses consist of opportunistic infections and immunodeficiency-associated malignancies.
- It is important to note that each illness in itself is not specific to HIV/AIDS.

Appendix A The World Health Organization Clinical Staging System for HIV

Clinical Stage 1 (Asymptomatic)
Asymptomatic
Persistent generalized lymphadenopathy

Clinical Stage 2 (Mild Symptoms)
Moderate unexplained weight loss (< 10% of presumed or measured body weight)
Recurrent respiratory tract infections, sinusitis, tonsillitis, otitis media, and pharyngitis)
Herpes zoster
Angular cheilitis
Recurrent oral ulceration
Papular pruritic eruptions
Seborrhoeic dermatitis
Fungal nail infections

Clinical Stage 3 (Advanced Symptoms)
Unexplained severe weight loss (> 10% of presumed or measured body weight)
Unexplained chronic diarrhea for longer than 1 month
Unexplained persistent fever (above 37.6°C intermittent or constant, for longer than 1 month)
Persistent oral candidiasis
Oral hairy leukoplakia
Pulmonary tuberculosis (current)
Severe bacterial infections (such as pneumonia, empyema, pyomyositis, bone or joint infection, meningitis or bacteremia)
Acute necrotizing ulcerative stomatitis, gingivitis, or periodontitis
Unexplained anaemia (< 8 g/dL), neutropenia (< 0.5×10^9/L), or chronic thrombocytopenia (< 50×10^9/L)

Clinical Stage 4 (Severe Symptoms)
HIV wasting syndrome
Pneumocystis pneumonia
Recurrent severe bacterial pneumonia
Chronic herpes simplex infection (orolabial, genital, or anorectal of >1-month duration or visceral at any site)
Esophageal candidiasis (or candidiasis of trachea, bronchi, or lungs)
Extrapulmonary tuberculosis
Kaposi sarcoma
Cytomegalovirus infection (retinitis or infection of other organs)

Central nervous system toxoplasmosis HIV encephalopathy
Extrapulmonary cryptococcosis including meningitis
Disseminated nontuberculous mycobacterial infection
Progressive multifocal leukoencephalopathy
Chronic cryptosporidiosis (with diarrhoea)
Chronic isosporiasis
Disseminated mycosis (coccidiomycosis or histoplasmosis)
Recurrent nontyphoidal *Salmonella* bacteremia
Lymphoma (cerebral or B-cell non-Hodgkin) or other solid HIV-associated tumors
Invasive cervical carcinoma
Atypical disseminated leishmaniasis
Symptomatic HIV-associated nephropathy or symptomatic HIV-associated cardiomyopathy

Appendix B AIDS-Defining Illnesses

- Bacterial infections, multiple or recurrent*
- Candidiasis of bronchi, trachea, or lungs
- Candidiasis of esophagus[†]
- Cervical cancer, invasive[§]
- Coccidioidomycosis, disseminated or extrapulmonary
- Cryptococcosis, extrapulmonary
- Cryptosporidiosis, chronic intestinal (> 1-month duration)
- Cytomegalovirus disease (other than liver, spleen, or nodes), onset at age >1 month
- Cytomegalovirus retinitis (with loss of vision)[†]
- Encephalopathy, HIV related
- Herpes simplex: chronic ulcers (> 1-month duration) or bronchitis, pneumonitis, or esophagitis (onset at age > 1 month)
- Histoplasmosis, disseminated or extrapulmonary
- Isosporiasis, chronic intestinal (> 1-month duration)
- Kaposi sarcoma[†]
- Lymphoid interstitial pneumonia or pulmonary lymphoid hyperplasia complex*[†]
- Lymphoma, Burkitt (or equivalent term)
- Lymphoma, immunoblastic (or equivalent term)
- Lymphoma, primary, of brain
- *Mycobacterium avium* complex or *Mycobacterium kansasii,* disseminated or extrapulmonary[†]
- *Mycobacterium tuberculosis* of any site, pulmonary[†§], disseminated[†], or extrapulmonary[†]
- *Mycobacterium*, other species or unidentified species, disseminated[†] or extrapulmonary[†]
- *Pneumocystis jirovecii* pneumonia[†]
- Pneumonia, recurrent[†§]

- Progressive multifocal leukoencephalopathy
- *Salmonella* septicemia, recurrent
- Toxoplasmosis of brain, onset at age > 1 month[†]
- Wasting syndrome attributed to HIV

[*]Only among children aged < 13 years. (CDC. 1994 revised classification system for human immunodeficiency virus infection in children < 13 years of age. *MMWR*. 1994;43[RR-12]: 1-10.)
[†]Condition that might be diagnosed presumptively.
[§]Only among adults and adolescents aged ≥13 years. (CDC. 1993 revised classification system for HIV infection and expanded surveillance case definition for AIDS among adolescents and adults. *MMWR*. 1992;41[RR-17]: 1-12.)

Bibliography

Antman K, Chang Y. Kaposi's Sarcoma. *New Eng J Med*. 2000;342:1027-1038.

Cooley TP. Non-AIDS-defining cancer in HIV-infected people. *Hematol Oncol Clin North*. 2003;17:889.

Marsot-Dupuch K, Quillard J, Meyohas MC. Head and neck lesions in the immunocompromised host. *Eur Radiol*. 2004;14:E155-E167.

Patton LL. Oral lesions associated with human immunodeficiency virus disease. *Dent Clin N Am*. 2013;57:673-698.

World Health Organization. *WHO Case Definitions of HIV for Surveillance and Revised Clinical Staging and Immunological Classification of HIV-Related Diseases in Adults and Children*. Switzerland: World Health Organization; 2007.

Questions

1. Which malignancy has the weakest association with HIV?
   A. Kaposi sarcoma
   B. Burkitt lymphoma
   C. Plasmablastic lymphoma
   D. Hodgkin lymphoma

2. Which is the most common type of oral candidiasis?
   A. Pseudomembranous
   B. Atrophic
   C. Erythematous
   D. Hyperplastic

3. Which is generally not considered a treatment option for benign lymphoepithelial cysts?
   A. HAART
   B. Serial needle aspiration
   C. Sclerotherapy
   D. Surgical excision

4. Which diagnosis does not require subsequent investigation into HIV status?
   A. Oral histoplasmosis
   B. Oral hairy leukoplakia
   C. Necrotizing gingivostomatitis
   D. Oral candidiasis

5. HIV can be transmitted through all of the following except:
   A. Blood
   B. Semen
   C. Saliva
   D. Vaginal fluid
   E. Breast milk

Chapter 12
Granulomatous Diseases of the Head and Neck

Overview

- What is a granuloma?/Histology
  - (a) A granuloma is created by a chronic immunologic process mediated by monocytes and macrophages. Macrophages can give rise to epithelioid cells which can secrete extracellular enzymes. Multinucleated giant cells are often found in granulomas and are thought to arise from the fusion of macrophages.
  - (b) These cells are surrounded by lymphocytes and eosinophils.
  - (c) A granuloma is complete with a fibroblastic proliferation occurring around the cells.
- What is the differential diagnosis of a granuloma in the head and neck?
  - (a) There is a significant range of symptoms caused by granulomatous diseases, not limited to the head and neck. A full history and physical examination should be considered for all patients with a granulomatous biopsy.

Differential Diagnosis

See Table 12-1.

Autoimmune

Granulomatosis With Polyangiitis (GPA, Renamed From Wegener Granulomatosis)
- Small and medium-vessel vasculitis.
- Belongs to a larger group of necrotizing vasculopathy syndromes, all of which involve an autoimmune attack by abnormal circulating ANCA antibodies (anti-neutrophil cytoplasmic antibodies).
- Initially named after Friedrich Wegener, a German pathologist whose Nazi past was discovered, leading to the eponym being abandoned and renaming in 2011.

Incidence/Epidemiology
- Cause unknown.
- 10 to 20 cases per million per year.
- 5-year survival is over 80% with adequate treatment.
- Commonly occurs in whites, in third to fifth decades.

Table 12-1 Differential Diagnosis: Granulomatous Diseases of the Head and Neck

Autoimmune	Unknown origin	Neoplastic	Infectious	Fungal/parasitic	Congenital
Granulomatosis with polyangiitis	Sarcoidosis	Langerhan histiocytosis	Cat scratch disease	Histoplasmosis	Chediak-Higashi syndrome
Churg-Strauss (eosinophilic granulomatosis with polyangiitis)		Eosinophilic granulomatosis	Rhinoscleroma	Blastomycosis	Job syndrome
Relapsing polychondritis		Han-Schuller-Christian disease	Leprosy	Rhinosporidiosis	
Systemic lupus erythematous		Letterer-Siwe disease	Nontuberculous mycobacteria		
Behcet disease		Fibrous histiocytoma	Tuberculosis		
		Lobular capillary hemangioma	Actinomycosis		
			Syphilis		

Presentation
- Extremely variable.
- *Classic triad*: Airway necrotizing granulomas, systemic vasculitis, and focal glomerulonephritis.
- Most common presenting symptom is rhinitis.
- *Renal*: Rapidly progressive glomerulonephritis (75%).
- *Sinonasal*: Nasal congestion, crusting, rhinitis, epistaxis, septal perforation, and possible saddle nose deformity.
- *Otologic*: Conductive hearing loss from Eustachian tube dysfunction, possible sensorineural hearing loss.
- *Oral cavity*: Gingivitis, tooth decay, nonspecific ulcerations.
- *Ocular*: Pseudotumors, conjunctivitis, scleritis, episcleritis, uveitis.
- Subglottic stenosis.
- *Pulmonary*: Cavitary lesions, nodules, infiltrates, pulmonary hemorrhage.

Histology
- Characteristic patchy necrosis surrounded by giant cells, causing necrotizing granuloma formation in nonspecific inflammatory background
- Macrophages, inflammatory cells and giant cells
- A true vasculitis, demonstrating granulomatous inflammation of vessel wall in arteries and veins

Workup/Diagnosis
- cANCA (cytoplasmic staining ANCAs) that react with proteinase are associated with Wegener but are not definitely sensitive or specific.
- Elevated erythrocyte sedimentation rate (ESR) and C-reactive protein (CRP).

- Anemia, CXR, urine sediment.
- Must have tissue biopsy.

Treatment
- Induce remission with cyclophosphamide or rituximab in addition to high-dose corticosteroids.
- Maintenance with less toxic immunosuppressant therapy, such as methotrexate, azathioprine, leflunomide, or mycophenolate mofetil. Trimethoprim/sulfamethoxazole may help prevent relapse.

Churg-Strauss (Eosinophilic Granulomatosis With Polyangiitis [EGPA])
- Allergic, granulomatous, small and medium-vessel vasculitis
- Necrotizing vasculopathy syndrome, in same group as GPA

Presentation
- Extremely variable.
- *Classic triad*: Asthma, systemic vasculitis, eosinophilia.
- Occurs in patients with history of airway allergic hypersensitivity, with asthma developing 3 to 9 years prior to onset of other signs and symptoms.
- 70% have nasal involvement (allergic rhinitis, polyps, obstruction, rhinorrhea, crusting).
- Usually manifests in three stages:
  - (a) *Allergic stage*: Prodromal, allergic rhinitis and asthma, polyps, nasal obstruction
  - (b) *Eosinophilic stage (aka Loeffler syndrome)*: Hypereosinophilia causes damage to respiratory and GI tracts, may experience weight loss, night sweats, asthma, cough, abdominal pain, GI bleeding
  - (c) *Vasculitic stage*: Inflammation of vessels causes decreased perfusion of tissues and organs, may be severe and life-threatening. May develop thrombi, peritonitis or perforation, or heart disease

Histology
- Fibrinoid, epithelioid, and eosinophilic extravascular granulomas with necrosis

Workup/Diagnosis
- Associated with pANCA (perinuclear anti-neutrophil cytoplasmic antibodies that bind myeloperoxidase), positive in 50%
- Elevated eosinophils and granulomas in affected tissues
- American College of Rheumatology Criteria (1990); require 4/6
  - (a) Asthma
  - (b) Eosinophils > 10% of complete blood count with differential
  - (c) Mononeuropathy or polyneuropathy
  - (d) Nonfixed pulmonary infiltrates
  - (e) Paranasal sinus abnormalities
  - (f) Histological evidence of extravascular eosinophils

Treatment
- High-dose corticosteroids and immunosuppressive agents such as azathioprine or cyclophosphamide are the mainstays of treatment.

Relapsing Polychondritis
- Rare disorder characterized by episodic recurrent inflammation and deterioration of cartilage and tissues containing glycosaminoglycans; eventually replaced by granulation and fibrosis

Incidence/ Epidemiology
- Often presents in fifth or sixth decades, and no gender predilection

Presentation
- Recurrent episodes of sudden, painful chondritis that resolve within 7 days.
- Nasal chondritis 15%.
- Auricular chondritis 50%, and "Lobule sparing."
- Nonerosive polyarthritis 50%.
- Respiratory tract chondritis 15%.
- Ocular inflammation 15%.
- Sequelae can include saddle nose deformity, auricular deformity, collapse of laryngotracheal cartilage framework and airway compromise, visual disturbance.
- Often presents with other autoimmune disorders.

Histology
- Inflammatory cells infiltrate perichondrium and are destructive.
- Gross appearance is nonspecific thickening of cartilages.

Workup/Diagnosis
- Elevated inflammatory markers (ESR or CRP) during disease activity
- Testing for autoantibodies to type II collagen, found only in cartilage
- McAdam criteria (6) most often used for clinical diagnosis
  - (a) Recurrent chondritis of both auricles
  - (b) Chondritis of nasal cartilages
  - (c) Laryngotracheal chondritis
  - (d) Nonerosive seronegative polyarthritis
  - (e) Ocular inflammation
  - (f) Cochleovestibular damage
- Grounds for diagnosis
  - (a) 3+ of 6 McAdam criteria alone
  - (b) 1+ criteria and histopathological confirmation with biopsy
  - (c) Chondritis in two or more separate anatomical locations with response to steroids and/or dapsone

Treatment
- Immunosuppressive agents, primarily corticosteroids.
- Colchicine, dapsone, nonsteroidal anti-inflammatory drugs (NSAIDs).
- Upper airway collapse may require tracheostomy.

Lupus

- Caused by deposition of antibodies and immune complexes, Type 3 hypersensitivity reaction

Incidence/Epidemiology
- Typically occurs in young, black female patients.
- Human leukocyte antigen DR2 (HLA-DR2) and DR3 have genetic predisposition.

Presentation
- Three subtypes.
- *Discoid lupus erythematosus (DLE)*: Least aggressive type, only affecting superficial tissues. Oral or cutaneous erythematous plaque lesions, alopecia. May develop scarring.
- *Subacute cutaneous lupus (SCL)*: Papulosquamous lesions that do not scar; mild systemic involvement.
- *Systemic lupus erythematosus (SLE)*: The most severe form of lupus. Typically present with malar butterfly rash. Hoarseness and pain may result from laryngotracheal

perichondritis and true vocal fold thickening. May have nasal crusting, dryness, or septal perforation.

Workup/Diagnosis
- *DLE*: Clinical diagnosis alone (serology negative)
- *SCL*: Clinical diagnosis, inconsistent results from anti-nuclear antibodies (ANA), SS-A, and SS-B
- *SLE*: Nonspecific tests are typically positive and used to establish initial diagnosis (ANA, SS-A, SS-B). Specific markers include antidouble-stranded DNA (ds-DNA) and Sm Antigen (SmAg).
  - (a) ACR diagnostic criteria require 4/11 for SLE (acronym is "SOAP BRAIN MD"); **S**erositis, **O**ral ulcers, **A**rthritis, **P**ulmonary fibrosis, **B**lood cells, **R**aynaud/renal, **A**NA, **I**mmunologic (anti-Sm or anti-dsDNA), **N**europsychiatric, **M**alar rash, **D**iscoid rash

Treatment
- Typically consists of NSAIDs and corticosteroids.
- Other options include azathioprine, cyclophosphamide, and antimalarial agents such as hydroxychloroquine.

Behcet Disease

Presentation
- Recurrent aphthous ulcers on the oral mucosa and genitalia.
- Uveitis and ocular inflammation also present.
- May experience neurologic disease, brainstem or spinal cord involvement.
- Sensorineural hearing loss.
- Vasculitis; affects vessels of all sizes, even as large as pulmonary arterial.
- Venous thromboembolic events, arthritis, and renal and cardiac involvement are all possible.

Workup/Diagnosis
- Recurrent oral ulcers (three or more episodes per year) and two of genital ulcers, uveitis, skin lesions (erythema nodosum), or positive pathergy test

Treatment
- Interferon alpha-2a is effective in long-term treatment of severe uveitis.
- Steroid cream for topical treatment.
- Colchicine or Dapsone.
- Eye drops.

Idiopathic

Sarcoidosis

- Idiopathic, systemic noncaseasting granulomatous disease of unknown origin; commonly affects lungs and hilar lymph nodes and upper respiratory tract
- Most cases clear without treatment

Incidence/Epidemiology
- Predominates in females, third to fifth decades.
- 10 to 20 times more common in black patients in North America.

Presentation
- Often presents with hilar adenopathy on chest radiography or cervical adenopathy.
- 90% of patients have pulmonary involvement (hilar adenopathy, cough, dyspnea).
- Laryngeal sarcoid presents as supraglottic submucosal mass, usually in epiglottis, and possible with vocal cord paralysis.
- Sinonasal sarcoid may present with crusting, "cobblestone" mucosa, epistaxis, synechiae, stenosis, or cartilage destruction.
- Salivary gland involvement can range from asymptomatic parotid mass to "Heerfordt syndrome" or uveoparotid fever, an extrapulmonary manifestation of sarcoid consisting of uveitis, parotitis, fever, facial palsy, and sensorineural hearing loss.
- Cutaneous findings include erythema nodosum, Darier-Roussy (subcutaneous) nodules, and "lupus pernio."
- *Lupus pernio*: Chronic, red or purple indurated cutaneous plaques on nose, cheeks, ears, and hands that is pathognomonic for sarcoidosis.
- Cardiac arrhythmia, neuropathy, sensorineural hearing loss, renal and hepatic involvement may also be present.

Histology
- Discrete noncaseating, epitheliod granulomas
- Accumulation of T cells, mononuclear macrophages, and Langhans giant cells containing laminated mucopolysaccharide
- *Schaumann bodies*: Calcium and protein inclusion inside giant cells

Workup/Diagnosis
- *Lab*: Elevated angiotensin-converting enzyme (ACE) and urine/serum calcium levels are associated with sarcoidosis.
- Serum protein electrophoresis (SPEP) may show polyclonal gammopathy.
- Biopsy.
- *Stage 0*: No intrathoracic involvement; stage I: bilateral hilar adenopathy; stage II: pulmonary parenchyma involved; stage III: pulmonary infiltrates with fibrosis; stage IV: end-stage lung disease with fibrosis and honeycombing.

Treatment
- Most cases clear without medical treatment but may progress to long-term or even life-threatening disease.
- Average mortality rate is 5% in untreated cases.
- Usually treated with NSAID therapy.
- Corticosteroids can be used for exacerbations of pulmonary and sinonasal disease.
- Severe disease may be treated with azathioprine, methotrexate, or leflunomide.
- Sinonasal surgery may improve symptoms but recurrence likely.
- Supraglottic lesions monitored conservatively; surgery reserved for obstruction lesions.

Neoplastic

Langerhans Cell Histiocytosis
- Classification for this group of disease is not well established; previously referred to as "Histiocytosis X."
- Rare disorders involve clonal proliferation of Langerhans cells, which are epidermal macrophages or dendritic cells.

Incidence/Epidemiology
- Poor prognosis if presenting in young patients

Presentation
- Most commonly present as otitis media.
- Finding on nasal examination can include a mass, septal perforation, or epistaxis.

Histology
- Sheets of polygonal histiocytes
- Variable number of eosinophils, plasma cells, and lymphocytes
- Langerhans cell nucleus is pale and deeply grooved, and cytoplasm may demonstrate Birbeck granules on electron microscopy (tennis racket-shaped organelles with the nuclear cytoplasm)

Workup/Diagnosis
- Histological diagnosis by tissue biopsy
- Immunohistochemistry–CD1 positive, S100 positive

Treatment
- *Solitary lesion*: May be excised or treated with limited radiotherapy.
- *Multiple lesions*: Chemotherapy often employed, agents include alkylating compounds, antimetabolites, or vinca alkaloids. Can be combined with steroids.

Eosinophilic Granuloma

- Also known as pulmonary histiocytosis X or pulmonary Langerhans cell histiocytosis X

Incidence/Epidemiology
- Rare presentation, usually in third to fourth decade.
- Exposure to cigarette smoke is a potential risk factor.

Presentation
- Usually present in single organ, most commonly the lung.
- 4% to 20% have cystic lesions in bones and can be mono-ostotic or polyostotic.
- In the head and neck it can affect the temporal and frontal bones.
- May present with similar symptoms as acute mastoiditis, middle ear granulation tissue, tympanic membrane perforations, proptosis, and facial nerve paralysis.
- Other bones affected include femur, pelvis, vertebrae, and ribs.

Histology
- Parenchymal infiltration of lungs by activated Langerhans cells
- Normally found in skin, reticuloendothelial system, heart, pleura, and lungs
- Granulomas include Langerhan cells, eosinophils, lymphocytes, macrophages, plasma cells, fibroblasts

Workup/Diagnosis
- Histological diagnosis by tissue biopsy

Treatment
- Surgical curettage
- Radiation therapy for inaccessible lesions, recurrence in high-risk patients

Hand-Schuller-Christian Disease

Incidence/Epidemiology
- Children and young adults

Presentation
- Chronic disseminated form of Langerhan histiocytosis.
- More commonly polyostotic.
- Classic presentation in the head and neck include: skull lesions, exophthalmos, diabetes insipidus from erosion of sella turcica. This occurs in approximately 10% of cases.

Treatment
- Surgical excision, chemotherapy and/or radiation therapy
- Mortality rate approximately 30%

Letterer-Siwe Disease

Incidence/Epidemiology
- Infants and young children (< 3 years) mostly affected

Presentation
- Acute and disseminated form for Langerhan histiocytosis
- Rapidly progressive
- Usually extra-skeletal bony lesions
- Fever, proptosis, adenopathy, splenomegaly, hepatomegaly, dermatitis

Treatment
- Radiation and chemotherapy in combination
- Uniformly fatal

Fibrous Histiocytoma

Incidence/Epidemiology
- Males
- Occurring at any age

Presentation
- Slow growing, painless mass.
- Commonly found in sun-exposed skin and orbital tissues in dermis and hypodermis.
- In the head and neck can be found in aerodigestive tract, salivary glands, layers of the scalp and face.
- Nasal obstruction, epistaxis, dysphagia, and dyspnea, most commonly.
- Metastasis is rare.
- One-third of patients present with multiple lesions.

Histology
- Fibroblasts and histiocytes
- Spindle-shaped cells with elongated nuclei in cartwheel pattern
- May demonstrate a degree of atypia and mitotic activity

Treatment
- Local excision with clear margins

Lobular Capillary Hemangioma

- Also known as pyogenic granuloma

Incidence/Epidemiology
- Prepubescent males, post-pubescent females, pregnancy
- Can be related to trauma and local irritation

Presentation
- Painless, friable, benign lesion
- Can occur anywhere in the head and neck region commonly in the oral cavity including gingiva, lips, and tongue but also the face and nasal cavity
- May present with epistaxis
- Usually hormone responsive

Histology
- Capillaries arranged in lobules

Treatment
- If pregnancy related, it will resolve.
- Surgical excision, electrocautery or laser.
- Recurrence can occur if incompletely excised.

Infectious

Cat Scratch Disease

Incidence/Epidemiology
- Caused by *Bartonella henselae*an intercellular, pleomorphic, gram-negative bacteria
- Often seen in children

Presentation
- Patients have a history of cat exposure (scratch or bite).
- Tender adenopathy occurring within 3 to 14 days in the region of exposure (axillary, cervical, or submandibular).
- May or may not present with a vesicle or pustule at site of scratch within a week.
- *Parinaud oculoglandular syndrome*: Occurrence of granuloma on the eye after contact with cornea after cat exposure (petting) with or without regional lymphadenopathy.
- In rare cases, course of infection may be complicated by liver, spleen, bone marrow, lower respiratory involvement, and CNS involvement.
- *Bacillary angiomatosis*: May occur in patients with HIV. It is caused by *B henselae* or *B quintana*. Patients present with cutaneous papules and subcutaneous nodules or on mucous membranes. Other organs such as the spleen, bone, and liver may be affected.

Histology
- Necrotizing granulomatous lymphadenitis with stellate microabscesses will be seen on biopsy.
- *Bacillary angiomatosis*: Ectatic vessels lined by plump endothelial cells with pleomorphism and mitotic activity.

Workup/Diagnosis
- (1) History of cat exposure with (2) presence of inoculation site and (3) lymphadenopathy; (4) Warthin-Starry silver stain will show intracellular, gram-negative bacteria (will turn black or brown); (5) Excisional biopsy showing suppurative and granulomatous lymphadenitis.
- Polymerase chain reaction (PCR) may confirm presence of bacteria.
- Enzyme-linked immunosorbent assay can be used for detecting early antibodies to the bacteria.

Treatment
- Usually self-limited, supportive treatment.
- Azithromycin, rifampin, or trimethoprim-sulfamethoxazole may be used in immunocompromised patients.
- Bacillary angiomatosis should be treated as this disease is progressive and fatal.

Rhinoscleroma

Incidence/Epidemiology
- Caused by *Klebsiella rhinoscleromatis*, a gram-negative bacterium
- Seen most commonly in the Middle East, Latin America, and Eastern Europe

Presentation
- 3 stages over years:
  - (a) *First stage*: Catarrhal; purulent rhinorrhea, honeycombed crusting. This stage may last weeks to months.
  - (b) *Second stage*: Granulomatous or hypertrophic stage; granulomatous nodules on head and neck, most commonly glottis and subglottis. Can lead to bleeding and cartilage destruction.
  - (c) *Third stage*: Cicatricial; fibrotic reaction that may stenose the nasal cavity, larynx, or tracheobronchial tree
- Usually involves the nose and paranasal sinuses but also larynx, ear, and trachea

Histology
- Pseudoepitheliomatous hyperplasia
- Presence of Russell bodies (birefringent inclusions found in eosinophilic plasma cells) and Mikulicz cells (multinucleated macrophages containing bacteria and foamy cytoplasm)

Workup/Diagnosis
- Clinical diagnosis based on presence of honeycomb crusting in the nose.
- Diagnosis is usually made in the granulomatous stage.

Treatment
- Debridement
- Long-term streptomycin or tetracycline
- Dilatation for stenosis

Leprosy

Incidence/Epidemiology
- Caused by *Mycobacterium leprae*: Obligate intracellular parasitic, acid-fast bacillus

Presentation
- Slow evolution of bacterial infection.
- Bacteria are thermolabile and grow optimally at 27°C to 33°C.
- Common areas of infection include cold peripheral tissues including fingers, nose, testicles, feet, and earlobes.
- Patients present with loss of peripheral sensation.
- Skin lesions can be hypopigmented or erythematous macules; eyebrow and eyelash loss can also occur.
- Early symptoms may include nasal and paranasal sinus involvement including saddle nose deformity, epistaxis, and nasal congestion.
- Late symptoms may include CNS (nerve paralysis), eye (pain, photophobia, glaucoma, blindness), laryngeal (stridor, hoarseness, ulceration) involvement.

Workup/Diagnosis
- Biopsy is required for diagnosis.
- PCR may be performed on nasal smears, skin biopsy, and blood specimens.

Treatment
- Long-term dapsone alone or in combination with clofazimine and rifampin

Nontuberculous Mycobacteria

Incidence/Epidemiology
- Caused by *Mycobacterium avium-intracellulare* complex, *M scrofulaceum, M kansasii, M fortuitum,* and *M bohemicum.*
- It is the most common cause of non-TB infection in children; *M scrofulaceum* is the most common cause of lymphadenitis in children younger than 6 years.

- It is transmitted via oral or ocular contact with soil as they are ubiquitous in the environment.
- Strains of bacteria are often less virulent than *M tuberculosis.*

Presentation
- Patients present with corneal ulceration, cervical lymphadenopathy, and possibly mastoiditis.
- Adenitis is slow growing in the submandibular or periauricular region without systemic signs of infection.
- This mass is often nontender and does not respond to antibiotics.
- It may cause overlying skin changes or spontaneous fistulalization.

Work up/Diagnosis
- Stains for acid-fast are only positive in 20% to 50% of patients.
- Diagnosis is typically suggested by clinical course and physical findings.

Treatment
- Excision of lymph node.
- Recurrence may occur with incision and drainage.

Tuberculosis

Incidence/Epidemiology
- Caused by *Mycobacterium tuberculosis*: acid-fast positive bacillus
- Inhaled into lungs and rarely affected head and neck
- Common in areas where AIDS is prevalent
- Inner city African American and Hispanic males, 25 to 35 years of age

Presentation
- Most common head and neck presentation is cervical lymphadenopathy.
- Nodes are firm, matted, bilateral, and nontender.
- Nodes are most commonly found in the posterior triangle and supraclavicular area.
- Can also present in the larynx, typically in the posterior glottis as granulation and ulceration cause hoarseness, odynophagia, dysphagia and stridor.
- Laryngeal involvement can present with edema, hyperemia, nodularity, ulcerations, and obliteration of anatomic landmarks.
- Epiglottis can become characteristically turban shaped.
- Otologic manifestation includes painless, odorless, watery to thick cheesy otorrhea with multiple, small tympanic membrane perforations.
- Ossicular chain may or may not be eroded by granulation tissue.
- Other manifestations include septal perforation, involved salivary gland, and tonsillar tissue.

Workup/Diagnosis
- Purified protein derivative test (positive if 15-mm or larger induration).
- Chest X-ray or chest CT.
- PCR of sputum or cultures or biopsy can also be diagnostic.
- Consider excisional biopsy if others tests are negative.

Treatment
- Respiratory isolation should be started.
- Consider contacting the local public health department.
- Isoniazid, rifampin, pyrazinamide, and ethambutol for 2 months, followed by repeat smear and culture to determine remainder of treatment course which can last for up to 9 months.
- *En bloc* lymph node excision may be needed for chronically draining nodes.

Actinomycosis

Incidence/Epidemiology
- Caused by *Actinomyces* species, most commonly *Actinomyces israelii* in humans-branching, filamentous anaerobic rods

Presentation
- Chronic granulomatous and suppurative disease.
- Results most commonly following dental manipulation, trauma, or infection.
- 50% have head and neck or cervicofacial manifestation is consistent with a mass.
- May also present in the thorax, abdomen, or pelvis.
- In the head and neck it can present as a mass in the sinuses, mastoid, major salivary glands, and thyroid.
- Mass often have purple discoloration to overlying skin and may spontaneously fistualize.
- Mass is slow growing or may present rapidly as a suppurative infection and abscess formation.

Histology
- Multifilamented, anaerobic.
- Sulfur granules can be present and represent neutrophils and organisms.

Treatment
- Surgical debridement.
- IV penicillin G for 2 to 6 weeks followed by 6 to 12 months of oral penicillin.
- Tetracycline or clindamycin is used in penicillin-allergic patients.

Syphilis

Incidence/Epidemiology
- Caused by *Treponema pallidum*-spirochete
  - (a) *Primary stage:* Presents with a painless chancre at inoculation site approximately 3 weeks after exposure.
  - (b) *Second stage*: Contagious stage approximately 4 to 10 weeks after primary lesion. General malaise, fever, arthralgias, and skin and mucosal lesions.
  - (c) One-third remain latent, one-third go into remission, one-third progress to tertiary syphilis. The latent phase may last up to 30 years.
  - (d) *Tertiary stage*: May occur years after infection, may involve CNS (neurosyphilis), major vessels (aortitis) or produce gumma in various places including the temporal bone.
- Spreads via sexual transmission

Presentation
- Gumma are inflammatory granulomas with an intervening zone of epithelioid and multinucleate cells and a peripheral zone with fibroblasts and capillaries.
- Gumma develop in bone, skin, and the liver.
- Head and neck symptoms include generalized lymphadenopathy, laryngitis, vocal fold paralysis, dysphasia, and oral ulcers.
- Granulomas may also be found in the oral cavity and nasal cavity.
- Septal perforation can be found in the bony septum.
- May cause fluctuating high-frequency sensorineural hearing loss, tinnitus, and vertigo (otosyphilis). Hearing loss may progress to profound levels. Patients may present with a positive Hennebert sign and may exhibit Tulio phenomenon.

Histology
- Dense chronic inflammation with many plasma cells.

Workup/Diagnosis
- Serologic tests such as rapid plasma reagin (RPR) on serum or Venereal Disease Research Laboratory (VDRL) on cerebrospinal fluid (CSF) can be sensitive for screening patients. Seroreactivity can correlate with disease progression.
- Specific fluorescent treponemal antibody absorption (FTA-ABS) testing.
- Direct visualization of spirochetes through dark-field examination.

Treatment
- IM Benzathine penicillin, one dose is used for early syphilis; three weekly injections are used to treat late latent stage syphilis; 10 to 14 days of IV penicillin is recommended for treatment of tertiary syphilis.
- Steroids if otologic symptoms present.
- Cases should be reported to the public health department.

Fungal

Histoplasmosis

Incidence/Epidemiology
- Caused by *Histoplasma capsulatum,* a dimorphic fungus found in the Ohio and Mississippi River Valleys
- Airborne transmission of avian or bat droppings

Presentation
- Will affect those immunocompromised patients.
- Presents with painful ulceration of the lips, gingiva, tongue, pharynx, and larynx in the head and neck.
- Sore throat, painful mastication, hoarseness, gingival irritation, and weight loss can be experienced by patients.
- Pulmonary histoplasmosis may present with acute pneumonitis and mediastinal lymphadenopathy.
- The disease may progress to involve the heart and CNS.

Workup/Diagnosis
- Cultures are performed on Sabouraud medium.
- Skin testing.
- Complement fixation.
- Latex agglutination.
- Urine antigen detection via complement fixation.

Treatment
- Itraconazole is used for the treatment of mild disease.
- Amphotericin B is used for severe disease including CNS involvement.

Blastomycosis

Incidence/Epidemiology
- Caused by *Blastomyces dermatitidis* endemic to central United States and southern parts of the Canadian prairie provinces.
- This organism is inhaled in soil dust or in old homes.

Presentation
- Patients may be asymptomatic.
- Triad of symptoms are cutaneous disease, pulmonary involvement, and constitutional symptoms in immunocompromised patients.

- Genitourinary symptoms may also be present.
- Skin lesions are commonly found on the face and limbs and are initially verrucous with scarring.
- Rarely can blastomycosis present in the larynx, parotid, and paranasal sinuses.

Histology
- Pseudoepitheliomatous hyperplasia
- Single birefringent, broad-based bud

Workup/Diagnosis
- Sputum culture on Sabouraud medium
- Urine antigen detection tests
- Enzymatic and antigenmediated radioimmunoassay can be used for diagnosis.

Treatment
- Itraconazole is the general treatment option.
- Amphotericin B is used for immunocompromised patients or those with CNS involvement.

Rhinosporidiosis

Incidence/Epidemiology
- Caused by *Rhinosporidium seeberi*, a parasite found in southern India
- Spread by contaminated water

Presentation
- Painless, wart-like lesions on mucous membranes of head and neck called strawberry lesions.
- Most commonly found in the nasal cavity producing painless, enlarging mucosal papules. These lesions enlarge and easily bleed with touch.

Treatment
- Surgical excision and oral antifungal agents

Congenital

Chronic Granulomatous Disease (CGD)

Incidence/Epidemiology
- Due to hereditary defects in the immune system. These typically involve neutrophils and monocytes (phagocytes).
- 66% are X linked, 33% are autosomal recessive.
- Within this spectrum of disorders, Chediak-Higashi and Job syndrome is included.
- Chediak-Higashi syndrome is an autosomal recessive disorder presenting with neuropathy, neutropenia, oculocutaneous albinism, and malignancy.
- Job syndrome is characterized by increased levels of IgE and eosinophilia. Patient usually present with multiple *Staphylococcus* abscesses.

Presentation
- Multiple, chronic infections by catalase-positive organisms, gram-negative bacteria and fungi.
- Patients present with eczema, osteomyelitis, abscesses, and granulomas.
- Can affect single- or multiple-organ systems. The lung is the most common site of involvement; however, lymphatic, hepatic, skeletal, gastrointestinal, and genitourinary can also be affected.

Treatment
- Multiple courses of antibiotics
- Surgical debridement
- Other treatments include interferon gamma, granulocyte colony-stimulating factor (G-CSF), and granulocyte-macrophage colony-stimulating factor to stimulate neutrophils.

Bibliography

Flint D, Mahadevan M, Barber C, et al. Cervical lymphadenitis due to non-tuberculous mycobacteria: surgical treatment and review. *Int J Pediatr Otorhinolaryngol.* 2000;53:187-194.

Gulati S, Krossnes B, Olofsson J, Danielsen A. Sinonasal involvement in sarcoidosis: a report of seven cases and review of literature. *Eur Arch Otorhinolaryngol.* 2012;269(3):891-896.

Lynch JP 3rd, Hoffman GS. Wegener's granulomatosis: controversies and current concepts. *Compr Ther.* 1998;24(9):421-440.

Montone KT. Infectious diseases of the head and neck. *Am J Clin. Pathol.* 2007;128:35-67.

Thompson LD. Rhinoscleroma. *Ear Nose Throat J.* 2002;81(8):506.

Questions

1. Which disease is often associated with a bony septal perforation?
   A. Tuberculosis
   B. Leprosy
   C. Syphilis
   D. Blastomycosis
   E. Langerhan histiocytosis

2. An 8-year-old patient presents with a history of several weeks of a violaceous, submandibular mass showing sulfur granules on fine needle aspiration. What is your definitive management?
   A. PO antibiotics only
   B. IV antibiotics only
   C. Surgical curettage only
   D. Surgical curettage and IV, then PO antibiotics
   E. Conservative management

3. "Heerfordt's Syndrome" is a variant of what condition?
   A. HIV
   B. Sjogren
   C. Lyme disease
   D. Melkersson-Rosenthal syndrome
   E. Sarcoidosis

4. Which of the following facts about Churg-Strauss is incorrect?
   A. A small- and medium-vessel necrotizing vasculitis
   B. aka eosinophilic granulomatosis with polyangiitis

    C. Classic triad of airway necrotizing granulomas, systemic vasculitis, and focal glomerulonephritis

    D. Associated with pANCA

    E. Can be divided into allergic, eosinophilic, and vasculitic stages

5. Which of the following is not one of the five diagnostic criteria for cat scratch disease?

    A. History of exposure to a cat

    B. Inoculation site

    C. Fever

    D. Adenopathy

    E. Biopsy showing necrotic granuloma

    F. Warthin-Starry-Sky stain showing intracellular pleomorphic gram-negative bacillus

Chapter 13
Anatomy of the Ear

A. The temporal bone forms part of the side and base of the skull. It constitutes two-thirds of the floor of the middle cranial fossa and one-third of the floor of the posterior fossa. There are four parts to the temporal bone:

   i. Squamosa

   ii. Mastoid

   iii. Petrous

   iv. Tympanic

B. The following muscles are attached to the mastoid process:

   i. Sternocleidomastoid

   ii. Splenius capitis

   iii. Longissimus capitis

   iv. Digastric

   v. Anterior, superior, posterior, auricular (The temporalis muscle attaches to the squamosa portion of the temporal bone and not to the mastoid process.)

C. The auricle (Figure 13-1) is made of elastic cartilage, the cartilaginous canal of fibrocartilage. The cartilaginous canal constitutes one-third of the external auditory canal (whereas the eustachian tube is two-thirds cartilaginous), the remaining two-thirds is osseous. Innervation of auricle is outlined in Figure 13-2.

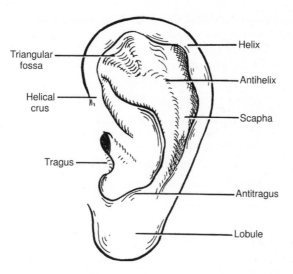

Figure 13-1 Auricle.

D. The skin over the cartilaginous canal has sebaceous glands, ceruminous glands, and hair follicles. The skin over the bony canal is tight and has no subcutaneous tissue except periosteum.

E. Boundaries of the *external auditory canal* are:

Anterior	Mandibular fossa
	Parotid
Posterior	Mastoid
Superior	Epitympanic recess (medially)
	Cranial cavity (laterally)
Inferior	Parotid

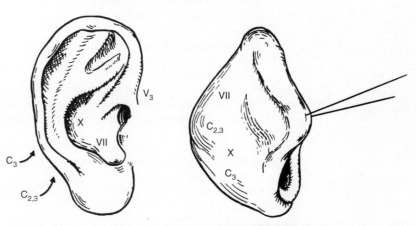

Figure 13-2 Sensory innervation of the auricle. C_3, via greater auricular nerve; $C_{2,3}$ via lesser occipital nerve; X, auricular branch; V_3, auriculotemporal nerve; VII, sensory twigs.

The anterior portion, floor, and part of the posterior portion of the bony canal are formed by the tympanic part of the temporal bone. The rest of the posterior canal and the roof are formed by the squamosa.

F. Boundaries of the *epitympanum* are

Medial	Lateral semicircular canal and VII nerve
Superior	Tegmen
Anterior	Zygomatic arch
Lateral	Squamosa (scutum)
Inferior	Fossa incudis
Posterior	Aditus

G. Boundaries of the *tympanic cavity* are

Roof	Tegmen
Floor	Jugular wall and styloid prominence
Posterior	Mastoid, stapedius, pyramidal prominence
Anterior	Carotid wall, eustachian tube, tensor tympani
Medial	Labyrinthine wall
Lateral	Tympanic membrane, scutum (laterosuperior)

H. The *auricle* is attached to the head by
   i. Skin
   ii. An extension of cartilage to the external auditory canal cartilage
   iii. Ligaments
      a. Anterior ligament (zygoma to helix and tragus)
      b. Superior ligament (external auditory canal to the spine of the helix)
      c. Posterior ligament (mastoid to concha)
   iv. Muscles
      a. Anterior auricular muscle
      b. Superior auricular muscle
      c. Posterior auricular muscle
I. Notch of Rivinus is the notch on the squamosa, medial to which lies Shrapnell membrane. The tympanic ring is not a complete ring, with the dehiscence superiorly.
J. *Meckel cave* is the concavity on the superior portion of the temporal bone in which the gasserian ganglion (V) is located.
K. *Dorello canal* is between the petrous tip and the sphenoid bone. It is the groove for the VI nerve. *Gradenigo syndrome,* which is secondary to petrositis with involvement of the VI nerve, is characterized by
   i. Pain behind the eye
   ii. Diplopia
   iii. Aural discharge

L. The suprameatal triangle of *Macewen triangle* is posterior and superior to the external auditory canal. It is bound at the meatus by the spine of Henle, otherwise called the *suprameatal spine*. This triangle approximates the position of the antrum medially. *Tegmen mastoideum* is the thin plate over the antrum.

M. *Trautmann triangle* is demarcated by the bony labyrinth, the sigmoid sinus, and the superior petrosal sinus or dura.

Citelli angle is the *sinodural* angle. It is located between the sigmoid sinus and the middle fossa dura plate. Others consider the superior side of Trautmann triangle to be Citelli angle.

Solid angle is the angle formed by the three semicircular canals.

Scutum is the thin plate of bone that constitutes the lateral wall of the epitympanum. It is part of the squamosa.

Mandibular fossa is bound by the zygomatic, squamosa, and tympanic bones.

Huguier canal transmits the chorda tympani out of the temporal bone anteriorly. It is situated lateral to the roof of the protympanum.

Huschke foramen is located on the anterior tympanic plate along a nonossified portion of the plate. It is near the fissures of Santorini.

Porus acusticus is the "mouth" of the internal auditory canal. The canal is divided horizontally by the *crista falciformis*.

N. There are three parts to the inner ear (Figure 13-3).

   i. *Pars superior*: Vestibular labyrinth (utricle and semicircular canals)

   ii. *Pars inferior*: Cochlea and saccule

   iii. Endolymphatic sac and duct

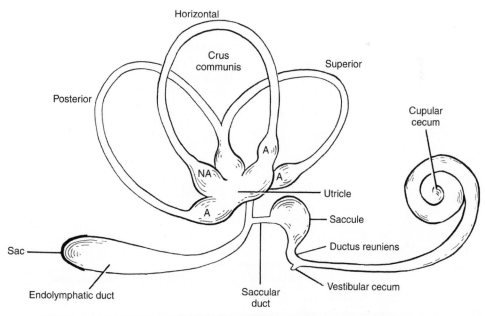

Figure 13-3 Membranous labyrinth. A, ampulated end; NA, nonampulated end.

O. There are four small outpocketings from the perilymph space:
   i. Along the endolymphatic duct
   ii. Fissula ante fenestram
   iii. Fossula post fenestram
   iv. Periotic duct
P. There are four openings into the temporal bone:
   i. Internal auditory canal
   ii. Vestibular aqueduct
   iii. Cochlear aqueduct
   iv. Subarcuate fossa
Q. The *ponticulum* is the ridge of bone between the oval window niche and the sinus tympani.
R. The *subiculum* is a ridge of bone between the round window niche and the sinus tympani.
S. *Körner septum* separates the squamosa from the petrous air cells.
T. Only one-third of the population has a pneumatized petrous portion of the temporal bone.
U. *Scala communis* is where the scala tympani joins the scala vestibuli. The helicotrema is at the apex of the cochlea where the two join (Figure 13-4).
V. The *petrous pyramid* is the strongest bone in the body.
W. The upper limit of the internal auditory canal diameter is 8 mm.
X. The *cochlear aqueduct* is a bony channel connecting the scala tympani of the basal turn with the subarachnoid space of the posterior cranial cavity. The average adult cochlear aqueduct is 6.2-mm long.

Middle Ear

Tympanic plexus = V_3, IX, and X
$V_3 \rightarrow$ Auriculotemporal nerve
$IX \rightarrow$ Jacobson's nerve
$X \rightarrow$ Auricular nerve

Inner Ear

See Figure 13-5.

Superior and horizontal semicircular canals.
Superior vestibular nerve — Utricle
— Voit nerve
Inferior vestibular nerve — Saccule
— Posterior semicircular canal

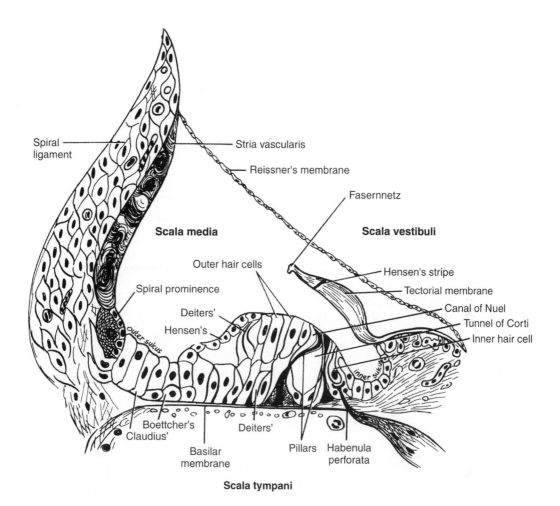

Figure 13-4 Organ of Corti.

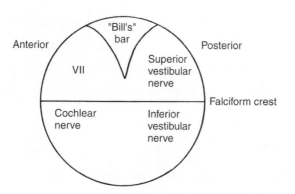

Figure 13-5 Cross-section of internal auditory canal.

Blood Supply

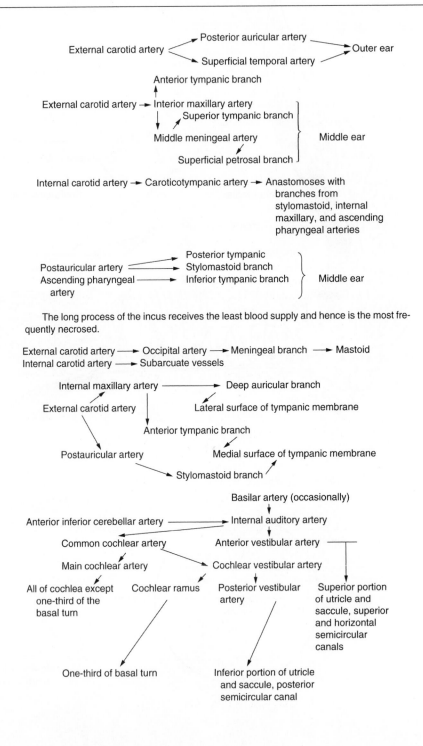

External carotid artery
- Posterior auricular artery → Outer ear
- Superficial temporal artery → Outer ear

Anterior tympanic branch
↑
External carotid artery → Interior maxillary artery
↓ → Superior tympanic branch
Middle meningeal artery
Superficial petrosal branch
} Middle ear

Internal carotid artery → Caroticotympanic artery → Anastomoses with branches from stylomastoid, internal maxillary, and ascending pharyngeal arteries

Postauricular artery → Posterior tympanic
→ Stylomastoid branch
Ascending pharyngeal artery → Inferior tympanic branch
} Middle ear

The long process of the incus receives the least blood supply and hence is the most frequently necrosed.

External carotid artery → Occipital artery → Meningeal branch → Mastoid
Internal carotid artery → Subarcuate vessels

Internal maxillary artery → Deep auricular branch
External carotid artery → Lateral surface of tympanic membrane
Anterior tympanic branch
Postauricular artery → Medial surface of tympanic membrane
→ Stylomastoid branch

Basilar artery (occasionally)
↓
Anterior inferior cerebellar artery → Internal auditory artery
Common cochlear artery   Anterior vestibular artery
Main cochlear artery   Cochlear vestibular artery
All of cochlea except one-third of the basal turn   Cochlear ramus   Posterior vestibular artery   Superior portion of utricle and saccule, superior and horizontal semicircular canals
One-third of basal turn   Inferior portion of utricle and saccule, posterior semicircular canal

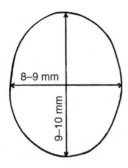

Figure 13-6 Measurements of tympanic membrane.

Tympanic Membrane

See Figure 13-6.

The tympanic membrane has four layers:
(A) Squamous epithelium
(B) Radiating fibrous layer
(C) Circular fibrous layer
(D) Mucosal layer

Average total area of tympanic membrane: 70 to 80 mm^2
Average vibrating surface of tympanic membrane: 55 mm^2

Venous Drainage

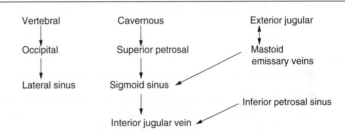

Ossicles

Malleus

A. Head
B. Neck
C. Manubrium
D. Anterior process
E. Lateral or short process

Incus

A. Body
B. Short process
C. Long process (lenticular process)

Stapes

A. Posterior crus
B. Anterior crus
C. Footplate (average 1.41 mm × 2.99 mm)

Ligaments

Malleus

A. Superior malleal ligament (head to roof of epitympanum)
B. Anterior malleal ligament (neck near anterior process to sphenoid bone through the petrotympanic fissure)
C. Tensor tympani (medial surface of upper end of manubrium to cochleariform process)
D. Lateral malleal ligament (neck to tympanic notch)

Incus

A. Superior incudal ligament (body to tegmen)
B. Posterior incudal ligament (short process to floor of incudal fossa)

Stapes

A. Stapedial tendon (apex of the pyramidal process to the posterior surface of the neck of the stapes)
B. Annular ligament (footplate to margin of vestibular fenestram)
    i. *Malleal*: Incudal joint is a diarthrodial joint.
    ii. *Incudo*: Stapedial joint is a diarthrodial joint.
    iii. *Stapedial*: Labyrinthine joint is a syndesmotic joint.

Middle Ear Folds of Significance

There are five malleal folds and four incudal folds:

A. *Anterior malleal fold*: Neck of the malleus to anterosuperior margin of the tympanic sulcus
B. *Posterior malleal fold*: Neck to posterosuperior margin of the tympanic sulcus
C. *Lateral malleal fold*: Neck to neck in an arch form and to Shrapnell membrane
D. *Anterior pouch of von Troeltsch*: Lies between the anterior malleal fold and the portion of the tympanic membrane anterior to the handle of the malleus
E. *Posterior pouch of von Troeltsch*: Lies between the posterior malleal fold and the portion of the tympanic membrane posterior to the handle of the malleus

Prussak space (Figure 13-7) has the following boundaries:

A. *Anterior*: Lateral malleal fold
B. *Posterior*: Lateral malleal fold
C. *Superior*: Lateral malleal fold
D. *Inferior*: Lateral process of the malleus
E. *Medial*: Neck of the malleus
F. *Lateral*: Shrapnell membrane

The *oval window* sits in the sagittal plane.
    The *round window* sits in the transverse plane and is protected by an anterior lip from the promontory. It faces posteroinferiorly as well as laterally.

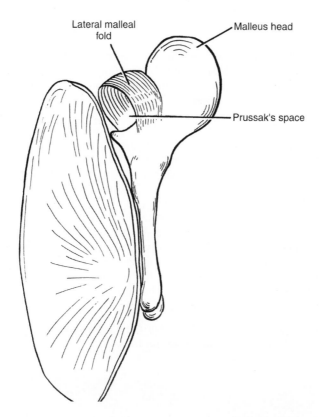

Figure 13-7 Prussak space.

The tensor tympani inserts from the cochleariform process onto the medial surface of the upper end of the manubrium. It supposedly pulls the tympanic membrane medially, thereby tensing it. It also draws the malleus medially and forward. It raises the resonance frequency and attenuates low frequencies.

The stapedius muscle most frequently attaches to the posterior neck of the stapes. Occasionally, it is attached to the posterior crus or head and rarely to the lenticular process. It is attached posteriorly at the pyramidal process. It pulls the stapes posteriorly, supposedly increases the resonant frequency of the ossicular chain, and attenuates sound.

Eustachian Tube

A. It is 17 to 18 mm at birth and grows to about 35 mm in adulthood.
B. At birth, the tube is horizontal and grows to be at an incline of 45° in adulthood. Thus, the pharyngeal orifice is about 15 mm lower than the tympanic orifice.
C. It can be divided into an anteromedial cartilaginous portion (24 mm) and a posterolateral bony (11 mm) portion. The narrowest part of the tube is at the junction of the bony and the cartilaginous portions. (Reminder: The external auditory canal is one-third cartilaginous and two-thirds bony.)
D. The cartilaginous part of the tube is lined by pseudostratified columnar-ciliated epithelium, but toward the tympanic orifice, it is lined by ciliated cuboidal epithelium.

E. It opens by the action of the tensor palati (innervated by the third division of the V nerve) acting synergistically with the levator veli palatini (innervated by the vagus). In children, the only muscle that works is the tensor palati because the levator palati is separated from the eustachian tube cartilage by a considerable distance. Therefore, a cleft palate child with poor tensor palati function is expected to have eustachian tube problems until the levator veli palatini starts to function.

F. In a normal individual, a pressure difference of 200 to 300 mm H_2O is needed to produce airflow.

G. It is easier to expel air from the middle ear than to get it into the middle ear (reason for more tubal problems when descending in an airplane).

H. A pressure of -30 mm Hg or lower for 15 minutes can produce a transudate in the middle ear. A pressure differential of 90 mm Hg or greater may "lock" the eustachian tube, preventing opening of the tube by the tensor palati muscle. It is called the critical pressure difference.

I. If the pressure differential exceeds 100 mm Hg, the tympanic membrane may rupture.

J. A Valsalva maneuver generates about 20 to 40 mm Hg of pressure.

K. The lymphoid tissues within the tube have been referred to as the tonsil of Gerlach.

L. The tympanic ostium of the tube is at the anterior wall of the tympanic cavity about 4 mm above the most inferior part of the floor of the cavity. The diameter of the ostium is 3 to 5 mm. The size of the pharyngeal ostium varies from 3 to 10 mm in its vertical diameter and 2 to 5 mm in its horizontal diameter.

Figures 13-8 to 13-22 are temporal bone horizontal sections from HF Schuknecht's Research Laboratory at the Massachusetts Eye and Ear Infirmary.

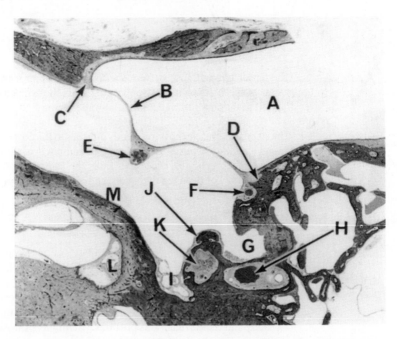

Figure 13-8 A, external auditory canal; B, tympanic membrane; C, fibrous annulus; D, tympanic sulcus; E, malleus handle; F, chorda tympani; G, facial recess; H, facial nerve; I, sinus tympani; J, pyramidal process; K, stapedius muscle; L, round window; M, promontory.

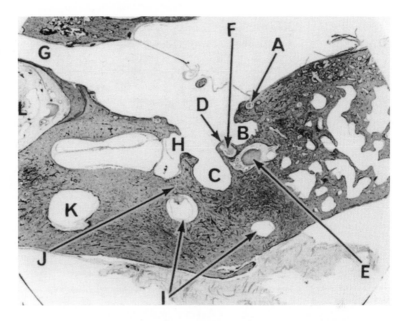

Figure 13-9 A, chorda tympani; B, facial recess; C, sinus tympani; D, pyramidal process; E, facial nerve; F, stapedius muscle; G, eustachian tube; H, round window niche; I, posterior semicircular canal; J, microfissure with no known significance; K, internal auditory meatus; L, carotid canal.

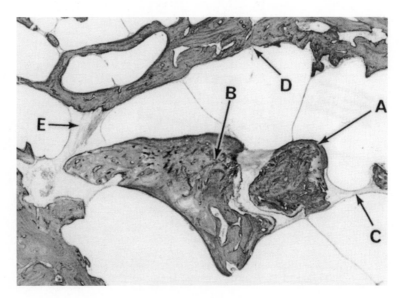

Figure 13-10 A, malleus head; B, incus body; C, anterior malleal ligament; D, lateral wall of the attic; E, posterior incudal ligament.

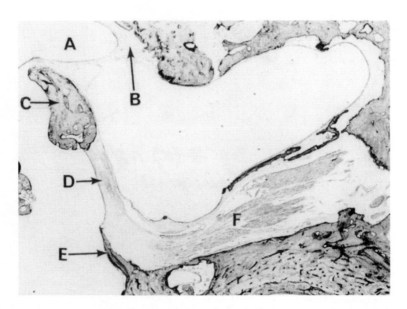

Figure 13-11 A, external auditory canal; B, fibrous annulus; C, malleus; D, tendon of tensor tympani; E, cochleariform process; F, tensor tympani muscle.

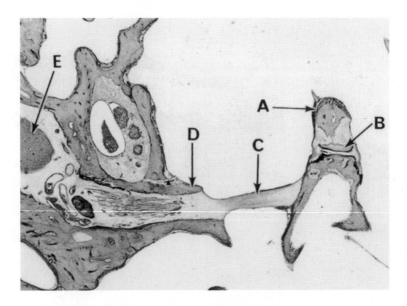

Figure 13-12 A, incus; B, lenticular process; C, stapedius tendon; D. pyramidal process; E, facial nerve.

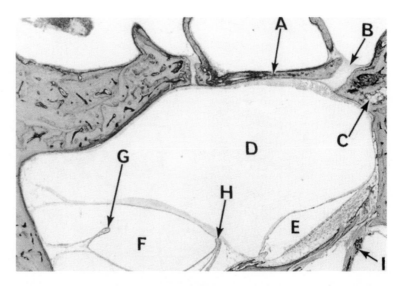

Figure 13-13 A, stapes footplate; B, annular ligament; C, fissula ante fenestram; D, vestibule; E, saccule; F, utricule; G, inferior utricular crest; H, utriculoendolymphatic valve; I, saccular nerve.

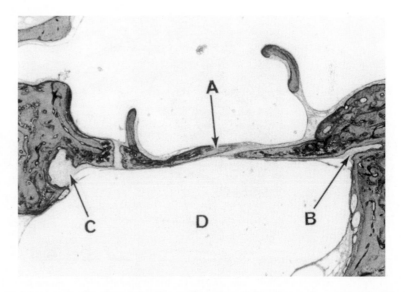

Figure 13-14 A, stapes footplate; B, fissula ante fenestram; C, fossula post fenestram; D, vestibule.

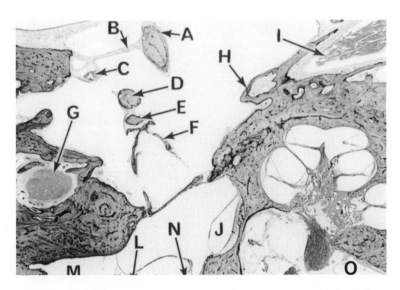

Figure 13-15 A, malleus; B, tympanic membrane; C, chorda tympani; D, incus; E, lenticular process; F, stapes; G, facial nerve; H, cochleariform process; I, tensor tympani; J, saccule; L, inferior utricular crest; M, lateral semicircular canal; N, sinus of endolymphatic duct; O, internal auditory canal.

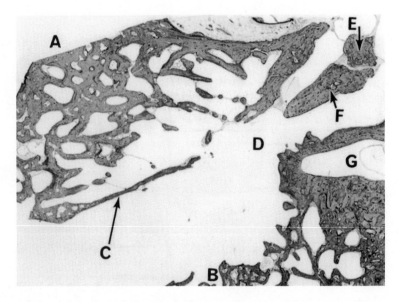

Figure 13-16 A, squamosa part of the temporal bone; B, petrous part of the temporal bone; C, Körner septum; D, aditus; E, malleus; F, incus; G, lateral semicircular canal.

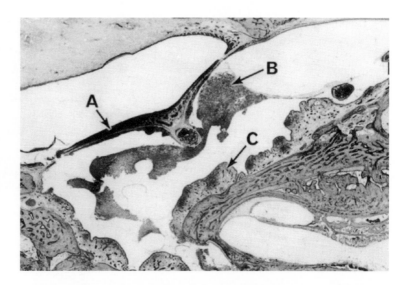

Figure 13-17 Acute otitis media. A, tympanic membrane; B, purulent material; C, thickened middle ear mucosa.

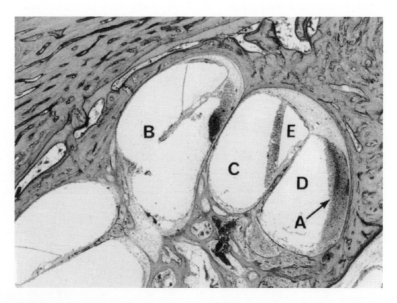

Figure 13-18 Acute labyrinthitis. A, leukocytes; B, helicotrema; C, scala vestibuli; D, scala tympani; E, scala media.

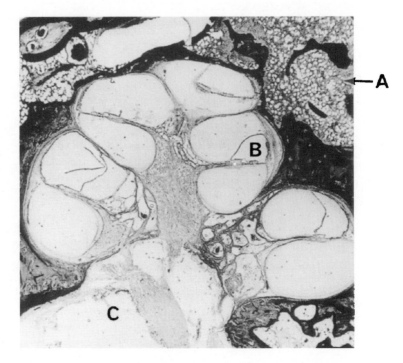

Figure 13-19 Congenital syphilis. A, leutic changes in the otic capsule; B, endolymphatic hydrops; C, internal auditory canal.

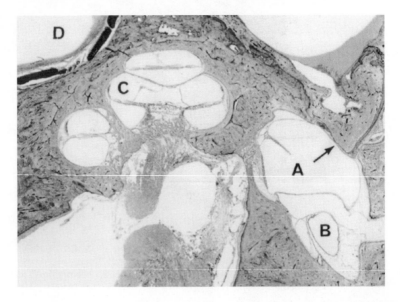

Figure 13-20 Ménière disease. A, enlarged saccule against footplate; B, utricule; C, "distended" cochlear duct; D, carotid artery.

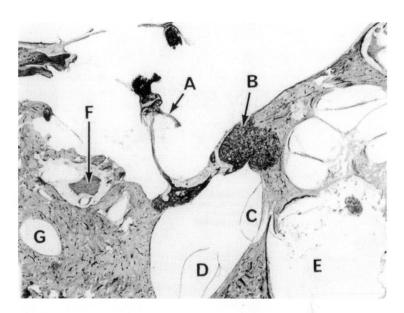

Figure 13-21 Otosclerosis. A, stapes; B, otosclerotic bone; C, saccule; D, utricle; E, internal auditory canal; F, facial nerve; G, lateral semicircular canal.

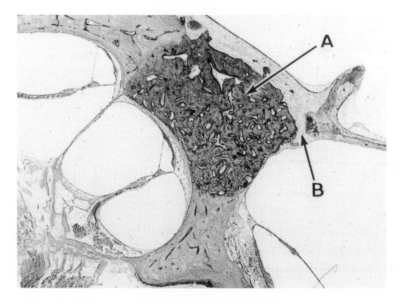

Figure 13-22 Otosclerosis. A, histologic otosclerosis without involving the footplate; B, annular ligament.

Embryology of the Ear

Auricle

During the sixth week of gestation, condensation of the mesoderm of the first and second arches occurs, giving rise to six hillocks (hillocks of His). The first three hillocks are derived from the first arch, and the second arch contributes to the last three (Figure 13-23).

First arch:	First hillock → Tragus (1)
	Second hillock → Helical crus (2)
	Third hillock → Helix (3)
Second arch:	Fourth hillock → Antihelix (4)
	Fifth hillock → Antitragus (5)
	Sixth hillock → Lobule and lower helix (6)

Seventh week: Formation of cartilage is in progress.

Twelfth week: The auricle is formed by fusion of the hillocks.

Twentieth week: It has reached adult shape, although it does not reach adult size until age 9.

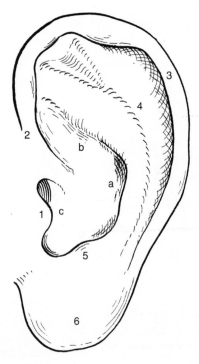

Figure 13-23 Embryology of the auricle.

The concha is formed by three separate areas from the first groove (ectoderm) (see Figure 13-23).

A. *Middle part of the first groove*: Concha cavum
B. *Upper part of the first groove*: Concha cymba
C. *Lowest part of the first groove*: Intertragus incisor

External Auditory Canal

During the eighth week of gestation, the surface ectoderm in the region of the upper end of the first pharyngeal groove (dorsal) thickens. This solid core of epithelium continues to grow toward the middle ear. Simultaneously, the concha cavum deepens to form the outer one-third of the external auditory canal. By the 21st week, this core begins to resorb and "hollow out" to form a channel. The innermost layer of ectoderm remains to become the superficial layer of the tympanic membrane. Formation of the channel is completed by the 28th week. At birth, the external auditory canal is neither ossified nor of adult size. Completion of ossification occurs around age 3, and adult size is reached at age 9.

Eustachian Tube and Middle Ear

During the third week of gestation, the first and second pharyngeal pouches lie laterally on either side of what is to become the oral and pharyngeal tongue. As the third arch enlarges, the space between the second arch and the pharynx (first pouch) is compressed and becomes the eustachian tube. The "outpocketing" at the lateral end becomes the middle ear space. Because of the proximity to the first, second, and third arches, the V, VII, and IX nerves are found in the middle ear. By the 10th week, pneumatization begins. The antrum appears on the 23rd week. It is of interest that the middle ear is filled with mucoid connective tissue until the time of birth. The 28th week marks the appearance of the tympanic membrane, which is derived from all three tissues.

> Ectoderm → Squamous layer
>
> Mesoderm → Fibrous layer
>
> Entoderm → Mucosal layer

Between the 12th and the 28th weeks, four primary mucosal sacs emerge, each becoming a specific anatomic region of the middle ear.

> Saccus anticus → Anterior pouch of von Troltsch
>
> Saccus medius → Epitympanum and petrous area
>
> Saccus superior → Posterior pouch of von Troltsch, part of the mastoid, inferior incudal space
>
> Saccus posterior → Round window and oval window niches, sinus tympani

At birth, the embryonic subepithelium is resorbed, and pneumatization continues in the middle ear, antrum, and mastoid. Pneumatization of the petrous portion of the temporal bone, being the last to arise, continues until puberty.

The middle ear is well formed at birth and enlarges only slightly postnatally. At age 1, the mastoid process appears. At age 3, the tympanic ring and osseous canal are calcified.

The eustachian tube measures approximately 17 mm at birth and grows to 35 mm in adulthood.

Malleus and Incus

During the sixth week of embryonic development, the malleus and incus appear as a single mass. By the eighth week, they are separated, and the malleoincudal joint is formed. The head and neck of the malleus are derived from Meckel cartilage (first arch mesoderm), the anterior process from the process of Folius (mesenchyme bone), and the manubrium from Reichert cartilage (second arch mesoderm). The body and short process of the incus originate from Meckel cartilage (first arch mesoderm) and the long process from Reichert cartilage (second arch mesoderm). By the 16th week, the ossicles reach adult size. On the 16th week, ossification begins and appears first at the long process of the incus. During the 17th week, the ossification center becomes visible on the medial surface of the neck of the malleus and spreads to the manubrium and the head. At birth, the malleus and incus are of adult size and shape. The ossification of the malleus is never complete, so that part of the manubrium remains cartilaginous. (The lenticular process is also known as "sylvian apophysis" or "os orbiculare.")

Stapes

At 4.5 weeks, the mesenchymal cells of the second arch condense to form the blastema. The VII nerve divides the blastema into stapes, interhyale, and laterohyale. During the seventh week, the stapes ring emerges around the stapedial artery. The lamina stapedialis which is of the otic mesenchyme appears to become the footplate and annular ligament. At 8.5 weeks, the incudostapedial joint develops. The interhyale becomes the stapedial muscle and tendon; the laterohyale becomes the posterior wall of the middle ear. Together with the otic capsule, the laterohyale also becomes the pyramidal process and facial canal. The lower part of the facial canal is said to be derived from Reichert cartilage.

During the 10th week, the stapes changes its ring shape to the "stirrup" shape. During the 19th week, ossification begins, starting at the obturator surface of the stapedial base. The ossification is completed by the 28th week except for the vestibular surface of the footplate, which remains cartilaginous throughout life. At birth, the stapes is of adult size and form.

Inner Ear

During the third week, neuroectoderm and ectoderm lateral to the first branchial groove condense to form the otic placode. The latter invaginates until it is completely submerged and surrounded by mesoderm, becoming the otocyst or otic vesicle by the fourth week. The fifth week marks the appearance of a wide dorsal and a slender ventral part of the otic vesicle. Between these two parts, the endolymphatic duct and sac develop. During the sixth week, the semicircular canals take shape, and by the eighth week, together with the utricle, they are fully formed. Formation of the basal turn of the cochlea takes place during the seventh week, and by the 12th week the complete 2.5 turns are developed. Development of the saccule follows that of the utricle. Evidently, the pars superior (semicircular canals and utricle) is developed before the pars inferior (sacculus and cochlea). Formation of the membranous labyrinth without the end organ is said to be complete by the 15th week of gestation.

Concurrent with formation of the membranous labyrinth, the precursor of the otic capsule emerges during the eighth week as a condensation of mesenchyme precartilage. The 14 centers of ossification can be identified by the 15th week, and ossification is completed during the 23rd week of gestation. The last area to ossify is the fissula ante fenestram, which may remain cartilaginous throughout life. Other than the endolymphatic sac which continues to grow until adulthood the membranous and bony labyrinths are of adult size at the 23rd week of embryonic development. The endolymphatic sac is the first to appear and the last to stop growing.

At the third week, the common macula first appears. Its upper part differentiates into the utricular macula and the cristae of the superior and lateral semicircular canals, whereas its lower part becomes the macula of the saccule and the crista of the posterior semicircular canal. During the eighth week, two ridges of cells as well as the stria vascularis are identifiable. During the 11th week, the vestibular end organs, complete with sensory and supporting cells, are formed. During the 20th week, development of the stria vascularis and the tectorial membrane is complete. During the 23rd week, the two ridges of cells divide into inner ridge cells and outer ridge cells. The inner ridge cells become the spiral limbus; the outer ones become the hair cells, pillar cells, Hensen cells, and Deiters cells. During the 26th week, the tunnel of Corti and canal of Nuel are formed.

The neural crest cells lateral to the rhombencephalon condense to form the acoustic-facial ganglion, which differentiates into the facial geniculate ganglion, superior vestibular ganglion (utricle, superior, and horizontal semicircular canals), and inferior ganglion (saccule, posterior semicircular canal, and cochlea).

At birth, four elements of the temporal bone are distinguishable: petrous bone, squamous bone, tympanic ring, and styloid process. The mastoid antrum is present, but the mastoid process is not formed until the end of the second year of life; pneumatization of the mastoid soon follows. The tympanic ring extends laterally after birth, forming the osseous canal.

Clinical Information

    A. Congenital microtia occurs in about 1:20,000 births.

    B. The auricle is formed early. Therefore, malformation of the auricle implies a malformation of the middle ear, mastoid, and VII nerve. On the other hand, a normal auricle with canal atresia indicates abnormal development during the 28th week, by which time the ossicles and the middle ear are already formed.

    C. Improper fusion of the first and second branchial arches results in a preauricular sinus tract (epithelium lined).

    D. Malformation of first branchial arch and groove results in:
        i. Auricle abnormality (first and second arches)
        ii. Bony meatus atresia (first groove)
        iii. Abnormal incus and malleus (first and second arches)
        iv. Abnormal mandible (first arch)

    E. When the maxilla is also malformed, this constellation of findings is called Treacher Collins syndrome (mandibular facial dysostosis).
        i. Outward–downward slanted eyes (antimongoloid)
        ii. Notched lower lid
        iii. Short mandible
        iv. Bony meatal atresia
        v. Malformed incus and malleus
        vi. Fishmouth

    F. Abnormalities of the otic capsule and labyrinth are rare because they are phylogenetically ancient.

    G. An incidence of 20% to 30% dehiscent tympanic portion of the VII nerve has been reported.

    H. The incidence of absent stapedius tendon, muscle, and pyramidal eminence is estimated at 1%.

    I. Twenty percent of preauricular cysts are bilateral.

    J. In very young infants, Hyrtl fissure affords a route of direct extension of infection from the middle ear to the subarachnoid spaces. The fissure closes as the infant grows. Hyrtl fissure extends from the subarachnoid space near the glossopharyngeal ganglion to the hypotympanum just inferior and anterior to the round window.

Bibliography

Anson B, Donaldson JA. *Surgical Anatomy of the Temporal Bone.* 3rd ed. Philadelphia, PA: WB Saunders; 1980.

Eggston AA, Wolff D. *Histopathology of the Ear, Nose and Throat.* Baltimore, MD: Williams & Wilkins; 1947.

May M. Anatomy of the facial nerve (spacial orientation of fibres in the temporal bone). *Laryngoscope.* 1973;83:1311.

Moore GF, Ogren FP, et al. Anatomy and embryology of the ear. In: Lee KJ, ed. *Textbook of Otolaryngology and Head and Neck Surgery.* New York, NY: Elsevier Science Publishing Co, Inc; 1989.

Schuknecht HF. *Pathology of the Ear.* 2nd ed. Philadelphia, PA: Lea & Febiger; 1993.

Questions

1. Development of the membranous portion of the inner ear is complete by which embryologic time frame?
   A. Week 8
   B. Week 15
   C. Week 28
   D. Week 34

2. Which of the following nerves does not innervate the middle ear?
   A. V_3
   B. IX
   C. X
   D. VII

3. Which structure may be responsible for the spread of infection from the middle ear to the subarachnoid space in infants?
   A. Huguier canal
   B. Petrotympanic fissure
   C. Hyrtl fissure
   D. Foramen of Huschke

4. Normal development of the auricle with external canal atresia suggests a developmental abnormality during which embryologic time frame?
   A. Week 8
   B. Week 28
   C. Week 14
   D. Week 34

5. Which of the following attaches to the mastoid process?
   A. Sternocleidomastoid
   B. Splenius capitis
   C. Longissimus capitis
   D. Digastric
   E. All of the above

Chapter 14
Audiology

[handwritten: 20 - 20,000 Hz = human hearing]

Acoustics

- *Sound:* energy waves of particle displacement, both *compression* (more dense) and *rarefaction* (less dense) within an elastic medium; triggers sensation of hearing.
- *Amplitude of sound:* extent of vibratory movement from rest to farthest point from rest in compression and rarefaction phases of energy waves.
- *Intensity of sound:* amount of sound energy through an area per time; refers to sound strength or magnitude; psychoacoustic correlate is loudness.
- *Sound pressure:* sound force (related to acceleration) over a surface per unit time.
- *Decibel (dB):* unit to express intensity of sound; more specifically the logarithm of the ratio of two sound intensities. One-tenth of a Bel (named for Alexander Graham Bell).
- *Frequency:* number of cycles (complete oscillations) of a vibrating medium per unit of time; psychoacoustic correlate is pitch. Time of one cycle is period.
- *Hertz (Hz):* in acoustics, unit to express frequency (formerly cycles per second or cps). Human ear capable of hearing from approximately 20 to 20,000 Hz.
- *Pure tone:* single-frequency sound; rarely occurs in nature.
- *Complex sound:* sound comprising more than one frequency.
- *Noise:* aperiodic complex sound. Types of noise frequently used in clinical audiology are white noise (containing all frequencies in the audible spectrum at average equal amplitudes), narrow band noise (white noise with frequencies above and below a center frequency filtered out or reduced), and speech noise (white noise with frequencies > 3000 and < 300 Hz reduced by a filter). However, the term "noise" can also mean any unwanted sound.
- *Resonant frequency:* frequency at which a mass vibrates with the least amount of external force. Determined by elasticity, mass, and frictional characteristics of the medium. Natural resonance of external auditory canal is 3000 Hz; of middle ear, 800 to 5000 Hz, mostly 1000 to 2000 Hz; of tympanic membrane, 800 to 1600 Hz; of ossicular chain, 500 to 2000 Hz.

[handwritten: EAC = 3000 Hz; middle ear = 800-5000 Hz (1-2K)]

The Decibel

The decibel scale is listed as follows:

- A logarithmic expression of the ratio of two intensities.
- Nonlinear (eg, the energy increase from 5-7 dB is far greater than the increase from 1-3 dB because it is a logarithmic scale).

- A relative measure (ie, 0 dB does not indicate the absence of sound).
- Expressed with different reference levels, such as, sound pressure level (SPL), hearing level (HL), and sensation level.

Sound Pressure Level (SPL) The referent of SPL is the most common measure of sound strength.

- Decibels SPL are currently usually referenced to micropascals (but can be referenced to dynes per centimeter squared or microbars).
- Sound pressure is related to sound intensity.
- The formula for determining the number of decibels is

$$dB\ Intensity = 10 \log I_o/I_r$$

where

$$I_o = \text{intensity of output sound being measured}$$

$$I_r = \text{intensity of reference}$$

However, intensity is proportional to pressure squared, as

$$I \propto p^2$$

$$\therefore dB\ SPL = 10 \log (p_o^2/p_r^2)$$

or

$$dB\ SPL = 10 \log (p_o/p_r)^2$$

$$= 10 \times 2 \log (p_o/p_r)$$

$$= 20 \log (p_o/p_r)$$

where

$$p_o = \text{pressure of the output of sound being measured}$$

$$p_r = \text{pressure of the reference, usually 20 } \mu Pa$$

Hearing Level When the reference is hearing level (HL).

- 0 dB HL at any frequency is the average lowest intensity perceived by normal ears 50% of the time.
- This scale (dB HL) was developed because the ear is not equally sensitive to all frequencies. The human ear, for example, cannot perceive 0 dB SPL at 250 Hz; rather, a 250 Hz sound must be raised to 26.5 dB SPL before it is heard. This level is assigned the value 0 dB HL. The referent is to normal ears (Table 14-1).
- This scale takes into account differences in human sensitivity for the various frequencies: normal hearing is 0 dB HL across the frequency range rather than 47.5 dB SPL at 125 Hz, 26.5 dB SPL at 250 Hz, 13.5 dB SPL at 500 Hz, 7.5 dB SPL at 1000 Hz, and so on.
- HL is the reference used on clinical audiometers.

Sensation Level When the reference is sensation level (SL).

- The referent is an individual's threshold.
- 0 dB SL is the level of intensity at which an individual can just perceive a sound in 50% of the presentations (ie, "threshold").
- For example, if a person has a threshold of 20 dB HL at 1000 Hz, 50 dB SL for that individual would equal 70 dB HL.

Table 14-1 **Number of dB SPL Needed to Equal 0 dB HL at Different Frequencies for TDH-49 and TDH-50 Earphones**

Frequency (Hz)	dB SPL
125	47.5
250	26.5
500	13.5
1000	7.5
1500	7.5
2000	11.0
3000	9.5
4000	10.5
6000	13.5
8000	13.0

Adapted with permission from American National Standard Specifications for Audiometers. ANSI S3.6–1996. New York, NY: American National Standards Institute, Inc.; 1996.

It is important to state a reference level when speaking of decibels. Table 14-2 lists typical SPLs for various environmental noises.

The Auditory Mechanism

Outer Ear

- The outer ear comprises the auricle or pinna (the most prominent and least useful part), the external auditory canal or ear canal (it is ~1 inch or 2.5 cm in length and 1/4 inch in diameter, and it has a volume of 2 cm^3), and the outer surface of the tympanic membrane or eardrum.
- The pinna is funnel-shaped and collects sound waves. The ear canal directs the sound waves, which vibrate the eardrum.
- The pinna also aids in the localization of sound and is more efficient at delivering high- than low-frequency sounds.
- The external auditory canal is a resonance chamber for the frequency region of 2000 to 5500 Hz. Its resonant frequency is approximately 2700 Hz but varies by individual ear canal.

Middle Ear

- The middle ear is an air-filled space approximately 5/8 inch high (15 mm), 1/8 to 3/16 inch wide (2-4 mm), 1/4 inch deep, and 1 to 2 cm^3 in volume.
- Sound waves from the tympanic membrane travel along the ossicular chain, which comprises three bones (the malleus, incus, and stapes), to the oval window. The displacement of the ossicular chain varies as a function of the frequency and intensity of the sound.
- The malleus and incus weigh approximately the same, but the stapes is about one-fourth the mass of the other ossicles. This difference facilitates the transmission of high frequencies.

Table 14-2 Decibel Levels (dB SPL) of Some Environmental Sounds

Sound	Decibels (dB SPL)	
Rocket launching pad	180	Noises > 140 dB SPL may cause pain
Jet plane	140	
Gunshot blast	140	
Riveting steel tank	130	
Automobile horn	120	
Sandblasting	112	
Woodworking shop	100	Long exposure to noises > 90 dB SPL may eventually harm hearing
Punch press	100	
Boiler shop	100	
Hydraulic press	100	
Can manufacturing plant	100	
Subway	90	
Average factory	80-90	
Computer printer	85	
Noisy restaurant	80	
Adding machine	80	
Busy traffic	75	
Conversational speech	66	
Average home	50	
Quiet office	40	
Soft whisper	30	

- The tympanic membrane and ossicular chain most efficiently transmit sound between 500 and 3000 Hz. Thus, the ear has greatest sensitivity at those frequencies most important to understanding speech.
- The middle ear transforms acoustic energy from the medium of air to the medium of liquid. It is an impedance-matching system that ensures energy is not lost. This impedance matching is accomplished by the following four factors:
  (a) *The area effect of the tympanic membrane:* Although the area of the adult tympanic membrane is between 85 and 90 mm^2, only about 55 mm^2 effectively vibrates (the lower two-thirds of the tympanic membrane); the stapes footplate is 3.2 mm^2. Thus, the ratio of the vibrating portion of the tympanic membrane to that of the stapes footplate results in a 17:1 increase in sound energy by concentrating it into a smaller area.
  (b) *Lever action of the ossicular chain:* As the eardrum vibrates, the ossicular chain is set into motion about an axis of rotation from the anterior process of the malleus

through the short process of the incus. Because the handle of the malleus is approximately 1.3 times longer than the incus long process, the force (pressure) received at the stapes footplate, through the use of leverage, is greater than that at the malleus by about 1.3:1. Thus, the transformer ratio of the middle ear is approximately 22:1 (the combination of the area effect of the tympanic membrane and the lever action of the ossicles: $17 \times 1.3 = 22$) which translates to approximately 25 dB.

(c) *The natural resonance and efficiency of the outer and middle ears* (500-3000 Hz).

(d) *The phase difference between the oval window and the round window*: When sound energy impinges on the oval window, a traveling wave is created within the cochlea progressing from the oval window, along the scala vestibuli and the scala tympani, to the round window. The phase difference between the two windows results in a small change (~4 dB) in the normal ear.

Inner Ear

- Once the sound signal impinges on the oval window, the cochlea transforms the signal from mechanical energy into hydraulic energy and then ultimately, at the hair cells, into bioelectric energy. As the footplate of the stapes moves in and out of the oval window, a traveling wave is created in the cochlea (Bekesy's traveling wave theory). As the wave travels through the cochlea, it moves the basilar and tectorial membranes. Because these two membranes have different hinge points, this movement results in a "shearing" motion that bends the hair cell stereocilia. This bending depolarizes the hair cells, which, in turn, activates afferent electrical nerve impulses.

- The energy wave travels from base to apex along the basilar membrane until the wave reaches a maximum. The basilar membrane varies in stiffness and mass throughout its length. The point of maximum displacement of the traveling wave is determined by the interaction of the frequency of the sound and the basilar membrane's physical properties. The outer hair cells (OHCs) are motile, reacting mechanically to the incoming signal by shortening and lengthening according to their characteristic (best) frequency. Under strong efferent influence, the OHCs are part of an active feedback mechanism, adjusting the basilar membrane's physical properties so that a given frequency maximally stimulates a specific narrow group of inner hair cells (IHCs). This effect is the "cochlear amplifier." The IHCs trigger the preponderance of afferent nerve responses; 95% of all afferent fibers innervate the IHCs.

- The cochlea is organized spatially according to frequency, that is, tonotopic arrangement. For every frequency there is a highly specific place on the basilar membrane where hair cells are maximally sensitive to that frequency, the basal end for high frequencies, and the apical end for low frequencies. Frequency-selective neurons transmit the neural code from the hair cells through the auditory system. For multiple frequencies (complex sound), there are several points of traveling wave maxima, and the cochlear apparatus constantly tunes itself for best reception and encoding of each component frequency. The auditory mechanism's superb frequency resolution is mostly secondary to the highly tuned hair cell response rather than on processing at higher auditory centers.

- The cochlea is nonlinear, acting like a compression circuit by reducing a large range of acoustic inputs into a much smaller range. The compression mainly occurs around the OHC's characteristic frequency. This nonlinearity allows the auditory system to process a very wide range of intensities, which is represented by the nonlinear, logarithmic decibel scale. The perception of pitch and loudness is based on complex processes from the outer ear up through the higher auditory centers. However, the major factor is the periphery, where the cochlea acts as both a transducer and analyzer of input frequency and intensity.

Central Pathway

- Once the nerve impulses are initiated, the signals continue along the auditory pathway from the spiral ganglion cells within the cochlea to the modiolus, where the fibers form the cochlear branch of the eighth nerve. The fibers pass to the cochlear nucleus at the pontomedullary junction of the brain stem, the first truly central connection. The fibers and nucleus are tonotopically organized. All fibers synapse at the ipsilateral cochlear nucleus. The majority of fibers cross through the acoustic stria and trapezoid body to the contralateral superior olivary complex in the lower pons of the brain stem. This crossing is the first point of decussation where signals from both ears first interact to allow binaural function. Fibers ascend to the nuclei of the lateral lemniscus in the pons and to the inferior colliculus in the midbrain. The medial geniculate body in the thalamus is the last auditory nucleus before the cortex. From there, the nerve fibers radiate to the auditory cortex. Tonotopic organization is largely maintained throughout the auditory pathway from the cochlea to the cortex.
- The central pathway is a complex system with several crossovers and nuclei. Not all neuronal tracts synapse with each auditory nucleus sequentially in a "domino" fashion but rather may encounter two to five synapses. There is a proliferation of fibers ranging from about 25,000 in the eighth nerve to millions from the thalamus. In addition to the various nuclei, there are afferent and efferent fibers, all exerting a mutual influence on one another. It would be an enormous task to examine all of the possible pathways, nuclei, and processing involved in this neural transmission. A mnemonic for the general sequence of these auditory structures is ECOLI: *E*ighth nerve, *C*ochlear nucleus, *O*livary complex, *L*ateral lemniscus, and *I*nferior colliculus. However these pathways, nuclei and processing are complex and still active areas of ongoing research.
- Labyrinthine biochemistry is an ongoing area of research but Tables 14-3 and 14-4 provide basic information.

Tuning Fork Tests

The most useful fork is the 512-Hz fork. A 256-Hz fork may be felt rather than heard. In addition, ambient noises are also stronger in the low frequencies, around 250 Hz. It is essential to striking the fork gently to avoid creating overtones. See Table 14-5 for a summary of these tests.

Table 14-3 Enzymes in the Organ of Corti and Stria Vascularis
Succinate dehydrogenase
Cytochrome oxidases
Diaphorases (DPN, TPN)
Lactic dehydrogenase
Malic dehydrogenase
α-Glycerophosphate dehydrogenase
Glutamate dehydrogenase

Table 14-4 Normal Labyrinthine Fluid Values

	Perilymph				Endolymph		
	Serum	CSF	Scala tymp.	Scala vestibuli	Cochlea	Vestibule	Endolymph sac
Na (mEq/L)	141	141	157	147	6	14.9	153
K (mEq/L)	5	3	3.8	10.5	171	155	8
Cl (mEq/L)	101	126	—	—	120	120	—
Protein (mg/dL)	7000	10-25	215	160	125	—	5200
Glucose (mg/dL)	100	70	85	92	9.5	39.4	—
pH	7.35	7.35	7.2	7.2	7.5	7.5	—

Table 14-5 Summary of Tuning Fork Tests

Test	Purpose	Fork Placement	Normal Hearing	Conductive Loss	Sensorineural Loss
Weber	To determine conductive versus sensorineural loss in unilateral loss	Midline	Midline sensation; tone heard equally in both ears	Tone louder in poorer ear	Tone louder in better ear
Rinne	To compare patient's air and bone conduction hearing	Alternately between patient's mastoid and entrance to ear canal	Positive Rinne: tone louder at ear	Negative Rinne: tone louder on mastoid	Positive Rinne: tone louder by ear
Gellé	To determine if tympanic membrane and ossicular chain are mobile and intact	Mastoid	Decrease in intensity when pressure is increased	No decrease in intensity when pressure is increased if tympanic membrane and/or ossicular chain are not mobile or intact	Decrease in intensity when pressure is increased
Bing	To determine if the occlusion effect is present	Mastoid	Positive Bing: tone is louder with ear canal occluded	Negative Bing: tone is not louder with ear canal occluded	Positive Bing: tone is louder with ear canal occluded
Schwabach	To compare patient's bone conduction to that of a person with normal hearing	Mastoid	Normal Schwabach: patient hears tone for about as long as the tester	Prolonged Schwabach: patient hears tone for longer time than the tester or normal Schwabach	Diminished Schwabach: patient stops hearing the tone before the tester

Weber Test

- The Weber test is a test of lateralization.
- The tuning fork is set into motion and its stem is placed on the midline of the patient's skull. The patient must state where the tone is louder: in the left ear, in the right ear, or the midline.
- A patient with normal hearing or equal amounts of hearing loss in both ears (conductive, sensorineural, or mixed loss) will experience a midline sensation.
- A patient with a unilateral sensorineural loss will hear the tone in the better ear.
- A patient with a unilateral conductive loss will hear the tone in the poorer ear.

Rinne Test

- The Rinne test compares a patient's air and bone conduction hearing.
- The tuning fork is struck and its stem placed first on the mastoid process (as closely as possible to the posterosuperior edge of the canal without touching it), then approximately 2 inch (5 cm) lateral to the opening of the external ear canal. The patient reports whether the tone sounds louder with the fork on the mastoid or just outside the ear canal.
- Patients with normal hearing or sensorineural hearing loss will perceive the tone as louder outside the ear canal (positive Rinne).
- Patients with conductive hearing loss will perceive the sound as louder when placed on the mastoid (negative Rinne).
- A negative Rinne with the 512-Hz fork indicates a 25-dB or greater conductive hearing loss. A negative Rinne with a 256-Hz fork implies an air–bone gap of at least 15 dB. A negative Rinne with a 1024-Hz fork suggests an air–bone gap of 35 dB or more.

Bing Test

- The Bing test examines the occlusion effect.
- The tuning fork is set into motion and its stem placed on the mastoid process behind the ear while the tester alternately opens and closes the patient's ear canal with a finger.
- Patients with normal hearing or mild sensorineural hearing loss report that the tone becomes louder when the canal is closed and softer when it is open (positive Bing).
- Patients with conductive hearing loss will notice no change in the tone's loudness (negative Bing).

Schwabach Test

- The Schwabach test compares the patient's bone conduction hearing to that of a normal listener (usually the examiner).
- The tuning fork is set into motion and its stem placed alternately on the mastoid process of the patient and that of the examiner. When the patient no longer hears the sound, the examiner listens to the fork to see whether the tone is still audible.
- Patients with normal hearing will stop hearing the sound at about the same time as the tester (normal Schwabach).
- Patients with sensorineural hearing loss will stop hearing the sound before the examiner (diminished Schwabach).
- Patients with conductive hearing loss will hear the sound longer than the examiner (prolonged Schwabach).

Standard Audiometric Testing

Typical Equipment

- Audiometer to test hearing for pure tone thresholds and speech recognition
- Immittance analyzer to assess middle ear function and acoustic reflex
- A sound-isolated or acoustically treated room adequate for measuring 0-dB HL thresholds by air and by bone conduction

The main controls on a diagnostic audiometer include the following:

- Stimulus selector (pure tone; warbled tone; pulsed or alternating tones; narrow band, white, or speech noise; microphone)
- Output selector (right, left, or both headphones; bone oscillator; right or left speaker; insert earphone)
- Frequency selector (125-8000 Hz) or up to 20,000 Hz for high-frequency audiometry
- Attenuator dial (−10 to +110 dB HL) with maximum intensity limit indicator
- Stimulus mode selector (tone or microphone—either continuously on or off)
- Volume unit (VU) meter to monitor speech or external signal
- Adjustment dials to maintain proper input and output levels of speech, noise, tape, and compact disc stimuli
- Interrupter switch/bar to present or interrupt the stimulus
- Talk forward switch and dial enabling one to speak to the patient at a comfortable intensity level without requiring the microphone mode
- Talk back dial enabling one to hear the patient from the booth at a comfortable level

The immittance analyzer usually has the following minimum components:

- Probe tip
- Frequency selector (for acoustic reflex and reflex decay testing)
- Intensity selector (for acoustic reflex and reflex decay testing)
- Earphone (for stimulating the contralateral ear reflex)
- Pressure control (to increase or decrease manually the pressure in the ear canal during tympanometry)

A test will be valid only if the equipment used is appropriate and calibrated. Therefore, selection and maintenance of equipment, including care in use and at least annual calibrations, are vital.

Routine Test Battery

The purposes of the basic audiologic evaluation are to determine the following:

- Degree and configuration of hearing loss (eg, moderate, flat hearing loss)
- Site of lesion (conductive, sensorineural, or mixed)
- Possible nonsurgical intervention, such as hearing aids, speech-reading, and communication strategies
- Need for further testing

A test-battery approach allows cross-checking results to judge reliability and validity. Inconsistencies may be secondary to pseudohypacusis (nonorganic hearing loss), an inattentive or uncooperative patient, or a patient who does not understand the instructions. Results of a single test must be interpreted with caution.

A typical test battery for an audiologic evaluation includes the following:

- Pure tone audiometry (air conduction, and, if needed, bone conduction)
- Speech audiometry (speech reception threshold and word recognition score)
- Immittance/impedance measures (tympanometry and acoustic reflexes)

Pure Tone Audiometry

Pure tone audiometry is the foundation of audiometric testing. Thus, its reliability and validity are paramount. Influencing factors include the following:

- Test location (quiet enough to measure 0-dB HL thresholds; a sound-treated booth is usually required for both examiner and patient rooms)
- Equipment calibration (complete calibration at least annually)
- Personnel (generally a licensed/certified audiologist)
- Clear instructions
- Proper placement of headphones and bone oscillator
- Patient comfort

Aspects of Pure Tone Testing

- Test of sensitivity to pure tones as measured by air conduction; and by bone conduction if air conduction thresholds are 15 dB HL or greater.
- Determines thresholds: lowest levels at which patient responds at least 50% of time
- Octave frequencies 250 to 8000 Hz; interoctave frequencies (eg, 1500 Hz) if 25 dB or more difference between octave frequency thresholds
- 3000 and 6000 Hz for baseline audiograms, for example, persons exposed to high-intensity sound or receiving ototoxic medication

Masking

- Noise introduced into nontest ear to prevent that ear from detecting signals intended for test ear.
- Necessary when signal to test ear strong enough to vibrate skull and travel to nontest ear: *crossover.*
- Reduction in sound energy from one side of skull to other is *interaural attenuation.*
- Interaural attenuation for air conduction with most supra-aural headphones is 40 to 65 dB depending on frequency and patient characteristics; over 70 dB for insert earphones; for bone conduction 0 to 10 dB.
- Crossover in air conduction can occur as low as 40-dB HL and in bone conduction as low as 0-dB HL.
- For pure tones, masker is narrow-band noises; for speech, masker is speech-spectrum noise.
- Insert earphones allow much higher interaural attenuation, and thus there is much less chance of crossover. Interaural attenuation may be 70 to 90 dB, which often eliminates the need for masking during air conduction testing.

Two rules of when to mask (pure tone or speech audiometry):

A. *Air conduction*: Mask the nontest ear whenever the air conduction level to the test ear exceeds the bone conduction level of the nontest ear by 40 dB or more for circumaural earphones, 70 dB or more for insert earphones.

B. *Bone conduction*: Mask the nontest ear whenever there is an air–bone gap greater than 10 dB in the test ear. See examples in Figure 14-1.

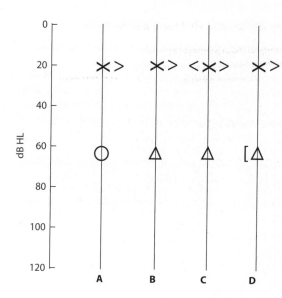

Figure 14-1 Examples of applying the rules that determine the need for masking and the results after having masked. A. Right air conduction threshold, unmasked, is 45 dB poorer than left bone conduction threshold and must be verified by masking. B. Right air conduction threshold masked (no change with masking). C. Right bone conduction threshold, unmasked, shows an air–bone gap greater than 10 dB. D. Right bone conduction threshold, masked (shifted with masking).

Air–Bone Comparisons

- *Air conduction*: earphones—hearing sensitivity from auricle to brain stem
- *Bone conduction*: bone oscillator on mastoid or forehead—hearing sensitivity only from cochlea to brain stem; bypasses outer and middle ears
- Bone conduction results show degree of hearing loss due to inner ear, nerve or central damage; air conduction results show degree of hearing loss of any conductive or sensorineural disorder. The difference or air–bone gap reflects the loss secondary to reduced transmission or conduction of sound through outer and/or middle ears.

The thresholds for air and bone conduction are recorded on an audiogram, a graphic representation of a person's sensitivity to pure tones as a function of frequency. For each frequency, indicated by numbers across the top of the audiogram, the individual's threshold in decibels HL (dB HL), indicated by numbers along the side of the audiogram, is plotted where the two numbers intersect. The most commonly used audiogram symbols are shown in Table 14-6.

Table 14-6 Commonly Used Audiogram Symbols

Left Ear	Interpretation	Right Ear
X	Unmasked air conduction	O
□	Masked air conduction	Δ
>	Unmasked bone conduction	<
]	Masked bone conduction	[
↘	No response (NR)	↙
S	Sound field	S

Data from Guidelines for audiometric symbols. Committee on Audiologic Evaluation. American Speech-Language-Hearing Association, *ASHA Suppl.* 1990 Apr;(2):25-3.

Pure tone testing yields one of several audiogram types:

- *Normal hearing*: All air conduction thresholds in both ears are within normal limits (≤ 25-dB HL; Figure 14-2).
- *Conductive hearing loss*: Hearing loss only by air conduction, with normal bone conduction thresholds, indicating outer or middle ear pathology (Figure 14-3).
- *Sensorineural hearing loss*: Hearing loss by air and by bone conduction of similar degree, indicating pathology of the cochlea (sensory) or of the nerve (neural) (Figure 14-4).
- *Mixed hearing loss*: Hearing loss by both air and bone conduction, but air conduction hearing is worse than bone conduction, indicating a conductive pathology overlaid on sensorineural pathology (Figure 14-5).

When describing a hearing loss plotted on an audiogram, configuration of the loss is important information. The audiogram may be

- Flat (see Figure 14-5)
- Rising (see Figure 14-3)
- Sloping (see Figure 14-4)
- Falling (Figure 14-6)
- Notched (Figure 14-7)
- Saucer-shaped (Figure 14-8)

Thus, pure tone air and bone conduction threshold testing provides a good profile of an individual's hearing. However, pure tone results should be interpreted in conjunction with speech audiometry, tympanometry, and acoustic reflexes.

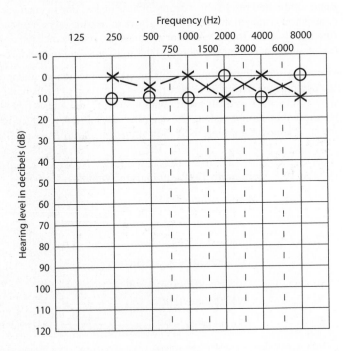

Figure 14-2 Normal hearing.

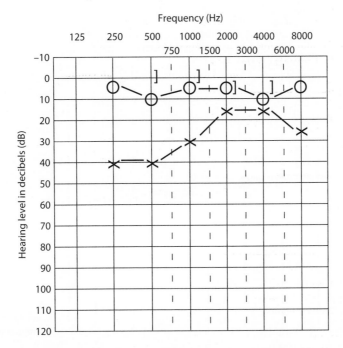

Figure 14-3 Conductive loss in the left ear in rising configuration.

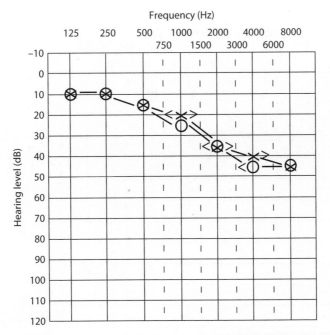

Figure 14-4 Sensorineural hearing loss in sloping configuration.

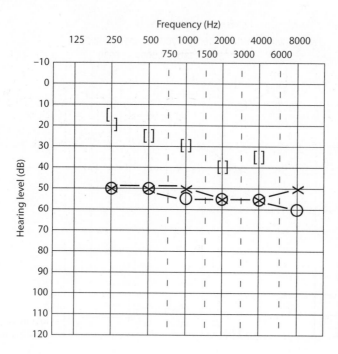

Figure 14-5 Bilateral mixed hearing loss in flat configuration.

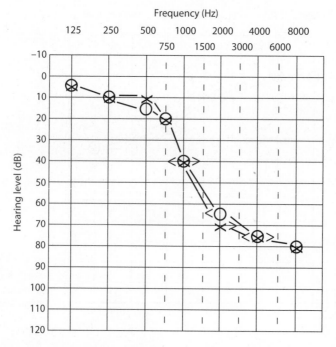

Figure 14-6 Sensorineural hearing loss in falling configuration.

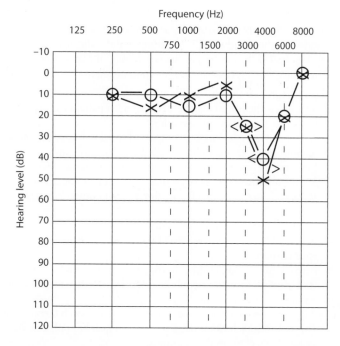

Figure 14-7 Sensorineural hearing loss in notched configuration.

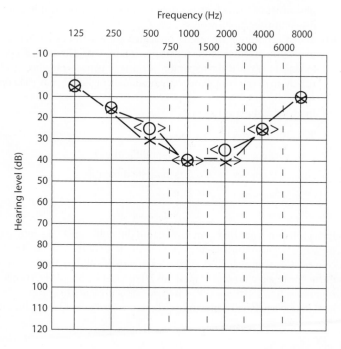

Figure 14-8 Sensorineural hearing loss in saucer-shaped configuration.

Speech Audiometry

Routine speech audiometry measures speech recognition threshold (SRT) (formerly speech reception) and suprathreshold word recognition ability reflected in the word or speech recognition score (WRS/SRS) (formerly speech discrimination). Speech stimuli may be presented by monitored live voice (MLV), cassette tape, or compact disc.

- Speech recognition threshold (SRT)
  - (a) The SRT is the lowest level in dB at which a patient can repeat spondaic words (spondees) in 50% of presentations.
  - (b) A spondee is a two-syllable compound word that is pronounced with equal stress on both syllables (eg, railroad, sidewalk, and eardrum).
  - (c) Measured primarily to confirm pure tone thresholds, SRT should be within 10 dB of the pure tone average (PTA, the average of air conduction thresholds at 500, 1000, and 2000 Hz). In a falling or rising audiometric pattern, a best two-frequency PTA may better corroborate the SRT.
- Speech awareness/detection threshold (SAT/SDT)
  - (a) An SAT/SDT is the lowest level in dB at which an individual responds to the presence of speech.
  - (b) An SAT/SDT is sometimes appropriate when assessing small children, persons with physical or mental disabilities, or those with a language barrier or any time an SRT cannot be obtained.
- Word (speech) recognition score (formerly called speech discrimination)
  - (a) This test reflects how clearly a patient can hear suprathreshold speech, usually assessed at a comfortable loudness.
  - (b) The percentage of phonetically balanced (PB) words that a patient repeats correctly is the WRS/SRS.
  - (c) A PB word list has 50 monosyllabic words; the list contains the same proportion of phonemes as that which occurs in connected (American English) discourse; a half-list comprises 25 PB words.
  - (d) The speech stimuli are usually presented at a sensation level 30 to 40 dB above SRT in order to obtain the individual's maximum score. However, if a person has reduced loudness tolerance, the maximum score is sometimes obtained at a lower SL. Conversely, in sloping or falling configurations, a higher SL may yield one's maximum score.
  - (e) Interpretation is as follows:

90%-100% correct	Normal
76%-88% correct	Slight difficulty
60%-74% correct	Moderate difficulty
40%-58% correct	Poor
40% correct	Very poor

- Interpretation regarding communication difficulty must take into account not only the score but also the absolute presentation level of the stimuli. The level of average conversational speech is 50 to 60-dB HL. In a 25-dB hearing loss, 30-dB SL means that the test words are presented at 55 dB HL, a level we are likely to encounter in most situations. In a 45-dB loss, 30-dB SL means a presentation level of 75-dB HL, a higher level than we normally encounter. Therefore, two individuals with different degrees of hearing loss may have the same score but have marked differences in how well they understand daily conversation.

Immittance/Impedance Measures Measures of middle ear function can be based on the amount of energy rejected (impedance) or the amount of energy accepted (admittance) by the middle ear. Impedance and admittance are opposite sides of the same phenomenon and yield the same information. The term "immittance" was coined to encompass both approaches, although nowadays most measurements are in admittance.

The tests performed on an immittance/impedance meter in a routine test battery are tympanometry and acoustic (stapedial) reflexes. Tympanometry is an objective test that measures the mobility (loosely termed "compliance") of the middle ear at the tympanic membrane as a function of applied air pressure in the external ear canal. Compliance is typically expressed as acoustic admittance in millimho (mMho) (or as the admittance of an equivalent volume of air in cm³ or mL), and pressure is expressed in dekapascals (daPa). As the pressure changes, the point of maximum compliance of the middle ear is identified as a peak on the tympanogram. The point of maximum compliance indicates the pressure at which the eardrum is most mobile and occurs when the pressure in the external ear canal equals the pressure in the middle ear.

There are five types of tympanograms, illustrated in Figure 14-9.

- *Type A*: normal middle ear pressure and mobility. Peak is in a normal range of compliance with pressure between −100 to +100 daPa (see Figure 14-9A).
- *Type A$_s$*: type A with abnormally shallow or low peak; restricted mobility. This type may be seen in otosclerosis, scarred tympanic membrane, or fixation of the malleus (see Figure 14-9D).

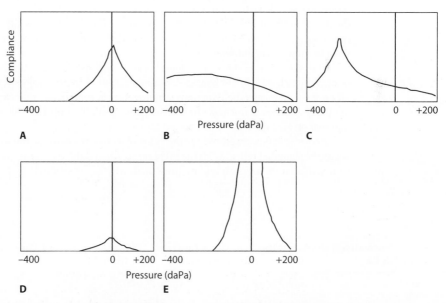

Figure 14-9 A. Type A, normal range of compliance and pressure, normal middle ear function. B. Type B, poor middle ear compliance across pressures. C. Type C, abnormal negative middle ear pressure. D. Type A$_s$, abnormally low compliance. E. Type A$_d$, abnormally high compliance.

- *Type A$_d$*: type A with abnormally deep or high peak; "loose" or hypercompliant middle ear system. This type may be seen in flaccid tympanic membrane or in disarticulation, even partial, of the ossicular chain (see Figure 14-9E). In the case of a flaccid eardrum, there may be little or no hearing loss while in the case of disarticulation; there is a substantial conductive hearing loss, which, unlike most conductive hearing losses, may be worse at the high frequencies. A type A$_d$ might be redrawn on an expanded compliance scale.
- *Type B*: flat or very low, rounded peak, but the indicated ear canal volume is within the normal range. This suggests little or no mobility and is consistent with fluid in the middle ear. In contrast, when there is no or low peak but the indicated ear canal volume is large, there probably is a patent pressure equalizing (PE) tube or a perforation in the tympanic membrane (see Figure 14-9B). If the volume reading for the canal is very low, the probe may be plugged or against the ear canal.
- *Type C*: compliance peak in region of negative pressure greater than –150 daPa; negative middle ear pressure. This finding may be consistent with a retracted tympanic membrane and a malfunctioning eustachian tube or simply a child sniffling (see Figure 14-9C). A tympanogram with extreme negative pressure might be redrawn on an expanded pressure scale.
- *Type A versus type A$_s$*: tympanometric widths (TW) distinguish between normal and abnormally low compliance.

Whereas a tympanogram gives a qualitative depiction of middle ear function, results can be quantified through normative values of (a) static acoustic admittance (compliance), (b) TW, and (c) equivalent ear canal volume shown in Table 14-7. Static acoustic admittance is a metric of middle ear mobility. Tympanometric width (TW) denotes the gradient or steepness of the tympanogram. A horizontal line is drawn at one-half the height of the compliance peak, and the points where it intersects with the tympanogram describe its width in daPa. The poorer the compliance, the broader the TW. In practice, the values overlap by age and ear condition, and must be viewed as guidelines.

One should note the scale values, because dimensions may vary by manufacturer or with tympanometric result. For example, if a middle ear is hypercompliant and the peak is clipped off on the usual scale, the tympanogram might be automatically redrawn on a larger scale making the result appear normal. Or, if the negative peak lies beyond –400 daPa, pressure might be redrawn on an expanded scale and not look as severe.

Acoustic reflex threshold testing is an objective measure of the lowest stimulus level that elicits the stapedial reflex. With the pressure set to hold the tympanic membrane at its maximum compliance, pure tone stimuli are presented; whether the signals go to one ear or to both, the

Table 14-7 Normative Values of Static Acoustic Admittance, TW, and Equivalent Ear Canal Volume for Children and Adults

Age (year)	Admittance (mL)	TW (daPa)	EC Vol (mL)
3-10	0.25-1.05	80-160	0.3-0.9
Adults (>18)	0.3-1.7	50-114	0.9-2.0

Data from Margolis RH, Hunter LI. Acoustic immittance measurements. In: Roeser RJ, Valente M, Hosford-Dunn H, eds. *Audiology Diagnosis.* New York, NY: Thieme; 2000.

stapedial reflex occurs bilaterally in response to loud sounds. Testing is performed with either ipsilateral or contralateral recording, or both.

The acoustic reflex pathway is determined by the stimulation-recording arrangement.

A. Ipsilateral recording (stimulus and recording in same ear)
    i. Acoustic nerve
    ii. Ipsilateral ventral cochlear nucleus
    iii. Trapezoid body
    iv. Ipsilateral facial motor nucleus *or* ipsilateral medial superior olive
    v. Ipsilateral facial nerve
    vi. Ipsilateral stapedius muscle
B. Contralateral recording (stimulus and recording in opposite ears)
    i. Acoustic nerve
    ii. Ipsilateral ventral cochlear nucleus
    iii. Contralateral medial superior olive
    iv. Contralateral facial motor nucleus
    v. Contralateral facial nerve
    vi. Contralateral stapedius muscle

Normal acoustic reflex thresholds range from 70- to 100-dB HL for pure tones. In the presence of any significant conductive pathology or hearing loss in the recording ear, the reflex will likely be absent; also if there is a hearing loss, whether conductive or sensorineural, in the stimulated ear greater than 65-dB HL, the reflex will likely be absent (Figure 14-10).

Hearing Impairment and Disorders of Hearing

Hearing impairments are generally characterized by degree, type, and audiometric configuration.

Degree of Hearing Loss

- Based on pure tone thresholds, hearing loss may be described according to various scales of hearing impairment. See Table 14-8 for examples of such scales. It should be noted that depending on which scale is used, the same hearing loss may be qualified

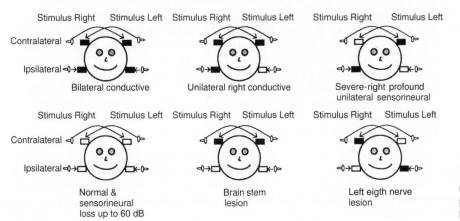

Figure 14-10 Acoustic reflex patterns. A. Reflex present at normal level. B. Reflex absent/elevated.

Table 14-8 **Scales of Hearing Impairment and Impact on Communication**

Degree of Hearing Loss	
A common classification system for use with children	
0-15 dB HL	Within normal limits
15-25 dB HL	Slight
25-30 dB HL	Mild
30-50 dB HL	Moderate
50-70 dB HL	Severe
70+	Profound

Data from Northern JL, Downs MP. *Hearing in Children.* 5th ed. Hagerstown, MD: Lippincott-Raven; 2002.

A common classification system for use with adults	
0-25 dB HL	Within normal limits
26-40 dB HL	Mild
41-55 dB HL	Moderate
56-70 dB HL	Moderate to severe (or moderately severe)
71-90 dB HL	Severe
91+	Profound

Data from Roeser R, Buckley KA, Stickney GS. Pure tone tests. In: Roeser RJ, Valente M, Hosford-Dunn H, eds. *Audiology Diagnosis.* New York, NY: Thieme; 2000.

differently (eg, a 25-dB loss may be called "hearing within normal limits" on one scale and a "mild hearing loss" on another). The discrepancy is generally because of different scales for children, who are still developing speech and language, and adults who have already acquired speech and language. The most commonly used scales for children (Northern and Downs 2002) and adults (Roeser et al 2000) are in Table 14-8.

- The degree of impairment may also be expressed as a percentage of hearing loss. Formulas for percentages of hearing loss are often based on an individual's thresholds at the speech frequencies of 500, 1000, 2000, and 3000 Hz. One such formula is used by the American Medical Association (see Table 14-9). An advantage to using a percentage is that it is a single number as opposed to a phrase, such as "mild sloping to severe." Its utility is in medicolegal cases. However, descriptive terminology is more useful in most other situations, such as communication (see Table 14-10). When portraying a loss for the purpose of rehabilitation, for example, "mild, sloping to severe hearing loss" would be more useful than "40% loss" because a percentage is an absolute number that gives no indication of the configuration of the hearing loss.

Note: If a percentage score is used to quantify degree of loss, it is important that the patient does not confuse the percentage hearing loss number with their word recognition score, which is often obtained at 40 dB above the SRT (resulting in a presentation level above that of average conversation). Few comparisons can be directly made between percent of hearing loss and a word recognition score. For example, one patient may have a word recognition score of 92%

Table 14-9 AMA Formula for Percentage of Hearing Loss

For each ear

1. Average the thresholds at 500, 1000, 2000, and 3000 Hz. If a threshold is better than 0 dB, take the threshold as 0 dB; if the threshold is poorer than 100 dB, take the threshold as 100 dB.

2. Subtract 25 from this number.

3. Multiply by 1.5. This is the percentage of hearing loss for one ear.

For binaural hearing impairment

1. Multiply the percentage of hearing impairment for the better ear by 5.

2. Add to this number the percentage of hearing impairment for the poor ear.

3. Divide this sum by 6. This is the percentage of binaural hearing impairment.

---

at 60-dB HL with a 17% hearing loss and another patient may have a word recognition score of 68% at 60-dB HL with a 4% hearing loss, particularly in a steeply sloping loss. The amount of difficulty that one may have for a given hearing loss is individual and cannot be generalized among patients.

- The difference between "hearing impaired" and "deaf" should be noted. Whereas hearing impaired refers to anyone with a hearing loss, deaf applies only to those with profound, sensorineural hearing loss (usually > 90-dB HL and for whom hearing is nonusable even with a hearing aid). The term "hard-of-hearing" refers to the wide range of hearing loss between normal and deaf.

Table 14-10 Degree of Communication Difficulty as a Function of Hearing Loss

Communication Difficulty	Level of Hearing Loss (Pure Tone Average 500-1000-2000 Hz)	Degree of Loss
Demonstrates difficulty understanding soft-spoken speech; good candidate for hearing aid(s); children will need preferential seating and resource help in school.	25-40	Mild
Demonstrates an understanding of speech at 3-5 ft; requires the use of hearing aid(s); children will need preferential seating, resource help, and speech therapy.	40-55	Moderate
Speech must be loud for auditory reception; difficulty in group settings; requires the use of hearing aid(s); children will require special classes for hearing-impaired, plus all of the above	55-70	Moderate to severe
Loud speech may be understood at 1 ft from ear; may distinguish vowels but not consonants; requires the use of hearing aid(s); children will require classes for hearing impaired, plus all of the above.	70-90	Severe
Does not rely on audition as primary modality for communication; may benefit from hearing aid(s); may benefit from cochlear implant; children will require all of the above plus total communication.	90+	Profound

Data from Goodman A. Reference zero levels for pure tone audiometers. *ASHA.* 1965;7:262-263. As in Roeser R, Buckley KA, Stickney GS. Pure tone tests. In: Roeser RJ, Valente M, Hosford-Dunn H, eds. *Audiology Diagnosis.* New York, NY: Thieme; 2000.

Types of Hearing Loss

Sample audiograms of the types of hearing loss—conductive, sensorineural and mixed—can be found on pages 251-255.

Conductive

- Caused by a disorder of external and/or middle ear.
- Generally cannot exceed 60-dB HL.
- Pathologies that increase middle ear stiffness, for example, effusion, primarily affect low frequencies.
- Pathologies that decrease middle ear stiffness, for example, ossicular interruption, produce a flat loss (exception: partial ossicular discontinuity can produce a predominantly high frequency loss).
- Pathologies that only alter mass are infrequent and primarily affect high frequencies.
- Sufficient effusion combines stiffness and mass, producing a loss in both low and high frequencies, often with a characteristic peak at 2000 Hz.

Sensorineural

- Caused by a disorder of the cochlea and/or eighth nerve.
- Can range from mild to profound.
- Great majority of cases are cochlear rather than retrocochlear; thus the term "sensorineural" should be used instead of "nerve" loss.

Mixed

- Combination of conductive and sensorineural hearing losses

Central

- Caused by a disorder of the auditory system in brain stem or higher
- May or may not appear as hearing loss on pure tone audiogram or yield abnormal results on conventional speech audiometric tests
- May cause patients to report disproportionate difficulty in understanding or processing speech relative to the audiogram

Other Auditory Tests: Behavioral and Physiologic Site-of-Lesion Testing

In cases of sensorineural hearing loss, there are tests that can help identify whether the site of lesion is cochlear or retrocochlear. The tests are both behavioral and physiologic, the latter being far more efficient. The objective physiologic procedures along with improved radiologic imaging have rendered the behavioral approaches virtually obsolete. As in routine audiologic evaluations, site-of-lesion testing involves a battery approach.

Because behavioral tests for peripheral site of lesion are primarily of historical interest, they are presented here in brief summary.

Alternate Binaural Loudness Balance Test

Alternate binaural loudness balance (ABLB) test checks for recruitment, an abnormally rapid loudness growth. In unilateral or asymmetrical sensorineural hearing loss, the listener balances the loudness of a suprathreshold tone alternated between ears. A loudness balance achieved at equal intensity levels (dB HL), rather than at equal sensation levels (dB SL), indicates recruitment and suggests a cochlear site of damage.

Short Increment Sensitivity Index

Short increment sensitivity index (SISI) assesses whether the listener detects small momentary increases in intensity. If a patient identifies only 30% or less of the brief 1-dB increments in a continuous high-intensity tone, that is characteristic of an eighth nerve lesion. Conversely, a high detection score of 70% or more is inconsistent with a neural insult, thereby supporting a cochlear site.

Bekesy Audiometry

Bekesy audiometry assesses auditory adaptation or fatigue. A patient plots one's threshold using a Bekesy audiometer. The person raises or lowers the intensity with a hand switch to keep the signal near threshold while the audiometer automatically sweeps across frequency. The patient plots thresholds for a pulsed tone and then for a continuous tone. A continuous signal is more likely to induce fatigue than an interrupted one. For normal listeners, threshold plots will be nearly identical (Békésy type I), and for persons with cochlear lesions, tracings for the continuous tone will be poorer than those for the pulsed tone only by approximately 20 dB (type II). Patients with a neural lesion tend to produce continuous tone tracings more than 20 dB poorer than pulsed tracings, sometimes dramatically worse in the high frequencies (type III) or consistently across the spectrum (type IV). The excessive auditory fatigue shown by type III or IV is a sign of a neural lesion.

Tone Decay Test

Tone decay test assesses auditory adaptation or fatigue. The patient listens to a continuous tone slightly above threshold and indicates when the tone is no longer audible. If the patient cannot hear it for 60 seconds, tone intensity is increased 5 dB and a new timing period is begun, until the patient hears the tone for the full minute. Decay or fatigue beyond 25 dB is a sign of neural lesion. Tone decay tests may have usefulness in screening for eighth nerve lesions. Evaluating acoustic reflex decay is a superior test of auditory fatigue and is less time consuming.

Performance Intensity Function

Performance intensity function assesses degradation in word recognition at high levels. Word recognition scores are obtained for successive lists of PB words at increasing intensities to create a performance intensity function (PI-PB). Persons with normal hearing or conductive hearing losses will have functions that rise to a high score and remain high. In sensorineural hearing losses, the function will peak and then decrease ("rollover"). Typically, rollover is slight in cochlear lesions and marked in eighth nerve lesions. The rollover ratio = (PB max − PB min [beyond peak score])/PB max. A rollover ratio of 0.30 or greater is indicative of an eighth nerve lesion; however, sensitivity is poor.

Acoustic Reflex Decay

The acoustic reflex decay test measures whether or not the stapedius muscle contraction is maintained during a continuous signal 10 dB above acoustic reflex threshold for 10 seconds. As in the acoustic reflex threshold test, both ipsilateral and contralateral stimulations are used. Inability to maintain the contraction (loss of half of the amplitude of the reflex in 5 seconds at 1000 Hz and especially at 500 Hz) is considered positive for retrocochlear involvement.

Auditory Brain Stem Response

The auditory brain stem response (ABR) is an acoustically evoked series of bioelectrical potentials of the eighth nerve and brain stem. ABR testing is the most effective diagnostic tool to assess the integrity of the auditory system from the eighth nerve up through the midbrain, but results can be affected by conductive and cochlear disorders because they reduce the level of the signal activating the auditory pathway. The ABR is not a direct test of hearing in that it does not measure the perception of sound. Rather, the waveform of the ABR is a representation of the synchronous discharge of onset-sensitive activity of the first- through sixth-order peripheral and central neurons in the auditory system. Clinical applications are neonatal hearing screening, estimating hearing thresholds in patients who cannot or will not comply with behavioral measures, neurodiagnostic assessment of retrocochlear pathology, and intraoperative monitoring. (See Chapter 15 for information on setup, administration, and interpretation of the ABR.)

There are a number of variables that must be considered when performing the ABR.

Subject Variables

- *Age*: The ABR is incomplete at birth; generally, only waves I, III, and V are observed; the absolute latencies of wave III and especially wave V are longer than those of adults rendering their interpeak latency values (especially wave I-V) prolonged relative to adult values. The delay is secondary to the immaturity of the central auditory system. During the first 18 months, other wave components develop and the absolute latencies and resultant interpeak latencies of the waves shorten to adult values.
- *Gender*: Females often have shorter latencies (0.2 millisecond) and larger amplitudes (waves IV and V) than males, and may also have shorter interwave latencies.
- *Temperature*: Temperatures exceeding ± 1°C (< 36°C or > 38°C) may affect latencies. A temperature reading is necessary only on seriously ill patients. A correction factor of −0.2 millisecond for every degree of body temperature below normal and −0.15 millisecond for each degree of body temperature above normal can be used for the wave I-V interpeak latency.
- *Medication and drugs*: The ABR is affected by a number of drugs as well as acute or chronic alcohol intoxicants. However, as opposed to longer-latency evoked potentials, the ABR is not markedly affected by the usual sedation/anesthesia so often necessary with difficult-to-test patients when seeking thresholds.
- *Attention and state of arousal*: Muscular (neck or jaw muscles) and movement artifacts are unwanted noise in an ABR assessment. It is important to encourage a natural sleeplike state or medically induce a drowsy or sleep state, if necessary, in order to obtain the best wave forms. Metabolic or toxic coma and natural sleep do not appear to affect the ABR. If sedation is needed, as is common in pediatric patients, the usual involvement of anesthesia and recovery personnel and equipment are required and must be arranged in advance.
- *Hearing loss*: In conductive or mixed hearing losses, subtract the amount of the air–bone gap from the signal level and compare results to norms for that level. In cochlear impairments, low-frequency losses have negligible effect on the click ABR, and flat losses above 75-dB HL usually preclude the ABR. High-frequency cochlear losses yield essentially normal click ABRs, provided the loss is no more than moderate and that the signal is 20 dB above the pure-tone threshold at 4000 Hz. Otherwise, cochlear losses can degrade waveform morphology, alter latency, and decrease amplitude but not in a perfectly predictable way. When an ABR is abnormal, one must consider the type, degree, and configuration of hearing loss, before presuming retrocochlear involvement.

Stimulus Variables

- *Click polarity*: In most patients rarefaction stimuli result in shorter latency, higher amplitude for early components, and a clearer separation of wave IV and V components than do condensation clicks.
- *Rate*: Stimulus rates of over 30 clicks per second begin to increase latency of all components. Fast click rates greater than 55 per second tend to reduce waveform clarity. Rate has more of an effect on premature than term newborns, on children younger than 18 months than on older children, and on older children than on adults. Rate influences wave V the most and, therefore, the III-V and I-V intervals.
- *Intensity*: As intensity increases, amplitude increases and latency decreases. As intensity decreases, amplitude decreases and latency increases. Wave V latency increases about 2 milliseconds when going from a high level (80 dB) to a low level (20 dB) (ie, the absolute latency may shift from 5.5 to 7.5 milliseconds).
- *Stimulus frequency*: Higher-frequency stimuli result in shorter latencies than do lower-frequency stimuli, such as a 500-Hz tone pip because they emanate primarily from the more basal turn of the cochlea. It requires more time for a signal to travel to the lower-frequency regions of the cochlea.

Recording Parameters

- *Electrode montage*: Waves IV and V are better separated in contralateral recordings; waves I and III are more prominent in ipsilateral recordings. A horizontal montage (ie, ear to ear as opposed to vertex to ear) results in an increase in wave I amplitude. Electrode placement on the earlobe results in less muscle potential and greater amplitude of wave I than does placement on the mastoid.
- *Filter settings*: Up to 3000 Hz, high-frequency information results in increased amplitude and decreased latency. Below 1500 Hz, low-frequency information results in rounded peaks and longer latencies.

Otoacoustic Emissions

Otoacoustic emissions (OAEs) are acoustic signals generated by the cochlear OHCs and transmitted out through the middle ear to the ear canal where they can be recorded by a sensitive microphone in a quiet, but not usually sound treated, environment. The subject needs to be relatively quiet and calm and have normal middle ear function for good recordings. As a measure of OHC function, OAEs can be used to screen hearing, to estimate cochlear sensitivity by frequency, and to differentiate between sensory and neural hearing losses. OAEs do not require any behavioral response from the patient. Thus they can be used even in neonates and comatose patients.

Either spontaneous or evoked OAEs can be recorded clinically, but the evoked emissions are more useful. Spontaneous otoacoustic emissions (SOAEs) are generated with no external stimulus. Evoked otoacoustic emissions (EOAEs) are generated in response to an acoustic stimulus. Two types of EOAEs are in common clinical use: transient otoacoustic emissions (TEOAEs) and distortion product otoacoustic emissions (DPOAEs). Sustained frequency otoacoustic emissions (SFOAEs), occurring in response to ongoing stimuli, exist but have no clinical application.

Characteristics of all OAEs:

- Can be detected as acoustic energy within external auditory canal.
- Pathway of energy transfer is: OHC, basilar membrane, cochlear fluids, oval window, ossicles, and tympanic membrane, which acts as a loudspeaker to external ear canal.

- OAEs are an epiphenomenon, that is, not a process of hearing but a byproduct of it.
- Efficient, objective, noninvasive "window" into cochlear function.
- Limited and can be precluded by conductive hearing loss, which inhibits sound energy both from being transmitted from external ear canal to cochlea and from cochlea to external ear canal; present OAEs indicate intact OHC function, but absent OAEs do not necessarily indicate OHC malfunction, unless normal middle ear status is confirmed.

Three types of OAEs recorded clinically

A. *SOAEs:* Approximately 35% to 60% of normally hearing individuals have spontaneous otoacoustic emissions, that is, generated with no external stimulus. When present, SOAEs can indicate good OHC function, but because they are absent even in many normally hearing individuals, their absence is nondiagnostic. In general, SOAEs do not correlate to tinnitus although exceptions exist.

B. *TEOAEs:* TEOAEs occur in response to transient signals such as clicks or very brief tone bursts. The normal TEOAE response has the same frequency components of the stimulus. In a confirmed sensorineural hearing loss of greater than 30 to 40 dB, TEOAEs are absent in cochlear lesions but present in purely neural lesions. However, an acoustic neuroma, if it impairs cochlear blood supply, can affect OAEs.
   i. Low-level stimuli below 30-dB SPL, therefore must be measured in quiet environment with sensitive microphone, spectral analysis, and computer averaging..
   ii. A sign that the cochlea has either normal function through the OHCs or has no more than approximately a 30-40-dB HL sensorineural hearing impairment.
   iii. TEOAEs can be analyzed by octave band for presence or absence of cochlear response across the frequency range but only provides a present or absent response for whether cochlear hearing is better or worse than the 30 to 40 dB range at each octave band up through 4000 Hz.

C. *DPOAEs:* DPOAEs occur in response to two simultaneous brief pure tones of different frequencies (F_1 and F_2). In response to F_1 and F_2 stimuli, the healthy cochlea then produces several distortion products at frequencies different from the stimuli. The most prominent distortion product is usually at the frequency $2F_2$-F_1.
   i. A DPOAE is a single tone evoked by two simultaneously presented pure tones.
   ii. Stimulus levels typically 55 to 65-dB SPL but intensity functions may be tested.
   iii. Usually easiest to obtain a distortion product (DP) from the human cochlea when the stimulus (or primary) frequencies, F1 and F2, are separated by ratio of 1:1.2, for example, 2000 and 2400 Hz.
   iv. By using different combinations of primary tones, different distortion-product frequencies can be generated, thereby allowing objective assessment of a large portion of the basilar membrane.
   v. Of the several interactions of the stimulus tones, the interaction 2F1-F2 (or the cubic difference tone), usually produces the most detectable distortion product whose frequency is lower than either of the two stimulus frequencies.
   vi. Reflects cochlear status nearer F2 as opposed to F1 or the DP.
   vii. DPOAEs can be obtained in persons with more OHC loss and in response to higher frequency stimuli than can TEOAEs.
   viii. Help estimate presence of hearing loss by frequency, but not precise thresholds, in the 1000 to 8000 Hz range; absent DPOAEs with normal middle ear function generally indicate at least a 40-dB cochlear hearing loss depending on stimulus intensity. Research is continuing on threshold predictions with DPOAEs.

Clinical applications of both TEOAES and DPOAEs:

- Neonatal, ear-specific, hearing screening via automated DPOAE instruments (although vernix in outer ear canal or mesenchyme in middle ear may preclude recording OAEs in first few days of extrauterine life).
- Part of test battery for *auditory neuropathy/dyssynchrony*, a rare condition in which there are sensorineural hearing loss, abnormal ABR, absent acoustic reflexes (ipsilateral and contralateral), and poorer word recognition ability than expected based on the pure-tone audiogram, but OAEs are present.
- Useful in patients who are difficult to test because they are unable or unwilling to respond validly during conventional audiometry; part of a test battery and the cross-check principle.
- Differentiating between cochlear and eighth nerve lesions in sensorineural hearing impairments (including idiopathic sudden loss and candidacy for cochlear implant). Because OAEs are preneural events, absent EOAEs in losses 40 dB or greater point to the cochlea as a site of lesion whereas present OAEs support an eighth nerve site of lesion; part of a battery of tests. However an acoustic neuroma, if affecting cochlear blood flow, may reduce OAEs.
- Intraoperative monitoring of cochlear function during surgical removal of neoplasms involving the eighth nerve if OAEs are present.
- Monitoring for ototoxicity or exposure to high sound levels; DPOAEs and/or TEOAEs may be lost or diminished for high frequencies before there are changes in pure tone thresholds. However, high-frequency audiometry is more commonly used and readily interpreted for ototoxicity monitoring and generally provides the first indication of ototoxic change.
- In cases of suspected pseudohypacusis; present TEOAEs ensures no significant conductive hearing loss and no cochlear loss greater than approximately 40-dB HL and probably less than 30-dB HL. DPOAEs can also contribute objective information of possible audiometric configuration and cochlear sensitivity.

Evaluation of Difficult-to-Test and Pediatric Patients

For patients who are difficult to test, there are specialized behavioral techniques as well as physiologic measures. Behavioral testing, when achievable, is generally preferable to physiologic procedures alone, because behavioral approaches test hearing, whereas the latter test some aspect of auditory function. However, conducting both types of tests follows the cross-check principle.

Behavioral Observation Audiometry

A. The patient is situated in center of the test room.
B. Speech, warbled tones, or other signals are presented into the sound field through loudspeakers located on either side.
C. Responses may vary but typically include eye widening, pause in activity, or (subtle) head turn toward the side of the sound.
D. Intensity of the signals is varied until lowest level of response obtained.
E. Reliance on behavioral observation audiometry (BOA) should be minimal because, if not reinforced, responses fade quickly, and reliability and validity are poor.

Visual Reinforcement Audiometry

A. Set up the same as for BOA.

B. When patient makes some response, a darkened toy on the same side as the sound source is lighted or moves.

C. If there is not a spontaneous head turn toward the sound, the light usually elicits a head turn, or the clinician points and prompts a head turn; in any case, the toy reinforces the behavior of looking in the direction of the sound.

D. Repeat until sound alone elicits head turn toward the correct side; the visual reinforcer toy is then lighted or activated; after a few times, reinforcement converts the reflexive reaction into a conditioned response.

E. Noting patient's ability to localize sound accurately on one side or the other permits some estimation of binaural hearing in the absence of earphone testing, because to localize sound, hearing must be symmetrical within 30 dB.

F. Intensity of the various signals is varied until lowest conditioned response level obtained.

G. Ultimately, discrete frequencies are preferable signals to speech, because a broadband signal could miss a loss in part of the frequency range.

H. Visual reinforcement audiometry (VRA) is appropriate for children of 6 to 30 months of age. Normative data are given in Table 14-11.

Table 14-11 Normative Data and Expected Response Levels for Infants[a]

Age	Noisemakers (~SPL)	Warbled Pure Tones (dB HL)	Speech (dB HL)	Expected Response	Startle to Speech (dB HL)
0-6 wk	50-70	75	40-60	Eye widening, eye blink, stirring or arousal from sleep, startle	65
6 wk-4 mo	50-60	70	45	Eye widening, eye shift, eye blinking, quieting; beginning rudimentary head turn by 4 mo	65
4-7 mo	40-50	50	20	Head turn on lateral plane toward sound; listening attitude	65
7-9 mo	30-40	45	15	Direct localization of sounds to side, indirectly below ear level	65
9-13 mo	25-35	38	10	Direct localization of sounds to side, directly below ear level, indirectly above ear level	65
13-16 mo	30-25	30	5	Direct localization of sound on side, above and below	65
16-21 mo	25	25	5	Direct localization of sound on side, above and below	65
21-24 mo	25	25	5	Direct localization of sound on side, above and below	65

[a] Testing done in a sound room.

Data from Northern J, Downs M. *Hearing in Children.* 5th ed. Hagerstown, MD: Lippincott-Raven; 2002.

Conditioned Play Audiometry

- By 36 months, most children can be conditioned to make a voluntary response through a game.
- In conditioned play audiometry (CPA), a game is made of listening for the "beeps"; each time a tone is presented, the child responds by playing the game, for example, dropping blocks in a bucket.
- The game activity itself is the reinforcer.
- Intensity of the various signals is varied until lowest response level obtained.
- By this age many children will accept a headset, allowing air-conduction threshold testing of each ear and bone conduction testing.

Speech Audiometry

- SRT may be obtained by using spondee picture cards or objects (eg, an airplane or toothbrush) for responses; the child points to the object or to the picture of the word presented.
- Word recognition may be tested using a standardized picture-pointing task.

Immittance Measures

- Tympanometry and acoustic reflexes are objective measures that assess middle ear status without relying on a behavioral response, but some cooperation is necessary.
- Struggling and vigorous crying can complicate obtaining an acoustic seal, make recording and interpreting a tympanogram difficult, produce a peak at high positive pressures, and obscure the acoustic reflex.
- With infants below 6 months of age, the usual 220-Hz probe tone may produce false-normal tympanograms due to compliant external canal walls and also underestimate the acoustic reflex; a higher probe tone, particularly 1000 Hz, is more sensitive to middle ear changes and produces more valid results.
- Gross impressions of hearing can be formed on the basis of the tympanogram and reflexes. A flat tympanogram suggests a slight to moderate conductive hearing loss but provides no information on sensorineural status; given a normal tympanogram, finding an acoustic reflex rules out a severe sensorineural hearing loss, whereas an absent reflex suggests a severe-profound sensorineural hearing loss or central problem.

Auditory Brain Stem Response

- Auditory brain stem response helps estimate hearing sensitivity for frequencies 1000 to 4000 Hz. Frequency-specific tone bursts are generally employed. Click stimuli are sometimes used for a quick estimate of threshold in the 2000- to 4000-Hz range.
- A 500-Hz tone burst helps estimate sensitivity in low frequencies, but estimation is not as accurate as for high frequencies.
- It can be performed by bone conduction, if AC results abnormal, but information is more limited than by behavioral testing.
- It is complicated by need for sedation in older infants and toddlers and its requisite life support and recovery services.

Otoacoustic Emissions

- OAEs only test cochlear function (ie, specifically OHC function). Thus if a retrocochlear lesion exists that impacts auditory function, OAEs would still be normal.
- Presence of TEOAEs ensures that cochlear hearing could not be worse than about 30 to 40-dB HL and results can be interpreted by octave band analysis.

- DPOAEs can be recorded sometimes in the presence of even moderate to severe hearing loss depending on stimulus levels but provide more frequency specific information.
- Requires substantially less time than ABR.
- As with ABR, OAE testing requires that the patient be relatively still and quiet but only for 5 to 10 minutes per ear. Because OAEs take so little time, sedation and its requisite life support are rarely needed.
- A common limitation in children is presence of a middle-ear disorder, which usually precludes recording any type of OAE.
- In rare cases, persons may have hearing loss on behavioral testing, normal middle ear function, abnormal ABR, but normal OAEs; these findings may indicate auditory neuropathy/dyssynchrony.

History Interview

An important component of evaluating the pediatric patient is the history interview. The following should be addressed:

- Does the child respond as well as other children of the same age, ask "what?" excessively, or turn TV on loud or sit close?
- Is communication development as good as that of same-age children?
- Has the child had more than the usual number of ear, nose, or throat problems? Does any hearing loss, speech, or language delay seem disproportionate to the amount of the child's ear trouble? (The concern is that recurrent OME can mask a sensorineural hearing loss.)

Identification of Infant Hearing Impairment

Early hearing loss detection and intervention (EHDI) in infants is crucial, because otherwise children will lag behind in communicative, cognitive, and social-emotional development, and likely have lower educational and occupational levels later in life. An EHDI program includes universal neonatal hearing screening, particularly valuable because nearly 50% of congenital hearing losses have no associated risk indicator (many presumably recessive traits) (Table 14-12). EHDI programs target congenital permanent bilateral, unilateral sensory, or permanent conductive hearing loss, neural hearing loss (eg, "auditory neuropathy/dyssynchrony") in infants admitted to the NICU, and late-onset, progressive hearing loss. In 2007, the Joint Committee on Infant Hearing endorsed these principles for an EHDI program:

- All neonates have hearing screening via a physiologic measure (ABR and/or OAE) during their birth admission, and if not possible then, before 1 month of age.
- For those who do not pass the birth admission screen or subsequent rescreenings (either before discharge or as outpatients), appropriate audiologic and medical evaluations to confirm the presence of hearing loss should be in progress before 3 months of age.
- Infants with confirmed permanent hearing impairment must receive intervention services before 6 months of age.
- All infants who pass newborn screening but who have a risk indicator (see Table 14-12) for hearing loss or communicative delays should have ongoing audiologic and medical surveillance and monitoring. These include indicators associated with late-onset, progressive, or fluctuating hearing loss or auditory neural dysfunctions.

Table 14-12 **Risk Indicators Associated With Permanent Congenital, Delayed-Onset, or Progressive Hearing Loss in Childhood**

1. §Caregiver concern regarding hearing, speech, language, or developmental delay.

2. §Family history of permanent childhood hearing loss.

3. Neonatal intensive care of > 5 days or any of the following regardless of length of stay: ECMO, §assisted ventilation, exposure to ototoxic medications (gentamycin and tobramycin) or loop diuretics (furosemide/Lasix), and hyperbilirubinemia that requires exchange transfusion.

4. §In utero infections, such as CMV, herpes, rubella, syphilis, and toxoplasmosis.

5. Craniofacial anomalies, including those that involve the pinna, ear canal, ear tags, ear pits, and temporal bone anomalies.

6. Physical findings, such as white forelock, that are associated with a syndrome known to include a sensorineural or permanent conductive hearing loss.

7. §Syndromes associated with hearing loss or progressive or late-onset hearing loss, such as neurofibromatosis, osteopetrosis, and Usher syndrome; other frequently identified syndromes include Waardenburg, Alport, Pendred, and Jervell and Lange-Nielson syndromes.

8. §Neurodegenerative disorders, such as Hunter syndrome, or sensory motor neuropathies, such as Friedreich ataxia and Charcot-Marie-Tooth syndrome.

9. Culture-positive postnatal infections associated with sensorineural hearing loss, §including confirmed bacterial and viral (especially herpes viruses and varicella) meningitis.

10. Head trauma, especially basal skull/temporal bone fracture§ that requires hospitalization.

11. §Chemotherapy.

Risk indicators marked with a "§" are of greater concern for delayed-onset hearing loss.
Data from Joint Committee on Infant Hearing, 2007.

Pseudohypacusis

Pseudohypacusis means false or exaggerated hearing loss (FEHL), that is, hearing behaviors discrepant with audiologic test results, inconsistent/invalid test results, or an alleged loss of hearing sensitivity in the absence of organic pathology. The terms "functional" and "nonorganic" hearing loss are not synonymous with pseudohypacusis. When applied to other complaints, "functional" and "nonorganic" mean no organic disorder of the organs involved, but they do not mean the absence of any problem whatsoever (eg, irritable bowel syndrome). However, when applied to hearing, they mean that there is not a problem with the hearing system or not as great as presented. As with other diagnostic questions, a battery approach is advisable.

Pseudohypacusis can be deliberate, unintentional, or a mix of both; the difference is difficult to know because those are states of mind. Thus, psychological labels, such as malingering or conversion disorder, as well as a judgmental posture should be avoided. FEHL is twice as common in children as in adults, and, among children, twice as prevalent in females as in males. The typical age in children is 11 years. An FEHL should not be dismissed lightly, particularly in children, because it is often associated with a psychosocial disorder and may require prompt intervention.

Signs of possible pseudohypacusis are as follows:

- *Pretest interview*: Patient seems to have no difficulty understanding but presents a moderate, bilateral hearing loss during testing.

- *Referral source*: A compensation case; eligibility determination for goods or services.
- *Patient history*: Patient can name a specific incident that caused the hearing loss and stands to gain in some way as a result, for example, money, avoidance of some burdensome duty or task, or excuse for poor performance.
- Performance on routine tests.
  - (a) Certain behaviors, such as leaning or cocking the head to the side of the signal, straining, looking confused or wondering, especially upon signal presentation, half-word responses during the SRT ("ear" for "eardrum"), and responding during speech audiometry with a questioning intonation as if uncertain.
  - (b) *Test–retest reliability worse than 5 dB*: However, inattentiveness on the part of the patient must first be ruled out and reinstruction and retesting may be necessary. Factors affecting attention can be pain, mental confusion, advanced age, or other substantial psychomotor limitation.
  - (c) Disparity between the PTA and the SRT greater than 10 dB is one of the most common inconsistencies in pseudohypacusis. Agreement of the two measures should be within 10 dB. However, before pseudohypacusis is suspected, SRT–PTA disagreement due to audiogram configuration must be ruled out. In markedly rising or sloping patterns, the two-frequency average (the average of the two best/lowest thresholds of 500, 1000, and 2000 Hz) or even the one best speech frequency may better agree with the SRT.
  - (d) An invalidly elevated SRT may be detected by obtaining a word recognition score at or near the voluntary SRT (eg, SRT + 10 dB). If a good word recognition score is obtained at threshold, the SRT was invalid.
  - (e) Presence of acoustic reflexes with audiometric air–bone gaps.
  - (f) In unilateral or asymmetrical hearing losses, a difference greater than 65 dB between test ear and nontest ear results or absence of response (unmasked) in the poorer ear. In air conduction testing, cross-hearing (crossover) should occur at no more than about 65 dB (may be 75 dB for insert earphones) above opposite-ear bone conduction thresholds; in bone conduction testing, no air–bone gap in the worse ear even without masking the better ear, because cross-hearing should occur at no worse than 10 dB above opposite-ear bone conduction thresholds.

Tests for Suspected Pseudohypacusis

For a patient with possibility of pseudohypacusis, such as noise-induced hearing loss (NIHL) for compensation, OAEs are a valuable and objective tool for measuring OHC function. Often when these results are presented to the patient, the patient begins to cooperate. It is generally best to avoid alienating the patient by using a gentle approach such as "These tests suggest that maybe I didn't make it clear to you that you had to respond even if you barely heard the sound rather than when it was easy to hear. Let's try that test again." The ABR, while more expensive and time consuming, can also be very useful as it requires no behavioral response from the patient and can give a good estimate of actual threshold. OAES and ABRs are not described in detail here because they are discussed elsewhere in this chapter and in Chapter 15. Acoustic reflex thresholds may also be helpful. In addition some behavioral tests are fairly quick and inexpensive although they do not have the objectivity of OAEs and ABRs.

Physiologic Tests for Pseudohypacusis

Acoustic Reflex Testing The presence of the acoustic reflex at a level 5 dB or less above voluntary auditory thresholds strongly suggests some degree of pseudohypacusis (see Immittance Measures under Evaluation of Difficult-to-Test and Pediatric Patients).

Otoacoustic Emissions OAEs can be very helpful by providing objective information about cochlear function. The presence of TEOAEs indicates that cochlear hearing could not be worse than approximately 30- to 40-dB HL for each octave band response present. DPOAEs can help determine probable audiometric configuration including higher-frequency information.

Auditory Brain Stem Response Because it is an objective test, the ABR is a powerful tool for determining the presence or absence of hearing loss and for estimating degree of genuine hearing loss. However, it is far more time consuming than most of the other procedures but can be helpful if the other approaches are not sufficient.

Behavioral Tests for Pseudohypacusis

Stenger Test

- Excellent test for unilateral or asymmetrical hearing losses in which the difference between ears is at least 30 dB.
- Based on the Stenger effect: when two tones of the same frequency are presented simultaneously to both ears, the patient will perceive the tone only in the ear in which the tone is louder.
- To perform the Stenger test, simultaneously present a tone 5 dB above threshold to the good ear and an identical tone 5 dB below the voluntary threshold to the poor ear.
- If the patient responds, the test is negative because the patient heard the tone in the good ear. If the patient does not respond, the test is positive. The patient should respond, because the tone presented to the good ear is 5 dB above its threshold; if the patient does not respond, it must be because the tone was perceived in the poorer ear and the patient chooses not to respond.
- To help estimate thresholds, simultaneously present a tone at 5-dB SL to the good ear and 0-dB HL to the poor ear. The patient should respond. Increase the presentation level in the poor ear by 5 dB steps until the patient ceases to respond. This level should be within 15 dB of the patient's actual threshold in the poor ear.
- A speech Stenger may be performed in the same manner using spondee (SRT) words in place of pure tones.

Behavioral Tests of Historical Interest

Delayed Auditory Feedback With the advent of OAEs and ABRs, delayed auditory feedback (DAF) is almost never used, and most clinics no longer have the equipment for this test. DAF is based on the principle that individuals monitor the loudness and rate of their speech by auditory self-monitoring. An individual hearing their speech with a slight delay will alter their speech (eg, speed, increased vocal intensity, hesitations, prolongations, or stuttering). The patient reads aloud while speech is played back with a delay of 0.1 to 0.2 second at 0 dB HL. The task is repeated with an increase of 10 dB each time until a positive result is observed. Changes are evidence that patients can hear themselves. This test is applicable to monaural/binaural losses, has good sensitivity, and can provide an estimate of SRT. However, it requires proper tape recording and is seldom used now that better physiologic measures are available.

Doerfler–Stewart Test Individuals with either normal hearing or with genuine hearing loss can repeat SRT words in the presence of a masking noise that is as loud as the speech signal. In contrast, persons with pseudohypacusis stop responding at lower masking noise levels. An SRT is first established in quiet and then with the masking noise on. The intensity of the masking is increased with each word until the patient no longer responds. Next, a threshold for just the masking noise is determined, followed by obtaining a second SRT in noise. These measures are compared to normative data. This procedure is involved and time consuming and has only fair accuracy; hence it is rarely used. However, it is applicable to one- or two-ear hearing losses if OAEs and ABRs are not available as in field work in other countries.

Lombard Test This test is based on the Lombard effect, the phenomenon that a person increases the volume of one's voice in the presence of loud background noise because the noise interferes with self-monitoring. To perform the test, masking noise is introduced through the headphones as the patient reads aloud. The tester monitors the volume of the patient's voice. With a true hearing loss, there is no change in the volume because the patient does not hear the masking noise, but in pseudohypacusis, the patient speaks louder. Although applicable to monaural and binaural hearing losses, sensitivity is fair at best, and it affords only a rough estimate of the SRT; as a result, this test is hardly ever used.

Bekesy Audiometry A type V Bekesy tracing is suggestive of pseudohypacusis. It can be used in either monaural or binaural losses. Even in modified Bekesy versions, a type V pattern is fair at best, both in sensitivity and in specificity. It is also a lengthy procedure; moreover, the equipment is generally not available. Hence, audiologists use Bekesy audiometry infrequently in cases of suspected pseudohypacusis.

Ototoxicity Monitoring

For patients receiving ototoxic medications (eg, cisplatin, long-term aminoglycosides) high-frequency audiometry generally for stimuli 10,000 to 20,000 is performed along with pure tone audiometry in the conventional frequency range. Detecting threshold changes in the high-frequency threshold range provides the physician the opportunity to change the medication protocol before the hearing loss affects the conventional frequency range and the patient's communication. If the medication protocol cannot be changed, the audiologist can work with the patient and their family on communication strategies and possibly amplification as the hearing loss progresses. Significant ototoxic change is either (1) a threshold shift of 20 dB or greater at any one test frequency, (2) threshold shifts of 10 dB or greater at any two adjacent frequencies, or (3) loss of response at any three consecutive frequencies where thresholds were previously obtained. It is also critical that a change in middle ear status be ruled out and the noted changes be replicated within 24 hours (frequently the replication occurs on the same test appointment). These criteria can be applied to both the conventional and high-frequency ranges. OAEs may also be helpful in detecting early ototoxic changes, but no standardized significant change criteria have been established. Ototoxicity monitoring may include a variety of considerations, including patient age, baseline hearing status, general health status, specific drug and dosing employed, concomitant medications, treatment schedule, and kidney and liver function.

Central Auditory Processing

Central auditory processing (CAP) is the active, complex set of operations performed by the central nervous system on auditory inputs. Auditory processing is not only central; auditory signals are acted upon throughout the auditory system, including the peripheral portion from the outer ear through the cochlea and eighth nerve. Certain behaviors are typical of persons, especially children, who have central auditory disorders. The behaviors associated with central auditory disorders overlap with those of peripheral hearing impairment. Examples include frequently misunderstanding or misinterpreting what is said, attention deficiency, difficulty discriminating among speech sounds leading to reading, spelling, and other academic problems, unusual difficulty in background noise, reduced auditory memory, reduced receptive and expressive language skills, and, in general, difficulty learning through the *auditory* channel. History taking regarding hearing might well include consideration of these behaviors.

Before testing for a CAP disorder, one must rule out peripheral hearing impairment. Conventional audiologic assessment should include pure tone audiometry (many CAP tests are presented at suprathreshold levels that are above the PTA) and speech audiometry, especially recognition ability. Additional procedures are the ipsilateral and contralateral acoustic reflexes and ABR, which help to assess the integrity of the brain stem. Since no single test can assess the several aspects of auditory processing, a battery of CAP tests is mandatory. Which tests to administer depends on a test's efficacy for the patient's symptomatology and age. The CAP tests are presented monotically (stimulation of one ear at a time) or dichotically (stimulation of both ears by different stimuli). The tests are designed to make demands on the auditory system, for example, understanding degraded speech (filtered; time-altered; competing speech or noise in the ipsilateral, contralateral, or each ear; part of the signal to one ear and another to the opposite ear), identifying auditory patterns, or requiring effective interaction of the two hemispheres.

If a CAP disorder is found, management should be based on the pattern of results from the test battery. In general, management includes optimizing the auditory experience, that is, good signal-to-noise ratio (signal well above noise), good acoustic environment (low noise and reverberation), and enhanced speech input (strong, clear, and somewhat slowed). These are strategies that also are called for when there is peripheral hearing loss. In short, whether an auditory disorder is peripheral or central, intervention is most effective with a high-quality speech signal in quiet surroundings. Some patients may benefit from assistive listening devices (FM, infrared), which provide good signal versus noise characteristics (see "Assistive Devices").

Management

There are a number of ways to help persons with permanent hearing loss. They include providing high-quality amplification, maximizing auditory skills, enhancing use of visual cues, counseling, appropriate education, and vocational assistance. The goal is to have the individual function to the best of their abilities and be a full, productive, independent, well-adjusted member of society.

Instrumentation

Hearing Aids

Function

Hearing aids amplify sound to make speech more audible to enable an individual to communicate more effectively.

Terms of hearing aid function are listed as follows:

Frequency response range: the range of useful amplification across frequency.

Gain: amplification or the acoustic energy added to input sound, the difference between the input and output.

Maximum power output: the highest sound level a hearing instrument can produce; also known as saturation SPL (SSPL) and output SPL (OSPL 90).

Components

All hearing instruments have a microphone, amplifier, and output receiver powered by a battery. Hearing aids may have additional components or features.

Styles

There are five styles of hearing aids: body worn, behind-the-ear (BTE), in-the-ear (ITE), in the canal (ITC), and completely in canal (CIC) aids. Size is not an indicator of sound quality or of the latest technology; rather the larger the instrument, the greater the array of circuit capabilities that can be incorporated.

General Classes

- *Peak clipping*: constant gain until the hearing aid's maximum power output is reached above which the amplitude peaks are "clipped off." Peak clipping limits output to prevent sound from being too loud, but it also results in distortion.
- *Compression limiting*: automatic gain reduction (compression) at a preset level; whether input or output compression, the purpose is to limit the output with less distortion.
- *Wide dynamic range compression*: gain decreases as input increases over a relatively wide range of sound input. The purpose of WDRC is to compensate for the loss of cochlear OHCs. OHCs act as compressors to accommodate a large range of sound intensity; damage to OHCs curtails this "biologic compression."
- *Programmable*: gain, frequency response, and SSPL are programmed into the hearing aid according to the individual's audiometric data and preferences. Most programmable instruments have multiband compression, that is, different gain and output for separate frequency bands, because hearing loss often differs across frequencies. The boundary between frequency bands is also adjustable. Thus, programmable instruments are highly flexible and more tunable to one's hearing loss.
- *Digital*: the hearing aid's signal processing is entirely digital. The great advantage of digital circuitry is the array of features and capabilities that can be incorporated in a small housing.
  - (a) Great flexibility in setting all parameters, especially helpful for unusual audiometric configurations
  - (b) Robust feedback reduction
  - (c) *Multimemory*: different sets of performance saved in the hearing aid from which the wearer can select for different listening situations
  - (d) *Datalogging*: accumulating information, such as percentage of time spent in different acoustic environments and the user's preferred manual settings, which can be used to fine tune the hearing aid for that particular patient

Additional Considerations

- A vent (allowing sound in the ear canal to escape) decreases low frequencies, giving relatively more boost to high frequencies, reduces sense of pressure in the ear, and lessens the occlusion effect so the user's voice sounds more natural, but it also increases the chance of feedback (whistling).
- *"Open fit" hearing aids*: sit over the pinna, and a thin tubing delivers the sound into the ear canal leaving the canal open; excellent for hearing loss in high frequencies and good hearing in low and mid frequencies, because open fittings amplify just the high frequencies while allowing other sound to pass into the canal normally without amplification; they also eliminate the plugged "booming" sound of one's own voice.
- Directional microphones that improve signal-to-noise ratio.
- A "telecoil" for telephone listening without feedback whistle.
- Unaidable ear:
  - (a) CROS (contralateral routing of signal) is for unaidable hearing loss in one ear and good hearing in the other ear. Sound on the poor side is picked by a microphone and routed to the good ear.
  - (b) BiCROS (bilateral CROS) is for bilateral hearing loss, but one ear is unaidable. A CROS system on the unaidable side is combined with a conventional aid on the

better side, that is, the aidable ear receives inputs from the microphones on each side of the head.

(c) *Bone conduction hearing aid*: when an air-conduction, canal-occluding aid not possible, such as in atresia, chronic purulent drainage, or otitis externa. A bone-anchored hearing aid (BAHA) is a BC aid in which the output is connected to a metal post embedded through skin into the skull. BAHAs have slightly higher gain than conventional bone conduction hearing aid because of closer mechanical coupling.

(d) *Middle ear implant hearing aid*: a hearing aid is worn externally and coupled via magnet to a signal processor implanted under the skin; output driver connected to ossicles. This topic is covered in Chapter 19.

(e) *Disposable hearing aids*: characteristics are permanently preset and battery is non-replaceable; when the battery is exhausted, the entire unit is discarded and replaced with another instrument.

(f) *Tinnitus*: a tinnitus masker has a noise generator in a hearing aid case to drown out the tinnitus. For persons with tinnitus and hearing loss, a hearing aid itself may help mask the tinnitus. Masker-hearing aids combine a hearing aid and a noise generator.

Real-Ear Measurements and Fitting Formulas

The performance of a hearing aid in an analyzer chamber differs from that in an individual's ear canal. In real ear measurements, a probe tube microphone measures sound very close to the tympanic membrane, thereby including the (real ear) effects of the outer ear and canal and the loss of the natural gain produced by the ear canal resonance near 2700 Hz, when a hearing aid is put in place. By making unaided and aided test runs, real-ear measurements help in assessing the suitability of a hearing aid, in setting controls for optimal output, and in finding the basis for a wearer's complaints. Real-ear instruments include fitting formulas or "prescriptions" of gain and output for maximum audibility of speech without being uncomfortable. The instruments display a formula's target of optimum gain and frequency response for a particular patient's hearing loss; then one can see if the desired target is reasonably well approximated with the hearing aid in place. The formulas have minor differences, and no one formula is best.

Cochlear Implants

This topic is covered in Chapter 20.

Assistive Devices

- A hearing-impaired individual's lifestyle may be improved by a variety of assistive devices, whether or not hearing aids are used. Some are auditory—assistive listening devices (ALDs)—and others are visual or vibratory devices.
- Some of the major ALDs are listed as follows:
  (a) Telephone amplifiers
  (b) FM or infrared television listening systems
  (c) FM systems for large areas, such as classrooms, conference halls, and houses of worship.
- Some visual or vibratory assistive devices are listed as follows:
  (a) Alarm clocks, smoke detectors, security systems, baby-cry detectors, and doorbells.
  (b) Closed-caption television decoders (TV, and recorded or DVD movies).
  (c) Text telephones (TT, also known as TTD and TTY); persons who cannot use a telephone can type and receive messages via telephone. TTs also allow access to many public services, medical care, governmental agencies, and businesses. TTs can be used by persons with severe voice or speech limitations as well as by those with severe hearing disorders.

Intervention, Training, and Education

When hearing loss is present before communication is established, early intervention is crucial to take advantage of the "sensitive" period" of fastest communication growth from birth to age three. From 3 to 21 years of age, federal and state mandates require that children have a "free, appropriate education" in the "least restrictive environment."

Communicative and educational options overlap and include auditory-oral, visual (sign and finger spelling), or a combination ("total communication"). Factors other than hearing loss must be considered, such as the family's communicative system and desires and presence of other limiting conditions. Provided there is usable hearing, auditory training promotes listening skills, such as sound recognition and comprehension. Speech reading is the integrating of another person's lip movements, facial expressions, body gestures, situational cues, and linguistic factors. School-age children can be taught specific speech (articulation, voice) and language (vocabulary, grammar) skills.

Adults who become hard of hearing may benefit from auditory training and speech reading lessons. Adventitiously deafened adults can be helped to minimize the usual deterioration in speech and voice (due to absent auditory self-monitoring) and to become better users of visual cues.

Counseling and vocational guidance may be invaluable to individuals with hearing impairment. Counseling should not only give information (facts about communication, hearing loss, hearing aids, etc) but also address psychosocial issues (acceptance of one's situation, parental guilt and anger, one's self-image, social adjustment, and so on). States have agencies that can help with career choices and preparation.

Noise-Induced Hearing Loss and Industrial Audiology

Exposure to excessively strong sounds may destroy auditory cells, resulting in hearing loss. Such losses are often described as "noise-induced," but any sound—noise, speech, music—of sufficient intensity can damage hearing. Since noise is the most common cause of hearing loss due to exposure to high sound level, the *term noise-induced hearing loss* (NIHL) is the usual designation. The effects of noise on hearing may be classified as temporary threshold shift (TTS), permanent threshold shift (PTS), or acoustic trauma resulting from one or relatively few exposures to a very high sound level, such as an explosion. Typically, the hearing loss begins in a notch pattern in the 3000- to 6000-Hz region but with repeated exposure broadens to the other frequency regions giving a shallower notch.

Hazardous noise exposure can be occupational and/or recreational. Occupational noise is not inherently more hazardous to hearing than recreational noise. The public tends to discount the dangers of noise, deny their degree of exposure, and disdain means to protect hearing. Shooters, in particular, are unaware of or minimize the risk involved. A sign of early damage in shooters is an asymmetrical 4000-Hz notch loss, which is worse in the ear opposite the shoulder from which the gun is fired. By informing, counseling, and motivating persons to protect their hearing, otolaryngologists can make an enormous impact on preventing hearing impairment.

Four factors contribute to the effects of noise: sound level (in dB SPL), spectral composition, time distribution of the exposure during a working day, and cumulative noise exposure over days, weeks, or years. OSHA has established guidelines for permissible noise exposure levels for a working day, assuming constant, steady-state noise and a 20-year work life (Table 14-13). However, since occupational noise is not always constant, a time-weighted average takes

Table 14-13 **OSHA Permissible Noise Exposures**

Duration (h/day)	SPL (on dBA scale, slow response)
8	90
6	92
4	95
2	100
1	105
0.5	110
≤ 0.25	115

Reproduced with permission from United States Department of Labor, Occupational Safety and Health Administration. 29 CFR. Part 1910.95. Occupational noise exposure, 1981.

into account both level and duration, and that average is a level that, if constant for an 8-hour day, would have the same effect as the measured dose.

A hearing conservation program has four main components:

- Assess the level and cumulative dose of noise exposure in a given setting using a sound level meter and dosimeter.
- Control the amount of overexposure in a given setting by reducing the amount noise created by the source, reducing the amount of noise reaching an individual's ears by constructing barriers, or by changing job procedures or schedule.
- If sound cannot be brought within safe levels, provide ear protection devices and information to motivate their proper use.
- *Monitor hearing*: preemployment testing with periodic follow-up tests, usually annually.

Ear protection devices act as barriers to sound. Earmuffs, custom-fitted earplugs, or disposable earplugs provide 20 to 40 dB of sound attenuation, more in high frequencies than in low frequencies. Proper fit, comfort, and motivation are equally important.

There are passive ear protection devices (nonelectric) and active devices (electric). Some passive devices, such as valves, are amplitude sensitive to allow relatively normal hearing. They pass moderate sound levels but reduce high sound levels although not always to a safe level. For some occupations, notably musicians, the greater sound reduction for high frequencies of hearing protectors is objectionable because it alters sound quality. Thus, "musicians' plugs" have a uniform or flat attenuation across the sound spectrum. While effective, they do not ensure complete protection against damage to hearing.

Active devices typically limit output to 85-dB SPL. However, to offset the blockage effect of the ear protectors, some units include slight amplification in order to hear usual conversation and environmental sounds. Nevertheless, the low level of peak clipping tends to distort speech. Thus, the best application of active devices is brief use for intermittent and impulse noise (gunfire). Another strategy is "active noise reduction," in which the sound phase is inverted 180° to cancel the noise. ANR is effective below 1000 Hz. Combining the low-frequency attenuation of ANR with the high-frequency reduction of muffs provides a good overall result. ANR systems are advantageous in noisy communication situations (eg, pilot), but give no better hearing protection than well-fitted earplugs or muffs.

Bibliography

American National Standard Specifications for Audiometers. ANSI S3.6-1996. New York, NY: American National Standards Institute, Inc.; 1996.

American Speech-Language-Hearing Association. Guidelines for audiometric symbols. *Asha* 20. 1990;(suppl 2):225-230.

Joint Committee on Infant Hearing. Year 2007 Position Statement: Principles and Guidelines for Early Hearing Detection and Intervention Programs. *Pediatrics.* 2007;120:898-921.

Martin FN. Nonorganic hearing loss. In: Katz J, Medwetsky L, Burkhard R, Hood L, eds. *Handbook of Clinical Audiology.* 6th ed. Baltimore, MD: Lippincott Williams & Wilkins; 2009:699-711.

Peck JE. *Pseudohypacusis: False and Exaggerated Hearing Loss.* San Diego, CA: Plural Publishing; 2011.

Questions

1. Which of the following statements is true regarding the decibel?
   A. It is a logarithmic expression of the ratio of two intensities.
   B. It is nonlinear.
   C. It is a relative measure.
   D. It is expressed with different reference levels.
   E. All of the above are true.

2. Otoacoustic emission types include all of the following *except*:
   A. DPOAEs
   B. TEOAEs
   C. SOAEs
   D. LOAEs

3. Normal conversational speech is typically in what range in dB SPL?
   A. 30-40
   B. 100-110
   C. 60-70
   D. 90-100

4. All of the following tests require voluntary patient responses *except*:
   A. ABR
   B. DPOAEs
   C. Tympanometry
   D. Conditioned play audiometry

5. The active, complex set of operations performed by the central nervous system on auditory inputs is termed:
   A. Auditory steady state
   B. Central auditory processing
   C. Auditory neuropathy
   D. Pseudohypacusis

Chapter 15
Electrical Response Audiometry

Basic Concepts of Electrical Response Audiometry

Electrical response audiometry (ERA) is a description used for an assortment of procedures in which electrical potentials are recorded while being evoked by a sound stimulus. The presence of the response or the response characteristic allows us to surmise the subjects' hearing capability or the performance of their auditory pathways. ERA techniques are considered an "objective" evaluation because the subject is not required to actively participate in the assessment. The short-latency automatic components are favored for threshold estimation, as they are modestly affected by the brain state of the subject. The long-latency components are generally used to surmise the cognitive processing capacity of the brain and are often called event-related potentials (ERPs). Auditory evoked potentials (AEPs) is another term used for tests within the ERA category.

Types of Electrical Response Audiometry

Electrical response audiometry is an objective testing method commonly employed in both clinical and research settings. Following is a list of available electrical response testing techniques:

- Electrocochleography (ECoG or ECochG)
- Auditory brain stem response (ABR), brain stem evoked response audiometry (BERA), brain stem auditory evoked response audiometry (BAER)
- Cortical electric response audiometry (CER or CERA), N1-P2 response
- Auditory steady-state response (ASSR), auditory steady-state evoked potential (ASSEP)
- Middle-latency response (MLR)
- Cervical vestibular evoked myogenic potentials (cVEMP)
- Occular vestibular evoked myogenic potentials (oVEMP)
- Somatosensory evoked potential (SSEP)
- Electroneurography (ENoG)
- Electromyography (EMG)
- Neural response telemetry (NRT)
- P300

Classification of AEPs by Latency

AEPs are primarily based on peak response latency and include short-latency (ie, ABR), middle-latency response (MLR), and long-latency (auditory late responses—ALR) AEPs.

- ABR peaks are indicated by roman numerals:
  - (a) Waves I, II, III, IV, and V.
  - (b) The most reliable peaks are waves I, III, and V.
- MLR:
  - (a) Po, Na, Pa, Nb, and Pb
- ALR:
  - (a) P1, N1, P2, and N2

Generators of Auditory Evoked Responses

There is ongoing debate over the generation sites of a number of evoked responses and it is commonly accepted that there is more than one neural origin involved in creating each response. Following are the presently recognized generator sites of the AEPs:

Sensory Function

- ABR
  - (a) Cochlea, eighth nerve and brain stem
    - Wave I = distal end of the eighth nerve (near cochlea)
    - Wave II = proximal end of the eighth nerve
    - Wave III = caudal (lower) brain stem near trapezoid body and superior olivary complex
    - Wave IV = superior olivary complex
    - Wave V = lateral lemniscus as it enters the inferior colliculus
    - Waves VI and VII = inferior colliculus
- MLR
  - (a) Early cortical
    - Na = possibly thalamus
    - Pa = Primary auditory cortex (measured over temporal lobe)
    - Pa = Subcortical generator (measured with a midline electrode)
- ALR
  - (a) P2 (Cortical) = primary or secondary auditory complex

Processing Potential

- Auditory P300
  - (a) P3 (cortical) = auditory regions of hippocampus in medial temporal lobe
- Mismatched negativity response (MMN)
  - (a) Subcortical and primary cortical auditory regions

Electrocochleography

Electrocochleography (ECoG) has an array of clinical applications and is beneficial in the evaluation of the inner ear and auditory nerve function. This is a method that is used to record the potentials produced from the cochlea and the auditory nerve. Knowledge of the electrophysiology of the cochlea and the electrical potentials in the cochlea are needed to fully comprehend the measurements of ECoG. ECoG requires analysis of the electrical potentials occurring in response to sound stimuli. These include the summating potential, action potential, and the cochlear microphonic. Detailed descriptions of these events are numerous; however for the scope of this chapter, this section will assess the key features related to clinical ECoG application.

- Resting potential (RP):
  - (a) Present without sound input
  - (b) Not presently used clinically in the interpretation of an ECoG
- Summating potential (SP):
  - (a) Outer hair cells
  - (b) Organ of Corti
  - (c) Inner hair cells (> 50%)
- Compound action potential (CAP):
  - (a) Spiral ganglion
  - (b) Distal eighth cranial nerve afferent fibers
- Cochlear microphonic (CM):
  - (a) Outer hair cells
  - (b) Receptor potentials

Cochlear Microphonic

The CM is an alternating current (AC) voltage primarily occurring from the outer hair cells and the organ of Corti. The CM literally reflects the acoustic stimulus at low to moderate levels which causes difficulty in differentiating between the CM response and stimulus artifacts in clinical settings using noninvasive techniques. Alternating stimuli for phase cancellation of the CMs is used for ECoG tests. Recently, however, there has been a greater focus on the use of CMs for the evaluation of site of lesion via ECoG for diagnosing auditory neuropathy. For this reason, there has been increasing interest in distinguishing CMs for use in clinical and research settings.

Summating Potential

The SP is seen as a direct current (DC) voltage that reflects the time-displacement pattern of the cochlear partition in response to the stimulus envelope. Depending on the interaction between the location of the recording electrodes and the stimulus parameters, a positive or negative shift in the CM baseline occurs, causing the DC shift. Some components of the SP are believed to reflect the nonlinear distortion in the transduction product when DC voltage reacts to AC voltage. There is much debate over the specific pathophysiology, however it is suggested that an enlarged SP is an indication of endolymphatic hydrops/Ménière disease.

Compound Action Potential

The action potential (AP) is an action potential occurring at the onset of a click stimulus that represents the summed response of the synchronous firing of several thousand auditory nerve fibers that excite the basilar membrane. The AP is an AC voltage that primarily appears as negative deflections called N1 and N2 that are synonymous with waves I and II, respectively, of an ABR.

Recording Techniques

There are currently three methods of recording an ECoG, including both invasive (transtympanic [TT]) and noninvasive (extratympanic [ET]) techniques. The distance of the electrode site from the source of the impulse, in this case the cochlea, affects the amplitudes and the reliability of the ECoG. It is also important to note that the normative data is altered by the electrode site when analyzing the results.

- Transtympanic:
  - (a) *Transtympanic electrode*: A needle electrode is used to penetrate the tympanic membrane at the inferior portion and is placed over the cochlear promontory. This is an invasive technique that requires the tympanic membrane to be anesthetized prior to placement. This technique produces ECoG recording with optimal quality and amplitudes.
- Extratympanic:
  - (a) *TIPtrode or intrameatal electrode*: An insert earphone that is covered in gold foil is inserted into the external auditory canal making contact with the canal walls. This far-field placement produces low amplitudes that require significantly more signal averaging.
  - (b) *Tymptrode electrode*: The electrode is placed in direct contact with the tympanic membrane without penetrating. This method yields better amplitudes than the TIPtrode method, because of the fact that the electrode is closer to the cochlea.

Clinical Applications of Electrocochleography

- Ménière disease and endolymphatic hydrops
  - (a) Diagnosis, assessment, and monitoring through the measurement of the SP/AP ratio resulting in a prevalence of approximately 60% of Ménière patients having positive results for endolymphatic hydrops. The SP/AP ratio percentages differ depending on the electrode used for the test:
    - ○ TIPtrode: > 50% = abnormal
    - ○ Tymptrode: > 35% = abnormal
    - ○ Transtympanic: > 30% = abnormal
- Enhancing ABR wave I amplitude in individuals whose wave I may be absent or difficult to identify
- Intraoperative monitoring of the peripheral auditory system
- Objective assessment of audiometric thresholds:
  - (a) However, the ABR has become more widely used than ECoG for threshold evaluation.
- Acoustic neuroma: ABR has replaced ECoG as the standard because it is a more accurate test in this application
- Auditory neuropathy (AN):
  - (a) Diagnosis of AN by comparing an ABR tracing to an ECoG tracing
    - ○ Absent neural function (ie, abnormal ABR) in the presence of normal cochlear (ie, normal CM) function

Auditory Brain stem Response Audiometry

An ABR is an objective test that elicits brain stem potentials in response to click or tone burst/tone pip stimuli. A computer system filters and averages the response of the auditory pathway to the auditory stimuli, resulting in a waveform with peaks that represent generator sites: waves I, II, III, IV, and V. ABRs can be performed via air conduction using supra-aural earphones/insert earphones or via bone conduction.

It is generally agreed that ABRs can be affected by the subjects' sex, age, body temperature, and degree of hearing loss, but are not acutely affected by most sedatives, anesthesia, drugs, or state of arousal. The ABR should be used in conjunction with other audiologic procedures.

Neurologic ABR

The neurologic ABR evaluates the integrity of the auditory neural pathways as a diagnostic tool used primarily to indicate auditory nerve and brain stem lesions. The use of a high stimulus level is required (80-90 dB nHL). Depending on the subject's hearing loss, a higher level may be required to elicit a response; masking noise may also be needed. The audiometric region important in generating an ABR is chiefly the 2000- to 4000-Hz range since the click-generated response is dependent on activation of the basal portion of the cochlea.

The most popular usage is as a screening instrument to rule out acoustic neuromas/vestibular schwannoma. In some cases, ABRs can be surprisingly accurate in determining the precise site of lesion; however, this is not always the case and ABRs should not be used primarily in this manner. The principal use of an ABR is to determine whether there is retrocochlear involvement and not a specific site of lesion. However, an ABR can be used in lieu of an MRI when conditions preclude (such as in the presence of an implanted magnetic device).

There is a 90% sensitivity and 80% specificity for eighth nerve tumor detection with click ABR. However, ABRs are not known to be sensitive to small eighth nerve tumors. For this reason, a newer method to enhance small tumors was developed, called a stacked ABR.

Stacked ABR

It covers essentially all regions of the cochlea with a more thorough evaluation of auditory nerve fibers by combining synchronous activity from octave-wave regions.

Research indicates promising results. Subjects with small eighth nerve tumors that were not found using conventional click ABR had a stacked ABR which detected 95% of abnormalities with an 88% specificity.

Threshold ABR

The threshold ABR is used to estimate hearing thresholds in pediatric populations, difficult-to-test populations, and those that are suspected of a nonorganic hearing loss. The wave V peak is identified at each intensity level in a descending method with either a click or a tone burst stimuli until it is no longer identifiable. Wave V will no longer be identifiable at or near the subject's hearing threshold. The click stimuli will give an estimated hearing sensitivity threshold for the 1000- to 4000-Hz region. With the use of high-pass masking techniques, a click stimulus can be used to gather frequency-specific information.

Tone burst ABR uses a brief tone stimulus and is becoming the standard procedure for gathering frequency-specific and ear-specific information at 500, 1000, 2000, and 4000 Hz. This uses the same descending intensity method to track wave V. It is used to estimate hearing threshold, but a reminder is required that evoked potentials analyze auditory function; they do not provide an exact threshold measure.

It is generally accepted that ABR thresholds are about 10 to 20 dB above behavioral responses, with slight variation in the different ABR computer systems that are in use.

Clinical Applications

- Newborn infant auditory screening
- Estimation of auditory sensitivity
- Neurodiagnosis:

(a) Eighth nerve
(b) Auditory brain stem dysfunction
- Intraoperative monitoring:
  (a) Eighth nerve and auditory brain stem status during posterior fossa surgery
  (b) Auditory brain stem implant
  (c) Vestibular nerve sectioning
  (d) Acoustic tumor removal
  (e) Eighth nerve vascular decompression

Parameters Used to Evaluate an ABR

Age-correlated normative data is used to analyze the parameters; these parameters can be affected by stimulus presentation level.

- Absolute latencies
  (a) Primarily waves I, III, and V
    ○ Wave I
      – Small or not present—indication of high-frequency (cochlear) hearing loss
      – Delayed latency—indication of conductive hearing loss
    ○ Wave II and/or III
      – Cannot be identified or absent—indication of hearing loss or brain stem dysfunction
    ○ Wave V
      – Delayed latency—indication of peripheral or brain stem auditory dysfunction
- Interpeak intervals (interwave latencies)
  (a) Waves I-III, III-V, and I-V
    ○ I-III
      – Useful descriptor of eighth nerve tumor
    ○ III-V
      – Not usually influenced by eighth nerve tumors unless they compromise the brain stem
    ○ I-V
      – Delayed latency can indicate brain stem dysfunction
      – Short latency can indicate brain stem dysfunction
- Interaural wave V latency (ITV difference)
  (a) Abnormal = 0.4 ms or greater
    ○ Sensitive for eighth nerve tumor detection
    ○ Not effective for indicating brain stem involvement
- Rate latency shift for wave V
  (a) Abnormal = 0.8 ms or greater
    ○ Indicator of retrocochlear pathology
- Morphology
  (a) Poor morphology—indication of high-frequency sensory (cochlear) hearing loss
- Amplitude ratio
  (a) 1.0 ms or greater
  (b) Highly variable
  (c) Not a primary factor in ABR, more so in ECoGs

ABR Interpretation as a Function of Type of Hearing Loss
- Normal hearing
  (a) All parameters within normal limits

- Conductive hearing loss
  - (a) Delayed absolute latencies; specifically delayed wave I latency
  - (b) All other parameters and morphology within normal limits
- Sensory hearing loss
  - (a) Wave I diminished or absent
  - (b) Delayed absolute latencies
  - (c) Poor morphology
  - (d) Interpeak intervals within normal limits
  - (e) And/or reduced I-V
- Neural hearing loss
  - (a) Wave I latency within normal limits; delay of all other absolute latencies
  - (b) Delayed interpeak intervals
    - ○ And/or prolonged I-V
    - ○ Poor morphology

Auditory Steady-State Evoked Potentials

ASSR uses a continuous (steady-state) frequency-specific, pure tone stimulus that activates the cochlea and CNS. It is generated by a mixture of amplitude modulation and rapid modulation of carrier frequencies (CF) of 500, 1000, 2000, and 4000 Hz. The theoretical assumption is that the part of the cochlea that is being stimulated by the carrier frequency (eg, 1000 Hz) must be intact for the cochlea to respond to the modulation rate (eg, 80 Hz, cycle of change in the CF) producing an ASSR. A complex and sophisticated algorithm is performed that is specific to the manufacturer and ASSR unit to analyze the electrophysiological response.

Clinical Application

- Audiometric threshold estimations that are frequency specific
- Assessment of severe/profound hearing loss

Advantages and Disadvantages of ASSR Testing

Advantages

- Estimates severe to profound hearing loss. This information cannot be obtained using click or tone burst ABR
- Reasonably frequency specific
- Automated analysis
- Objective for both the subject and the examiner
- Records simultaneous responses, allowing faster assessment

Disadvantages

- Requires quiet patient state (sleep or sedation)
- Possible artifactual response
- Limited anatomic site information
- Difficult with bone conduction stimulation and may require masking
- Questionable results at near-normal threshold levels; possible overestimation of actual thresholds
- Cannot distinguish between profound hearing loss and auditory neuropathy
- More research needed in areas including, but not limited to, normative data and effects of sedatives on test results

There are multiple terms used from auditory steady-state evoked potentials:

- Auditory steady-state response (ASSR)
- 40-Hz response
- Steady-state evoked potentials (SSEP)
- Amplitude-modulating-following response (AMFR)
- Envelope-follow response (EFR)
- Frequency-following response (FFR)

Cortical Auditory Evoked Responses

Middle-Latency Response Potentials

The auditory evoked potential termed middle-latency response (MLR) occurs within 10 to 50 ms after the onset of a stimulus that includes transient evoked potentials and the 40-Hz steady-state potentials (Table 15-1). The consensus today is that the responses are chiefly neurogenic in makeup, not myogenic as previously thought. However, the myogenic potentials within the latency range of Na and Pa can distort the MLRs and steps must be taken to avoid this when performing MLR studies.

MLRs are currently the subject of much research in applications such as binaural hearing because of the fact that they are believed to be useful in gathering processing information and auditory language functioning.

MLRs are known to be affected by age, sedation, and alertness/state of the person being tested.

Table 15-1 AEPs Compared and Contrasted

| | *Latency Range* | | |
	Early	*Middle*	*Later*
Examples	ECoG, ABR	AMLR	ALR, P300, MMN
Stimulus rate	Faster (< 30/s)	< 10/s	Slower (< 2/s)
Stimulus type	Transient	Transient	Tonal
Stimulus duration	Very brief (< 5 ms)	Brief (5 ms)	Longer (> 10 ms)
Spectral content	High (100-2000 Hz)	20-40 Hz	Low (< 30 Hz)
Filter settings	30-3000 Hz	10-200 Hz	1-30 Hz
Amplitude	0.5 µV	About 1 µV	> 5 µV
Number of repetitions-averages	> 1000	About 500	< 250
Preamplification	> 75,000	About 75,000	< 50, 000
Effects of sedation	None	Slight	Pronounced

Reproduced with permission from Hall III, JW, Mueller III HG. Audiologists' Desk Reference Volume 1 Diagnostic Audiology Principles, Procedures and Practices. San Diego California: Singular Publishing Group; 1997.

Clinical Applications

- Evaluation of the auditory pathway above the brain stem
- Documentation of auditory CNS dysfunction
- Localize lesions at the thalamocortical and primary auditory cortex
- Evaluate functional integrity of the auditory pathway
- Approximate frequency-specific auditory sensitivity up to the cortical level
- Evaluate effectiveness of electrical stimulation for cochlear implants

P300

- An *endogenous* response which indicates a response dependent on the test subject's state or attention.
- Perhaps the most extensively used AEP to study age-related declines in central processing.
- An oddball or unpredictable and random acoustic stimuli is the test paradigm and latencies are examined using age-related normative data.
- Prolonged latencies = abnormal. However, there are several reports of prolonged latencies in normal aging adults.
- Can be recorded with speech stimuli.
- Assesses auditory temporal processing and hemispheric asymmetry.
- More frequently used to assess higher-level changes in cognition and memory and age-related decline in central processing.
- Current research occurring in the application of P300 evaluation in patients with Alzheimer and dementia.

Mismatch Negativity Response

- An endogenous response.
- As stated previously in this chapter, the MMN is believed to be generated from the supratemporal plane of primary auditory cortex (AI), or Heschl gyrus.
- Also contributing is the frontal cortex, the thalamus, and hippocampus.
- Potential clinical applications.
  (a) Speech perception information
  (b) Confirm neural dysfunction in certain population
  (c) Assessment of high-level auditory processing in infants
  (d) Cortical auditory organization
- Said to reflect acoustic discrimination and auditory sensory memory; assess temporal resolution in the aging population.
- Like earlier responses, this is a passive paradigm and does not require patient to participate in a task like P300.
- Can be affected by sensorineural hearing loss, for the reason low frequency stimulus is most commonly used.

Recording Parameters

Recording parameters can vary from clinic to clinic and from tester to tester. Each tester may have individual preferred parameters for all the AEP testing that is performed. This takes into account not only a tester's preference, but also the subject that is being tested and the machines that are being used. Most commercially available AEP machines have set protocols and parameters that are recommended, however, these can be adjusted by the tester.

Cervical Vestibular Evoked Myogenic Potentials

Cervical vestibular-evoked myogenic potentials (cVEMP) test the vestibulo-collic reflex, a righting reflex from the vestibular system to the sternocleidomastoid muscle (SCM) and the trunk. The vestibular system can be activated with high-intensity sound and a myogenic response can be measured at the ipsilateral SCM. Studies suggest the anatomic pathway for cVEMP starts at the saccular macula, afferent inferior vestibular nerve, brain stem vestibular nuclei, the descending medial vestibulospinal tract, and the motoneurons of the SCM muscle. The SCM must sustain contraction since the cVEMP is a result of brief inhibition of electromyogram activity caused by an acoustic stimulus.

A repetitive click or tone burst stimuli is presented at a frequency between 500 and 1000 Hz resulting in an evoked potential that can be used to determine the functionality of the saccule, inferior vestibular nerve, and central connection. There is also research going into VEMPs evoked from bone conductions or skull taps and by galvanic response; however these methods are not being routinely used. The click-induced cVEMP not only requires sound stimuli, but also activation of the subject's anterior neck muscles. No cVEMP will be elicited without the tension and activation of their neck muscles. cVEMP is generally an ipsilateral response resulting from either a supine flexion which is when the patient raises their head against gravity while lying in the supine position (bilateral response) or via a head rotation which has the patient turn their head away from the stimulus ear while sitting upright (unilateral response). cVEMPs are not affected by the degree of sensorineural hearing loss a patient may have. However, they are affected by the middle ear status, so any conductive hearing loss even as little as a 5-dB nHL air bone gap can obliterate a response; background activity of the SCM, stimulus level, stimulus frequency, spinal cord injuries, muscular atrophy, thickness of neck and patients on valium or other muscle relaxants. It is also important to note that research has shown that cVEMPs can be absent in normal patients 60 years or older, so this should be accounted for during analysis.

- Response characteristics
  (a) P1 (P13): occurs around 12 ms (SD=2.5 ms)
  (b) N1 (P23): occurs around 19 ms (SD=1.5 ms)
- Interpretation
  (a) P1 and N1 absolute latencies: more than 2 standard deviations above or below the average
  (b) P1-N1 amplitude
    ○ Click: 16-179 μV.
    ○ Tone burst: 15-337 μV.
    ○ Amplitude may be decreased in patients > 60 years old.
  (a) Asymmetry ratio = $100 \, (A_L - A_S)/(A_L + A_S)$
    ○ A_L = P1-N1 of larger amplitude
    ○ A_S = P1-N1 of smaller amplitude
    ○ Normal = 0-~40%
  (a) Threshold: stimulus level
    ○ In a "normal" patient, this response will only be present around and above 90-dB nHL. It should not be present with intensities < 80-dB nHL.
    ○ Patients with superior canal dehiscence have a much lower threshold for this response. At intensities < 80-dB nHL, P1 and N1 will still be visible.

Results are indicative of such pathologies as: Otologic Meniere' Disease, superior canal dehiscence syndrome, vestibular neuritis, labrynthitis; neurologic–multiple sclerosis, lower brain stem stroke, spinocerebellar degeneration, and migraine.

Diagnostic Applications
- Saccule disorder
  (a) Higher than normal thresholds or low amplitudes
  (b) Amplitude asymmetry

- Conductive hearing loss:
  (a) Can obliterate cVEMP responses.
  (b) An intact middle ear is required.
- Sensorineural hearing loss:
  (a) Little or no effect on cVEMPs
- Vestibular nerve disturbance/vestibular neuritis:
  (a) Absent or reduced amplitudes.
  (b) Response may recover in a small number of patients within 6 months to 2 years.
- Tullio phenomenon:
  (a) Asymmetrical amplitudes
  (b) Lower than normal thresholds
- Superior canal dehiscence syndrome (SCDS)
  (a) Lower than normal thresholds
  (b) Presence of cVEMPs in subject with an air–bone gap
  (c) Enhanced amplitudes
- Acoustic neuroma/ Vestibular Schwannoma
  (a) Absent or reduced cVEMPs
- Bilateral vestibular loss
  (a) Reduced or absent cVEMPs are expected.
- Otosclerosis
  (a) Expected to be absent due to abnormal middle ear status
- Meniere Disease
  (a) Absent response; more prevalent during an attack.
  (b) Reduced or enhanced amplitudes.
  (c) Current research indicates abnormally large amplitude in suspected ear and asymmetrical ratio.
- Migraine
  (a) Absent response
  (b) Reduced Amplitudes
  (c) Delayed latencies
  (d) Normally a unilateral abnormality
- Brain stem stroke, multiple sclerosis, and spinocerebellar degeneration
  (a) Absent response
  (b) Delayed latencies

Ocular Vestibular Evoked Myogenic Potentials

Cervical vestibular-evoked myogenic potentials (oVEMPs) are used to measure functioning of the saccule and inferior branch of the vestibular nerve, but the end organ (utricle, saccule, or both) responsible for ocular vestibular-evoked myogenic potentials is still under debate. The general though is that oVEMPs evaluate the functional integrity of the utricle and superior branch of the vestibular nerve. oVEMPs elicited via bone conduction or vibratory stimulus are generally accepted as emanating from the utricle, but whether or not the utricle is responsive to air conduction stimuli is still the matter of intense research. oVEMPs are currently being used primarily on a research basis with few clinics performing them. However, once standardization of stimuli, responses and equipment become more widely available and agreed upon, it is predicted that this test will become widely used along with cVEMPs since it can be used to evaluate the function of the utricle. VEMPs, both ocular and cervical, represent a clinically useful extension to the prevailing vestibular battery which currently focuses on the canal rather than the otolith function.

Response Characteristics
- N1 (N10) – median latency of 10 ms
- P1 (P15) – median latency of 15-17 ms
- Amplitude – 5 μV ± 3
    - (a) Very small compared to cVEMP response
    - (b) The largest magnitude responses are gathered when the patient is looking 30 degrees above the midline during signal averaging since the upward gaze brings the inferior oblique muscle closer to the location of the infraorbital active electrode.

Diagnostic Application
- When oVEMP results are analyzed in conjunction with cVEMP and bithermal caloric results, research has shown that certain patterns of abnormality have started to become apparent that can indicate site of lesion or impairment. The oVEMP is also currently the only test available that can analyze the function of the utricle. One primary application is if a patient has normal calorics, normal cVEMP, and an abnormal oVEMP; this is indicative of impairment in the patient's utricle.
- Abnormal oVEMPS can also indicate an impairment of the saccule, superior vestibular nerve, inferior vestibular nerve, horizontal semicircular canal or indicate superior semicircular canal dehiscence when analyzed alongside cVEMPs and calorics.

Electroneuronography

Electroneuronography (ENoG) is a neurophysiological evaluation that involves the use of supramaximal electrical stimulation at or near the stylomastoid foramen and is recorded at the nasolabial fold. It is the most commonly used objective evaluation of the integrity of the facial nerve and measurement of facial nerve function. In the setting of Bell palsy, it may help differentiate patients who will spontaneously recover to a satisfactory grade (House-Brackmann facial nerve grading system) versus those that will have poor outcomes without intervention. The ENoG has been shown to be 50% to 91% accurate in identifying patients that would require medical/surgical intervention and 80% to 100% accurate in predicting spontaneous recoveries.

Purpose
- Whether or not the facial nerve is neurophysiologically intact
- Measure the amount of degeneration of the nerve on the affected side
- Monitor and chart progression of facial nerve function
- An objective measure used to decide if surgical or medical intervention is required

Types of Facial Nerve Injuries with ENoG Responses
- *Neuropraxia*: ENoG–Normal or reduced responses; indicates nerve fiber and sheath intact
- *Axonotmesis*: ENoG–No response; intact epineurium with inner nerve fiber disruption
    - (a) ENoG results cannot differentiate between neurotmesis and axonotmesis. There is a > 50% chance of an incomplete recovery when the ENoG is reduced by ≥ 90%.
- *Neurotmesis*: ENoG–No response; total separation

Timing of ENoG
- Test valid from 3 to 21 days after presentation of symptoms
- Never performed before a minimum of 72 hours after initial presentation of symptoms
    - (a) Patients should be tested in acute phase, day 3 or later
    - (b) Wallerian degeneration must occur (which takes 72 hours)
- Monitor during recovery
    - (a) Patient should be tested every 3 to 5 days until a plateau occurs
- No guidelines established for after 21 days and is thought to be of little clinical value

Analysis

- Latency of response is not vital, however N1 latencies are customarily less than 6 ms.
- Amplitude comparison of uninvolved to the involved side.
  - (a) Response is
    - ○ (amplitude of involved side/amplitude of uninvolved side) × 100 = % response
    - ○ 100 − % response = % denervation
- If involved side is ≤ 10% of uninvolved side (> 90% denervation), significant degeneration has occurred and medical/surgical intervention is recommended.
- If involved side is ≥ 10% of uninvolved side (< 90% denervation), spontaneous recovery is more likely.
- Some studies suggest using a 75% denervation criteria, however the 90% denervation is the standard performed by most clinics.

Bibliography

Burkard RF, Don M, Eggermont JJ, eds. *Auditory Evoked Potentials: Basic Principles and Clinical Application*. Baltimore, MD: Lippincott Williams & Wilkins; 2007.

Dallos P, Schoeny ZG, Cheatham MA. Cochlear summating potentials: descriptive aspects. *Acta Otolaryngologica*. 1972;301(Suppl):1-46.

Don M, Masuda A, Nelson R, Brackmann D. Successful detection of small acoustic tumors using the stacked derived-band auditory brain stem response amplitude. *Am J Otol*. 1997;18:608-621.

Jacobson JT, ed. *Principles & Applications in Auditory Evoked Potentials*. Needham Heights, MA: Allyn and Bacon; 1994.

Hall JW III, Mueller HG III. *Audiologists' Desk Reference Volume 1 Diagnostic Audiology Principles, Procedures and Practices*. San Diego, CA: Singular Publishing Group; 1997:395.

Questions

1. The primary anatomic site responsible for Wave V in an ABR is the
   A. Cochlear nucleus
   B. Lateral lemniscus/ inferior colliculus
   C. Superior olivary complex
   D. Cochlea/VIII nerve (distal)

2. Auditory brain stem response studies are performed for the following reason(s):
   A. Indicate integrity of the auditory nerve and/or brain stem lesions
   B. Intraoperative monitoring of VIII nerve vascular decompression
   C. Estimate hearing sensitivity thresholds
   D. All of the above

3. Auditory steady state potentials
   A. Are not affected by artifact
   B. Can distinguish between profound hearing loss and auditory neuropathy
   C. Are an active test paradigm
   D. Are used in assessment of severe/profound hearing loss

4. Which of the following is true concerning cervical vestibular evoked myogenic potentials (cVEMP)?

   A. It cannot be performed on patients of any age.

   B. It cannot indicate patients with superior canal dehiscence syndrome.

   C. It is affected by the middle ear status.

   D. It is affected by the degree of sensorineural hearing loss.

5. Which of the following is true concerning electroneuronography?

   A. It should be performed prior to the onset of Wallerian degeneration.

   B. If ≤ 10% response or > 90% denervation is present, there is a possible indication for medical/surgical intervention.

   C. It can be used to tell the difference between neurotmesis and axonotmesis.

   D. It is 50% to 91% accurate in predicting spontaneous recoveries.

Chapter 16
Vestibular and Balance Disorders

Essential Principles of Vestibular Physiology

Principle 1

Traditionally there have been five "senses," namely vision, hearing, smell, touch and taste. It is entirely reasonable to name balance as the true "sixth sense." What sets balance apart from the other senses is that it is not used to actively "investigate" our surroundings in the same way the others are. Balance is automatic and subconscious until there is a disruption of the vestibular system and symptoms develop. These symptoms are often substantial.

Principle 2

The vestibular system has two broad functions — the maintenance of balance and the maintenance of stable gaze. The vestibular end organs comprise the otolith organs (the utricle and saccule) and the three semicircular canals (lateral, superior, and posterior). The semicircular canals are activated during rotational movements and the otolith organs during linear movements.

The semicircular canals are paired structures. While the lateral canals are paired with each other, the superior canal on the left is functionally paired with the posterior canal on the right and vice versa. Eye movements are produced in the plane of the canal being stimulated. Stimulation of the semicircular canal occurs when the cupula is deflected as a result of endolymph within the canal remaining relatively still, as a result of its inertia, as the head is moved.

Principle 3

The vestibulo-ocular reflex serves to maintain the visual field in a stable fashion on an area of interest. The area of high visual acuity afforded by the fovea centralis is relatively small when compared to the entire visual field and must be kept accurately directed toward the area of interest even during head and body movements. Systems of smooth pursuit are not sufficiently fast to allow this to be undertaken voluntarily and thus the vestibulo-ocular reflex (VOR) is used to ensure that eye movements are produced that are equal and in an opposite direction to head movements. Defects in this reflex cause reduced dynamic visual acuity owing to the "retinal slip" caused by an image not being held consistently over the fovea.

Principle 4

Although there is substantial crossover between the function of these systems, the otolith organs play the greatest role in the maintenance of an upright posture through the detection of body or head tilt while the semicircular canals play the greatest role in the vestibulo-ocular reflex.

Principle 5

Hair cells within the semicircular canals fire at a baseline rate when at rest with no head movement. When the head is moved in a rotational fashion, one of the pair of canals will increase its firing rate while the other will decrease. This differential will signal a head movement in the plane of that semicircular canal. In the case of the lateral canal, there will be an increased rate of firing of the hair cells on the side to which the head is being rotated and a decrease in the contralateral side. The eye movement produced by the vestibulo-ocular reflex will be the vector of the signals produced by the vestibular end organs, primarily the semicircular canals.

Principle 6

In most physiological conditions of head movement there is no clinically relevant upper limit on the rate of firing whereas the reduction in the rate of firing in the contralateral ear can reach easily zero, below which there is no further reduction possible. This limit results in the principle that, although the canals are paired, at higher peak velocities of head movement, the contralateral ear cannot provide accurate velocity signals alone. As a result, a unilateral lesion will affect the VOR if sufficient acceleration is applied to the affected ear.

Principle 7

The difference in firing rates of the semicircular canals is the determinant of the signal received by the central nervous system (CNS) when detecting head movement. In the case of a sudden, pathological loss of vestibular function there will be a sudden difference in firing rates between the paired canals. In the case of the lateral semicircular canal, the affected baseline rate would be zero, whereas the contralateral side would be still firing at its baseline rate. This differential would be interpreted by the CNS as the head being rotated in the direction of the unaffected ear. The VOR then produces a slow phase eye movement in the direction of the affected ear and a fast phase movement in the direction of the unaffected ear to reset.

Principle 8

The vestibulo-ocular reflex is velocity/acceleration dependent. To maintain an equal and opposite eye movement, the central nervous system must receive signals from the vestibular system that are capable of delivering information on the velocity of the head movement, not just the direction. This is of importance when considering the results of caloric testing that assign a single value to a loss of vestibular function.

Principle 9

Over time the CNS can compensate for changes in the baseline firing rate of an affected vestibular end organ, but the weakness will remain and, owing to the fact that the contralateral ear cannot compensate at higher velocities for the affected semicircular canal to which it is paired and the VOR will remain pathological.

Principle 10

Testing of vestibular function is by no means reliable, exhaustive or complete. The semicircular canals are most easily assessed, but the otolith organs are not easy to test and the tests that are currently available produce a very crude assessment of function. It is worth considering that the amount of neuroepithelium contained in the otolith organs is similar to that contained by the cochlea, yet current tests of otolithic function produce an output that determines whether a response is either "absent" or "present." Clearly an audiogram that presented hearing in those terms would be unacceptable. No test provides a "gold standard" and no test is indicative of overall vestibular function. Normal vestibular function testing does not exclude vestibular pathology and all abnormal test results should be viewed in a clinical context.

Physiology

Peripheral Vestibular System

A. Three paired semicircular canals (SCCs) and the otolithic (macular) organs within the otic capsule
    i. SCCs (superior, posterior, and lateral): for angular acceleration perception
    ii. Otolithic organs (utricle, saccule): for linear acceleration perception
B. Cristae = end organs containing hair cells; located within the ampullated portion of the membranous labyrinth
C. Cupula = a gelatinous matrix that the cilia of hair cells are embedded into; acts as a hinged gate between the vestibule and the canal itself
D. Otoliths = a blanket of calcium carbonate crystals on a supporting matrix; found only in the otolithic end organs (not in SCCs)
E. Vestibular nerve = the afferent connection to the brain stem nuclei for the peripheral vestibular system
    i. Superior vestibular nerve: superior, lateral SCCs and utricle
    ii. Inferior vestibular nerve: posterior SCC and saccule
    iii. Each vestibular nerve consists of approximately 25,000 bipolar neurons whose cell bodies are located in the Scarpa ganglion within the internal auditory canal

Hair Cells

A. The fundamental units for vestibular activity inside the inner ear.
    i. Type I hair cells
      a. Flask-shaped
      b. Surrounded by the afferent nerve terminal at its base in a chalice-like fashion
      c. High amount of both tonic and dynamic electrical activity
      d. Largely stimulatory effect
    ii. Type 2 hair cells
      a. Cylindrical
      b. Surrounded by multiple nerve terminals
      c. Predominately inhibitory effect
B. Each hair cell contains 50 to 100 stereocilia and one long kinocilium that project into the gelatinous matrix of the cupula or macula.
C. The location of the kinocilium relative to the stereocilia gives each hair cell an intrinsic polarity that can be influenced by angular or linear accelerations.
    i. The hair cells of the ampulla within the lateral SCC all have the kinocilia located closest to the utricle.
    ii. The hair cells within the superior and posterior SCC all have the kinocilia located away from the utricle or on the crus commune side of the ampulla.
    iii. In the otolithic membranes, the hair cells are lined up with the kinocilia facing a line which almost bisects the membrane, called the striola.
D. Displacement of the stereocilia toward/away from the kinocilium alters calcium influx at the apex of the cell → release/inhibition of neurotransmitters

Central Vestibular System

    A. Four distinct second-order neurons within the vestibular nuclei
       i. Superior (Bechterew nucleus): major relay station for conjugate ocular reflexes mediated by the SCCs
       ii. Lateral (Deiters nucleus): control of ipsilateral vestibulospinal (the so-called "righting") reflexes
       iii. Medial (Schwalbe nucleus): coordination of eye, head, and neck movements with connections to the medial longitudinal fasciculus
       iv. Descending (spinal vestibular nucleus): integration of signals from the vestibular nuclei, the cerebellum, and reticular formation
    B. Neural integrator = amorphous area in the reticular formation responsible for the final velocity and position command for conjugate eye movements
    C. Vestibulocerebellum = the phylogenetically oldest parts of the cerebellum (the flocculus, nodulus, ventral uvula, and the ventral paraflocculus) into which the vestibular nerve directly projects
    D. Responsible for
       i. Conjugate eye movements, VOR, smooth pursuit
       ii. Holding the image of a moving target within a certain velocity range on the fovea of the retina
       iii. Cancelling the effects of VOR (eg, figure skater can twirl without getting dizzy)
       iv. Compensation process for a unilateral vestibular loss

Evaluation of Patients

Describe Dizziness

    A. Vertigo: illusion of rotational, linear, or tilting movement, either of self (subjective) or the environment (objective)
    B. Disequilibrium: sensation of instability of body positions, walking, or standing
    C. Oscillopsia: inability to focus on objects during head movement
    D. Lightheadedness: sense of impending faint, presyncope
    E. Physiologic dizziness: motion sickness, dizziness in heights
    F. Multisensory dizziness: cumulative loss from deterioration/degeneration in the multiple sensory systems responsible for balance (ie, vision, proprioception, vestibular and central integration) often related to age, diabetes, stroke, etc.

History

A minimum vertigo history should address the following (Figure 16-1):

    A. Duration of individual attack (seconds/minutes/hours/days)
    B. Frequency (daily vs weekly vs monthly)
    C. Effect of head movements (worse, better, or no effect)
    D. Inducing position or posture (eg, rolling onto right side of bed)
    E. Associated aural symptoms such as hearing loss, tinnitus and aural pressure
    F. Concomitant or prior ear disease and/or ear surgery
    G. Family history (eg, neurofibromatosis, diabetes, or other factors)
    H. Head trauma, medications, comorbidities

Physical Examination

See Table 16-1.

Special Clinical Tests of Vestibular Function

    A. Head shake test
       i. High-frequency vestibular test (2 Hz; 15 seconds).

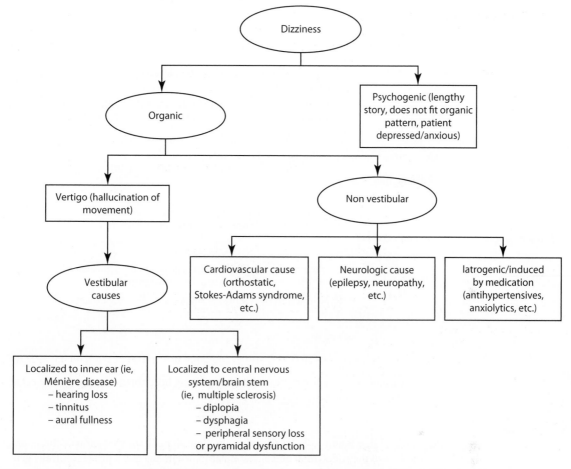

Figure 16-1 Flow-chart of the history of a dizzy patient. (*Reproduced with permission Blitzer A: Office based surgery in otolaryngology. New York, NY: Thieme; 1998.*)

    ii. Presence of post head shake nystagmus (HSN) correlates well with increasing right/left excitability difference on caloric testing.

    iii. Fast-phase of HSN usually directed (but not always) away from the involved ear. The presence of atypical nystagmus (either vertical or rotatory) after horizontal head shaking is called cross coupling and requires exclusion of a CNS disorder.

  B. Halmagyi (horizontal high-velocity/acceleration head thrust) maneuver

    i. High-velocity/acceleration test of VOR function.

    ii. VOR deficit suspected if refixation saccades (to stabilize eyes on a target following fast head movement) are present.

    iii. Deficit can be unilateral or bilateral.

  C. Oscillopsia test

    i. Loss of dynamic visual acuity: loss of visible lines on Snellen or LogMAR chart (more than five lines) with rapid horizontal head shaking (> 2 Hz) suggests a bilateral vestibular loss

Table 16-1 **The Otoneurologic Examination**

Examination Component	Purpose
Ears Otoscopic and fistula test	Identify middle ear pathology (eg, labyrinthine fistula, cholesteatoma)

Neurologic
  Central function
  Cranial nerves (I-XII)
  Cerebellar (midline, hemispheric)
  Oculomotor testing (saccade, pursuit, convergence, fixation)
  Spontaneous/gaze-evoked nystagmus
	Brainstem lesions or tumors in the cerebellopontine angle
	Assesses vestibulospinal pathways and the posterior fossa
	
	CNS pathology often involves oculomotor function; pursuit pathways most often involved
	Cardinal sign of a vestibular lesion (except congenital nystagmus)

General balance function
  Romberg test
  Tandem gait test (eyes open and closed)
	General test of proprioception, vestibulospinal/cerebellar tracts
	Assessment of balance and corresponding tracts

Diagnostic Hallpike maneuver	Confirmation of typical benign paroxysmal positional vertigo (BPPV) or atypical positioning nystagmus
Hyperventilation for 60s	Reproduction of symptoms suggests underlying anxiety

    D. VOR suppression test
       i. Inability to visually suppress nystagmus during head rotation suggests a defect at the level of the vestibulocerebellum.

Nystagmus

    A. Cardinal sign for a vestibular disorder. The slow phase of the nystagmus = direction of the flow of the endolymph and is vestibular in origin; the quick phase (centrally generated) = compensatory mechanism. Types are as follows:
       i. Physiologic: end-point nystagmus noted on lateral gaze > 30 degree
      ii. Spontaneous: nystagmus present without positional or other labyrinthine stimulation
     iii. Induced: nystagmus elicited by stimulation, that is, caloric, rotation, etc.
     iv. Positional: nystagmus elicited by assuming a specific position
    B. Ewald laws
       i. Eye and head movements occur in the plane of the canal being stimulated and in the direction of the endolymph flow.
      ii. Ampullopetal flow causes a greater response than ampullofugal flow in the lateral canal.
     iii. The reverse is true in the posterior and superior canals.
    C. Alexander's law: The slow-phase velocity of the nystagmus increases when the eyes look in the direction of the fast phase (commonly observed in peripheral lesions).
       i. First-degree: present only when gazing in the direction of the fast component
      ii. Second-degree: present when gazing in the direction of the fast component and on straight gaze
     iii. Third-degree: present in all three directions

Laboratory Vestibular Testing

Formal balance function testing indicated when:

A. Site/side of lesion not identified through history or physical examination
B. To ascertain who is likely to benefit from vestibular rehabilitation
C. To assess recovery of vestibular function
D. To assess contralateral function if destructive procedure is contemplated
E. To determine if intervention (ie, gentamicin ablation, vestibular neurectomy, etc) has been successful

Electronystagmography/Videonystagmography (ENG/VNG)

A. Electronystagmography (ENG)
　i. Horizontal and vertical eye movements are recorded indirectly using electrodes measuring changes in the corneoretinal potential (dipole).
　ii. Electrodes are typically placed at each lateral canthus and above and below at least one eye with a common electrode on the forehead.
B. Videonystagmography (VNG)
　i. Eye movements are recorded directly using infrared video cameras and digital video image technology.
　ii. Eye movements can be observed in real-time and/or recorded.
C. ENG/VNG testing
　i. Vestibular subsets
　　a. Spontaneous nystagmus
　　b. Gaze nystagmus
　　c. Positional nystagmus
　　d. Positioning nystagmus
　　e. Fistula test
　　f. Bithermal caloric tests
　ii. Oculomotor subsets
　　a. Pursuit system evaluation
　　b. Saccadic system
　　c. Optokinetic system evaluation
　　d. Fixation system evaluation
D. ENG/VNG interpretation
　i. Findings suggestive of central pathology
　　a. Spontaneous/positional nystagmus with normal calorics
　　b. Direction-changing nystagmus; failure of fixation suppression
　　c. Bilateral reduced or absent caloric responses without a history of labyrinthine, middle ear disease, or ototoxicity
　　d. Abnormal saccades or saccadic pursuit results, especially with normal caloric results
　　e. Hyperactive caloric responses (ie, loss of cerebellum-generated inhibition, in absence of TM defect or mastoid cavity)
　ii. Findings suggestive of peripheral pathology
　　a. Unilateral caloric weakness
　　b. Bilateral caloric weakness with history of labyrinthine disease or ototoxicity
　　c. Fatiguing positional nystagmus
　　d. Intact fixation suppression response
　　e. Direction-fixed nystagmus

E. Bithermal caloric test
    i. A bithermal stimulus (eg, water or air) is used to irrigate ears to evaluate function of lateral SCCs in caloric test position (CTP)
        a. Water = body temperature ±7°C (30°C and 44°C) for 30 seconds
        b. Air = body temperature ±13°C (24°C and 50°C) for 60 seconds
        * Irrigation parameters based on BSA (1999) recommendation
    ii. Nystagmus response: "COWS"- "Cold-Opposite," "Warm-Same" responses
        a. cool water/air → endolymphatic fluid drops → ampullofugal flow in the lateral SCC → deflection of hair cells away from kinocilium → inhibition of involved side → slow drift of eyes toward involved side and compensatory (fast) saccades in the opposite direction
        b. warm water/air → endolymphatic fluid rises → ampullopetal flow in the lateral SCC → deflection of hair cells toward kinocilium → excitation on the involved side → slow drift of eyes toward opposite side and compensatory saccades in same direction as stimulus
        c. Unilateral weakness (UW)

$$\frac{(RW + RC) - (LW + LC)}{(RW + RC + (LW + LC)} \times 100\%$$

        d. Directional preponderance (DP)

$$\frac{(RW + LC) - (LW + RC)}{(RW + RC + LW + LC)} \times 100\%$$

where
    RW = the peak slow-phase eye velocity of the response following right ear-warm temperature irrigation
    RC = right ear-cool
    LW = left ear-warm
    LC = left ear-cool
        e. UW > 15% to 30% (lab dependent) difference = abnormal
        f. Bilateral weakness = when the total added maximum slow phase velocity for the left **and** for the right are <12 degree/s (ie, LW+LC <12 degree/s **and** RW+RC <12 degree/s; lab dependent)
        g. DP > 30% difference = significant but its clinical value remains questionable (some believe that DP is directed toward the side of a central lesion and away from side of a peripheral lesion)
    iii. Practical considerations
        a. Cursory otoscopic inspection should be completed before ordering caloric test.
        b. Use of water as stimulus is contraindicated when tm perforation is present; heightened response expected on perforated side (using air as stimulus).
        c. Excess cerumen can impede accuracy of test results and should be removed; many labs are not equipped to do cerumen management on site.

Rotational Chair Testing

A. Offers higher frequency and more physiologic testing conditions than the calorics (typically 0.01-2 Hz with maximum velocity of 50 degree/s) for evaluating VOR function of lateral SCCs

B. Off-vertical axis rotation (OVAR) available in newer rotational chairs; used to assess otolithic organs

C. Reproducible and tests both ears simultaneously (integrated function)

D. Multiple tests used clinically (eg., sinusoidal harmonic acceleration, constant angular acceleration, impulse angular acceleration, velocity step test)

E. Useful for:
  i. Identifying residual function for patients with no caloric response
  ii. Monitoring changes in vestibular function over time

F. Measurements are:
  i. Phase
    a. Leading/lagging of maximum chair velocity vs maximum slow-phase velocity of nystagmus
    b. Often exaggerated in patients with peripheral vestibular disease but can be central (damage in vestibular nuclei within the brainstem)
  ii. Gain
    a. Ratio of maximum eye velocity to maximum chair velocity
    b. Gain of 1 indicates that slow-phase eye velocity equals chair velocity and is opposite in direction; gain of 0 when there is no eye movement
    c. Depressed bilateral gains under good testing conditions suggest bilateral vestibular loss
  iii. Symmetry
    a. Compares left and right peak slow-wave velocitycannot be used alone to localize lesion
    b. Shows weakness on the affected side in acute unilateral weakness
    c. Improves after insult; useful for monitoring recovery

Video Head Impulse Test (vHIT)

A. Lightweight goggles with built-in high-speed camera (> 250 Hz) for capturing eye movements; gyroscope measures head rotation

B. Used to evaluate VOR function when performing Halmagyi (head thrust) maneuver

C. Reduced gain values (normal ~1) expected when head is rotated toward impaired side(s); indication of reduced VOR function of lateral SCCs

D. Not ideal for measuring very fast head impulses (200-300 degree/s) due to issues with artifact and goggle slippage; maximum head impulse velocity ~150 to 200 degree/s

E. Re-fixation saccades are also captured for analysis
  i. Overt ("catch-up") saccades: occur after head rotation (visible to naked eye); common during acute phase
  ii. Covert saccades: occur during head rotation (very difficult to see); indicate compensated lesion

F. Assessment of VOR function for superior and posterior canals also possible on some devices (ie, left superior/right posterior, right superior/left posterior)

Magnetic Scleral Search Coil

A. Silicone annulus with embedded copper wire

B. Direct contact with the globe of the eye, contrary to the noncontact techniques of ENG/VNG, vHIT

C. Detects changes in its orientation relative to surrounding alternating-current magnetic field

D. Gold standard technique for measuring eye movement, though less-invasive video-capture techniques (described previously) are improving rapidly

E. Capable of accurately capturing very fast eye movements (> 300 degree/s)

       i. Ideal for detecting high-velocity vestibular loss (HVVL)
          a. HVVL: reduced VOR function resulting from high velocity head impulses when performing Halmagyi maneuver
          b. Useful measurement of high-frequency oscillations (> 2 Hz) during rotational chair testing

Vestibular Evoked Myogenic Potentials (VEMPs)

    A. Brief (0.1 ms), loud (SPL > 90 dB) 500 Hz tone burst presented in ear to evoke short latency myogenic potentials for evaluating otolith function (utricle and saccule)
       i. Cervical VEMP (cVEMP)
          a. Ipsilateral response from tonically contracted sternocleidomastoid (SCM) muscle; air-conducted stimuli typically used
          b. Tracing: positive (inhibitory) peak ~13 ms followed by negative trough ~23 ms
          c. Evaluates saccule (sensitive to vertical linear accelerations) and inferior branch of vestibular nerve
          d. Pathway: saccule → inferior vestibular nerve → vestibular nuclei → medial vestibulospinal tract (ipsilateral) → spinal accessory nuclei (CN XI) → sterno-cleidomastoid muscle
       ii. Ocular VEMP (oVEMP)
          a. Contralateral response from inferior oblique/rectus muscles during upward gaze; air- and bone-conducted stimuli used (research ongoing)
          b. Tracing: negative (excitatory) peak ~10 ms, positive peak ~16 ms
          c. Evaluates utricle (sensitive to horizontal accelerations) and the superior branch of the vestibular nerve
          d. Pathway: utricle → superior vestibular nerve → vestibular nuclei → medial longitudinal fasciculus → oculomotor nuclei (iii) → inferior oblique muscle
    B. VEMPs typically evaluated for amplitude (peak-to-peak) asymmetry, threshold, and latency
       i. Rectification can be used to remove muscle bias (eg, differences in muscle tone or effort) from resultant waveforms, making asymmetry calculations more reliable (> 40% difference is abnormal)
    C. Increased threshold/absent response: middle ear pathology or ossicular chain abnormalities, may also be age-related
    D. Decreased threshold: superior canal dehiscence syndrome (SCDS), perilymphatic fistula
    E. Response is dependent on pressure changes derived from the presented stimulus only; response can be obtained in absence of cochlear function

Subjective Visual Vertical (SVV)

    A. Detects patients whose perception of vertical is significantly offset from true vertical (normal range = ± 2-3 degree)
    B. Highly sensitive for detection of damage to utricle and its central connections, particularly during acute stage; can also detect brainstem lesions
    C. Expensive computer-based equipment available in specialized labs; reliable results can also be produced inexpensively (eg, bucket method)

Computerized Dynamic Posturography (CDP)

    A. Determines functional limitations by quantifying and isolating impairments due to visual, somatosensory, or vestibular inputs; correlates well with dizziness handicap inventory (DHI)

B. Centre of pressure (COP) data used to evaluate performance
C. Three tests
    i. Sensory organization test (SOT): evaluates the anterior-posterior body sway under conditions with eyes-opened (eo) or eyes-closed (ec)
        a. eo: fixed surface and visual surrounding
        b. ec: fixed surface
        c. eo: fixed surface, sway referenced visual surrounding
        d. eo: sway referenced surface, fixed visual surrounding
        e. ec: sway referenced surface
        f. eo: sway referenced surface and visual surrounding
    ii. Motor control test (MCT): assesses patient's ability to recover from external provocation
        a. Tested with a series of translational movements (horizontal forward/backward motions increasing in magnitude)
        b. Evaluation based on subject's ability to make automatic postural adjustments to remain stable
    iii. Adaptation test (ADT): assesses motor adjustments made by subject when platform rotates in "toes up" or "toes down" direction
        a. Subject's score based on force needed to overcome unexpected movement

Central vs Peripheral Pathology

See Table 16-2.

Differential Diagnosis

See Table 16-3.

Table 16-2 Characteristics of Nystagmus/Oculomotor Abnormalities in Peripheral Vestibular vs Central Pathology

	Acute Unilateral Peripheral Loss	*Bilateral Peripheral Loss*	*Central*
Direction of nystagmus	Mixed horizontal torsional (arching)	None	Mixed or pure torsional or vertical
Fixation/suppression	Yes	Yes	No
Slow phase of nystagmus	Constant	No nystagmus expected	Constant or increasing/decreasing exponentially
Smooth pursuit	Normal	Normal	Usually saccadic
Saccades	Normal	Normal	Often dysmetric
Caloric tests	Unilateral loss	Bilateral loss	Intact/direction of nystagmus often perverted (reverse direction)
CNS symptoms	Absent	Absent	Often present
Symptoms	Severe motion aggravated vertigo/vegetative symptoms	Oscillopsia/imbalance/gait ataxia, vertigo not a complaint	Vertigo not as severe as in acute unilateral loss

Table 16-3 **Five Common Causes of Inner Ear Dysfunction**

Disorder	Duration of Vertigo	Hearing Loss	Tinnitus	Aural Fullness
BPPV	Seconds	–	–	–
Meniere disease	Minutes to hours	Fluctuant SNHL	+	+
Recurrent vestibulopathy	Minutes to hours	–	–	+/–
Vestibular neuronitis (VN)	Days to weeks	–	–	–
Acoustic neuroma	"Imbalance"	Progressive with poor speech discrimination	+	–

Vertigo Lasting Seconds

Benign Paroxysmal Positional Vertigo (BPPV)
Pathophysiology
  A. Posterior semicircular canal (PSCC) most commonly involved
  B. Early theory of cuplolithiasis is now replaced with canalolithiasis theory for most cases of BPPV
  C. Utricular degeneration or trauma liberates otoconia→ float downward toward ampulla of PSCC (inferior-most region of vestibule) → head movement stimulation→ motion of otolithic fragments within canal endolymph→ deflection of the cupula of the PSCC

HISTORY
Severe vertigo with change in head position lasting on order of seconds

RISK FACTORS
Head injury, history of vestibular neuronitis, infections, ear surgery
PHYSICAL FINDINGS
Classic nystagmus patterns in Hallpike maneuver
  A. Nystagmus is rotational and geotropic that crescendos then decrescendos
  B. Latency of onset (seconds)
  C. Short duration (< 1 minute)
  D. Fatigues on repeated testing
  E. Reverses on upright positioning of the head (ageotropic reversal)
TREATMENT
Spontaneous resolution within a few months in most cases
  A. Conservative
    i. Epley maneuver
    ii. Brandt exercise for habituation
    iii. Semont liberatory maneuvers
  B. Surgical
    i. Posterior canal occlusion
    ii. Singular neurectomy (rarely done)
    iii. Vestibular neurectomy
    iv. Labyrinthectomy (recalcitrant cases or in a deafened ear)

Vertigo Lasting Minutes to Hours

Meniere Disease

Pathophysiology

A. Idiopathic endolymphatic hydrops
   i. Possible causes: endolymphatic sac inflammation and fibrosis (autoimmune, infectious, ischemic), accumulation of glycoproteins, or altered endolymph production rates as possible etiologies for sac dysfunction → blockage of endolymph reabsorption
   ii. Most commonly seen in pars inferior (cochlea and saccule)
   iii. Characterized by bowing and rupture of Reissner membrane → leakage of potassium rich fluid (endolymph) into perilymph → interference with generation of action potential (Na^+/K^+ intoxication theory)
   iv. Bulging of membranous labyrinth expands into scala vestibuli, distorting SCCs, utricle and occasionally impinging under stapes footplate (vestibulofibrosis)

DEFINITIONS

A. Certain Meniere disease: Definite Meniere disease plus histopathologic confirmation (only detected at necropsy)
B. Definite Meniere disease: two or more episodes of spontaneous rotational vertigo that last 20 minutes or longer, with tinnitus or aural fullness in the affected ear; audiometric hearing loss documented on at least one occasion; other causes excluded
C. Probable Meniere disease: one definitive episode of vertigo and fulfillment of other criteria
D. Possible Meniere disease: episodic vertigo of the Meniere type without documented hearing loss

PRESENTATION

A. Variable frequency for recurrent attacks of vertigo, tinnitus, aural fullness and sensorineural hearing loss in the affected ear
B. Otolithic crisis of Tumarkin = sudden unexplained falls without loss of consciousness or associated vertigo
C. Lermoyez variant = resolution of hearing loss and tinnitus with onset of vertigo
D. Cochlear hydrops = fluctuating hearing loss, aural fullness, tinnitus without vertigo

PHYSICAL FINDINGS

Direction of nystagmus varies over time course of attack Phases of nystagmus:
A. Irritative phase: early in attack nystagmus beats toward the affected ear
B. Paralytic (deafferentative) phase: later in disease the nystagmus beats toward healthy ear
C. Recovery phase: as attack subsides and vestibular function improves, nystagmus often reverses toward the affected ear

INVESTIGATIONS

A. Audiogram: low frequency sensorineural loss which fluctuates over time
B. ECoG: increased SP/AP ratio (typically > 0.35 is considered abnormal)
C. ENG/VNG: unilateral weakness

TREATMENT

A. Conservative
   i. Dietary modification (low salt diet, avoidance of caffeine, etc)
   ii. Diuretics

   iii. Antivertiginous medication (vestibular sedatives)
   iv. Vasodilators
   v. Ca^{2+} channel blockers
B. Hearing conservative, vestibular non-ablative
   i. Endolymphatic sac decompression (controversial)
   ii. Tenotomy of tensor tympani and stapedial tendons (controversial)
   iii. Intratympanic steroid injections
C. Hearing conservative, vestibular ablative
   i. Intratympanic gentamicin ablation
   ii. Vestibular neurectomy
D. Hearing and vestibular ablative
   i. labyrinthectomy

Secondary Endolymphatic Hydrops
Otologic Syphilis
A. Early syphilis
   i. Vestibular symptoms are less frequent, vary from mild to protracted vertigo with vegetative features lasting days
B. Late syphilis
   i. Can present up to 50 years after initial exposure
   ii. High rate of fluctuating sensorineural hearing loss, vertigo plus interstitial keratitis
C. Diagnosis established by serologic testing
   i. VDRL (nontreponemal test)-less sensitive for late stage patients
   ii. FTA-ABS (fluorescent treponemal antibody)-test of choice for tertiary otologic syphilis
D. Treatment: long course of penicillin (> 6 weeks), short course of high-dose steroid administered simultaneously; recovery of hearing possibly up to 30% to 50%

Delayed Endolymphatic Hydrops
A. Characterized by attacks of vertigo identical to those of Meniere disease in patients with a prior history of profound loss of hearing in one or both ears
B. Causes of initial hearing loss vary
   i. trauma (acoustic and physical head trauma)
   ii. infections, for example, viral labyrinthitis (influenza, mumps), mastoiditis, meningitis

Cogan syndrome (see Chapter 1: Syndromes and Eponyms)
A. Autoimmune disease characterized by interstitial keratitis (nonsuppurative corneal inflammation), bilateral rapidly progressive audiovestibular dysfunction and multisystem involvement from vasculitis
B. Progressive to complete absence of vestibular function manifested by ataxia and oscillopsia
C. Hearing loss is bilateral and progressive, often without spontaneous improvement and can become profound
D. Ocular and otologic findings tend to occur within 6 months of one another
E. Treatment: high dose steroids, if no improvement further immunosuppression with cyclophosphamide (or other immunosuppressive agents) is indicated

Recurrent Vestibulopathy (RV)

A. Recurrent attacks of episodic vertigo similar to Meniere without auditory or focal neurological dysfunction. Synonymous with vestibular Meniere, episodic vertigo, vertigo without hearing loss, etc.

B. Longitudinal studies over 8.5 years showed that 60% of patients went on to remission, 15% developed Meniere, 10% continued with active attacks, 10% developed BPPV and 5% had other suspected peripheral vestibular symptoms

C. Treatment: symptomatic control only given its good clinical outcomes

Vertigo Lasting Days to Weeks

Vestibular Neuronitis

A. Typically presents with dramatic, sudden onset of vertigo and vegetative symptoms lasting days to weeks with gradual improvement throughout time course.

B. Complete absence of auditory dysfunction (in contrast to a complete labyrinthitis).

C. Instability with certain head movements is present for months and BPPV can occur subsequently in up to 15% of patients.

D. Fast phase of nystagmus is directed away from the involved side and hypofunction is observed on caloric responses in majority of affected individuals.

E. Treatment is supportive for vertigo and vegetative symptoms.

F. Failure to improve over a 2 to 3 week timeframe requires a CNS lesion to be excluded (ie, cerebellar infarction).

Vertigo of Variable Duration

Traumatic Perilymphatic Fistula

Pathophysiology

Abnormal communication between perilymphatic space and middle ear or an intramembranous communication between endolymphatic and perilymphatic spaces

Mechanism of trauma can vary.

A. Barotrauma

B. Penetrating trauma

C. Surgical trauma such as stapedectomy, cholesteatoma surgery, penetrating middle ear trauma

D. Physical exertion

PRESENTATION

A. Symptoms vary from mild and inconsequential to severe and incapacitating; include episodic vertigo equivalent to a Meniere attack, positional vertigo, motion intolerance, or occasional disequilibrium

B. Disequilibrium following increases in CSF pressure (Valsalva) such as nose blowing or lifting (Hennebert sign), exposure to loud noises (Tullio phenomenon)

PHYSICAL FINDINGS

A. Introduce positive pressure, either by rapid pressure on tragus, compressing external canal, or via pneumatic otoscope, while eyes observed.

B. Positive fistula sign: conjugate contralateral slow deviation of eyes followed by three or four ipsilaterally directed beats of nystagmus (high false-negative rate).

C. Increased SP/AP ratios (> 0.35) on ECoG with straining would be expected.

TREATMENT

A. Conservative: bed rest with head elevation, laxatives

B. Monitoring of both hearing and vestibular function

C. Surgical exploration if hearing loss worsens/vestibular symptoms persist

Superior Canal Dehiscence Syndrome (SCDS)

A. A form of inner ear fistula where there is communication between the middle cranial fossa and the superior SCC, creating a third mobile window within the canal and produces abnormal endolymphatic flow.

B. The cause of dehiscence of the bone covering the superior SCC is unknown-may be congenital or acquired.

C. Classic sound- and pressure-evoked vertigo, hyperacusis, gaze-evoked tinnitus, with chronic disequilibrium.

D. Diagnosis based on history, vestibular examination (positive fistula sign), positive VEMP (decreased threshold and increased amplitude), CT scan temporal bone (oblique view) showing absent bone over canal.

E. Treatment: surgical repair by resurfacing or plugging the site of dehiscence via a transmastoid or middle cranial fossa approach.

Differential Diagnosis for Vertigo Associated With Positive Fistula Test (Hennebert sign or Tullio Phenomenon)

A. Meniere disease (vestibulofibrosis-hydropic saccule)

B. Superior canal dehiscence syndrome

C. Neurosyphilis affecting otic capsule

D. Perilymphatic fistula

Controversial Causes for Vertigo

Migraine-Associated Vertigo (Vestibular Migraine)

A. Association of migraine and vertigo commonly mentioned in literature.

B. Controversial:

  i. Pathogenesis remains unclear

  ii. Difficult to know if association is related to the commonality of both conditions in the general population

C. Correlation requires close temporal association of vertiginous attack with migraine.

D. Successful treatment with anti-migraine therapy provides most reasonable hypothesis that the two conditions are related.

Cervicogenic vertigo

A. Abnormalities in the cervico-ocular reflex (COR) following trauma (specifically whiplash associated disorders (WAD)) have been postulated to cause episodic vertigo.

B. Controversial:

  i. COR activity is thought to be rudimentary in humans.

  ii. No specific diagnostic test available.

  iii. Pathology is not well defined etc.

C. Treatment: physiotherapy for neck related issues.

Spontaneous Perilymphatic Fistula

A. Symptoms similar to traumatic perilymphatic fistula with episodic attacks of vertigo to extraneous pressure.

B. Unlike traumatic perilymphatic fistula, formation controversy exists for its occurrence. Probably overdiagnosed.

C. Differential diagnosis: a variant of Meniere disease, superior canal dehiscence syndrome (SCDS).

D. Surgical exploration for confirmation of diagnosis: perilymphatic leak from oval or round window membranes. Successful obliteration of leak should result in clinical improvement.

Central Nervous System Disorders That Can Cause Dizziness (See Table 16-4)

A. Vertebrobasilar insufficiency
B. Wallenberg syndrome (lateral medullary infarction)
C. Head trauma
D. Cervical vertigo (controversial)
E. Vestibulocerebellar degeneration
F. Brainstem encephalitis
G. Demyelination (ie, multiple sclerosis)
H. Chiari malformation
I. Pseudotumor cerebri
J. Normal pressure hydrocephalus

Cerebellar Ataxia With Bilateral Vestibulopathy (CABV) and Cerebellar Ataxia With Neuropathy and Bilateral Vestibular Areflexia Syndrome (CANVAS)

Distinct syndrome of progressive imbalance from cerebellar atrophy and bilateral vestibular loss. Requires exclusion of other multisystem spinocerebellar (SPA) degenerations (ie, Friedriech ataxia, paraneoplastic syndromes, multisystem atrophy of the cerebellar type, etc)

A. Cerebellar ataxia with bilateral vestibulopathy (CABV)
B. Cerebellar ataxia with neuropathy and bilateral vestibular areflexia syndrome (CANVAS), that is, CABV associated with non-length dependent sensory deficit in legs =CANVAS

Pathophysiology

Suspected late onset recessive disorder with cerebellar degeneration of anterior and dorsal vermis, progressive ganglionopathy of vestibular (strial) ganglion cells and sensory peripheral neuropathy

Table 16-4 Signs and Symptoms Seen With Infarction in the Territories of the Posterior Inferior, Anterior Inferior, and Superior Cerebellar Arteries

Symptoms and Signs	Lateral Medullary (PICA)	Lateral Pontomedullary (AICA)	Superior Lateral Pontine (SCA)
Vertigo, nystagmus	+	+	+
Gait and ipsilateral limb ataxia	+	+	+
Tinnitus, hearing loss (ipsilateral)	-	+	-
Facial paralysis (ipsilateral)	+/-	+	-
Facial pain or numbness (ipsilateral)	+	+	+
Body hemianesthesia (contralateral)	+	+	+
Horner syndrome	+	+	+
Dysphagia, hoarseness, decreased gag, vocal cord weakness (ipsilateral)	+	-	-
Impaired vibration and position sense (contralateral)	-	-	+

CLINICAL PRESENTATION
  A. Progressive gait ataxia/imbalance
  B. Oscillopsia

PHYSICAL FINDINGS FOR CABV
  A. Significant dynamic visual acuity loss (DVA)
  B. Oculomotor abnormalities (ie, poor pursuit, abnormal optokinetic eye movements, inability to suppress residual VOR function)
  C. Nystagmus (gaze evoked, downbeat)
  D. Gait ataxia
  E. a-d + peripheral neuropathy = CANVAS

INVESTIGATIONS
  A. MR imaging
  B. Sensory neural action potential (SNAP) testing
  C. ENG/VNG and vHIT/scleral coil

TREATMENT
  A. Vestibular rehabilitation
  B. Avoidance to known cerebellar toxins (ie, alcohol, solvents, antiepileptics)
  C. Assistive devices as balance worsens

Bibliography

Handelsman JA, Shepard NT. Rotational chair testing. In: Goebel JA, ed. *Practical Management of the Dizzy Patient.* 2nd ed. Philadelphia, PA: Lippincott; 2008:137-152.

Konrad HR, Bauer CA. Peripheral vestibular disorders. In: Bailey BJ, ed. *Head and Neck Surgery-Otolaryngology.* 4th ed. Philadelphia, PA: Lippincott; 2006:2295-2302.

LeLiever W, Barber HO. Recurrent vestibulopathy. *Laryngoscope.* 1981;91:1-6.

Rutka JA. Physiology of the vestibular system. In: Roland PS, Rutka JA, eds. *Ototoxicity.* 1st ed. Hamilton, ONT; BC Decker; 2004:20-27.

Thorp MA, Shehab ZP, Bance ML, Rutka JA. AAO-HNS Committee on Hearing and Equilibrium. The AAO-HNS Committee on Hearing and Equilibrium guidelines for the diagnosis and evaluation of therapy in Meniere disease: have they been applied in the published literature of the last decade? *Clin Otolaryngol Allied Sci.* 2003;28:173-176.

Questions

1. Acute loss of labyrinthine function on the right side creates:
   A. Left-beating nystagmus and veering right
   B. Right-beating nystagmus and veering right
   C. Left-beating nystagmus and veering to the left
   D. Right-beating nystagmus and veering to the left
   E. Vertical downbeat nystagmus

2. Bilateral loss of vestibular input is clinically manifested as:
   A. Vertigo
   B. Oscillopsia
   C. Disconjugate eye movements

      D. Gaze-evoked nystagmus

      E. None of the above

3. What conclusion can be made about a patient with no warm, cool, and ice water caloric responses for right ear irrigation?

      A. The right peripheral vestibular system has no residual function.

      B. It must be a technical error.

      C. There is a central lesion.

      D. There is severe low-frequency loss for the right peripheral vestibular system. A rotational chair testing is recommended to test for higher frequency function.

      E. None of the above.

4. Superior canal dehiscence syndrome is a cluster of symptoms that may include all of the following except:

      A. Noise-induced vertigo

      B. Hyperacusis

      C. Gaze-evoked tinnitus

      D. Oscillopsia

      E. Autophony

5. Which is not a feature of cerebellar ataxia with bilateral vestibulopathy (CABV)?

      A. Impaired smooth pursuit

      B. Intranuclear ophthalmoplegia

      C. Bilateral positive head thrust manoeuvre

      D. Gait ataxia/imbalance

      E. Gaze evoked nystagmus

Chapter 17
Congenital Hearing Loss

Introduction

Deafness is the most common sensory defect (1 in 1000-2000 births)
- Early identification allows appropriate intervention as soon as indicated.
- Fifty percent is due to environmental factors.
- Fifty percent of congenital hearing loss is due to genetic factors.
- Seventy percent is nonsyndromic.
- Usually caused by mutation in single gene.
- Thirty percent syndromic causes of congenital hearing loss (Alport, Pendred, Usher).
- Seventy-five percent to 80% of genetic deafness is due to autosomal recessive (AR) genes.
- Eighteen percent to 20% is due to autosomal dominant (AD) genes.
- One percent to 3% is classified as X-linked, or chromosomal, disorders.

Environmental Factors

Common risk factors to consider include TORCH (toxoplasmosis, other agents, rubella, cytomegalovirus [CMV], Herpes Simplex), meningitis, extracorporeal membrane oxygenation (ECMO), hypoxia, and prenatal alcohol or ototoxic medication exposure.

Cytomegalovirus Infection

Most prevalent environmental cause of prelingual hearing loss in the United States (10%). Hearing loss can be unilateral, fluctuating and onset can be delayed for months or years. The diagnosis of congenital CMV infection at birth is usually by the detection of the virus in urine or saliva within the first three weeks of life.

Rubella Syndrome

- Congenital cataract.
- Cardiovascular anomalies.
- Mental retardation.
- Retinitis.
- Deafness.
- Five percent to 10% of mothers with rubella in first trimester give birth to baby with deafness.

- The eye is the most commonly affected organ, followed by the ears, and then the heart.
- Identification of fluorescent antibody, serum hemagglutination, and viral cultures from stool and throat confirm the diagnosis.
- Deafness of viral etiology shows degeneration of the organ of Corti, adhesion between the organ of Corti and Reissner membrane, rolled-up tectorial membrane, partial or complete stria atrophy, and scattered degeneration of neural elements (cochlea–saccule degeneration).

Kernicterus

- Twenty percent of kernicteric babies have severe deafness secondary to damage to the dorsal and ventral cochlear nuclei and the superior and inferior colliculi nuclei.
- High-frequency hearing loss occurs.
- Indication for exchange transfusion is usually a serum bilirubin greater than 20 mg/dL.

Syphilis

Tamari and Itkin estimated that hearing loss occurred in
- Seventeen percent of congenital syphilis
- Twenty-five percent of late latent syphilis
- Twenty-nine percent of asymptomatic patients with congenital syphilis
- Thirty-nine percent of symptomatic neurosyphilis

Karmody and Schuknecht reported 25% to 38% of patients with congenital syphilis have hearing loss. There are two forms of congenital syphilis: early (infantile) and late (tardive). The infantile form is often severe and bilateral. These children usually have multisystem involvement and hence a fatal outcome.

Late congenital syphilis has progressive hearing loss of varying severity and time of onset. Hearing losses that have their onset during early childhood are usually bilateral, sudden, severe, and associated with vestibular symptoms. The symptom complex is similar to that of Méniére disease. The late-onset form (sometimes as late as the fifth decade of life) has mild hearing loss. Karmody and Schuknecht also pointed out that the vestibular disorders of severe episodic vertigo are more common in the late-onset group than in the infantile group. Histopathologically, osteitis with mononuclear leukocytosis, obliterative endarteritis, and endolymphatic hydrops is noticed. Serum and cerebrospinal fluid (CSF) serology may or may not be positive. Treatment with steroids and penicillin seems to be of benefit. Other sites of congenital syphilis are:
A. Nasal cartilaginous and bony framework
B. Periosteitis of the cranial bones (bossing)
C. Periosteitis of the tibia (saber shin)
D. Injury to the odontogenous tissues (Hutchinson teeth)
E. Injury to the epiphyseal cartilages (short stature)
F. Commonly, interstitial keratitis (cloudy cornea)

Two signs are associated with congenital syphilis: Hennebert sign consists of a positive fistula test without clinical evidence of middle ear or mastoid disease, or a fistula. It has been postulated that the vestibular stimulation is mediated by fibrous bands between the footplate and the vestibular membranous labyrinth. Hennebert sign may also be present in Méniére disease. Another explanation is that the vestibular response is due to an excessively mobile footplate. The nystagmus in Hennebert sign usually is more marked upon application of a negative pressure.

Tullio phenomenon consists of vertigo and nystagmus on stimulation with high-intensity sound, such as the Bárány noise box. This phenomenon occurs not only in congenital syphilis but also in patients with a semicircular canal fistula or dehiscence and in postfenestration patients if the footplate is mobile and the fenestrum patent. It also can be demonstrated in chronic otitis media should the patient have an intact tympanic membrane, ossicular chain, and a fistula—a rare combination.

For Tullio phenomenon to take place, a fistula of the semicircular canal and intact sound transmission mechanism to the inner ear (ie, intact tympanic membrane, intact ossicular chain, and mobile footplate) must be present. The pathophysiology is that the high-intensity noise energy transmitted through the footplate finds the course of least resistance and displaces toward the fistula instead of the round window membrane.

Hearing loss may occur in the secondary or tertiary forms of acquired syphilis. Histopathologically, osteitis with round cell infiltration is noticed. With tertiary syphilis, gummatous lesions may involve the auricle, mastoid, middle ear, and petrous pyramid. These lesions can cause a mixed hearing loss. Because penicillin and other antibiotic therapies are quite effective in treating acquired syphilis, this form of deafness is now rare.

Hypothyroidism

Cretinism consists of retarded growth, mental retardation, and mixed hearing loss; is seen in conjunction with congenital deafness.

Nonsyndromic

Accounts for 70% of congenital hearing loss.
- Autosomal recessive (AR) inheritance is the most common form (80%).
- Autosomal dominant (AD) loci are called DFNA ("DeaFNess").
- ARs are DFNB, X-linked are DFN.
- Approximately 40 loci for AD deafness, 30 loci for AR, and 7 loci for X-linked have been mapped and 50 genes have been cloned.

Population analysis suggests that there are over 100 genes involved in non-syndromic hearing impairment. The mutation in connexin 26 molecule (gap junction protein, gene *GJB2*) accounts for about 49% of patients with nonsyndromic deafness and about 37% of sporadic cases.
- Assays for connexin 26 are commercially available.
- One in thirty-one individuals may be carriers of this mutation. One mutation is particularly common, namely the 30delG.

Autosomal Dominant

AD: 15% of cases of nonsyndromic hearing loss.
- DNFA loci.
- Congenital, severe, non-progressive hearing impairment usually represents more than one disorder, with several different genes having been localized.

Examples of AD deafness:

Missense mutation in *COL11A2* (DFNA13), encodes a chain of type XI collagen. It is a progressive, sensorineural hearing loss resulting in a flat sensorineural deafness.

The DFNA6/14-WFS1 mutation presents as a progressive low-frequency sensorineural hearing impairment caused by a heterozygous *WFS1* mutation. Mutations in the *WFS1* gene are the most common form of dominant low-frequency sensorineural hearing loss.

Autosomal Recessive

Genetic linkage studies have identified at least 30 gene loci for recessive nonsyndromic hearing loss. The gene *DFNB2* on chromosome 13q may be the most common and has been identified as connexin 23. *DFNB1*, also found on chromosome 13, codes for a connexin 26 gene gap junction protein. The connexin 26 protein plays an important role in auditory transduction. Expression of connexin 26 in the cochlea is essential for hearing.

Although many genes may be implicated in recessive nonsyndromic hearing loss, it is likely that most of them are rare, affecting one or a few inbred families.

Nonsyndromic X-Linked Hearing Loss

X-linked nonsyndromic hearing impairment is even more uncommon than X-linked syndromic deafness. Most of the X-linked genes responsible for hereditary hearing impairment have yet to be elucidated. At least six loci on the X-chromosome for nonsyndromic hearing loss are known.

Two types of non-syndromic, X-linked severe sensorineural hearing loss have been described: an early onset, rapidly progressive type and a moderate, slowly progressive type.

X-linked fixation of the stapes with perilymphatic gusher associated with mixed hearing impairment has been localized to the *DNF3* locus, which encodes the *POU3F4* transcription factor. This gene is located close to a gene causing choroideremia, and deletion of these genes produces the contiguous gene syndrome of choroideremia, hearing loss, and mental retardation. Preoperative CT scanning can be used to detect predictive findings, such as an enlarged internal auditory canal with thinning or absence of bone at the base of the cochlea. X-linked forms of hearing impairment may also involve congenital sensorineural deafness. Both forms of nonsyndromic hearing impairment have been linked to Xq13-q21.2. Researchers have also identified an X-linked dominant sensorineural hearing impairment associated with the Xp21.2 locus. The auditory impairment in affected males was congenital, bilateral, sensorineural, and profound, affecting all frequencies. Adult carrier females demonstrated bilateral, mild to moderate high-frequency sensorineural hearing impairment of delayed onset.

Syndromic

More Common Autosomal Dominant Syndromic Disorders

Branchio-oto-renal syndrome Branchio-oto-renal syndrome is estimated to occur in 2% of children with congenital hearing impairment. The syndrome involves branchial characteristics including ear pits and tags or cervical fistula and renal involvement ranging from agenesis and renal failure to minor dysplasia. Seventy-five percent of patients with branchio-oto-renal syndrome have significant hearing loss. Of these, 30% are conductive, 20% are sensorineural, and 50% demonstrate mixed forms. Mutations in *EYA1*, a gene of 16 exons within a genomic interval of 156 kB, have been shown to cause the syndrome. The encoded protein is a transcriptional activator. The gene has been located on chromosome 8q.

Neurofibromatosis Neurofibromatosis (NF) presents with café-au-lait spots and multiple fibromas. Cutaneous tumors are most common, but the central nervous system, peripheral nerves, and viscera can be involved. Mental retardation, blindness, and sensorineural hearing loss can result from central nervous system (CNS) tumors.

Neurofibromatosis is classified as types 1 and 2. NF type 1 is more common with an incidence of about 1:3000 persons. Type 1 generally includes many café-au-lait spots, cutaneous neurofibromas, plexiform neuromas, pseudoarthrosis, Lisch nodules of the iris, and optic gliomas. Acoustic neuromas are usually unilateral and occur in only 5% of affected patients. Hearing loss can also occur as a consequence of a neurofibroma encroaching on the middle or inner ear, but significant deafness is rare. The expressed phenotype may vary from a few café-au-lait spots to multiple disfiguring neurofibromas. Type 1 is caused by a disruption of the *NF1* gene (a nerve growth factor gene) localized to chromosome 17q11.2.

NF type 2, which is a genetically distinct disorder, is characterized by bilateral acoustic neuromas, café-au-lait spots, and subcapsular cataracts. Bilateral acoustic neuromas are present in 95% of affected patients and are usually asymptomatic until early adulthood. Deletions in the *NF2* gene (a tumor suppressor gene) on chromosome 22q12.2 cause the abnormalities associated with neurofibromatosis type 2. Both types of neurofibromatosis demonstrate AD inheritance with high penetrance but variable expressivity. High mutation rates are characteristic of both types of disorder.

Osteogenesis imperfecta Osteogenesis imperfecta is characterized by bone fragility, blue sclera, conductive, mixed, or sensorineural hearing loss, and hyperelasticity of joints and ligaments. This disorder is transmitted as AD disorder with variable expressivity and incomplete penetrance. Two genes for osteogenesis imperfecta have been identified, *COLIA1* on chromosome 17q and *COLIA2* on chromosome 7q. The age at which the more common tarda variety becomes clinically apparent is variable. van der Hoeve syndrome is a subtype in which progressive hearing loss begins in early childhood.

Otosclerosis Otosclerosis is caused by proliferation of spongy type tissue on the otic capsule eventually leading to fixation of the ossicles and producing conductive hearing loss. Hearing loss may begin in childhood but most often becomes evident in early adulthood and eventually may include a sensorineural component.

Otosclerosis appears to be transmitted in an AD pattern with decreased penetrance, so only 25% to 40% of gene carriers show the phenotype. The greater proportion of affected females points to a possible hormonal influence. Recent statistical studies suggest a role for the gene *COLIA1* in otosclerosis, and measles viral particles have been identified within otosclerotic foci, raising the possibility of an interaction with the viral genome.

Stickler syndrome Cleft palate, micrognathia, severe myopia, retinal detachments, cataracts, and marfanoid habitus characterize stickler syndrome clinically. Significant sensorineural hearing loss or mixed hearing loss is present in about 15% of cases, whereas hearing loss of lesser severity may be present in up to 80% of cases. Ossicular abnormalities may also be present.

Most cases of Stickler syndrome can be attributed to mutations in the *COL2A1* gene found on chromosome 12 that causes premature termination signals for a type II collagen gene. Additionally, changes in the *COL 11A2* gene on chromosome 6 have been found to cause the syndrome.

Treacher Collins syndrome Treacher Collins syndrome consists of facial malformations such as malar hypoplasia, downward slanting palpebral fissures, coloboma of the lower eyelids (the upper eyelid is involved in Goldenhar syndrome), hypoplastic mandible, malformations of the external ear or the ear canal, dental malocclusion, and cleft palate. The facial features are bilateral and symmetrical in Treacher Collins syndrome.

Conductive hearing loss is present 30% of the time, but sensorineural hearing loss and vestibular dysfunction can also be present. Ossicular malformations are common in these patients. Inheritance is AD with high penetrance. However, a new mutation can be present in as many as 60% of cases of Treacher Collins syndrome.

The gene responsible for Treacher Collins syndrome is *TCOF1* which is located on chromosome 5q and produces a protein named treacle, which is operative in early craniofacial development. There is considerable variation in expression between and within families, suggesting other genes can modify the expression of the treacle protein.

Waardenburg syndrome Waardenburg syndrome (WS) accounts for 3% of childhood hearing impairment and is the most common form of AD congenital deafness. There is a significant amount of variability of expression in this syndrome. There may be unilateral or bilateral sensorineural hearing loss in patients and the phenotypic expressions may include pigmentary anomalies and craniofacial features. The pigmentary anomalies include: white forelock (20%-30% of cases), heterochromia irides, premature graying, and vitiligo. Craniofacial features that are seen in Waardenburg syndrome include dystopia canthorum, broad nasal root, and synophrys. All of the above features are variable.

There are four different forms of Waardenburg syndrome, which can be distinguished clinically. Type 1 is characterized by congenital sensorineural hearing impairment, heterochromia irides, white forelock, patchy hypopigmentation, and dystopia canthorum. Type 2 is differentiated from type 1 by the absence of dystopia canthorum, whereas type 3 is characterized by microcephaly, skeletal abnormalities, and mental retardation, in addition to the features associated with type 1. The combination of recessively inherited WS type 2 characteristics with Hirschsprung disease has been called Waardenburg-Shah syndrome or WS type 4.

Sensorineural hearing loss is seen in 20% of patients with type 1 and in more than 50% of patients with type 2. Essentially all cases of type 1 and type 3 are caused by a mutation of the *PAX3* gene on chromosome 2q37. This genetic mutation ultimately results in a defect in neural crest cell migration and development. About 20% of type 2 cases are caused by a mutation of the *MITF* gene (microphthalmia transcription factor) on chromosome 3p. Waardenburg syndrome has also been linked to other genes such as *EDN3*, *EDNRB*, and *SOX10*.

More Common Autosomal Recessive Syndromic Disorders

The most common pattern of transmission of hereditary hearing loss is autosomal recessive (AR), compromising 80% of cases of hereditary deafness. Half of these cases represent recognizable syndromes.

Jervell and Lange-Nielsen syndrome Jervell and Lange-Nielsen syndrome is a rare syndrome consisting of profound sensorineural hearing loss and cardiac arrhythmias. The genetic defect is caused by a mutation affecting a potassium channel gene that leads to conduction abnormalities in the heart.

Electrocardiography reveals large T waves and prolongation of the QT interval, which may lead to syncopal episodes as early as the second or third year of life. The cardiac component of this disorder is treated with beta-adrenergic blockers such as propranolol. An electrocardiogram should be performed on all children with early onset hearing loss of uncertain etiology.

Genetic studies attribute one form of Jervell and Lange-Nielsen syndrome to homozygosity for mutations affecting a potassium channel gene (*KVLQT 1*) on chromosome 11p15.5, which is thought to result in delayed myocellular repolarization in the heart. The gene *KCNE1* has also been shown to be responsible for the disorder.

Pendred syndrome Pendred syndrome is believed to be the most common syndromic form of congenital deafness. It includes thyroid goiter and profound sensorineural hearing loss. Hearing loss may be progressive in about 10% to 15% of patients. The majority of patients present with bilateral moderate to severe high-frequency sensorineural hearing loss, with some residual hearing in the low frequencies.

The hearing loss is associated with abnormal iodine metabolism (defect in tyrosine iodination) resulting in a euthyroid goiter, which usually becomes clinically detectable at about 8 years of age. The perchlorate discharge test shows abnormal organification of nonorganic iodine in these patients and is needed for definitive diagnosis. Radiological studies reveal that most patients have Mondini aplasia or enlarged vestibular aqueduct.

Mutations in the *PDS* gene, on chromosome 7q31, have been shown to cause this disorder. The *PDS* gene codes for the pendrin protein, which is a sulfate transporter. Recessive inheritance is seen in many families, whereas others show a dominant pattern with variable expression. Treatment of the goiter is with exogenous thyroid hormone.

Usher syndrome Usher syndrome has a prevalence of 3.5 per 100,000 people; it is the most common type of autosomal recessive syndromic hearing loss. This syndrome affects about one half of the 16,000 deaf and blind persons in the United States. It is characterized by sensorineural hearing loss and retinitis pigmentosa (RP). Genetic linkage analysis studies demonstrate three distinct subtypes, distinguishable on the basis of severity or progression of the hearing loss and the extent of vestibular system involvement.

Usher type 1 describes congenital bilateral profound hearing loss and absent vestibular function; type 2 describes moderate hearing losses and normal vestibular function. Patients with type 3 demonstrate progressive hearing loss and variable vestibular dysfunction and are found primarily in the Norwegian population.

Ophthalmologic evaluation is an essential part of the diagnostic workup, and subnormal electroretinographic patterns have been observed in children as young as 2 to 3 years of age, before retinal changes are evident fundoscopically. Early diagnosis of Usher syndrome can have important rehabilitation and educational planning implications for an affected child. These patients may benefit from a cochlear implant.

Linkage analysis studies reveal at least five different genes for type 1 and at least two for type 2. Only type 3 appears to be due to just one gene.

Sex-Linked Disorders

X-linked disorders are rare, accounting for only 1% to 2% of cases of hereditary hearing impairment. **Alport syndrome** Alport syndrome affects the collagen of the basement membranes of the kidneys and the inner ear, resulting in renal failure and progressive sensorineural hearing loss. The renal disease may cause hematuria in infancy, but usually remains asymptomatic for several years before the onset of renal insufficiency. The hearing loss may not become clinically evident until the second decade of life. Dialysis and renal transplantation have proven important therapeutic advances in the treatment of these patients.

COL4A5, which codes for a certain form of type IV collagen, has been identified as the gene locus for this syndrome. Genetic mutation results in fragile type IV collagen in the inner ear and kidney resulting in progressive hearing impairment and kidney disease.

These collagens are found in the basilar membrane, parts of the spiral ligament, and stria vascularis. Although the mechanism of hearing loss is not known, in the glomerulus there is focal thinning and thickening with eventual basement membrane splitting. Assuming a similar process occurs in the ear, it has been suggested that mechanical energy transmission is likely affected by loss of integrity of the basilar and tectorial membranes.

Norrie syndrome Classic features of Norrie syndrome include specific ocular symptoms (pseudotumor of the retina, retinal hyperplasia, hypoplasia and necrosis of the inner layer of the retina, cataracts, phthisis bulbi), progressive sensorineural hearing loss, and mental disturbance. One-third of the affected patients have onset of progressive sensorineural hearing loss beginning in the second or third decade.

A gene for Norrie syndrome has been localized to chromosome Xp11.4, where studies have revealed deletions involving contiguous genes. A number of families have shown variable deletions in this chromosomal region.

Otopalatodigital syndrome Otopalatodigital syndrome includes hypertelorism, craniofacial deformity involving supraorbital area, flat midface, small nose, and cleft palate. Patients are short statured with broad fingers and toes that vary in length, with an excessively wide space between the first and second toe. Conductive hearing loss is seen due to ossicular malformations. Affected males manifest the full spectrum of the disorder and females may show mild involvement. The gene has been found to be located on chromosome Xq28.

Wildervanck syndrome Wildervanck syndrome is comprised of the Klippel-Feil sign involving fused cervical vertebrae, sensorineural hearing or mixed hearing impairment, and cranial nerve VI paralysis causing retraction of the eye on lateral gaze. This syndrome is seen most commonly in females because of the high mortality associated with the X-linked dominant form in males. Isolated Klippel-Feil sequence includes hearing impairment in about one-third of cases. The hearing impairment is related to bony malformations of the inner ear.

Mohr-Tranebjaerg syndrome (DFN-1) Mohr-Tranebjaerg syndrome (DFN-1) is an X-linked recessive syndromic hearing loss characterized by postlingual sensorineural deafness in childhood followed by progressive dystonia, spasticity, dysphagia, and optic atrophy. The syndrome is caused by a mutation thought to result in mitochondrial dysfunction.

It resembles a spinocerebellar degeneration called Friedreich ataxia, which also may exhibit sensorineural hearing loss, ataxia, and optic atrophy. The cardiomyopathy characteristic of Friedreich ataxia is not seen in Mohr-Tranebjaerg.

X-linked Charcot-Marie-Tooth (CMT) X-linked CMT is inherited in a dominant fashion and is caused by a mutation in the connexin 32 gene mapped to the Xq13 locus. Usual clinical signs consist of a peripheral neuropathy combined with foot problems and "champagne bottle" calves. Sensorineural deafness occurs in some.

Multifactorial Genetic Disorders

Some disorders appear to result from a combination of genetic factors interacting with environmental influences. Examples of this type of inheritance associated with hearing loss include clefting syndromes, involving conductive hearing loss, and the microtia/hemifacial microsomia/Goldenhar spectrum.

Goldenhar syndrome or oculoauriculovertebral dysplasia Oculoauriculovertebral dysplasia (OAVD) has an incidence of 1 in 45,000. It includes features such as hemifacial micro, otomandibular dysostosis, epibulbar lipodermoids, coloboma of upper lid, and vertebral anomalies that stem from developmental vascular and genetic field aberrations. It has diverse etiologies and is not attributed to a single genetic locus.

Autosomal Chromosomal Syndromes

Trisomy 13 can have significant sensorineural hearing loss.

Turner syndrome, monosomic for all or part of one X chromosome, presents generally in females as gonadal dysgenesis, short stature, and often webbed neck or shield chest. They will also have sensorineural, conductive, or mixed hearing loss, which can be progressive and may be the first evidence of the syndrome in prepubertal females.

Mitochondrial Disorders

Hearing loss can occur as an additional symptom in a range of mitochondrial syndromes. Mutation in the mitochondrial genome can affect energy production through adenosine triphosphase (ATP) synthesis and oxidative phosphorylation. Tissues that require high levels of energy are particularly affected. Typically, mitochondrial diseases involve progressive neuromuscular degeneration with ataxia, ophthalmoplegia, and progressive hearing loss.

Disorders such as Kearns-Sayre; mitochondrial encephalopathy, lactic acidosis, and stroke (MELAS); myoclonic epilepsy with ragged red fibers (MERRF); and Leber hereditary optic neuropathy are all mitochondrial disorders. All of these disorders have varying degrees of hearing loss.

Several other mitochondrial mutations have been found to produce enhanced sensitivity to the ototoxic effects of aminoglycosides. Screening for these mutations would be indicated in maternal relatives of persons showing hearing loss in response to normal therapeutic doses of aminoglycosides.

Inner Ear Structural Malformations

By week 9 of gestation, the cochlea reaches adult size (2¾ turns). Arrest in normal development or aberrant development of inner ear structures may result in hearing impairment. Depending on the timing and nature of the developmental insult, a range of inner ear anomalies can result. Computerized temporal bone imaging techniques reveal that about 20% of children with congenital sensorineural hearing loss have subtle or severe abnormalities of the inner ear. About 65% of such abnormalities are bilateral; 35% are unilateral. On the basis of temporal bone histopathologic studies inner ear malformations have typically been classified into five different groups.

Michel aplasia Complete agenesis of the petrous portion of the temporal bone occurs in Michel aplasia although the external and middle ear may be unaffected. This malformation is thought to result from an insult prior to the end of the third gestational week. Normal inner structures are lacking, resulting in anacusis. Conventional amplification or cochlear implantation offers little assistance. Vibrotactile devices have proven beneficial in some patients. Autosomal dominant inheritance has been observed, but recessive inheritance is also likely.

Mondini aplasia Mondini aplasia involves a developmentally deformed cochlea in which only the basal coil can be identified clearly. The upper coils assume a cloacal form and the interscalar septum is absent. The endolymphatic duct is also usually enlarged. It is postulated that the deformity results from developmental arrest at approximately the sixth week gestation because of the underdeveloped vestibular labyrinth. This anomaly can be inherited in an autosomal dominant fashion and may not be bilateral. It has been described in several other disorders including Pendred, Waardenburg, Treacher Collins, and Wildervanck syndromes. Association of Mondini aplasia with nongenetic etiologies, such as congenital cytomegalovirus (CMV) infection, has been reported. CMV infection may account for more than 40% of deafness of unknown etiology.

A related anomaly and more severe syndrome, the CHARGE association consists of coloboma, heart disease, choanal atresia, retarded development, genital hypoplasia, ear anomalies including hypoplasia of the external ear and hearing loss. These individuals have a Mondini type deformity and absence of semicircular canals.

Often accompanying the Mondini dysplasia is abnormal communication between the endolymphatic and perilymphatic spaces of the inner ear and subarachnoid space. It is usually caused by a defect in the cribriform area of the lateral end of the internal auditory canal. Presumably because of this abnormal channel, perilymphatic fistulae are more common in this disorder.

The presence of neurosensory structures in most cases warrants an aggressive program of early rehabilitative intervention, including conventional amplification.

Scheibe aplasia (cochlearsaccular dysplasia or pars inferior dysplasia) The bony labyrinth and the superior portion of the membranous labyrinth, including the utricle and semicircular canals, are normally differentiated in patients with Scheibe aplasia. The organ of Corti is generally poorly differentiated with a deformed tectorial membrane and collapsed Reissner membrane, which compromises the scala media. Scheibe aplasia is the most common form of inner ear aplasia and can be inherited as an autosomal recessive nonsyndromic trait.

The deformity has been reported in temporal bones of patient with Jervell and Lange-Nielsen, Refsum, Usher, and Waardenburg syndromes as well as in congenital rubella infants.

Conventional amplification with rehabilitative intervention is beneficial in many of these children.

Alexander aplasia In Alexander aplasia, cochlear duct differentiation at the level of the basal coil is limited with resultant effects on the organ of Corti and the ganglion cells. Audiometrically these patients have a high-frequency hearing loss with adequate residual hearing in the low frequencies to warrant the use of amplification.

Enlarged vestibular aqueduct syndrome An enlarged vestibular aqueduct has been associated with early onset sensorineural hearing loss, which is usually bilateral and often progressive and may be accompanied by vertigo or incoordination. This abnormality may also accompany cochlear and semicircular canal deformities. The progressive hearing loss is apparently the result of hydrodynamic changes and possibly labyrinthine membrane disruption. Familial cases have been observed, suggesting autosomal dominant inheritance, but recessive inheritance is also possible. The deformity has also been found in association with Pendred syndrome.

Enlarged vestibular aqueduct syndrome (EVAS) is defined as a vestibular aqueduct measuring 1.5 mm or greater as measured midway between the operculum and the common crus on CT scan. Coronal CT scan is the best view for evaluating it in children. Enlarged vestibular aqueducts can also be seen on high-resolution magnetic resonance imaging (MRI).

EVAS may present as fluctuating sensorineural hearing loss. Conservative management, including avoidance of head trauma and contact sports, has been the mainstay of treatment. Surgery to close the enlarged structure frequently results in significant hearing loss and is not indicated. Patients with EVAS who develop profound hearing loss are suitable cochlear implant candidates.

Semicircular canal malformations Formation of the semicircular canals begins in the sixth gestational week. The superior canal is formed first and the lateral canal is formed last. Isolated lateral canal defects are the most commonly identified inner ear malformations identified on temporal bone imaging studies. Superior semicircular canal deformities are always accompanied by lateral semicircular canal deformities, whereas lateral canal deformities often occur in isolation.

These types of abnormalities account for roughly 20% of congenital deafness. In general, these disorders can be associated with genetic disorders, but more often occur independently.

Hereditary Deafness

Hereditary deafness can also be classified as follows:
- A. Hereditary (congenital) deafness without associated abnormalities (AD, AR, or sex linked)
- B. Hereditary congenital deafness associated with integumentary system disease (AD, AR, or sex linked)
- C. Hereditary congenital deafness associated with skeletal disease (AD, AR, or sex-linked)
- D. Hereditary congenital deafness associated with other abnormalities (AD, AR, or sex linked)

Hereditary Deafness Without Associated Abnormalities

Stria Atrophy (Hereditary, Not Congenital)
- A. Autosomal dominant.
- B. The sensorineural hearing loss begins at middle age and is progressive.
- C. Good discrimination is maintained.

     D. Flat audiometric curve.
     E. Positive short increment sensitivity index (SISI) test.
     F. Bilaterally symmetrical hearing loss.
     G. Patient never becomes profoundly deaf.

Otosclerosis (Hereditary, Not Congenital)

Described in Chapter 23.

Hereditary Congenital Deafness Associated With Integumentary System Disease

Albinism With Blue Irides

     A. Autosomal dominant or recessive
     B. Sensorineural hearing loss

Ectodermal Dysplasia (Hidrotic)

Note that anhidrotic ectodermal dysplasia is sex-linked recessive, with a mixed or conductive hearing loss.

     A. Autosomal dominant
     B. Small dystrophic nails
     C. Coniform teeth
     D. Elevated sweat electrolytes
     E. Sensorineural hearing loss

Forney Syndrome

     A. Autosomal dominant
     B. Lentigines
     C. Mitral insufficiency
     D. Skeletal malformations
     E. Conductive hearing loss

Lentigines

     A. Autosomal dominant
     B. Brown spots on the skin, beginning at age 2
     C. Ocular hypertelorism
     D. Pulmonary stenosis
     E. Abnormalities of the genitalia
     F. Retarded growth
     G. Sensorineural hearing loss

Leopard Syndrome

     A. Autosomal dominant with variable penetrance
     B. Variable sensorineural hearing loss
     C. Ocular hypertelorism
     D. Pulmonary stenosis
     E. Hypogonadism
     F. Electrocardiographic (ECG) changes with widened QRS or bundle branch block

G. Retardation of growth
H. Normal vestibular apparatus
I. Lentigines
J. Skin changes progressively over the first and second decades

Piebaldness

A. Sex linked or autosomal recessive
B. Blue irides
C. Fine retinal pigmentation
D. Depigmentation of scalp, hair, and face
E. Areas of depigmentation on limbs and trunk
F. Sensorineural hearing loss

Tietze Syndrome

A. Autosomal dominant
B. Profound deafness
C. Albinism
D. Eyebrows absent
E. Blue irides
F. No photophobia or nystagmus

Waardenburg Disease (Also Described Earlier)

A. Autosomal dominant with variable penetrance
B. Contributes 1% to 7% of all hereditary deafness
C. Widely spaced medial canthi (present in all cases)
D. Flat nasal root in 75% of cases
E. Confluent eyebrow
F. Sensorineural hearing loss—unilateral or bilateral (present in 20% cases)
G. Colored irides
H. White forelock
I. Areas of depigmentation (10% of the patients)
J. Abnormal tyrosine metabolism
K. Diminished vestibular function (75% of the patients)
L. Cleft lip and palate (10% of the patients)

Hereditary Congenital Deafness Associated With Skeletal Disease

Achondroplasia

A. Autosomal dominant
B. Large head and short extremities
C. Dwarfism
D. Mixed hearing loss (fused ossicles)
E. Saddle nose, frontal and mandibular prominence

Apert Disease (Acrocephalosyndactyly)

A. Autosomal dominant
B. Syndactylia
C. Flat conductive hearing loss secondary to stapes fixation

D. Patent cochlear aqueduct histologically
E. Frontal prominence, exophthalmos
F. Craniofacial dysostosis, hypoplastic maxilla
G. Proptosis, saddle nose, high-arched palate, and occasionally spina bifida
H. Occurs in about 1:150,000 live births

Atresia Auris Congenital

A. Autosomal dominant
B. Unilateral or bilateral involvement
C. Middle ear abnormalities with seventh nerve anomaly
D. Internal hydrocephalus
E. Mental retardation
F. Epilepsy
G. Choanal atresia and cleft palate

Cleidocranial Dysostosis

A. Autosomal dominant
B. Absent or hypoplastic clavicle
C. Failure of fontanelles to close
D. Sensorineural hearing loss

Crouzon Disease (Craniofacial Dysostosis)

A. Autosomal dominant
B. Hearing loss in one-third of cases
C. Mixed hearing loss in some cases
D. Cranial synostosis
E. Exophthalmos and divergent squint
F. Parrot-beaked nose
G. Short upper lip
H. Mandibular prognathism and small maxilla
I. Hypertelorism
J. External auditory canal sometimes atretic
K. Congenital enlargement of the sphenoid bone
L. Premature closure of the cranial suture lines, sometimes leading to mental retardation

Engelmann Syndrome (Diaphyseal Dysplasia)

A. Autosomal dominant; possible recessive
B. Progressive mixed hearing loss
C. Progressive cortical thickening of diaphyseal regions of long bones and skull

Hand–Hearing Syndrome

A. Autosomal dominant
B. Congenital flexion contractures of fingers and toes
C. Sensorineural hearing loss

Klippel-Feil (Brevicollis, Wildervanck) Syndrome

A. Autosomal recessive or dominant
B. Incidence in female subjects greater than in male subjects

C. Sensorineural hearing loss along with middle ear anomalies

D. Short neck due to fused cervical vertebrae

E. Spina bifida

F. External auditory canal atresia

Madelung Deformity (Related to Dyschondrosteosis of Leri-Weill)

A. Autosomal dominant

B. Short stature

C. Ulna and elbow dislocation

D. Conductive hearing loss secondary to ossicular malformation with normal tympanic membrane and external auditory canal

E. Spina bifida occulta

F. Female to male ratio of 4:1

Marfan Syndrome (Arachnodactyly, Ectopia Lentis, Deafness)

A. Autosomal dominant

B. Thin, elongated individuals with long spidery fingers

C. Pigeon breast

D. Scoliosis

E. Hammer toes

F. Mixed hearing loss

Mohr Syndrome (Oral-Facial-Digital Syndrome II)

A. Autosomal recessive

B. Conductive hearing loss

C. Cleft lip, high-arched palate

D. Lobulated nodular tongue

E. Broad nasal root, bifid tip of nose

F. Hypoplasia of the body of the mandible

G. Polydactyly and syndactyly

Osteopetrosis (Albers-Schonberg Disease, Marble Bone Disease)

A. Autosomal recessive (rare dominant transmission has been reported)

B. Conductive or mixed hearing loss

C. Fluctuating facial nerve paralysis

D. Sclerotic, brittle bone due to failure of resorption of calcified cartilage

E. Cranial nerves II, V, VII involved sometimes

F. Optic atrophy

G. Atresia of paranasal sinuses

H. Choanal atresia

I. Increased incidence of osteomyelitis

J. Widespread form: may lead to obliteration of the bone marrow, severe anemia, and rapid demise

K. Hepatosplenomegaly possible

Oto-Facial-Cervical Syndrome

A. Autosomal dominant

B. Depressed nasal root

    C. Protruding narrow nose
    D. Narrow elongated face
    E. Flattened maxilla and zygoma
    F. Prominent ears
    G. Preauricular fistulas
    H. Poorly developed neck muscles
    I. Conductive hearing loss

Oto-Palatal-Digital Syndrome

    A. Autosomal recessive
    B. Conductive hearing loss
    C. Mild dwarfism
    D. Cleft palate
    E. Mental retardation
    F. Broad nasal root, hypertelorism
    G. Frontal and occipital bossing
    H. Small mandible
    I. Stubby, clubbed digits
    J. Low-set small ears
    K. Winged scapulae
    L. Malar flattening
    M. Downward obliquity of eye
    N. Downturned mouth

Paget Disease (Osteitis Deformans)

    A. Autosomal dominant with variable penetrance
    B. Mainly sensorineural hearing loss but mixed hearing loss as well
    C. Occasional cranial nerve involvement
    D. Onset usually at middle age, involving skull and long bones of the legs
    E. Endochondral bone (somewhat resistant to this disease)

Pierre Robin Syndrome (Cleft Palate, Micrognathia, and Glossoptosis)

    A. Autosomal dominant with variable penetrance (possibly not hereditary but due to intrauterine insult)
    B. Occurs in 1:30,000 to 1:50,000 live births
    C. Glossoptosis
    D. Micrognathia
    E. Cleft palate (in 50% of cases)
    F. Mixed hearing loss
    G. Malformed auricles
    H. Mental retardation
    I. Hypoplastic mandible
    J. Möbius syndrome
    K. Subglottic stenosis not uncommon
    L. Aspiration a common cause of death

Pyle Disease (Craniometaphyseal Dysplasia)

    A. Autosomal dominant (less often autosomal recessive).
    B. Conductive hearing loss can begin at any age. It is progressive and secondary to fixation of the stapes or other ossicular abnormalities. Mixed hearing loss also possible.

    C. Cranial nerve palsy secondary to narrowing of the foramen.

    D. Splayed appearance of long bones.

    E. Choanal atresia.

    F. Prognathism.

    G. Optic atrophy.

    H. Obstruction of sinuses and nasolacrimal duct.

Roaf Syndrome

    A. Not hereditary

    B. Retinal detachment, cataracts, myopia, coxa vara, kyphoscoliosis, retardation

    C. Progressive sensorineural hearing loss

Dominant Proximal Symphalangia and Hearing Loss

    A. Autosomal dominant

    B. Ankylosis of proximal interphalangeal joint

    C. Conductive hearing loss early in life

Treacher Collins Syndrome (Mandibulofacial Dysostosis; Franceschetti-Zwahlen-Klein Syndrome)

    A. Autosomal dominant or intrauterine abuse

    B. Antimongoloid palpebral fissures with notched lower lids

    C. Malformation of ossicles (stapes usually normal)

    D. Auricular deformity, atresia of external auditory canal

    E. Conductive hearing loss

    F. Preauricular fistulas

    G. Mandibular hypoplasia and malar hypoplasia

    H. "Fishmouth"

    I. Normal IQ

    J. Usually bilateral involvement

    K. May have cleft palate and cleft lip

    L. Arrest in embryonic development at 6 to 8 weeks to give the above findings

van Buchem Syndrome (Hyperostosis Corticalis Generalisata)

    A. Autosomal recessive

    B. Generalized osteosclerotic overgrowth of skeleton including skull, mandible, ribs, and long and short bones

    C. Cranial nerve palsies due to obstruction of the foramina

    D. Increased serum alkaline phosphatase

    E. Progressive sensorineural hearing loss

van der Hoeve Syndrome (Osteogenesis Imperfecta)

    A. Autosomal dominant with variable expressivity.

    B. Fragile bones, loose ligaments.

    C. Blue or clear sclera, triangular facies, dentinogenesis imperfecta.

    D. Blue sclera and hearing loss are seen in 60% of cases and are most frequently noted after age 20. The hearing loss is conductive and is due to stapes fixation by otosclerosis. Hearing loss also can be due to ossicular fracture. (Some use the term van der Hoeve syndrome to describe osteogenesis imperfecta with otosclerosis. Others use the term interchangeably with osteogenesis imperfecta regardless of whether or not otosclerosis is present.)

E. The basic pathologic defect is "abnormal osteoblastic activity."

F. When operating on such a patient, it is important to avoid fracture of the tympanic ring or the long process of the incus. It is also important to realize that the stapes footplate may be "floating."

G. The sclera may have increased mucopolysaccharide content.

H. These patients have normal calcium, phosphorus, and alkaline phosphatase in the serum.

I. Occasionally, capillary fragility is noted.

Hereditary Congenital Deafness Associated With Other Abnormalities

Acoustic Neurinomas (Inherited)

A. Autosomal dominant

B. Progressive sensorineural hearing loss during the second or third decade of life

C. Ataxia, visual loss

D. No café au lait spots

Alport Syndrome (Also Described Earlier)

A. Autosomal dominant.

B. Progressive nephritis and sensorineural hearing loss.

C. Hematuria, proteinuria beginning the first or second decade of life.

D. Men with this disease usually die of uremia by age 30. Women are less severely affected.

E. Kidneys are affected by chronic glomerulonephritis with interstitial lymphocytic infiltrate and foam cells.

F. Progressive sensorineural hearing loss begins at age 10. Although it is not considered sex linked, hearing loss affects almost all male but not all female subjects. Histologically, degeneration of the organ of Corti and stria vascularis is observed.

G. Spherophalera cataract.

H. Hypofunction of the vestibular organ.

I. Contributes to 1% of hereditary deafness.

Alström Syndrome

A. Autosomal recessive

B. Retinal degeneration giving rise to visual loss

C. Diabetes, obesity

D. Progressive sensorineural hearing loss

Cockayne Syndrome

A. Autosomal recessive

B. Dwarfism

C. Mental retardation

D. Retinal atrophy

E. Motor disturbances

F. Progressive sensorineural hearing loss bilaterally

Congenital Cretinism (See Earlier)

Congenital cretinism must be distinguished from Pendred syndrome.

A. About 35% present with congenital hearing loss of the mixed type (irreversible).
B. Goiter (hypothyroid).
C. Mental and physical retardation.
D. Abnormal development of the petrous pyramid.
E. This disease is not inherited in a specific Mendelian manner. It is restricted to a certain geographic locale where a dietary deficiency exists.

Duane Syndrome

A. Autosomal dominant (some sex-linked recessive)
B. Inability to abduct eyes, retract globe
C. Narrowing of palpebral fissure
D. Torticollis
E. Cervical rib
F. Conductive hearing loss

Fanconi Anemia Syndrome

A. Autosomal recessive
B. Absent or deformed thumb
C. Other skeletal, heart, and kidney malformations
D. Increased skin pigmentation
E. Mental retardation
F. Pancytopenia
G. Conductive hearing loss

Fehr Corneal Dystrophy

A. Autosomal recessive
B. Progressive visual and sensorineural hearing loss

Flynn-Aird Syndrome

A. Autosomal dominant
B. Progressive myopia, cataracts, retinitis pigmentosa
C. Progressive sensorineural hearing loss
D. Ataxia
E. Shooting pains in the joints

Friedreich Ataxia

A. Autosomal recessive
B. Childhood onset of nystagmus, ataxia, optic atrophy, hyperreflexia, and sensorineural hearing loss

Goldenhar Syndrome (Also Described Earlier)

A. Autosomal recessive
B. Epibulbar dermoids
C. Preauricular appendages
D. Fusion or absence of cervical vertebrae
E. Colobomas of the eye
F. Conductive hearing loss

Hallgren Syndrome

    A. Autosomal recessive
    B. Retinitis pigmentosa
    C. Progressive ataxia
    D. Mental retardation in 25% of cases
    E. Sensorineural hearing loss
    F. Constitutes about 5% of hereditary deafness

Hermann Syndrome

    A. Autosomal dominant
    B. Onset of photomyoclonus and sensorineural hearing loss during late childhood or adolescence
    C. Diabetes mellitus
    D. Progressive dementia
    E. Pyelonephritis and glomerulonephritis

Hurler Syndrome (Gargoylism)

    A. Autosomal recessive
    B. Abnormal mucopolysaccharides are deposited in tissues (when mucopolysaccharides are deposited in the neutrophils, they are called Adler bodies); middle ear mucosa with large foamy gargoyle cells staining PAS-positive
    C. Chondroitin sulfate B and heparitin in urine
    D. Forehead prominent with coarsening of the facial features and low-set ears
    E. Mental retardation
    F. Progressive corneal opacities
    G. Hepatosplenomegaly
    H. Mixed hearing loss
    I. Dwarfism
    J. Cerebral storage of three gangliosides: GM_3, GM_2, and GM_1
    K. Beta-galactosides deficient

Hunter Syndrome

Signs are the same as for Hurler syndrome, except that they are sex linked.

Jervell and Lange-Nielsen Syndrome (Also Described Earlier)

    A. Autosomal recessive
    B. Profound bilateral sensorineural hearing loss (high frequencies more severely impaired)
    C. Associated with heart disease (prolonged QT interval on ECG) and Stokes-Adams disease
    D. Recurrent syncope
    E. Usually terminates fatally with sudden death
    F. Histopathologically, PAS-positive nodules in the cochlea

Laurence-Moon-Bardet-Biedl Syndrome

    A. Autosomal recessive
    B. Dwarfism
    C. Obesity

    D. Hypogonadism

    E. Retinitis pigmentosa

    F. Mental retardation

    G. Sensorineural hearing loss

(Recessive) Malformed Low-Set Ears and Conductive Hearing Loss

    A. Autosomal recessive

    B. Mental retardation in 50% of cases

(Dominant) Mitral Insufficiency, Joint Fusion, and Hearing Loss

    A. Autosomal dominant with variable penetrance

    B. Conductive hearing loss, usually due to fixation of the stapes

    C. Narrow external auditory canal

    D. Fusion of the cervical vertebrae and the carpal and tarsal bones

Möbius Syndrome (Congenital Facial Diplegia)

    A. Autosomal dominant, possible recessive

    B. Facial diplegia

    C. External ear deformities

    D. Ophthalmoplegia

    E. Hands or feet sometimes missing

    F. Mental retardation

    G. Paralysis of the tongue

    H. Mixed hearing loss

(Dominant) Saddle Nose, Myopia, Cataract, and Hearing Loss

    A. Autosomal dominant

    B. Saddle nose

    C. Severe myopia

    D. Juvenile cataract

    E. Sensorineural hearing loss that is progressive, moderately severe, and of early onset

Norrie Syndrome (Also Described Earlier)

    A. Autosomal recessive

    B. Congenital blindness due to pseudotumor retini

    C. Progressive sensorineural hearing loss in 30% cases

Pendred Syndrome (Also Described Earlier)

    A. Autosomal recessive.

    B. Variable amount of bilateral hearing loss secondary to atrophy of the organ of Corti. A U-shaped audiogram is often seen.

    C. Patients are euthyroid and develop diffuse goiter at the time of puberty. It is said that the metabolic defect is faulty iodination of tyrosine.

    D. Positive perchlorate test.

    E. The goiter is treated with exogenous hormone to suppress thyroid-stimulating hormone (TSH) secretion.

    F. Normal IQ.

    G. Unlike congenital cretinism, the bony petrous pyramid is well developed.

    H. Constitutes 10% of hereditary deafness.

Refsum Disease (Heredopathia Atactica Polyneuritiformis)

A. Autosomal recessive
B. Retinitis pigmentosa
C. Polyneuropathy
D. Ataxia
E. Sensorineural hearing loss
F. Visual impairment usually beginning in the second decade
G. Ichthyosis often present
H. Elevated plasma phytanic acid levels
I. Etiology: neuronal lipid storage disease and hypertrophic polyneuropathy

(Recessive) Renal, Genital, and Middle Ear Anomalies

A. Autosomal recessive
B. Renal hypoplasia
C. Internal genital malformation
D. Middle ear malformation
E. Moderate to severe conductive hearing loss

Richards-Rundel Syndrome

A. Autosomal recessive
B. Mental deficiency
C. Hypogonadism (decreased urinary estrogen, pregnanediol, and total 17-ketosteroids)
D. Ataxia
E. Horizontal nystagmus to bilateral gazes
F. Sensorineural hearing loss beginning during infancy
G. Muscle wasting during early childhood and absence of deep tendon reflexes

Taylor Syndrome

A. Autosomal recessive
B. Unilateral microtia or anotia
C. Unilateral facial bone hypoplasia
D. Conductive hearing loss

Trisomy 13 to 15 (Group D); Patau Syndrome

A. Low-set pinnae
B. Atresia of external auditory canals
C. Cleft lip and cleft palate
D. Colobomas of the eyelids
E. Micrognathia
F. Tracheoesophageal fistula
G. Hemangiomas
H. Congenital heart disease
I. Mental retardation
J. Mixed hearing loss
K. Hypertelorism
L. Incidence is 0.45:1000 live births
M. Usually die early in childhood

Trisomy 16 to 18 (Group E)

    A. Low-set pinnae
    B. External canal atresia
    C. Micrognathia, high-arched palate
    D. Peculiar finger position
    E. Prominent occiput
    F. Cardiac anomalies
    G. Hernias
    H. Pigeon breast
    I. Mixed hearing loss
    J. Incidence is 0.25:1000 to 2:1000 live births
    K. Ptosis
    L. Usually die early in life

Trisomy 21 or 22 (Down Syndrome; G Trisomy)

    A. Extra chromosome on no. 21 or no. 22
    B. Mental retardation
    C. Short stature
    D. Brachycephaly
    E. Flat occiput
    F. Slanted eyes
    G. Epicanthus
    H. Strabismus, nystagmus
    I. Seen in association with leukemia
    J. Subglottic stenosis not uncommon
    K. Decreased pneumatized or absent frontal and sphenoid sinuses
    L. Incidence is 1:600 live births

Turner Syndrome

    A. Not inherited; possibly due to intrauterine insult
    B. Low hairline
    C. Webbing of neck and digits
    D. Widely spaced nipples
    E. XO; 80% sex-chromatin negative
    F. Gonadal aplasia
    G. Incidence is 1:5000 live births (Klinefelter syndrome is XXY)
    H. Ossicular deformities
    I. Low-set ears
    J. Mixed hearing loss
    K. Large ear lobes
    L. Short stature
    M. Abnormalities in the heart and kidney
    N. Some with hyposmia

(Dominant) Urticaria, Amyloidosis, Nephritis, and Hearing Loss

    A. Autosomal dominant
    B. Recurrent urticaria
    C. Amyloidosis

D. Progressive sensorineural hearing loss due to degeneration of the organ of Corti, ossification of the basilar membrane, and cochlear nerve degeneration
E. Usually die of uremia

Usher Syndrome (Recessive Retinitis Pigmentosa With Congenital Severe Deafness) (Also Described Earlier)

A. Autosomal recessive.
B. Retinitis pigmentosa giving rise to progressive visual loss. The patient is usually completely blind by the second or third decade.
C. These patients usually are born deaf secondary to atrophy of the organ of Corti. Hearing for low frequencies is present in some patients.
D. Ataxia and vestibular dysfunction are common. Usher syndrome, among all congenital deafness syndromes, is most likely to include vestibular symptoms.
E. It constitutes 10% of hereditary deafness.
F. Usher syndrome is classified as 4 types:
   i. *Type I*: Profound congenital deafness with the onset of retinitis pigmentosa by age 10; has no vestibular response; constitutes 90% of all cases of Usher syndrome
   ii. *Type II*: Moderate to severe congenital deafness with the onset of retinitis pigmentosa in late teens or early twenties; normal or decreased vestibular response; constitutes 10% of all cases
   iii. *Type III*: Progressive hearing loss; retinitis pigmentosa begins at puberty; constitutes less than 1% of all cases (types I, II, and III are autosomal recessive)
   iv. *Type IV*: X-linked inheritance; phenotype similar to that of type II

Well Syndrome

A. Nephritis
B. Hearing loss
C. Autosomal dominant

External Ear Deformities

Middle and external congenital deformities have been classified, but this classification is less commonly used than that for inner ear development anomalies.

Class I

A. Normal auricle in shape and size
B. Well-pneumatized mastoid and middle ear
C. Ossicular abnormality
D. Most common type

Class II

A. Microtia
B. Atretic canal and abnormal ossicles
C. Normal aeration of mastoid and middle ear

Class III

A. Microtia
B. Atretic canal and abnormal ossicles

C. Middle ear and mastoid poorly aerated
   i. The external deformity does not necessarily correlate with middle ear abnormality.
   ii. Patients with a congenitally fixed footplate have the following characteristics that differentiate them from patients with otosclerosis:
      a. Onset during childhood
      b. Nonprogressive
      c. Negative family history
      d. Flat 50 to 60 dB conductive hearing loss
      e. Carhart notch not present
      f. Schwartz sign not present

Evaluation and Genetic Counseling

Obtain a detailed family history. Look for hereditary traits that may be associated with syndromic hereditary hearing impairment, such as white forelock of hair, premature graying, different colored eyes, kidney abnormalities, night blindness, severe farsightedness, childhood cardiac arrhythmias, or a sibling with sudden cardiac death.

Audiologic evaluation should be undertaken in all cases of suspected hereditary hearing impairment. For infants and younger patients, electrophysiologic tests such as the sleep deprived or sedated auditory brain stem response (ABR), stapedial reflex, and otoacoustic emission (OAE) can be done. An audiogram that is U-shaped or cookie bite should alert the clinician to hereditary hearing loss. Vestibular function tests can be helpful in the diagnosis of patients with Usher syndrome.

Depending on the history and physical findings, further evaluations, such as imaging or laboratory studies, may be indicated. All children diagnosed with hearing loss should have a urinalysis to assess for proteinuria and hematuria. Other tests should be ordered as appropriate, for example, thyroid function tests, electrocardiogram, electroretinograms, and perchlorate discharge test.

Radiographic studies should be ordered on a case-by-case basis. A CT scan can help to visualize cochlear abnormalities, internal auditory canal aberrations, and cochlear dysplasia. MRI with gadolinium enhancement is the study of choice in patients with a family history of NF type 2. MR is also used when the hearing loss is progressive but the CT scan is normal. Risk of radiation from CT scanning needs to be taken into account as well. At completion of an intensive and sometimes expensive evaluation, the specific etiology of a hearing loss still may remain uncertain.

The range of recurrence risk for future offspring cited for a family with an only child, who has an unexplained hearing loss, is 10% to 16%. Each additional normal hearing child born to such a family would decrease the probability that the disorder has a genetic etiology and thus decrease the recurrence risk. Likewise if another child is born to the same family and has a hearing impairment, then the recurrence risk increases because the possibility of a genetic component causing the hearing loss is increased.

Conclusion

Diagnosis, prognosis, and estimation of recurrence risk are components of a complete genetic evaluation of a child with suspected genetic hearing loss. Precise diagnosis with a diligent search for etiology should be undertaken. Review of clinical and laboratory data by a clinician skilled in pattern recognition can lead to identification of a syndrome or family pattern useful in predicting the likely clinical course of the disorder. An accurate diagnosis also enhances the accuracy of recurrence-risk estimates. Future studies of genetic basis of hearing loss may lead to treatment options, such as gene therapy, in order to provide auditory rehabilitation to these patients.

Bibliography

Karmody C, Schuknecht HF. Deafness in congenital deafness. *Arch Otolaryngol.* 1966;83:18.

Loundon N, Marlin S, Busquet D, et al. Usher syndrome and cochlear implantation. *Otol Neurotol.* 2003;24:216-221.

Merchant SN, McKenna MJ, Nadol JB Jr, et al. Temporal bone histopathologic and genetic studies in Mohr-Tranebjaert Syndrome (DFN-1). *Otol Neurotol.* 2001;22:506-511.

Morton NE. Genetic epidemiology of hearing impairment. *Ann NYAS.* 1991;630:16-31.

Tamari M, Itkin P. Penicillin and syphilis of the ear. *Eye Ear Nose Throat Mon.* 1951;30:252, 301, 358.

Questions

1. Which of the following is false regarding congenital hearing loss?
   A. Waardenburg syndrome is the most common AD syndromic cause of deafness.
   B. Usher syndrome is the most common AR syndromic cause of deafness.
   C. Most congenital types of hearing loss are inherited in an autosomal dominant pattern.
   D. Perchlorate discharge test may be found abnormal in patients with a Mondini deformity.
   E. Congenital syphilis can lead to hearing loss and dizziness with similar presentation as Meniere disease.

2. A 17-year-old male patient presents with sudden decrease in hearing of right ear (moderate hearing loss) after being hit in head with basketball. No loss of consciousness, or other symptoms noted. Audiogram confirms a new onset of hearing loss in right ear without prior history of hearing issues. No family history of hearing loss. Next appropriate step in order to make the most likely diagnosis is
   A. Order renal ultrasound
   B. Order MRI of internal auditory canal (IAC) to rule out retrocochlear pathology
   C. Order CT to rule out enlarged vestibular aqueduct syndrome
   D. Order Connexin 26 bloodwork
   E. Refer for genetic testing

3. What percentage of patients with NF type 1 have acoustic neuromas and what percentage of patients with NF type 2?
   A. Five percent and 95%
   B. Twenty percent and 20%
   C. Fifty percent and 50%
   D. Twenty-five percent and 100%
   E. Twenty-five percent and 5%

4. What is the basic defect that causes Alport syndrome?
   A. Abnormal renal tubules
   B. Abnormal collagen IV in glomerulus

  C. Abnormal collagen I in glomerulus

  D. Abnormal renal arteries

  E. Abnormal gap junction protein in cochlea and glomerulus

5. All of the following can be treated with hearing devices or cochlear implants except

  A. Mondini aplasia

  B. Michel aplasia

  C. Enlarged vestibular aqueduct

  D. Alexander aplasia

  E. Scheibe aplasia

Chapter 18
Tinnitus

Two categories based on whether observer can hear the tinnitus (objective) or not (subjective).

- Objective—much less common than subjective
  - (a) Vascular—typically corresponds to pulse (aka pulse synchronous tinnitus); may be venous, arterial, or combination (arteriovenous) source or secondary to high output cardiac state, tumors, other; (pulse synchronous tinnitus may be subjective also)
    - ○ Pathogenesis:
      - – Venous sources
        - ◊ Jugular bulb: High riding and large, turbulent flow, dehiscent jugular plate at level of middle ear
        - ◊ Sigmoid sinus: diverticulum, turbulent flow, dehiscent sigmoid plate
        - ◊ Other venous structures: aberrant condylar vein, superior petrosal sinus, inferior petrosal sinus; aberrant vein contacting labyrinthine structures
      - – Arterial sources
        - ◊ Carotid artery: cervical carotid dissection, aneurysm, or stenosis; aberrant carotid artery; carotid body tumor; dehiscent carotid plate within the middle ear
        - ◊ Persistent stapedial artery: derived from internal carotid artery, passes through obturator foramen of stapes superstructure
      - – Arteriovenous (AV) malformations and dural AV fistulas
        - ◊ May be associated with venous drainage leading to enlarged cortical veins (high rate of bleeding)
        - ◊ Often associated with sigmoid/transverse sinus
      - – Tumors
        - ◊ Paraganglioma, middle ear adenoma, choristoma, facial nerve neuroma, hemangioma
        - ◊ Any tumor (or encephalocele) contacting the ossicular chain or tympanic membrane (TM) may lead to pulse synchronous tinnitus (subjective or objective)
      - – High cardiac output states: anemia, thyrotoxicosis, pregnancy, beriberi, etc.
    - ○ Diagnosis: Auscultation with stethoscope, Toynbee tube, palpation of peri-auricular tissue
      - – CT angiography
      - – MRA/MRV
      - – Formal cerebral angiography (small risk of stroke)

○ Treatment: based on etiology and severity of symptoms
  – Selective embolization, surgical resection/clipping, and radiosurgery are options for dural AV fistulas and malformations.
  – Surgical excision or combination of surgery and radiosurgery may be used for tumors.
  – High output states should be medically corrected.
  – Anatomic vascular abnormalities may or may not be amenable to intervention.

(b) Nonvascular—typically presents as clicking sensation
  ○ Palatal myoclonus—rapid (50-200 beats/min) irregular clicking caused by eustachian tube opening and closing from palatal musculature contraction.
    – Symptoms often worse during times of stress.
    – Diagnosed by prolonged tympanogram showing movement with palatal contraction; may visualize palate with nasopharyngoscope as well; Toynbee tube may be used to auscultate rhythmic sound.
    – Treated with muscle relaxants or botox in refractory cases.
    – Often associated with central nervous system disease; MRI of posterior fossa should be performed to assess.
  ○ Stapedial or tensor tympani muscle spasm
    – Can be heard as clicking or crackling noise
    – Diagnosis similar to above, but without observed palatal muscle contractions
    – Treated with muscle relaxants or sectioning of tendons if refractory
  ○ Patulous eustachian tube—symptoms worsen with respiration and are often described as roaring sensation; autophony
    – Can be diagnosed by TM movement with respiration, but not always visualized. Prolonged tympanometry may be helpful also.
    – Placement of head in dependent position for relief of symptoms.
  ○ May be associated with temporomandibular joint disorders, normal swallowing that leads to TM movement (latter may be heard as single click with Toynbee tube)

• Subjective
  (a) Incidence: 10% of population
  (b) Can arise due to numerous conditions, many of which are poorly understood
  (c) Most commonly occurs secondary to hearing loss
    ○ Presbycusis, noise-induced hearing loss, acoustic neuroma, and Meniere disease are common associated problems
  (d) Most pharmacologic agents that induce tinnitus are reversible
    ○ Partial list includes aspirin, aminoglycosides, loop diuretics, caffeine, and alcohol
  (e) Characteristics:
    ○ Buzzing, clicking, humming, chirping or hissing type sounds are commonly described.
    ○ Roaring quality may be associated with Meniere disease.
    ○ Pulsatile or pulse-synchronous sounds may be described, despite not being audible to observer.
      – Encephalocele against ossicles may cause pulsatile tinnitus.
      – Idiopathic intracranial hypertension.
        ◊ Common in obese, middle-aged females
        ◊ Associated visual disturbances and headache
    ○ Sounds may be intermittent or continuous.
      – SBUTT: Sudden, brief, unilateral, tapering tinnitus; common in normal individuals

(f) Pathogenesis
  ○ Most likely occurs due to functional abnormalities of the auditory portion of the central nervous system (CNS)
  ○ Neural plasticity may cause reorganization in the auditory nuclei in response to a more peripheral event. This may then induce a hyperactive state causing tinnitus. Possible peripheral events include
    – Decreased or abnormal peripheral input (hair cell loss, etc).
    – A pathological insult may lead to decreased or abnormal spontaneous time pattern firing of auditory nerve fiber.
      ◊ This may be the cause in cases of nerve compression in acoustic neuromas and vascular loops.
  ○ Other CNS centers likely play a role in the perception of tinnitus
    – Cranial nerve centers (trigeminal) influence the auditory system
    – Amygdala, the limbic system, and other centers dealing with emotion may play a role as well
    – May explain why some individuals with normal audiograms may develop tinnitus
(g) Diagnosis
  ○ Complete history to evaluate for potential sources of trauma, ototoxicity, noise exposure, etc.
  ○ Otomicroscopy to evaluate the ear canal, tympanic membrane, and middle ear space.
    – Debris, wax, hair, foreign body, and other materials may cause tinnitus.
  ○ Standard audiometric testing should be done to evaluate hearing thresholds and word recognition scores.
  ○ Otoacoustic emission testing may be performed to document outer hair cell function.
  ○ Tinnitus matching may be performed in contralateral ear to characterize frequency and volume of tinnitus.
    – No correlation between tinnitus characteristics and patient aggravation level
    – Approximately 50% of patients studied have tinnitus amplitude of 5 dB
  ○ If vascular etiology is considered, workup as above.
(h) Treatment
  ○ Avoidance of noise/medication/other source of potential injury.
  ○ Counseling patients plays a major role in tinnitus treatment.
    – Patients should be screened for anxiety and depression as these often exacerbate tinnitus symptoms.
    – All medications should be reviewed.
    – Dietary triggers such as high salt diet, alcohol intake, and caffeine should be discussed.
  ○ Over time, approximately 25% of patients have near symptom resolution, 50% report significant improvement, and 25% remain stable.
  ○ Bedside masking (whether actual masking device versus fan or radio between stations) should be used in those bothered by bedtime symptoms.
  ○ Hearing aid—first line of treatment in patients with associated hearing loss.
    – Return of previously lost sounds may mask tinnitus.
    – If tinnitus refractory, can use masking device (or tinnitus instrument) in hearing aids.
      ◊ Creates sound stimulus in hopes of masking tinnitus
      ◊ Can also be used independent of hearing aids

- – Use of masking device in hearing aid increases likelihood of tinnitus control from 25% to 55%.
  - ○ Tinnitus retraining therapy—combination of counseling and broadband sound exposure habituate patient to tinnitus.
    - – Patients are exposed to 16 hours of broad-band noise per day.
    - – Noise is initially presented low but slowly increased to a level where the tinnitus is just still audible to the patient.
    - – Ideally over a year a patient will either no longer hear tinnitus or be undisturbed by it.
  - ○ Biofeedback therapy—requires patient cooperation in undergoing therapy with psychologist.
    - – Uses various triggers such as increased temperature or pulse for patient to recognize increased focus on tinnitus. Using these triggers patients can learn to focus attention away from tinnitus.
    - – Significant overlap with stress reduction.
  - ○ Neuromodulators—special auditory devices that deliver a combination of tones, music and other sounds, based on a patient's unique tinnitus characteristics, in an effort to effect change in auditory neural pathways
  - ○ Transcranial magnetic stimulation—repetitive treatments, designed to alter perception of tinnitus; still investigational with little supportive data in terms of efficacy
  - ○ Cochlear implant placement—unilateral placement is being offered in some centers for disabling tinnitus; in conjunction with single-sided deafness, may represent emerging treatment option; still investigational with limited data
  - ○ Medication
    - – Treatment of underlying anxiety and depression can help patients contend with tinnitus
    - – Various supplements, such as melatonin, lipoflavinoids, niacin, among others, have been suggested for tinnitus treatment
    - – Psychotropic medications, including low dose anti-depressants, anti-anxiety medications, SSRIs, and benzodiazepines have also been used for tinnitus treatment

Bibliography

Galazyuk AV, Wenstrup JJ, Hamid MA. Tinnitus and underlying brain mechanisms. *Curr Opin Otolaryngol Head Neck Surg.* 2012;20(5):409-415.

Moller A. Tinnitus. In: Jackler R, Brackmann D, eds. *Neurotology.* 2nd ed. Philadelphia, PA: Elsevier Mosby; 2005:182-193.

Sismanis A. Pulsatile tinnitus: contemporary assessment and management. *Curr Opin Otolaryngol Head Neck Surg.* 2011;19(5):348-357.

Snapp HA, Schubert MC. Habilitation of auditory and vestibular dysfunction. *Otolaryngol Clin North Am.* 2012;45(2):487-511.

Questions

1. Which of the following is true with regard to tinnitus matching?
   A. Tinnitus frequency is correlated with patients' aggravation with symptoms.
   B. Tinnitus intensity is correlated with patients' aggravation with symptoms.

C. Tinnitus frequency is correlated with likelihood of resolution.

D. Tinnitus intensity is correlated with likelihood of resolution.

E. None of the above.

2. What percentage of patients with tinnitus notice symptom improvement over time?

A. 75%

B. 50%

C. 25%

D. <1%

3. Which of the following best describes tinnitus retraining therapy?

A. Continuous sound stimulus to eliminate perception of tinnitus

B. Use of an amplification device to amplify previous hearing loss frequencies

C. Broadband sound exposure for portions of the day to habituate patient to tinnitus

D. Use of various physiological triggers to help focus attention away from tinnitus

4. Which of the following is NOT a potential cause of objective pulsatile tinnitus?

A. Dural AV fistula

B. Idiopathic intracranial hypertension

C. Carotid dissection

D. Persistent stapedial artery

5. What is the primary treatment for stapedius muscle spasm?

A. Surgical sectioning

B. Beta-blockers

C. Botox

D. Muscle relaxants

Chapter 19
Hearing Rehabilitation: Surgical and Nonsurgical

Part 1: Hearing Amplification

Hearing Aid Basics

Components of a Hearing Aid

- **Microphone** picks up sound and converts it into electrical signals.
- **Amplifier/signal processor** is the heart of a digital hearing aid. A variety of digital signal processing (DSP) techniques can be used to process sound, identify and selectively amplify speech, and recognize and suppress ambient noise, etc.
- **Receiver** converts the processed electrical signals back to acoustic energy and delivers it to the ear, acting as a loudspeaker.
- **Power source** is usually a zinc-air battery.

Hearing aid components are housed in a custom-made acrylic shell. Hearing aids can be analog, digital, or hybrid (analog-digital combinations). Analog and hybrid models are obsolete. Nearly all hearing aids dispensed today are purely digital.

Electroacoustic Properties of Hearing Aids

- Hearing aid is characterized by three parameters: frequency response, gain, and OSPL-90.
- Frequency response of a typical hearing aid extends up to 3 to 4 kHz; however, some hearing aids have an extended high-frequency response.
- Gain is the ratio of output power to input power. Gain depends on the input frequency and input intensity.
- OSPL-90 (SSPL-90)—output or saturated sound pressure level. Describes how much sound energy is generated by the hearing aid when the input level is high at 90 dB.
- Linear processing—hearing aid amplified by the same factor regardless of the input level. This technique is now obsolete.
- Nonlinear processing (compression)—hearing aid amplifies softer sounds more and louder sounds less. This method is utilized in digital hearing aids and allows for more comfortable listening in ears with sensorineural hearing loss with much recruitment (narrowed dynamic range).
- Directional microphones enhance the signal-to-noise ratio and allow better understanding of speech in noisy environments. Many hearing aids allow the user to switch between directional and omnidirectional microphones.
- Some digital hearing aids use DSP techniques to recognize different listening environments and optimize their performance in real time. These devices can suppress feedback and amplify speech selectively while suppressing ambient noise.

- Two major parameters predict patients' success with hearing aids. These are *word recognition scores* and *dynamic range*. Patients with word recognition scores of at least 50% and a wide dynamic range are usually successful hearing aid users.
- Dynamic range is the difference between the uncomfortable loudness level (UCL) and the speech reception threshold (SRT).
- Dynamic range = UCL − SRT.
- MCL (most comfortable level) approximately bisects the dynamic range.
- The narrower the dynamic range of an ear, the more difficult to fit a comfortable hearing aid.

Styles of Hearing Aids

- The four basic styles of hearing aids are
  - (a) **BTE** (behind the ear)
  - (b) **ITE** (in the ear)
  - (c) **ITC** (in the canal)
  - (d) **CIC** (completely in the canal)
- Several variations of these basic styles are offered by various manufacturers, such as mini-BTE, invisible in the canal (IIT), half-shell (HS; a smaller version of the ITE), and others.
- Each of these styles incorporates some degree of venting. Large venting makes a hearing aid more comfortable by eliminating the occlusion effect and enhancing hearing in noise. Occlusion effect results from reverberation of low frequencies in a closed ear canal. Large venting allows low frequencies to escape the ear canal. Large venting unfortunately is contraindicated in ears with significant low-frequency hearing loss. (Table 19-1).
- Open-fit hearing aid is essentially a BTE style aid with a modified earmold that is open, soft, and not custom fitted and eliminates the occlusion effect, making it a comfortable first choice for new hearing aid wearers. Because of the large venting, it is not suitable for patients with significant low-frequency hearing loss.
- RITE (receiver in the ear) is a BTE style aid with the receiver (speaker) positioned through the acoustic tube into the ear canal. This design takes advantage of the general principle that sound is perceived as more natural if delivered closer to the tympanic membrane. This feature is common today and can be recognized by the narrow acoustic tube with a wire inside.
- Extended-wear hearing aids. These CIC style hearing aids are placed in the ear canal by an audiologist and worn continuously for a few months. When the battery needs to be replaced, the device is removed and replaced by the audiologist.

Implantable Hearing Devices

- Implantable hearing systems have been used primarily for rehabilitation of sensorineural hearing loss, but also for conductive and mixed hearing loss. These systems can be partially or fully implantable. Two technologies are currently available: electromagnetic and piezoelectric.
- In **electromagnetic** implantable hearing devices, a floating mass transducer is attached surgically to the ossicular chain, usually incus. Examples are the partially implantable Vibrant Soundbridge (Med-El, GmbH, Innsbruck, Austria) FDA approved in 2000, and the partially implantable MAXUM (offered by Ototronix, Inc, Houston, TX) FDA approved in 2009.
- In **piezoelectric** implantable hearing devices, a driver is implanted to mechanically vibrate the ossicular chain. A piezoelectric crystal changes shape (bends) in response

to a changing electric field. A driver containing a piezoelectric crystal can convert electrical signals into mechanical vibrations of the ossicular chain. Example is the fully implantable Esteem (Envoy Medical Corp, St Paul, MN), which requires partial removal of the incus and was FDA approved in 2010.

- Most patients perceive a benefit in sound fidelity of implantable hearing devices over conventional hearing aids. Occlusion effect is eliminated and feedback problems are significantly reduced. Hearing while bathing, swimming or sleeping carries a clear advantage.
- Disadvantages of implantable hearing systems are the complexity of the surgical procedure for device placement, high cost, lack of insurance coverage, need for surgical battery replacement, and limited magnetic resonance imaging (MRI) compatibility. Some systems require an iatrogenic ossicular discontinuity to reduce feedback problems.
- The *osseointegrated bone conduction hearing device* (Ponto by Oticon Inc, Somerset, NJ, and Baha by Cochlear Corp, Sydney, Australia) is indicated for rehabilitation of mixed and conductive hearing loss. It can also be used for unilateral deafness which is discussed separately. The titanium implant/abutment complex is surgically placed in the bone behind the affected ear, near the temporal line, and is allowed to osseointegrate for 6 weeks to 3 months. The abutment protrudes through an opening in the skin. The processor is then attached to the abutment. The system collects sound as a hearing aid, processes the sound electronically, and delivers it to the cochlea via the **bone conduction** mechanism (Figure 19-1). The advantage of this system over conventional hearing aids is that any conductive hearing loss component is effectively bypassed while amplification is provided only for the sensorineural component. The greater the conductive component of hearing loss, the greater the advantage of this bone conduction system over conventional hearing aids. A bone conduction system is a good hearing rehabilitation method for mixed hearing losses with a significant conductive component, for ears with mastoid cavities which may be draining, and for ears with conductive losses which are not amenable to surgical correction (ie, congenital atresia with severe ossicular malformations).

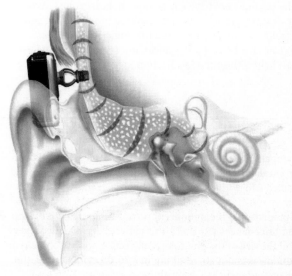

Figure 19-1 This osseointegrated system (Baha) delivers sound to the cochlea via the bone conduction mechanism. *(Used with permission of Cochlear™ Americas, © 2012 Cochlear Americas.)*

- Baha Attract (Cochlear Corp, Sydney, Australia) is a magnetic bone conduction system, with the same indications as a direct connect osseointegrated system that FDA approved in 2013. The internal portion consists of a titanium osseointegrated implant and magnet, all placed under an intact skin flap. The external processor has a magnet as well, attaching to the internal components similar to a cochlear implant. The internal magnet is MRI safe up to 1.5 tesla.

Options for Single-Sided Deafness

- In patients with unilateral hearing loss, which is not aidable by conventional hearing aids because of the severity of hearing loss and poor word recognition, several hearing rehabilitation options still exist. These strategies depend on various mechanisms to transfer acoustic energy from the deaf ear to the contralateral healthy cochlea where sound is perceived.
- *CROS (contralateral routing of signal)*: A microphone is worn on the deaf ear. Sound information is transferred to the receiver worn on the normal ear, historically through a wire behind the neck or more recently via radio waves. A system with some additional amplification delivered to the better hearing ear is termed Bi-CROS. Although effective, the disadvantage of CROS and Bi-CROS systems is that devices have to be worn in both ears.
- *t-CROS (transcranial contralateral routing of signal)*: This BTE style device is worn solely on the deaf ear. Sound is processed in the usual manner and delivered to the bony portion of the external auditory canal through a long earmold. From that point, sound energy is delivered through bone conduction to the contralateral healthy cochlea. Smaller ear canals are difficult to fit and a long earmold is sometimes uncomfortable.
- *SoundBite* (Sonitus Medical, Inc, San Mateo, CA) is a bone conduction hearing rehabilitation system for single-sided deafness. It consists of a BTE microphone unit worn on the deaf ear and a removable dental-worn appliance. The dental appliance picks up sound signals from the BTE microphone and through a small actuator, converts sound signals into vibrations which are heard in the contralateral healthy cochlea.
- *Osseointegrated bone conduction hearing device* (Baha or Ponto) is indicated for rehabilitation of single-sided deafness when the pure tone average in the better ear is 20-dB HL or better. The only-hearing ear must not have any significant hearing loss. Acoustic signals are collected from the deaf side, processed, and delivered through bone conduction to the contralateral healthy cochlea. When used for single-sided deafness, this bone conduction device eliminates the head shadow effect, improves speech understanding in noise, but does not help with sound localization.

Part 2: Ossiculoplasty

Mechanics of the Ossicular Chain

- The middle ear structures (tympanic membrane, ossicular chain, oval and round windows) collectively provide an **impedance matching** mechanism between the air-filled external canal and the fluid-filled labyrinth, ensuring that acoustic energy is not attenuated as it enters the inner ear.
- The *ideal transformer model* predicts that the middle ear provides about 28 dB of gain, which offsets the losses due to impedance mismatch. This gain results from two lever mechanisms. First, the ratio of the size of the physiologically active portion of the tympanic membrane and oval window is about 20, resulting in a 26-dB gain. Second, the ratio of the length of the malleus and incus is 1.3, resulting in a modest 2-dB gain.

- Actual experimental measurements of middle ear pressure gains average only about 23 dB. Middle ear gain is frequency dependent and peaks around 1 kHz.
- Ideal middle ear prosthesis is lightweight; made of a biocompatible material; easy to trim, handle, and adjust; stable in the middle ear; and MRI compatible.
- Common ossicular prosthesis materials are: plastipore, hydroxyapatite, HAPEX (hydroxyapatite with polyethylene), and titanium.

Malleus-Incus Defect

- A prosthesis designed to replace the malleus-incus complex is termed *partial ossicular reconstruction prosthesis* (PORP). This prosthesis spans the distance between the stapes superstructure and the tympanic membrane.
- To reduce the chance of prosthesis extrusion, many surgeons recommend placement of a layer of cartilage between the prosthesis and the tympanic membrane. The tragus is a common source of cartilage for ossicular reconstruction. Some argue that such cartilage interposition is not necessary if the prosthesis head is made of hydroxyapatite.
- Generally good hearing results are obtained with partial prostheses with most studies reporting at least two-thirds of patients reaching air–bone gaps of 20 dB or less.

Total Ossicular Defect

- A prosthesis designed to replace the entire ossicular chain is termed *total ossicular reconstruction prosthesis* (TORP). This prosthesis spans the entire middle ear cleft between the stapes footplate and the tympanic membrane (Figure 19-2).
- A thin layer of cartilage is often placed between the prosthesis head and the tympanic membrane to reduce the chance of extrusion.
- A *footplate shoe* is often used to stabilize the total prosthesis on the stapes footplate. The shoe can be built-in or added by the surgeon prior to the implantation.
- Generally good hearing results are obtained with total ossicular prostheses, with most studies reporting at least half of patients reaching a postoperative air–bone gap of 20 dB or less.

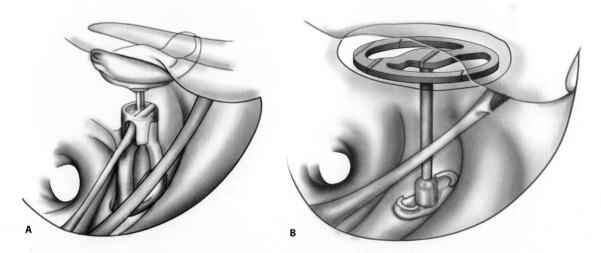

Figure 19-2 A. Partial prosthesis placed over the stapes capitulum. B. Total prosthesis placed on the footplate. (*Used with permission of Grace Medical, Inc.*)

Incus Defect

- Incus defect can be reconstructed using native incus interposition or a synthetic prosthesis. A variety of prostheses are available to span the gap between the malleus and stapes (Figure 19-3).
- The most common native ossicle reconstruction technique is *incus interposition*, generally used in cases involving discontinuity at the incudostapedial joint. The native incus is removed, turned, and replaced to reestablish continuity between the malleus and stapes. Incus can be sculpted as desired before repositioning. Generally good hearing results are obtained in experienced hands, with 66% of ears brought to within 20 dB of the bone conduction line, with hearing results remaining stable over time.

Stapes Defect

- When the stapes become fixed due to otosclerosis, it can be replaced with a prosthesis to restore mobility to the ossicular chain.
- Stapedectomy—removal of stapes superstructure and all or most of the stapes footplate.
- Stapedotomy—removal of stapes superstructure and fenestration of the footplate to accommodate the prosthesis.
- *Indications for stapedectomy*: (A) conductive hearing loss with an air-bone gap of at least 25 to 30 dB, sufficient to produce a negative Rinne test with the 512-Hz tuning fork; (B) normal otoscopic examination; and (C) acoustic reflex either biphasic or absent.
- Stapedectomy is performed on the worse-hearing ear. If hearing is similar in both ears, the patient is asked to identify which ear is better and again, stapedectomy is performed on the worse-hearing ear as identified by the patient.

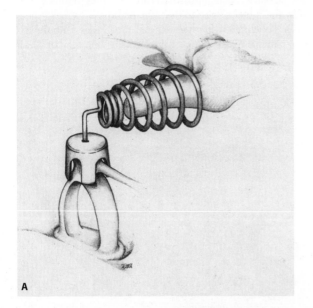
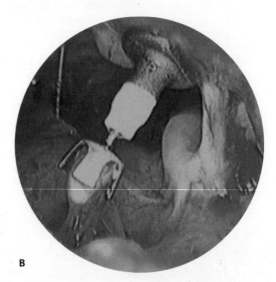

A

B

Figure 19-3 Examples of incus replacement prostheses: **A.** K-Helix reestablishes continuity between the eroded incus and healthy stapes. **B.** Wedge incus strut replaces the entire incus. *(Used with permission of Grace Medical, Inc.)*

Special Situations

- Patients with osteogenesis imperfecta have brittle bones. While stapedectomy can improve hearing, care must be taken not to fracture the tympanic ring while curetting the scutum or fracture the incus while crimping the prosthesis.
- In rare patients with otosclerosis and Ménière disease, there is endolymphatic hydrops and increased risk that the saccule may be punctured as stapedectomy is performed, resulting in a degree of sensorineural hearing loss or a completely deaf ear. A hearing aid or osseointegrated bone conduction system should be considered.
- A blind patient may have more trouble compensating for minor vestibular complications that can occur with stapedectomy. Similarly, a patient with contralateral peripheral vestibulopathy may not tolerate even minor vestibular complications. A hearing aid should be considered. If peripheral vestibulopathy is suspected, caloric testing is indicated before considering stapedotomy.
- Patient with a mixed hearing loss should be counseled that hearing aids will likely be necessary even if the stapedectomy is successful in closing the air-bone gap.
- **Stapedectomy surgical steps** generally include: elevation of the tympanomeatal flap, curetting the scutum for exposure, testing mobility of ossicles, dividing the stapedius tendon, separating the incudostapedial joint, removing the stapes superstructure, removing or fenestrating the footplate, placing an oval window covering, placing and securing the prosthesis, testing prosthesis mobility, and replacing the tympanic membrane to its normal anatomic position. Order of steps varies among surgeons.

Stapedectomy Intraoperative Complications

- If a tympanic membrane perforation occurs, it is repaired with an underlay fascia graft.
- A markedly thickened footplate can complicate the surgery, but can be drilled out and a prosthesis safely placed. A floating footplate can occur during efforts to remove it and can make the task near impossible. Options include fenestrating the floating footplate using a laser, or aborting the procedure, allowing the footplate to refixate, and then attempting the surgery again at a later date.
- The tympanic segment of the facial nerve is examined before stapes surgery as it courses superior to the oval window. Mild dehiscence and overhang of the facial nerve can be managed by bending the prosthesis wire. If severe facial nerve overhang is encountered, it is prudent to abort the procedure and recommend a hearing aid.
- Rarely a persistent stapedial artery is seen coursing between the stapes crura. Surgery may proceed only if this artery appears vestigial, otherwise surgery is aborted.

Stapedectomy Delayed Complications

- Persistent conductive hearing loss may be due to unrecognized malleus or incus ankylosis in the epitympanum, incus subluxation, prosthesis that is too short, inadequately crimped prosthesis, or rarely superior canal dehiscence syndrome.
- Recurrent conductive hearing loss can occur due to necrosis and shortening of the long process of incus, displaced prosthesis, or reparative granuloma (1-2 weeks after surgery).
- Vertigo is sometimes seen for a few days after stapedectomy. This may be due to perilymph loss from suctioning. If vertigo persists, the ear may be reexplored. A perilymph fistula or an excessively long prosthesis may be the cause.
- Sensorineural hearing loss can occur after stapedectomy. Historically, incidence is about 1% to 2% after primary stapedectomy and higher after revisions. Temporary threshold shifts can occur after stapes surgery as well.

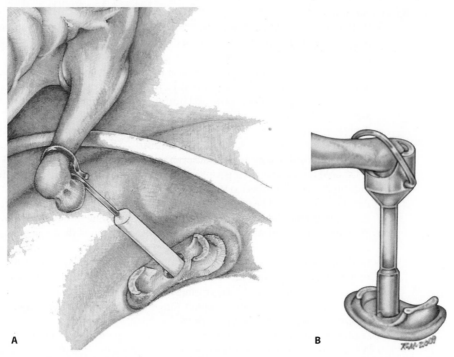

Figure 19-4 Designs of stapes prostheses: **A.** Piston-style. **B.** bucket handle. *(Used with permission of Grace Medical, Inc.)*

- Serous labyrinthitis is thought to occur during the healing process after stapedectomy. Sensorineural hearing loss above 2 kHz and mild dysequilibrium may occur. This type of postop labyrinthitis usually resolves within a few days without permanent sequelae.
- Stapes prosthesis designs are either *piston style* or *bucket handle* (Figure 19-4). The bucket handle is simply flipped over the distal incus for stability, and the piston prosthesis has to be mechanically crimped to the incus. Stapes pistons made of nitinol can be crimped using a specialized heating tool or a laser.
- Large series show comparable hearing results with stapedectomy and stapedotomy, with results stable over time. Air-bone gap closure within 10 dB is expected in the majority of primary stapedectomies, and closure within 20 dB in nearly all cases.

Ossicular Chain Reconstruction in a Modified Mastoid Cavity
- Same principles are generally applied to ossicular reconstruction in a modified mastoid cavity.
- Middle ear volume in a mastoid cavity is smaller and the middle ear cleft is shallower, making ossicular reconstruction more challenging.
- Ossicular chain reconstruction in a mastoid cavity can be done at the time of creation of the cavity or it can be staged, depending on the extent of disease and surgeon preference.
- There is a variety of shorter prostheses available to span the distance between the stapes and tympanic membrane (ie, Goldenberg cap), or if stapes suprastructure is absent, between the footplate and the tympanic membrane.

Bibliography

House HP, Hansen MR, Al Dakhail AA, House JW. Stapedectomy versus stapedotomy: comparison of results with long-term follow-up. *Laryngoscope*. 2002;112(11):2046-2050.

Luetje CM, Brackman D, Balkany TJ, et al. Phase III clinical trial results with the Vibrant Soundbridge implantable middle ear hearing device: a prospective controlled multicenter study. *Otolaryngol Head Neck Surg*. 2002;126(2):97-107.

Slater PW, Rizer FM, Schuring AG, Lippy WH. Practical use of total and partial ossicular replacement prostheses in ossiculoplasty. *Laryngoscope*. 1997;107(9):1193-1198.

Truy E, Naiman AN, Pavillon C, Abedipour D, Lina-Granade G, Rabilloud M. Hydroxyapatite versus titanium ossiculoplasty. *Otol Neurotol*. 2007;28(4):492-498.

Yuen HW, Bodmer D, Smilsky K, Nedzelski JM, Chen JM. Management of single-sided deafness with the bone-anchored hearing aid. *Otolaryngol Head Neck Surg*. 2009;141(1):16-23. Epub 2009 May 5.

Questions

1. Which of the following parameters best predict successful use of hearing aids?
   A. MCL and word recognition scores
   B. MCL and UCL
   C. SRT and UCL
   D. Word recognition scores and dynamic range
   E. SRT and MCL

2. Which of the following can be used for rehabilitation of single-sided deafness? Choose all that apply.
   A. Conventional hearing aid
   B. CROS
   C. Bi-CROS
   D. Osseointegrated bone conduction system (Ponto, Baha)
   E. Piezoelectric implantable hearing device

3. All of the following are advantages of behind-the-ear (BTE) style hearing aids compared to other styles, except
   A. It can accommodate directional microphones.
   B. It can allow larger venting and accommodates a wide range of hearing losses.
   C. It is easy to manipulate controls and easy to incorporate switches and volume control.
   D. It is preferred in children because only the earmold has to be replaced as the child grows.
   E. It is invisible.

4. All of the following statements regarding hearing amplification are true, except
   A. OSPL-90 measures the output of a hearing aid when the input is low at a mere 10 dB.
   B. The larger the dynamic range of an ear, the easier it is to fit a comfortable hearing aid.
   C. Large venting improves hearing in noise but is contraindicated in ears with significant low-frequency hearing loss.

    D. Methods for rehabilitation of single-sided deafness depend on transferring sound energy from the deaf ear to the contralateral healthy cochlea.

    E. Patients with implantable hearing devices generally report increased sound fidelity (compared to their conventional hearing aids), reduced feedback problems, and no occlusion effect.

5. The following statements regarding ossiculoplasty are true, except

    A. Postoperative hearing results are generally better with partial prostheses (PORP) than with total prostheses (TORP)

    B. The middle ear provides an impedance matching mechanism between the air-filled external canal and the fluid-filled labyrinth.

    C. The middle ear cleft in a modified mastoid cavity is deeper and has a larger volume than in a normal ear.

    D. Footplate shoe can be used to stabilize the total prosthesis on the stapes footplate.

    E. In stapedectomy, closure of the air-bone gap within 10 dB can be expected in a majority of cases, without significant widening of the air-bone gap over time.

Chapter 20
Cochlear Implants

Cochlear Implant System

A. Electronic devices which provide hearing to patients with severe to profound hearing loss.
B. Replace nonfunctional inner ear hair cell transducer system by converting mechanical sound energy into electrical signals.
C. Stimulate cochlear ganglion cells and cochlear nerve in deaf patients.
D. Damaged or missing hair cells of cochlea are bypassed and signal is delivered to brain.

Multichannel, Multielectrode Cochlear Implant Systems
A. Take advantage of tonotopic (place) organization of cochlea.
B. Different electrical signals sent to different sites in the cochlea (high pitches heard at cochlear base and low pitches at apex).
C. Incoming speech signals filtered into frequency bands which correspond to a given electrode in the array (spectral information transferred).
D. Temporal coding (timing) of information limited to frequencies below 500 Hz.
E. Amplitude (loudness) coded by altering the intensity cues of speech.
F. Stimuli may be presented simultaneously or sequentially.

Processed Speech Signal
A. Amplified and compressed to match narrow electrical dynamic range of ear (typical response range of deaf ear to electrical stimulation is on the order of only 10-20 dB, even less in high frequencies).
B. Transmission of electrical signal across the skin from the external unit to the implanted electrode array accomplished with electromagnetic induction or radio frequency transmission.
C. Spiral ganglion cells or axons appear to be the critical residual neural elements that are stimulated.

Components of Cochlear Implant
A. Microphone picks up acoustic information.
B. Processor produces stimuli for electrode array.
C. Transmission link.
D. *Electrode array*: current emphasis on small, soft, flexible arrays of varying lengths to protect cochlear structures.

Patient Selection

Medical Assessment

    A. Otologic history and physical examination (precise etiology of deafness cannot always be determined but is identified whenever possible).

    B. Stimulable auditory neural elements nearly always present regardless of cause. Three exceptions: (i) *Michel deformity*, congenital agenesis of the cochlea; (ii) narrow *internal auditory canal syndrome*, cochlear nerve may be congenitally absent; and (iii) neurofibromatosis type 2, bilateral vestibular schwannomas.

Radiologic Evaluation

    A. Determines whether cochlea is present and patent.

    B. High resolution, thin-section computed tomography (CT) of the cochlea identifies congenital deformities of the cochlea. Congenital malformations of cochlea not contraindications to cochlear implantation. Cochlear dysplasia occurs in approximately 20% of children with congenital sensorineural hearing loss.

    C. Intracochlear bone formation resulting from labyrinthitis ossificans usually can be demonstrated by CT; however, when soft tissue obliteration occurs after sclerosing labyrinthitis, CT may not detect the obstruction. In these cases, T_2-weighted magnetic resonance imaging (MRI) is an effective adjunctive procedure providing additional information regarding cochlear patency. The endolymph/perilymph signal may be lost in sclerosing labyrinthitis. Intracochlear ossification is not a contraindication to cochlear implantation but can limit the type and insertion depth of the electrode array that can be introduced into the cochlea.

    D. Anomalous facial nerve may be associated with temporal bone dysplasia which may increase the surgical risk.

    E. MRI may determine the status (or absence) of the cochlear nerve.

    F. A thin cribriform area between the modiolus and a widened internal auditory canal is often observed and is thought to be the route of egress of cerebrospinal fluid (CSF) during surgery or postoperatively.

Otoscopic Evaluation of Tympanic Membrane

    A. Otologic condition should be stable before implantation (free of infection or cholesteatoma).

    B. Tympanic membrane should be intact.

    C. Middle ear effusions in children under consideration for cochlear implantation or who already have a cochlear implant deserves special consideration. Conventional antibiotic treatment usually accomplishes this goal, but when it does not, myringotomy and insertion of tympanostomy tubes may be required. Removal of the tube several weeks before cochlear implantation usually results in a healed, intact tympanic membrane. When an effusion occurs in an ear with a cochlear implant, no treatment is required as long as the effusion remains uninfected.

    D. Chronic otitis media, with or without cholesteatoma, must be resolved before implantation. This is accomplished with conventional otologic treatments. Prior ear surgery that has resulted in a mastoid cavity does not contraindicate cochlear implantation, but this situation may require mastoid obliteration with closure of the external auditory canal or reconstruction of the posterior bony ear canal.

Audiologic Assessment

A. Primary means of determining suitability for cochlear implantation.
B. The first patients to undergo implantation were postlingually deafened adults with no hearing and who received no benefit from conventional amplification. Many or all aspects of spoken language had developed before the onset of their deafness. There was no likelihood that their hearing could worsen with cochlear implantation. Knowledge gained from these patients and with improved technology, candidacy criteria have broadened to include prelingually deafened children and patients with some minimal residual hearing.
C. Patients who become deaf at or after age 5 are classified as postlingually deafened.
D. Once access to auditory input and feedback is lost, rapid deterioration of speech intelligibility often occurs. Implantation soon after the onset of deafness potentially can ameliorate this rapid deterioration.
E. Cochlear implantation may be less successful in postlingually deafened patients if there is a long delay between the onset of deafness and implantation.
F. A postlingual onset of deafness is an infrequent occurrence in the pediatric population.

Current Selection Criteria

A. Aided speech recognition scores are the primary determinants for adults and older children.
B. For very young children and those with limited language abilities, parent questionnaires are used to determine hearing aid benefit.

Adults

A. Pure tone average greater than 70 dB
B. Aided HINT (hearing in noise test) sentences less than 60%

Children

A. 12 months of age
B. Bilateral profound hearing loss for 12 to 18 month olds, severe to profound for the older than 18 months; LNT (lexical neighborhood test) less than 40%
C. Little to no benefit from hearing aids (trial period waived for postmeningitis children with radiographic evidence of ossification)
D. No medical contraindications
E. Educational program that emphasizes auditory development
F. Appropriate family support and expectations

Implantation of Congenitally or Early Deafened Adolescents

A. Electrical stimulation of the auditory system has not led to high levels of success.
B. Adolescents with profound hearing loss with a history of consistent hearing aid use who communicate through audition and spoken language are among the best candidates in this age group.
C. Conversely, adolescents with little previous auditory experience and those who rely primarily on sign language for communication may have difficulty learning to use the sound provided by an implant and may find it disruptive. Such adolescents are at high risk for nonuse of a cochlear implant.
D. With both groups, implantation can be successful if time is spent counseling about potential outcomes.

Implantation of Young Children and Infants

A. Currently, most children who receive cochlear implants have congenital or prelingually acquired hearing loss. They must use the sound provided by a cochlear implant to acquire speech perception, speech production, and spoken language skills.

B. With the advent of Universal Newborn Hearing Screening, infants with profound hearing loss are being identified and fitted with hearing aids. Current FDA guidelines permit the implantation of children as young as 12 months. However, a lower age limit even younger than 12 months is being explored and may ultimately prove to be advantageous.

C. There is mounting evidence that the age at which a child receives a cochlear implant is one of the most important predictors of speech and language outcomes.

D. Early implantation may also be important when the cause of deafness is meningitis as progressive intracochlear ossification can occur and preclude standard electrode insertion. The window of time during which this advancing process can be circumvented is short. Thus, infants with deafness secondary to meningitis may undergo implantation before the age of 1 year if they have completed a brief hearing aid trial with no evident benefit.

Psychological Assessment

A. Performed for exclusionary reasons to identify subjects who have organic brain dysfunction, mental retardation, undetected psychosis, or unrealistic expectations.

B. Valuable information related to the family dynamics and other factors in the patient's milieu that may affect implant acceptance and performance are assessed.

Surgical Technique

A. Cochlear implantation performed under general endotracheal anesthesia with continuous facial nerve monitoring.

B. Skin incision designed to provide access to the mastoid process and coverage of the external portion of the implant package while preserving the blood supply of the postauricular skin.

C. With the introduction of infants into the patient population, modifications to the standard surgical approach have been made and generalized to our entire implant subject group.

D. The retroauricular skin incision has been reduced to a 4 to 5 cm extending from the mastoid tip posterosuperiorly. A subperiosteal pocket above the level of the linea temporalis is created for positioning the implant induction coil.

E. A shallow bone is well developed extending only through the outer cortex with no dural exposure.

F. The previously used tie-down sutures have been eliminated.

G. A groove is drilled for the electrodes.

H. A mastoidectomy is performed maintaining a cortical bone overhang to protect the electrode.

I. The horizontal semicircular canal is identified in the depths of the mastoid antrum, and the short process of the incus is identified in the fossa incudis.

J. The facial recess is opened using the fossa incudis as an initial landmark. The facial recess is a triangular area bound by (1) the fossa incudis superiorly, (2) the chorda tympani nerve laterally and anteriorly, and (3) the facial nerve medially and posteriorly. The facial nerve usually can be visualized through the bone without exposing it.

K. The round window niche is visualized through the facial recess about 2 mm inferior to the stapes. Occasionally, the round window niche is posteriorly positioned and is not well visualized through the facial recess or is obscured by ossification. In these situations, it is important not to be misdirected by hypotympanic air cells.

L. Entry into the scala tympani is accomplished through a cochleostomy created anterior and inferior to the annulus of the round window membrane. A small fenestra slightly larger than the electrode to be implanted (usually 0.5 mm) is developed. A small diamond burr is used to "blue line" the endosteum of the scala tympani, and the endosteal membrane is removed with small picks. This approach bypasses the hook area of the scala tympani, allowing direct insertion of the active electrode array. After insertion of the active electrode array, the cochleostomy area is sealed with small pieces of fascia. Alternatively, when visualization permits, the electrode may be positioned directly through the round window.

M. At the completion of the implantation, bone pate which was collected during the mastoidectomy is packed along the lower margin of the implant package in the subperiosteal pocket.

Complications

Complications infrequent with cochlear implant surgery and largely avoided by careful preoperative planning and meticulous surgical technique.

A. Postauricular flap breakdown
   i. Most common problem encountered in the past
   ii. Eliminated by the current incision

B. Facial nerve injury
   i. In patients with malformations of the labyrinth (occasionally in patients with normal anatomy), the facial nerve may follow an aberrant course.
   ii. Care must be taken in opening the facial recess and in making the cochleostomy. Steroids will treat nerve swelling.

C. Cerebrospinal fluid leak
   i. Eliminated by drilling shallow well for implant package not exposing dura and eliminating control holes for tie-down sutures.
   ii. CSF gushers have occurred in children with a Mondini deformity and major inner ear malformations as well in several patients with the large vestibular aqueduct syndrome.
   iii. The flow of CSF has been successfully controlled by entry into the cochlea through a small fenestra, allowing the CSF reservoir to drain off, insertion of the electrode into the cochleostomy, and tight packing of the electrode with fascia at the cochleostomy site.
   iv. It is postulated that the source of the leak is through the lateral end of the internal auditory canal.
   v. In addition, the eustachian tube is occluded with tissue and fibrin glue is placed in the middle ear. Supplementally, a lumbar drain can be placed to reduce the spinal fluid reservoir until tissue is satisfactorily sealed although this is rarely necessary.

D. Infection
   i. Because children are more susceptible to otitis media than adults, justifiable concern has been expressed that a middle ear infection could cause an implanted device to become an infected foreign body, requiring its removal.
   ii. Two children in our series experienced delayed mastoiditis (several years after the implant surgery) resulting in a postauricular abscess. These cases were treated by incision and drainage and intravenous antibiotics without the need to remove the implant.
   iii. An even greater concern is that infection might extend along the electrode into the inner ear, resulting in a serious otogenic complication, such as meningitis or further degeneration of the central auditory system. (A previously used positioner, a small silicone rubber wedge inserted next to the implanted electrode to improve transmission, has been removed from the market because of a possible relation to meningitis).
   iv. Although the incidence of otitis media in children who have received cochlear implants parallels that in the general pediatric population, no serious complications related to otitis media have occurred in our patients.
E. Intracochlear ossification
   i. Ossification at round window common in postmeningitic patients (encountered in approximately one-half of children deafened by meningitis)
   ii. In these patients, a cochleostomy is developed anterior to round window. New bone is drilled. If an open scala tympani is entered, a full insertion is performed.
   iii. Less frequently, the scala tympani is completely obliterated by bone. Our preference is to drill open the basal turn and create a tunnel approximately 6 mm in depth and partially inert a straight electrode. This allows implantation of 10 to12 active electrodes which has proven satisfactory.
   iv. Alternately, specially designed split electrodes have been developed by the Med-El and Nucleus Corporations. One branch of the electrode array is placed into the tunnel described earlier and the second active electrode is inserted into a second cochleostomy developed just anterior to the oval window.

Initial Fitting of Cochlear Implant

A. External processor and transmitter fit approximately 1 month after surgery.
B. Magnet strength for transmitter determined.
C. Electrical threshold and comfort levels determined.
D. Map created.
E. Water resistant external equipment has been developed to allow swimming and showering.

Results

Expectations concerning speech perception, production and language development for patients with cochlear implants are higher than ever before, although these skills may develop over time. Improvements have been documented in

A. Auditory-only word recognition
B. Auditory-only sentence recognition
C. Audiovisual speech recognition

Other demographic factors which influence cochlear implant performance are

A. Duration of implant use
B. Age at time of implantation
C. Communication method (oral vs sign)
D. Educational environment
E. Age at the time of implantation

New Sensory Aid Configurations

In recent years, there has been a move toward providing bilateral auditory input to cochlear implant recipients. Binaural auditory input yields improved sound localization and higher levels of spoken word recognition especially in noise. This has taken the form of

A. Bilateral cochlear implantation
B. Monaural cochlear implantation combined with hearing aid use in the contralateral ear (With the broadening of cochlear implant candidacy criteria to include individuals with severe hearing loss, many people with cochlear implants have the potential to benefit further from hearing aid use in the non-implanted ear)
C. Cochlear implant and hearing aid in the same ear

When possible, acoustic stimulation provided by a hearing aid provides the listener with finer spectral and temporal pitch cues that are not well conveyed by a cochlear implant.

Conclusions

A. Cochlear implants are appropriate sensory aids for selected deaf patients who receive minimal benefit from conventional amplification.
B. Improvements in technology and refinements in candidacy criteria have secured a permanent role for cochlear implantation.
C. With improved postoperative performance, implantation is clearly justified not only in patients with bilateral profound sensorineural hearing loss but also in patients with severe sensorineural hearing loss.
D. Patients as young as 12 months may undergo implantation under current FDA guidelines, and experience with even younger children is accumulating.

Bibliography

Dettman SJ, Pinder D, Briggs RJ, Dowell RC, Leigh JR. Communication development in children who receive cochlear implant younger than 12 months: risks versus benefits. *Ear Hear.* 2007;20(Suppl):S11-S18.

Gifford RH, et al. Cochlear implantation with hearing preservation yields significant benefit for speech recognition in complex listening environments. *Ear Hear.* 2013;34(4):413-425.

Houston DM, Miyamoto RT. Effects of early auditory experience on word learning and speech perception in deaf children with cochlear implants: implications for sensitive periods of language development. *Otol Neurotol.* 2010;31(8):1248-1253.

Jiang ZY, Odiase E, Isaaacson B, Roland PS, Kutz JW Jr. Utility of MRIs in adult cochlear implant evaluations. *Otol Neurotol.* 2014;35(9):1533-1535. Epub June 2, 2014.

Kuhn H, Schon F, Edelmann K, Brill S, Muller J. The development of lateralization abilities in children with bilateral cochlear implants. *ORL J Otorhinolaryngolo Relat Spec.* 2013;75(2):55-67.

Questions

1. Low Pitches are heard in the
   A. Cochlear apex
   B. Reissner membrane
   C. Outer hair cells
   D. Cochlear base
   E. Supporting cells

2. Temporal coding (timing) of information is limited to frequencies
   A. Above 8000 HZ
   B. Below 500 HZ
   C. Beyond the range of audio ability
   D. Ultra high frequencies
   E. At uncomfortable levels

3. Cochlear implants are not appropriate for
   A. Postlingual deafness
   B. Ossified cochleas
   C. Congenitally deformed cochleas
   D. Prelingual deafness
   E. Michel deformity

4. When low-frequency hearing is present, spectral information is best transmitted by
   A. Telephone
   B. Hearing Aid
   C. Cochlear Implant
   D. Tactile Aid
   E. Middle ear implant

5. Essential components of a cochlear implant system are
   A. Microphone
   B. Processor
   C. Electrode array
   D. Transmission link
   E. All of the above

Chapter 21
Facial Nerve Paralysis

Embryology

Development of the Intratemporal Facial Nerve

- *Week 3 of gestation:* fascioacoustic primordium appears. This eventually gives rise to the VII and VIII cranial nerves.
- *Week 4 of gestation:* facial and acoustic nerves become distinguishable. The facial nerve splits into two parts:
  - (a) *Chorda tympani nerve:* courses ventrally to enter the first (mandibular) arch.
  - (b) *Main trunk:* enters mesenchyme of the second (hyoid) arch.
- *Week 5 of gestation:* geniculate ganglion, nervus intermedius, and greater superficial petrosal nerve are visible. The predominantly sensory fibers of nervus intermedius develop from the geniculate ganglion and course to the brain stem between the VII and VIII cranial nerves.
- *Week 6-7 of gestation:* muscles of facial expression develop within the second arch. During this time the facial nerve courses across the region that will become the middle ear toward its destination to provide innervation to these muscles.
- Month 5 of gestation: fallopian canal forms as the otic capsule ossifies.

Development of the Extratemporal Facial Nerve

- *Week 8 of gestation:* the five major extratemporal branches of the facial nerve (temporal, zygomatic, buccal, marginal mandibular, and cervical) are formed. Extensive connections between the peripheral branches of the facial nerve continue to develop as the face expands.
- *Week 12 of gestation:* peripheral branches of facial nerve are completely developed.
- *At term:* the anatomy of the facial nerve approximates that of the adult, with the exception of its superficial location as it exits the temporal bone since the mastoid process is absent (Figure 21-1).
- *Age 1-3:* mastoid process develops and displaces the facial nerve medially and inferiorly.

Development of the Ear

- Development of the external ear correlates with that of the facial nerve.
- Because the facial nerve is the nerve to the second branchial arch, any malformations in the derivatives of Reichert cartilage make the nerve suspect for variation in its anatomic course.
- *Week 6 of gestation:* the first and second arches give rise to small condensations of mesoderm known as Hillocks of His. These eventually coalesce to form the auricle around the 12th week.

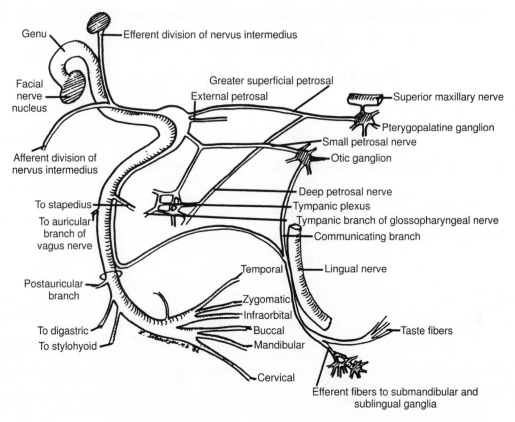

Figure 21-1 Branches of the facial nerve. (*Reproduced with permission from Sataloff RT:* Embryology and Anomalies of the Facial Nerve and Their Surgical Implications. *New York, NY: Lippincott Williams & Wilkins; 1991.)*

- *Week 8 of gestation*: the first pharyngeal groove begins to invaginate and grow toward the middle ear.
- *Week 28 of gestation*: the external auditory canal (EAC) and tympanic membrane appear.
- *At birth*: the shape of the auricle is complete, the tympanic ring is small, and the EAC has yet to ossify.
- The presence of a congenitally malformed external ear warns the clinician of the possibility of additional abnormalities. The clinician may be able to predict the anomalous course of the nerve by determining the age at which development arrested. Other findings that alert the clinician to possible facial nerve abnormalities include ossicular anomalies, craniofacial anomalies, and the presence of a conductive hearing loss.

Anatomy

- The facial nerve is a mixed nerve containing motor, sensory, and parasympathetic fibers.
- It has four functional components: two efferent and two afferent:

Efferent Components

A. Efferent motor fibers from the motor nucleus innervate the platysma, posterior belly of the digastric muscle, the stylohyoid muscle, the stapedius muscle, and the muscles of facial expression.
   i. The upper motor neuron tracts to the upper face cross and re-cross before reach- ing the facial nerve nucleus in the pons, sending bilateral innervation to the upper face. However, tracts to the lower face only cross once. Therefore, lesions proximal to the facial nerve nucleus spare the upper face of the involved side, allowing forehead movement and eyelid closure, whereas distal lesions produce complete paralysis of the affected side.
B. Efferent parasympathetic fibers originating from the superior salivatory nucleus are responsible for lacrimation and nasal secretions (via greater superficial petrosal nerve to lacrimal and nasal glands) and salivation (via chorda tympani nerve to subman- dibular and sublingual glands).

Afferent Components

A. Taste from the anterior two-thirds of the tongue is transmitted by afferent fibers to the nucleus tractus solitarius by way of the lingual nerve, the chorda tympani, and even- tually the nervus intermedius, the sensory root of the facial nerve.
B. A second set of afferent fibers conducts sensation from specific areas of the face, including the postauricular area, concha, earlobe, EAC, and tympanic membrane via nervus intermedius to the spinal trigeminal nucleus.

The course of the facial nerve is divided into six segments (Figure 21-2):

A. *Intracranial segment*: 23 to 24 mm, brain stem to porus of the internal auditory canal (IAC).
B. *Meatal segment*: 8 to 10 mm, porus of the IAC to the meatal foramen. The nerve runs anterior to the superior vestibular nerve and superior to the cochlear nerve.

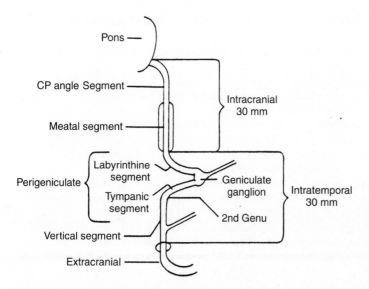

Figure 21-2 Segments of the facial nerve. (*Adapted with permission from Coker N, et al: Traumatic intratemporal facial nerve injury: Man- agement rationale for preservation of function,* Otolaryngol Head Neck Surg. *Sept;97(3):262-269, 1987.)*

C. *Labyrinthine segment*: 3 to 5 mm, meatal foramen to geniculate ganglion. The nerve gives rise to its first branch, the greater superficial petrosal nerve. The fallopian canal is narrowest within the labyrinthine segment, particularly at its entrance (meatal foramen).

D. *Tympanic segment*: 8 to 11 mm. At the geniculate ganglion the nerve makes a 40° to 80° turn to proceed posteriorly across medial wall of the tympanic cavity, medial to the cochleariform process, then above the oval window, and then under the lateral semicircular canal to the pyramidal eminence. The majority of intratemporal facial nerve injuries result from trauma to the nerve in the tympanic and mastoid segments.

E. *Mastoid (vertical) segment*: 10 to 14 mm, pyramidal process/second genu to stylomastoid foramen. Fascicular arrangement is thought to occur in this segment. Three branches arise from this segment: nerve to the stapedius muscle, chorda tympani nerve, and nerve from auricular branch of the vagus nerve (Arnold nerve).

F. *Extratemporal segment*: from stylomastoid foramen to facial muscles. After emerging from the stylomastoid foramen, the nerve courses anteriorly and slightly inferiorly, lateral to the styloid process and external carotid artery, to enter the posterior surface of the parotid gland. At this point the nerve lies on the posterior belly of the digastric muscle. Once it enters the substance of the parotid gland, it bifurcates into an upper *temporozygomatic division* and a lower *cervicofacial division*. The extensive network of anastomoses that develops between the various limbs is called the *pes anserinus*. By the time it exits the anterior border of the parotid, the five branches of the facial nerve can be identified: the temporal, zygomatic, buccal, marginal mandibular, and cervical branches (Figure 21-3).

Surgical Anatomy

- Landmarks for identification of the extratemporal facial nerve:
  - (a) *Tragal pointer*: nerve identified 1 to 1.5 cm deep to and just anterior and inferior to the lateral edge of the external canal cartilage.
  - (b) *Tympanomastoid fissure*: nerve can be identified 6 to 8 mm below the inferior "drop-off" of the fissure.
  - (c) *Posterior belly of the digastric muscle at its insertion to the mastoid process*: nerve exits stylomastoid foramen just anterior to this.
  - (d) *Proximal dissection of peripheral facial nerve branches through the parotid gland*: allows the surgeon to localize the nerve when its proximal extratemporal anatomy is distorted or parotid neoplasm is present.
- Landmarks for identification of the intratemporal facial nerve:
  - (a) *Cochleariform process*: tympanic segment located just deep to this.
  - (b) *Lateral semicircular canal*: second genu lies inferior and medial to this.
  - (c) *Digastric ridge*: stylomastoid foramen located at anterior end of ridge.
- A prominence of the nerve posterior and lateral to the lateral semicircular canal makes the nerve more susceptible to injury in this area. This is the most common site of facial nerve injury during mastoid surgery.
- Dehiscence of the fallopian canal is extremely common, with a reported incidence of 30%. The most common location of dehiscence, and also the most common site of iatrogenic injury during middle ear surgery, is the tympanic segment adjacent to the oval window.

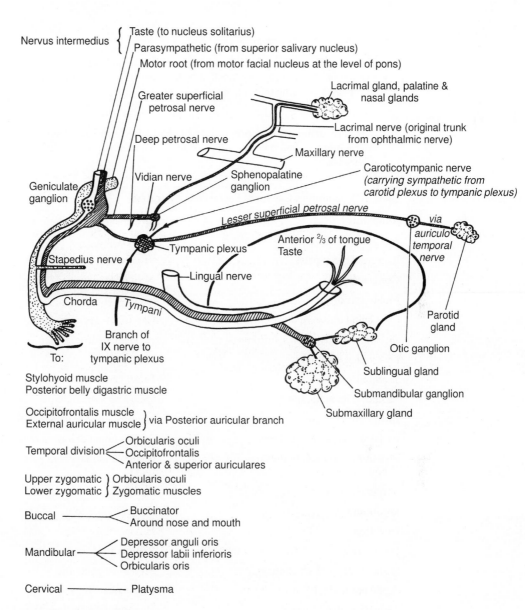

Figure 21-3 Course of the facial nerve.

Evaluation

- The common causes of facial paralysis are listed in Table 21-1.
- Evaluation should include a detailed history, physical examination, audiogram, and, in select cases, imaging or electrophysiologic testing.

History

- Any palsy demonstrating progression beyond 3 weeks or lack of any sign of recovery after 6 months should be considered due to an underlying neoplasm until proven otherwise.

Table 21-1 Common Causes of Facial Nerve Paralysis

Idiopathic	Influenza
Bell palsy	Encephalitis
Recurrent facial palsy	Sarcoidosis
Congenital	**Neoplasia**
Möbius syndrome	Cholesteatoma
Congenital unilateral lower lip paralysis	Carcinoma (primary or metastatic)
Melkersson-Rosenthal syndrome	Acoustic neuroma
Dystrophic myotonia	Meningioma
Traumatic	Facial neuroma
Temporal bone fractures	Ossifying hemangioma
Birth trauma	Glomus jugulare or tympanicum
Facial contusions/lacerations	Schwannoma of lower cranial nerves
Penetrating wounds to the face or temporal bone	Benign and malignant parotid tumors
Iatrogenic injury	Leukemia
Barotrauma	Hemangioblastoma
Infection	Histiocytosis
Herpes zoster oticus (Ramsay Hunt syndrome)	Rhabdomyosarcoma
Otitis media with effusion	**Metabolic/systemic**
Acute mastoiditis	Diabetes mellitus
Malignant otitis externa	Hyperthyroidism/hypothyroidism
Acute suppurative otitis media	Pregnancy
Tuberculosis	Autoimmune disorders
Lyme disease	**Neurologic**
Acquired immunodeficiency syndrome	Guillain-Barré syndrome
Infectious mononucleosis	Multiple sclerosis
	Millard-Gubler syndrome

- Coexistence of this indolent course with facial twitching, additional cranial nerve involvement, sensorineural hearing loss, or obvious mass is also highly suggestive of a tumor.
- Numbness in the middle and lower face, otalgia, hyperacusis, diminished tearing, and an altered taste are common findings in Bell palsy and herpes zoster oticus.
- Herpes zoster oticus (Ramsay Hunt syndrome) will also manifest as vesicular eruptions of the face/ear, sensorineural hearing loss, and vertigo.
- A previous history or family history of facial paralysis is suggestive of Bell palsy.
- The patient should be questioned in detail regarding other medical conditions, including Lyme disease, sarcoidosis, carcinoma, diabetes mellitus, immune suppression, and pregnancy; previous ear disease, hearing loss, or otologic surgery; and present medications.
- Tick exposure should be questioned in tick-endemic areas.

Physical Examination

- The initial evaluation should determine if the weakness is complete or partial.
- Extent of paralysis should be documented using a standardized grading system such as the House-Brackmann functional recovery grading system (Table 21-2).
- A common mistake is to interpret upper eyelid movement as partial facial nerve integrity. Remember that eyelid elevation is a function of the levator palpebrae muscle, which is innervated by the oculomotor nerve, and will remain intact despite a total facial nerve paralysis.
- Differentiate between central versus peripheral involvement of the facial nerve. Central unilateral facial paralysis usually involves only the lower face, as the innervation of the upper face is derived from bilateral upper facial motor neurons. Lesions of the peripheral nerve involve the upper and lower face. In addition, the presence of emotional facial expression as well as lacrimation, taste, and salivation on the ipsilateral side suggest a central lesion. These functions are not governed by the motor cortex of the precentral gyrus and, therefore would be unaffected by lesions in these areas.
- Include a thorough otologic examination; an evaluation of the remaining cranial nerves; and an assessment of cutaneous involvement, signs of trauma, or associated systemic findings (Table 21-3).

Imaging Studies

- The need for radiologic evaluation is based on the history and clinical course of each individual case.
- High-resolution computed tomography (CT) scan of the temporal bone:
  (a) This scan is the study of choice for assessment of the intratemporal facial nerve; provides the best assessment of the integrity of the fallopian canal.
  (b) This scan is the imaging study of choice for skull base trauma or when temporal bone disease is clinically evident.
- Magnetic resonance imaging (MRI) of the facial nerve (include brain and parotid) with gadolinium enhancement:
  (a) MRI is the study of choice for soft tissue assessment and instrumental in detecting neuronal enhancement from infection or neoplasia.
  (b) It is necessary for evaluation of the facial nerve at the level of the cerebellopontine angle.
  (c) Imaging is *not* routinely indicated for typical Bell palsy. Gadolinium-enhanced MRI of the brain in Bell palsy has been shown to demonstrate intense enhancement

Table 21-2 House-Brackmann Facial Nerve Grading System

Grade	Characteristics
I. Normal	Normal facial function in all areas.
II. Mild dysfunction	**Gross**
	Slight weakness noticeable on close inspection. May have very slight synkinesis. At rest, normal symmetry and tone.
	Motion
	Forehead: moderate-to-good function.
	Eye: complete closure with minimal effort.
	Mouth: slight asymmetry.
III. Moderate dysfunction	**Gross**
	Obvious, but not disfiguring difference between the two sides. Noticeable but not severe synkinesis, contracture, or hemifacial spasm. At rest, normal symmetry and tone.
	Motion
	Forehead: slight-to-moderate movement.
	Eye: complete closure with effort.
	Mouth: slightly weak with maximum effort.
IV. Moderately severe dysfunction	**Gross**
	Obvious weakness and/or disfiguring asymmetry. At rest, normal symmetry and tone.
	Motion
	Forehead: none.
	Eye: incomplete closure.
	Mouth: asymmetric with maximum effort.
V. Severe dysfunction	**Gross**
	Only barely perceptible motion. At rest, asymmetry.
	Motion
	Forehead: none.
	Eye: incomplete closure.
	Mouth: slight movement.
VI. Total paralysis	No movement.

of the labyrinthine facial nerve. However, the presence and degree of enhancement have not been shown to correlate with the severity of paralysis, electrophysiologic test results, and prognosis for recovery.

(d) In the absence of any clinically identifiable cause for facial palsy, MRI scan of the brain and parotid gland should be obtained when recovery of function has not begun 6 months after onset of paralysis.

Table 21-3 **Diagnosis of Lesions From Level of Impairment**

Level of Impairment	Signs	Diagnosis
Supranuclear	Good tone, intact upper face, presence of spontaneous smile, associated neurologic deficits	Cerebrovascular accident, trauma
Nuclear	Involvement of the VI and VII cranial nerves, corticospinal tracts	Vascular or neoplastic, poliomyelitis, multiple sclerosis, encephalitis
Cerebellopontine angle	Involvement of vestibular and cochlear portions of the VIII cranial nerve (facial nerve, particularly taste, lacrimation, and salivation may be altered); the V and later IX, X, and XI cranial nerves may become impaired	Schwannoma, meningioma, epidermoid tumor, glomus jugulare
Geniculate ganglion	Facial paralysis, hyperacusis, decreased lacrimation and salivation, altered taste	Herpes zoster oticus, temporal bone fracture, Bell palsy, cholesteatoma, schwannoma, arteriovenous malformation, meningioma
Tympanomastoid	Facial paralysis, decreased salivation and taste, lacrimation intact	Bell palsy, cholesteatoma, temporal bone fracture, infection
Extracranial	Facial paralysis (usually a branch is spared), salivation and taste intact	Trauma, tumor, parotid carcinoma, pharyngeal carcinoma

Facial Nerve Testing

- Prognosis for recovery is dependent on degree of facial nerve injury.
- Classification of nerve injury and prognostic implications:
  - (a) *Neuropraxia*: blockage of axonal transport due to local compression. The nerve does not sustain permanent damage and no wallerian degeneration occurs. Normal function will be restored when the compression is relieved. All electrophysiologic tests will be within normal limits.
  - (b) *Axonotmesis*: axonal integrity has been disrupted, but endoneural sheaths are preserved. Wallerian degeneration distal to the lesion occurs. Electrophysiologic tests will reveal rapid and complete degeneration 72 hours after injury. As long as the endoneurium is preserved, there will be complete recovery with return of normal function.
  - (c) *Neurotmesis*: destruction of the axon and surrounding support tissue. Characterized by wallerian degeneration, an unpredictable regeneration potential, and the likelihood of significant resultant dysfunction and synkinesis. Early electrophysiologic testing mimics that of axonotmesis.
- Any significant injury to the facial nerve with violation of its neural support structures is likely to result in neural degeneration with aberrant neural regeneration and reinnervation, which results in synkinesis.
- *Synkinesis*: defined as the loss of discrete facial movements after facial nerve injury. Results from a single axon or a small group of axons innervating motor end units of numerous and separated muscles.
- *Bogorad syndrome* (crocodile tear syndrome): occurs when regenerating nerve fibers originally destined for the salivary glands innervate the lacrimal gland. This causes profuse lacrimation during eating.

- *Topodiagnostic testing*: the concept of testing specific neuronal function corresponding to the numerous branches of the facial nerve in an attempt to localize the site of injury and to predict functional outcome. Commonly used examples include the Schirmer test, the submandibular flow test, and the stapedial reflex test. These tests have been found to correlate poorly with the site of injury and are unreliable in predicting recovery. While they are included in this discussion, they are rarely used in clinical practice today and indicated only if information about a specific function is required.
- Not all patients with facial paralysis require prognostic tests because the outcome may already be predictable (acoustic tumor surgery) or because the underlying cause is the indication for treatment (chronic otitis media with facial nerve paralysis).
- Testing is indicated primarily for prognosticating recovery in complete facial paralysis. In some cases, these tests may have diagnostic value. Functional recovery for incomplete facial paralysis is good and therefore prognostic testing is not required in when paralysis is incomplete.
- Since all electrodiagnostic tests used for evaluating facial nerve function measure downfield electrical activity distal to the site of lesion, neural degeneration will only be measurable 3 days after the onset of complete paralysis.

Nerve Excitability Test

- First described by Hilger in 1964.
- Compares current thresholds required to elicit minimal muscle contraction on the normal side of the face to those of the paralyzed side.
- The current, measured in milliamperes (mA), is delivered percutaneously with a DC current while the face is monitored for the slightest movement. The electrodes are then placed in corresponding locations on the involved side, and the same procedure is performed.
- A difference of 3.5 mA or greater is considered significant and suggests degeneration.
- Since measured results are subjective and variable, this test is unreliable clinically and rarely used in clinical practice when objective testing is not available to the clinician.

Maximum Stimulation Test

- Similar to nerve excitability test (NET) except that it uses maximal rather than minimal stimulation.
- The main trunk as well as each major branch of the nerve on the normal and abnormal sides is stimulated at an intensity that produces maximal muscle contraction of the nonparalyzed side without discomfort.
- Results of the maximum stimulation test (MST) are expressed as the difference in facial muscle movement between the normal and paralyzed sides using the same suprathreshold electrical stimulus.
- A maximal stimulus elicits a response from the entire nerve and, therefore serves as a better prognostic indicator of muscle denervation compared to the NET. However, as with the NET, results are subject to interobserver variability and therefore clinically unreliable. As with NET, MST is performed with the Hilger nerve stimulator only when electroneurography (EnoG) testing is not available.

Electroneurography

- Unlike the NET and MST, electroneurography (EnoG) provides quantitative analysis of the extent of degeneration without being dependent on observer quantification.
- Currently the most reliable prognostic indicator of all the electrodiagnostic tests in the first 2 weeks following onset of complete facial paralysis.

- A suprathreshold electrical stimulus is used to elicit facial contraction on the normal and paralyzed side. Instead of visual observation of the degree of response (as performed for the MST), the compound muscle action potential (CMAP) generated is measured using an electromyography (EMG) recording device.
- The normal side is compared to the paralyzed side, and the degree of degeneration is inferred by the difference between the amplitudes of the measured CMAPs.
- Surgical decompression of the facial nerve may be considered when 90% or greater degeneration has occurred. Absence of early neural regeneration in these cases must be confirmed on EMG testing.
- ENoG is valuable when used between 3 and 14 days after the onset of complete facial paralysis.
- Both extent and time course of neural degeneration is used to prognosticate functional recovery.

Electromyography

- Determines the activity of the muscle itself.
- A needle electrode is inserted into the muscle, and recordings of individual motor unit action potentials are taken at rest and on voluntary contraction.
- Degeneration of a lower motor nerve with muscle denervation is followed in 14 to 21 days by spontaneous muscle electrical activity called *fibrillation potentials*.
- Six to 12 weeks prior to clinical return of facial function, polyphasic reinnervation potentials are detected with voluntary muscle contraction and provide the earliest evidence of nerve recovery.
- Electromyography (EMG) is valuable as a diagnostic and prognostic test at anytime after the onset of complete facial paralysis. It is also used in conjunction with ENoG to confirm the absence of recovery (voluntary motor unit action potentials absent on EMG testing).

Lacrimation (Schirmer Test)

- Evaluates greater superficial petrosal nerve function (ie, tear production).
- Filter paper strips are placed in the conjunctival fornix of both eyes and the eyes are closed for 5 minutes. After 5 minutes the length of paper moistened is compared.
- Significant abnormalities (positive Schirmer test) include reduction of tearing of greater than 50% of the healthy side or reduction in total lacrimation to less than 25 mm after a 5-minute period.
- Schirmer II test is a modification of this test with the addition of nasal mucosal stimulation.
- The clinical utility of this test includes the ability to evaluate the protective mechanism of the eye in patients with significant facial dysfunction.

Stapedial Reflex

- The stapedius muscle contracts reflexively in both ears when one ear is stimulated with a loud tone. This alters the reactive compliance of the middle ear, which can be measured with impedance audiometry.
- If the lesion involves the nerve proximal to the branch to the stapedius muscle, the muscle will not contract and no change in impedance will be recorded (absent stapedial reflex).
- CT and MR imaging have largely surpassed the utility of this test for localization of facial nerve lesions.
- The presence of an acoustic reflex on the affected side is a good prognostic indicator for recovery.

Trigeminofacial (Blink) Reflex

- Percutaneous electrical stimulation of the supraorbital nerve elicits a blink reflex that is recorded by electrodes placed over the orbicularis oculi muscle. This is the electrical correlate of the corneal reflex test.
- The afferent limb of the reflex arc is mediated by the trigeminal nerve (ophthalmic division) and efferent limb is mediated by the facial nerve.
- This test is helpful in differentiating peripheral facial palsy from trigeminal and central causes of facial palsy.

Salivary Flow Testing

- By cannulating Wharton papillae, a measurement of salivary flow to gustatory stimulation can be obtained.
- A reduction of 25% as compared to the uninvolved side is considered abnormal.
- This test is difficult to perform and is subject to a significant level of inaccuracy. It is no longer used clinically.

Idiopathic Facial Paralysis (Bell Palsy)

- The most common cause of acute facial paralysis, accounting for 70% of cases.
- Annual estimated incidence ranges from 15 to 40 per 100,000.
- Occurs in any age group but most common between ages 15 and 45.
- No sexual or racial predilection.
- Both sides of the face are affected equally. Bilateral simultaneous palsy is rare.
- Recurrent paralysis occurs in approximately 10% to 12% of patients and is more common on the contralateral side.
- Positive family history is reported in up to 14% of cases.
- Herpes simplex virus (HSV) has been implicated in the etiopathogenesis of Bell palsy. The viral infection induces an inflammatory response that results in neural edema and vascular compromise of the facial nerve within the fallopian canal. This entrapment neuropathy is most evident in the labyrinthine segment of the facial nerve where the fallopian canal is narrowest in diameter.
- Presents with unilateral facial weakness of sudden onset, involving all branches of the nerve, which may progress to complete paralysis in two-thirds of patients over the course of 3 to 7 days.
- Bell palsy is a diagnosis of exclusion. However, minimum diagnostic criteria for Bell palsy include the following:
  - (a) Paralysis or paresis of all muscle groups on one side of the face
  - (b) Rapid onset within 72 hours
  - (c) Absence of signs of central nervous system disease, ear disease, or cerebellopontine angle disease
- *Additional characteristics*: viral prodrome (60%); ear pain (60%), numbness or pain of the ear, face, or neck (60%); dysguesia (57%); hyperacusis (30%); and decreased tearing (17%).
- The majority of patients with Bell palsy demonstrate onset of recovery by 6 months, and 85% of patients will have good functional recovery (House-Brackmann grade I-II).
- An audiogram is obtained to provide a good general screening of the auditory system although hearing loss is unlikely with Bell palsy.
- If complete paralysis is identified, electrophysiologic tests should be performed to prognosticate recovery.

- Imaging is not routinely obtained for Bell palsy patients. However, in cases of total paralysis with sensorineural hearing loss on the affected side, recurrent ipsilateral facial paralysis, atypical presentation, or polyneuropathy, a gadolinium-enhanced MRI scan of the facial nerve is recommended. Absence of onset of clinical recovery 6 months after onset of paralysis, progressive paralysis beyond 3 weeks, and the presence of facial twitching also constitute clinical indicators for imaging of the facial nerve.
- The prognosis for recovery in Bell palsy is very good regardless of treatment. All patients recover to some extent. Patients with incomplete paralysis almost always have complete recovery. In patients with complete paralysis, over two-thirds have a complete recovery and 15% have a good clinical recovery with mild residual palsy. The remaining 15% have a fair to poor recovery and is the group that would benefit most from aggressive medical or surgical intervention.
- Oral steroids administered early in the course of the disease (within 72 hours of onset) have been shown to improve functional recovery. With steroid therapy alone, 65% to 85% of patients regain good facial function.
- Concomitant antiviral therapy (acyclovir, valacyclovir, or famciclovir) early in the course of the disease is controversial and of questionable added benefit compared to oral steroids alone. Gastrointestinal complaints are the most common side effects associated with antiviral medications.
- Surgical decompression for Bell palsy has been advocated by some for cases of complete facial paralysis with electrical evidence of extensive nerve degeneration. When ENoG testing indicates greater than 90% neural degeneration within the first 2 weeks following onset of facial paralysis, the patient has a 50% chance of residual facial weakness and synkinesis. For Bell palsy patients who have 90% or greater degeneration on ENoG testing within the first 14 days of onset of complete paralysis and absence of motor unit action potentials on voluntary EMG testing, surgical decompression of the facial nerve at the meatal foramen, labyrinthine segment, and geniculate ganglion resulted in a 91% chance of good outcome seven months after paralysis compared to a 42% chance of good recovery in those patients with the same ENoG and EMG parameters who were treated with steroids only. In individuals with good hearing, a middle cranial fossa approach is used for surgical decompression of the facial nerve. In those with poor or no hearing in the affected ear, a translabyrinthine approach is used.
- Surgical decompression of the facial nerve for Bell palsy remains very controversial and scientific studies to support this are limited.
- Physical therapy and other adjuvant therapies for Bell palsy including acupuncture, massage, and facial exercises are of questionable benefit.

Trauma

- Second most common cause of facial paralysis.
- Diagnosis is usually apparent due to the mechanism of injury, related injuries, or recent surgical history.
- Traumatic injuries to the facial nerve are subdivided into iatrogenic and noniatrogenic causes. Each has its typical presentation and management objectives.

Iatrogenic Injury

- Facial nerve injury during mastoid or middle ear surgery is uncommon (~1%-3%).
- The most common site of iatrogenic injury to middle ear surgery is the tympanic segment.

- Extratemporal resections, including parotid or neck tumors, may necessitate the sacrifice of part of the nerve. Usually, these injuries are identified at the time of surgery and appropriate repair (ie, end-to-end anastomosis or cable grafting) is performed.
- The clinical challenge arises when there is unexpected postoperative facial paralysis. Local anesthetics (ie, lidocaine) may result in residual weakness or paralysis and should be given appropriate time to wear-off (few hours). If paralysis persists, middle ear and mastoid packing that may be compressing a dehiscent segment of the nerve should be removed.
- The decision to explore the nerve is dependent on the surgeon's confidence of the status of the nerve.
  (a) If the nerve was not identified during the procedure or if injury is felt to be a possibility, the nerve should be explored and decompressed or repaired as soon as possible.
  (b) If the surgeon is convinced that the nerve was not compromised, it is safe to follow the paralysis with electrical tests and surgically explore only if there is electrical evidence of significant neural degeneration. Systemic steroids may be used to reduce neural edema.
  (c) EMG testing in the immediate postoperative setting is very valuable in determining the anatomic continuity of the nerve. If no voluntary motor unit action potentials are detected, a severe contusion or disruption of the nerve can be inferred and surgical exploration is warranted.
  (d) A postoperative paresis is almost always the result of minor trauma and edema, and rarely progresses to paralysis. Systemic steroids may be administered to reduce the extent of neural edema associated with the traumatic injury.

Noniatrogenic Intratemporal Injury

- Results from temporal bone fractures, which are classified as longitudinal or transverse with respect to the long axis of the petrous ridge.
- Eighty to 90% of temporal bone fractures are *longitudinal* and usually result from blunt trauma to the temporoparietal area. They almost always involve the middle ear, but only 20% will have concomitant facial nerve injury. Common presentations include bleeding from the middle or external ear, laceration of the tympanic membrane, and conductive hearing loss. Facial nerve injury, if present, is usually the result of compression and ischemia as opposed to neural disruption.
- *Transverse* fractures account for a much smaller proportion of temporal bone injuries, but an associated facial nerve injury is present in up to half of the cases. It is usually the result of trauma to the occiput. Common presentations include hemotympanum, vestibular symptoms, and severe sensorineural or mixed hearing loss. Nerve severance is the typical form of injury.
- Gunshot wounds make up a much smaller proportion of intratemporal injuries but are equally challenging. When the nerve is injured, it is usually in the tympanic and mastoid segments, and is often the result of thermal and compression injury as opposed to disruption. Even with surgical decompression, recovery of facial function is often incomplete. In addition, blast injuries are often accompanied by significant central nervous system or vascular injury.
- Regardless of the type of trauma, if paralysis is incomplete, conservative management is indicated since spontaneous recovery occurs in most individuals. Delayed-onset facial paralysis associated with temporal bone trauma is also likely to recover without surgical intervention.

- Serial examination is important to assess for any progressive paralysis and electrical testing should be performed if complete paralysis occurs.
- The use of steroids remains controversial. As long as there are no contraindications to short-course steroid use, there is some evidence to suggest that this may assist in shortening the recovery phase by reducing neural edema.
- All patients should be evaluated with a coronal and axial high-resolution CT scan and audiometric testing.
- In cases of penetrating injury, arteriography may be indicated if vascular injury is suspected.
- ENoG testing is performed once paralysis is complete. If degeneration of greater than 90% is identified on the affected side within 2 weeks after the injury, surgical decompression of the facial nerve at the affected site should be considered.
- If paralysis is complete and CT imaging demonstrates an obvious bone fragment impinging on the intratemporal facial nerve, surgical decompression is indicated even beyond the 2-week window period.
- More than 90% of temporal bone fractures with complete facial paralysis involve the region of the geniculate ganglion, especially the labyrinthine segment. If surgical exploration of the facial nerve is undertaken, the decompression should extend beyond this region.
- The surgical approach is dependent on the hearing status of the patient. A middle cranial fossa approach should be employed in a patient with intact hearing. Often, this procedure can be combined with a transmastoid approach if decompression of the distal tympanic and mastoid segments is indicated. In the case of a nonhearing ear, a translabyrinthine approach is used.
- Decompression of the nerve, including incision of the epineurium, is adequate in cases where obvious impingement was present and the nerve is otherwise intact; however, if the injury to the nerve is significant, despite its apparent continuity, resection and reanastomosis or nerve grafting will offer a better surgical result than decompression alone. In cases of complete transection, the decision to reanastomose the nerve should be based on the ability to approximate the nerve edges with negligible tension at the anastamotic site.
- The great auricular nerve is well suited for facial nerve cable grafting based on its size and location. If a longer segment of nerve is required, the sural nerve is the graft of choice.

Noniatrogenic Extratemporal Injury

- The extracranial nerve is susceptible to trauma, especially penetrating injuries, and an immediate assessment should be done to evaluate the status of nerve function, the extent of soft tissue injury, and the amount of contamination.
- Electrical testing can be of significant value in evaluating peripheral injuries of the facial nerve. A transected or severely injured nerve will show no response to stimulation proximal to the injury. In addition, electrical testing is instrumental in identifying nerve branches intraoperatively.
- An extensive examination should also include a survey of surrounding soft tissues, including the globe, the parotid duct, and the mouth.
- Injuries to the trunk or main branches of the facial nerve are extremely debilitating. Because of the extensive network of branching and anastomoses, peripheral injuries are associated with much less morbidity.
- All facial nerve injuries associated with loss of function should be explored and repaired as soon as possible. Injuries occurring distal to the lateral canthus and the oral facial crease are left to recover spontaneously.

- The decision to repair the nerve primarily versus nerve grafting is dependent on the ability to achieve a tension-free anastamosis. Two exceptions to immediate repair include (1) the presence of significant soft tissue loss and (2) extensive gross contamination of the wound. Under these circumstances, immediate exploration with wound debridement and tagging of the nerve branches is initially performed. A second-stage procedure for nerve repair can be achieved safely within 30 days from the time of the injury.

Infection

Viral

- Herpes zoster is the most common cause of facial nerve paralysis after Bell palsy.
- Herpes zoster is easily distinguishable from Bell palsy because of
  - (a) *Associated findings*: intense otalgia, vesicular eruptions involving the external ear (occasionally extending onto the tympanic membrane), sensorineural hearing loss, and vertigo. The combination of vesicular eruptions on the ear and facial paralysis is referred to as *Ramsay Hunt syndrome*.
  - (b) Unlike facial paresis in Bell palsy, which peaks within 2 weeks, progressive paresis may occur up to 3 weeks following onset.
- Incidence of Herpes zoster infection increases dramatically after age 60, presumably because of decreased cell-mediated immunity in this age group.
- Serologic and epidemiologic data suggest that the reactivation of a latent varicella zoster virus, as opposed to a reinfection, is the mechanism of infection.
- The diagnosis is rarely in question but can be confirmed by rising titers of antibodies to the varicella zoster virus.
- Enhancement patterns of the facial nerve by gadolinium-enhanced MRI are similar to those observed in Bell palsy, but again there is no correlation between the degree of enhancement and the severity of the paralysis, electrophysiologic test results, and prognosis for recovery.
- Compared to Bell palsy, nerve degeneration tends to be progressive and more severe, and therefore the overall prognosis for recovery is worse.
- Systemic corticosteroids are thought to relieve the acute pain, reduce vertigo, and minimize postherpetic neuralgia despite their questionable role in reversing the disease process. Antiviral medication, steroids, or the combination of the two have been reported to improve outcome. Postherpetic neuralgia is known to occur and can be prolonged and incapacitating. It can be managed with opioid analgesics, nortriptyline, amitriptyline, and gabapentin.

Bacterial

- Infections involving the ear that may cause facial paralysis include acute suppurative otitis media, chronic otitis media, mastoiditis, and malignant otitis externa (MOE).
- A natural dehiscence in the fallopian canal serves as a portal of entry for bacterial invasion and inflammatory products to cause neural edema in acute suppurative otitis media.
- Facial paralysis progresses rapidly over the course of 2 to 3 days and is usually preceded by severe otalgia with or without otorrhea.
  ### Acute Otitis Media
  - (a) Treatment: (1) intravenous antibiotic therapy for gram-positive cocci and Haemophilus, (2) wide-field myringotomy for middle ear evacuation, if a CT scan

of the temporal bone shows coalescent mastoiditis or intracranial extension of the infection, and (3) a cortical mastoidectomy should be performed.

(b) Prognosis for recovery of facial function is good without surgical decompression of the facial nerve.

Chronic Otitis Media

(a) Facial nerve paralysis most commonly associated with cholesteatoma or chronic inflammatory tissue involving the tympanic and mastoid segments of the facial nerve.

(b) Facial nerve dysfunction may be caused by inflammation, edema, and subsequent entrapment neuropathy. Alternatively, extraneural and intraneural compression may also result from an enlarging cholesteatoma or abcess.

(c) Treatment: (1) surgical removal of cholesteatoma or inflammatory tissue, (2) antibiotic therapy, and (3) corticosteroid therapy.

(d) Prognosis for recovery of facial function is usually favorable and related to time of intervention. Patients with chronic suppurative otitis media without cholesteatoma appear to have a better functional outcome compared to those with cholesteatoma.

Malignant Otitis Externa

(a) Requires rapid and aggressive management.

(b) Usually affects older patients with a long-standing history of diabetes and can result in multiple cranial nerve palsies. May also occur in immunocompromised individuals.

(c) Presents with severe, painful inflammation of the EAC with purulent otorrhea and fleshy granulation tissue along the inferior aspect of EAC at the bony-cartilaginous junction.

(d) *Pseudomonas aeruginosa* is the most common pathogen, accounting for up to 98% of documented cultures.

(e) The nidus of disease originates in the EAC but spreads into adjacent tissues. The temporal bone, parotid gland, and lower cranial nerves may become involved.

(f) Diagnosis is made by physical findings and can be confirmed with a CT scan of the temporal bone demonstrating erosive bony changes involving and extending beyond the EAC or gadolinium-enhanced MR imaging of the skull base revealing inflammatory disease in the area.

(g) Further evidence of osteomyelitis can be obtained on a *technetium radioisotope scan*, which identifies increased osteogenic activity. Once positive, the bone scan will remain positive for an indefinite period. A *gallium scan* detects inflammatory response (granulocyte binding) and is useful in following the course of the disease. A reduction in uptake on the gallium scan correlates with clinical improvement.

(h) Treatment consists of a 6-week course of high-dose intravenous antipseudomonal antibiotic regimen. Ciprofloxacin is typically administered in conjunction with a third- or fourth-generation cephalosporin. Surgical debridement is not usually indicated and is performed only to remove any obvious necrotic bone.

(i) Recovery of facial function with MOE is poorer than that for other lower cranial nerves involved with the infection.

Lyme Disease

- Facial nerve palsy occurs in only 10% of infected patients but remains the most common neurologic sign of Lyme disease.
- Bilateral involvement is not uncommon.

- It can be distinguished from Bell palsy by its flu-like symptoms and characteristic cutaneous manifestation—erythema chronicum migrans (a rash that starts as a flat reddened area and extends with central clearing).
- Serum antibody titers to the spirochete *Borrelia burgdorferi* are unreliable in the early phases of the disease and are therefore of limited value in the diagnostic workup. Intrathecal antibody production is found in a high proportion of patients presenting with facial paralysis.
- The prognosis for recovery of facial function is excellent, with almost 100% achieving a complete recovery.
- Treatment with a 4-week course of doxycycline is necessary to prevent late complications of the infection.

Systemic Diseases

- Various systemic diseases may result in facial nerve paralysis but should remain relatively low in the differential diagnosis.
  (a) *Guillain-Barré syndrome*: should be considered when facial paralysis accompanies an ascending motor paralysis, autonomic dysfunction, or central nervous system involvement. Along with Lyme disease, it is a common cause of facial diplegia.
  (b) *Infectious mononucleosis*: resulting from Epstein Barr viral infection. Characterized by a prodrome of headache, malaise, and myalgia. Subsequently, a fluctuating fever develops along with a sore throat, exudative tonsillitis, and lymphadenopathy. The diagnosis is confirmed on a positive mono spot test for rising titers of heterophil antibodies.
  (c) *Sarcoidosis*: is an idiopathic, chronic noncaseating granulomatous disease. Bilateral facial nerve paralysis is present in 50% of patients with a variant of sarcoidosis, also referred to as *uveoparotid fever* or *Heerfordt disease*.
  (d) *HIV infection: may cause facial paralysis in later stage of disease*; however, it must be emphasized that this is a rare sequela of the disease. The palsy may be a direct result of the virus infection, or it may be secondary to the immunodeficiency. The palsy often mimics that of Bell and has the same general recovery pattern.
  (e) *Others*: listed systemic in Table 21-1. In general, the prognosis for recovery of facial function with systemic diseases is good.

Neoplasms

- Tumors resulting in facial paralysis may involve the facial nerve itself or may originate from surrounding structures and eventually compromise nerve function.
- Of patients presenting with new-onset paralysis, only 5% are due to a neoplastic process.
- Features of facial nerve paralysis that suggest the possibility of tumor involvement include the following:
  (a) Progression of paresis beyond 3 weeks
  (b) Associated facial twitching
  (c) Absence of functional recovery 6 months after onset of paralysis
  (d) Ipsilateral recurrence of a facial paralysis
  (e) Facial paralysis with concurrent sensorineural hearing loss or vestibular symptoms
  (f) Presence of multiple cranial nerve deficits

(g) Presence of a parotid mass

(h) History of carcinoma

Intratemporal and Intracranial Neoplasms

- These are generally benign but can be extremely debilitating due to the mass effect on surrounding neurovascular structures.
- Commonest benign tumors originating from the facial nerve are facial neuromas and hemangiomas.
  - (a) Facial neuromas:
    - Rare, slow-growing tumors that arise from the facial nerve at any point along its course, but most frequently involve the geniculate ganglion.
    - Facial paralysis is the most common presenting complaint, although hearing loss is not uncommon.
  - (b) Hemangiomas of the facial nerve:
    - Tend to cause facial paralysis early in the disease process despite their small tumor size.
  - (c) Other intracranial tumors:
    - Acoustic neuromas (91%), meningiomas (2.5%), congenital epidermoids (2.5%), adenoid cystic carcinomas, and arachnoid cysts.
- Any suspicion of a neoplastic process requires an extensive neurotologic workup, including audiometry and imaging. When tumor is suspected, a gadolinium-enhanced MRI is the best means of assessing neural structures and continuity. If the tumor is intratemporal, additional unenhanced CT imaging of the temporal bone is helpful in localizing the tumor and visualizing the anatomy surrounding it.
- If the facial paralysis is of acute onset, reduced CMAP amplitude in combination with prolonged conduction latency on ENoG testing supports the diagnosis of an underlying tumor. Additionally, the presence of both fibrillation and polyphasic reinnervation potentials on EMG testing is characteristic of tumor disease due to simultaneous ongoing degeneration and regeneration of the nerve.
- Regardless of the histologic diagnosis, definitive management of tumors causing facial paralysis involves surgical excision. The surgical approach used is determined by the hearing status of the involved ear and the location of the tumor. Since surgical excision of primary tumors of the facial nerve results in complete facial paralysis, surgery is generally deferred until significant functional loss has occurred. In the best case scenario, facial nerve repair with a cable graft following tumor resection will result in a House-Brackmann grade III function. Surgical decompression of facial neuromas may be offered as a treatment option in those wishing to preserve facial function, although surgical removal of the tumor is eventually necessary.
- Stereotactic radiation treatment has been offered as an alternative treatment modality for enlarging facial neuromas with no or minimal facial dysfunction.

Extracranial Neoplasms

- Almost exclusively of parotid origin.
- They can be classified into benign and malignant lesions. Benign neoplasms constitute approximately 85% of parotid masses, of which pleomorphic adenomas make up the vast majority.

Benign Parotid Lesions

- Typical presentation is that of a slowly growing, nontender mass in the parotid region. Although uncommon, benign lesions may cause compression of surrounding soft tissues, resulting in facial nerve dysfunction and salivary flow obstruction.

- Fine-needle aspiration biopsies are an acceptable and commonly used method to evaluate salivary gland neoplasms.
- Treatment consists of surgical excision with a cuff of normal salivary gland tissue. This is best accomplished with a superficial or total parotidectomy, depending on the nature, location, and extent of the neoplasm. Great care must be taken to preserve the facial nerve, as the normal anatomy may be somewhat distorted due to the mass effect and surrounding edema from the tumor.

Malignant Neoplasms Involving the Facial Nerve
- May be of parotid origin or more rarely; may arise from the facial nerve itself.
- These lesions are often clinically indistinguishable from benign masses and must be confirmed by fine-needle aspiration biopsy.
- Approximately 12% to 15% of malignant parotid neoplasms cause facial nerve paralysis.
- Mucoepidermoid carcinoma is the most common malignancy of the parotid gland; however, adenoid cystic carcinoma has a higher predilection for facial nerve involvement.
- Regardless of the histologic type, facial nerve paralysis is a poor prognostic sign.
- Malignancy involving the nerve requires excision for a tumor-free margin. This should be confirmed intraoperatively with frozen section analysis of tumor and facial nerve margins.
- Reconstruction of the nerve should take place during the initial ablative procedure and often requires a nerve graft. The remainder of cases is treated with surgical excision of the gland with sparing of the nerve.
- Adjunctive radiotherapy and chemotherapy may also be indicated.

Pediatric

- Incidence of facial nerve paralysis in the newborn is approximately 1 in 2000 deliveries.
- It is important to determine the etiology of the paralysis in this population because prognosis and treatment differ for traumatic and developmental causes.

Birth Trauma

- Accounts for the majority of cases.
- Characterized by unilateral complete facial nerve dysfunction, a prolonged or complicated delivery, ecchymosis of the face or temporal region, and hemotympanum.
- While the use of forceps is still considered to be the most common insulting agent, often paralysis is present after an uncomplicated low or outlet forceps delivery.
- As discussed previously, the mastoid tip is poorly developed in the newborn infant, and the facial nerve lies in a superficial location. This makes the nerve vulnerable to compression and injury.

Congential Paralysis

- Accounts for the remainder of cases.
- Typically associated with other findings, including contralateral facial paralysis, additional cranial nerve deficits, and other congenital aberrances, particularly in the head and neck region.
- The most common anomalies affecting facial muscle function are *Möbius syndrome* and *agenesis of the depressor anguli oris muscle.*

    (a) Möbius syndrome:
- Hereditary condition.
- Presents with congenital facial diplegia and unilateral or bilateral abducens palsy.
- May also affect cranial nerves IX, X, and XII, as well as other extraocular motor nerves.
- Abnormalities of the extremities may also occur, including the absence of the pectoralis major muscle in Poland syndrome.
- Controversy exists as to the specific site of lesion. The lack of a functional neuromuscular unit may result from nuclear agenesis, muscular agenesis, or both.
- Surgical rehabilitation should include transposition of healthy muscle, along with its nerve supply.

    (b) Hypoplasia or aplasia of the depressor anguli oris muscle:
- Also termed *congenital unilateral lower lip paralysis* (CULLP).
- Thought to be a brain stem lesion that results in a lack of development of the depressor anguli oris muscle.
- Usually affects one side and is noted by facial asymmetry when crying.
- Associated anomalies occur in up to 70% of children, most commonly involving the head and neck and cardiovascular system.

- In any neonate in whom facial nerve paralysis is identified, a complete physical examination should be performed, including an assessment of partial versus complete paralysis, an otoscopic evaluation, and a survey of other traumatic sequelae, additional anomalies, or both.
- Serial electrophysiologic testing (EMG and ENoG) is extremely important in diagnosing the etiology of paralysis, documenting the extent of the lesion and following the clinical course. Emphasis is placed on differentiating between a traumatic versus a congenital etiology since management and prognosis for recovery differ between the two. ENoG and EMG testing may be normal at birth in traumatic cases and subsequently demonstrating declining responses on ENoG testing and fibrillation potentials on EMG testing. When facial paralysis is the result of a developmental disorder, ENoG and EMG responses are reduced or absent at birth, and show no progression or recovery with time. Tests that attempt to localize the site of disruption are usually of limited value in the neonate.
- Spontaneous recovery rate for traumatic neonatal facial nerve paralysis approaches 90% and is usually complete.
- Prognosis is worse for congenital lesions. Many of these children will have persistent asymmetrical function, but most will adapt well and not require surgical intervention.
- Surgical intervention for congenital facial paralysis is generally deferred until adolescence when facial development is nearly mature and the child is able to cope with the psychosocial aspects of facial reanimation.
- Management of traumatic neonatal facial nerve paralysis is considerably more controversial. Recommended criteria for surgical intervention are limited to
  - (a) Unilateral complete paralysis at birth
  - (b) Hemotympanum with displace temporal bone fracture
  - (c) Electrophysiologic studies demonstrating complete absence of voluntary and evoked motor unit responses in all muscles innervated by the facial nerve by 3 to 5 days
  - (d) No return of facial nerve function clinically or electrophysiologically by 5 weeks of life
- In addition to traumatic and congenital facial nerve disorders, children are subject to the same etiologic factors that result in adult facial nerve paralysis. Infection, trauma, and systemic disease have all been implicated in pediatric cases.

- *Bell palsy* is generally less common in children but is the most common diagnosis when facial paralysis occurs in older children. It has a characteristic prodrome of an upper respiratory illness and presents as unilateral facial paralysis associated with ear pain, altered taste, and reduced tearing. The prognosis for functional recovery is excellent. Treatment consists of eye protection and close observation. The benefit of steroids in children with Bell palsy is unclear due to the lack of inclusion of this population group in large controlled trials. If there is no evidence of recovery by 6 months, the diagnosis of Bell palsy should be reconsidered.

Eye Care

- The most common complication of facial nerve paralysis, regardless of cause, is corneal desiccation and exposure keratitis.
- In addition to lagophthalmos, lower lid ectropion, and diminished lacrimation, there is often altered corneal reflex. The result is a significant risk of corneal ulceration, scarring, and permanent visual loss, especially in the absence of a normal Bell phenomenon.
- Management of facial paralysis should include liberal eye lubrication, use of a protective moisture chamber at night, and use of a protective eyewear during the day.
- If recurrent ophthalmologic conditions warrant treatment or recovery of facial function is likely to be delayed, early eyelid reanimation is recommended.
- Eye closure may be restored using a temporary eyelid weight, an implanted upper eyelid weight, a palpebral spring, or lateral tarsorrhaphy.
  - (a) Upper eyelid weights and palpebral springs provide better eye protection, are easily reversible, and have become the procedures of choice. Temporary upper lid weights applied with adhesive tape may be used if short-term corneal protection is needed.
  - (b) Palpebral springs are technically more difficult to insert than upper eyelid implants.
  - (c) Tarsorrhaphy is avoided when possible as it limits the visual field, provides incomplete corneal coverage, and results in a significant additional cosmetic deformity.

Facial Reanimation

- Complete recovery of facial motor function is the goal for all patients with facial nerve paralysis; however, many will be left with significant dysfunction and will require further intervention.
- Knowledge of the etiology of the paralysis, as well as the status of the nerve and distal musculature, is crucial for appropriate management decision making.
- The ideal rehabilitative procedure for facial nerve injuries provides symmetrical appearance at rest and discrete movement of all facial musculature, both voluntary and involuntary. In addition, it eliminates or prevents mass movement and other motor deficits.

Direct Nerve Repair/Grafting

- (a) The most successful outcome is obtained with direct neural anastomosis, *neurorrhaphy*, or using interpositional grafts when tension-free primary anastomosis is not possible.

(b) Requires early recognition of the injury and assumes that the distal portion of the nerve and facial musculature are intact.

(c) Best surgical results are obtained when an endoneural anastomosis is performed.

Nerve Crossover Anastomosis

(a) Excellent technique to provide neural input to an intact distal facial nerve when the proximal nerve is not available.

(b) Most often employed in situations where damage to the proximal aspect of the nerve precludes primary neurorrhaphy.

(c) Requires intact facial musculature that is documented by EMG or muscle biopsy.

(d) Hypoglossal facial anastomosis provides the best result and is the only crossover anastomosis that has been reproducible. Resting muscle tone and protection are recovered in up to 95% of patients. Facial hypertonia and synkinesis are expected shortcomings of the surgery. The hemitongue paralysis that occurs as a result of a classic hypoglossal-facial nerve crossover procedure can result in profound functional deficits in speech, mastication, and swallowing. A hypoglossal-facial interposition jump graft will retain some hypoglossal function on the grafted side. This procedure involves interposing a nerve graft between a partially severed but functionally intact twelfth cranial nerve and the degenerated seventh cranial nerve, and is often combined with other reanimation procedures.

Neuromuscular Transfers and Facial Slings

(a) Indicated when there is irreversible atrophy of facial musculature.

(b) Confer static as well as dynamic support to oppose the activity of the contralateral facial musculature.

(c) Results are usually cosmetically inferior to that of neural reconstitution but provide important protective function to the eye and mouth.

- *Botox*: Hemifacial spasm and hyperkinetic blepharospasm are common side effects of facial nerve injury that can be extremely debilitating. *Clostridium botulinim* A toxin (Botox) is a potent neurotoxin that interferes with acetylcholine release from terminal ends of motor nerves. Botox is an effective temporary treatment for blepharospasm and hemifacial spasm. Repeated injections are generally required at 3- to 6-month intervals. Its long-term applicability is still under investigation. Complications related to the use of Botox for control of hyperkinetic activity in patients with facial dysfunction include ptosis, diplopia, corneal exposure, facial weakness, and epiphora.

Miscellaneous Notes

A. Blood supply of the facial nerve
External carotid artery (ECA) → postauricular artery → stylomastoid artery
ECA → middle meningeal artery → greater superficial petrosal artery

B. Pons to IAC = 23 to 24 mm
IAC = 8 to 10 mm
Labyrinthine = 3 to 5 mm
Tympanic = 8 to 11 mm
Mastoid = 10 to 14 mm
Parotid before branching = 15 to 20 mm

C. In parotid surgery, the facial nerve can be identified at 6 to 8 mm below the inferior "drop-off" of the tympanomastoid fissure.

D. The chorda tympani branches off at about 5 to 7 mm before the stylomastoid foramen.

E. *Bell phenomenon*: The globe turns up and out during an attempt to close the eyes.

F. Facial paralysis of central origin is characterized by
   i. Intact frontalis and orbicularis oculi
   ii. Intact mimetic function
   iii. Absence of Bell phenomenon

G. Bilateral simultaneous facial paralysis is a sign of central generalized disease and is rare in Bell palsy. The most common cause of bilateral facial paralysis is Guillain-Barré syndrome.

H. Facial nerve paralysis not involving the greater superficial petrosal nerve would give a "tearing" eye because of:
   i. Paralysis of Horner muscle that dilates the nasolacrimal duct orifice
   ii. Ectropion that produces malposition of the puncta
   iii. Absence of blinking (ie, lack of the pumping action)

I. Patients with slowly progressive facial paralysis of more than 3 weeks' duration and those with no evidence of recovery after 6 months should be suspected of having a neoplasm involving the facial nerve. Other indicators of underlying neoplastic etiology include facial twitching and ipsilateral recurrence. MRI should be obtained in these patients. Remember that progression of facial paresis in Ramsay Hunt syndrome may continue for 14 to 21 days.

J. Nearly 100% of patients with Ramsay Hunt syndrome as the cause of facial paralysis have associated pain, and 40% have sensorineural hearing loss. Vertigo, a red pinna, and vesicles in the area of sensory distribution of the facial nerve (pinna, face, neck, or oral cavity) are other signs and symptoms seen with herpes zoster oticus (Ramsay Hunt syndrome); however, the presence of pain does not rule out Bell palsy, as 60% of patients with Bell palsy will also complain of ear pain.

K. Hitzelberger sign, involving decreased sensitivity in the posterior-superior aspect of the concha corresponding to the sensory distribution of the VII nerve, suggests a space-occupying lesion in the IAC.

L. The incidence of severe neural degeneration with Bell palsy approximates 15%, whereas with herpes zoster oticus, the incidence approximates 40%.

M. Ten percent of patients with Bell palsy have a positive family history. Recurrent facial paralysis is seen in 15% of patients with Bell palsy and is more common on the contralateral side. Recurrent facial paralysis is also seen in Melkersson-Rosenthal syndrome. Other clinical features of Melkersson-Rosenthal syndrome include recurrent facial/lip swelling and fissuring of the tongue.

N. Tumors occur in 30% of patients with recurrent ipsilateral facial paralysis.

O. Twenty-five percent of longitudinal fractures involve the facial nerve; 50% of transverse fractures involve the facial nerve.

P. Bell palsy is more common in diabetics and outcomes are generally poorer compared to nondiabetics.

Q. The most likely area of compression in Bell palsy is the labyrinthine segment of the facial nerve where the fallopian canal is narrowest.

R. *Melkersson-Rosenthal syndrome*: recurrent unilateral or bilateral facial palsy of unknown etiology. It is associated with chronic or recurrent edema of the face with fissuring of the tongue. The peak age group is the 20s. Histologically, dilated lymphatic channels, giant cells, and inflammatory cells are seen.

S. *Crocodile tears*: regenerating fibers innervate the lacrimal gland instead of the salivary glands.
T. The facial nerve regenerates at 3 mm/day.
U. ENoG and EMG are the most clinically useful electrical tests for prognosticating functional recovery in patients with complete facial paralysis. ENoG testing is of value between days 3 and 14 after onset of complete paralysis. EMG is of prognostic value at anytime although spontaneous fibrillation potentials associated with muscle denervation are detected only after 10 to 21 days.

A Guideline for Management of Facial Nerve Paralysis

Bell Palsy

A. A complete otologic and audiometric evaluation is required.
B. All patients should be treated with a 10-day course of tapering oral steroids within 72 hours of onset. Antiviral therapy alone has no benefit in Bell palsy. The benefit of antiviral therapy administered in combination with oral steroids is unclear.
C. *Partial paralysis*: observe.
D. *Complete paralysis*: determine level of involvement.
  i. Electrical testing days 3 to 14 every other day until
    a. ENoG declines to less than 10% of normal side
    b. There is evidence of some return of facial function
  ii. If a. is found, lack of neural regeneration should be confirmed with the absence of voluntary motor unit action potentials on EMG testing.
  iii. Surgical decompression for Bell palsy is controversial. Decompression of the labyrinthine facial nerve has been suggested when the above electrical test criteria are met within the first 14 days following onset of complete facial paralysis.

Iatrogenic Following Ear Surgery

A. Rule out effects of local anesthetics and compressive effects of the mastoid packing.
B. EMG testing can be used to determine neural integrity immediately following surgery.
C. *Delayed onset (partial or complete)*: steroids and observe
D. *Immediate onset (complete)*: explore the nerve immediately if no improvement with A.
E. *Immediate onset (incomplete)*: observation with steroids. Consider surgical exploration if progresses rapidly to complete and intraoperative trauma suspected.

Traumatic (Head Injury)

A. *Delayed onset (partial or complete)*: observe and steroids unless contraindicated.
B. *Immediate onset (partial)*: observe and steroids unless contraindicated.
C. *Immediate onset (complete)*: consider exploring the nerve when the patient is stabilized.

Herpes Zoster Oticus

A. The most common motor nerve involved is the VII nerve, and the next are III, IV, and VI.
B. Treat with steroids and antiviral medication.

Chronic Otitis Media

Partial or complete: tympanomastoidectomy, removal of cholesteatoma and/or granulation tissue, and possible facial nerve decompression.

Acute Otitis Media/Mastoiditis

    A. Myringotomy and tube placement

    B. Systemic and topical antibiotics

    C. Mastoidectomy if coalescent mastoiditis or associated intracranial extension of infection

Bibliography

Baugh RF, Basura GJ, Ishii LE, et al. Clinical practice guideline: Bell's palsy. *Otolaryngol Head Neck Surg.* 2013;149(3 suppl)S1-S27.

Gantz BJ, Rubenstein JT, Gidley P, et al. Surgical management of Bell's palsy. *Laryngoscope.* 1999;109:1177-1188.

Gronseth GS, Paduga R. Evidence-based guideline update: steroids and antivirals for Bell's palsy: report of the Guideline Development Subcommittee of the American Academy of Neurology. *Neurology.* 2012;79:2209-2213.

McAllister K, Walker D, Donnan PT, et al. Surgical interventions for the early management of Bell's palsy. *Cochrane Database Syst Rev.* 2011;(2):CD007468.

Teixeira LJ, Valbuza JS, Prado GF. Physical therapy for Bell's palsy (idiopathic facial paralysis). *Cochrane Database Syst Rev.* 2011;7(12):CD006283.

Questions

1. What is the most common site injury to the facial nerve following blunt head trauma with fracture of the temporal bone?

    A. Mastoid segment

    B. Meatal foramen

    C. Perigeniculate area

    D. Tympanic segment

    E. Second genu

2. Which is the most common site for congenital dehiscence of the fallopian canal?

    A. Tympanic segment

    B. Mastoid segment

    C. Labyrinthine segment

    D. Geniculate ganglion

    E. Stylomastoid foramen

3. Which of the following characteristic is not consistent with Bell palsy?

    A. Complete facial paralysis

    B. Facial hyperkinesis

    C. Otalgia

    D. Hyperacusis

    E. Viral prodrome

4. Which of the following is the most appropriate treatment option for Bell palsy?

    A. Decompression of the labyrinthine segment

    B. Physical therapy

    C. Oral steroids

    D. Antiviral therapy

    E. Observation

5. A 17-year-old male patient presents with a chronic draining ear and new-onset progressive facial palsy. Which of the following imaging study would be most valuable in determining the appropriate management for this patient?

    A. High-resolution CT scan of the temporal bone

    B. Enhanced MRI of the skull base

    C. Gallium scan

    D. Technetium scan

    E. PET-CT scan

Chapter 22
Infections of the Temporal Bone

Bacterial

- Spectrum of disease from mild superficial skin infection to chondritis
  - (a) Superficial infections are commonly related to *Staphylococcus* and *Streptococcus* species.
  - (b) Any infection of deeper depth should include treatment for *Pseudomonas* species.

Etiology
  - A. Trauma—most common cause
    - i. Blunt trauma resulting in hematoma and secondary infection
    - ii. Ear piercing
  - B. Burn
  - C. Extension of otitis externa (OE)
    - i. Woody induration of the pinna can be seen with malignant otitis externa (MOE)
  - D. Extension of subperiosteal abscess
  - E. Postoperative complication of otology surgery
  - F. Rule out:
    - i. Relapsing perichondritis—autoimmune condition that involves the cartilage and spares the lobule from inflammation
    - ii. Cutaneous lymphoma
    - iii. Gouty tophus

Signs and Symptoms
  - A. Pain
  - B. Erythema
  - C. Induration or edema
  - D. Fluctuation may be seen when abscess formation occurs
  - E. Cartilage deformity in advanced or untreated cases

Diagnosis and Pathogens
  - A. *Pseudomonas* species most commonly cultured organism from abscess contents.
    - i. Antibiotic sensitivity is variable, so perform testing on any isolated organism.
  - B. *Staphylococcus aureus* also commonly cultured.
  - C. *Escherichia coli* and *Proteus* species are also common.

Treatment
  - A. Superficial infections
  - B. Mild infections
    - i. Oral anti-staphylococcal and anti-streptococcal antibiotics

C. Severe or immunocompromised
   i. Intravenous (IV) antibiotics to cover *Staphylococcus*, *Streptococcus*, and *Pseudomonas*
D. Perichondritis or chondritis
   i. Involvement of the cartilage with inflammation or abscess formation frequently results in cosmetic deformity (cauliflower ear).
   ii. Goal of treatment is to eradicate infection and maximize the aesthetic outcome.
   iii. No abscess—IV antibiotics with pseudomonal coverage, such as fluoroquinolone or aminopenicillin.
   iv. Abscess—incision and drainage with debridement of necrotic cartilage as necessary.
   v. Antibiotic therapy indicated for 2 to 4 weeks.
   vi. Tissues must be handled gently.
   vii. Place bolsters as necessary.

Viral

Herpes Zoster

Etiology
- Thought to occur following viral reactivation within the ganglion nerve cells following insult (direct trauma, dental work, upper respiratory infection) or immunosuppression.

Signs and Symptoms
- Pain in distribution of the affected nerve precedes the development of vesicular eruption.
- When associated with facial paralysis known as Ramsay Hunt syndrome.
  (a) May be associated with auditory or vestibular symptoms.
  (b) Other cranial neuropathies (V, IX, X, XI, and XII) can be seen.
  (c) Prognosis for facial nerve recovery worse than Bell palsy (60% regain normal function).

Diagnosis and Pathogens
- Tzanck smear to look for multinucleated giant cells at the base of the ruptured vesicle
  (a) Positive in herpes zoster, herpes simplex, cytomegalovirus (CMV), and pemphigus vulgaris
- Viral antibody titers
- Magnetic resonance imaging (MRI) with contrast to rule out other cause of facial paralysis in Ramsey Hunt syndrome

Treatment
- High-dose oral steroids (1 mg/kg/d × 14 days) + antiviral (acyclovir, valacyclovir).
- Surgical decompression not generally advocated as the neural degeneration is widespread rather than localized to geniculate and labyrinthine segment as seen in Bell palsy.

Fungal

Etiology
- May be localized infection or manifestation of disseminated fungal infection.
- Geographic location, particular hobbies (rose handling, etc) may aid in diagnosis.
- More common in immunocompromised patient.

Signs and Symptoms
- Erythematous, edematous skin as seen in bacterial cellulitis.
- If disseminated fungal disease, multisystem symptoms may be present.

Diagnosis
- High index of suspicion—consider if cellulitis is unresponsive to oral or IV antibiotics
- Fungal smears and cultures—may require tissue biopsy to identify organisms
- Fungal serologic titers and chest x-ray if systemic disease is suspected

Pathogens
- *Aspergillus* species
- *Histoplasma*
- *Mucormyces*
- *Candida*
- *Coccidiomyces*
- *Blastomyces*
- *Dermatophyses*
- *Sporothrix* species

Treatment
- Topical antifungals for mild infection.
- IV therapy for severe or disseminated disease.
- Consider infectious disease consultation.

Rare Pinna Infections

Parasites
- Cutaneous leishmaniasis.
- Scabies.

Mycobacterial Infection
- Leprosy—*Mycobacterium leprae*
- Cutaneous tuberculosis

External Auditory Canal

Bacterial

Acute Otitis Externa
BACTERIAL CELLULITIS OF THE EXTERNAL AUDITORY CANAL
- Furuncle is a localized abscess of the apopilosebaceous unit.
  - (a) Rupture of furuncle may result in more diffuse cellulitis and acute otitis externa (AOE).
- Carbuncle is a confluence of multiple furuncles.

ETIOLOGY
- Associated with warm, humid climates.
- Common in swimmers.
- Maceration of the ear canal skin allows invasion of skin commensal bacteria to the apopilosebaceous unit.
- Trauma to skin from cotton tip applicators or other instrumentation.
- Chronic skin conditions including eczema, psoriasis, and seborrhea dermatitis.

- Risk factors
  - (a) Immunosuppression
  - (b) Long narrow canal with poor self-cleaning capability
  - (c) Obstructive exostosis
  - (d) Lack of cerumen
    - ○ Cerumen is antibacterial.
    - ○ Acidic.
    - ○ Contains lysozyme.
    - ○ Antibodies.

SIGNS AND SYMPTOMS

- Pain—usually severe, frequently requires narcotic analgesia.
- Pruritus.
- Edema—may be severe and result in occlusion of the external auditory canal (EAC).
- Erythema.
- Otorrhea.
- Normal tympanic membrane mobility—used to distinguish from acute otitis media with perforation and subsequent otorrhea.
- Fever is rare unless there is significant periauricular cellulitis.

DIAGNOSIS

- Culture of debris is typically unhelpful as most bacteria are susceptible to the high doses of medication available in otologic drops.

PATHOGENS

- Pseudomonas species
- *S aureus*
- Other gram-negative rods (GNR)

TREATMENT

- Pain control.
- Debridement of ear canal allows topical medication to penetrate to affected tissues.
  - (a) Otowick may be necessary in severe infection with obstructive edema.
    - ○ Allows antibiotic drops to treat medial tissues
    - ○ Should be replaced every 3 to 5 days to avoid toxic shock syndrome
- Acidification—prevents bacterial overgrowth and fungal secondary infection.
  - (a) For mild infection dilute vinegar irrigation may be all that is needed.
- Dry ear precautions.
  - (a) Prevent water entry during bathing.
  - (b) Use of a hairdryer on low setting 12 to 18 in from the ear for 2 to 3 minutes following bath.
- Topical antibiotics.
  - (a) Provide high concentrations of medication to the canal without systemic toxicity.
  - (b) Frequently effective in treating periauricular cellulitis as well.
  - (c) Neomycin may cause a dermatitis in some patients that is indistinguishable from AOE. Consider switching agents if patient does not respond to neomycin containing drop.
- Oral antibiotics.
  - (a) Not used for uncomplicated AOE.
  - (b) May be considered for patients with severe periauricular cellulitis and immunocompromise.
- Incision and drainage.
  - (a) Used for furuncles or carbuncles, then treat with topical antibiotics.
  - (b) Otowick can be placed following incision and drainage.

Myringitis
Uncommon infection of the tympanic membrane
- Two percent of patients with acute otitis media (AOM) will develop bullous myringitis.
- Chronic myringitis is one-tenth as common as chronic otitis media (COM).

Acute (Bullous Myringitis)
- Less than 1 month

ETIOLOGY
- Primary—no middle ear (ME) pathology
- Secondary—associated with AOM

SIGNS AND SYMPTOMS
- Severe pain lasting for 3 to 4 days then subsiding.
- Blisters on the lateral surface of tympanic membrane (TM) or medial EAC.
- Hemorrhagic myringitis demonstrates no blisters but extravascular blood in the middle layer of the TM.

DIAGNOSIS
- Diagnosis is made on physical examination.

PATHOGENS
- *Streptococcus pneumoniae.*
- Nontypable *Hemophilus influenzae.*
- *Moraxella catarrhalis.*
- *Mycoplasma pneumoniae* is no long felt to be a primary pathogen for primary bullous myringitis.

TREATMENT
- Topical antibiotics
- Lance the bullae for pain control
- If secondary then treat AOM with oral antibiotics
- Dry ear precautions

Chronic (Granular) Myringitis
- Uncommon, prolonged, and difficult to treat infection of the lateral surface of the TM.
- Characterized by loss of epithelium of the TM and replacement with granulation tissue.
- Relapsing and recurring symptoms are common.

ETIOLOGY
- Unclear. No, predisposing factors have been identified.

SIGNS AND SYMPTOMS
- Painless otorrhea.
- Pruritus.
- Severe cases can result in conductive hearing loss due to TM thickening and blunting.
- Late stages—scarring of the anterior angle resulting blunting or acquired canal stenosis or obliteration.
- Replacement of epithelium with beefy, weeping granulation tissue.
- Thirty-three percent of patients develop TM perforation at some time during the disease process, frequently heals spontaneously (Blevins).
- Lack of ME pathology.

DIAGNOSIS
- Diagnosis based on history and physical examination
- May require computed tomography (CT) of temporal bone to rule out COM

PATHOGENS
- *Pseudomonas aeruginosa*
- *S aureus*
- *Proteus mirabilis*

TREATMENT
- Numerous treatment regimens in the literature
- Topical antibiotics
- Drying agents
- Chemical cautery (silver nitrate or trichloroacetic acid [TCA])
- Laser cautery with CO_2 laser
- Acidification with dilute vinegar irrigation
- Tympanoplasty with canaloplasty reserved for severe or obliterative disease
  - (a) Surgery frequently exacerbates the condition.
  - (b) Recurrence is common.

Chronic Bacterial Otitis Externa

Etiology
- Associated with chronic skin conditions such as seborrhea dermatitis and atopic dermatitis
- Chronic inflammation within the dermis and surrounding the apocrine glands resulting in increased depth of rete pegs
- Loss of normal sebaceous glands

Signs and Symptoms
- Thickened skin of the cartilaginous canal
- Keratosis—adherent skin debris
- Lichenification
- Pruritus
- Lack of otalgia
- Canal obliteration in late stage disease

Diagnosis
- Biopsy, especially if granulation is present

Pathogens
- Gram-negative species, especially *Proteus*

Treatment
- Frequent debridement
- Treatment of underlying skin condition
- Topical antibiotics
- Topical steroids
- Canaloplasty with split thickness skin graft for obliterative cases

Skull base Osteomyelitis (Aka Malignant Otitis Externa or Necrotizing Otitis Externa)
- Primarily in immunocompromised patients
- Severe infection of the EAC and skull base
- Still highly morbid even in the antibiotic era
  - (a) Mortality rates between 5% and 20%
- Must have a high index of suspicion
  - (a) Most patients delay in treatment up to 6 months from the onset of symptoms.

Etiology
- Diabetics with microangiopathy and cellular immune dysfunction allows bacterial invasion of the vessel walls.
  - (a) Vessel thrombosis
  - (b) Coagulative necrosis of surrounding tissue

- Other immune dysfunction such as malignancy or human immunodeficiency virus (HIV) or acquired immunodeficiency syndrome (AIDS) or transplant recipients may have a rapid progression of disease.
- Proposed to begin as AOE but microorganisms then invade bone through fissures of Santorini and progress medially.

Signs and Symptoms
- Deep-seated aural pain (pain out of proportion to examination findings).
- Otorrhea.
- Granulation tissue along the tympanomastoid suture line.
- Edema.
- Cranial nerve palsy.
  (a) CN VII most commonly affected.
  (b) CN VI, IX, X, XI, and XII may be affected.
    ○ Multiple cranial neuropathies are indicative of worse prognosis.
- Involvement of the cavernous sinus and CN III, IV, and VI.
- Thrombosis of the sigmoid and transverse sinuses then propagating to the internal jugular vein.
- Intracranial abscess and meningitis are usually terminal events.

Diagnosis
- Biopsy of granulation tissue used to rule out noninfectious (malignant) process
- Imaging
  (a) Nuclear imaging
    ○ Technetium Tc99 scintigraphy (bone scan) is imaging of choice to confirm diagnosis.
      – Concentrates in areas of osteoblastic activity
      – Can detect inflammation in bone before bony destruction seen on CT
      – Used in diagnosis only as remains positive indefinitely
    ○ Gallium 67 is used to follow treatment response.
      – Should be scanned every 4 weeks of therapy to assess response
  (b) CT
    ○ Useful for evaluating extent of bony destruction.
    ○ Contrasted studies can be used to identify associated abscess or cellulitis.
  (c) MRI
    ○ Used if intracranial extension is suspected

Pathogens
- *P aeruginosa* most common pathogen.
- *S aureus*, *Klebsiella* species, and *P mirabilis* are also reported.
- Fungal MOE 15% of cases.
  (a) Aspergillus fumigatus.
  (b) Mucormycoses have been reported.

Treatment
- Aggressive diabetic control.
- Gentle EAC debridement.
- Correct immunodeficiency if possible (decrease immunosuppressant medication or stimulate bone marrow production).
- Long antibiotic therapy.
  (a) Monotherapy with oral fluoroquinolone is first-line therapy.
    ○ Have been increasing reports of quinolone-resistant *Pseudomonas*
  (b) IV antipseudomonal aminopenicillins is second-line therapy for those who cannot take quinolones.

- Parenteral antifungal therapy required for invasive fungal disease (amphotericin B).
- Surgical intervention warranted for drainage of associated abscesses and debridement of bony sequestrum.

Fungal

Acute Fungal Otitis Externa (Otomycosis)
Etiology
- Warm wet ear canal (swimmers, surfers, divers, tropical environment)
- Trauma to ear canal
- Fungal overgrowth in patients with postsurgical mastoid cavities
- Immunocompromised patients

Signs and Symptoms
- Indistinguishable from acute bacterial OE.
- Fungal hyphae may be visible.
- Pruritus is a more common complaint than in bacterial infections.

Diagnosis
- Cultures not usually helpful
- Biopsy with tissue culture in immunocompromised patients or atypical presentations

Pathogens
- *Candida, Aspergillus,* and *Penicillium* are the most common species.

Treatment
- Meticulous canal debridement
- Dry ear precautions
- Acidify and drying agents
  - (a) Boric acid
  - (b) Gentian violet
  - (c) Many others
- Topical antifungal agents
  - (a) Clotrimazole
  - (b) CFS-H powder (requires a compounding pharmacy)
    - ○ Chloromycetin
    - ○ Amphotericin B (Fungizone)
    - ○ Sulfanilamide
    - ○ Hydrocortisone
- Systemic antifungal therapy
  - (a) Reserved for severely immunocompromised with suspicion of invasive fungal disease

Infections of the Middle Ear and Mastoid

Suppurative Otitis Media

Acute Otitis Media
Epidemiology
- Most common cause for pediatrician visits in the United States
- Significant direct and indirect costs of the disease
  - (a) Physician visits and prescription medication
  - (b) Lost days of work and school
- Risk factors
  - (a) Cleft palate

(b) Genetic predisposing—Down syndrome
(c) Indigenous people
  ○ Native American
  ○ Inuit
  ○ Native Australians
(d) Lower socioeconomic status
(e) Premature birth
(f) Presence of siblings
(g) Attendance at day care facility
(h) Second hand smoke exposure
(i) Lack of breastfeeding in the first 6 months of life
(j) Supine bottle feeding

Etiology

- Frequently associated with upper respiratory tract infection (URI) symptoms implicate obstruction of eustachian tube (ET).
  (a) ET lined by Gerlach tonsil which may become inflamed during URI and compromise ET function
- Adenoid pad harbors reservoir of bacteria that can reflux into the ME.
- Combination of poor ME clearance and refluxed bacteria leads to acute inflammation of the ME and TM.

Signs and Symptoms

- Otalgia
- Irritability
- Fever
- Bulging of the TM—best indicator of AOM
- Limited or absence of movement of the TM
- Air–fluid level behind the TM
- Otorrhea if TM is ruptured
- Erythema of the TM

Diagnosis

- Acute onset of symptoms.
- Presence of a ME effusion (MEE).
- Signs and symptoms of ME inflammation.
- Clinical history of ear pulling, fever, and irritability is nonspecific for AOM.
- Physical examination with pneumatic otoscopy is required to make the diagnosis.
- If physical examination is still equivocal, adjunctive testing such as tympanometry or acoustic reflex testing may be used to determine the presence of a MEE.

Pathogens

- *S pneumoniae* is the most common organism.
  (a) Introduction of prior 7-valent and current 13-valent pneumococcal vaccine has altered the prevalence of certain serotypes.
    ○ Introduction of the vaccine has decreased the absolute number of invasive complications related to pneumococcal infection.
    ○ Serotype 19A is a highly multidrug-resistant strain that has become more prevalent since introduction of the pneumococcal vaccine.
      – Unclear if this change is due to a decrease in the strains covered by the vaccine or natural change in resistance patterns
  (b) Mechanism of pneumococcal penicillin resistance is due to alterations of the penicillin-binding proteins in the cell wall.

- *H influenzae* and *M catarrhalis* are the other most common pathogens.
  - (a) *Haemophilus influenzae* strains are predominantly nonserotypable since the introduction of the *H influenzae* type b (HIB) vaccine.
  - (b) Fifty percent of *H influenzae* and 100% of *M catarrhalis* are beta-lactamase positive.
- Viruses are likely a significant contributor to AOM.
  - (a) Respiratory syncytial virus (RSV)
  - (b) Rhinovirus
  - (c) Coronavirus
  - (d) Parainfluenza virus
  - (e) Enterovirus
  - (f) Adenovirus
  - (g) Virus has been identified in up to 75% of AOM aspirates

Treatment

- Recommendations for treatment of AOM were published in 2004 by the American Academy of Pediatrics (AAP) in conjunction with the American Academy of Family Practice (AAFP) and the American Academy of Otolaryngology–Head and Neck Surgery (AAO–HNS); recent revised guidelines for diagnosis and management of AOM in children aged 6 months to 12 years were published in 2013 by the AAP/AAFP
  - (a) Guidelines for children without underlying medical conditions (immunodeficiencies), genetic conditions (Down syndrome), cochlear implants (CIs), recurrent AOM, or AOM with underlying chronic otitis media with effusion (COME).
- Pain control
  - (a) Very important component of therapy
  - (b) Frequently overlooked by treating clinician
  - (c) Oral analgesic or antipyretics
    - ○ Acetaminophen
    - ○ Ibuprofen
    - ○ Narcotics
      - − Respiratory depression is a problem with this class of medication and should be used sparingly.
  - (d) Topical analgesics
    - ○ Benzocaine drops
      - − Short-lived effect
      - − May be useful in patients elder than 5 years
  - (e) Myringotomy or tympanostomy
    - ○ Relieves the pressure within the ME space which causes the pain
    - ○ Requires sedation in children
    - ○ Requires access to specialty equipment
    - ○ Risk of chronic perforation
- Antibiotics should be prescribed for bilateral or unilateral AOM in children aged at least 6 months with severe signs or symptoms (moderate or severe otalgia or otalgia for 48 hours or longer or temperature 39°C or higher) and for nonsevere, bilateral AOM in children aged 6 to 23 months
- Option for observation for 48 to 72 hours without antibiotic intervention.
  - (a) May be advised in certain situations as the natural history of AOM is resolution of symptoms and effusion over time in the majority of patients.
  - (b) Patients should still be treated for pain.

(c) Children younger than 2 years should be treated with antibiotics as the rates of failure are high in this group when not treated.

(d) Children elder than 2 years can be observed if the symptoms are mild or the diagnosis is uncertain.

(e) If the child fails to improve, antibiotic therapy is instituted.

   ◦ Requires compliant parents with ready access to health care provider

(f) Does not appear to result in increased rates of mastoiditis.

(g) Institution of antibiotic therapy decreases symptomatic infection by 1 day compared to observation.

   ◦ Does not decrease missed school or work days

- 2010 analysis of data suggests that there is a benefit to immediate antibiotic treatment.

(a) If 100 otherwise healthy children are assessed for AOM, 80 will improve within 3 days without antibiotics.

(b) Immediate institution of antibiotics would increase the improvement to 92 children.

(c) However, 3 to 10 children would develop a rash and 8 to 10 children would develop diarrhea.

(d) Clinician and parents must decide if risk of gastrointestinal (GI) side effects justifies the use of antibiotic treatment.

- Guidelines for otherwise healthy children are:

(a) Amoxicillin 90 mg/kg/d divided tid

   ◦ Provides high enough tissue concentrations to overcome bacterial resistance in most intermediate-resistant (> 0.1-1 µg/mL minimal inhibitory concentration [MIC]) pneumococcal strains and *H influenzae* and *M catarrhalis* strains.

   ◦ Length of treatment is controversial.

   – Patients receiving therapy for less than 7 days have higher rates of recurrence but less GI side effects.

   – Patients receiving standard 10-day course of therapy have lower rates of recurrence but higher rates of nausea, vomiting, and diarrhea.

   – Current recommendations are:

     ◊ Children under 2 years—10 days of therapy

     ◊ Children 2 to 5 years—10 days of therapy

     ◊ Children greater than 6 years—5 to 7 days of therapy if mild to moderate disease

   ◦ Children harboring highly resistant *Pneumococcus* (MIC > 2 µg/mL) will not respond to this regimen.

   – Children in group day care or those with older siblings are at risk for these strains.

   ◦ Patients with severe illness (fever > 39°C, severe otalgia) or in whom *H influenzae* or *M catarrhalis* are suspected should be started on amoxicillin-clavulanate (90 mg/kg/d of amoxicillin and 6.4 mg/kg/d of clavulanate).

(b) Penicillin-allergic patients

   ◦ Type I hypersensitivity (ie, urticaria and anaphylaxis)

   – Azithromycin 10 mg/kg for 1 day then 5 mg/kg for 4 days

   – Clarithromycin

   – Erythromycin—sulfisoxazole

   ◦ Those known to harbor highly resistant *Pneumococcus* should receive clindamycin 30 to 40 mg/kg/d divided tid

- (c) AOM treatment failure
  - ○ Failure if symptoms do not improve within 48 to 72 hours of starting antibiotic therapy
  - ○ If started on amoxicillin, then switch to amoxicillin–clavulanate
  - ○ If on amoxicillin–clavulanate, 3-day course of parenteral ceftriaxone (IM or IV)
    - – Pneumococcal resistance to erythromycin and trimethoprim–sulfasoxazole is high enough to warrant parenteral therapy with a third-generation cephalosporin.
  - ○ Tympanocentesis with cultures
    - – Should be considered when patients fail second-line therapies.
  - ○ Treatment failure more common in younger patients, those in group day care, geographic regions with highly resistant bacteria
- Special populations
  - (a) Cochlear implant recipients
    - ○ CI patients should be vaccinated with 13-valent pneumococcal vaccine at least 2 weeks prior to implantation.
    - ○ Close contacts (family members and care givers) should also receive this vaccine.
    - ○ After age 24 months, the 23-valent pneumococcal vaccine can be given.
    - ○ Children with CI are at higher risk for development of meningitis.
      - – Many CI patients who develop meningitis also have AOM at the time of diagnosis.
    - ○ The presumed pathogens are the same that cause AOM in the general population; however, no study is available to confirm this.
    - ○ CI patients should not undergo a period of observation if a diagnosis of AOM is made.
      - – AOM within the first 2 months after implantation should be treated aggressively with parenteral antibiotics to prevent both meningitis and device infection.
      - – AOM developing greater than 2 months after implantation can be treated with high-dose oral amoxicillin or amoxicillin-clavulanate.
        - ◊ Patients must be closely monitored.
        - ◊ If any sign of treatment failure, parenteral antibiotic therapy should be instituted.
        - ◊ Tympanocentesis is appropriate in this population to guide antimicrobial therapy.
    - ○ Possible meningitis should be aggressively worked up.
      - – Lumbar puncture for cerebrospinal fluid (CSF) cultures.
      - – Within first 2 months of implantation, higher rates of GNR.
      - – Greater than 2 months, same organisms as meningitis caused by AOM.
      - – Broad-spectrum antibiotic coverage is warranted.
    - ○ Tympanostomy tubes in CI patients.
      - – Controversial topic.
      - – If child has history of recurrent AOM prior to implantation, consider subtotal petrosectomy, eustachian tube ablation with ear canal closure, and second-stage CI.
      - – Exposure of the electrode within the ME may put patient at risk for biofilm infection.
      - – Preliminary data suggest that tubes in CI patients do not increase the risk of infectious complications but randomized controlled trial (RCT) data are lacking.

Recurrent Acute Otitis Media

Most commonly seen in children younger than 2 years with highest incidence in the 6- to 12-month age group.

Etiology
- Viral and bacterial disease
- Similar risk factors as AOM (see earlier)

Signs and Symptoms
- Same as for AOM
- May have effusion between episodes without evidence of inflammation of the TM or ME

Diagnosis
- *Definition*: Three or more episodes of AOM in a 6-month period or four or more episodes in a 12-month period
  (a) Must be asymptomatic between episodes

Pathogens
- Same as AOM

Treatment
- Prophylactic antibiotics
  (a) Not recommended
  (b) Increases rates of antibiotic resistance
  (c) Increases incidences of GI complications
  (d) Requires 9 months of treatment to prevent one episode of AOM
- Tympanostomy tubes (grommets)
  (a) Significantly decrease the number of AOM episodes.
  (b) Children with grommets who develop AOM will develop painless otorrhea that can be treated with topical antibiotics.
- Adenoidectomy
  (a) Cochrane review demonstrated no benefit in decreased number of AOM events following adenoidectomy.
- Risk reduction

Chronic Suppurative Otitis Media (With or Without Cholesteatoma)

Etiology
- Biofilms
  (a) Relatively new theory on etiology of COM.
  (b) Sessile highly organized networks of bacteria.
    ○ Different from bacterial colonization in that biofilms illicit a host inflammatory response
    ○ Unclear what causes conversion between colonization and biofilm infection as many patients are colonized with pathologic bacteria but few proceed to clinically significant infection (ie, COM)
  (c) Significantly different characteristics from free-floating (planktonic) bacteria.
    ○ Decreased metabolic rate
    ○ Different gene expression
    ○ Encased within matrix containing oligopolysaccarides
      – Inhibits innate host immune response as leukocytes are unable to penetrate the matrix
    ○ Innate antibiotic resistance
      – Production of efflux pumps not seen in planktonic bacteria
  (d) Most bacteria can form biofilms.

- ○ All major OM pathogens readily form biofilms.
- ○ Biofilms frequently polymicrobial.
  - (e) Biofilm matrix contains bacterial endo- and exotoxins that illicit host response.
  - (f) Biofilms may be adherent to respiratory epithelium, organized within mucus, or intracellularly within the respiratory epithelium.
    - ○ Intracellular aggregates have been found in clinical specimens from OM patients.
    - ○ May be reservoir for reinfection.
    - ○ Multiple locations within the same patient have been identified.
      - – Multiple areas for persistent infection
- ET dysfunction
  - (a) Abnormal function of ET leads to reduced aeration of the ME space.
  - (b) Nitrogen-absorbing cells within the mastoid antrum reduced the volume of air within the ME cleft resulting in negative pressure.
  - (c) TM retracts as a result of negative pressure.
    - ○ Most susceptible area for retraction is pars flacida due to inherent weakness in this area.
  - (d) Localized areas of negative pressure and retraction can occur.
    - ○ Isolated pars flacida retraction with normal ME aeration
- Risk factors
  - (a) Genetic
    - ○ Higher incidence in native populations (native Americans, Inuit, native Australian, or native New Zealanders)
  - (b) Nasopharyngeal reflux
  - (c) Chronic ME or TM dysfunction
    - ○ Tympanostomy tube or perforation resulting in exposure of the ME mucosa to contamination from the EAC

Signs and Symptoms
- TM perforation
- Hearing loss
  - (a) Typically conductive hearing loss (HL) confirmed by tuning fork examination
    - ○ Aural fullness.
    - ○ Chronic or intermittent otorrhea.
    - ○ Middle ear mucosa inflamed.
    - ○ Granulation tissue or aural polyps may be visible and obscure normal landmarks.
    - ○ TM retraction pockets +/− keratin debris.

Diagnosis
- Directed at identifying cholesteatoma.
  - (a) Otomicroscopy with pneumatic insufflation
- Audiometry.
- Routine cultures are unhelpful.
  - (a) Biofilms are frequently culture negative.
  - (b) Can typically identify bacteria via reverse transcriptase polymerase chain reaction (RT-PCR) for bacterial messenger ribonucleic acid (mRNA).
- Imaging
  - (a) High-resolution CT temporal bone
    - ○ Used if complications of COM or cholesteatoma are suspected
    - ○ Treatment failures
    - ○ Revision procedures

(b) MRI with contrast
  ○ Used if intracranial complications are suspected
- Biopsy
  (a) Persistent granulation tissue should be biopsied after an appropriate course of topical antibiotics to rule out malignancy or other pathology (ie, Wegener granulomatosis, tuberculosis [TB]).

Pathogens
- Nonserotypable *H influenzae* is the most common pathogen found within OM biofilms.
- Pneumococcus, *M catarrhalis, S aureus,* and *P aeruginosa* can all be found within OM biofilms.

Treatment
- Goal is to create a dry, safe ear
  (a) Dry = no otorrhea
  (b) Safe = no collection of keratin debris, reduce risk of suppurative complications
- Antibiotics
  (a) Used to stop otorrhea and decrease the likelihood of suppurative complication.
  (b) Bacteria within biofilms are frequently resistant to both topical and systemic antibiotics.
    ○ Although concentrations within topical antibiotics are high enough to overcome resistance in planktonic bacteria, biofilms have adapted multicellular strategies to overcome even elevated antibiotic levels.
      – Efflux pumps
    ○ However, current standard is to treat with topical antibiotics in cases with perforated TM.
      – 4- to 6-week course following debridement
      – Polymyxin b or neomycin or hydrocortisone
        ◊ Theoretical risk of inner ear injury from neomycin
      – Fluoroquinolone
  (c) Adenoids may serve as reservoir for bacteria causing biofilms in the ME.
    ○ Adenoidectomy is not routinely advocated in this patient population but may be considered on an individual basis.
- Surgery
  (a) Tympanoplasty
    ○ Majority of patients will have successful surgery (60%-90% closure rates).
    ○ Likelihood of successful surgery increased if air can be insufflated through the perforation and felt by the patient in the nasopharynx.
    ○ Indicated for patients with recurrent suppuration due to water exposure.
  (b) Tympanomastoidectomy
    ○ Used in cases with suspected or diagnosed cholesteatoma or otorrhea refractory to medical treatment
    ○ Goals of surgery
      – Identify and remove all cholesteatoma.
      – Removal of granulation tissue.
      – Restoration of continuity between ME cleft and mastoid cavity.
        ◊ Epitympanum and aditus ad antrum are frequently obstructed by disease.
        ◊ Reestablishes more physiologic aeration patterns.
    ○ Multiple approaches

  - Canal wall up
  - Canal wall reconstruction with mastoid obliteration
  - Canal wall down
  ○ Details of these procedures are beyond the scope of this chapter. The reader is directed to *Brackmann, Shelton and Arriaga's Otologic Surgery*, third edition for a more detailed description of these procedures.
- Eustachian tube treatment
  (a) Many remedies have been tried but none have demonstrated long-term efficacy in providing a functional ET.
    ○ Balloon tuboplasty
    ○ Laser tuboplasty
    ○ Finger manipulation of ET orifice
    ○ ET implants
    ○ Many others

Chronic OM With Effusion
A. Extremely common in children
  i. Sixty percent of children will have had an MEE by the age of 6 years.
  ii. Highest incidence in 1- to 2-year-old children.

Etiology
- ET dysfunction as a result of viral URI or allergy causes reduced middle ear clearance.
  (a) Unilateral MEE in adult necessitates examination of the nasopharynx to rule out nasopharyngeal mass or malignancy.
- Transudate from middle ear mucosa forms.
  (a) Secretion of glycoproteins from middle ear mucosa increases fluid viscosity and may slow transit out of the ME cleft.
- Bacterial infection of the ME effusion then results in clinical infection.
  (a) Likely from adenoid reservoir
- Biofilms
  (a) Direct connection between biofilms and COME less clear than in COM.
  (b) However, biofilms can form in less than 3 days on a mucosal surface after inoculation by pathogenic bacteria.
- In children, COME can usually be linked to an episode of AOM.

Signs and Symptoms
- Aural fullness
- Hearing loss
  (a) Conductive
- Visible ME effusion
- Intact TM
- Frequently asymptomatic, especially in children

Diagnosis
- *Definition*: inflammation within the ME space resulting in a collection of fluid behind an intact TM.
- This diagnosis implies a lack of otalgia and systemic symptoms such as pyrexia and malaise.
- Pneumatic otoscopy is key for making the diagnosis.
  (a) Tympanometry may assist when physical examination is equivocal.
- Unilateral effusion should be further investigated to rule out nasopharyngeal pathology.
  (a) Nasopharyngoscopy
  (b) CT or MRI if direct examination is impossible

Treatment
- Goals to restore hearing and prevent further complications within the ME space (ossicular damage or TM atelectasis or cholesteatoma).
- Seventy percent of children will clear an ME effusion within 3 months.
- Ninety percent of children will clear an MEE within 3 months when associated with a treated episode of AOM.
- 2004 clinical practice guidelines published by a joint committee of the AAO–HNS, AAP, AAFP, updated in 2013
  - (a) Watchful waiting is appropriate in children without evidence of hearing loss, speech delay, developmental disability, or TM complication.
    - If these complications occur, surgery recommended.
    - Observation can be continued until the effusion resolves spontaneously.
  - (b) Antibiotics, corticosteroids, antihistamines, and decongestants do not have long-term benefit in eradicating the MEE and should not be used routinely.
  - (c) Tympanostomy tube should be used for those with hearing loss, speech delay, developmental disability, and TM complications.
- Adenoidectomy.
  - (a) Cochrane review demonstrated reduction in rate of COME following adenoidectomy.
    - Clinical significance of this reduction was unclear as there was no statistically significant change in hearing.
    - Possible benefits would include reduction of TM retraction, atelectasis, and chronic perforation but no study has looked at these outcomes.
  - (b) Tonsillectomy is not effective for treating COME.

Special Populations
- Cleft palate
  - (a) Nearly all children with this condition will develop COME.
  - (b) Comprehensive treatment by cleft palate team should include an otolaryngologist to assess for TM and ME status.
  - (c) Etiology is ET dysfunction.
  - (d) Most children will require tympanostomy tubes.
  - (e) Some will require reconstructive techniques for TM and ossicular damage.
- Down syndrome
  - (a) High incidence of COME in this population due to mid-face hypoplasia, ET dysfunction, and immune system immaturity.
  - (b) Indications for intervention are same as advised in 2004 recommendations.
  - (c) Higher rate of tympanostomy tube placement due to developmental delay and speech delay confounded by conductive hearing loss.
  - (d) Patients with chronic ET dysfunction may require cartilage tympanoplasty procedures to prevent recurrence of TM atelectasis or perforation.

Tuberculous Otitis Media
- In early 20th century it was responsible for up to 20% of COM.
  - (a) Rates declined as antibiotic therapy and living conditions improved.
  - (b) Increasing incidence again due to multidrug-resistant strains, rise of immuno-compromised patients (HIV or AIDS, transplant recipients, malignancy, etc), and immigration from endemic regions.

Etiology
- Hematogenous spread from a primary lung infection

- Direct inoculation of the bacillus through the ear canal from respiratory droplets
- Direct extension from nasopharynx and ET

Signs and Symptoms
- Thin, cloudy, painless otorrhea
- Thickened TM
- Multiple perforations within the TM in early disease
- Subtotal or total TM perforation in late disease
- Hearing loss—usually conductive
- Polypoid granulation tissue in the ME cleft
- Pale thickened mucosa within the antrum or mastoid
- Facial paresis or paralysis in 10%
- COM that is unresponsive to standard antibiotics
- History of failed ME or mastoid surgery

Diagnosis
- Biopsy
  - (a) Positive staining for acid-fast bacilli (AFB)
    - ○ AFB may be negative due to fastidious nature of the organism.
  - (b) Caseating granulomas
  - (c) Consider PCR for *Mycobacterium tuberculosis* DNA if high index of suspicion
- Chest x-ray
- Skin testing with purified protein derivative (PPD)
- CT temporal bone
  - (a) Findings consistent with chronic OM
    - ○ Mucosal thickening with mastoid opacification.
    - ○ Normal septations in 50%.
    - ○ 25% will demonstrate bony erosion.
    - ○ Ossicular erosion.

Pathogen
- *M tuberculosis*
- Atypical *Mycobacterium* uncommon

Treatment
- Medical therapy is first line.
  - (a) Multidrug antituberculous regimen.
    - ○ Isoniazid
    - ○ Rifampin
    - ○ Ethambutol
    - ○ Pyrazinamide
  - (b) Surgery indicated for TM and ossicular chain repair or for biopsy.
    - ○ Following medical therapy, successful surgery is possible in up to 90% of patients.
  - (c) Return of facial function is good following medical therapy.

Complications of Otitis Media and Mastoiditis

Intratemporal

Hearing Loss
- A. Conductive HL
  - i. Occurs to some extent in all cases of AOM and most COM.

ii. ME effusion decreases TM compliance.
    a. Resolves as effusion clears
iii. Erosion of the ossicular chain in COM
    a. Fibrous union at incudostapedial joint is the most common finding.
    b. Does not resolve spontaneously.
B. Sensorineural HL (SNHL)
  i. Unusual complication
  ii. Usually mediated by bacterial exotoxins and inflammatory cytokines
    a. See the section Infections of the Inner Ear.

Vestibular Dysfunction
A. Usually mediated by bacterial exotoxins and inflammatory cytokines
  i. See the section Infections of the Inner Ear.

Tympanic Membrane perforation
A. AOM
  i. Spontaneous rupture of the TM.
    a. Occurs in approximately 5% of cases.
  ii. Typically heals rapidly without intervention.
    a. Ninety percent of spontaneous ruptures healed without intervention.
B. COM
  i. Hallmark of chronic disease.
  ii. Successful repair depends on ET function.

Mastoiditis

Complication of AOM
- Distinction must be made between radiographic and clinic mastoiditis.
  (a) Clinic disease results in:
    ◦ Postauricular skin changes
    ◦ Mastoid tenderness
    ◦ Auricular protrusion
    ◦ Fullness of the posterior-superior EAC skin
    ◦ Peripheral blood leukocytosis
    ◦ Systemic toxicity (ie, fever, lethargy etc)
- Likely that some degree of subclinical mastoiditis accompany most cases of AOM.
  (a) Mastoid opacification can be seen routinely on CT of temporal bone during acute infection.
  (b) Clinically relevant disease is more common in partially or untreated AOM.
  (c) Coalescent mastoiditis.
    ◦ Purulent fluid collection within the mastoid
    ◦ Results in above-mentioned signs of clinical mastoiditis in addition to radiographic evidence of bony erosion on CT
      – Irregular bony destruction of mastoid air cells
    ◦ Indication for immediate or urgent surgical intervention
  (d) Can progress to involve other contiguous areas.

Pathogens
- In patients with previously treated AOM, 30% to 50% will not yield an organism on cultures.
- *S pnuemoniae* is the most common cultured organism.
  (a) Following introduction of pneumococcal vaccine absolute incidence of pneumococcal AOM has decreased.
  (b) However, now seeing rise in number of cases of more virulent organisms not covered by vaccine which may lead to increase in rates of complicated infections.

- *Pseudomonas* species
- *S aureus*
- Polymicrobial infection
- *S pyogenes*
- Other GNR

Treatment
- Infection limited to temporal bone
  - (a) Depends on the toxicity of the patient
    - ○ Severely ill patients may require earlier surgical intervention.
  - (b) IV antibiotics—first line
    - ○ Empiric therapy with third-generation cephalosporin or antipseudomonal aminopenicillin
    - ○ If no improvement after 24 to 48 hours of therapy consider surgical intervention
  - (c) Surgery
    - ○ Tympanostomy with tube placement
    - ○ Mastoidectomy
      - – Indicated in coalescent mastoiditis as primary therapy followed by antibiotics
      - – Performed if cholesteatoma suspected
      - – Failure of tympanostomy and antibiotics
- Infection beyond the mastoid
  - (a) IV antibiotics
  - (b) Mastoidectomy
  - (c) Incision and drainage of any abscess
  - (d) If intracranial complication, may require intracranial procedure to address suppuration
- Following symptom resolution, continue on 14 days of oral antibiotics

Acquired Cholesteatoma
- Occurs in COM.
- Believed to occur due to retraction pocket of TM as a result of ET dysfunction.
- Secondary infection of the cholesteatoma debris results in painless otorrhea.
- A full discussion of cholesteatoma, its etiology, and treatment is beyond the scope of this chapter.

Facial Nerve Dysfunction
- Mediated by bacterial exotoxins and inflammatory mediators
- Access the nerve through dehiscent fallopian canal
  - (a) Up to 20% of population have bony dehiscence in the tympanic segment.
- AOM with facial paralysis
  - (a) Myringotomy
  - (b) IV and topical antibiotics
  - (c) Recovery rate is high
- COM with facial paralysis
  - (a) Frequently associated with infected cholesteatoma.
  - (b) Tympanomastoidectomy should be performed.
    - ○ Remove matrix and granulation tissue from the epineurium.
    - ○ Bony decompression without neurolysis for the remaining tympanic and mastoid segments.
  - (c) IV antibiotics acutely with transition to oral antibiotics based on cultures.
  - (d) Recovery to House-Brackmann grades I to II in 52% to 83% of patients.

Labyrinthine Fistula

- COM with cholesteatoma
  (a) Occurs in up to 10% of patients.
  (b) May be asymptomatic.
    ○ Must have a high index of suspicion when removing matrix from the surface of the lateral canal
  (c) Any balance canal or cochlea can be affected.
  (d) Treatment is controversial.
    ○ Complete matrix removal with fistula repair
      – Usually recommended for small fistulae.
      – Larger fistulae of balance canals can be safely exenterated with obliteration of the open bony channel using bone wax or pâté then resurfaced with fascia.
      – Can leave canal wall intact.
      – Conflicting data if there is increased risk of SNHL if matrix is completely removed.
    ○ Exteriorization
      – Leave matrix over the exposed canal
      – Requires a canal wall down mastoidectomy
    ○ Fistula of the cochlea associated with high rates of profound SNHL when manipulated

Petrous Apicitis

- Rare in the antibiotic era.
- Triad of symptoms (Gradenigo syndrome).
  (a) Otorrhea
  (b) Retro-orbital pain
  (c) Diplopia caused by CN VI palsy
- IV antibiotics first line of therapy.
- Petrous apicectomy should be considered if infection does not improve or intracranial complications are suspected.
- If due to COM with cholesteatoma:
  (a) IV antibiotics first
  (b) Surgical management of the cholesteatoma when acute infection resolved

Extratemporal

Extracranial

A. Typically extension of acute mastoiditis
  i. Subperiostial abscess
    a. Usually associated with mastoiditis.
    b. Treatment varies in the literature.
      1. Needle aspiration with IV antibiotics may be used in small children.
      2. Incision and drainage with cortical mastoidectomy generally recommended for older children and adults.
  ii. Citelli abscess
    a. Involvement of the occipital bone
  iii. Bezold abscess
    a. Erosion of the mastoid tip
    b. Fluid collection within the substance of the sternocleidomastoid (SCM) muscle

    iv. Luc abscess
        a. Subperiosteal abscess of the temporal area
        b. Distinct from extension of abscess of the zygomatic root
    v. Zygomatic root abscess
        a. Bony erosion of the zygoma associated with OM
        b. May cause temporal soft tissue infection as well

Intracranial

Meningitis

- Most common intracranial complication of AOM and COM

ETIOLOGY

- Hematogenous spread
- Direct extension via bony erosion
- Direct extension through bony channels (ie, Hyrtl fissures)

SIGNS AND SYMPTOMS

- Fever
- Meningismus
- Photo or phonophobia
- Positive Brudzinski and Kernig signs
- Severe headache

DIAGNOSIS

- CT temporal bone
- CT brain to rule out mass effect
- Lumbar puncture

PATHOGEN

- Same as those for AOM and COM
- In patients with COM, more likely to be GNR or polymicrobial than in AOM

TREATMENT

- Broad-spectrum antibiotics with good CSF penetration.
- Cultures of CSF to direct antibiotic therapy.
- 7 to 10 days of IV antibiotics followed by 2 to 3 weeks of oral antibiotics.
- Administration of IV steroids in the acute period decreases long-term neurologic sequalae.
- Monitor hearing for post meningitic hearing loss
  - (a) Audiogram
  - (b) CT temporal bone to evaluate for ossification of the cochlea
    - ○ Indication for urgent cochlear implantation

Lateral Sinus Thrombosis

Etiology

- Infection or inflammation of dura around sinus results in coagulation of the blood within.

Signs and Symptoms

- "Picket-fence" fevers
  - (a) Spiking fevers that tend to cluster at a particular time of day
- Severe headache
- Otorrhea
- Edema and tenderness of mastoid (Griesinger sign)
- Papilledema
- Septic emboli to lungs

- Jugular vein thrombosis
  - (a) Lower cranial nerve deficits if inflammation spreads to the pars nervosa of the jugular bulb

Diagnosis
- CT brain with contrast
  - (a) Delta sign
    - ○ Rim enhancement of the sinus with central hypodensity
- Magnetic resonance venography (MRV)
  - (a) Flow void in affected sinus
- Intraoperative
  - (a) Needle aspiration of the sinus
    - ○ If blood returns, no intervention
    - ○ If no blood returns, sinus ligation and clot evacuation

Treatment
- Multimodality therapy
  - (a) Broad-spectrum antibiotics
  - (b) Mastoidectomy with possible sinus ligation
    - ○ If clot extends into the neck, may require neck exploration with intrajugular (IJ) ligation as well.
  - (c) Anticoagulation
    - ○ Controversial
    - ○ May be indicated in patients with propagating infected clot
    - ○ Conflicting evidence if it improves neurologic outcomes

Subdural Empyema
- High mortality rate even in the antibiotic era (5%-30%).
- Long-term neurologic deficits are common.

Etiology
- Severe infection of the leptomeninges of the brain
- Presumed same possible routes of spread that cause meningitis

Signs and Symptoms
- Altered mental status
- Focal neurologic deficits
- Increased intracranial pressure (ICP) common and must be ruled out prior to lumbar puncture to prevent tonsillar herniation

Diagnosis
- MRI with contrast
  - (a) Enhancing fluid collections within the subdural space
- Lumbar puncture if normal ICP

Treatment
- Urgent neurosurgical evaluation for surgical drainage
- High-dose broad-spectrum antibiotics

Epidural Abscess
- Good prognosis when treated in a timely fashion

Etiology
- Pus between the temporal bone and the dura.
- Middle fossa or posterior fossa may be affected.

Signs and Symptoms
- Those of coalescent mastoiditis

Diagnosis
- CT temporal bone with contrast
- High index of suspicion

Treatment
- Surgical drainage
  - (a) Middle fossa
    - ○ Limited subtemporal approach (also known as middle fossa approach)
    - ○ Do not remove tegmen mastoideum unless already eroded by disease
      - – Risk of encephalocele
      - – If eroded consider repair to prevent encephalocele
  - (b) Posterior fossa
    - ○ Removal of bony plate
    - ○ No risk of clinically significant encephalocele
- Culture-directed antibiotics

Intraparenchymal Abscess

Etiology
- Most likely due to direct spread of infection.
- Patients will usually present with several weeks of otologic symptoms.
- Otogenic brain abscesses are located within the cerebellum or temporal lobe.

Signs and Symptoms
- Three stages of brain abscess:
  - (a) Encephalitis—headache, mental status change, fever, seizures, and increased ICP
  - (b) Coalescence—may be relatively asymptomatic at this stage
  - (c) Rupture—increasing headache, meningeal signs, systemic collapse
- Focal deficits are seen eventually in 70% of patients.
  - (a) Cerebellum—ataxia, dysmetria, nystagmus, nausea, or vomiting
  - (b) Temporal lobe—if dominant hemisphere results in aphasia, visual defects, and headache

Diagnosis
- Contrast-enhanced CT or MRI brain

Pathogens
- *S aureus* most common
- Polymicrobial infection particularly common in COM
- GNR such as *Klebsiella, Proteus, E coli*, and *Pseudomonas*
- Anaerobic bacteria—bacteroides

Treatment
- Urgent neurosurgical intervention for abscess drainage.
- When patient is stable, surgical management of the otologic disease is warranted.
- Broad-spectrum, high-dose antibiotics with coverage for anaerobes.
  - (a) Mortality rate is 10% but as high as 80% if abscess ruptures into the ventricular system.

Otitic Hydrocephalus

Etiology
- Associated with lateral sinus thrombosis
  - (a) Impedes venous drainage and consequently CSF reabsorption through the arachnoid granulations
  - (b) Particularly if clot propagates to the transverse sinus
- May occur without evidence of sinus thrombosis
  - (a) Mechanism for this is unclear.

Signs and Symptoms
- Headache
- Photo or phonophobia
- Increased ICP
- Evidence of AOM or COM

Diagnosis
- Papilledema on fundoscopic examination.
- Do no perform lumbar puncture (LP) as there is a risk of tonsillar brain herniation with elevated ICP.

Treatment
- Acute lowering of ICP
  (a) Mannitol and diuretics
- Mastoidectomy and eradication of disease
  (a) Serial ophthalmologic examination to assess for increased papilledema and visual compromise.
  (b) Worsening ophthalmologic examination is indication for optic nerve decompression.

Infections of the Inner Ear

Bacterial
- Difficult to make a definitive distinction between serous and suppurative labyrinthitis on symptoms alone.
  (a) Temporal bone histopathology (postmortem) may be the only way to make definitive diagnosis.

Serous Labyrinthitis
Most common in pediatric population as this age group is mostly at risk for AOM.

Etiology
- Bacterial toxins and inflammatory mediators from otitis media enter the labyrinth by crossing the round window (RW) membrane or via labyrinthine fistula.
  (a) Animal models suggest that RW membrane permeability is increased by inflammatory mediators in the middle ear.
- No bacteria in the inner ear.
- Possible that labyrinthine dysfunction is related to changes in ionic potentials induced by inflammatory mediators rather than destruction of neuroepithelium or neural elements.
  (a) As endocochlear or labyrinthine electrical potentials are regenerated, end-organ function can return which implies preservation of viable cochlear and vestibular hair cells.

Signs and Symptoms
- Typically unilateral, unless there is bilateral AOM
- Variable involvement of the cochlea and balance organs
  (a) Mild to severe SNHL with or without vestibular symptoms
    ○ Typically the symptoms are reversible and resolve gradually with time.

Diagnosis and Pathogens
- Culture of middle ear effusion
- Audiogram
- Vestibular testing

- Imaging only if other complications of OM are suspected
- Pathogens that cause otitis media—*S pneumoniae*, *H influenzae*, and *M catarrhalis*

Treatment

- Directed at the infectious source.
- Oral antibiotics are typically effective.
- Steroids may improve outcomes but data are lacking.
- Myringotomy if ear is not draining.
- Tympanomastoidectomy if cholesteatoma is the source.

Suppurative Labyrinthitis

- Uncommon in the antibiotic era

Etiology

- Otogenic infections result from infections of the middle ear or mastoid.
  - (a) Most commonly associated with cholesteatoma in the modern era.
  - (b) Bacterial entry usually occurs through labyrinthine fistula or congenital abnormality.
- Meningitic labyrinthitis results from infection transmitted via CSF through the internal auditory canal to the cochlear modiolus or cochlear aqueduct.

Signs and Symptoms

- Profound hearing loss, frequently bilateral in meningitic labyrinthitis
- Severe vestibular symptoms
- Fever
- Meningeal signs
- Evidence of OM or cholesteatoma
- May develop cranial neuropathies if disease spreads outside of otic capsule

Diagnosis

- Cultures via myringotomy or lumbar puncture
- Audiogram
- Vestibular testing
- CT to evaluate for evidence of cholesteatoma, congenital inner ear abnormalities, or intracranial complications
  - (a) Post meningitis hearing loss should prompt urgent evaluation of labyrinthitis ossificans.
    - ○ MRI if other intracranial complications suspected or suggested on CT

Pathogens

- *S pneumoniae (most common)*, *H influenzae*, and *Neisseria meningitidis*
  - (a) Polymicrobial or GNR may be found in otogenic suppurative labyrinthitis.
  - (b) *S pneumoniae* is the most common pathogen associated with hearing loss.

Treatment

- Directed at primary source
  - (a) Parenteral antibiotics with good meningeal penetration
  - (b) Myringotomy with tube if non-cholesteatoma otogenic infection
  - (c) Tympanomastoidectomy if due to cholesteatoma
    - ○ Steroids have been shown to improve hearing outcomes in meningitic labyrinthitis caused by *H influenzae* and *S pneumoniae*.
    - ○ Patients must be monitored for labyrinthitis ossificans with serial CT.

Spirochetes

- A. **Otosyphilis**
  - i. May be acquired or congenital
  - ii. Great masquerader—otologic symptoms may present at any stage of disease

a. Workup for many inner ear disorders should include screen for syphilis.

b. Increasing incidence of syphilis after many years of declining rates of infection.

B. Congenital syphilis

    i. Thirty percent of patients will have hearing loss.

C. Acquired tertiary disease

    i. Constellation of symptoms associated with neurosyphilis.

    ii. Eighty percent of patients with neurosyphilis have SNHL.

Etiology

- Initially is a meningoneurolabyrinthitis.
- Late congenital, latent, and tertiary syphilis.
  - (a) Osteitis of the temporal bone
  - (b) Obliterative endarteritis
  - (c) Microgummata
  - (d) Endolymphatic hydrops
  - (e) Ossicular involvement
  - (f) Degeneration of the organ of Corti
  - (g) Cochlear neuron loss

Signs and Symptoms

- Variable patterns of hearing loss
  - (a) Sudden onset
  - (b) Fluctuating
  - (c) Slowly progressive
- May have symptoms consistent with endolymphatic hydrops
  - (a) Fluctuating SNHL
  - (b) Aural fullness
  - (c) Episodic vertigo
  - (d) Tinnitus
  - (e) May be unilateral
- Positive Tullio phenomenon
  - (a) Induction of vertigo with visible nystagmus with loud sound
- Positive Hennebert sign
  - (a) False-positive fistula test.
  - (b) Thought to be due to scar band between the saccule and the footplate.
  - (c) Positive Hennebert sign may be due to third window phenomenon in non-syphillitic patients.

Diagnosis and Pathogen

- Caused by Treponema pallidum.
- Venereal disease research laboratory (VDRL) or rapid plasma regain (RPR) can be used for screening.
  - (a) Eighty percent to 85% sensitive in primary syphilis
  - (b) Ninety percent to 100% sensitive in secondary syphilis
  - (c) Can be false positive
- Confirmatory testing required if VDRL or RPR are positive.
  - (a) Fluorescent treponemal antigen absorption (FTA-ABS)
    - 85% sensitive for 1-degree syphilis
    - 95%-100% sensitive for 2-degree syphilis
    - 95% sensitive for 3-degree syphilis
- Ancillary testing
- Slit lamp examination to evaluate for interstitial keratitis

- Lumbar puncture
  - (a) Test CSF for VDRL, if positive indicates active infection
- Imaging
  - (a) May be useful to diagnose other complications of the disease
  - (b) CT of the temporal bone
    - ○ Luetic osteitis of the otic capsule

Treatment
- Prolonged parenteral penicillin G therapy (qid × 3 weeks).
- Steroids (high dose for 2 weeks).
- 35% to 50% of patients will have improvement in hearing and balance function following treatment.
  - A. **Lyme disease**
    - i. Extremely rare cause of neurosensory hearing loss.
    - ii. Caused by *Borreila burgdorferi* carried by the deer tick *Ixodes* species in endemic areas.
    - iii. Hearing loss is late symptom of disease; other systemic symptoms usually present.
    - iv. Routine testing for Lyme titers not warranted for unilateral sudden hearing loss unless risk factors present or living within endemic areas.

Mycobacterium
  - A. Rare cause of SNHL or vestibular pathology
  - B. May be asymmetric

Etiology
- Associated with tuberculous meningitis
- Rare reports in literature of histopathology
  - (a) Inflammatory infiltrates in the perilymphatic spaces, cochlear modiolus, Rosenthal canal
  - (b) Degeneration of organ of Corti and spiral ganglion cells

Signs and Symptoms
- Signs and symptoms of meningitis
  - (a) Fever
  - (b) Nuchal rigidity
  - (c) Positive Kernig and Brudzinski signs
  - (d) Photophobia or phonophobia
- SNHL
- Vertigo

Diagnosis and Pathogen
- Caused by *M tuberculosis* or atypical *Mycobacterium* rarely
- Audio or electronystagmography (ENG)
- Lumbar puncture with AFB

Treatment
- Multiple drug therapy (high rates of multidrug-resistant strains).
- Hearing restoration may be difficult given the loss of spiral ganglion cells.

Viral

  - A. Causation very difficult to prove as labyrinthine tissues are not routinely available for viral cultures or histopathology.
  - B. Serologic studies are indirect method of evaluating infection.

        i. Many of the suspected viruses are responsible for latent infection (herpes simplex virus type 1 [HSV-1], CMV, herpes zoster virus [HZV], etc) and are presumed to result in pathology when reactivated.

        ii. Serology is not useful in evaluating these viruses because once the virus is acquired (usually in childhood) the patient will have immunoglobulin G (IgG) to the virus.

C. Animal models may not accurately represent human disease as viruses may affect species differently.

D. Broad-spectrum of symptoms because viruses affect different areas of the membranous labyrinth differently.

E. Sudden sensory hearing loss and acute vestibular dysfunction (aka vestibular neuritis, neuronitis, labyrinthitis, etc) may be a spectrum of disease depending on the specific end-organ affected.

F. Proposed causative viruses are as below.

CMV

A. Most common cause of nonsyndromic congenital SNHL.

        i. One percent of infants are born with CMV infection.

        ii. Ten percent of these will have symptomatic infections.

        iii. Seven percent of asymptomatic patients will develop hearing loss.

        iv. Median age for identification of HL in asymptomatic patients is 18 months.

           a. Most are not detected on newborn screening.

B. Spectrum of disease with severely affected infants having cytomegalic inclusion disease (CID).

        i. Thirty-five percent to 50% of patients with CID will have bilateral deafness.

C. Patients with less severe manifestations may also have SNHL (10% of patients).

Etiology

- Acute changes include viral inclusion cysts in neuroepithelium, stria vascularis, and supporting cells.
- Late changes include hydrops, extracellular calcifications, strial atrophy, loss of sensory, and support cells in the organ of Corti.

Signs and Symptoms

- CID.
  - (a) Deafness
  - (b) Hepatosplenomegaly
  - (c) Jaundice
  - (d) Microcephaly
  - (e) Intracerebral calcifications
- Hearing loss in asymptomatically infected patients is variable.
  - (a) Patterns
    - ◦ Improvement in plasma thromboplastin antecedents (PTAs)
    - ◦ Stable PTA
    - ◦ Progressive loss
    - ◦ Fluctuating loss
- Patients with symptomatic infection have worse hearing loss and higher likelihood of progression.

Diagnosis

- Isolation of viral particles from urine.
- IgM and IgG levels are useful in acute infection.

- Antibody titers not useful in distinguishing primary infection versus reactivation.
- Viral particles have been identified in perilymph samples taken from patients undergoing cochlear implantation but causal relationship difficult to prove.

Pathogen

- Caused by CMV
- Herpesvirus family
  (a) DNA virus

Treatment

- Antiviral therapy (ganciclovir) for symptomatic infection in neonates demonstrated improved hearing outcomes compared to no therapy.
- Currently no recommendations for asymptomatic infections.
- Hearing aid use for those with aid-able losses.
- Cochlear implantation should be considered for profoundly deafened patients.

Mumps

A. May be very common cause of unilateral hearing loss in childhood.
B. Hearing loss can occur during asymptomatic infection.
C. Hearing loss affects 1 in 2000 patients with mumps infection.

Etiology

- Predominantly affects the cochlear duct.
- Atrophy of organ of Corti and stria vascularis.
- Vestibular dysfunction is rare but reported.
- Vestibular testing in subjects with balance dysfunction suggests there may also be injury to the neural components of the balance system.
- Demyelination of the eighth nerve.
- Route of spread is either hematogenous viral invasion of the cochlea or through CSF viremia through the cochlear aqueduct or modiolus.
- May result in delayed endolymphatic hydrops years after infection.

Signs and Symptoms

- Range of hearing impairment—mild to severe or profound
- Usually sudden in onset
- Usually unilateral but bilateral loss has been reported
- Mild losses may be recoverable
- Severe loss is usually permanent
- Unilateral caloric weakness
- Salivary adenitis
- Orchioepididymitis
- Meningitis
  (a) Occurs in 10% of patients

Diagnosis

- Audiogram
- Vestibular testing
- Isolation of the virus from saliva or CSF

Pathogen

- Mumps virus
- Paramyxovirus family
  (a) RNA virus

Treatment

- Primary prevention with MMR vaccine (measles, mumps, rubella).
- Supportive.

- Oral steroids may be used with varied success for sudden hearing loss.
- No antiviral therapy currently available.

Rubeola (Measles)

A. Highly contagious infection spreads by respiratory droplets.
B. Incidence of hearing loss following infection or vaccination is unknown but literature supports the association.
C. Congenital infection has high mortality rate.
D. Chronic infection of the otic capsule with measles virus has been implicated as one cause of otosclerosis.
   i. Viral particles found in the footplates of surgical patients
   ii. Perilymphatic titers of IgG for measles virus higher than in serum

Etiology
- Inflammation, fibrous infiltration, and ossification of the basal turn of the cochlea
- Degeneration of the organ of Corti, stria, and vestibular neuroepithelium
- Eighth nerve demyelination

Signs and Symptoms
- Koplik spots—pathognomonic
  (a) "Grain of rice" on red base of the oral mucosa
- Three Cs—cough, coryza, conjunctivitis
- Maculopapular rash
- High fever
- Encephalitis
- Subacute sclerosing panencephalitis (SSPE)
  (a) Rare, delayed neural degeneration
  (b) Fatal, unless diagnosed early

Diagnosis
- Typically involves in measles outbreak and diagnosis is based on symptoms alone.
- Audiogram to document hearing change.
- Lumbar puncture if intracranial complications suspected.

Pathogen
- Measles virus
- Paramyxovirus family
  (a) RNA virus

Treatment
- Supportive in general.
- Vitamin A has been shown to decrease morbidity and mortality.
- Hearing aid for mild to moderate HL.
- Cochlear implant for bilaterally deafened patients.

Herpes Simplex Virus 1

A. Role as causative agent in sudden SNHL (SSNHL) and vestibular neuritis is postulated but controversial.
   i. Has been used to create an animal model of SSNHL but causative role in humans has yet to be proven

Signs and Symptoms
- SSNHL
- Vertigo
- May have flu-like prodrome

Diagnosis
- Viral particles have been found in the endolymphatic system.
- Perilymph specimens from CI patients failed to show viral DNA.

Pathogen
- Human HSV-1
- Herpesvirus family
  (a) DNA virus

Treatment
- Acyclovir and valacyclovir are frequently used.
- Several randomized controlled trials including antiviral therapy with steroids have failed to show added benefit of antivirals in improving hearing outcomes.

Herpes Zoster

Etiology
- Latent infection within the spiral or vestibular ganglion may result in labyrinthine infection.

Symptoms and Signs
- When associated with facial paralysis known as Ramsey Hunt syndrome (herpes zoster oticus)
  (a) Typically severe unilateral hearing loss.
  (b) Vestibular symptoms are common.
  (c) Vesicular eruption in the conchal bowl, ear canal, or tympanic membrane.

Diagnosis
- Tzanck smear of ruptured vesicles to identify multinucleated giant cells

Pathogen
- Herpes zoster
- Herpesvirus family
- DNA virus

Treatment
- A. High-dose oral steroids.
- B. Antiviral therapy effective in treatment when zoster affects other tissues but trials involving herpes zoster oticus is lacking.
  (a) Recovery of hearing is poor despite recovery of facial nerve function.

Rubella (German measles)

- A. Incidence is low in developed world due to widespread use of the MMR vaccine.
- B. Congenital rubella associated with HL in 50% of patients.
  - i. May develop months to years after the acute infection
- C. Acquired infection generally not associated with the hearing loss.

Etiology
- Congenital infection (Gregg syndrome)
  (a) Maternal infection during first trimester of pregnancy
- Cochlear and saccule degeneration
- Atrophy of the stria vascularis
- Utricle and semicircular canals not generally involved

Signs and Symptoms
- Congenital rubella
  (a) Cataracts
  (b) Microphthalmia
  (c) Cardiac defects
  (d) "Blueberry muffin" skin lesions
  (e) Developmental delay
  (f) Hearing loss
    ○ Usually severe to profound

Diagnosis
- Viral isolation from nasopharyngeal swab or urine is diagnostic procedure of choice.
- Serologies are very difficult to interpret in congenital rubella due to transplacental transmission of IgG.

Pathogen
- Togavirus family
- RNA virus

Treatment
- No current medication used to treat congenital rubella
- Supportive
- Hearing aid or cochlear implantation as indicated

Other viruses that may Cause Membranous Labyrinthine Pathology
- Influenza A
- Parainfluenza
- Adenovirus
- Coxsackievirus
- RSV

Bibliography

Coker TR, Chan LS, Newberry SJ, et al. Diagnosis, microbial epidemiology and antibiotic treatment of acute otitis media in children: a systematic review. *JAMA*. 2010;304(19): 2161-2169.

Lieberthal AS, Carroll AE, Chonmaitree T, et al. The diagnosis and management of acute otitis media. *Pediatrics*. 2013:131(3):e964-e999.

Merchant SN, Durand ML, Adams JC. Sudden deafness: is it viral? *ORL J Otorhinolaryngol Relat Spec.* 2008;70(1):52-60.

Rosenfeld RM, Culpepper L, Doyle KJ, et al. American Academy of Pediatric subcommittee on otitis media with effusion, American Academy of Family Physicians; American Academy of Otolaryngology-Head and Neck Surgery. Clinical practice guideline: otitis media with effusion. *Otolaryngol Head Neck Surg.* 2004;130(5 Suppl):S95-S118.

Rubin LG. Prevention and treatment of meningitis and acute otitis media in children with cochlear implants. *Otol Neurotol.* 2010;31(8):1331-1333.

Questions

1. Appropriate first-line therapy for acute bacterial otitis externa would include
   A. Daily irrigation with normal saline
   B. Topical antibiotic drops
   C. Oral antibiotics
   D. Canaloplasty

2. Otosyphilis may present with which of the following signs and symptoms?
   A. Hydropic pattern hearing loss
   B. Positive Tullio phenomenon
   C. Positive Hennebert sign
   D. All of the above

3. An abscess is identified within the substance of the SCM in a patient with mastoiditis. This is called a
   A. Citelli abscess
   B. Subperiosteal abscess
   C. Bezold abscess
   D. Luc abscess

4. Most common cause of nonsyndromic congenital SNHL is
   A. CMV
   B. Rubella
   C. Mumps
   D. Herpes simplex virus type 1

5. A patient presents to the emergency room with a draining ear, diffuse headaches, "picket-fence" fevers, and postauricular tenderness. The clinician should be concerned for
   A. Intraparenchymal abscess
   B. Lateral sinus thrombosis
   C. Meningitis
   D. Malignant otitis externa

Chapter 23
Noninfectious Disorders of the Ear

External Ear

- Trauma
  - (a) Lacerations: Simple with or without involved cartilage; stellate from blunt trauma; partial or total avulsion
    - ○ Treatment: Deep cleaning, debridement, surgical repair; may require stage or flap reconstruction; dressing, systemic antibiotics. Consider bolster to prevent hematoma.
    - ○ Complications: Perichondritis, cartilage necrosis.
  - (b) Hematoma—typically occur from blunt trauma
    - ○ Treatment: Incision and drainage with through-and-through sutures and bolster dressing
      - – Systemic antibiotics (consider fluoroquinolones)
    - ○ Complications: fibrosis, cauliflower/wrestler's ear, perichondritis
  - (c) Frostbite—exposure to subfreezing temperature and wind leading to disruption of endothelial layer with extravasation of erythrocytes, platelet aggregation, and sludging
    - ○ Symptoms: pain, burning, discoloration; reduced pliability; loss of sensation.
    - ○ Treatment: slow warming; antibiotics; anticoagulants; debridement of necrotic tissue after demarcation. No pressure or pressure dressing to the ear.
  - (d) Bites—lobe of ear is most common site
    - ○ Treatment: Meticulous cleaning; systemic antibiotics; surgical repair and/or debridement.
      - – Human bites have greater propensity for infection.
  - (e) Keloids and hypertrophic scars—increased rates in African American and Hispanic population (up to 30%)
    - ○ Treatment: Steroid injection, surgical excision, pressure dressing, rarely radiation therapy
- Carcinoma of the external ear
  - (a) 6% of skin cancers involve the ear
  - (b) Lymphatic drainage—Anterior auricular nodes: lateral pinna and anterior canal wall; postauricular nodes: superior and upper posterior pinna, posterior canal wall; superficial and deep cervical nodes: lobule and floor of external ear canal.
  - (c) Metastasis assocaited with depth of invasion
  - (d) Staging:

       ○ Skin and Pinna
- TX—Primary tumor cannot be assessed.
- T0—No evidence of primary tumor.
- Tis—Carcinoma in situ.
- T1—Tumor 2 cm or less.
- T2—Tumor larger than 2 cm but smaller than 5 cm.
- T3—Tumor larger than 5 cm.
- T4—Tumor invades deep extradermal structures (bone, muscle, cartilage).

       ○ University of Pittsburgh staging system for SCC involving the temporal bone
- T1—Tumor limited to external auditory canal without bone or soft tissue extension
- T2—Tumor with limited external auditory canal bony erosion or < 0.5 cm soft tissue involvement
- T3—Tumor eroding full thickness bony external auditory canal with < 0.5 cm soft tissue involvement, or tumor involving the middle ear and/or mastoid
- T4—Tumor eroding the medial wall of middle ear or beyond, or > 0.5 cm soft tissue involvement, or patient with facial nerve paresis or paralysis

       ○ Regional lymph nodes:
- NX—Regional lymph nodes cannot be assessed.
- N0—No regional lymph node metastasis.
- N1—Regional lymph node metastasis.

(e) Basal cell carcinoma—most common malignancy of the ear (45%)
    ○ Symptoms: Erythematous lesion with raised margins; silvery scales common, occurs on the pinna and in the external canal.
    ○ Treatment: Biopsy, topical agents, wide local excision; may require cartilage excision, skin graft, or local flaps

(f) Squamous cell carcinoma
    ○ Symptoms: Pain, bloody discharge, polyp with granular appearance, facial nerve paralysis, hearing loss
    ○ Treatment: Biopsy, wide surgical excision, may require parotidectomy, sleeve resection of ear canal or temporal bone resection; postoperative radiation for advanced cases

(g) Malignant melanoma—7% of head and neck sites involve the ear

(h) Other tumors of the ear: Adenoid cystic carcinoma, adenocarcinoma, adenoma, and pleomorphic adenoma

External Ear Canal

- Seborrheic dermatitis, psoriasis
  (a) Psoriasis affects 2% to 5% of the population. In 18% with systemic psoriasis, ear is affected. Scalp and postauricular sulcus affected often.
  (b) Eczema—External otitis, the most common dermatologic condition of the external canal, may be associated with dandruff.
  (c) Symptoms: Itching; weeping; dry, scaly, fissured skin; crusting and flaking; recurrent external otitis; canal stenosis.
  (d) Treatment: Frequent cleaning to prevent accumulation, 1% hydrocortisone solution or lotion, betamethasone for acute treatment.

- Keratosis obturans
  - (a) Rapid accumulation of keratin debris; wax casts; plugged external auditory canal; painless erosion and expansion of external canal; may be associated with drainage, foul odor, and secondary external otitis
  - (b) Pathology: Chronic inflammation and poor epithelial migration
  - (c) Treatment: Frequent cleaning; topical 1% hydrocortisone; betamethasone for acute treatment
- Cholesteatoma of the ear canal
  - (a) Keratin accumulation in the external canal associated with osteitis and bone necrosis; usually occurs on the floor of the external canal; commonly associated with pain and keratin invasion of bone.
  - (b) Treatment: Frequent cleaning of the external auditory canal; topical steroids; may require surgical debridement of osteitic bone. May require canal wall down mastoidectomy if extensive bone erosion.
- Osteoma
  - (a) Pedunculated bone mass developing along tympanosquamous and tympanomastoid suture lines; occluding osteoma may require surgical removal.
- Exostoses
  - (a) Lamellar thickening of bone of external ear canal associated with cold air/water exposure, commonly involving the anterior and posterior canal wall. Exostoses may cause canal stenosis, cerumen impaction, retention of moisture and skin, and rarely hearing loss.
  - (b) Treatment: Canaloplasty and possible skin graft.
- Foreign bodies
  - (a) Insects, nuts, beans, gum, putty, beads, toys, etc. Avoid irrigation—vegetable matter will expand; blind instrumentation may cause bleeding or swelling of the ear canal and may impale the foreign material through the eardrum.
  - (b) Treatment: Local anesthetic block, microscopic examination, and instrumentation for removal of foreign body; mineral oil or antibiotic solution may facilitate removal. Depending on status of canal after removal, topical antibiotic may be required.

Middle Ear and Mastoid

- Trauma
  - (a) Temporal bone fractures, basilar skull fractures
    - ○ Epidemiology: Most common cause is motor vehicle accidents followed by assault.
      - – 70% occur in second to fourth decades of life with a male/female ratio of 3:1.
    - ○ Classification: Traditionally classified as transverse, longitudinal, and mixed based on orientation of fracture line to the petrous ridge axis.
      - – Modern classification is based on whether the fracture involves or spares the otic capsule.
        - ◊ Created due to poor correlation between temporal bone sequelae and traditional fracture classification. For example: transverse fractures originally thought to be associated with (SNHL) but modern data show longitudinal fractures are three times more likely to have associated SNHL.

◊ Only 5.8% of temporal bone fractures involve the otic capsule.
◦ Diagnosis
   – Otoscopic evaluation often reveals hemotympanum, which is the most common cause of initial conductive hearing loss.
      ◊ If present, audiometric evaluation should be repeated in 6 to 8 weeks to allow resolution.
   – Ability to perform bedside tuning fork exam is dependent on the level of patient consciousness.
   – CT temporal bone to evaluate fracture location, ossicular integrity, and otic capsule involvement.
   – Ultimately audiometry is required for diagnosis.
      ◊ Conductive hearing loss can occur from hemotympanum, tympanic membrane (TM) perforation, and ossicular discontinuity. Incudostapedial joint subluxation followed by incus dislocation and stapes crura fracture are most common ossicular disruptions.
      ◊ SNHL is most severe with otic capsule involvement. Nonotic capsule fractures involving SNHL have been suggested to occur from intralabyrinthine hemorrhage and membranous labyrinth injury.
      ◊ Hearing loss pattern is often mixed.
(b) Middle ear trauma
   ◦ Foreign body can puncture TM resulting in a wide variety of injuries.
      – Simple TM perforation without ossicular injury leads to temporary CHL; these typically heal without surgical intervention.
      – Ossicular injury can occur from incudostapedial joint subluxation, incus dislocation, and stapes subluxation.
         ◊ Middle ear exploration is warranted after recovery from any vestibular insults.
         ◊ On pneumatic otoscopy TM may be hypermobile.
      – Penetrating trauma can also enter the vestibule through the oval window.
         ◊ When acute vestibular complaints occur with hearing loss, perilymphatic fistula should be considered. This can also occur with stapes subluxation.
         ◊ Treated with bed rest, minimization of straining (stool softeners), and antivertiginous agents. Surgery is avoided if possible during the healing phase.
   ◦ Audiometric evaluation is required to determine type and severity of hearing loss.
   ◦ CT is often imaging modality of choice to determine the integrity of the ossicles and labyrinth.
• Congenital cholesteatoma—develops from rest of embryonic epithelial cells in middle ear
(a) Occur in anterosuperior quadrant of mesotympanum and tympanic membrane or adjacent to malleus and posterior mesotympanum
(b) Presentation: 2 to 6 years of age—white mass beneath drum, usually adjacent to malleus
(c) Imaging: CT to evaluate extent of disease
(d) Treatment: Surgical removal
• Otosclerosis
(a) Epidemiology: Caucasians 8% to 12%, clinical disease 0.5% to 2%; African American population 1%, clinical disease 0.1%.
   ◦ Female:male ratio 2:1

(b) Genetics: Approximately 50% have positive family history; 70% autosomal dominant with 25% to 40% penetrance.

(c) Pathology:
- Early phase—vascular, spongy bone progressing to fibrosis
- Late phase—new bone replaced with sclerotic bone
- Anterior oval window (fissulae ante fenestrum): Most common location, 70% to 90%. Round window: 30% to 70%; cochlear: 14%; extensive involvement: 10% to 12%
- Measles virus associated with otosclerotic foci

(d) Symptoms: Progressive conductive or mixed hearing loss; typical presentation age of 30 to 50; associated with pregnancy in 30% to 63%; paracusis of willis (hearing better in noise), 36% to 85%; tinnitus, 75% to 100%; imbalance, 22%; vertigo, 26%; Schwartz sign (promontory hyperemia), 10%.

(e) Audiometry: Progressive, low frequency, conductive or mixed hearing loss; maximum conductive component, 60 dB; Carhart notch is depressed bone threshold at 2000 Hz; word discrimination often 70% or better.

(f) Acoustic reflex: No reflex suggests fixed stapes.
- *Biphasic reflex (on-off)*: Occurs in 94% with symptoms of less than 5 years and in 9% greater than 10 years (40% of normals have biphasic acoustic reflexes.)
- If normal reflex consider other possible etiologies (superior semicircular canal dehiscence syndrome)

(g) Tuning Forks: Weber lateralizes to affected ear; Rinne is negative—bone greater than air, masking the opposite ear with unilateral hearing loss. Applying the tuning forks to the teeth rather than the forehead will increase the sensitivity 5 to 10 dB.

Tuning fork	Air-bone gap
Negative 256 Hz Rinne	15 dB or more
Negative 512 Hz Rinne	25 dB or more
Negative 1024 Hz Rinne	35 dB or more

(h) Computed Tomography:
- Thin section (0.5 mm) of labyrinth, axial and coronal views; areas of reduced bone density, cochlear deformity. CT Indications—rapid loss of bone threshold, cochlear otosclerosis, questionable conductive hearing loss, vestibular complaints.

(i) Surgical Indications:
- Conductive hearing loss 20 dB or greater; negative Rinne test, 256 Hz and 512 Hz (good candidate); if also negative 1024 Hz (excellent candidate); good bone conduction threshold; speech discrimination 70% or better; stable middle and inner ear
- Poorer-hearing ear always operated first

(j) Other Considerations:
- Hearing disability; occupation; hobbies (scuba diving); inability to use a hearing aid at air conduction thresholds but aidable bone thresholds

(k) Surgical Contraindications: Only or better-hearing ear; ear with better speech discrimination; perforated tympanic membrane; active middle ear disease; active Ménière's disease

    (l) Relative Contraindications:
- Child less than 18 years of age; poor eustachian tube function; air conduction threshold less than 30 dB; air–bone gap less than 15 dB; aidable hearing with bone conduction greater than 40 dB:
- *Occupation*: roofer, acrobat, scuba diver; sommelier (chorda)

    (m) Medical Treatment
- Sodium fluoride, calcium, vitamin D (widely accepted but not FDA approved)

    (n) Surgical Results
- Dependent on surgeon's experience more than prosthesis.
- *Experienced surgeon*: closure of air–bone gap, less than 10 dB, 90% to 95%;
- Revision surgery (lifetime): 5%
- Significant sensorineural hearing loss, less than 5%
- Mild transient vertigo, 5%
- Severe persistent vertigo, less than 5%
- Preservation of chorda tympani nerve, 95%
- Dysgeusia, 5% to 10%

    (o) Intraoperative complications:
- Torn tympanomeatal flap; dislocation of incus; fractured long process of incus; perilymph gusher (1/300); vertigo; sensorineural hearing loss; floating footplate

    (p) Revision stapes surgery:
- Up to 5% of cases.
- Displaced prosthesis from incus necrosis is most common.
- Other causes: displaced prosthesis, perilymph fistula, tympanic membrane perforation or retraction, reparative granuloma.

- Congenital ossicular fixation—stapes fixation is most common followed by malleus fixation
  - (a) 35-50 dB air–bone gap
  - (b) CT important to evaluate for ossicular deformity or fixation
  - (c) X-linked stapes fixation: surgery contraindicated (stapes gusher)
    - Widened cochlear aperture at internal auditory canal

- Systemic diseases
  - (a) Wegener granulomatosis—ear involvement 30% to 50% of patients
    - Overall 10% have SNHL.
    - CHL from chronic serous otitis media is most common. 30% of patients with middle ear involvement will have associated SNHL.
  - (b) Sarcoidosis—associated with facial nerve paralysis and cochlear-vestibular neuropathy
  - (c) Paget Disease—*osteitis deformans*
    - Male:female ratio 4:1; inherited autosomal dominant
    - Symptoms: thickening of the skull; mixed conductive hearing loss; thickening of the ossicles with fixation
    - Pathology: vascular, spongy bone, thick or enlarged ossicle, and otic capsule
    - Radiology: CT shows thickening of cortical bone, ossicles, and otic capsule
    - Treatment: consider stapedectomy in patients with CHL versus hearing aid

Inner Ear

- Idiopathic sudden sensorineural hearing loss (ISSNHL).
  - (a) Epidemiology: 5 to 20 per 100,000 per year, median age 40 to 54 years, male=female
  - (b) Generally defined as 30 dB loss over three frequencies within a 3-day period

     (c) Presentation: May initially present with aural fullness and tinnitus prior to hearing complaints. Typically unilateral.

     (d) Pathophysiology remains unclear.

     (e) Treatment: High-dose oral steroid regimen.
- Intratympanic steroids have been suggested for use as first-line treatment and salvage therapy.
- No evidence for antiviral therapy.

     (f) Factors associated with low likelihood of hearing recovery.
- Flat and high frequency hearing loss.
- More severe hearing loss
- Presence of vertigo
- Advanced age

- Perilymphatic fistulas.

     (a) Presentation: Sudden or progressive hearing loss (SNHL or mixed) associated with roaring tinnitus, dysacusis, dysequilibrium
- May be seen in setting of stapes surgery or trauma (especially barotrauma)

     (b) Diagnosis:
- Hennebert sign (vertigo with pneumatic otoscopy) on physical examination
- Serial audiograms and imaging to rule out retrocochlear pathology

     (c) Treatment: Observation 7 to 10 days with bed rest and minimized straining (stool softeners)
- Surgery is considered with progressive hearing loss and persistent symptoms
  - In nonoperated patient, perilymph leak around annular ligament of stapes is most common.

- Autoimmune inner ear disease (AIED)

     (a) Classically defined as rapidly progressive bilateral SNHL that responds to immunosuppressive agents

     (b) Now separated into:
- Primary AIED—symptoms only involving the inner ear
- Secondary AIED—inner ear and systemic involvement

     (c) Primary AIED—poorly defined with no gold standard for diagnosis
- Pathophysiology: Theorized to occur from localized labyrinthine immune reaction to antigen resulting in physiologic changes leading to symptoms. Response is likely initiated in the endolymphatic sac as it contains the only immunocompetent cells in the labyrinth.
- Symptoms: Patients typically develop bilateral SNHL that worsens over weeks to months.
  - Hearing may fluctuate, but overall trend is toward worse hearing.
  - 50% of patient have vestibular complaints.
- Treatment: Corticosteroid use is mainstay of treatment but with highly variable results.
  - Typically started on 60 mg for 4 weeks in adults. If pure tone thresholds improve 15 dB in a single frequency or 10 dB or more in two or more consecutive frequencies, patients are considered steroid-responders.
  - Responders continue steroid therapy at full dose until audiometric recovery plateaus. Then steroids are slowly tapered over 8 weeks to maintenance dose (5-20 mg every other day).
  - No clear understanding of how and when to discontinue maintenance dose. Non-responders are tapered off steroids.

- Alternative and adjuvant therapies include methotrexate, cyclophosphamide, etanercept, and intratympanic steroids.
  - (d) Secondary AIED
    - Cogan syndrome—classic symptoms include SNHL, vertigo, tinnitus, and interstitial keratitis
      - Atypical Cogan syndrome includes patients with non-keratitic ocular inflammation
    - Wegener granulomatosis—(see above)
    - Antiphospholipid antibody syndrome—autoimmune disorder that causes coagulopathy. Patients suffer from recurrent thrombi and spontaneous abortions
      - Have antiphospholipid, antilupus anticoagulant, or anticardiolipin antibody
      - Can develop SNHL likely due to labyrinthine thrombus formation
    - Systemic lupus erythematosus—necrotizing vasculitis with chronic otitis media, SNHL, and/or vestibular symptoms
- Presbycusis—SNHL related to age without other identifiable cause
  - (a) Progressive hearing loss, typically in high frequencies first.
  - (b) More severe hearing loss in men.
  - (c) Four classifications of presbycusis.
    - Neural presbycusis—loss of auditory nerve fibers results in worse than expected speech discrimination based on pure tone thresholds
    - Strial presbycusis—atrophy of stria vascularis results in relatively flat audiograms
    - Sensory presbycusis—progressive loss of hair cells beginning in the basal turn of the cochlea, leads to high frequency loss
    - Cochlear conductive presbycusis—theorized that increase basilar membrane stiffness results in gradually descending hearing loss
  - (d) Treatment: Hearing aids when word recognition scores are good. Cochlear implantation is considered with poor word recognition.
- Noise induced hearing loss
  - (a) Temporary threshold shift (TTS)—loud noise exposure that causes SNHL that resolves within 24 hours
    - Level of injury is dependent on sound level (decibel) and sound frequency (high frequency causing more injury).
    - Continuous and longer sound exposure cause a greater threshold shift than interrupted noise.
  - (b) Permanent threshold shift (PTS)—noise exposure that leads to SNHL lasting > 24 hours
    - Can results from single loud noise exposure or repeated noise exposure over time.
    - Like TTS, level of injury is related to sound level and frequency.
    - Controversial whether injury continues after sound insult ceases or stops with sound.
    - Diagnosis:
      - Typically see hearing loss around 3 to 6 kHz with recovery at higher frequencies
        ◊ Greatest hearing loss seen at 4 kHz
        ◊ 3 to 6 kHz notch is often lost over time
      - Acoustic reflex (tensor tympani and stapedius muscle) likely plays a protective role
        ◊ Given delay (40-150 ms) between noise and reflex, not entirely protective
        ◊ Most protective at frequencies <2 kHz

– Calculating binaural hearing impairment (BHI)
  ◊ Determine PTA for each ear at 0.5, 1, 2, and 3 kHz
  ◊ Monoaural impairment (MI) = 1.5(PTA−25)
  ◊ Better and worse hearing ears are not equally weighed.
  ◊ BHI=[5(MI of better ear) + (MI of worse ear)]/6
○ Pathophysiology
  – Injury occurs initially at level of the outer hair cells (OHC). OHC stereocillia become stiffened by injury and less responsive to noise.
○ In TTS, stereocilia likely recover normal mobility and hearing subsequently recovers. However in PTS, repetitive injury or louder noise exposure causes more significant damage leading to loss of stereocilia and OHC and inner hair cell death.
○ Prevention:
  – There is a clear susceptibility difference for noise-induced hearing loss between individuals, but no clear genetic or predictive causes have been found.
  – Occupational Safety and Health Administration has clear allowances for duration of noise exposure.

OSHA Noise Level Standards	
dB level	*Duration (h)*
90	8
92	6
95	4
97	3
100	2
102	1.5
105	1
110	0.5
115	< 0.25

  ◊ Exposure to sound greater than 90 dB for 8 hours a day requires hearing protection.
    * For each 5 dB increase the allowed exposure time is halved (ie, for 90-95 dB the allowed time decreased from 8 hours to 4 hours)
  ◊ Sound greater than 115 dB is only allowed for less than one second.
  – Animal models have demonstrated possible benefit of N-acetyl cysteine (NAC) against noise induced hearing loss, but no definitive evidence in humans.
• Ototoxicity
  (a) Aminoglycosides—individual drugs vary in impact on cochlear and vestibular system
    ○ Kanamycin, amikacin, neomycin, and tobramycin are most cochleotoxic.
    ○ OHCs in the basal turn are first area injured (high-frequency SNHL), but with continued insult, spiral ganglion cells involved.

  - ○ Hearing loss typically occurs during treatment but may arise 1 to 3 weeks after completion.
  - ○ Ribosomal mitochondrial 12S mutations increase patient susceptibility to aminoglycoside induced hearing loss.
- (b) Cisplatin—dose-dependent SNHL
  - ○ Advanced age or children < 5 year old and noise exposure also increase likelihood and severity of SNHL.
  - ○ Hearing loss is permanent and bilateral.
  - ○ Injury occurs initially at outer hair cell, but may ultimately effect stria vascularis and ganglion cell.
- (c) Loop diuretics (furosemide)—results in transient SNHL
  - ○ Stria vascularis is the most common site of injury.
- (d) Salicylates—bilateral flat SNHL
  - ○ Dose dependent and typically reversible.
  - ○ Injury occurs initially at outer hair cells, but spiral ganglion can be affected with prolonged treatment.
- (e) Ototopicals
  - ○ Both gentamicin and neomycin/polymyxin have reports of ototoxicity when used with perforated TM.
  - ○ Chlorhexidine has been shown to be ototoxic if enters the middle ear.

Bibliography

Harris JP, Nguyen QT, eds. Meniere's disease. *Otolaryngol Clinic North Am.* 2010;43(5):965–1139.

Little SC, Kesser BW. Radiographic classification of temporal bone fractures: clinical predictability using a new system. *Arch Otolaryngol Head Neck Surg.* 2006;132:1300-1304.

Poliquin JF. Immunology of the ear. In: Alberti PW, Ruben RJ, eds. *Otologic Medicine and Surgery.* Vol 1. New York, NY: Churchill Livingstone; 1988:813-829.

Schucknecht HF. Trauma. In: Schucknecht HF, ed. *Pathology of the Ear.* Cambridge, MA: Harvard University Press; 1974:291-316.

Shea CR. Dermatologic disorders, diseases of the external ear canal. *Otolaryngol Clin North Am.* 1996;29:783-794.

Questions

1. A patient is referred to you for management of otosclerosis. Which of the following findings should be present before considering stapes surgery?

    A. Present acoustic reflexes

    B. Carhart notch at 2000 Hz

    C. Reversal of the 512-Hz tuning fork

    D. Mixed hearing loss

    E. None of the above

2. Last week, immediately after diving into a pool, a patient had severe pain in one ear and loss of hearing. There is no previous history of ear problems. On examination you notice some

dried blood in the ear canal and a 20% central perforation. How would you manage this patient?

A. Antibiotic drops

B. Observation

C. Emergent tympanoplasty

D. Office patch

3. A patient presents to the emergency room with vertigo and hearing loss after a stick went in his ear. The ear canal is filled with blood. How would you manage this patient?

A. Antibiotic drops

B. Bed rest and labyrinthine sedatives

C. Emergency surgery—tympanoplasty and ossicular reconstruction

D. Emergency surgery—tympanoplasty, tissue seal of the oval window, and secondary reconstruction

E. Reevaluate in 6 weeks

4. Patient presents to the emergency department after falling asleep while ice fishing. You notice his ear is has decreased sensation, no capillary refill, and is deep blue. You recommend

A. Immediate debridement of nonviable tissue

B. Rapid rewarming of the ear

C. Slow rewarming of the ear

D. Hyperbaric oxygen

5. According to OSHA standards, a patient who works in a factory regularly exposed to 100-dB noise can work for how long before requiring hearing protection?

A. 1 hour

B. 2 hours

C. 4 hours

D. 6 hours

Chapter 24
Tumors of the Temporal Bone

Selected Benign Tumors

See Table 24-1.

Glomus Tumor (Paraganglioma)

A. Most common neoplasm of the middle ear and second most common neoplasm of the temporal bone/cerebellopontine angle (CPA)
   i. Glomus tympanicum (GT)
   ii. Glomus jugulare (GJ)
   iii. Glomus vagale (GV)
B. Caucasians more commonly affected
C. Also known as chemodectoma
D. M:F—1:5
E. May be multicentric (10%)
F. Majority are sporadic; 10% are familial
G. Rarely malignant—(2%-4%)
   i. Diagnosis requires metastasis to non-neuroendocrine tissue.
   ii. Most common sites are nodal, bone, lung, liver, and spleen.
H. Rarely functional—5% or less secrete neuroactive peptides
   i. May result in catastrophic hypertension upon induction of anesthesia if not identified and treated preoperatively.
   ii. If secretory treat with phentolamine (nonselective reversible alpha-adrenergic agent).
   iii. Functional tumors are rare in extra-adrenal locations.
I. Biology
   i. Arise from chemoreceptor cells of the neuroendocrine system
      a. Cells located along the sympathetic chain
      b. Found in the jugular dome, tympanic promontory, along Jacobson and Arnold nerves
   ii. Genetics
      a. Familial tumors are caused by genetic defect in mitochondrial DNA encoding for succinyl dehydrogenase subunit B, C, or D (SDHB, SDHC, SDHD) of mitochondrial complex II.
         1. Thought to be the mutation in sporadic tumors as well
      b. Phenotype is maternally imprinted but passed via male carriers.
         1. Explains why phenotype can skip a generation

Table 24-1 **Tumors of the temporal bone**

	Benign	*Malignant*
EAC	Osteoma	SCCA
	Adenoma	BCCA
		Adenocarcinoma (ceruminous)
		Melanoma
		Direct extension of tumors from surrounding areas
ME/Mastoid	Lipoma/choristoma	SCCA
	Glomus tympanicum	Adenoid cystic carcinoma
	Hemangioma	Acinic cell carcinoma
	Endolymphatic sac tumor	Rhabdomyosarcoma
Petrous Apex	Schwannoma (facial/vestibular)	SCCA
	Meningioma	Osteosarcoma
	Hemangioma	Chondrosarcoma
	Glomus jugulare	Lymphoma
	Chordoma	Metastatic carcinoma to the temporal bone (TB)
		Direct extension of tumors of the surrounding area

BCCA, basal cell carcinoma; SCCA, squamous cell carcinoma

    J. Classification schemes (Table 24-2)
       i. Fisch
      ii. Glasscock-Jackson
        a. Glomus tympanicum
        b. Glomus jugulare
    K. Diagnosis
       i. Symptoms
        a. Pulsatile tinnitus (80%) (GT and GJ)
        b. Hearing loss, conductive or mixed (60%) (GT and GJ)
        c. Otalgia (13%) (GT and GJ)
        d. Aural fullness (32%) (GT and GJ)
        e. Hoarseness/dysphagia (15%) (GJ)
        f. Facial weakness (15%) (GT and GJ)
        g. Functional tumors will present with palpitations, unexplained weight loss, poorly controlled hypertension
      ii. Physical examination
        a. Middle ear mass
          1. For diagnosis GT must be able to see 360 degree around mass otherwise adjunctive imaging required for diagnosis.
          2. Brown sign—blanching of middle ear mass with pneumatic otoscopy

Table 24-2 Glomus Tumor Classification Schemes

Fisch	
Type A	Limited to the middle ear
Type B	Limited to the tympanomastoid area with no involvement of the infralabyrinthine compartment
Type C	Involves the infralabyrinthine compartment and petrous apex
	C1—limited involvement of carotid canal
	C2—invasion of the vertical portion of carotid canal
	C3—invasion of the horizontal portion of the carotid canal, does not involve the foramen lacerum
	C4—involves the entire course of the intrapetrous carotid
Type D	Intracranial extension
	De1—extradural, extension of < 2 cm
	De2—extradural, extension of > 2 cm
	Di1—intradural, extension of < 2 cm
	Di2—intradural, extension of > 2 cm
	Di3—intradural, unresectable

Glasscock-Jackson

Glomus tympanicum

Type I	Limited to the promontory
Type II	Completely filling the middle ear
Type III	Filling middle ear and extending into the mastoid
Type IV	Filling middle ear, into the mastoid, tympanic membrane (TM) and into the external auditory canal (EAC) (may extend anterior to the internal carotid artery)

Glomus jugulare

Type I	Small tumor involving the jugular bulb, middle ear, and mastoid
Type II	Extending under the internal auditory canal (IAC); may have intracranial extension
Type III	Extending into petrous apex, may have intracranial extension
Type IV	Extending beyond the petrous apex into the clivus or infratemporal fossa, may have intracranial extension

  b. EAC mass
  c. Neck mass or pharyngeal fullness
  d. Cranial nerve deficits including lower cranial nerve examination
    1. Audiogram (GT and GJ)
    2. Laryngoscopy (GJ)
  iii. Diagnostic workup
    a. Urine for vanillylmandelic acid (VMA), metanephrines

1. Must be 5× higher than normal to be symptomatic
2. Used to exclude a functional component

b. Radiography
1. Computed tomography (CT) IAC—imaging modality of choice.
   - Use to evaluate extent of lesion
   - GT—used to classify tumor as GT or GJ if diagnosis is unclear from physical examination
   - Evaluate extent of carotid canal involvement for GJ
   - Differentiate mass from high-riding jugular bulb or aberrant carotid
   - Infiltrative and erosive into the bone
2. Magnetic resonance imaging (MRI) with contrast.
   - Identify the extent of the lesion and assess intracranial extension
   - Classic "salt and pepper" appearance due to flow voids within the tumor
3. CT and MRI are complementary in the skull base.
4. Angiography.
   - Four-vessel angiography to identify feeding vessels.
   - Embolization of the feeding vessels should be performed 24 to 48 hours prior to surgical resection.
   - Significantly improves intraoperative blood loss.
   - Preoperative balloon occlusion testing using ^{99Tm}Tc-HMPAO SPECT scanning or Xenon CT of the ipsilateral carotid should be performed if imaging suggests arterial invasion.

L. Treatment
   i. Surgical
      a. Glomus tumors are a surgical disease unless patient's comorbidities prevent operation.
      b. GT
         1. Small tumors limited to the promontory can be removed via a transcanal or anterior tympanostomy approach.
         2. Larger tumors require wider exposure via mastoidectomy and posterior tympanostomy.
      c. GJ
         1. Requires proximal control of the great vessels in the neck and the sigmoid sinus.
         2. Large tumors may require transposition of the facial nerve to expose the tumor anteriorly.
         3. Infratemporal fossa approach (Fisch type A) is method of choice for removal.
         4. Considerable care is required to preserve the lower cranial nerves (CNIX-XII).
         5. For very large tumors—may need to stage the procedure if blood loss is greater than 3 L during removal of tumor from the neck and temporal bone. Intracranial resection can proceed at a later date.
   ii. Radiation
      a. Used in patients who cannot withstand surgery or refuse surgery.
      b. Used to prevent further tumor growth.
      c. Likely efficacious due to fibrosis of the arterioles rather than direct effect on tumor cells.
      d. Lower doses are used (15 Gy) for malignancies.

        e. Stereotactic radiosurgery (SRS) has reported 80% rate of tumor control.

           1. *Risks of SRS*: radiation-induced malignancy, osteoradionecrosis of the skull base, temporal lobe necrosis, cranial nerve injury

Endolymphatic Sac Tumor

A. Locally aggressive tumors of the endolymphatic sac.

B. Histologically described as a destructive papillary cystic adenomatous tumor of the temporal bone.

C. Can be sporadic or associated with von Hippel-Lindau (VHL) disease.

    i. Patients with VHL can have bilateral tumors and should be screened for this entity.

    ii. VHL caused by loss of function of tumor suppressor gene located on chromosome 3p25.

D. Typically involves the sac and the endolymphatic duct.

E. Symptoms are that of endolymphatic hydrops, likely due to obstruction of the normal flow and resorption patterns of endolymph.

    i. Sensorineural hearing loss (SNHL).

    ii. Tinnitus.

    iii. Aural fullness.

    iv. Vertigo.

    v. Late symptoms include facial paralysis, symptoms of brainstem compression, and lower cranial neuropathies.

F. Imaging

    i. CT—bony destruction of the posterior fossa plate with central calcifications. May extend into the mastoid as well

    ii. MRI

        a. T1—isointense to hyperintense when compared to cerebellar white matter

        b. T2—heterogeneous (suggesting its highly vascular nature)

        c. T1 with contrast—strongly enhancing

G. Treatment

    i. Surgery is the method of choice.

        a. Should involve removal of both surfaces of the dura to ensure complete removal.

        b. Hearing sparing approaches for small tumors.

           1. Retrolabyrinthine—transdural

        c. Patients with nonserviceable hearing.

           1. Translabyrinthine approach

        d. Large tumors can be preoperatively embolized to minimize blood loss.

Hemangioma

A. Benign tumors that arise from blood vessels

B. Typically associated with the facial nerve, particularly the geniculate ganglion

    i. Less common are lesions of the IAC facial nerve.

        a. Symptoms similar to vestibular schwannoma

C. Results in slowly progressive or recurrent facial weakness with twitching

D. Locally aggressive resulting in bony destruction

    i. Erosion into the cochlea results in SNHL

    ii. Dilation of the fallopian canal

E. Imaging

      i. CT—infiltrative erosive lesion centered at the geniculate ganglion
        a. May erode into cochlea or labyrinth
        b. Intratumor calcifications are common
      ii. MRI—on T1 imaging hypo- to isointense to brain and enhance avidly with contrast.
   F. Treatment
      i. Small lesions can be meticulously dissected free from the nerve when centered at the geniculate with full preservation of facial function.
      ii. For IAC lesions, unless face is paralyzed, surgical treatment involves decompression of the IAC as resection requires resection and nerve grafting.
      iii. For larger lesions or those with complete facial paralysis, treatment is resection with nerve grafting.

Chordoma

A. Unusual locally aggressive neoplasms of the clivus
B. Metastases are reported but are unusual
C. Impacts the temporal bone due to lateral extension of the tumor into the CPA or lower cranial nerves
D. Develops from the notochord remnant
E. Histology: physaliferous cells
F. Presents with diplopia due to involvement of CN VI as it passes through Dorello canal and headache
      i. Involvement of CN V is also common.
G. Treatment
      i. Surgical resection is the gold standard.
        a. Incomplete resection should be followed with adjuvant radiation.
        b. Bioactive chemotherapeutic agents are in clinical trials (tyrosine kinase inhibitors).
        c. Approaches include Fisch infratemporal fossa B and C.
        d. Can also be managed with transnasal endoscopic resections in combination with lateral skull base approaches.
H. Five-year survival, 51%

Lipoma/Choristoma

A. Rare middle ear masses.
B. Presents with conductive hearing loss and middle ear effusion.
C. Choristoma is defined as histologically normal tissue in an abnormal location.
      i. Salivary tissue is most common histologic type.
      ii. Fat within the middle ear may be due to choristoma development or neoplastic process. Etiology is unclear.
      iii. Other tissue types reported include glial choristoma.
D. Treatment is surgical excision.

Selected Malignant Tumors

See Table 24-1.

Squamous Cell Carcinoma

A. Most common malignancy of the temporal bone

B. Most common histology of EAC and middle ear carcinoma (basal cell carcinoma [BCCA] most common histology of the pinna/conchal bowl)

    i. All different subtypes of squamous cell carcinoma (SCCA) have been reported in the ear.

        a. Most commonly well or moderately differentiated SCCA.

        b. Poorly differentiated, spindle cell, basaloid SCCA, and verrucous carcinoma have all been described.

C. Epidemiology

    i. Rare tumor representing less than 0.2% of head and neck (HN) malignancies.

    ii. M:F—1:1.

    iii. Caucasians are most commonly affected.

    iv. Sixty-six percent affected patients are greater than 55 years old.

D. Biology

    i. Older literature reference association with chronic inflammation/otorrhea of the EAC or middle ear as in chronic otitis externa (OE) or chronic otitis media (COM).

    ii. Human papillomavirus (HPV) has been found in some tumors of the middle ear.

    iii. May be associated with prior radiation for unrelated disease (ie, nasopharyngeal carcinoma).

E. Diagnosis

    i. Symptoms

        a. Otorrhea—most common complaint (60%-80%)

        b. Otalgia (50%-60%)

        c. Bleeding (5%-20%)

        d. Hearing loss (20%-60%)

    ii. Physical examination

        a. Mass in EAC (10%-25%)

        b. Facial paresis/paralysis (10%-15%)

        c. Preauricular mass (10%)

        d. Neck/nodal examination (1%-5%)

    iii. Adjunctive testing

        a. Audiogram

        b. CT IAC/temporal bone study

            1. Evaluate the extent of involvement of the EAC, middle ear structures, and petrous apex

            2. Does not differentiate between retained secretions and tumor

        c. MRI with contrast if extratemporal and/or intracranial involvement is suspected

F. Classification

    i. T stage—Based on physical examination and radiographic findings (Table 24-3).

    ii. T staging as described in Table 24-3 applies to both EAC and middle ear (ME)/mastoid lesions. Therefore, any patient with primary SCCA of the ME/mastoid is automatically in advanced-stage disease (T3 or T4).

    iii. Vast majority of lesions (80%) originate in the EAC and less than 10% originate in the ME. Approximately 10% of the site of origin cannot be determined.

    iv. Nodal staging.

Table 24-3 T-Staging for Squamous Cell Carcinoma of the Temporal Bone

T Stage	Extent of Disease
T1	Tumor limited to EAC without evidence of bony erosion or soft tissue involvement
T2	Tumor causes limited bony erosion (not full thickness) or < 0.5cm of soft tissue involvement
T3	Tumor erodes through the bony EAC with limited (< 0.5cm) soft tissue involvement; or involves middle ear and/or mastoid
T4	Tumor erodes into the medial wall of the middle ear to involve the cochlea, labyrinth, petrous apex, jugular foramen, carotid canal, or dura; soft tissue involvement of > 0.5cm (temporomandibular joint [TMJ], styloid or parotid); evidence of facial paresis/paralysis

Reproduced with permission from Moody SA, Hirsch BE, Myers EN. Squamous cell carcinoma of the external auditory canal: an evaluation of a staging system, *Am J Otol.* 2000 Jul;21(4):582-588.

    a. Nodal metastasis (met) occurs in approximately 10% of patients.
    b. EAC nodal basins.
       1. First echelon—superficial parotid lymph nodes (LNs), postauricular LN
       2. Second echelon—level 2 in the neck
    c. Presence of nodal disease indicates advanced stage (IV).
    d. N stage.
       1. N0—no nodal mets
       2. N1—single ipsilateral node less than 3 cm in diameter
       3. N2— (a) single ipsilateral node 3 to 6 cm in diameter, (b) multiple ipsilateral nodes not greater than 6 cm, (c) contralateral nodal metastasis
       4. N3—any node greater than 6 cm in diameter
  v. Distant metastasis
    a. Presents in less than 10% of patients
    b. Lungs, bone, liver
G. Patterns of spread
  i. Anteriorly into the TMJ, parotid via direct bony erosion, invasion of the fissures of Santorini (cartilaginous EAC) or patent foramen of Huscke (bony EAC)
  ii. Laterally into the meatus and conchal bowl
  iii. Medially through the tympanic membrane/annulus in the middle ear and attic
  iv. Posteriorly into the mastoid via direct bony erosion
  v. Inferiorly into the mastoid and stylomastoid foramen usually through direct bony erosion but may have perineural spread along the facial nerve into the foramen
  vi. Superiorly into the root of zygoma and intracranial space through direct bony erosion
H. Prognosis
  i. Overall survival for all patients with SCCA of the temporal bone is reported between 30% and 45% at 5 years.
    a. Disease-free survival (DFS) at 5 years reported at 60%.
  ii. Higher T stage correlates with worse prognosis.
    a. T1-2 tumors have 80% to 100% 5-year DFS following definitive treatment.
       1. Many succumb to comorbid conditions.
    b. T3-4 tumors have 28% DFS at 5 years.

  iii. Poor prognostic findings.
   a. Nodal disease
   b. Recurrence of disease following definitive treatment
    1. Most patients recur within 12 months of treatment.
   c. Facial nerve involvement
   d. Positive surgical margins
 I. Treatment
  i. Surgery (Table 24-4)
   a. Should be considered the treatment modality of choice with addition of adjuvant therapies as needed
   b. Sleeve resection only appropriate for clear tumor margins of primary pinna tumors
    1. Not indicated for primary lesions of the EAC
   c. T1
    1. Lateral temporal bone resection (LTBR).

Table 24-4 Temporal Bone Resection

Surgery	Tissues Removed	Limits of Dissection
LTBR	En bloc removal of cartilaginous and bony EAC, TM, malleus, incus	A: capsule of TMJ
	Optional: parotidectomy, neck dissection, mandibular condyle	S: epitympanum, root of zygoma
		P: mastoid cavity
		I: facial nerve, hypotympanic bone, infratemporal fossa
		M: stapes
STBR	LTBR + contents of ME and mastoid, otic capsule, medial wall of ME	A: anterior capsule of TMJ, mandibular ramus
	Optional: facial nerve, dura, infratemporal fossa, sigmoid, brain parenchyma	S: middle fossa dura
	May be piecemeal or en bloc resection	P: dura of posterior fossa
		I: infratemporal fossa
		M: IAC, petrous apex with neurovascular structures
TTBR	STBR + petrous apex and neurovascular bundle	A: anterior capsule of TMJ, mandibular ramus
	Piecemeal resection used when carotid and lower CN preserved; en bloc resection requires sacrifice of carotid and lower CN	S: temporal lobe
		P: cerebellum
		I: Infratemporal fossa
		M: +/− carotid, clivus

A, anterior; I, inferior; M, medial; P, posterior; S, superior

2. Superficial parotidectomy can be considered to assess for microscopic nodal metastasis.
3. Routine postoperative radiation is not necessary if surgical margins are negative; there is no evidence of nodal spread and there is no perineural/lymphovascular invasion.

d. T2
1. LTBR or extended LTBR.
2. Parotidectomy.
3. Consider condylectomy particularly for anterior EAC tumors.
4. Ipsilateral selective neck dissection involving levels 2-4.
5. Locoregional versus free tissue transfer reconstruction.
6. Adjuvant radiation has been shown to significantly improve survival in T2 patients.

e. T3
1. Subtotal temporal bone resection (STBR)
2. Parotidectomy—superficial versus total
3. Neck dissection—levels 2-4 and to identify vessels for microvascular reconstruction
4. Consider mandibulectomy
5. Free tissue transfer for reconstruction
6. Adjuvant radiation

f. T4
1. STBR versus total temporal bone resection (TTBR)
2. Parotidectomy
3. Mandibulectomy
4. Neck dissection
5. Free tissue transfer for reconstruction
6. Adjuvant radiation
7. Consider neoadjuvant or adjuvant chemotherapy

g. Patients with distant metastatic disease at the time of presentation may still be considered candidates for palliative surgical resection to decrease the morbidity of the locoregional disease. Alternatively, metastatic tumors may be treated with palliative chemoradiation.

ii. Radiation
a. Radiation alone used for patients who cannot tolerate surgery.
b. Survival rates after radiation alone are low (10%).
c. Radiation does not penetrate bone well and thus does not sufficiently affect the tumor.
d. Improves local control and DFS when used as adjuvant therapy with surgery.

iii. Chemotherapy
a. Platinum-based therapies (cisplatinum) have been used as neoadjuvant and adjuvant treatment.
b. Given alone for palliation only.
c. No trials demonstrating addition of chemotherapy improves local control or survival.

J. Controversies
i. Extent of surgery
a. En bloc total temporal bone resection is rarely performed due to significant operative mortality and postoperative morbidity.

b. Reports of treatment of advanced disease with LTBR with postoperative chemoradiation with overall survival (OS) of 30% to 40% (similar to STBR and TTBR).

Rhabdomyosarcoma

A. Epidemiology
   i. Most common malignancy of the temporal bone in childhood.
   ii. Rhabdomyosarcoma (RMS) involves the HN in 30% of cases.
      a. Orbit 25%
      b. Parameningeal, 50%
         1. Nasopharynx (NP), nasal cavity, sinuses, ME/mastoid, pterygoid fossa
      c. Nonparameningeal, 25%
B. Biology
   i. Arises from mesenchymal cells
   ii. Associated with loss of material from chromosome 11p15
C. Histology
   i. *Subtypes*: embryonal (most common), alveolar, boytroid, spindle cell, and anaplastic
   ii. Diagnosis can be made by identifying striated muscle fibers within the tumor cells
   iii. *Immunohistochemistry staining*: desmin, MyoD1, myogenin, and muscle-specific actin
   iv. Electron microscopy—Z bands and intermediate filaments
D. Diagnosis
   i. Symptoms and physical examination
      a. Hearing loss
      b. Bloody otorrhea
      c. Otalgia
      d. Aural polyp
      e. Cranial neuropathies
   ii. Adjunctive testing
      a. Biopsy
      b. Audiogram
      c. CT
         1. Demonstrates locally destructive process within the ME and mastoid, loss of septation, and bony erosion
         2. If facial nerve is involved may widen the fallopian canal
      d. MRI
         1. T1—isointense to muscle
         2. T2—iso- to hyperintense to muscle
         3. T1 + contrast—strongly enhancing lesion
      e. Bone studies
         1. Used to identify bony metastasis
      f. Bone marrow biopsy
         1. Marrow involvement worsens prognosis
E. Classification
   i. Intergroup RMS study group (IRSG) presurgical staging system.
      a. TNM staging system (Table 24-5)
         1. T
            • T1—confined to anatomic site of origin

Table 24-5 TNM Staging System for Rhabdomyosarcoma

Stage	Site	T	N	M
I	Orbit, HN (× parameningeal), genitourinary (GU) nonbladder/nonprostate	T1 or T2a or b	N0 or N1	M0
II	Bladder/prostate, extremity, cranial, parameningeal	T1 or T2a or b	N0	M0
III	Bladder/prostate, extremity, cranial, parameningeal	T1 or T2a or b	N1	M0
IV	All sites	T1 or T2a or b	N0 or N1	M1
Group 1	Localized disease, completely excised, no microscopic residual			
	A. Confined to site of origin, completely resected			
	B. Infiltrating beyond the site of origin, completely resected			
Group 2	Total gross resection			
	A. Gross resection with evidence of microscopic local residual			
	B. Regional disease with involved lymph nodes, completely resected with no microscopic residual			
	C. Microscopic local and/or nodal residual			
Group 3	Incomplete resection or biopsy with gross residual			
Group 4	Distant metastasis			

          (a) T1a—less than 5 cm in diameter
          (b) T1b—greater than 5 cm in diameter
       • T2—extension and/or fixation to surrounding tissue
          (a) T2a—less than 5 cm in diameter
          (b) T2b—greater than 5 cm in diameter
    2. N
       • N0—no regional nodal metastasis
       • N1—regional nodes clinically involved
       • Nx—clinical status of regional nodes unknown
    3. M
       • M0—no distant metastasis
       • M1—metastasis present
  ii. IRSG postsurgical classification (used for study groups I-IV).
  iii. Patients with ME/mastoid RMS are at high risk for leptomeningeal involvement.
    a. Usually occurs through tumor invasion of the fallopian canal, erosion of the tegmen, or posterior fossa plates
    b. Portends a poor prognosis (considered M1)
F. Treatment
  i. Surgery
    a. Used for diagnostic biopsy
    b. Extent of surgery is dictated by predicted postoperative morbidity

1. Current recommendation is to remove as much tumor as possible without causing significant morbidity.
2. Radical resection in the head and neck is difficult due to complex anatomy of the skull base.
- ii. Chemotherapy
  a. Mainstay of treatment
  b. Currently multiple clinical trials evaluating various chemotherapy regimens for patients with RMS
  c. Given intrathecally for patients with parameningeal sites
- iii. Radiation
  a. Used in conjunction with chemotherapy.
  b. Long-term side effects such as effect on skeletal growth centers and radiation-induced malignancy must be considered when using this therapy.
- G. Prognosis
  - i. Steadily improved since 1970s
  - ii. OS 5 years (postsurgical IRSG classification)
    a. Stage I—80%
    b. Stage II—70%
    c. Stage III—52%
    d. Stage IV—20%

Metastasis to or Direct Invasion of the Temporal Bone

- A. Mets to the tempotal bone (TB)
  - i. Most common temporal origin in order of frequency
    a. Breast
    b. Lung
    c. Gastrointestinal tract
    d. Renal cell
    e. Prostate
    f. Salivary gland
  - ii. Most common histology in order of frequency
    a. Adenocarcinoma
    b. Squamous cell carcinoma
    c. Small cell carcinoma
    d. Lymphoma
    e. Melanoma
    f. Sarcoma
- B. Direct invasion of the TB
  - i. Nasopharyngeal carotic artery (CA)
  - ii. Adenoid cystic CA
    a. May be direct extension via stylomastoid foramen or skip lesions of perineural invasion of the facial nerve
  - iii. Clival tumors
    a. Chordoma
    b. Chondrosarcoma
  - iv. Meningeal sarcoma
  - v. Squamous cell carcinoma of the pharynx

Bibliography

Barrs DM. Temporal bone carcinoma. *Otolaryngol Clin North Am.* 2001;34:1197-1218.

Chen PG, Nguyen JH, Payne SC, Sheehan JP, Hashisaki GT. Treatment of glomus jugulare tumors with gamma knife radiosurgery. *Laryngoscope.* 2010;120:1856-1862.

Gidley PW, Robers DB, Sturgis EM. Squamous cell carcinoma of the temporal bone. *Laryngoscope.* 2010;120:1144-1151.

Horn KL, Hankinson HL. Tumors of the jugular foramen. In: Jackler RK, Brackmann DE, eds. *Neurotology.* 2nd ed. Philadelphia, PA: Elsevier Mosby; 2005:1037-1046.

Janecka IP, Kapadia SB, Mancuso AA, Prasad S, Moffat DA, Pribaz JJ. Cancers involving the skull base and temporal bone. In: Harrison LB, Sessions RB, Hong WK, eds. *Head and Neck Cancer: A Multidisciplinary Approach.* 3rd ed. Philadelphia, PA: Wolters Kluwer; 2009:629-654.

Megerian CA, Semaan MT. Evaluation and management of endolymphatic sac and duct tumors. *Otolaryngol Clin North Am.* 2007;40:463-478.

Questions

1. A patient presents with pulsatile tinnitus of 6 months duration and a reddish colored mass that is incompletely seen through the tympanic membrane. What is the next best diagnostic test to assist in making the diagnosis?

    A. MRI brain with/without contrast

    B. CT temporal bone without contrast

    C. Tissue biopsy

    D. Urine VMA and metanephrines

2. Patients with von Hippel-Lindau disease should be screened for which of the following conditions?

    A. Squamous cell carcinoma of the external ear canal

    B. Chondrosarcoma of the petrous apex

    C. Endolymphatic sac tumors

    D. Glomus jugulare tumors

3. A 5-year-old child presents with a history of hearing loss and otalgia. On examination he has an aural polyp and a mass visible behind the tympanic membrane. A biopsy of the mass is performed. Immunohistochemical studies are likely to show

    A. Positive desmin

    B. Positive epithelial membrane antigen

    C. Positive tyrosinase

    D. Positive neuron-specific enolase

4. In a lateral temporal bone resection, the medial margin is the

    A. Tympanic annulus

    B. Fundus of the internal auditory canal

    C. Stapes

    D. Carotid artery

5. Which of the following findings is not indicative of poor prognosis in squamous cell carcinoma of the EAC?

A. Nodal disease

B. Extension into the petrous apex

C. Gender

D. Facial nerve involvement

Part 3
Rhinology

Chapter 25
Nasal Function and the Evaluation of Taste/Smell

Nasal Function

A. Warming and humidification
   i. Air is humidified to high relative humidity
   ii. Air is warmed through heat diffusion and convection
   iii. Optimum mucociliary clearance is facilitating by temperature of 37°C
B. Regulation of nasal secretions and airway resistance
   i. Proteins in nasal secretions
   a. Plasma proteins
      1. Albumin
      2. Immunoglobulins (IgG, IgM, IgA)
   b. Serous cell products
      1. Antibacterial defense molecules
         • Lysozymes
         • Lactoferrin
         • Secretory component
   c. Mucous cell products
      1. Mucoglycoproteins
      2. Mucins
   d. Epithelial goblet cell products
      1. Macromolecules and ions

      ii. Proteins are dissolved or suspended in epithelial lining fluid
- a. Modified by epithelial ion pumps
- b. Plasma extravasation controlled by interepithelial tight junctions
  1. Dependent on rate of blood flow and plasma transudation
     - Arterial vasodilation and filling of venous sinusoidal vessels results in plasma extravasation, thickened nasal mucosa, increased airway resistance.
     - Vasoconstriction reduces mucosal blood flow, reduces plasma extravasation, relieves venous sinusoidal congestion.

    iii. Autonomic innervation
- a. Vidian nerve
  1. Formed at junction of greater petrosal (preganglionic parasympathetic fibers) and deep petrosal nerves (postganglionic sympathetic fibers)
  2. Postganglionic sympathetic and parasympathetic fibers carried in the nerve of the vidian canal and join branches of sphenopalatine nerve
     - Parasympathetic neurons
       - (a) Cotransmitter to acetylcholine (vasointestinal peptide (VIP))
         - ○ Vasodilation at arterial and sinusoidal vessels
         - ○ Enhanced secretory activity
         - ○ Mast cell degranulation
           - – Release of histamine, bradykinin, arachidonic acid metabolites, ions
     - Sympathetic fibers join branches of sphenopalatine nerve and artery
       - (a) Cotransmitter to noradrenaline (neuropeptide Y)
         - ○ Vasoconstriction of venous sinusoidal vessels

    iv. Nonadrenergic, noncholinergic responses
- a. Trigeminal sensory neurons use peptides as neurotransmitters
  1. Secreted by macrophages, eosinophils, lymphocytes, dendritic cells
  2. Substance P, neurokinin A, calcitonin gene-related peptide (CGRP)
     - Induce vasodilation
     - Increase vascular permeability
     - Increase nasal resistance
     - Stimulate glandular secretion
     - Leukocyte chemotaxis
     - Mast cell degranulation

    v. Nasal cycle
- a. Cyclical vascular phenomenon that occurs in 80% of normal individuals
- b. Alternating congestion/decongestion every 3 to 7 hours
- c. Centrally-mediated autonomic tone of capacitance vessels of erectile mucosa

    vi. Other influences on nasal resistance
- a. Exercise decreases nasal resistance
- b. Irritants (dust, smoke), cold/dry air, alcohol, pregnancy, hypothyroidism and drugs cause congestion of capacitance vessels
  1. Drugs that cause nasal congestion
     - Antihypertensives (alpha and beta blockers)
     - Oral contraceptives
     - Antidepressants
     - Nonsteroidal anti-inflammatory medications
     - Decongestants in excess may result in rhinitis medicamentosa

     c. Atrophic rhinitis
       1. Chronic, degenerative disorder characterized by nasal crusting, malodorous discharge, and nasal obstruction
- Atrophy of serous and mucinous glands
- Loss of cilia and goblet cells
- Inflammatory cell infiltrates

       2. Possible causes
- Underlying chronic inflammatory disease
    (a) Granulomatous disorders
- Irradiation
- Bacterial and viral infection
- Excessive nasal surgery

C. Nasal airflow
  i. At low flow rates, airflow is laminar
  ii. Maximum velocity occurs in the nasal valve region
     a. Bernoulli principle
       1. Airflow velocity is greatest at the narrowest segment
       2. Increased airflow velocity leads to negative pressure and nasal valve collapse
     b. Poiseuille's law
       1. Airflow resistance is inversely proportional to fourth power of the radius
       2. Small decrease in cross-sectional area produces large increase in airway resistance
  iii. Relatively slow flow rates found in olfactory region with quiet breathing
  iv. During inspiration, main flow stream occurs in the lower and middle airway (space between middle meatus and nasal septum)
  v. During expiration, maximum velocity is lower but expiratory air is evenly distributed across inferior, middle, and olfactory regions
  vi. Diagnostic testing of nasal airflow
     a. Nasal inspiratory peak flow
       1. Objective, physiologic measurement of nasal airflow
       2. Advantages: portable equipment, easy to use
       3. Disadvantages: test-retest variability, influenced by the lower airway
     b. Rhinomanometry
       1. Pressure sensors placed with and without decongestion to develop flow-pressure curves
       2. Measurements calculated to determine airflow resistance
       3. Advantages: functional test, may be done on both sides simultaneously
       4. Disadvantages: time, expense, inability to identify site of obstruction
     c. Acoustic rhinometry
       1. Sound waves transmitted into nasal cavity, which is reflected back and converted into digital impulses constructed on a rhinogram
       2. Detects variances in cross-sectional area along predetermined points in the nasal cavity
       3. Advantages: fast test, localizes area of obstruction
       4. Disadvantages: technically challenging, unable to accurately measure beyond narrow apertures
D. Immunology/mucociliary clearance
  i. First line of defense against bacteria/viruses.
  ii. Mucociliary transport of microorganisms and noxious particles.

a. Mucus travels along ciliated columnar epithelial cells of nasal mucosa at a rate of 2 to 10 mm/h.
iii. Seromucinous glands and goblet cells secrete mucus.
iv. Periciliary fluid contains immunomodulating cells/proteins: macrophages, neutrophils, basophils, eosinophils, mast cells, B and T leukocytes, immunoglobulins A, G, M E, lysozymes, lactoferrin, interferon.
v. Particles >12 μm may be filtered.
vi. Evaluation of mucociliary transport.
  a. Saccharin test
    1. 0.5 mm saccharin particle placed approximately 1cm behind the anterior end of the inferior turbinate.
    2. Measure time elapsing until the first experience of sweet taste at posterior nasopharynx.
  b. 99Tc-macroaggregated albumin scintigraphy
    1. Radiolabeled droplet placed in anterior nasal floor.
    2. Gamma camera systems obtain dynamic images over 10 to 20 minutes to measure transport time between a reference point and the distance traveled to nasopharynx.
  c. Electron microscopy
    1. Absent or shortened outer dynein arms of ciliary ultrastructure observed in patients with ciliary dyskinesia
  d. Nasal nitric oxide measurements
    1. Reduced in patients with primary ciliary dyskinesia and cystic fibrosis
E. Olfaction
  i. Basic terminology
    a. Smell—the perception of an odor
    b. Taste—the perception of salty, sweet, sour, bitter
    c. Flavor—the complex interaction of smell, taste, and somatic sensation
      1. Mediated by CNs I, V, VII, IX, and X in the nose, oral cavity, pharynx and larynx
    d. Anosmia—the inability to detect odors
    e. Hyposmia—decreased ability to detect odors
    f. Dysosmia/parosmia—altered perception of odors
    g. Parosmia—incorrectly identifying odors
      1. Often mistaking pleasant or neutral odors for unpleasant ones
    h. Phantosmia—smell in the absence of a corresponding stimulus
    i. Ageusia—inability to taste
    j. Hypogeusia—decreased ability to taste
    k. Dysgeusia—distorted sense of taste

Anatomy and Physiology of Olfaction

A. Peripheral elements of the olfactory system consist of approximately 6 million bipolar receptor cells.
B. Bipolar receptor cell bodies, dendrites, axons located within the olfactory neuroepithelium (ON).
  i. ON found at superior-posterior septum, superior turbinate, superior and medial aspect of middle turbinate
    a. Pseudostratified columnar epithelium
    b. Basal cells—capable of undergoing continuous regeneration throughout life and following injury

    c. Sustentacular/supporting cells—secrete mucopolysaccharides into mucus that degrades odorants for transport across the epithelium

    d. Olfactory sensory neurons

    e. Bowman glands are interspersed and secrete mucus

C. Olfaction plays a primary role in the regulation of food intake, the perception of flavor and in detection of irritating and toxic substances.

D. Olfactory mucosa is sheltered during normal respiration.

    i. Sniffing redistributes airflow to the upper portion of the nasal cavities to the olfactory organ (orthonasal olfaction)

E. Humans can discriminate more than 1 trillion olfactory stimuli.

F. Olfactory transduction:

    i. Movement of odors from the air phase of the nasal cavity into the aqueous phase of the olfactory mucus.

    ii. Odorants are transported through aqueous medium to olfactory receptor proteins of the cilia.

    iii. Action potentials induced in receptor cells.

    iv. Receptor neurons are unique in that each cell serves as both a receptor cell and first-order neuron.

        a. Axons are projected directly from the nasal cavity into the brain without an intervening synapse.

    v. Olfactory transduction involves a G protein-mediated cascade.

        a. Results in membrane depolarization through the influx of calcium, outflow of chloride and activation of a sodium/calcium exchanger

    vi. Action potential travels down the axon of the olfactory receptor cell.

        a. Meets with axons of other olfactory receptor cells to form the olfactory nerve.

        b. Axons traverse the cribriform plate of the ethmoid bone to form the olfactory bulb.

        c. Axons make their first synapse in the glomeruli of the bulb.

        d. Axons branch and synapse on second order neurons which merge to form olfactory tract.

    vii. Olfactory tract travels to the piriform cortex.

        a. Encodes representations of odor quality, identity, memory and the coordination of olfaction, vision, and taste.

        b. Thalamus is further involved in the interpretation of odors.

        c. Amygdala responds to the intensity of emotionally significant pleasant or unpleasant odors.

        d. Entorhinal cortex preprocesses information entering the hippocampus, which is involved in learning and memory.

        e. Orbitofrontal cortex provides interpretive processing.

            1. Corresponds to brodmann areas 10,11,25

    viii. While sight and hearing are processed by a relay center in the cerebral hemisphere, smell has a direct route to many parts of the brain

        a. Sight and hearing more closely connected with higher functioning

        b. Smell is associated with emotion

    ix. Trigeminal system (fifth nerve) delivers somatosensory information from within the nasal cavity through branches of the ophthalmic and maxillary divisions

        a. Stinging, burning, pungent sensations mediated by trigeminal afferents

        b. Cell bodies of trigeminal afferents located in gasserian ganglion within Meckel cave

      c. Axons project to the trigeminal nucleus in the brain stem, thalamus, and insula and cingulate cortices (both part of the limbic system)

G. Taste
    i. Taste refers to sensations arising from the taste buds.
    ii. Flavor is the combination of taste and smell.
    iii. Retronasal olfaction occurs when food is chewed and swallowed.
      a. Tastants contact the taste buds on the tongue, oropharynx and larynx.
      b. Odorants pumped behind the palate into the nasal cavity.
    iv. Mediated by CNsVII, IX, and X
      a. Chorda tympani receives taste information from the anterior 2/3 of the tongue.
        1. Runs along lingual nerve
      b. Greater superficial petrosal nerve receives input from posterior tongue and junction of the hard and soft palate.
      c. Both arise from the nervus intermedius.
    v. Glossopharyngeal nerve receives taste information from posterior 1/3 of the tongue.
    vi. Superior laryngeal nerve innervates taste buds on the laryngeal surface of the epiglottis.

H. Taste map myth
    i. Although studies have shown that thresholds for certain sensations are lower at certain areas of the tongue, the differences are very small.

Olfactory and Taste Disorders

A. 200,000 patient visits a year for smell and taste disturbances.
B. Men are more commonly affected than women.
    i. Men begin to lose the ability to smell earlier in life.
C. Chemosensory loss is age-dependent.
    i. 80 years of age, 80% have olfactory impairment, nearly 50% are anosmic.
    ii. Age 65 to 80 years, 60% have major olfactory impairment and nearly 25% are anosmic
    iii. < 65years, 1% to 2% have smell impairment
D. Prevalence: estimated 2 million people are affected in the US.
E. Risk factors include advanced age, poor nutritional status and smoking.
F. Etiology:
    i. Since olfactory dysfunction can result from pathologic processes at any level along the olfactory pathway, from the nasal cavity to the brain, they can be thought of as conductive or sensorineural defects.
      a. Transport loss refers to conditions that interfere with access of odorants to the olfactory neuroepithelium.
        1. Viral infections, bacterial rhinitis and sinusitis, allergic rhinitis, nasal polyposis, congenital abnormalities, septal deviation
          • Kallmann syndrome—x-linked disorder characterized by congenital anosmia and hypogonadotropic hypogonadism
      b. Sensory loss refers to injury at the receptor region.
        1. Viral infections, drugs, neoplasms, radiation therapy, toxin exposure
          • Post-viral smell dysfunction not well understood.
          • Virus may damage ON.

- Parainfluenza virus type 3 is especially detrimental to olfaction.
- HIV is associated with subjective distortion of smell and taste.

   c. Neural loss refers to damage of the central olfactory pathways.

     1. Trauma, alcoholism, neurodegenerative disease, cigarette smoking, depression, diabetes mellitus, drugs/toxins, hypothyroidism, Kallman syndrome, malnutrition, neoplasms, neurosurgery, AIDS, vitamin B12/zinc deficiency, temporal lobe seizures, pregnancy

- Head trauma induces smell impairment in up to 15% of cases
  - (a) Anosmia more common than hyposmia.
  - (b) Olfactory dysfunction is more common when the trauma is associated with loss of consciousness, moderately severe head injury and skull fracture.
  - (c) Frontal injuries, fractures and shearing injury disrupt the olfactory axons that perforate the cribriform plate.
  - (d) Sometimes associated with CSF rhinorrhea, resulting from tearing of the dura overlying the cribriform plate.
  - (e) Traumatic anosmia is usually permanent.
  - (f) Only 10% of patients ever improve.
  - (g) Dysosmia may occur as a transient phase in the recovery process.
- Neoplasms
  - (a) Meningiomas of the inferior frontal region are the most frequent neoplastic cause of anosmia.
  - (b) Others: pituitary adenoma, craniopharyngioma, glioma, sinonasal tumors.
- Neurodegenerative disorders
  - (a) Alzheimer, PD, MS, ALS.
  - (b) Olfactory loss may be the first clinical sign of disease.

Evaluation of Olfactory Function

A. History

   i. Focus on targeting an underlying cause

     a. URI, allergies, dental problems, cognitive deficits, weight change, increased use of salt/sugar, medications

   ii. Clarify the taste-smell distinction

     a. Patients with olfactory dysfunction may present with taste complaints.

B. Physical examination

   i. Thorough head and neck, neurologic examination

   ii. Cognition and mood

   iii. Signs of systemic disease

   iv. Nasal endoscopy

     a. 4 mm zero or 30 degree scope

     b. Endoscopy without decongestant

     c. Topical anesthetic + decongestant applied

     d. Color of mucosa, presence of inflamed or hypertrophic mucosa, presence of nasal polyps or secretions, anatomic abnormalities (septal deviation, spur, concha bullosa, accessory ostia, middle meatus, sphenoethmoid recess, olfactory cleft)

C. Labs
  i. CBC, CMP, TSH, IgE levels in the appropriate patient
D. Smell threshold and identification tests
  i. Odor stix—odor-producing magic marker waved about 6 in from the nose
  ii. 12-in alcohol test—open alcohol packet, wave it in front of the nose, the patient is normally able to detect odor at approximately 12 in
  iii. Scratch and sniff card containing three odors
  iv. University of Pennsylvania Smell Identification Test
    a. Self-administered 40-item, multiple choice scratch and sniff test
    b. Quantitative measurement of olfaction
    c. High test-retest reliability
    d. Most widely used clinical test
    e. Adjusts for age and gender
    f. Patient's characterized as normal, mild, moderate or severe microsmia, anosmia or probable malingering
      1. Malingering appears as the reporting of fewer correct responses than expected on the basis of chance
      2. Present strong CN V stimulant (ammonia) to test for malingering
E. No convenient standardized tests for taste function
  i. Solutions containing sweet, salty, bitter, and sour components may be used.
F. Imaging
  i. CT scan is the most useful, cost-effective technique.
  ii. High resolution coronal MRI images from frontal sinus to posterior corpus callosum.
    a. Coronal MRI is technique of choice to image the olfactory bulbs, tracts and cortical parenchyma.

Treatment of Olfactory Dysfunction

A. Address underlying cause
  i. Inflammatory disease, polyps addressed with medical or surgical management
    a. Olfactory outcomes following ESS for CRS variable and challenging to predict.
    b. Presence of nasal polyposis is predictive of postoperative olfactory improvement.
  ii. Several medical therapies under investigation for postviral, posttraumatic and idiopathic anosmia
    a. Topical and systemic steroids
      1. Local effects on mucosa in the form of membrane stabilization, alteration of mediator release, inhibition of cell migration
      2. Central effects: excitability increases and thresholds for stimulus qualities are lowered
      3. Additional effect of topical therapy after pretreatment with oral steroids
    b. Alpha lipoic acid
      1. Fatty acid derivative that acts as an antioxidant
      2. May be helpful in patients with olfactory loss after URI
    c. Theophylline (topical and oral administration)
      1. Phosphodiesterase inhibitor thought to increase olfactory sensitivity due to interaction with signal transduction in the olfactory epithelium

       2. Chronic use is associated with the need for repeated serum monitoring due to narrow therapeutic range and potential toxicities (seizures, MI)

  B. Olfactory training

    i. Retrain the brain in odor detection and discrimination with repeated exposure to stimuli

    ii. Frequent short-term exposure to odors

    iii. Used in patients with olfactory loss due to URI, head trauma and neurodegenerative disorders

Bibliography

Barunjuk JN, Kaliner M. Neuropeptides and nasal secretion. *Am J Physiol.* 1991;261:L223-L235.

Geurkink N. Nasal anatomy, physiology, and function. *J Allergy Clin Immunol.* 1983;72:123-128.

Hummel, Rissom K, Reden J, et al. Effects of olfactory training in patients with olfactory loss. *Laryngoscope.* 2009;119:496-499.

Papon JF, Coste A. Physiology of the nose. European Manual of Medicine. *Otolaryngol Head Neck Surg.* 2010;173-175.

Stenner M, Vent J, Hüttenbrink KB, Hummel T, Damm M. Topical therapy in anosmia: relevance of steroid-responsiveness. *Laryngoscope.* 2008;118(9):1681-1686.

Questions

1. Which of the following contributes to the parasympathetic response in the nasal cavity?
   A. Substance P
   B. Vasointestinal peptide
   C. Neuropeptide Y
   D. Neurokinin A
   E. Calcitonin gene-related peptide

2. Which diagnostic test of nasal function allows for the localization of an area of obstruction?
   A. Rhinomanometry
   B. Nasal nitric oxide measurements
   C. Acoustic rhinometry
   D. Nasal inspiratory peak flow
   E. 99Tc-macroaggregated albumin scintigraphy

3. Which of the following decreases nasal resistance?
   A. Exercise
   B. Oral contraceptives
   C. Cold air
   D. Beta blockers

    E. Nonsteroidal anti-inflammatory medications

4. Which of the following is particularly detrimental to olfaction?
   A. IV
   B. Rhinovirus
   C. Paramyxovirus
   D. Adenovirus
   E. Parainfluenza virus type 3

5. Anosmia is associated with intranasal preparations containing
   A. Fluticasone
   B. Phenylephrine
   C. Azelastine
   D. Zinc
   E. Budesonide

Chapter 26
Paranasal Sinuses: Embryology, Anatomy, Endoscopic Diagnosis, and Treatment

Introduction

- Basic techniques for the treatment of inflammatory disease have evolved as a result of increasing recognition of the importance of mucoperiosteal preservation and improving knowledge of disease pathogenesis and management.
- Endoscopic approaches are now widely utilized for the management of mucoceles, benign tumors, skull base defects, orbital and optic nerve decompression, and dacryocystorhinostomies.
- The boundaries of the endoscopic approach to the sinuses have now expanded to include endoscopic or endoscopic-assisted resection of appropriately selected paranasal sinus, skull base, and intracranial tumors.
- Because of the variability of the anatomy and the critical relationships of the sinuses, endoscopic surgical techniques require a detailed knowledge of the anatomy and embryology to avoid potentially disastrous complications.
- The introduction of balloon technology combined with local or systemic medical therapy creates the opportunity for office-based procedures for more limited disease, but further studies need to be performed to compare these approaches to medical therapy.

Embryology of the Paranasal Sinuses

Traditional Teaching
Ethmoturbinals
- Development heralded by the appearance of a series of ridges or folds on the lateral nasal wall at approximately the eighth week.
- Six to seven folds emerge initially but eventually only three to four ridges persist through regression and fusion.
- Ridges that persist throughout fetal development and into later life are referred to as *ethmoturbinals*. These structures are all considered to be ethmoid in origin.
  - (a) First ethmoturbinal—rudimentary and incomplete in humans
    - ○ Ascending portion forms the agger nasi.
    - ○ Descending portion forms the uncinate process.
  - (b) Second ethmoturbinal—forms the middle turbinate

(c) Third ethmoturbinal—forms the superior turbinate
(d) Fourth and fifth ethmoturbinals—fuse to form the supreme turbinate
- Furrows form between the ethmoturbinals and ultimately establish the primordial nasal *meati* and *recesses.*
  (a) First furrow (between the first and second ethmoturbinals)
    ○ Descending aspect forms the ethmoidal infundibulum, hiatus semilunaris, and middle meatus. (The primordial maxillary sinus develops from the inferior aspect of the ethmoid infundibulum.)
    ○ Ascending aspect can contribute to the frontal recess.
  (b) Second furrow (between the second and third ethmoturbinals)
    ○ Forms the superior meatus
  (c) Third furrow (between the third and fourth ethmoturbinals)
    ○ Forms the supreme meatus

Frontal Sinus
- Originates from the anterior pneumatization of the frontal recess into the frontal bone
- A series of one to four folds and furrows arise within the ventral and caudal aspect of the middle meatus. Typically
  (a) The first frontal furrow forms the agger nasi cell.
  (b) The second frontal furrow forms frontal sinus (usually).
  (c) The third and fourth furrows form other anterior ethmoid cells.

Sphenoid Sinus
- During the third month, the nasal mucosa invaginates into the posterior portion of the cartilaginous nasal capsule to form a pouch-like cavity referred to as the cartilaginous cupolar recess of the nasal cavity.
- The wall surrounding this cartilage is ossified in the later months of fetal development and the complex is referred to as the ossiculum Bertini.
- In the second and third years the intervening cartilage is resorbed, and the ossiculum Bertini becomes attached to the body of the sphenoid.
- By the sixth or seventh year, pneumatization progresses.
- By the 12th year, the anterior clinoids and pterygoid process can become pneumatized.
- Sphenoid sinus pneumatization is typically completed between the 9th and 12th years.

Recent Contributions in Sinus Embryology

- In addition to the traditional ridge and furrow concept of development, a cartilaginous capsule surrounds the developing nasal cavity and plays a role in sinonasal development.
  (a) At 8 weeks, three soft-tissue elevations or preturbinates are seen that correlate to the future inferior, middle, and superior turbinates.
  (b) At 9 to 10 weeks a soft-tissue elevation and underlying cartilaginous bud emerges that corresponds to the future uncinate process.
  (c) By 13 to 14 weeks a space develops lateral to the uncinate anlagen that corresponds to the ethmoidal infundibulum.
  (d) By 16 weeks, the future maxillary sinus begins to develop from the inferior aspect of the infundibulum. The cartilaginous structures resorb or ossify as development progresses.
- All three turbinates arise and all the paranasal sinuses arise from the cartilaginous nasal capsule.
- The outpouching of the nasal mucous membranes is thought to be only a secondary phenomenon, rather than the primary force in sinonasal development.

- Certainly, all is not known about the complex mechanisms involved in sinus development.
- However, a basic grasp of sinonasal embryology will facilitate an understanding of the complex and variable adult paranasal sinus anatomy and the wide variations in pneumatization, which will be encountered in endoscopic sinus surgery.

Anatomy

The Lamellae

- The ethmoid sinus is commonly referred to as "the labyrinth" due to its complexity and intersubject variability.
- In this section, paranasal sinus anatomy is discussed with special emphasis on the ethmoid sinus and ethmoid structures important in endoscopic sinus surgery.
- The complex ethmoidal labyrinth of the adult can be reduced into a series of lamellae based on embryologic precursors.
- These lamellae are obliquely oriented and lie parallel to each other. They are helpful in maintaining orientation in ethmoid procedures.
  (a) The first lamella is the uncinate process.
  (b) The second lamella corresponds to the ethmoidal bulla.
  (c) The third is the basal or ground lamella of the middle turbinate.
  (d) The fourth is the lamella of the superior turbinate.
- The basal lamella of the middle turbinate is especially important as it divides the anterior and posterior ethmoids.
- The frontal, maxillary, and anterior ethmoids arise from the region of the anterior ethmoid and therefore drain into the middle meatus.
- The posterior ethmoid cells lie posterior to the basal lamella and therefore drain into the superior and supreme meati.
- The sphenoid sinus drains into the sphenoethmoid recess (medial to the superior turbinate).
- The lamellae are relatively constant features that can help the surgeon maintain anatomic orientation when operating within the ethmoid "labyrinth" of the ethmoid sinus.

Agger Nasi

- Mound or prominence on the lateral wall just anterior to the middle turbinate insertion.
- Frequently pneumatized by an agger nasi cell that arises from the superior aspect of infundibulum.
- The agger nasi cell is bordered by the following:
  (a) *Anteriorly*: frontal process of the maxilla
  (b) *Superiorly*: frontal recess or sinus
  (c) *Anterolaterally*: nasal bones
  (d) *Inferolaterally*: lacrimal bone
  (e) *Inferomedially*: uncinate process of the ethmoid bone

Uncinate Process

- Derived from the Latin *uncinatus*, which means hook-like or hook shaped.
- Approximately 3 to 4-mm wide and 1.5 to 2 cm in length and nearly sagittally oriented. It is best appreciated by viewing a sagittal gross anatomic specimen after reflecting the middle turbinate superiorly.

- Through most of its course, its posterior margin is free and forms the anterior boundary of the hiatus semilunaris.
- The uncinate process forms the medial wall of the ethmoidal infundibulum.
- Attaches anteriorly and superiorly to the ethmoidal crest of the maxillae. Immediately below this, it fuses with the posterior aspect of the lacrimal bone. The anterior inferior aspect does not have a bony attachment.
- Posteriorly and inferiorly the uncinate attaches to the ethmoidal process of the inferior turbinate bone. At its posterior limit, it gives off a small bony projection to attach to the lamina perpendicularis of the palatine bone.

The superior, middle, and inferior parts of the uncinate process are related to three different sinuses:

- Superior aspect most commonly bends laterally to insert on the lamina papyracea.
  - (a) Inferior and lateral to this portion of the uncinate lies the blind superior pouch of the infundibular airspace, the *recessus terminalis*.
  - (b) The floor of the frontal recess commonly lies superior and medial to this portion of the uncinate. This portion of the uncinate process is therefore important in frontal recess surgery.
  - (c) Alternatively, the uncinate process may occasionally attach superiorly to the ethmoid roof or even bend medially to attach to the middle turbinate.
- Mid aspect parallels the ethmoid bulla. For this reason, removal of the uncinate is one of the first steps in endoscopic sinus surgery as this allows surgical access of the ethmoid bulla and deeper ethmoid structures.
- Inferior aspect forms part of the medial wall of the maxillary sinus. The maxillary sinus ostium lies medial and superior to this part, and thus this portion of the uncinate must be removed to widen the natural ostium.

Nasal Fontanelles

- Lie immediately anterior (anterior fontanelle) and posterior (posterior fontanelle) to the inferior aspect of the uncinate where the lateral nasal wall consists only of mucosa.
- The posterior fontanelle is much larger and more distinct than its anterior counterpart.
- The fontanelles (especially posterior) may be perforated creating an accessory ostium into the maxillary sinus (20%-25% of patients). These accessory ostia may be indicators of prior sinus disease.

Ethmoid Bulla

- The ethmoid bulla is one of the most constant and largest of the anterior ethmoid air cells, located within the middle meatus directly posterior to the uncinate process and anterior to the basal lamella of the middle turbinate.
- Based on the lamina orbitalis, it projects medially into the middle meatus, and has the appearance of a "bulla," a hollow thin-walled rounded prominence.
- Superiorly, the anterior wall of the ethmoid bulla (or bulla lamella) can extend to the skull base and form the posterior limit of the frontal recess. If the bulla does not reach the skull base, a suprabullar recess is formed between the skull base and superior surface of the bulla.
- Posteriorly, the bulla may blend with the basal lamella or have a space between it and the basal lamella of the middle turbinate (retrobullar recess).
- The retrobullar recess may invaginate the basal lamella for a variable distance, occasionally extending the anterior ethmoid air cell system as far posteriorly as the anterior wall of the sphenoid sinus.

Hiatus Semilunaris

- The hiatus semilunaris is a crescent-shaped gap between the posterior free margin of the uncinate process and the anterior wall of the ethmoid bulla.
- It is through this two-dimensional sagittally oriented cleft or passageway that the middle meatus communicates with the ethmoid infundibulum.

Ethmoidal Infundibulum

- The ethmoidal infundibulum is the funnel-shaped passage through which secretions are transported or channeled into the middle meatus from various anterior ethmoid cells and the maxillary sinus.
- Depending on the anatomy of the frontal recess, the frontal sinus can also drain through the infundibulum.
- It has the following borders:
  - (a) *Medial*: uncinate process
  - (b) *Lateral*: lamina orbitalis
  - (c) *Posterior*: anterior wall of ethmoid bulla
  - (d) *Anterior and superior*: frontal process of the maxilla
  - (e) *Superior and lateral*: lacrimal bone
- The ethmoidal infundibulum communicates with the middle meatus through the hiatus semilunaris.

Ostiomeatal Unit

- The ostiomeatal unit is not a discrete anatomic structure but refers collectively to several middle meatal structures, including the middle meatus, uncinate process, ethmoid infundibulum, anterior ethmoid cells and ostia of the anterior ethmoid, and maxillary and frontal sinuses (Figures 26-1 and 26-2).
- The ostiomeatal unit is a functional, rather than an anatomic designation, identifying the drainage pathway of the maxillary sinus, frontal sinus, and anterior ethmoid sinus, and coined by Naumann as an aid in discussing the pathophysiology of sinusitis.

Frontal Recess and Sinus

- The frontal recess is the most anterior and superior aspect of the anterior ethmoid sinus that forms the connection with the frontal sinus.
- The boundaries of the frontal recess are as follows:
  - (a) *Lateral*: lamina papyracea
  - (b) *Medial*: middle turbinate
  - (c) *Anterior*: the posterior superior wall of the agger nasi cell (when present)
  - (d) *Posterior*: anterior wall of the ethmoid bulla (if it extends to the skull base)
- The frontal recess tapers as it approaches the superiorly located internal os of the frontal sinus.
- Above the os, it again widens as the anterior and posterior tables diverge to their respective positions.
- This gives the appearance of an hourglass, with the narrowest portion being the frontal ostium.
- There is tremendous variation regarding the pattern of the nasofrontal connection, but most frequently the recess opens just medial to the posterior aspect of the uncinate process.
- The nasofrontal connection has a very complex drainage pattern and does not resemble a true duct. Therefore, the "nasofrontal or frontonasal duct" is antiquated and obsolete terminology.

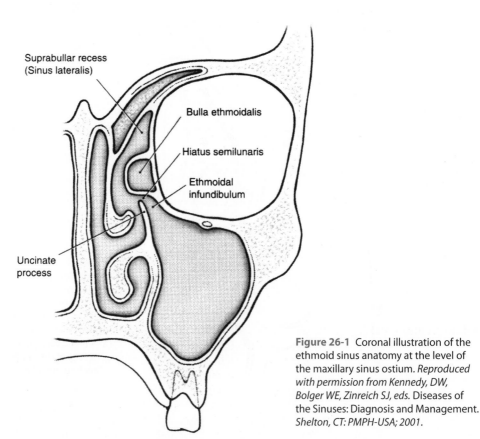

Suprabullar recess
(Sinus lateralis)

Bulla ethmoidalis

Hiatus semilunaris

Ethmoidal
infundibulum

Uncinate
process

Figure 26-1 Coronal illustration of the ethmoid sinus anatomy at the level of the maxillary sinus ostium. *Reproduced with permission from Kennedy, DW, Bolger WE, Zinreich SJ, eds.* Diseases of the Sinuses: Diagnosis and Management. *Shelton, CT: PMPH-USA; 2001.*

Middle Turbinate

- The middle turbinate of the ethmoid bone has several important features, which, if understood well by the surgeon, are helpful in safe, sophisticated surgical treatment.
- In its anterior aspect, the middle turbinate attaches laterally at the agger nasi region, specifically at the crista ethmoidalis maxillae (ethmoidal eminence of the maxilla).
- It courses superiorly and medially to attach vertically to the lateral aspect of the lamina cribrosa (cribriform plate). The anterior cranial fossa dura may invaginate into this attachment with the olfactory filae.
- The cribriform attachment is maintained for variable distance until the insertion courses horizontally across the skull base and inferiorly to attach to the lamina orbitalis and/or the medial wall of the maxillary sinus. This segment is oriented in a near coronal plane anteriorly and an almost horizontal plane more posteriorly. It divides the ethmoid labyrinth into its anterior and posterior components (basal lamella of the middle turbinate).
- The most posterior aspect of the middle turbinate is its inferior attachment to the lateral wall at the crista ethmoidalis of the perpendicular process of the palatine bone, just anterior the sphenopalatine foramen.
- Variability in the middle portion of the basal lamellae of the middle turbinate is important to appreciate. Various posterior ethmoid cells can indent the structure anteriorly and anterior ethmoid cells and the retrobulbar recess can indent the structure posteriorly.

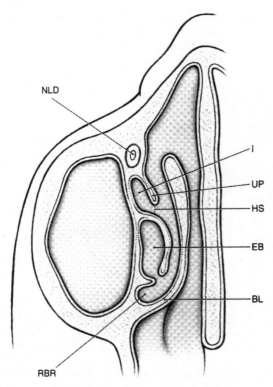

Figure 26-2 Axial illustration of the anterior nasosinus anatomy. EB, ethmoid bulla; HS, hiatus semilunaris; I, infundibulum; NLD, nasolacrimal duct; RBR, retrobullar recess; RBR, retrobullar recess; UP, uncinate process. *Reproduced with permission from Kennedy, DW, Bolger WE, Zinreich SJ, eds. Diseases of the Sinuses: Diagnosis and Management. Shelton, CT: PMPH-USA; 2001.*

- The shape of the middle turbinate is highly variable as it can be paradoxically curved (medially concave) or pneumatized.
- If the vertical portion or lamella of the middle turbinate is pneumatized, the cell that is formed is referred to as the intralamellar cell.
- Pneumatization of the head of the middle turbinate is referred to as a concha bullosa.

Ethmoid Roof and Cribriform Plate

- Typically, the ethmoid roof slopes inferiorly and medially, and is thinner medially than laterally (by a factor of 10×).
- Medially, the roof is formed by the lateral lamella of the cribriform, which is variable in its vertical height.
- A low-lying or asymmetric skull base must be recognized prior to surgery to avoid the potential complication of a CSF leak.

Keros described three types of formation of the ethmoid roof based on the vertical height of the lateral lamella:

- *Keros Type I*: 1- to 3-mm depth to the olfactory fossa
- *Keros Type II*: 4- to 7-mm depth to the olfactory fossa
- *Keros Type III*: 8- to 16-mm depth to the olfactory fossa

This is often regarded as the highest-risk configuration for inadvertent intracranial injury because of the long, thin lateral lamella adjacent to the ethmoid sinuses.

The Keros classification does not evaluate the skull base height in the posterior ethmoid. This should be carefully evaluated preoperatively by comparing the ratio of the ethmoid height to that of the height of the maxillary sinus.

Sphenoethmoidal (Onodi) Cell

- Onodi stressed that when the most posterior ethmoid cell was highly pneumatized, it could extend posteriorly along the lamina papyracea and superiorly into the anterior wall of the sphenoid sinus.
- If this occurred, the optic nerve and the internal carotid artery, both usually considered to border the lateral aspect of the sphenoid sinus, would actually become intimately related to the posterior ethmoid cell (Figure 26-3).
- Dissection in the posterior ethmoid could thus result in trauma to the optic nerve or carotid artery if the anatomic variation was not appreciated.

Sphenoid Sinus

- Located centrally within the skull, the sphenoid sinuses are separated by an intersinus septum that is highly variable in position.
- This septum may attach laterally to one side in the region of the carotid artery, an important consideration if it is being surgically removed.
- Like the other sinuses, pneumatization is highly variable. Laterally, the sinus may pneumatize for a variable distance under the middle cranial fossa (lateral recess), inferiorly it may pneumatize to a variable extent into the pterygoid processes, and posteriorly it may pneumatize for a variable distance inferior to the sella turcica.
- The sphenoid sinus is bordered by critical anatomy, which makes it important for both inflammatory disease and skull base endoscopic approaches:
  (a) Lateral to the sinus lie the carotid artery, the optic nerve, the cavernous sinus, and the third, fourth, fifth, and sixth cranial nerves.
  (b) Posterior and superior to the sinus lie the sella turcica and superior intercavernous sinus and the planum sphenoidale.

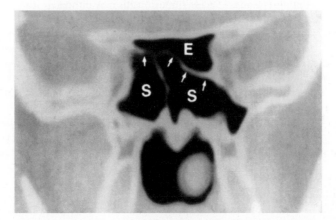

Figure 26-3 Coronal CT cut through the sphenoid sinus reveals a "horizontal septum" (arrows). The cell above the septum (E) represents a sphenoethmoidal cell (Onodi cell) that has pneumatized above the sphenoid sinus (S), bringing the ethmoid sinus into close proximity to the optic nerve and carotid artery. (*Reproduced with permission from Kennedy, DW, Bolger WE, Zinreich SJ, eds.* Diseases of the Sinuses: Diagnosis and Management. *Shelton, CT: PMPH-USA; 2001.*)

(c) In a well-pneumatized sphenoid, the vidian canal is often identified inferiorly and laterally within the sinus.

(d) The optic nerve and internal carotid artery can indent the sphenoid sinus covered only by a thin layer of bone.
   - The carotid canal may be dehiscent in up to 22% of specimens.
   - The optic canal may be dehiscent in up to 6% of specimens.

(e) In some cases, pneumatization of the posterosuperior lateral wall of the sphenoid extends between the optic nerve and carotid artery to create an opticocarotid recess.

Etiology and Pathophysiology of Chronic Rhinosinusitis

- Chronic rhinosinusitis (CRS) is a clinical disorder that encompasses a heterogeneous group of infectious and inflammatory conditions affecting the paranasal sinuses.
- Indeed, CRS may exist with or without nasal polyps and these entities may represent two points along a spectrum of disease.
- Its definition continues to evolve as we increase our understanding of the various etiologies and pathophysiologies that may result in a common clinical picture.
- CRS has multiple etiologies that include:
  (a) Environmental (eg, allergens, viruses, bacteria, biofilms, fungi, pollution)
  (b) Local host factors (eg, persistent localized ostiomeatal complex [OMC] inflammation, neoplasms, dental infections, and anatomic abnormalities)
  (c) General host factors (eg, immune deficiency, genetic predisposition or genetic disease, primary or acquired ciliary disorder, granulomatous diseases)
- The following sections describe several of the current theories behind the development of CRS.

Environmental

Progression of Acute Rhinosinusitis

- Multiple episodes of acute rhinosinusitis may ultimately lead to mucosal dysfunction and chronic infections.
- However, acute rhinosinusitis is histologically an exudative process characterized by neutrophilic inflammation and necrosis, while CRS is a proliferative process that is most often characterized by thickened mucosa and lamina propria.
- Acute rhinosinusitis is almost always infectious in etiology and is marked by inflammation that is associated with a recruitment of neutrophils as the predominant cell type to fight infection.
- While this type of infectious inflammation is certainly predominant in CRS when secondary to general and local host factors such as cystic fibrosis, ciliary dyskinesia, and rhinosinusitis of dental origin, most CRS has an inflammatory response where eosinophils are the predominant inflammatory cells in both atopic and nonatopic individuals with CRS.

Biofilms

- Bacterial biofilms are a complex organization of bacteria anchored to a surface.
- They can evade host defenses and demonstrate decreased susceptibility to systemic and local antibiotic therapy.
- The persistence of biofilms is largely due to their method of growth, whereby bacteria such as *Pseudomonas aeruginosa* grow in microcolonies surrounded by an extracellular matrix of the exopolysaccharide alginate.

- Biofilms elicit a considerable immunologic reaction and can be difficult to eradicate from the paranasal sinuses.
- Bacterial biofilm formation may explain the persistence of inflammation in some medically recalcitrant CRS, especially in patients who have undergone prior surgery.

IgE-Independent Fungal Inflammation

- Fungus may be a possible inflammatory trigger for CRS independent of a type I immunoglobulin E (IgE) allergic mechanism as seen in allergic fungal sinusitis (AFS).
- Eosinophils cluster around fungi, and there is evidence that they are recruited and activated as a response to fungi in patients with CRS, although this response is not seen in healthy patients.
- Furthermore, peripheral lymphocytes from CRS patients will produce large quantities of inflammatory cytokines when they are exposed to certain fungal antigens.
- The fungi in the nasal and sinus mucus may activate and induce inflammation independent from an allergic response. This is an area of continued investigation.

Bacterial Superantigen

- Bacteria possess the ability to elicit pathogenic exotoxins that can activate large subpopulations of the T-lymphocyte pool.
- These T-cell superantigens bind to human leukocyte antigen class II histocompatibility complexes on antigen-presenting cells and the T-cell receptors of T lymphocytes that are separate from the antigen-binding sites.
- The conventional antigen specificity is bypassed resulting in activation of up to 30% of the T-lymphocyte pool (normal < 0.01%) and a subsequent massive cytokine release.
- Individuals with major histocompatibility class II molecules, which allow this binding, would be more at risk for this upregulation by a superantigen.
- An example of this process is seen with the secretion of toxic shock syndrome toxin-1 by *Staphylococcus aureus* in toxic shock syndrome.
- The superantigen hypothesis has been proposed as a potential unifying theory for the pathogenesis of CRS.
- This theory proposes that microbial persistence, superantigen production, and host T-lymphocyte response are fundamental components unifying all common chronic eosinophilic respiratory mucosal disorders.
- This helps explain how a number of coexisting immune responses, including type 1 hypersensitivity, superantigen-induced T-lymphocyte activation, and cellular antigen-specific immune responses, could contribute to the heterogeneity of the disease.
- Nevertheless, it is likely that there are many additional mechanisms at work in CRS.

Local Host Factors

Anatomic Factors

- Certain anatomic variants may predispose to CRS, including infraorbital cells (Haller cells), silent sinus syndrome, or a narrow frontal sinus outflow tract from large agger nasi or frontal cells.
- The ostiomeatal unit can play a role in the development of sinusitis as this is immediately adjacent to the primary area of particulate deposition (anterior middle turbinate).
  - (a) Obstruction here predisposes toward chronic inflammation in the dependent sinuses.
  - (b) Once the ostium becomes occluded, a local hypoxia develops in the sinus cavity and sinus secretions accumulate.
  - (c) This creates an environment suitable for rapid bacterial growth.

(d) Bacterial toxins and endogenous inflammatory mediators can subsequently damage the highly specialized ciliated respiratory epithelium, resulting in a decrease in mucociliary clearance.

(e) A vicious cycle erupts with stasis of secretions and further infection.

Mucociliary Dysfunction

- Mucociliary clearance is especially important in maintaining the homeostasis of the paranasal sinuses.
- The ciliary beat of the epithelium removes allergens, bacteria, and pollutants trapped in the mucus or *gel* layer of the mucociliary blanket through natural drainage pathways.
- The mucus rests on a periciliary fluid or *sol* layer that enables the rapid elimination of viscous secretions.
- Defective mucociliary clearance can result from the interplay of environmental and local host factors.
- Mucociliary clearance can be disrupted by either defective ciliary function or alterations in the viscosity and production of mucus.
  (a) Environmental irritants, surgical trauma, and endogenous mediators of inflammation may all contribute to mucociliary dysfunction.
  (b) General host factors may also lead to ciliary dysfunction, including primary ciliary dyskinesia or Kartagener syndrome and cystic fibrosis.
  (c) Cystic fibrosis patients have high-viscosity mucus secondary to alterations in water and electrolyte transport. The gel and sol layers of the mucus blanket are severely affected, thereby hindering bacterial removal.
- All of these factors may lead to the accumulation of mucus in the sinuses, thereby decreasing the removal of bacteria and creating a favorable environment for bacterial growth.

Odontogenic Sinusitis

- Dental pathology can occasionally lead to maxillary sinusitis with subsequent spread to adjacent sinuses and should always be considered in unilateral sinusitis.
- This pathology can include dental infections, tooth root abscesses, oral antral fistula, and other oral surgery procedures that then incite a sinusitis.
- These patients typically require treatment of both the oral and the sinus pathology in order to eradicate the infection.

Bone Inflammation

- Recent work suggests that the bone may play an active role in the disease process and that, at a minimum, the inflammation associated with CRS may spread through the haversian system within the bone.
- The rate of bone turnover in CRS is similar to that seen in osteomyelitis.
- In animal studies, a surgically induced infection with either *S aureus* or *P aeruginosa* can induce all of the classic changes of osteomyelitis and induce chronic inflammatory changes in both the bone and the overlying mucosa at a significant distance from the site of infection.
- Bone inflammation may be a significant factor in the spread of chronic inflammatory changes in patients and may in part explain recalcitrance to medical therapy.
- It is still unclear, however, if the bone actually becomes infected with bacteria or if the observed changes simply occur as a reaction or extension of adjacent inflammation or infection.

Alteration in Sinus Microbiome

- There has been a significant amount of interest recently in the role of microbes in various health diseases (ie, *Clostridium difficile* colitis).

- The microbiome refers to the totality of all microbes in given environment.
- Recent advances in culture-independent bacterial analysis through 16s rRNA detection has allowed a new method of investigation into the role of the sinus microbiome in CRS.
- Early studies demonstrated that the sinuses are not sterile and have suggested that CRS may be characterized by a loss of microbial diversity compared to normal controls.
- Further studies are needed to substantiate the importance of microbiome homeostasis either in the etiology and pathogenesis of CRS.

General Host Factors

Allergic Fungal Rhinosinusitis

- Allergic fungal rhinosinusitis (AFS) is the most common form of fungal sinus disease, although the pathogenesis remains poorly understood.
- It was first recognized because of its histologic similarity to allergic bronchopulmonary aspergillosis (ABPA).
- Like ABPA, AFS is recognized as an IgE-mediated response to a variety of fungi, typically from the dematiaceous family, growing in the eosinophilic mucin of the sinuses.
- The classic diagnosis of AFS depends on five criteria: type I hypersensitivity, nasal polyposis, characteristic computed tomographic (CT) scan appearance (hyperdense material in the sinus cavity), positive fungal stain or culture, and the presence of thick, eosinophilic mucin.
- Eosinophilic mucin is typically thick, tenacious, "peanut butter"-like, brown-green mucus that contains eosinophils in sheets, Charcot-Leyden crystals, and fungal hyphae.
- The disease is often unilateral and can cause bony erosion and extension into orbital or intracranial contents.
- Fungal colonization of the nose and paranasal sinuses is a very common finding in both normal and diseased sinuses due to the ubiquitous nature of the organisms.
- Under some circumstances, fungal proliferation may lead to the development of fungus balls or saprophytic growth of fungus.
- In other cases, an intense inflammatory response to ubiquitous fungi results in the disease process of AFS.

Aspirin-Exacerbated Respiratory Disease

- If patients have nasal polyps in association with asthma and aspirin sensitivity, this is commonly referred to as Samter's triad (now known as aspirin-exacerbated respiratory disease [AERD])
- AERD represents a severe form of chronic hypertrophic eosinophilic sinusitis.
- Pathogenesis is postulated to be secondary to dysregulated eicosanoid synthesis.
- Arachidonic acid is normally cleaved from cellular membranes by phospholipase A2 and subsequently shunted to either the leukotriene pathway by the enzyme 5-lipoxygenase or the prostaglandin pathway by the enzyme cyclooxygenase.
- Leukotrienes, also known as the slow reacting substances of anaphylaxis, are a class of inflammatory mediators that increase vascular permeability, inflammatory cell chemotaxis, and smooth muscle constriction.
- Prostaglandin E2, a product of the cyclooxygenase pathway, inhibits 5-lipoxygenase in a feedback loop.
- In AERD patients, there is a baseline overproduction of leukotrienes.

- Aspirin and other nonsteroidal anti-inflammatories inhibit cyclooxygenase and decrease prostaglandin E2, resulting in a net increase in leukotrienes → results in acute acerbations of symptoms (ie, bronchoconstriction, mucus hypersecretion, vasodilation).
- Nasal polyps in AERD patients typically have a higher eosinophilic load and are generally more refractory to treatment (ie, higher recurrence rate) than other forms of CRS.

Airway Hyperactivity
- Although the nature of the relationship between the paranasal sinuses and the lungs is still unclear, the lungs and the upper airway share contact with inhaled pathogens and include many of the same epithelial properties.
- On histology, most CRS simulates the Th2-type inflammatory response seen in asthmatics where eosinophils are the predominant inflammatory cells in both atopic and nonatopic individuals.
- Thus, asthma and CRS are intimately related in many individuals even in the absence of aspirin sensitivity.
- CRS with nasal polyps is often considered "asthma of the upper airway."
- Furthermore, for asthmatic patients with CRS, a recent systematic review has demonstrated improved asthma control following functional endoscopic sinus surgery (FESS) and appropriate postoperative medical care.

Immune Barrier Hypothesis
- Recently, a unifying theory on the pathogenesis of chronic sinusitis has been proposed to help explain the plethora of potential etiologies as previously discussed.
- The interface between the nasal mucosa and the external environment contains both a mechanical and innate immune protective barrier that helps maintain the integrity and function of the respiratory epithelium.
- Defects in these protective mechanisms can allow antigen passage and processing which can lead to the chronic inflammation seen in chronic sinusitis.
- Genetic, epigenetic, and environmental (ie, allergens, *S. aureus*, fungi, biofilms) factors can all contribute to the development of these barrier defects.
- The wide spectrum of disease (CRS with and without polyps) that we see in patients may be explained by this complex interaction between genetics and environmental disease modifiers.
- This theory places chronic sinusitis in the same framework seen in other chronic mucosal inflammatory diseases (ie, inflammatory bowel disease, reactive airways disease).
- Further studies are needed to better understand the host immune response in chronic sinusitis and validate this hypothesis.

Etiology of CSF Leaks and Encephaloceles

- CSF leaks are broadly classified into traumatic (including accidental and iatrogenic trauma), tumor related, spontaneous, and congenital.
- The etiology of the CSF leak will influence the size and location of the bony defect, degree and nature of the dural disruption, associated intracranial pressure differential, and meningoencephalocele formation.
- In surgical traumatic leaks, any associated intracranial injury will influence timing and method of repair, but in general early closure is the clear goal.

- Spontaneous CSF leaks are frequently associated with elevated CSF pressure and empty sella; this increases hydrostatic force at the weakest sites of the skull base and may occur at another site when one area is repaired.
- The elevated CSF pressures seen in this subset of patients leads to the highest rate (50%-100%) of encephalocele formation, and may lead to a higher recurrence rate following surgical repair.
- The necessity of concurrent lumbar CSF drainage following surgical repair is controversial but appears to be most useful in patients with spontaneous CSF leaks.
- In some spontaneous CSF leaks, particularly in patients with significantly raised pressure or multiple leaks, long-term therapy to try to lower the CSF pressure (such as oral acetazolamide) may be advisable, and a ventriculoperitoneal shunt may be a consideration.

Evaluation, Diagnosis, and Preoperative Management

Patient Selection

- A decision to perform surgical intervention is relatively easy in the presence of a large mucocele, inflammatory complication, active CSF leak, or in the presence of diffuse nasal polyposis unresponsive to medical therapy.
- The surgical decision is considerably more difficult when the disease is more minor, or the primary complaint is recurrent sinusitis or headache.
- Some general *guidelines* are as follows:
  - (a) The patient should have had a trial of maximal medical therapy.
  - (b) The CT should be performed at least 4 weeks following the onset of medical therapy for the most recent episode of rhinosinusitis and at least 2 weeks following the most recent upper respiratory infection.
  - (c) There should be persistent evidence of mucosal disease (radiographic or endoscopic).
  - (d) Nasal congestion or obstruction, discolored nasal discharge, decreased olfaction, and nasal or sinus fullness are generally good signs of CRS.
  - (e) Headache correlates poorly with sinus disease and severe pain is unusual in CRS.
  - (f) Performing elective sinus surgery on patients who continue to smoke may result in increased scarring and worsening of symptoms.

Diagnostic Nasal Endoscopy

- The development of the modern rigid nasal endoscope represents a major advance in rhinologic diagnostic capability.
- Nasal endoscopy is more sensitive for the diagnosis of accessible disease than CT and provides essential complementary information for patient diagnosis.
- Endoscopy permits detailed evaluation of the critical areas for sinusitis, the OMC, and sphenoethmoidal recess.
- Equipment for diagnostic nasal endoscopy includes topical anesthesia, a 30° 4-mm endoscope, 30° 2.7-mm endoscope, freer elevator, light source, fiberoptic cable, and an assortment of suction tips.
- The 30° scope is the most useful endoscope as it provides an ample viewing field, and is well tolerated by most patients. A 45° or 70° telescope may be very helpful in some patients.

Diagnostic nasal endoscopy is typically performed in an orderly fashion, with the patient sitting or supine.

- The nasal cavities are sprayed with a topical decongestant and local anesthetic.
- Consider applying supplemental topical anesthetic on Farrell applicators to the infero-lateral surface of the middle turbinate and to other sites where passage of the endoscope may exert pressure.
- The examiner should always take appropriate precautions when dealing with secretions and blood. Gloves, mask, and eye protection are recommended.
- The 4-mm 30° telescope is usually selected first; the endoscope lens is treated with a thin film of antifog solution, held lightly in the left hand by the shaft with the thumb and first two fingers and introduced slowly, under direct vision.
- A complete examination can be successfully accomplished in an organized manner with three passes of the endoscope.
  - (a) First pass along the floor of the nose. The overall anatomy, presence of pathologic secretions or polyps, and the condition of nasal mucosa may be identified. In some cases it may also be possible to identify the nasolacrimal duct within the inferior meatus. Thereafter, the scope is advanced through the nasal cavity and toward the nasopharynx. As the scope is advanced into the nasopharynx, the entire nasopharynx, including the contralateral eustachian tube orifice, can be examined by rotating the telescope.
  - (b) Second pass of the telescope is made between the middle and inferior turbinates. While directing the scope posteriorly, the inferior portion of the middle meatus, fontanelles, and accessory maxillary ostia can be examined. The scope is then passed medial to the middle turbinate and advanced posteriorly to examine the sphenoethmoidal recess. Rotating the scope superiorly and slightly laterally allows for visualization of the superior turbinate and meatus as well as the slit-like or oval ostia of the sphenoid sinus.
  - (c) The Third pass of the examination is made as the telescope is withdrawn. As the scope is brought back anteriorly, it can frequently be rotated laterally under the middle turbinate into the posterior aspect of the middle meatus. The bulla ethmoidalis, hiatus semilunaris, and infundibular entrance are inspected. Withdrawing the telescope further can provide an excellent view of the middle turbinate, uncinate process, and surrounding mucosa. In selected patients this portion of the examination can be conducted from an anterior approach, if the anatomy is favorable. Alternatively, additional topical anesthesia may be placed within the middle meatus and in the region of the anterior insertion of the middle turbinate. The middle turbinate is then gently subluxed medially using a cotton-tipped applicator moistened with topical anesthetic, so as to allow insertion of a telescope into the middle meatus.

Diagnostic and Therapeutic Applications

- A crucial application of nasal endoscopy is to evaluate patient response to medical treatment, such as topical nasal steroids, antibiotics, oral steroids, and antihistamines.
- Equally or more important is the ability to examine and treat persistent asymptomatic disease following surgical intervention, so as to avoid revision surgery at a later time.
- Through serial endoscopic examinations, resolution of polyps, pathologic secretions, mucosal edema and inflammatory changes can be followed.

- These objective data are significantly more important than the patient's subjective response in determining the need for continued postoperative medical therapy because asymptomatic persistent disease is common postsurgery.
- Endoscopic examination provides early objective data regarding recurrence of polyps, hyperplastic mucosa, and chronic infection, often long before the symptoms occur.
- Endoscopy may greatly reduce, and in many cases eliminate, the need for repeated radiographic examination during and after medical or surgical therapy.
- An especially important diagnostic application of nasal endoscopy is to identify the causative organism in sinusitis. A small malleable Calgiswab is carefully directed to the middle meatus or other site of origin of purulent drainage and submitted for culture.
- Although diagnostic nasal endoscopy was originally used primarily for the evaluation of sinusitis, it has proved invaluable in postoperative surveillance following intranasal tumor resection and for the evaluation of CSF rhinorrhea.
- Postsurgery, nasal endoscopic examinations and sinus cavity debridement are important to promote consistent ethmoid cavity healing and decrease the risk of middle meatal synechiae.
- Under appropriate topical anesthesia, clot, mucus, and fibrin are removed from the nasal and sinus cavities, and the openings to the maxillary, sphenoid, and frontal sinuses are cleared of obstructive fibrin and forming scar tissue.
- Removal of osteitic bone can reduce foci of inflammation and promote healing.

Preoperative Patient Management

- Minimizing the risks for complications and optimizing surgical planning are of critical importance in patient management.
- Decreasing bleeding and systematically reevaluating the CT scans help accomplish these goals.

Preoperative Planning to Reduce Bleeding

- A screening history should include questions about bleeding during prior surgery, liver disease, use of antiplatelet or anticoagulant medications, or a family history of a bleeding disorder.
- Obtain screening coagulation studies or formal hematology consultation when appropriate.
- Discontinue aspirin and nonsteroidal anti-inflammatory agents, and restrict herbal dietary supplement use for an appropriate period prior to surgery.
- For patients with sinonasal polyposis, a course of oral corticosteroid therapy can reduce polyp size and vascularity if there are no contraindications (ie, prednisone 20-40 mg/d for 2-6 days)
- Oral steroids may also be useful in stabilizing the mucosa of patients with hyperreactive nasal lining.
- When chronic infection is present, a preoperative course of oral antibiotic therapy will help reduce tissue inflammation and vascularity.
- Utilize total intravenous anesthesia.

Preoperative Diagnosis of CSF Leak A number of tests to establish the diagnosis of a CSF leak are available and include the following:

- Beta-2 transferrin test of the nasal fluid.
  (a) Diagnostic, but nonlocalizing
- Nasal endoscopy with intrathecal fluorescein (0.1 mL of 10% intravenous fluorescein diluted in 10 mL of the patient's CSF and injected over 10 minutes). Not exceeding this

dosage is very important as seizures and other complications have been noted at higher dosage.

   (a) Fluorescein is not Food and Drug Administration (FDA) approved for intrathecal use, so patient consent and authorization is best obtained prior to injection.

   (b) Blue light and a blocking filter on the endoscope make the study significantly more sensitive.

- Fine-cut coronal and axial CT scans to identify any dehiscences in the skull base, but inability to distinguish CSF from other soft tissue limits its diagnostic accuracy.

   (a) Bony dehiscences may be present without a leak.

- Magnetic resonance imaging (MRI) or MR cisternography identifies brain parenchyma and CSF that have herniated into the sinus and is best obtained when there is sinus opacification adjacent to a skull base defect.

   (a) Poor at visualizing bony detail.

- Intrathecal injection of contrast medium or a radioactive tracer.

   (a) CT cisternogram can be diagnostic and aid in localization of the defect but requires a relatively rapid flow to be positive.

   (b) Radioactive cisternograms are less useful for localizing defects but can localize the side of the leak and identify low-volume or intermittent leaks. However, the study may have a significant false-positive rate.

   (c) Both studies are invasive and are used with less frequency.

CT Evaluation

- Regardless of the reason for surgery, all patients should have at least a coronal CT with 3-mm cuts.

- Triplanar reconstructions are particularly helpful in patients where frontal sinusotomy or sphenoidotomy is likely to be performed. In these latter situations, or in revision surgery, the use of computer-aided surgical navigation is also a reasonable consideration. In any case, the surgeon should have a 3D conceptualization of the anatomy before starting endoscopic sinus surgery.

- If the preoperative CT evaluation reveals an area of opacification adjacent to a skull base erosion, MRI should be performed to rule out a meningoencephalocele prior to surgery.

- Always identify potential landmarks on the CT in patients who have distorted anatomy due to prior surgery.

The *key points in reviewing the CT* scan prior to surgery are as follows:

- Shape slope and thickness of skull base
- Shape and dehiscences of medial orbital wall
- Vertical height of the posterior ethmoid (in relation to the posteromedial roof of the maxillary sinus) (Figure 26-4)
- Location of the anterior ethmoid artery
- Presence of a sphenoethmoidal (Onodi) cell
- Position of intrasinus sphenoid septae (in relation to carotid artery)
- The presence of maxillary sinus hypoplasia or infundibular atelectasis
- Conceptualization of the frontal sinus drainage pathway from the use of multiplanar CT

Extent of Surgery General guidelines for *chronic sinusitis* are as follows:

- Preserve the mucoperiosteum and try not to leave the exposed bone.
- Remove bony partitions and osteitic bone in the area of disease as completely as possible.

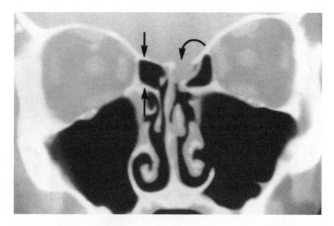

Figure 26-4 Coronal CT at the level of the posterior ethmoid sinuses demonstrating a narrow vertical height to the posterior ethmoid (arrows). On the left side the skull base has been violated (curved arrow), apparently as a result of the limited vertical height posteriorly. (*Reproduced with permission from Kennedy, DW, Bolger WE, Zinreich SJ, eds. Diseases of the Sinuses: Diagnosis and Management. Shelton, CT: PMPH-USA; 2001.*)

- Extend the dissection one step beyond the extent of disease (if possible).
- Preserve the middle turbinate if possible (ie, if not markedly diseased and covered with mucoperiosteum at the end of the surgery).
- More recently, full-house FESS (ie, complete sphenoethmoidectomy, maxillary antrostomy, and frontal sinusotomy) has been advocated for CRS patients with diffuse mucosal disease to facilitate the delivery of postoperative topical therapy and reduce the inflammatory burden

Anesthesia

- Endoscopic sinus surgery can be performed under local anesthesia with sedation but is generally performed under general anesthesia.
- Disadvantages of general anesthesia include the inability to monitor vision should an intraorbital hematoma occur, feedback regarding pain when the anterior or posterior ethmoid neurovascular bundles are approached.
- Mild hypotension is preferable.
- When performed correctly, total intravenous anesthesia provides an excellent method to decrease blood loss during the operation.
- CSF leak requires a rapid sequence intubation in order to minimize the risk of pneumocephalus from bag-mask ventilation and extubation without coughing.

Preparation of the Nasal Cavity

- Under local or general anesthesia, the nose is decongested prior to surgery with oxymetazoline.
- Prior to starting surgery on the first side, this decongestion can be supplemented with *either* 100 to 150 mg of topical cocaine on Farrell nasal applicators *or* topical epinephrine (1:1000) on nasal pledgets.

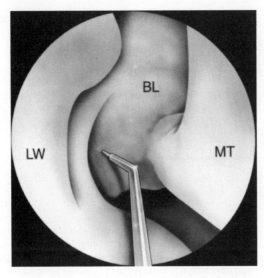

Figure 26-5 Endoscopic representation of the posterior middle meatus during transnasal injection of the sphenopalatine foramen. An angled tonsil needle is inserted in an upward and lateral direction through the inferior portion of the basal lamella (BL). The needle tip is used to feel for the foramen and the injection must be performed very slowly, after aspiration. LW, lateral wall; MT, middle turbinate. (*Reproduced with permission from Kennedy, DW, Bolger WE, Zinreich SJ, eds. Diseases of the Sinuses: Diagnosis and Management. Shelton, CT: PMPH-USA; 2001.*)

- The lateral wall is then infiltrated with 1% Xylocaine with 1:100,000 epinephrine as follows:
  - (a) Anterior to the attachment of the middle turbinate
  - (b) Anterior to the inferior portion of the uncinate process
  - (c) Inferior aspect of middle turbinate
  - (d) Mid point of the root of the inferior turbinate
- These injections may be augmented by a sphenopalatine block (transnasal or transoral) if the posterior ethmoid or sphenoid sinus requires dissection (Figure 26-5).
- However, sphenopalatine injection must be performed slowly and carefully following aspiration. Temporary diplopia can occur and visual loss has been reported.

Surgical Technique

Uncinectomy

- Anterior attachment recognized by a semilunar depression in the lateral nasal wall.
- May be incised with a sickle knife or elevator and removed with forceps. If site of attachment not evident, it is preferable to make the incision posterior to its attachment and remove any residual uncinate later.
- May also be identified and fractured medially with a ball-tipped seeker and removed with a backbiter, but care is required not to traumatize the middle turbinate.

Maxillary Antrostomy

- Identify the inferior cut edge of the uncinate process and pull it medially with a ball-tipped seeker.
- If the ostium is not visible lateral to uncinate remnant, press on the posterior fontanelle and look for a bubble.
- Resect the residual uncinate process with a back-biting forceps, and then extend the antrostomy inferiorly and posteriorly as necessary.
- In revision antrostomy, use a 45° of 70° telescope to ensure that the anterior portion of the natural ostium is opened.

Ethmoidectomy

- Use 0° telescope until the major landmarks have been identified (to avoid disorientation).
- Identify and open bulla (forceps or microdebrider).
- Identify medial orbital wall as early as possible during the procedure.
- Work close to the medial orbital wall (skull base thin and down-sloping medially).
- Identify the retrobullar and suprabullar recesses and basal lamella.

If the posterior ethmoid cells are to be entered:

- Withdraw telescope slightly to provide overview of basal lamella.
- Perforate the basal lamella immediately superior to its horizontal part (Figure 26-6).
- Use upbiting forceps to ensure that there is a space behind the bony lamella (Figure 26-7).
- Remove lamella laterally and posteriorly with microdebrider or forceps.
- Additional intercellular partitions are entered and removed in manner similar to the basal lamella.
- The most posterior ethmoid cell characteristically has a pyramidal shape with the apex pointing posteriorly, laterally, and superiorly toward the optic nerve. The sphenoid sinus lies inferiorly, medially, and posterior to this cell.
- If a superior ethmoid or frontal recess dissection is planned, the skull base should be identified when possible within the posterior ethmoid sinus. In general, the cells here are larger and the skull base is more horizontal, making identification significantly easier and safer than in the anterior ethmoid sinus.
- If disease extent makes identification of the skull base difficult at this time, sphenoid-otomy should be performed and the skull base identified within the sphenoid sinus.

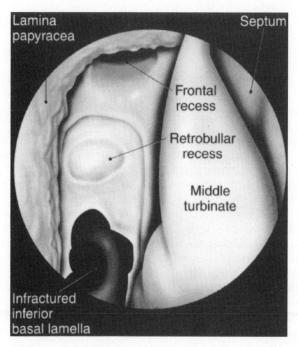

Figure 26-6 With lamina papyracea already identified, the basal lamella may be infractured with either forceps or a microdebrider, just superior to the horizontal portion. (*Reproduced with permission from Kennedy, DW, Bolger WE, Zinreich SJ, eds. Diseases of the Sinuses: Diagnosis and Management. Shelton, CT: PMPH-USA; 2001.*)

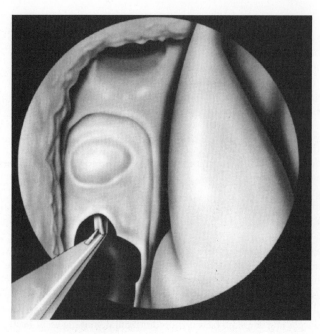

Figure 26-7 Upbiting forceps are utilized to feel for a space behind the bony partitions before they are taken down superiorly or toward the medial orbital wall. (*Reproduced with permission from Kennedy, DW, Bolger WE, Zinreich SJ, eds.* Diseases of the Sinuses: Diagnosis and Management. *Shelton, CT: PMPH-USA; 2001.*)

Sphenoidotomy With Ethmoidectomy

The safest method of entering the sphenoid from within the ethmoid sinus is as follows:

- Identify the superior meatus and the superior turbinate, by palpating medially between the middle and superior turbinate.
- Resect the most inferior part of the superior turbinate with a through-cutting forceps or with a microdebrider (Figure 26-8).
- Palpate the sphenoid sinus ostium just medial to where the superior turbinate was resected.
- Enlarge ostium with a Stammberger mushroom punch and Hajek rotating sphenoid punch.

Frontal Recess Surgery (Draf Type 1)

Because of the difficult anatomic relationships, it is very important to rereview the CT and have a 3D conceptualization of the anatomy before working in the region of the frontal sinus. The frontal sinus may then be accessed as follows:

- Dissect from posterior to anterior along the skull base, skeletonizing the medial orbital wall.
- Remember the anterior ethmoid vessel typically lies posterior to the supraorbital ethmoid cells and may cross up to 4 mm below the skull base.
- Remain laterally and close the medial orbital wall (thicker skull base).
- After opening the recess, carefully look for the opening to the frontal sinus—typically, the opening of the frontal sinus is medial, but this is variable.
- A small malleable probe may be used to palpate the opening and to confirm frontal sinus drainage pathway identified from the CT scans.
- A curette is then introduced and the bony roof of the agger nasi cell is fractured anteriorly or laterally, depending on whether the opening is posterior or medial (Figure 26-9).

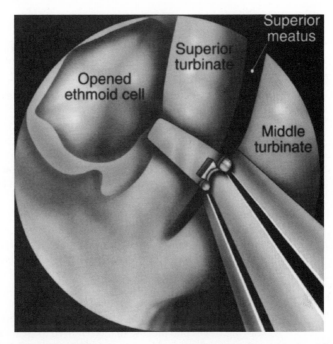

Figure 26-8 After identifying the superior meatus medially within the right ethmoid cavity, the inferior part of the superior turbinate is removed with a straight through-cutting forceps. (*Reproduced with permission from Kennedy, DW, Bolger WE, Zinreich SJ, eds.* Diseases of the Sinuses: Diagnosis and Management. *Shelton, CT: PMPH-USA; 2001.*)

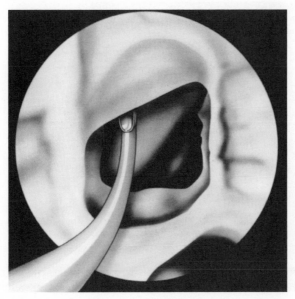

Figure 26-9 Using an angled telescope to view the frontal recess, a curved curette can be introduced posterior to the agger nasi cell and the roof of the cell fractured anteriorly ("uncapping the egg"). (*Reproduced with permission from Kennedy, DW, Bolger WE, Zinreich SJ, eds.* Diseases of the Sinuses: Diagnosis and Management. *Shelton, CT: PMPH-USA; 2001.*)

- The bone fragments are then painstakingly removed, taking care to avoid stripping mucosa.
- Document frontal sinus opening photographically for later comparison.

Draf Type 2 Frontal Sinusotomy

- In a Draf 2A, the frontal sinus is opened between the lamina papyracea and the insertion of the middle turbinate.
- In a Draf 2B, the frontal sinus is opened medial to the middle turbinate by removal of the most anterior attachment of the middle turbinate to the skull base.
- The Draf 2B procedure is best reserved for revision procedures where (1) the anterior portion of the middle turbinate has become osteitic and tends to scar laterally and (2) the internal os of the frontal sinus is small, it but can be extended medially.

Draf Type 3 Frontal Sinusotomy

- Also known as a trans-septal frontal sinusotomy or modified endoscopic Lothrop procedure, this operation removes part of the nasal septum and part of the frontal sinus septum to create one large opening accessible from both sides of the nose (Figure 26-10).
- Requires an adequate anterior and posterior (AP) diameter of the frontal recess on the CT scan. The minimum is approximately 5-6 mm.
- Given the degree of bone exposure, significant postoperative care is required to avoid scarring. The septal mucosa that is removed to create a window can be used as a free graft over the exposed bone anteriorly. However, this does somewhat narrow the AP diameter.
- Major complications such as CSF leak are reported to be less than 1%, but there is a failure rate of approximately 14%.

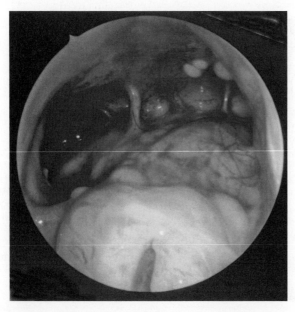

Figure 26-10 Endoscopic view of the frontal sinuses 5 years seen post Draf 3 procedure for extensive inverted papilloma (45° telescope). At the time of surgery, tumor was attached extensively to the anterior wall and was burred with a 70° diamond burr.

Surgical Steps

- Carefully evaluate the axial, coronal, and sagittal CT to evaluate anatomic suitability and the extent of bone that may need to be removed by drill.
- If one frontal sinuses open, perform an anterior ethmoidectomy on that side and identify the frontal sinus opening.
- Extend the frontal sinus ostium anteriorly into the "beak" and then medially to the midline.
- Identify the skull base, and the region of the ostium, on the opposite, closed, side.
- Resect the anterior portion of both middle turbinates and, after injection, create a window in the nasal septum.
- Using a 65° or 70° diamond burr, open the frontal sinus bilaterally working in a U-shaped fashion around the midline skull base. Use the open frontal sinus as a guide to the anatomy.
- The septal fenestration allows use of the telescope in one nostril and an instrument in the other.
- The mucosa of posterior wall of the frontal recess should not be traumatized.
- Remove the frontal sinus intersinus septum as widely as possible. The size of the frontal opening created will depend on the degree of bony thickening and mucosal inflammation present.

Management of the Nasal Septum

- The nasal septum is addressed during sinus surgery if it is markedly deviated to where it significantly interferes with nasal airflow or if the deviation is such that access to the anterosuperior attachment of the middle turbinate is not possible with the 0° telescope.
- Typically, the ethmoidectomy is performed on the wider side first, and the septum is then addressed, making the incision on the side of the previously performed ethmoidectomy, so as to avoid unnecessary bleeding onto the telescope during the second ethmoidectomy.
- Typically, septal corrections during FESS are best achieved with an endoscopic approach. This allows the deviated nasal septum to be addressed under excellent visualization, without the necessity to either change to a headlight or to change instrumentation.
- After making the incision using overhead lighting and initiating the flap elevation, the flaps are elevated with the use of a suction elevator and bony cartilaginous resection performed in the usual manner. We have found the 1-mm Acufex orthopedic punch particularly helpful in this regard.
- Septal reconstruction, if necessary, can be performed following the second ethmoidectomy by placing crushed cartilage into the septal pocket. The septal flaps are then quilted with a running chromic suture on a small straight needle.

Packing

- In general, postoperative packing is minimized following FESS and is generally not required for bleeding.
- A recent systematic review has demonstrated that the use of middle meatal spacers (such as Merocel sinus sponges) may be useful in preventing synechiae formation.
- More recently, steroid eluting stents have been shown to reduce inflammation in the postoperative ethmoid cavity and are a useful adjunct in disease control, especially in polypoid disease.

Balloon Catheter Sinus Surgery

- Over the last several years, the use of balloon technology has been developed as a tool to help surgically address diseased sinus ostia. The most common use is for the frontal sinus.
- Currently, there are three main types of balloon catheter devices: transnasal guide wire, transnasal malleable suction-based device, and transantral.
- All devices may be utilized in an office setting with local anesthesia in selected patients.
- The transnasal malleable suction-based device is primarily used for revision surgery and in conjunction with some endoscopic sinus surgery.
- Transnasal catheter-based devices:
  (a) Primarily treat the frontal sinus but may also be used for the maxillary or sphenoid sinus. In an unoperated maxillary sinus, it most frequently creates an accessory ostium.
  (b) With the aid of an endoscope, a guide catheter is used to direct a guide wire into the diseased sinus in question.
  (c) The guide wire has a light on its distal tip to provide transillumination and confirm localization within the sinus.
  (d) A balloon is passed over the guide wire and inflated with saline to dilate the sinus ostium.
- Transantral devices:
  (a) Only treat the maxillary sinus.
  (b) A canine fossa puncture is first created with a small trocar into the anterior wall of the maxillary sinus.
  (c) A flexible or rigid endoscope is placed through the canine fossa puncture to visualize the natural ostium.
  (d) A guide wire and balloon are then used to dilate the ostia under endoscopic visualization.
- Advantages:
  (a) The longest prospective nonrandomized study on transnasal balloon devices has demonstrated high ostial patency rates and improved SNOT-20 and Lund-MacKay scores 2 years after surgery.
  (b) Mucosal trauma is minimized.
  (c) May potentially decrease operative time and blood loss.
  (d) May be potentially performed in an office setting under local anesthetic.
  (e) As drug eluting stents become available, balloon technology should provide a viable method of both opening the sinus and reducing inflammation.
- Disadvantages:
  (a) Does not address the ethmoid sinuses.
  (b) Does not address polyps or bone that is thickened by chronic inflammation.
  (c) Does not currently address the issue of removing osteitic bone, which may play a significant role in persistent inflammatory disease.
  (d) Without drug eluting stents, they do not address the underlying inflammatory process.
  (e) Long-term outcome data are limited, and comparisons to medical therapy or the technique of antral irrigation have not been performed.
- Further prospective randomized trials comparing this technique with medical therapy and standard FESS are required to fully define the role of balloon catheter technologies in the management of chronic sinusitis.

Endoscopic Sinus Surgery for Neoplasms and Skull Base Defects

General guidelines for *mucoceles* are as follows:

- Identify skull base posteriorly (for frontal).
- Marsupialize widely, removing all osteitic bone from the opening.
- Make the opening flush with the surrounding bone.

General guidelines for *inverted papillomas* are as follows:

- Obtain permission to convert to an open procedure.
- Meticulously identify the site or sites of tumor attachment.
- Remove or burr the bone at the site(s) of tumor attachment.
- Convert to an open approach if you cannot adequately access the site(s) of attachment.
- Create a widely patent cavity that allows for easy long-term endoscopic surveillance.
- Do not compromise the tumor removal for the sake of an endoscopic approach.

General guidelines for *CSF leaks* are as follows:

- Consider a lumbar drain for spontaneous CSF leaks due to elevated intracranial pressure.
- Skeletonize the sinuses and skull base around the defect.
- Encephaloceles can be safely reduced with bipolar cautery.
- Strip mucosa around the defect to allow adherence of an overlay graft.
- If a lumbar drain has been placed preoperatively, draining 20 to 30 mL of CSF prior to graft placement will decrease flow through the defect and may help the graft seal the leak.
- Free mucoperiosteal grafts harvested from the nasal septum heal extremely well, but the pedicled Hadad-Bassagasteguy flap (based on the posterior septal artery) or other pedicled flaps may be used for larger skull base defects as an overlay graft.
- Multilayer closure may be employed, especially for larger high-flow defects, using septal bone or cartilage, mastoid bone or fascia or fat placed intracranially.
- Multiple layers of absorbable packing are placed, followed by a removable Merocel sponge.
- Access to inferior frontal sinus defects may be improved with a Draf 3 procedure. However, frontal sinus and supraorbital ethmoid defects may require an adjunctive external approach.
- Access to certain sphenoid sinus defects may be improved by resection of the posterior nasal septum and intersinus septum. Laterally placed defects may be approached with ligation or cauterization of the internal maxillary artery and a transpterygoid approach.

Avoiding and Managing Complications

Prevention of Bleeding

- Provide careful topical and infiltrative vasoconstriction.
- Minimize mucosal trauma, especially to the nasal mucosa anteriorly in the nose.
- Avoid trauma to the anterior ethmoid artery. Approximately 40% are dehiscent as the artery can travel beneath the ethmoid roof along a bony mesentery, in some cases 1 to 3 mm from the roof. Care must be taken not to mistake the artery for a bony septae of an ethmoid cell and attempt resection.

- Limit dissection in the region of the sphenopalatine artery and its branches. Care should be taken to avoid dissecting the basal lamella too far inferiorly when entering the posterior ethmoids. Bleeding can result as the sphenopalatine artery lies just behind the inferior aspect of the basal lamellae in most patients.
- If, during surgery, bleeding persists so that it interferes with visualization, it is safer to stop the procedure and, if necessary, return at a later time.

Management of Intraoperative Bleeding

- Pack the surgical cavity with cottonoid pledgets soaked in vasoconstrictive agents.
- Persistent bleeding or bleeding from the sphenopalatine, anterior or posterior ethmoid arteries, or their branches may require a small microfibrillar collagen pack or electrocautery.
- The use of an Endoscrub (Medtronic-Xomed Inc., Jacksonville, Florida) device to clear the endoscope lens of blood is extremely helpful in maintaining good visualization and thereby reducing complications from bleeding.

Management of Postoperative Epistaxis

- Application of topical hemostatic vasoconstrictive agents.
- Endoscopic localization of the bleeding site with treatment via electrocautery or direct packing of the bleeding site.
- Consider arterial ligation or embolization for refractory cases.

Prevention of Orbital Injury

- Identify the lamina orbitalis positively and do so early in the dissection.
- Initially, limit dissection in the lateral aspect of the most posterior ethmoid cells and the sphenoid to avoid trauma to the optic nerve. This is extremely important in cases where a sphenoethmoidal cell (Onodi cell) is present.
- Identify and preserve the anterior ethmoid artery. Should this artery be inadvertently divided during surgery, the lateral aspect of the vessel can retract within the orbit and bleed with a resultant and dramatic orbital hematoma.

Management of Orbital Complications

- If the lamina papyracea is entered during intranasal ethmoidectomy and orbital fat is exposed, further dissection should be terminated in the immediate region and the fat should not be removed or resected.
- Monitor for signs of an orbital hematoma such as lid edema, ecchymosis, and proptosis. Vision is checked if the patient is under local anesthesia.
- In all cases where the lamina papyracea has been violated, tight packing of the ethmoid cavity is prohibited as this can increase intraorbital pressure.
- When orbital hematoma is suspected and a sudden dramatic onset of progressive proptosis occurs, a "compartment syndrome" quickly results. To decrease the pressure within the orbit, initially perform a lateral canthotomy and cantholysis and then follow with orbital decompression and ophthalmology consult.
- For smaller orbital hematoma from capillary rather than arterial bleeding, remove nasal packing, check vision, and consult ophthalmology. Medical measures such as topical timolol; intravenous acetazolamide; mannitol; and high-dose steroids, globe massage, and CT scan should be considered.

Prevention of Skull Base Injury

- Conceptualize the CT anatomy. Identify the ethmoid roof positively and then work anteriorly feeling behind bony partitions before they are removed.
- Use through-cut instruments to remove partitions attached to the skull base.
- Use a 0° telescope to reduce the possibility of disorientation associated with the deflected angle endoscopes. After the skull base is identified, a 30° scope can be used more safely.
- When dissecting along the ethmoid roof, use caution clearing tissue from the medial aspect.

Management of Intraoperative Skull Base Injury/Cerebrospinal Fluid Rhinorrhea

- Inspect the area endoscopically to determine the site and size and determine if intradural injury has occurred.
- Consider neurosurgical and ID consultations.
- Remove the residual bony partitions to create a flat surface for graft placement.
- Remove the sinus mucosa adjacent to the leak site to create an area of denuded bone for the graft.
- Place a free overlay nasal mucosal graft over the leak site.
- Secure the graft with several layers of absorbable collagen based packing and Merocel sponges.
- Consider a postoperative head CT and MRI to rule out the possibility of intracranial bleeding and injury.

Postoperative Cerebrospinal Fluid Rhinorrhea

- We recommend early repair in all individuals who are identified as having a CSF leak postoperatively (Figure 26-11).
- Although conservative treatment such as bed rest and lumbar drainage has been attempted with small closed-head injury CSF leaks, there is a reported 29% incidence of meningitis with long-term follow-up of CSF leaks that are managed nonsurgically.

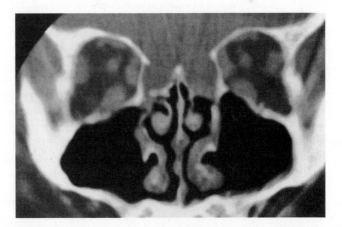

Figure 26-11 Coronal CT of a patient with complaint of anosmia, chronic nasal congestion, and discharge following prior sinus surgery at another institution. Nasal endoscopy demonstrated bilateral soft tissue masses and CT shows bilateral ethmoid roof defects. MR confirmed bilateral encephaloceles. (*Reproduced with permission from Kennedy, DW, Bolger WE, Zinreich SJ, eds. Diseases of the Sinuses: Diagnosis and Management. Shelton, CT: PMPH-USA; 2001.*)

Postoperative Care

Medical Therapy Following Surgery for CRS

- Antibiotic coverage is started in the operating room based either on preoperative culture or so as to provide coverage for the more frequently found organisms.
- Saline irrigations and topical steroids are instituted in the early postoperative period. The topical steroids are continued until the cavity is endoscopically normal.
- Oral steroids (if required) are tapered during the postoperative period based on the endoscopic appearance of the mucosa.
- If the cavity demonstrates evidence of increasing inflammation at any point during the postoperative healing period, it is recultured under endoscopic visualization and the antibiotics changed appropriately.
- Since the most common site for persistent disease is the frontal recess, when using steroid sprays, consider the use of one of the various positions that increase the dosage of steroid to that site. This includes Moffat's head-down kneeling position, Mygind's position (supine and head extended), or lying on the side head-down (LSHD) position.
- It is easier to instill drops in Mygind's position, but the LSHD position tends to have the least discomfort.
- Nasal saline irrigations are now a routine part of postoperative care and are usually started in the postoperative period. Adding budesonide (0.5 mg) to the saline reduces edema and may eliminate the necessity for oral steroids.
- During the first year or so postoperatively, patients with reactive mucosa may require both short courses of antibiotics and oral steroids in order to avoid recurrent mucosal disease and bacterial sinusitis following a viral upper respiratory infection.

Local Management of the Postoperative Cavity

- Merocel sponges are typically removed on the first postoperative day and the cavities suctioned free of blood under local anesthetic. In the case of a CSF leak repair, we typically wait 5 to 7 days before removing the packing.
- Nasal endoscopy and cleaning of the cavity is repeated on a weekly basis until the cavity is healed. At each visit, crusts are debrided, the cavity is examined for areas of persistent inflammation, and any residual fragments of exposed or osteitic bone are removed. Scars are divided and particular attention is paid to the all important frontal recess region.
- After CSF leak repair, minimal debridement of the area should be performed until the graft has healed. However, sinus cavities opened around the repair are debrided in the standard fashion.

Long-Term Management

- Symptoms, with the exception of postnasal discharge, usually resolve early following endoscopic sinus surgery.
- Pain and pressure in the postsurgical period is very uncommon and should be considered as a sign of persistent infection or inflammation requiring additional management.
- Olfaction is the symptom that appears to be the most sensitive indicator of persistent or recurrent disease. Indeed, patients should be instructed to follow their sense of smell and to obtain additional medical therapy and follow-up endoscopic examination, if they experience a significant decrease in their ability to smell.

- Advances in nasal endoscopy, radiologic imaging, medical treatments, and surgical technique have allowed for significant improvements in patient management. However, recalcitrant sinus disease is a particular problem and continues to await new therapeutic approaches.
- Since CRS is typically a multifactorial disease, surgery is only a small part of the overall management in the majority of patients.
- Following surgery and medical management in the postoperative period, patients require prolonged endoscopic surveillance for evidence of persistent or recurrent disease.
- In most cases, endoscopic evidence of disease is visible in the postoperative patient long before the return of patient symptoms.

Practice Guidelines

- A thorough understanding of paranasal sinus anatomy and embryology is required for successful and safe sinus surgery.
- CRS is a multifactorial inflammatory disease that is treated medically.
- ESS is indicated for CRS patients who have failed appropriate medical therapy.
- Ongoing postoperative care of the sinus cavity and continued medical treatment is necessary because all CRS patients have persistent asymptomatic disease following surgery.
- Endoscopic techniques have evolved to successfully treat a variety of skull base pathologies, including mucoceles, CSF leaks, and skull base tumors.

Bibliography

Abreu NA, Nagalingam NA, Song Y, et al. Sinus microbiome diversity depletion and *Corynebacterium tuberculostearicum* enrichment mediates rhinosinusitis. *Sci Transl Med.* 2012 Sep;4(151):151ra124.

Kennedy DW. Functional endoscopic sinus surgery: anesthesia, technique, and postoperative management. In: Kennedy, DW, Bolger WE, Zinreich SJ. *Diseases of the Sinuses: Diagnosis and Management.* Hamilton, ON: B.C. Decker Inc.; 2001:211-221.

Kennedy DW. The PROPEL steroid-releasing bioabsorbable implant to improve outcomes of sinus surgery. *Expert Rev Respir Med.* 2012 Nov;6(5):493-498.

Kern, RC, Consley DB, Walsh MD, et al. Perspectives on the etiology of chronic rhinosinusitis: an immune barrier hypothesis. *Am J Rhinol.* 2008;22(6):540-559.

Lee JM, Grewal A. Middle meatal spacers for the prevention of synechiae following endoscopic sinus surgery: a systematic review and meta-analysis of randomized controlled trials. *Int Forum Allergy Rhinol.* 2012;2(6):477-486.

Perloff JR, Gannon FH, Bolger WE, et al. Bone involvement in sinusitis: an apparent pathway for the spread of disease. *Laryngoscope.* 2000;110(12):2095-2099.

Varshita RJ, Soler ZM, Nguyen SA, et al. A systematic review and meta-analysis of asthma outcomes following endoscopic sinus surgery for chronic rhinosinusitis. *Int Forum Allergy Rhinol.* 2013 Oct;3(10):788-794.

Questions

1. Embryologically, the sphenoid sinus begins pneumatization at:
   A. Birth
   B. 6 weeks after birth
   C. 6 months after birth
   D. 6 years after birth
   E. 16 years after birth

2. The second lamella of the ethmoid complex corresponds to:
   A. The uncinate
   B. The middle turbinate
   C. The cribriform plate
   D. The middle meatus
   E. The ethmoidal bulla

3. Which one of the following structures is not part of the ostiomeatal complex (OMC)?
   A. Uncinate process
   B. Maxillary sinus ostium
   C. Inferior turbinate
   D. Ethmoidal bulla
   E. Middle meatus

4. If you were to consider using intrathecal fluorescein to help identify a suspected CSF leak, which of the following is an appropriate dosage and injection instruction?
   A. 0.1 mL of 10% fluorescein diluted in 10 mL of CSF injected over 10 minutes.
   B. 1 mL of 10% fluorescein diluted in 10 mL of CSF injected over 10 minutes.
   C. 0.1 mL of 10% fluorescein injected over 10 minutes.
   D. 0.1 mL of 10% fluorescein diluted in 10 mL of CSF injected over 1 minute.
   E. The dosage does not matter as long as you obtain consent prior to surgery.

5. Management of an acute orbital hematoma in the recovery room includes all of the following except:
   A. Lateral canthotomy and inferior cantholysis
   B. Urgent ophthalmology consult
   C. Mannitol
   D. High-dose intravenous steroids
   E. Topical steroids to the eye to decrease swelling and pressure on the optic nerve

Chapter 27
The Nose: Acute and Chronic Sinusitis

Nasal Embryology

- Nose develops from neural crest cells.
- Migration of neural crest cells around fourth week of gestation.
- Before closure, there are potential spaces forming between bone and cartilage.
  (a) *Fonticulus nasofrontalis*: space between frontal and nasal bone
  (b) *Prenasal space*: space between nasal bones and nasal capsule
  (c) *Foramen cecum*: space between frontal and ethmoid bone
- Two nasal placodes (thickenings of ectoderm that invaginate into nasal pits), one on each side of the area termed frontonasal process, develop inferiorly.
- Nasal pits (olfactory pits) divide each placode into medial and lateral nasal processes.
- Nasal pits become rudimentary nasal cavities.
- Rounded lateral angles of the medial processes form the globular processes of His; the globular processes extend backwards as nasal laminae, which fuse in the midline to form the septum.
- Medial processes fuse in the midline to form the philtrum and premaxilla.
- Lateral processes form the alae of the nose.
- The maxillary processes also form the lateral nasal wall.
- Nasobuccal membrane separates the nasal cavity from the oral cavity.
- As the olfactory pits deepen, the choanae are formed.

Anatomy of the Nose
Nasal Skeleton
- Bone
  (a) Two paired nasal bones, which attach laterally to nasal process of maxilla
- Cartilage
  (a) Paired upper lateral, lower lateral cartilages
  (b) Accessory sesamoid cartilages
Nasal Septum
- *Bone*: vomer, perpendicular plate of ethmoid bone, maxillary crest, palatine bone
- *Cartilage*: quadrangular cartilage
Lateral Nasal Wall
- Three turbinates and corresponding space (meatus)
- Inferior, middle, and superior turbinates
- *Inferior meatus*: drains nasolacrimal duct

- *Middle meatus*: drains maxillary, anterior ethmoid, and frontal sinuses
- *Superior meatus*: drains posterior ethmoid sinuses

Arterial Blood Supply
- External nose
  - (a) Primary supply from external carotid artery to facial artery
  - (b) *Superior labial artery*: columella and lateral nasal wall
  - (c) *Angular artery*: nasal side wall, nasal tip, and nasal dorsum
- Nasal cavity
  - (a) Both external and internal carotid artery
  - (b) External carotid artery system
    - Internal maxillary artery
      - *Sphenopalatine artery via sphenopalatine foramen*: divides into lateral nasal artery, supplying lateral nasal wall; and posterior septal artery, supplying posterior aspect of septum
      - *Descending palatine artery*: forms the greater and lesser palatine arteries; supplies lower portion of the nasal cavity
      - *Greater palatine artery*: passes inferiorly through greater palatine canal and foramen, travels within hard palate mucosa; bilateral arteries meet in midline and travel through single incisive foramen back into nasal cavity
  - (c) Internal carotid artery system
    - Ophthalmic artery enters orbit and gives off anterior and posterior ethmoid arteries; courses via anterior and posterior ethmoidal canal, takes an intracranial course and then turns inferiorly over the cribriform plate
    - *Anterior ethmoid artery*: supplies lateral and anterior one-third of nasal cavity; anastomoses with sphenopalatine artery (also known as nasopalatine artery; most common artery injured in septoplasty surgery, causing hematomas)
    - *Posterior ethmoid artery*: supplies small portion of superior turbinate and posterior septum
- Kiesselbach plexus (Little area)
  - (a) Confluence of vessels along the anterior nasal septum where the septal branch of sphenopalatine artery, anterior ethmoidal artery branches, greater palatine artery, and septal branches of superior labial artery anastomose
- Woodruff plexus (naso-nasopharyngeal plexus)
  - (a) Anastomosis of posterior nasal, posterior ethmoid, sphenopalatine, and ascending pharyngeal arteries along posterior lateral nasal wall inferior to the inferior turbinate

Venous Drainage
- Venous system is valveless.
- Sphenopalatine vein drains via sphenopalatine foramen into pterygoid plexus.
- Ethmoidal veins drain into superior ophthalmic vein.
- Anterior facial vein drains through common facial vein to internal jugular vein; also communicates with cavernous sinus via ophthalmic veins, infraorbital and deep facial veins, and the pterygoid plexus.
- Angular vein drains external nose via ophthalmic vein to cavernous sinus.

Lymphatic Drainage
- Anterior portion of nose drains toward external nose in the subcutaneous tissue to the facial vein and submandibular nodes.
- Others pass posterior to tonsillar region and drain into upper deep cervical nodes.
- Most drain into pharyngeal plexus and then to the retropharyngeal nodes.

Innervation

- Nasociliary nerve
  (a) Branch of ophthalmic division of cranial nerve (CN) V (CN V1)
  (b) Arises in the lateral wall of cavernous sinus and enters orbit and gives off two branches
    ○ Infratrochlear nerve
      – Supplies skin at the medial angle of eyelid
    ○ Anterior ethmoidal nerve
      – Leaves orbit with anterior ethmoidal artery
      – Supplies anterior superior nasal cavity, anterior ends of middle and inferior turbinate and corresponding septum; also region anterior to the superior turbinate
      – Leaves nasal cavity and supplies skin on dorsum of the tip of nose
- Maxillary nerve (CN V2)
  (a) Exits middle cranial fossa via foramen rotundum
    ○ Pterygopalatine (sphenopalatine) ganglion: contains parasympathetic, sympathetic, and sensory nerves
      – Lateral posterior superior nasal branch
      – Supplies posterior portion of superior and middle turbinates, posterior ethmoid cells
      – Medial posterior superior nasal branch
      – Crosses anterior surface of sphenoid; roof of nasal cavity; posterior septum
      – Nasopalatine nerve
      – Supplies anterior hard palate
      – Greater palatine nerve
      – Supplies mucous membrane over posterior portion of inferior turbinate and middle and inferior meatus
    ○ Infraorbital branch
      – Supplies portion of vestibule of the nose; anterior portion of inferior meatus; part of the floor of nasal cavity

Autonomic Innervation

- Derived from pterygopalatine ganglion
- Parasympathetic fibers of the nose
  (a) Derived from CN VII
  (b) Preganglionic fibers
    ○ From superior salivatory nucleus in medulla oblongata
    ○ Located in the nervus intermedius portion of facial nerve
    ○ Leave CN VII at the geniculate ganglion with greater superficial petrosal nerve and become vidian nerve and head to pterygopalatine ganglion
  (c) Postganglionic fibers
    ○ Arise in ganglion and join sympathetic and sensory fibers
    ○ Travel with branches of sphenopalatine nerve and provide secretomotor fibers to mucous glands in nasal mucosa
    ○ Vasodilation
- Sympathetic fibers of the nose
  (a) From thoracic spinal nerves (T1-T3)
  (b) Postganglionic fibers
    ○ From superior cervical ganglion and travel with internal carotid artery; leave this plexus as deep petrosal nerve and join the greater superficial petrosal nerve to form vidian nerve (nerve of pterygoid canal)
    ○ Mediate vasoconstriction

Histology

- Nasal vestibule:
  - (a) Keratinized squamous epithelium with vibrissae, sweat, and sebaceous glands
- Anterior one-third of nasal cavity, anterior portions of inferior and middle turbinates:
  - (a) Squamous and transitional cell epithelium
- Posterior two-thirds of nasal cavity:
  - (a) Pseudostratified columnar epithelium
  - (b) Contains ciliated, nonciliated columnar cells, mucin-secreting goblet cells, and basal cells (columnar to goblet cell ratio = 5:1)
  - (c) Each ciliated cell contains 50-200 cilia
  - (d) Each cilia is organized in "9+2" microtubules arranged in doublets; each doublet has dynein arms providing motion to cilia
- Respiratory epithelium:
  - (a) 20 to 30 nm
- Olfactory epithelium:
  - (a) Pseudostratified neuroepithelium containing primary olfactory receptors
  - (b) 60 to 70 nm; lacks dynein arms

Mucous Blanket

- *Two layers*: gel and sol phase
- *Gel phase*: superficial layer, produced by goblet and submucosal glands; layer to trap particulate matter
- *Sol phase*: deep layer, produced by microvilli; provides fluid that facilitates ciliary movement
- *Other components*: mucoglycoproteins, immunoglobulins, interferon, and inflammatory cells

Physiology of the Nose

Functions of the Nose

- *Airway*: conduit for air
- *Filtration*: trap and remove airborne particulate matter
- *Humidification*: increases relative humidity
- *Heating*: provides radiant heat of inspired air
- *Nasal reflex*: multiple that causes periodic nasal congestion, rhinorrhea, or sneezing
  - (a) *Postural reflex*: increased congestion with supine position; congestion on the side of dependence upon lying on the side
  - (b) *Hot or cold temperature reflex*: sneezing upon sudden exposure of skin to dramatic temperature extremes
- *Chemosensation*: detects irritants and temperature changes
- *Olfaction*: see later and Chapter 25

Nasal Airflow Resistance

- Contributes up to 50% of total airway resistance.
- Mucosal vasculature is under sympathetic tone; when tone decreases, vessels engorge, airflow resistance increases; change in tone is part of normal nasal cycle occurring every 2 to 7 hours.
- Three components of nasal resistance:
  - (a) Nasal vestibule
    - ○ First area of nasal resistance
    - ○ Also called as external nasal valve
    - ○ Skin lined area from nares to caudal upper lateral cartilage
    - ○ Collapses on inspiration

  (b) Nasal valve
  - ○ Referred to internal nasal valve
  - ○ Narrowest point
  - ○ *Borders:* lower edge of upper lateral cartilage, anterior end of inferior turbinates, and nasal septum
  - ○ Normal angle between nasal septum and upper lateral cartilage is 10 to 15 degree
  (c) Nasal cavum
  - ○ Located posterior to pyriform aperture
  - ○ Minor component of airway resistance
  - ○ Resistance determined by vascular engorgement of nasal tissues

Olfaction (See Chapter 25)
- Olfactory epithelium.
  (a) It is located in upper edge of nasal chamber adjacent to cribriform plates, superior nasal septum, and superior lateral nasal wall.
  (b) Pseudostratified neuroepithelium containing primary olfactory receptors.
  (c) Two layers separated by basement membrane.
  - ○ Olfactory mucosa
  - ○ Lamina propria
  (d) Different cell types:
  - ○ Bipolar receptor cell
  - ○ Sustentacular cell
  - ○ Microvillar cell
  - ○ Cells lining Bowman gland
  - ○ Horizontal basal cell
  - ○ Globose basal cell
- Unmyelinated axons from olfactory receptor neurons form myelinated fascicles which become olfactory fila that passes through the foramina of cribriform plate; each axon synapses in olfactory bulb.
- Olfactory bulb is highly organized with multiple layers (from outside in).
  (a) Glomerular layer
  (b) External plexiform layer
  (c) Mitral cell layer
  (d) Internal plexiform layer
  (e) Granule cell layer

Congenital Anomalies

Choanal Atresia
- 1 in 5000 to 8000 live births.
- Female to male ratio is 2:1.
- Unilateral greater than bilateral; right side more common in unilateral.
- The ratio of bony and membranous bony is 30%:70%.
- Four basic theories are:
  (a) Persistence of buccopharyngeal membrane
  (b) Abnormal persistence of bucconasal membrane
  (c) Abnormal mesoderm forming adhesions in nasochoanal region
  (d) Misdirection of neural crest cell migration

- Bilateral choanal atresia usually presents with airway distress at birth since newborns are obligate nasal breathers; classic presentation is cyclic cyanosis relieved by crying (paradoxical cyanosis).
- 20% to 50% with other associated congenital anomalies.
  - (a) CHARGE (coloboma, heart disease, choanal atresia, mental retardation, genital hypoplasia, ear anomalies)
  - (b) Apert syndrome, Crouzon disease, Treacher-Collins syndrome
- Unilateral choanal atresia presents usually between 5 and 24 months with unilateral obstruction and nasal discharge.
- Definitive diagnosis established by computed tomography (CT) scan.
- Treatment
  - (a) *Bilateral:* immediate management—airway stabilization with oral airway, McGovern nipple, intubation if ventilation is required
  - (b) Surgical correction
    - ○ Transpalatal approach
    - ○ Transnasal approach: puncture, most commonly with Fearon dilator
    - ○ Endoscopic approach

Congenital Midline Masses

Dermoid

- Epithelium-lined cavities or sinus tracts filled with keratin debris, hair follicles, sweat glands, and sebaceous glands.
- May present as intranasal, intracranial, or extranasal masses along the nasal dorsum.
- May also present as pit or fistulous tract.
- Mass is nontender, noncompressible, and firm; do not transilluminate.
- During development, projection of dura protrudes through fonticulus frontalis or inferiorly into prenasal space; the projection normally regresses and if it does not, the dura can remain attached to the epidermis, causing trapping of ectodermal elements.
- Have tendency for repeated infections, ranging from cellulitis to abscess.
- CT and magnetic resonance imaging (MRI) important for determining extent of lesion.
- Surgical excision is treatment of choice; incision and drainage are discouraged. Entire cyst and tract with bone and cartilage should be removed.

Glioma

- Comprised of ectopic glial tissue; 15% to 20% have intracranial connection.
- Abnormal closure of the fonticulus frontalis can lead to an ectopic rest of glial tissue if left extracranially.
- Sixty percent external; 30% unilateral intranasal; 10% combined.
- Mass is firm, nontender, noncompressible, does not transilluminate.
- Need to rule out intracranial connection by radiology.
- Complete surgical excision also is the treatment of choice.

Encephalocele

- Congenital herniation of central nervous system (CNS) tissue through skull base defect
  - (a) *Meningoceles:* contain only meninges
  - (b) *Meningoencephaloceles:* contain meninges and glial tissue
- Classified according to location of skull base defect
  - (a) *Occipital:* (most common; 75%)
  - (b) *Sincipital:*
    - ○ Also called as frontoethmoidal encephaloceles, defect at foramen cecum, just anterior to cribriform plate

- ○ Subtypes:
  - – Nasofrontal
  - – Nasoethmoidal
  - – Naso-orbital
- ○ Presents as external as mass over nose, glabella, or forehead
  - – Basal
  - – Defect in floor of anterior cranial fossa between cribriform plate and clinoid process
  - – Present as internal intranasal or nasopharyngeal mass
  - – Subtypes:
  - – Transethmoidal
  - – Trans-sphenoidal
  - – Sphenoethmoidal
  - – Sphenomaxillary
  - – Mass is often bluish or red, soft, compressible, and transilluminate
  - – Mass pulsatile, expand with crying or straining
  - – *Furstenberg test*: expand with compression of internal jugular veins
  - – CT and MRI important for diagnosis and surgical planning
  - – Should be surgically resected and repaired to prevent cerebrospinal fluid (CSF) leak, meningitis, or herniation

Teratoma

- Rare developmental tumors that comprise of all three germ layers.
- Head and neck teratomas account for 2% to 3% of all teratomas.
- Most common is cervical teratoma, followed by nasopharyngeal teratoma.
- Antenatal diagnosis by ultrasound is available in the United States.
- Secure the airway in cases of airway obstruction.
- Plain film radiograph showing calcification is pathognomonic.
- CT helpful in delineation of lesion extent and rule out intracranial connection.

Cysts

Rathke Pouch Cyst

- Rathke pouch is an invagination of the nasopharyngeal epithelium in the posterior midline; the anterior pituitary gland develops from this in fetal life.
- Remnants of this pouch may persist forming cyst or tumor.
- Rathke pouch cyst:
  - (a) Benign cyst in the sella turcica
  - (b) Usually present in fifth or sixth decades of life; females > males
  - (c) Usually asymptomatic but may compress adjacent structures such as the pituitary gland or optic chiasm
  - (d) MRI is modality of choice
- Tumor of Rathke pouch is craniopharyngioma.

Thornwaldt Cyst (Tornwaldt Cyst)

- Benign nasopharyngeal cyst
- Develops from remnant of notochord
- *Symptoms*: postnasal drainage, aural fullness, serous otitis media, and cervical pain
- *Examination*: smooth submucosal midline mass in nasopharynx
- *Treatment*: none if asymptomatic; if symptomatic, marsupialization through surgical correction via endoscopic approach

Intra-Adenoidal Cyst
- Occlusion of adenoid crypts, leading to retention cyst in adenoids; asymptomatic; in midline; rhomboid shape on imaging

Branchial Cleft Cyst
- Can be formed by either the first or second branchial arch
- Relative lateral position in nasopharynx
- Treatment is surgical excision

Allergic Rhinitis

- *Nasal symptoms*: nasal congestion, rhinorrhea (anterior and posterior), nasal pruritus, palate pruritus, postnasal drainage, anosmia, or hyposmia
- *Ocular symptoms*: ocular pruritus, watery eyes
- Pathophysiology:
  (a) Gell and Coombs type I hypersensitivity.
  (b) *Sensitization:* After initial exposure to an antigen, antigen-processing cells (macrophages, dendritic cells) present the processed peptides to T-helper cells. Upon subsequent exposure to the same antigen, these cells are stimulated to differentiate into either more T-helper cells or B cells. The B cells further differentiate into plasma cells and produce IgE specific to that antigen. Allergen-specific IgE molecules then bind to the surface of mast cells, sensitizing them.
  (c) Early phase response starts within 5 to 15 minutes.
    ○ Mast cells degranulate, releasing histamine, heparin, and tryptase; they produce symptoms of sneezing, rhinorrhea, congestion, and pruritus.
    ○ Degranulation also triggers formation of prostaglandin PGD2, leukotrienes LTC4, LTD4, LTE4, and platelet activating factor (PAF).
  (d) Late phase response begins 2 to 4 hours later.
    ○ Caused by newly arrived inflammatory cells recruited by cytokines.
    ○ Eosinophils, neutrophils, and basophils prolong the earlier reactions and lead to chronic inflammation.
      – *Seasonal allergies*: particular time of the year according to seasonal allergens (grass, trees, pollen, ragweed).
      – *Perennial allergies*: symptoms present all year around (insects, dust mites, dogs, cats).
      – Please refer to the Chapter 53 for further details of allergy testing and treatment.

Nonallergic Rhinitis

- Chronic symptoms of nasal congestion, rhinorrhea, posterior nasal drainage, may be distinguished from allergic rhinitis by consistent presence of symptoms, lack of nasal or ocular pruritus
- Possible triggers
  (a) Strong fragrances, tobacco smoke, changes in temperature, cleaning products
- Subclassification
  (a) *Infectious rhinitis*: most common is viral (rhinovirus, respiratory syncytial virus, parainfluenza virus, adenovirus, influenza virus, enterovirus)
  (b) *Vasomotor rhinitis (Nonallergic rhinopathy NAR)*: The Joint Task Force Rhinitis Practice Parameter defines it as: "a heterogeneous group of patients with chronic nasal symptoms that are not immunologic or infectious in origin and are usually not associated with nasal eosinophilia." It has been postulated to be an imbalance

in the autonomic system where the parasympathetic system predominates leading to vasodilation and mucosal edema. Changes in climate (temperature, humidity, barometric pressure), strong odors (perfume, cooking smells, flowers, chemicals), environmental tobacco smoke, pollutants, exercise, and alcohol ingestion have been found to exacerbate symptoms

(c) *Hormone-induced rhinitis*: associated with hormonal imbalance; usually due to pregnancy, puberty, menstruation, or hypothyroidism. Physiologic changes in pregnancy (expanded blood volume, vascular pooling, plasma leakage, and smooth muscle relaxation) exacerbate preexisting rhinitis. Rhinitis occurs in one-fifth of pregnancies.

(d) *Occupational rhinitis*: rhinitis at the workplace; usually due to inhaled irritant; frequently associated with concurrent occupational asthma

(e) Drug-induced rhinitis
   ○ *Antihypertensives*: angiotensin-converting enzyme (ACE) inhibitors, beta blockers
   ○ Nonsteroidal anti-inflammatory drugs (NSAIDs)
   ○ Oral contraceptives

(f) *Rhinitis medicamentosa*: tachyphylaxis associated with prolonged use of nasal sympathomimetics, over 5 to 7 days; alpha receptors in the nose are desensitized; rebound congestion due to overuse of decongestants; treat with intranasal steroids and stop decongestant. During the withdrawal process, sometimes a short course of systemic steroids is required.

(g) *Gustatory rhinitis*: watery rhinorrhea due to vasodilation after eating, especially with spicy or hot foods. It is mediated vagally. Preprandial treatment with topical ipratropium bromide is often effective.

(h) Nonallergic rhinitis of eosinophilia syndrome (NARES): a perennial disorder usually in middle aged adults.
   ○ Rhinitis with approximately 10% to 20% eosinophils on nasal smears in the setting of negative assessment for aeroallergen-specific IgE
   ○ Symptoms of nasal congestion, rhinorrhea, sneezing, pruritus, and hyposmia; usually responds well with topic nasal corticosteroids.

Atrophic Rhinitis

- Also called as rhinitis sicca or ozena
- Mucosal colonization with *Klebsiella ozaenae* and other organisms
- Nasal mucosa degenerates and loses mucociliary function
- Presents with foul smell as well as yellow or green nasal crusting with atrophy and fibrosis of mucosa, anosmia
- Primary atrophic rhinitis
  (a) Most prevalent in developing countries in subtropical and temperate climate zones. Etiology is unknown but bacterial infection is thought to be involved. These include *Klebsiella ozaenae*, *Staphylococcus aureus*, *Proteus mirabilis*, and *Escherichia coli*.
- Secondary atrophic rhinitis
  (a) More prevalent in developed countries, less severe and less progressive. Usually secondary to trauma or nasal surgery ("empty nose syndrome"). This may also result from underlying granulomatous disease.
- Management: nasal saline irrigation, antibiotics, surgical approach to reduce nasal cavity size

Granulomatosis With Polyangiitis (Wegener Granulomatosis) (See Chapter 12)

- Triad of necrotizing granulomas of respiratory tract, vasculitis, and glomerulonephritis
- Sinonasal symptoms usually manifest early with severe nasal crusting, epistaxis, rhinorrhea, and secondary rhinosinusitis
- Nasal biopsy usually nondiagnostic
- Cytoplasmic pattern (+C-ANCA) strongly associated with Wegener granulomatosis
- Anti-myeloperoxidase (MPO) and anti-proteinase 3 (PR3) testing for WG
- Consultation with rheumatology for systemic treatment
- Nasal treatment
    (a) Saline irrigation, nasal moisturization, topical antibiotics

Sarcoidosis (See Chapter 12)

- Multisystem inflammatory disease with noncaseating granulomas.
- *Sinonasal manifestations*: nasal obstruction, postnasal drainage, recurrent sinusitis.
- Serum ACE levels may be elevated.

Rhinoscleroma

- Chronic granulomatous disease due to *Klebsiella rhinoscleromatis*
- Endemic to Africa, central America, or Southeast Asia
- Usually affects nasal cavity, but may also affect the larynx, nasopharynx, or paranasal sinuses
- Three stages of disease progression
    (a) *Catarrhal or atrophic*: rhinitis, purulent rhinorrhea, and nasal crusting
    (b) *Granulomatous or hypertrophic*: small painless granulomatous lesions in upper respiratory tract
    (c) *Sclerotic*: sclerosis and fibrosis narrowing nasal passages
- Key pathologic findings:
    (a) *Mikulicz cells*: large macrophage with clear cytoplasm containing bacilli
    (b) Russell bodies in plasma cells
- *Treatment*: long-term antibiotics, biopsy, and debridement

Rhinosporidiosis

- Chronic granulomatous infection caused by *Rhinosporidium seeberi*
- Endemic to Africa, Pakistan, Sri Lanka, or India
- *Symptoms*: friable red nasal polyps, nasal obstruction, and epistaxis
- *Histopathology*: pseudoepitheliomatous hyperplasia, presence of *R. seeberi*
- *Treatment*: surgical excision

Epistaxis

- Over 90% of bleeds can be visualized anteriorly.
- Please refer to vascular anatomy earlier in the chapter.
- Causes.
    (a) Local
        ○ Trauma: digital, foreign body, fracture, surgery
        ○ Dessication
        ○ Drug-induced: cocaine, nasal steroids
        ○ Infectious: bacterial sinusitis
        ○ Inflammatory: allergic rhinitis, granulomatous disease
        ○ Neoplastic: angiofibroma, papillomas, carcinoma

(b) Systemic
- Intrinsic coagulopathy: von Willebrand disease, hemophilia, hereditary hemorrhagic telangiectasia (HHT)
- Drug-induced coagulopathy
- Hypertension
- Neoplastic
- Management:
(a) Airway breathing circulation (ABC); patient stabilization
(b) Cauterization under direct visualization
(c) Nasal packing:
  - Anesthetic: vasoconstrictor-solution-soaked cotton
  - Vaseline gauze
  - Merocel
  - Epistaxis balloon
  - Topical tranexamic acid application
  - Gelfoam or Surgicel in coagulopathic patient
  - Posterior packing (balloon or gauze) requires close monitoring
  - All patients with nasal packing should be on prophylactic antibiotics to prevent toxic shock syndrome
(d) Control of hypertension
(e) Correction of coagulopathies
(f) Greater palatine foramen block
(g) Saline sprays
(h) Humidity or emollients
(i) Surgical ligation
  - Continued bleeding despite nasal packing
  - IMAX ligation
    - Caldwell-Luc to enter maxillary sinus; enter posterior wall, vessels clipped
  - Endoscopic sphenopalatine ligation
    - Follow middle turbinate to posterior aspect
    - Make vertical incision approximately 7 to 8 mm anterior to the posterior end of middle turbinate
    - Crista ethmoidalis seen and marks anterior sphenopalatine foramen; vessels posterosuperior; clip or cauterize
  - Ethmoid artery ligation
    - Lynch incision; the distance between the anterior lacrimal crest of the maxilla's frontal process to anterior ethmoid artery foramen is 22 to 24 mm, distance between the anterior and posterior ethmoid artery foramina is 12 to 15 mm, distance between the posterior ethmoid artery foramen and optic canal is 3 to 7 mm.
  - External carotid artery ligation
    - Approach via anterior border of sternocleidomastoid (SCM) muscle
    - Identify bifurcation between internal and external arteries
(j) Embolization
  - Most commonly embolized vessel is IMAX (Internal maxillary artery) through a transfemoral approach
  - Pre-embolization angiograms of the ICA and ECA are performed to determine the location of the bleed as well as identify any vascular abnormality in the area.

○ Several types of embolic material are used: gelatin sponge, gelfoam powder, polyvinyl alcohol (PVA) particles, trisacryl gelatin particles, platinum coils, or a combination.
○ Indications: posterior epistaxis refractory to standard treatments
○ Contraindications: allergy to contrast material, renal insufficiency, access problems
○ Complications: Major: cerebrovascular accident, blindness, opthalmoplegia, soft tissue necrosis, seizures, anaphylaxis to contrast reagent. Minor: facial pain, facial edema, jaw pain, headache, paresthesia, mild palate ulceration, inguinal pain/hematoma.

Rhinosinusitis

- Inflammation of the nose and the paranasal sinuses
- Symptoms (two or more symptoms)
  (a) One of which should be nasal blockage or obstruction or congestion or nasal discharge (anterior or posterior nasal drip)
  (b) ± Facial pain or pressure
  (c) ± Hyposmia or anosmia

Classification of Rhinosinusitis

- The Rhinosinusitis Task Force (RSTF) in 2007 proposed a clinical classification system:
  (a) *Acute rhinosinusitis (ARS):* symptoms lasting for less than 4 weeks with complete resolution
  (b) *Subacute RS:* duration between 4 and 12 weeks
  (c) *Chronic RS (CRS) (with or without nasal polyps):* symptoms lasting for more than 12 weeks without complete resolution of symptoms
  (d) *Recurrent ARS:* ≥ 4 episodes per year, each lasting ≥ 7-10 days with complete resolution in between episodes
  (e) *Acute exacerbation of CRS:* sudden worsening of baseline CRS with return to baseline after treatment

Acute Rhinosinusitis

Acute Viral Rhinosinusitis

- Common cold
- Rhinovirus and influenzae are the most common agents
- Symptoms last for less than 14 days
- Symptoms self-limited

Acute Nonviral Rhinosinusitis

- Increase in symptoms after 5 days or persistent symptoms after 10 days
- Sudden onset of two or more symptoms
  (a) Nasal blockage or congestion
  (b) Anterior or posterior nasal drainage
  (c) Facial pain or pressure
  (d) Hyposmia or anosmia

Acute Bacterial Rhinosinusitis

- *Haemophilus influenzae, Streptococcus pneumoniae*, and *Moraxella catarrhalis* are the most common agents.

- Three cardinal symptoms for diagnosis.
  (a) Purulent nasal discharge
  (b) Face pain or pressure
  (c) Nasal obstruction
- Secondary symptoms that further support diagnosis.
  (a) Anosmia, fever, aural fullness, cough, and headache

Pathophysiology of ARS

- *Anatomic abnormalities may predispose one to ARS*: Septal deviation and spur, turbinate hypertrophy, middle turbinate concha bullosa; prominent agger nasi cell; Haller cells; prominent ethmoidal bulla; pneumatization and inversion of uncinate process.
- Acute viral respiratory infection affects nasal and sinus mucosa leading to obstruction of sinus outflow.
- *Other factors*: Allergies, nasal packing, sinonasal tumors, trauma, and dental infections.

Chronic Rhinosinusitis

- Four cardinal symptoms of CRS
  (a) Anterior or posterior purulent nasal discharge
  (b) Nasal obstruction
  (c) Face pain or pressure
  (d) Hyposmia or anosmia

Diagnosis of CRS

- At least two of the cardinal symptoms + one of the following:
  (a) *Endoscopic evidence of mucosal inflammation:* purulent mucus or edema in middle meatus or ethmoid region
  (b) Polyps in nasal cavity or middle meatus
  (c) Radiologic evidence of mucosal inflammation
- Three subtypes of CRS:
  (a) CRS with nasal polyps (20%-33%) (CRSwNP)
    ○ Predominantly neutrophilic inflammation
  (b) CRS without nasal polyps (60%-65%) (CRSsNP)
    ○ Predominantly eosinophilic inflammation; IL-5 and eotaxin involvement
  (c) Allergic fungal rhinosinusitis (8%-12%)

Factors Associated with CRS (See also Chapter 26)

- *Anatomic abnormalities*: Septal deviation and spur, turbinate hypertrophy, middle turbinate concha bullosa, prominent agger nasi cell, Haller cells, prominent ethmoidal bulla, pneumatization and inversion of uncinate process.
- *Ostiomeatal complex compromise*: The common drainage pathway for frontal, anterior ethmoid, and maxillary sinuses; blockage by inflammation or infection can lead to obstruction of sinus drainage, resulting in sinusitis.
- *Mucociliary impairment*: Ciliary function plays important role in clearance of sinuses; loss of ciliary function may result from infection, inflammation, or toxin; Kartagener syndrome (situs inversus, CRS, and bronchiectasis) may be associated with CRS.
- *Asthma*: Up to 50% of CRS patients have asthma.
- *Bacterial infection*: *Staphylococcus aureus,* coagulase-negative *Staphylococcus, Pseudomonas aeruginosa, Klebsiella pneumoniae, Proteus mirabilis, Enterobacter, Escherichia coli*; with chronicity, anaerobes develop *Fusobacterium, Peptostreptococcus, and Prevotella.*
- *Fungal infection*: May cause a range of diseases, from noninvasive fungus balls to invasive pathologies.

- *Allergy*: A contributing factor to CRS; there is increased prevalence of allergic rhinitis in patients with CRS.
- *Staphylococcal superantigen*: Exotoxins secreted by certain *S. aureus* strains; they activate T cells by linking T-cell receptors with MHC II surface molecule on antigen presenting cells (APCs).
- *Osteitis*: Area of increased bone density and thickening may be a marker of chronic inflammation.
- *Biofilms*: 3D structures of living bacteria encased in polysaccharide; have been found on sinus mucosa in CRS patients.
- *ASA or Samter triad*: Nasal polyposis, aspirin (ASA) sensitivity, and asthma; mediated by production of proinflammatory mediators, mainly leukotrienes.
- *Granulomatous vasculitis*: Churg-Strauss syndrome: CRSwNP, asthma, peripheral eosinophilia, pulmonary infiltrates, systemic eosinophilic vasculitis, and peripheral neuropathy (p-ANCA may be positive).

Fungal Rhinosinusitis

- Divided into invasive and noninvasive diseases
- *Invasive*: acute invasive, chronic invasive, and chronic granulomatous
- *Noninvasive*: fungal ball, saprophytic fungal, and allergic fungal rhinosinusitis
- Five types

Allergic Fungal Rhinosinusitis

- Five criteria of Bent and Kuhn
  - (a) Eosinophilic mucin (Charcot-Leyden crystals)
  - (b) Noninvasive fungal hyphae
  - (c) Nasal polyposis
  - (d) Characteristic radiologic findings
    - *CT*: rim of hypointensity with hyperdense central material (allergic mucin)
    - *CT*: speckled areas of increased attenuation due to ferromagnetic fungal elements
    - *MRI*: peripheral hyperintensity with central hypointensity on both T1 and T2
    - *MRI*: central "void" on T2
  - (e) Type 1 hypersensitivity by history, skin tests, or serology
- Dematiaceous fungi (*Alternaria*, *Bipolaris*, *Curvularia*, *Cladosporium*, and *Drechslera*)
- Typically unilateral but sometimes bilateral
- Dramatic bony expansion of paranasal sinuses
- High association with asthma

Fungal Ball

- Usually single sinus (maxillary sinus most common)
- *Most common fungus*: Aspergillus fumigates
- Immunocompetent patient
- Dense mass of fungal hyphae and secondary debris without mucosal invasion
- Pain over involved sinus
- Treatment is surgical removal

Acute Invasive Fungal Rhinosinusitis

- Also known as acute fulminant fungal rhinosinusitis
- *Symptoms*: nasal painless ulcer or eschar; periorbital or facial swelling, ophthalmoplegia
- Immunocompromised patient (diabetes mellitus [DM], HIV, chemotherapy, or transplant)

- Fungal invasion into mucosa, bone, soft tissues; angioinvasion, thrombosed vessels, necrotic tissue
- Sudden onset with rapid progression
- Organisms
  - (a) *Mucorales* (*Rhizopus, Rhizomucor, Absidia, Mucor, Cunninghamella, Mortierella, Saksenaea, Apophysomyces,* and *Zygomycosis*): nonseptate, 90-degree branching, necrotic background, serpiginous (most common in diabetic ketoacidosis patients)
  - (b) *Aspergillus:* septate, 45-degree branching, tissue background, and vermiform
- *Treatment:* aggressive surgical debridement, systemic antifungals, and correct underlying immunosuppressed states
- Poor prognosis

Chronic Invasive Fungal Rhinosinusitis
- Tissue invasion by fungal elements greater than 4 weeks duration, with minimal inflammatory responses
- Immunocompetent patients
- *Species: Aspergillus fumigates* common, *Mucor, Alternaria, Curvularia, Bipolaris, Candida,* or *Drechslera*
- *Treatment:* surgical debridement, systemic antifungals
- Poor prognosis

Chronic Granulomatous Fungal Rhinosinusitis
- Tissue invasion by fungal elements greater than 4 weeks duration, with mucosal inflammatory cell infiltrate
- Immunocompetent patients
- Onset gradual, symptoms caused by sinus expansion
- Multinucleated giant cell granulomas centered on eosinophilic material surrounded by fungus
- *Most common: Aspergillus flavus*
- Treatment is surgery for diagnosis and debridement; systemic antifungals

Complications of Rhinosinusitis
- *Hematogenous spread:* retrograde thrombophlebitis through valveless veins (veins of Breschet)
- *Direct spread:* through lamina papyracea, osteomyelitis
- Mucoceles
  - (a) Collection of sinus secretions trapped due to obstruction of sinus outflow tract; expansile process
  - (b) *Mucopyoceles:* infected mucocele
  - (c) Endoscopic marsupialization is treatment

Ophthalmologic
- Chandler classification
  - (a) *Preseptal cellulitis:* inflammatory edema; no limitation of extraocular movements (EOM)
  - (b) *Orbital cellulitis:* chemosis, impairment of EOM, proptosis, possible visual impairment
  - (c) C. *Subperiosteal abscess:* pus collection between medial periorbita and bone; chemosis, exophthalmos, EOM impaired, visual impairment worsening
  - (d) *Orbital abscess:* pus collection in orbital tissue; complete ophthalmoplegia with severe visual impairment

- ○ Superior orbital fissure syndrome (CN III, IV, V1, and VI)
- ○ Orbital apex syndrome (CN II, III, IV, V1, and VI)
  (e) Cavernous sinus thrombosis: bilateral ocular symptoms; worsening of all previous symptoms
- Treatment
  (a) Mild preseptal cellulitis: outpatient antibiotics, topical decongestants, saline irrigation with close follow-up
  (b) Hospital admission with low threshold for IV antibiotics, topical decongestants
  (c) Ophthalmology consultation
  (d) Surgical exploration if no improvement with IV antibiotics

Endoscopic decompression and external ethmoidectomy via Lynch incision are both options for surgical approach.

Neurologic
- *Meningitis*: severe headache, fever, seizures, altered mental status, and meningismus
- *Epidural abscess*: pus collection between dura and bone
- *Subdural abscess*: pus under dura
- *Brain abscess*: pus within brain parenchyma

Bony
- *Osteomyelitis*: thrombophlebitic spread via diploic veins
- *Pott puffy tumor*: subperiosteal abscess (frontal bone osteomyelitis to erosion of the anterior bony table)

Pediatric Rhinosinusitis

Symptoms
- Cold with nasal discharge, cough for more than 10 days
- Cold with severe symptoms includes high fever, purulent nasal discharge, periorbital pain or edema
- Cold that initially improves but worsens again

Pediatric ARS
- Children have approximately six to eight episodes of viral upper respiratory tract infections (URTIs) per year
- Five percent to 13% are complicated by bacterial sinusitis
- Pathogens:
  (a) Nontypable *H influenzae*
  (b) *S pneumoniae*
  (c) *M catarrhalis*
- Antibiotic treatment aims at the most common pathogens
- Topical decongestants
- Saline drops or sprays
- Topical nasal corticosteroids

Pediatric CRS (PCRS)
- defined as at least 90 continuous days of two or more symptoms of purulent rhinorrhea, nasal obstruction, facial pressure/pain, or cough and either endoscopic signs of mucosal edema, purulent discharge, or nasal polyposis and/or CT scan changes showing mucosal changes within the OMC and/or sinuses in pediatric patients aged 18 or younger
- Predisposing factors:
  (a) Viral URTIs
  (b) Day care attendance

(c) Allergic rhinitis
(d) Anatomic abnormalities
(e) Gastroesophageal reflux
(f) Immune deficiency
(g) Second-hand smoke
(h) Ciliary dysfunction
(i) Adenoiditis/tonsillitis
(j) Otitis media

- Similar to treatment of pediatric ARS, except antibiotic therapy of minimum of 10 days
- Medical therapy of pediatric CRS should include treatment for GERD when signs and symptoms of GERD are present
- Topical antibiotic therapy may have a role, as is antral irrigation in selected cases
- Daily topical nasal steroids are beneficial adjunctive medical therapy for PCRS
- Daily topical nasal saline irrigations are beneficial adjunctive medical therapy for PCRS
- Adenoidectomy is an effective first-line surgical procedure for children aged 13 or younger with CRS
- Balloon sinuplasty is a safe and effective treatment option for children with CRS
- Inferior turbinate reduction can benefit children with CRS by reducing nasal congestion and improving medication penetration topically
- Role of sinus surgery indicated in cases of failed medical therapy and adenoidectomy, mucocele, nasal polyposis, fungal rhinosinusitis, or orbital or intracranial complications

Treatment of Rhinosinusitis

Treatment of ARS

- Goals of treatment
  (a) Decrease time of recovery
  (b) Prevent chronic disease
  (c) Decrease exacerbations of asthma or other secondary diseases
- Objectives
  (a) Reestablish patency of ostiomeatal complex
  (b) Reduce inflammation and restore drainage of infected sinuses
  (c) Eradicate bacterial infection and minimize risk of complications or sequelae
- Medical treatment of ARS
  (a) Initial management should be symptomatic
  (b) Analgesics, decongestants, and mucolytics (saline irrigation) are recommended
  (c) Antibiotics and topical corticosteroids shown to be effective
  (d) Mild disease
    ○ Deferring antibiotics for up to 5 days in patients with nonsevere illness at presentation
    ○ Mild pain and temperature less than 38°C
    ○ Follow-up needs to be ensured
    ○ Reevaluate patient if illness persists or worsens
  (e) Moderate to severe disease (symptoms persistent or worsening after 5 days, temperature >38°C)
    ○ Empiric oral antibiotic
    ○ *First line*: amoxicillin or amoxicillin/clavulanate for 7-14 days; in penicillin-allergic patients: TMP/SMX, doxycycline, and macrolide

- Switch to respiratory quinolones (levofloxacin, moxifloxacin), high-dose amoxicillin/clavulanate if no improvement in 72 hours or if recent antibiotics use
- Nasal corticosteroids shown to be effective
- Decongestants should be used for less than 5 days
- Oral antihistamines in patients with allergic rhinitis
- Surgical treatment of ARS:
  - (a) Only limited to patients with complications of sinusitis (orbital or intracranial)

Treatment of CRS

- Controversial due to the spectrum of disease and underlying etiologies
- Many adjunct therapies have limited evidence to support their use: mucolytics, antihistamines, decongestants, leukotriene modifiers
- Medical treatment of CRS without nasal polyps:
  - (a) Level 1b evidence
    - Long-term oral antibiotics (>12 weeks), usually macrolide
    - Topical nasal corticosteroids
    - Nasal saline irrigation
- Medical treatment of CRS with nasal polyps:
  - (a) Level 1b evidence:
    - Topical nasal corticosteroids (drops better than sprays)
    - Systemic corticosteroids: 1 mg/kg initial dose and taper over 10 days
    - Nasal saline irrigation
    - Long-term oral antibiotics (>12 weeks), usually macrolide
- Surgical treatment of CRS (see Chapter 26)
  - (a) Endoscopic sinus surgery is reserved for small percentage of patients with CRS who fail medical management.
  - (b) Patients with anatomical variants often benefit from surgery to correct the underlying abnormality, reestablishing sinus drainage.
  - (c) Massive polyposis rarely responds to medical treatment and surgery will relieve symptoms and establish drainage as well as allow for use of topical corticosteroids.
  - (d) Other indications for surgery include mucocele formation, and suspected fungal rhinosinusitis.
  - (e) Continued use of medical therapy post surgery is key to success and is required for all patients.

Bibliography

Brietzke SE, Shin JJ, Choi S, et al. Clinical Consensus Statement: pediatric chronic rhinosinusitis. *Otolaryngol Head Neck Surg.* 2014;151(4):542-553.

Brown K, Rodriguez K, Brown OE. Congenital malformations of the nose. In: Cummings CW, Flint PW, Harker LA, et al, eds. *Cummings Otolaryngology Head & Neck Surgery.* 4th ed. Philadelphia, PA: Elsevier Mosby; 2005.

Chakrabarti A, Denning DW, Ferguson BJ, et al. Fungal rhinosinusitis: a categorization and definitional schema addressing current controversies. *Laryngoscope.* 2009;119(9):1809-1818.

Fokkens W, Lund V, Mullol J. European position paper on rhinosinusitis and nasal polyps. *Rhinol Suppl.* 2007;(20):1-136.

Melia L, McGarry GW. Epistaxis: update on management. *Curr Opin Otolaryngol Head Neck Surg.* 2011;19(1):30-35.

Rosenfeld RM et al. Clinical practice guidelines: adult sinusitis. *Otolaryngol Head Neck Surg.* 2007;137 (3 Suppl):S1-S31.

Chandra R, Chiu A, et al. Understanding Sinonasal Disease: A primer for medical students and residents. *Am J Rhinol Allerg.* 2013:27(Suppl):S1-S62.

Walsh WD, Kern RC. Sinonasal anatomy, function, and evaluation. In: Bailey BJ, Johnson JT, Newlands SD, et al, eds. *Head & Neck Surgery—Otolaryngology.* 4th ed. Philadelphia, PA: Lippincott Williams & Wilkins; 2006.

Questions

1. Which of the following is not a diagnostic criterion for allergic fungal sinusitis according to Bent and Kuhn?
   A. Characteristic radiologic findings
   B. Nasal polyposis
   C. Invasive fungal hyphae
   D. Eosinophilic mucin
   E. Type 1 hypersensitivity

2. Which is the bacterial organism responsible for atrophic rhinitis?
   A. *K rhinoscleromatis*
   B. *R seeberi*
   C. *S aureus*
   D. *K ozaenae*

3. All are the cell types found in olfactory epithelium except which one?
   A. Sustentacular cell
   B. Bipolar receptor cell
   C. Microvillar cell
   D. Monopolar receptor cell
   E. Globose basal cell

4. Which microorganism is not commonly implicated in acute rhinosinusitis?
   A. *S pneumoniae*
   B. *P aeruginosa*
   C. *H influenzae*
   D. *M catarrhalis*

5. All are the four cardinal symptoms of chronic rhinosinusitis except for which one?
   A. Anterior nasal drainage
   B. Nasal obstruction
   C. Posterior nasal drainage
   D. Hyposmia
   E. Cough

Chapter 28
Tumors of the Paranasal Sinuses

Paranasal and Anterior Skull Base Anatomy

- The paranasal sinuses develop from mesenchymal and ectodermal tissue.
- The sinuses define the spaces for tumor development and also the boney margins are barriers for spread to adjacent organs.
- The ventral skull base is often a direct route of spread for tumor invasion and this is what makes surgical treatment complex.

Margins for Tumor Spread	Anatomic Route
Anterior	Frontal sinus and septum
Superior lateral	Orbits and supraorbital dura
Inferior lateral	Pterygopalatine fossa
Posterior lateral	Fossa of rosenmuller
Inferior posterior midline	Clivus and arch of C1
Superior posterior midline	Sella
Superior	Cribriform plate

Paranasal Sinus Tumor Epidemiology

These tumors are a heterogeneous group of uncommon histopathologies. They vary from congenital malformations to benign tumors to high-grade cancers. The most common malignancy is squamous cell cancer (SCC), which occurs with frequency of <1:200,000 per year in the United States. Malignant tumors of the sinonasal tract comprise less than 1% of all cancers and 3% of cancers involving with upper aerodigestive tract. About 55% of cancers in the paranasal sinuses originate in the maxillary sinus, 35% in the nasal passage, 10% in the ethmoids, and rare tumors (<1%) in the frontal and sphenoid sinuses.

These tumors are a diagnostic and therapeutic challenge because they often present with symptoms that mimic common inflammatory sinonasal diseases. This often leads to a delayed diagnosis and higher stages at presentation. This combined with the sensitive surrounding structures (eyes, brain, cranial nerves, carotid artery, etc) makes surgery and comprehensive treatment complex with high risks.

History and Presentation

- **Most common** symptom: nasal obstruction
- Second **most common** symptom: neck lymphadenopathy
- Nasal: discharge, congestion, epistaxis, disturbance of smell
- Facial: infraorbital nerve hypoesthesia, pain
- Ocular: unilateral epiphoria, diplopia, fullness of lids, pain, vision loss
- Auditory: aural fullness, otalgia, hearing loss
- Oral: pain involving the maxillary dentition
- Constitutional symptoms: fever, malaise/fatigue, weight loss

Associated Causative Factors

Social and work exposures

- Squamous cell carcinoma (SCC): **nickel,** aflatoxin, chromium, mustard gas, volatile hydrocarbons, and organic fibers that are found in the wood, shoe, and textile industries
- Adenocarcinoma: **wood dust, woodworking,** furniture making, leather work

Human papillomas virus (HPV) may be a cofactor in some tumors; however, this finding may be an association and not a cause and effect situation. Tumor suppressor protein inhibition by viral E6 and E7 proteins has not been well studied in paranasal sinus tumors.

Physical Examination

- Head/Face: midface/periorbital edema
- Eye: proptosis, exophthalmoses
- Ear: middle ear effusion
- Nose: nasal cavity mass
- Oral cavity: loose dentition, palatal asymmetry, trismus, malocclusion, direct erosion into oral cavity
- Neurologic: cranial nerve deficits—commonly CN I, II, III, IV, V1, V2, VI

Diagnostic Nasal Endoscopy

- Evaluate extent of tumor and attempt to determine the origin or base
- Evaluate the potential vascular nature of the tumor
- Perform Valsalva maneuver under direct visualization —expansion implies intracranial or major venous extension
- Evaluate for ease and safety of biopsy

Diagnostic Biopsy

- Suspicious lesions can be biopsied during the endoscopic examination unless concern exists the mass is very vascular or there is concern for an encephalocele.
- Consider obtaining diagnostic imaging (CT and/or MRI) prior to biopsy since this will rule out brain pathologies and at times biopsy may confound the findings of the scans if bleeding or inflammation occurs.
- The safest method is a biopsy in the OR with the patient asleep. This allows for frozen section confirmation of neoplastic tissue and allows the surgeon to control bleeding. The down side is time and anesthesia risks.
- With experience most sinonasal tumors can be safely biopsied during sinonasal endoscopy in clinic.
- If nodal disease is noted, fine needle aspiration (FNA) is recommended.

- If distant metastatic disease is noted, at times CT or open biopsy is warranted to histologically confirm the presence of metastatic disease.

Imaging

Computed tomography (CT)

Advantages: Evaluating tumor involvement of the paranasal sinuses, the boney skull base and the retro-orbital and orbital apex region. The primary benefit is defining bone invasion and the initial anatomy of the tumor. CT Angiography can be of benefit if the tumor extents into the infratemporal fossa or near the carotid arteries in the ventral skull base.

Limitations: Defining soft tissue disease in areas of high contrast in tissue density (ie, dental fillings); evaluating orbital floor because of "partial volume averaging" of thin bone, demonstrating intracranial tumor extension; determining invasion of periorbita; and separating tumor from post obstructive sinus disease.

On CT most malignant lesions cause bony destruction; however, benign tumors, minor salivary gland carcinomas, extramedullary plasmacytomas, large cell lymphomas, hemangiopericytomas, and low-grade sinonasal sarcomas cause tissue remodeling. Some benign lesions (eg, JNAs, encephaloceles, fibrous dysplasia or osteomas) can be diagnostic on imaging; however, most tumors require tissue sampling for diagnosis. Often on CT imaging of inverted papillomas, hyperostotic bone can be found at the site of origin.

CT scanning with contrast of the neck and chest can be utilized instead of PET for staging of paranasal sinus cancers.

Magnetic resonance imaging (MRI)

Advantages: Delineating tumor from inflammatory mucosa/secretions (tumor is usually bright on T1 and will enhance with contrast whereas secretions are bright on T2), identifying perineural spread, and defining vascular anatomy. MRI is especially useful for evaluating intracranial tumor, dural invasion, nasopharyngeal invasion and infratemporal fossa extension. The primary limitation is anatomic resolution of bone.

Positron emission tomography (PET)

Due to low anatomic resolution and close proximity of sinus cancers to the high metabolic area of the brain, PET is not very useful for primary site disease evaluation. PET may be useful in assessing regional, retropharyngeal and distant metastatic disease.

Histopathologic Markers on Biopsy for Olfactory Groove Cancers

Pathologic sub categorization for skull base malignancies is imperative for management and prognostication of these aggressive tumors. The spectrum of tumors from esthesioneuroblastoma (ENB) to sinonasal neuroendocrine carcinoma (SNEC) to sinonasal undifferentiated carcinoma (SNUC) is important to understand. The immunohistochemical markers are listed below. The basics are: ENB is not a carcinoma (CK negative) and has significantly positive neuronal differentiation; SNEC maintains the neuronal differentiation; however, it is a carcinoma with CK positivity, and SNUC is a undifferentiated carcinoma made of small round blue cells without neural differentiation.

- SNUC: cytokeratin (CK), epithelial membrane antigen (EMA), weak neuron specific enolase (NSE)
- SNEC: express one or more of the neuroendocrine markers diffusely—chromogranin (CHR), NSE, synaptophysin (SYN) in additional to the epithelial markers (CK)
- ENB: CHR, SYN, absent CK and EMA

Differential Diagnoses of Paranasal Sinus Tumors

Anatomic/Structural

- Nasal/Sinus foreign body
- Mucocele
- Rhinolith: calcareous concretions around intranasal foreign bodies within the nasal cavity; usually in anterior nasal cavity
- Encephalocele

Infectious/Inflammatory Disorders

- Acute/chronic rhinosinusitis
- Invasive fungal sinusitis
- Allergic fungal sinusitis
- Fungal ball
- Nasal/sinus polyps

Granulomatous Disorders

- Wegener granulomatosis
- Sarcoid
- Midline lethal granuloma
- Syphilis
- Tuberculosis

Benign Neoplasms That Usually Are *Not* Destructive (Can Be Expansive)

- Osteoma
  - (a) Location: most commonly frontal sinus, then ethmoid and maxillary sinus
  - (b) Management: observation, unless obstructing sinus outflow tract or impinging on dura or rapidly growing
- Chondroma
- Schwannoma
- Neuromafibroma
- Fibroma
- Odontogenic tumors
- Fibrous dysplasia
- Sinonasal papillomas
  - (a) Septal papilloma (50%)
  - (b) Inverted papilloma (see below) (47%) from lateral nasal wall
  - (c) Cylindrical papilloma (3%) from lateral nasal wall

Intermediate Neoplasms That Can Be Destructive

- Inverting papillomas
  - (a) 5% to 9% chance of transformation to SCC
- Meningioma
- Pituitary tumors
- Hemangioma
- Angiofibroma (JNA)
  - (a) Presentation is usually unilateral bleeding in a teenage boy.
  - (b) Endoscopy shows a clear vascular lesion originating from the sphenopalatine area (do not biopsy in clinic).

(c) CT/MRI shows expansion of pterygopalatine fossa.
(d) Primary blood supply is the internal maxillary artery from the external carotid artery; however, the tumor can get blood supply from the internal carotid, ethmoid arteries, or the opposite side of the nose.
(e) Treatment is surgical resection after embolization. Endoscopic, midfacial degloving and transfacial (from least invasive to most) approaches can be performed.

- Hemangiopericytomas
    (a) Classified as a low-grade cancer with low metastatic potential.
    (b) Local recurrence rates can approach 30%.
    (c) Primary treatment is complete surgical resection with negative margins.
    (d) These tumors are vascular in nature and bleeding should be expected during surgery.

Malignant Neoplasms

- Squamous cell carcinoma (70%-80% of all paranasal sinus cancers)
- Adenocarcinoma
- Olfactory groove cancers: (from least aggressive to most)
    (a) ENB, SNEC, SNUC, SCC of the skull base
- Malignant salivary gland tumors
- Adenoid cystic carcinoma
    (a) Significant propensity to invade along nerve sheathes
    (b) Distant metastases are common; however, long-term survival (alive with disease) can be sustained.
- Sarcoma
- Sinonasal fibrosarcoma
- Septal desmoid tumor
- Osteosarcoma
- Chondrosarcoma
- Lymphoma
- Malignant mucosal melanoma
    (a) Surgery and radiation are mainstays of treatment.
    (b) 2-year survival is less than 25%.
    (c) Distant metastases are common.
    (d) Some tumors have c-kit over expression and can respond to Gleavec chemotherapy.
- Clival chordoma
    (a) Physaliferous cells with soap bubble appearance on pathology
- Primary nasopharyngeal cancer

Pediatric Paranasal Sinus Lesions

- Nasal glioma
- JNA
- Encephalocele
- Embryonal rhabdomyosarcoma (most common pediatric sinus cancer)

Staging

Staging is variable depending on site of origin and often individual histopathologies (see ENB below) can have their own prognostic and local staging systems.

Esthesioneuroblastoma (ENB) staging (reviewed in)

Kadish System

> A: tumors of the nasal fossa
> B: extension to paranasal sinuses
> C: extension beyond the paranasal sinuses
> D: extension into or beyond the dura

TNM ENB Staging System

> T1: tumor involving the nasal cavity and/or paranasal sinuses (excluding sphenoid), sparing the most superior ethmoid cells
> T2: tumor involving the nasal cavity and/or paranasal sinuses (including sphenoid) with extension to or erosion of the cribriform plate
> T3: tumor extending into the orbit or protruding into the anterior cranial fossa, without dural invasion
> T4: tumor involving the dura or brain
> N0: no cervical lymph node involvement
> N1: any cervical lymph node involvement
> M0: no metastases
> M1: distant metastases

ENB Hyams Histopathological Grading

- Grades 1-4
- Higher grades (3 and 4) associated with significant lower disease free survival
- Grading is based upon mitosis, necrosis, pleomorphism, and type of tissue architecture (Homor Wright pseudorosettes with grades 1 and 2; Flexner-Wintersteiner rosettes with grades 3 and 4)

American Joint Committee on Cancer (AJCC) Paranasal Sinus Cancer Staging (7th ed, 2010)

Primary Tumor Staging (T)

> Tx: cannot be accessed
> T0: no evidence of primary tumor
> Tcis: carcinoma in situ

Maxillary Sinus T Staging

> T1: Tumor limited to maxillary sinus mucosa without bone involvement.
> T2: Tumor causing erosion of bone including erosion of hard palate and extension of tumor into middle meatus. Posterior wall bone invasion including pterygopalatine fossa (PPF) is excluded.
> T3: Tumor invades any of the following: posterior wall of maxillary sinus, orbital floor, subcutaneous tissues, PPF or ethmoid sinuses.
> T4a: Moderately advanced local disease: tumor invades orbit, skin of face, pterygoid plates, IT Fossa, cribriform plate, sphenoid or frontal sinuses.
> T4b: Very advanced local disease: tumor invades orbital apex, dura, brain, nasopharynx, clivus, or any cranial nerves other than V2.

Nasal Cavity and Ethmoid Sinus T Staging

> T1: Tumor restricted to one subsite with or without boney invasion.
> T2: Tumor invading two adjacent subsites or extending to nasoethmoid complex.
> T3: Tumor invades orbital floor/medial wall, maxillary sinus, palate or cribriform plate.
> T4a: Moderately advanced local disease: tumor invades orbit, skin of face, pterygoid plates, IT Fossa, cribriform plate, sphenoid or frontal sinuses.
> T4b: Very advanced local disease: tumor invades orbital apex, dura, brain, nasopharynx, clivus, or any cranial nerves other than V2.

Nodal (N) and distant (M) staging *are the same as routine head and neck SCC.*

Factors Associated With Predicting Survival for Paranasal Sinus Cancer

   A. Histological findings of primary tumor:
      i. Worst: mucosal melanoma
      ii. Best: minor salivary gland tumors, low-grade sarcomas
   B. T stage
   C. Presence and extent of intracranial involvement
   D. Resection margins
   E. Previous radiation
   F. Previous incomplete resection (initial misdiagnosis)
   G. Nodal disease
   H. Distant metastasis

Treatment

Treatment of benign tumors ranges from observation, to partial resection for obstructive sino-nasal disease, to complete resection with margins (inverted papillomas). Radiation is reserved for symptomatic tumors in nonsurgical candidates or for radiation sensitive tumors such as plasmacytomas. Surgery for benign tumors must be match with the biology of the tumor and the specific patient. Clearly the acceptable risks with a JNA resection in a child are different that an osteoma in an elderly patient.

For sinonasal cancers, the acceptable risks of surgery are significant often putting the eyes and brain at risk. This is balanced with the issue of local tumor resection and the need to obtain nega-tive margins. However, the oncologic outcomes and treatment morbidity of patients with sinona-sal cancer has been improving over the last several decades. This is likely attributable to improved diagnostic imaging, more effective surgical treatment, the use of vascularized flaps for reconstruc-tion, and more effective adjuvant therapy. Obtaining local control is the most direct factor that impacts survival. For high-grade cancers, often tri-modality therapy provides the best cancer outcomes. While surgery is the mainstay of treatment, the need for excellent radiation treatment with IMRT advanced planning and concurrent chemotherapy cannot be understated. The same surgical risks to the vision, cranial nerves and the brain/brainstem are also risks with radiation therapy. Proton radiation therapy has the theoretical advantage of being more conformable with less dosage to nontumor involved sites such as the eye and brain. The limitation of proton radiation is its relative unavailability across the country, limited outcomes studies and overall higher cost.

Surgical Treatment of Maxillary Sinus Cancer

Determining surgical prognosis

   • Ohngren line (Anterior/inferior tumors have better outcomes)
   • Nodal disease should be managed with neck dissections and retropharyngeal dissections if possible.
   • Cranial base involvement should be managed by a skull base team to resect and recon-struct the cranial and dural defect.

Planning principles

   A. Assess bony and soft tissue extent of tumor/appropriately stage.
   B. Approach must allow adequate exposure while preserving functional tissue and cosmetic results, if possible.
   C. Repair should use prosthetics or vascularized reconstructions
      i. Prosthetics has the advantage of allowing for cavity visualization.
      ii. Vascular reconstructions heal well and do well in face of radiotherapy.
   D. Preoperative consultation with neurosurgery, maxillofacial prosthodontist (if obdurator required), plastic and reconstructive surgery and radiation oncology if needed.

Extirpative options

Maxillectomies should be individualized to the anatomy of the tumor and the need to obtain negative margins.

- From least to most extensive surgical options for maxillectomy
- Endoscopic medial maxillectomy
- Transfacial medial maxillectomy
- Inferior structure maxillectomy via midfacial degloving or transfacial approach
- Suprastructure maxillectomy without orbital exenteration
- Radical maxillectomy with infratemporal fossa resection
- Radical maxillectomy with orbital exenteration
- Radical maxillectomy with craniofacial resection

Paranasal sinus cancers other than low stage maxillary sinus tumors, such as those in the ethmoids, frontal and olfactory groove areas, usually need a resection of the involved sinuses as well as the surrounding cranial base and at times surrounding dura. Skull base tumor surgery, especially of the anterior cranial fossa, began with a combination of approaches via facial incisions and frontal craniotomies. These two approaches then collided with the standard anterior craniofacial resection, which provides excellent access to the entire anterior cranial fossa, orbits and sinonasal cavities. The craniofacial resection is the gold standard for this approach with the sinonasal portion of the tumor dissected via a transfacial approach and the dural/skull base portion of the tumor dissected via a frontal craniotomy, allowing for en-bloc removal of the skull base/sinuses and dura. The craniofacial resection also allows for direct access for reconstruction of the skull base and dural defect with a pericranial flap. Several modifications of the open anterior craniofacial approach have been modified to reduce brain retraction, facial scarring and minimize (but not eliminate) this morbidity. These include trans-brow approaches and sub-frontal approaches.

Over the last decade, there have been significant advances in the area of endoscopic cranial base surgery. These include an improved understanding of endoscopic anatomy, the development of new instrumentation, and the description of new endonasal surgical approaches and surgical techniques. Endoscopic approaches offer potential advantages such as no facial incisions, no need for craniotomy, no brain retraction, and excellent visualization and magnification using the endoscope. However, even through endoscopic skull base surgery does not have disfiguring incisions the risks of traditional skull base surgery and neurological complications are still very applicable. Also all patients undergoing endoscopic transcribriform craniofacial resections should have been counseled and informed consent obtained to convert to a standard open approach if needed to clear margins.

Open craniofacial resection (CFR)

- Mortality 4.7% (increased risk associated with presence of medical co-morbidities).
- Morbidity 33% to 36%, wound 20%, systemic 5%, orbital 1.5% (increased risk associated with presence of medical comorbidity, prior radiation therapy, dural and brain invasion).
- For all patients undergoing craniofacial resection for sinonasal cancer, the overall 5-year survival is approximately 50%.

Endoscopic transnasal transcribriform craniofacial resection

Indications: Initially thought to be only for those patients with low stage disease with no intracranial involvement; however, recent results with endoscopic dural and intradural resections have shown promise for highly experienced skull base surgery programs.

- Overall mortality 0.9%.
- Infectious complications/meningitis 2%.

- Kassam et al reported that transient neurological deficits occurred in 20/800 (all expanded endonasal endoscopic skull base cases, not just transcribriform) patients (2.5%) and permanent neurologic deficits in 14 patients (1.8%). Seven out of 800 patients died (0.9%); six died of systemic complications (eg, pulmonary embolism) and one of meningitis. Therefore, the overall permanent morbidity (14 patients) and mortality (7 patients) was 2.6% in that series.
- CSF leak rates have fallen to between 4% and 6% with the use of endoscopic vascularized reconstructions.
- 2-surgeon, 4-handed team surgery is required for optimal technical results.

Skull Base Reconstructive Goals and Options

The reconstructive goal (for open and endoscopic skull base surgery) is to completely separate the cranial cavity from the sinonasal tract, eliminate dead space, and preserve neurovascular and ocular function. The underlying principle of multilayered reconstruction to reestablish natural tissue barriers should be preserved. The use of vascularized reconstruction optimizes healing and minimizes postoperative complications (especially in the setting of radiotherapy).

Nonvascularized grafts

- Autologous nonvascularized tissue
  - (a) Tensor fascia lata
  - (b) Fat
  - (c) Temporalis fascia
- Nonvascularized bone grafts
- Cadaveric or Bovine allografts
- Titanium mesh (not routinely used or recommended for skull base repair other than for frontal cranioplasty/plating)

Vascular flaps for open craniofacial resection (Table 28-1)

- Pericranial flap (PCF)
  - (a) Supraorbital and supratrochlear arteries
  - (b) Primary option
  - (c) Ease of harvest and presence in surgical field
- Temporoparietal fascia flap (TPFF)
  - (a) Superficial temporal artery
- Temporalis muscle flap
  - (a) Deep temporal artery
- Free flap options
  - (a) Radial forearm free flap
  - (b) Anterior lateral thigh free flap

Paranasal Sinus Tumor Treatment Complications

Intraoperative complications	Most common site
Venous bleeding	Cavernous sinus or pterygoid plexus
Arterial bleeding	Ethmoid or internal maxillary arteries
Intradural nerve injury	CN II
Extradural nerve injury	CN I
Positive margins	Lateral supraorbital dura

Table 28-1 **Vascular Flaps Available for Anterior Skull Base Reconstruction**

Location	Vascular Tissue Flap	Pedicle	Comments/ Limitations
Intranasal vascular tissue flap	NSF	Sphenopalatine artery	• Ideal for all skull base reconstructions • Primary option if available • Must be free of cancer involvement for use during cancer surgery
	ITF	Inferior turbinate artery	• Good for small clival defects • Cannot reach ACF or sella
	MTF	Middle turbinate artery	• Good for small ACF or transphenoidal defects • Small in size • Thin mucosa • Difficult to elevate
Regional vascular tissue flap	PCF	Supraorbital and supratrochlear artery	• Hearty flap with versatile dimensions • Extends from ACF to sella, but not to posterior skull base • Ideal secondary option for transcribriform reconstruction when a NSF is not available
	TPFF	Superficial temporal artery	• Good for clival or parasellar defects • 90-degree pedicle rotation limits reconstruction of ACF

ACF: anterior cranial fossa; ITF: Inferior turbinate flap; MTF: Middle turbinate flap; NSF: Nasoseptal flap; PCF: Pericranial flap; TPFF: Temporoparietal fascia flap

Perioperative complications
- Wound: infection, dehiscence, flap necrosis
- Orbital: vision loss, diplopia, cellulitis/abscess, epiphoria/dry eye, retrobulbar hematoma, opthalmoplegia, nasolacrimal duct obstruction
- Intracranial: CVA, meningitis, CSF leak, pneumocephalus
- Neurologic: paresthesias/anesthesia, seizure, anosmia
- Vascular: life-threatening hemorrhage, cavernous sinus thrombosis
- Systemic: myocardial infarction, urinary tract infection, pulmonary emboli

Late complications
- Sinonasal mucocele
- Chronic rhinitis
- Skull base osteoradionecrosis

Bibliography

Fried DV, Zanation AM, Huang B, et al. Patterns of local failure for sinonasal malignancies. *Pract Radiat Oncol.* 2013;3(3):e113-120.

Ganly I, Patel SG, Singh B, et al. Craniofacial resection for malignant paranasal sinus tumors: report of an international collaborative study. *Head Neck.* 2005; 27(7):575-584.

Kassam AB, Prevedello DM, Carrau RL, et al. Endoscopic endonasal skullbase surgery: analysis of complications in the authors' initial 800 patients. *J Neurosurg.* 2011;114(6):1544-68.

Snyderman CH, Carrau RL, Kassam AB, et al. Endoscopic skull base surgery: principles of endonasal oncological surgery. *J Surg Oncol.* 2008;97(8):658-664.

Su SY, Kupferman ME, DeMonte F, Levine NB, Raza SM, Hanna EY. Endoscopic resection of sinonasal cancers. *Curr Oncol Rep.* 2014;16(2):369.

Questions

1. What is the nonepithelial cancer pathology of the paranasal sinuses?
   A. Squamous cell cancer
   B. Adenocarcinoma
   C. SNUC
   D. Esthesioneuroblastoma
   E. Sarcoma

2. What site of involvement within the paranasal sinuses pretends the worst prognosis?
   A. Ethmoids
   B. Sphenoid
   C. Frontal Sinus
   D. Cribriform plate
   E. Maxillary sinus

3. What would be an absolute contraindication for a solely endoscopic approach for sinonasal cancer resection?
   A. Dural invasion
   B. Nasopharyngeal involvement
   C. Posterior septal invasion
   D. Orbital muscle invasion
   E. Cribiform plate erosion

4. Which small round blue cell tumor is most correlated with the immunohistochemical staining pattern of cytokeratin positive, neuron specific immunomarker negative?
   A. Esthesioneuroblastoma
   B. Sinonasal neuroendocrine carcinoma
   C. SNUC
   D. SCC
   E. Adenocarcinoma

5. What is the stage of a maxillary sinus cancer whose tumor involves the pterygopalatine fossa and middle cranial fossa bone with two ipsilateral 2-cm level-2 nodes?
   A. T1 N1
   B. T4a N2b
   C. T3 N2b
   D. T3 N1
   E. T4b N2b

Chapter 29
Endoscopic Skull Base Surgery

Anatomy

Endoscopic Skull Base Surgery

- With the advent of the endoscopes in sinus surgery, the safety and number of endoscopic sinus surgeries has increased exponentially in the last two decades. This increase has led to an interest in surgical resection of tumors through an endonasal approach. Advantages such as improved surgical exposure, decreased duration of hospitalization, elimination of external incisions, and decreased overall morbidity have led to the insertion of endoscopic skull base surgery into mainstream practice.

Sellar Region

Boundaries

- Anterior: anterior wall of the sphenoid sinus
- Posterior: pituitary gland
- Superior: planum sphenoidale
- Inferior: clivus
- Lateral: optic nerve, cavernous sinus, parasellar carotid, and lateral optico-carotid recess
- Figure 29-1
  - (a) The sphenoid sinus has three types of pneumatization including sellar (80%), presellar (17%), and concha (3%).
  - (b) The sellar type has extensive anterior and inferior pneumatization, which makes dissection easier.
  - (c) The presellar type has decreased anterior pneumatization, which makes identification of landmarks more challenging during dissection.
  - (d) The concha type is minimally pnematized, which is typically seen in patients younger than 12.
  - (e) The sphenoid rostrum is formed by the nasal septum, anterior wall of the sphenoid sinus and the maxillary crest.
  - (f) The roof the sphenoid sinus is referred to as the planum sphenoidale. It articulates with the roof the ethmoid sinus anteriorly and the sella posteriorly.
  - (g) The area between the planum sphenoidale and the top of the sella is the tuberculum sellae. The optic chiasm is located just behind this section of bone.

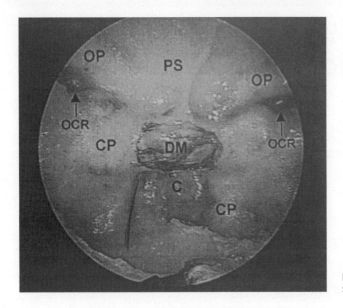

Figure 29-1 OCR: opticocarotid recess; CP: carotid protuberance; DM: duramater; C: clivus; PS: planum sphenoidale; OP: optic protuberance.

(h) Tuberculum recess is the junction between the planum sphenoidale and the anterior superior edge of the sella.

(i) Immediately lateral to the sella, the optic nerve, cavernous sinus, parasellar carotid artery, and lateral optico-carotid recess (OCR) can be found.

(j) The lateral OCR is located between the optic nerve superiorly and internal carotid artery (ICA) inferomedially.

(k) The lateral OCR corresponds to the anterior clinoid process. The oculomotor nerve can be found inferolateral to the OCR at the upper portion of the superior orbital fissure.

(l) The optic nerve, ICA, and the lateral OCR also help to identify the medial OCR which is the lateral extent of bone that can safely be removed above the sella. It coincides with the lateral portion of the tuberculum recess.

(m) The medial OCR is considered one of the most important landmarks in endoscopic resection of tuberculum sellae meningiomas.

(n) Figure 29-2.

(o) An onodi cell is a posterior ethmoid cell with superolateral pneumatization into the sphenoid sinus, creating a horizontal septation.

(p) Identification of an onodi cell is important in skull base surgery as this may be disorienting to the normal anatomy of the sphenoid sinus.

(q) Onodi cells are found in 7% to 25% of patients, and can be unilateral or bilateral.

(r) 25% of patients with onodi cells will have the optic nerve travel in the lateral superior part of the cell, increasing the risk of injury to the nerve.

Technique

(a) To access the sella the inferior, middle, and superior turbinates must be lateralized.

(b) The sphenoid ostium is identified just lateral and superior to the superior turbinate or 1.5 cm above the roof of the posterior choana.

(c) The sphenoid ostium is widened to allow easy identification with an endoscope.

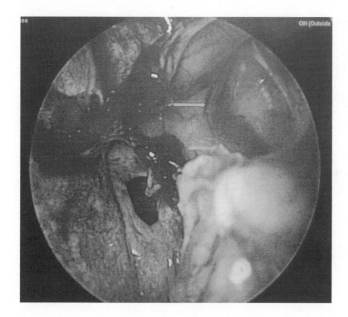

Figure 29-2 Arrow points toward onodi cell.

(d) The posterior septum is removed from the sphenoid rostrum to assist in two-nostril, four-handed surgery.

(e) The anterior wall of the sphenoid sinus is widely opened to provide adequate exposure of the sella, planum, floor of the sphenoid, paraclival carotid protuberance, optic nerve protuberance, lateral optico-carotid recess, and clivus.

(f) The keel which represents the fusion of the floor of the sphenoid and the rostrum is removed.

(g) During the exposure of the sella, the intersinus septum(s) is frequently encountered. This septum must be drilled prior to sellar dissection.

(h) Standard sellar exposure for endoscopic skull base surgery requires exposure to the lateral OCR bilaterally.

Anterior Cranial Fossa/Cribriform Plate

- Represents the roof of the nasal cavity

Boundaries

- Anterior: frontal sinus recess
- Posterior: planum sphenoidale
- Medial: perpendicular plate of the ethmoid in unilateral disease
- Lateral: lamina papyracea
  (a) The cribriform plate transmits olfactory fibers from the superior turbinate, the upper portion of the middle turbinate and nasal septum. This is done through approximately 40 foramina within the cribriform plate.
  (b) Lateral to the middle turbinate the ethmoid roof is referred to as the fovea ethmoidalis.
  (c) The fovea ethmoidalis attaches to the lamina papyracea laterally and lateral lamella medially.

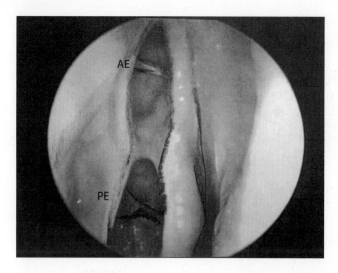

Figure 29-3 AE: anterior ethmoid artery; PE: posterior ethmoid artery.

(d) The vertical portion of the middle turbinate attaches to the skull base at the junction of the cribriform plate and fovea ethmoidalis. This junction is frequently the location of cerebrospinal fluid leaks.

(e) The anterior ethmoid artery (AEA) passes through the lamina papyracea before making an immediate turn posteriorly then anteriorly travelling in an anteromedial direction at a 45-degree angle.

(f) Figure 29-3.

(g) If the ethmoid bulla forms the posterior aspect of the frontal recess, the AEA typically sits directly behind this segment of the ethmoid.

(h) When a suprabullar recess is present, the AEA can be found in the frontal recess.

(i) The anterior ethmoid artery can be found within the bony canal or just inferior to it within the mesentery. The incidence of AEA in the mesentery is 14% to 43%.

(j) There is a pinching appearance of the lamina papyracea on coronal CT when the anterior ethmoid artery is within the mesentery.

(k) The posterior ethmoid artery (PEA) is located within a bony canal just anterior to the sphenoid roof.

Technique

(a) Begin with an anterior and posterior ethmoidectomy creating complete exposure of the skull base. This dissection should include the ethmoid bulla, suprabullar cells, and posterior ethmoid cells posterior to the basal lamella.

(b) The anterior and posterior ethmoid arteries are located, cauterized and divided.

(c) If the ethmoid arteries are covered by a bony canal, a diamond drill can be used to uncover the artery in the lateral aspect of the fovea ethmoidalis, after which cautery and division can commence.

(d) The frontal recess is identified and the upper portion of the nasal septum is removed to create a single cavity to facilitate bi-nostril surgery. A modified Lothrop procedure may be required if the lesion extends into the frontoethmoid region or an obstructing mucocele has formed. During this procedure the nasofrontal beak is drilled out and the intersinus septum is removed.

(e) Unilateral or bilateral middle turbinates are resected and the stump is cauterized with a suction bovie.

(f) Osteotomies are then performed with a diamond burr and Kerrison rongeur ensuring an appropriate margin around the tumor.

(g) The remaining attachment to the skull base will be the falx cerebri to the crista galli, which is transected with microscissors.

Suprasellar Region

Boundaries

- Anterior: ethmoid roof
- Posterior: third ventricle, basilar tip, mammary body
- Superior: frontal lobe gyri
- Inferior: sella
- Lateral: optic nerve

(a) The parameters for dissection in the suprasellar region are the optic nerves laterally and 1.5 to 2.0 cm anteriorly onto the planum sphenoidale.

(b) The suprasellar structures can be divided into suprachiasmal and subchiasmal.

(c) The suprachiasmal region includes the chiasmatic and lamina terminalis cisterns.

(d) The chiasmatic cistern contains the medial portions of the optic nerves and the anterior optic chiasm.

(e) The lamina terminalis contains the entire spectrum of anterior cerebral arteries and the gyri recti of the frontal lobes.

(f) The subchiasmal region contains the pituitary stalk just below the chiasm and the inferior and superior hypophyseal arteries.

(g) The floor of the third ventricle can be accessed by driving the scope between the pituitary stalk and the ICA and above the dorsum sellae.

Technique

(a) The sphenoid is opened in the same manner as the sellar technique.

(b) A portion of the posterior ethmoid may need to be removed to provide space for the endoscope during dissection of the suprasella.

(c) Exposure to the suprasella can be accomplished through removal of the superior half of the sellar bone, tuberculum sella, and the posterior portion of the planum sphenoidale.

(d) The dura is incised and the main neurovascular structures of the suprasellar area can be visualized.

(e) Neurosurgical dissection of the tumor may then commence.

Cavernous Sinus Region

- Lateral to the sella are multiple bony protuberances, which represent important anatomic structures.

Boundaries

- Superior: optic nerve
- Inferior: vidian nerve
- Medial: sella, clivus
- Lateral: CN III, IV, V2, V3, and VI
- Posterior: dorsum sellae

(a) The bony proturberance covering the carotid can be described as the parasellar and paraclival carotid.

(b) After removing the bony covering over the intracavernous carotid, its C-shaped structure can clearly be seen.

(c) The intercavernous carotid artery can be divided in multiple segments.

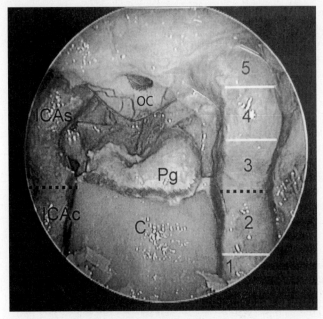

Figure 29-4 Course of the carotid artery. Segments 1 and 2 paraclival. Segments 3 and 4 parasellar, segment 5 cavernous sinus. Pg: pituitary gland; C: clivus; ICAc: Internal carotid artery—clival segment; ICAs: Internal carotid artery—sellar segment; OC: optic chiasm suprasellar segment of the pituitary gland.

(d) As described by Inoue et al, the intracavernous ICA was divided into five segments based on morphological features: (1) posterior vertical segment, (2) posterior bend, (3) horizontal segment, (4) anterior bend, and (5) anterior vertical segment.

(e) Figure 29-4.

(f) Laterally along the sphenoid wall, from superior to inferior, the cavernous sinus apex, trigeminal maxillary nerve, and trigeminal mandibular nerve can be found.

(g) The cavernous sinus apex is the cone shape swelling that sits at the inferior aspect of the lateral OCR.

(h) The depression between the second and third division of the trigeminal nerve is of importance because a congenital dehiscence or trauma in this area can lead to encephalocele formation from the middle cranial fossa or a cerebrospinal fluid leak.

(i) The oculomotor and trochlear nerves are seen coming from the C-shaped carotid superiorly toward the superior orbital fissure.

(j) Endoscopically, the oculomotor nerve appears to partially cover the trochlear nerve.

(k) Endoscopically, the abducen nerve partially covered the maxillary division of the trigeminal nerve.

Technique

(a) For lesions limited to the medial cavernous sinus, a sellar approach performed as previously described. If a supreme turbinate is present it should be removed and a posterior ethmoidectomy performed.

(b) If the tumor extends to the lateral cavernous sinus or lateral wall of the sphenoid sinus, an uncinectomy, total ethmoidectomy, as well as, a sphenoidotomy is performed. To access the lateral recess of the sphenoid, a portion of the posterior wall of the maxillary sinus and medial pterygoid plate is also removed. The bony covering over the carotid protuberance and lateral nasal wall are then removed using a diamond drill.

Clival Region

(a) The posterior cranial fossa from an endoscopic skull base prospective extends from the dorsum sellae to the craniovertebral junction.
(b) The clivus is composed of the basisphenoid (posterior portion of the sphenoid sinus) and basiocciptal (basilar part of the occipital bone).
(c) The clivus is divided into three levels: upper, middle, and lower clivus.
(d) The upper clivus is formed by the basisphenoid.
(e) The middle clivus represents the rostral part of the basisphenoid and is located superior to the line connecting caudal ends of the petroclival fissure.
(f) The lower clivus corresponds to the caudal basiocciput.

Boundaries

- Anterior: anterior wall of the sphenoid sinus, nasopharynx, and oropharynx
- Posterior: pons, basilar artery
- Lateral: vidian nerve, eustachian tube
- Superior: sellar floor
- Inferior: foramen magnum

(a) The upper two-thirds of the clivus is located anterior to the pons.
(b) The vidian nerve comes from the greater superior petrosal nerve and the deep petrosal nerve.
(c) Vidian nerve is the lateral extent of dissection of posterior skull base lesions, as it lies just medial to the intrapetrous carotid. When entering the pterygopalatine fossa this nerve is located inferior to the intrapetrous carotid artery.
(d) The lower clivus extends to the occipital condyles where the foramina lacerum lies.
(e) The abducens nerves can be visualized coming off the pontomedullary junction and extends through the basilar sinus in a superolaterally trajectory. The nerve enters Dorello canal medial to the paraclival carotid.

Technique

(a) The anterior wall of the sphenoid sinus is opened and a posterior septectomy is performed using the technique described above.
(b) Once this is completed the floor of the sella, carotid protuberance, and the upper clivus can be visualized.
(c) The sphenoid mucosa and vomer are removed and floor of the sphenoid is drilled away.
(d) This exposes the clivus from the pituitary gland to the Eustachian tubes.
(e) The clival bone is removed as superiorly as the sellar floor and inferiorly as the foramen magnum.
(f) At the level of the occipital condyles, the anterior third of the condyle can be removed. Beyond the anterior one-third of the condyles the hypoglossal canal is found.
(g) Mucosa of the nasopharynx is reflected and the atlanto-occipital membrane, longus capitis and longus colli muscles, the atlas, and axis are visualized.
(h) For intradural lesions, the external layer of the clival dura is incised and the abducens nerve is found along with the basilar venous plexus.
(i) Significant bleeding may occur during dissection in this layer which should be controlled with packing and coagulating agents, not cautery.

(j) Beyond the internal layer of the clival dura, the basilar artery, AICA, vertebral artery, cerebral arteries, and cranial nerves III-VI can be visualized.

(k) As the dissection extends inferiorly, the craniovertebral junction is reached.

Pterygopalatine Fossa

- The pterygopalatine fossa is an inverted cone-shaped space.

Boundaries

- Superior: infraorbital fissure, foramen rotundum, maxillary nerve
- Inferior: greater palatine canal
- Medial: palatine bone, sphenopalatine artery
- Lateral: pterygomaxillary fissure

    (a) Within the pterygopalatine fossa blood vessels are encountered before neural structures.

    (b) Structures entering the posterior wall of the pterygopalatine fossa include: the foramen rotundum, vidian nerve, and palatovaginal canal.

    (c) The infraorbital fissure runs between the infratemporal fossa and the pterygopalatine fossa.

Technique

(a) Begin with nasal decongestion and xylocaine 1% with 1:100,000 epinephrine injection of the uncinate, roof of the middle turbinate, and sphenopalatine artery. An inferior turbinectomy, uncinectomy, and maxillary antrostomy are performed. This is followed by completion of a total ethmoidectomy and wide sphenoidotomies.

(b) The ipsilateral middle turbinate may be partially amputated to improve exposure.

(c) The mucoperiosteum is removed from the lateral nasal wall posterior to the maxillary antrostomy to expose the crista ethmoidalis and identify the sphenopalatine artery (SPA) foramen.

(d) The SPA is cauterized and ligated and the mucosa of the posterior wall of the maxillary sinus is removed medially to the area of the infraorbital foramen.

(e) The bone of the posteromedial part of the maxillary sinus is removed exposing the soft tissue of the pterygopalatine fossa.

(f) The soft tissue of the pterygopalatine fossa is removed or lateralized and the neurovascular structures are dissected with possible ligation, which brings the medial pterygoid plate into view.

Infratemporal Fossa

Boundaries

- Superior: greater wing of the sphenoid bone and the squamous portion of the temporal bone
- Inferior: medial pterygoid muscles attaching to the mandible
- Medial: lateral pterygoid plate, lateral portion of clivus, and lower petrous apex
- Lateral: temporalis muscle and ramus of the mandible
- Posterior: tympanic and mastoid portion of the temporal bone
- Anterior: infratemporal surface of maxillary sinus

    (a) As the posterolateral wall of the sphenoid sinus is approached, the foramen ovale can be seen going into the quadrangular space of Meckel cave.

    (b) The lateral pterygoid muscle can be seen in the infratemporal fossa just beyond the fat.

    (c) The lateral pterygoid muscles lie against the middle cranial fossa.

    (d) The medial pterygoid plate is the lateral portion of the posterior choana.

Technique

(a) The initial approach is the same as the technique for lesions of the pterygopalatine fossa. However, the posterior maxillary sinus dissection extends to the lateral wall of the maxillary sinus.

(b) The vidian nerve can be found posterior and deep to the ligated SPA.

(c) The medial pterygoid plate can be drilled posteriorly, just inferior and medial to the vidian nerve, thus preventing ICA injury.

(d) The vidian nerve is drilled circumferentially to identify the ICA. The bone over the ICA genu, horizontal portion, and paraclival carotid are then removed.

(e) V2 is followed posteriorly through the pterygoid bone and pterygopalatine fossa.

(f) Once the pterygoid bone has been removed flush with the middle cranial fossa and the foramen rotundum, the dissection can be continued laterally through the lateral pterygoid plate.

(g) This access is ideal for trigeminal schwannomas, nasopharyngeal cancers, and meningiomas.

Petrous Apex

Boundaries

- Medial: posterior border of the greater wing of sphenoid bone
- Lateral: basilar portion of occipital bone
- Superior: middle cranial fossa
- Inferior: carotid canal

Technique

(a) The initial approach is the same as the technique for lesions of the pterygopalatine fossa.

(b) The sella and clivus are well exposed. The floor of the sphenoid sinus is drill flush with the clivus. Depending on the location of the tumor, the middle clivus may need to be exposed. In order to gain exposure to this area, an inverted U-shaped incision is made in the nasopharynx between the eustachian tubes. The mucosa, muscle, and fascia are dissected off the middle clivus.

(c) The vidian nerve is drilled circumferentially to identify the ICA. The bone over the ICA genu, horizontal portion, and paraclival carotid are then removed.

(d) The medial pterygoid plate can be drilled posteriorly, just inferior and medial to the vidian nerve, thus preventing ICA injury.

(e) This access is ideal for cholesterol granulomas and cholesteatomas.

Orbital Apex

Boundaries

- Superior: lesser wing of the sphenoid bone
- Inferior: pterygopalatine fossa, optic strut
- Medial: body of sphenoid sinus
- Lateral: anterior clinoid process
- Anterior: lamina papyracea at the foramen of the PEA
  (a) The optic strut separates the optic canal from the superior orbital fissure.
  (b) The optic canal is located in the superior medial aspect of the orbital apex and contains the optic nerve and ophthalmic artery.

(c) Approaching the orbital apex and sphenoid sinus, the lamina papyracea thickens to form the medial aspect of the infraorbital fissure, while the middle cranial fossa forms the lateral wall.
(d) Directly above the foramen ovale in the lateral wall is the cavernous sinus and above the cavernous sinus is the orbital apex.

Technique

(a) Posterior septectomy, uncinectomy, and sphenoethmoidectomy are performed. The lamina papyracea should clearly be visualized at this point.
(b) The optic nerve and carotid artery are identified within the sphenoid sinus.
(c) The medial wall of the orbital apex is identified. This typically is covered by thicken bone which must be drilled down.

Radiology

(a) Magnetic resonance imaging (MRI) is the imaging modality of choice for skull base lesions.
(b) MRI helps differentiate soft tissue lesions from inflammatory changes.
(c) Computerized tomography (CT) can be used as an adjunct for evaluation of bony defects or erosion.
(d) Early stages of malignant disease are typically difficult to distinguish from inflammatory disease on CT scan, especially because most patients attribute symptoms to sinusitis.
(e) Anterior skull base lesions typically require both a CT scan and MRI of the sinuses and skull base.
(f) Two key structures that need evaluation during review of imaging are the dura and periorbita. Invasion of either of these areas warrants more extensive resection and possibly changes the prognosis.
(g) Periorbital invasion must be confirmed intraoperatively, as bony destruction of the lamina papyracea on CT is not a definitive indication of periorbital involvement.
(h) Reliable signs of periorbital involvement includes enhancement or enlargement of extraocular muscles, stranding of periorbital fat, and nodularity of plane between the orbital tissue and the mass.
(i) The overall accuracy of determining the presence or absence of periorbital invasion is around 60% to 70%.
(j) Dural invasion is likely present when nodular or smooth thickening of the dura is more than 5 mm in length.
(k) Perineural invasion is better visualized with MRI.

Endoscopic Surgical Approaches

(a) Transsphenoidal: Surgical corridor is the sphenoid sinus. The sphenoid sinus is considered the "gateway" to endoscopic skull base surgery. It also can be used in combination with other approaches to reach lateral lesions.
(b) Transplanum/Transtuberculum: Surgical corridor is the planum sphenoidale. It requires a posterior ethmoidectomy and wide sphenoidectomy. This approach

is used for suprasellar lesions such as craniopharyngiomas and pituitary macroadenomas

(c) Transethmoid: Surgical corridor between the frontal sinus and sphenoid sinus. It requires completion of an uncinectomy and total ethmoidectomy. This approach can reach tumors such an encephalocele, ethmoid osteoma, esthesioblastoma, and meningioma. It can also be used in combination with the transsphenoidal approach for lesions in the medial cavernous sinus and orbital apex.

(d) Transpterygoid: Surgical corridor through the posterior wall of the maxillary sinus and the pterygoid plate. Performing this approach requires creation of a maxillary antrostomy, total ethmoidectomy, and sphenoidectomy. This approach can reach the cavernous sinus, lateral sphenoid sinus, infratemporal fossa, pterygopalatine fossa, and the petrous apex.

Lesions of the Sella and Suprasellar

Pituitary Adenoma

Epidemiology

(a) Most common sellar tumor, accounting for 90% of tumors in this region.

(b) 10% of all neurologic tumors.

(c) Prolactinomas are the most common hormone secreting pituitary tumor accounting for 30% of all pituitary adenomas and 50% to 60% of functional adenomas.

Clinical presentation

(a) Symptoms vary depending on size and functional status of the tumor.

(b) Mass effect from the tumor may lead to headache, visual changes with decline in peripheral vision, and hypopituitarism.

(c) Functional tumors present with systemic changes due to hypersecretion of hormone.

(d) Patients should be questioned about amenorrhea, galatorrhea, impotence, arthropathy, hyperhidrosis, changes in foot and hand size, weight gain or loss, polyuria, polydipsia, hirsutism, bruising, and stretch marks.

Workup

(a) In order to determine the functionality of the tumor and assess the integrity of the hypothalamic-pituitary axis (HPA), hormone labs should be drawn.

(b) These labs include prolactin, AM cortisol, ACTH, IGF-1, GH, TSH, free T4, LH, FSH, testosterone, and serum sodium level.

(c) Peripheral vision testing should be completed.

Radiograph studies

(a) Spherical versus dumbbell shaped tumor on MRI with homogenous enhancement on T2-weighted study.

(b) May have cystic or necrotic component.

(c) Two types of adenomas: microadenoma (< 10 mm in size) and macroadenoma (> 10 mm in size).

(d) Most microadenomas are hypointense on T1-weighted MRI in comparison to the rest of the gland.

(e) T1-weighed coronal images are best suited for visualization of microadenomas.

(f) An irregularly shaped pituitary gland without signal abnormality may have a microadenoma, which is only seen on postcontrast imaging.

    (g) Most microadenomas enhance less intensely than the normal portion of the pituitary gland after gadolinium contrast.

    (h) Macroadenomas have variable signal intensity; however, on T1-weighted imaging it is typically hypointense.

    (i) Suprasellar macroadenomas often take on a dumbbell shape due to constriction by the diaphragm sellae.

    (j) If a patient presents with symptoms consistent with Cushing disease but the MRI study is unremarkable, bilateral petrosal sinus sampling maybe used to confirm diagnosis by measuring adrenocorticotropic hormone (ACTH) levels.

Prolactinoma

    (a) A prolactinoma commonly presents as a microadenoma. Symptoms include amenorrhea, galactorrhea, and loss of libido with subsequent osteoporosis and infertility. Depending on the size of the lesion, mass effect may lead to headache, visual changes, cranial neuropathies, and hypopituitarism.

    (b) 1:1 male:female incidence; however, females are four times more likely to be symptomatic.

    (c) Normal laboratory findings for prolactin levels for women and men are below 25 ng/mL and 20 ng/mL, respectively.

    (d) Abnormal prolactin levels are 100 to 250 ng/mL for microadenomas and greater than 250 ng/mL for macroadenomas.

    (e) Can be associated with multiple endocrine neoplasia I.

    (f) Prolactinomas can be treated medically with dopamine agonist such as bromocriptine and cabergoline.

    (g) Surgical indications include preventing growth, recurrence of lesion, normalizing prolactin level, and decompressing visual apparatus, cranial nerves, and the pituitary gland.

    (h) Common approaches to this lesion include: transsphenoidal, transplanum, transtuberculum, sometimes clival or cavernous sinus.

Rathke Cleft Cyst
Origin/Epidemiology

    (a) Benign epithelium lined cyst, originating from the remnant Rathke pouch.

    (b) The incidence is approximately 15%, however most lesions are small and asymptomatic.

    (c) Only 2% to 9% of these lesions ultimately become symptomatic.

    (d) There is a female preponderance, with a peak in incidence between 40 and 50 years of age.

Clinical presentation

    (a) Symptoms include headache, visual changes, and hypopituitarism. However, hyperprolactinemia and growth hormone deficiency are also common.

Radiology

    (a) Well-circumscribed, centrally located spherical or ovoid shape cystic lesion, hypointense nonenhancing nodule on coronal T2-weighted MRI. Mucoid-filled cyst may be hyperintense.

    (b) These lesions are typically found in the sella and suprasellar region.

Treatment

(a) The majority of Rathke cleft cysts can be managed expectantly with yearly MRIs and/or clinical assessment.
(b) Surgical intervention is needed for lesion that results in visual changes or endocrinopathies.
(c) Clinical symptoms typically resolve after surgery; however, there is a 3% to 33% recurrence rate.
(d) Follow-up MRI should be performed at 3 months and yearly for 5 years.
(e) Common approaches to this lesion include: transsphenoidal, transplanum, transtuberculum.

Craniopharyngioma

Origin/Epidemiology

(a) Squamous epithelial remnant of Rathke pouch.
(b) There is a bimodal incidence peaking at 5 to 15 years old and again at 45 to 60 years old.
(c) Craniopharyngiomas account for 1% to 15% of pediatric brain tumors.
(d) Craniopharyngiomas have two types: adamantinomatous and papillary-squamous.
(e) The adamantinomatous type is typically seen in children. Adamantinomatous lesions are normally adherent to surrounding structures, encase vessels, and invade the brain.
(f) The papillary-squamous type is almost exclusively seen in adults.

Clinical presentation

(a) Symptoms include visual changes, endocrinopathies, and cranioneuropathies.

Radiology

(a) There is typically a prominent suprasellar component.
(b) Adamantinomatous lesions have a cystic component containing T1-weighted hyperintensity fluid and a solid heterogeneous component that contains calcifications or ossified elements.
(c) Papillary squamous is a solidly enhancing lesion within the suprasellar region.

Treatment

(a) There is controversy over appropriate aggressiveness of resection. If gross total resection (GTR) is not achieved radiation may be used as an adjunct therapy. Literature suggest the subtotal resection with radiation could be advantageous in order to prevent endocrinopathies for aggressive surgical resection.
(b) Common approaches to this lesion include: transsphenoidal, transplanum, transtuberculum.

Meningioma

Origin/Epidemiology

(a) Extra-axial tumor arising from the arachnoid cap cells.
(b) Meningioma account for 15% to 25% of primary intracranial tumors.
(c) These lesions are two times more common in women and the incidence increases with age peaking at 60 to 70 years old.
(d) 10% to 15% of meningiomas are located in the parasellar region.

Clinical presentation

(a) Symptoms typically occur because of visual changes from mass effect. These symptoms present as bitemporal hemianopsia.
(b) Risk factors including exposure to ionizing radiation and exogenous hormones.

Radiology

(a) Hypo- or isointense on T1- and T2-weighted MRI. Contrast enhancing lesion which is homogenous.

(b) Classic feature of "dural tails" are found in 60% to 70% of meningiomas.

(c) CT scan may show speckled calcifications, which are consistent with psammoma bodies and hyperostosis of the tuberculum sellae.

Treatment

(a) Indication for surgery include alleviation of neurologic deficit or progressive growth with threat of deficit.

(b) Remnant tumor from subtotal resection should be followed closely and radiated if significant growth occurs.

(c) Common approaches to this lesion include: transsphenoidal, transpterygoid, orbital apex, transethmoidal.

Empty Sella

(a) There is a primary and secondary type of empty sellae.

(b) The primary type is associated with a congenital dehiscence of the diaphragm sella with resultant herniation of arachnoid and CSF.

(c) The secondary type is associated with an underlying lesion causing spontaneous or iatrogenic reduction in pituitary gland volume.

(d) The chiasm may pull down into the enlarged sella.

Radiology

(a) The sella has an appearance of an absent pituitary gland because it is filled with cerebrospinal fluid (CSF).

Treatment

(a) If symptomatic the transsphenoidal approach can be used to open the sella and place gelfoam to lift the chiasm up.

Pituitary Apoplexy

Epidemiology/Pathophysiology

(a) The incidence ranges from 2% to 7% and is found more commonly in men.

(b) This condition is neurologic impairment due to acute hemorrhage or infarction of the pituitary gland. It typically occurs when infarction or hemorrhage extends laterally into cavernous sinus or superiorly to the optic chiasm.

(c) Pituitary apoplexy is typically seen with pituitary adenoma.

Clinical presentation

(a) Symptoms include sudden onset of headache, vomiting, nausea, meningismus, visual changes (ocular paresis, decreased visual fluids and acuity), altered mental status and hormonal dysfunction.

(b) Symptoms progress over a few hours to 3 days.

(c) Predisposing factors include head trauma, bromocriptine, anticoagulation, pregnancy, and recent surgery.

Radiology

(a) Variable degree of hyperintensity on T1-weighted MRI. Rim enhancement on T1-weighted MRI with contrast. Acute stage can be detected as hyperintensity on diffusion-weighted imaging.

Treatment
- (a) Prompt surgical decompression of the pituitary gland is required.
- (b) If decompression occurs within 1 week of symptoms near complete recovery of ophthalmologic function will occur.
- (c) Hormonal function may not recover completely and supplemental long-term hormones and steroids may be required.
- (d) Common approach is transsphenoidal.

Chordoma

Origin/Epidemiology
- (a) Arises from remnants of the notochord.
- (b) Chordomas account for 1% to 2% of intracranial tumors. One-third of these lesions arise from the sphenooccipital synchondrosis of the clivus.
- (c) Incidence is greatest in people between 30 and 40 years of age.

Clinical presentation
- (a) Symptoms include headache, diplopia caused by abducens nerve palsy, and trigeminal sensory deficit.
- (b) This tumor is a slow growing, low grade malignant tumor, with local aggressive invasion.

Radiology
- (a) Intense heterogeneous enhancement on T2-weighted MRI, hypo- to isointense on T1 imaging.
- (b) Nearly 100% of chordomas will exhibit bony destruction and expansion.

Treatment
- (a) The gold standard of treatment is surgical resection and postoperative radiation.
- (b) Common approaches are transsphenoidal and transclival.

Chondrosarcoma

Origin/Epidemiology
- (a) Arises from mesenchymal cells or embryonic rest of cartilaginous matrix.
- (b) This is a cartilaginous malignancy that typically arises from the nasal septum and extends to the skull base.
- (c) This tumor accounts for 5% to 15% of skull base tumors and generally occurs between the ages of 50 and 70 years.

Clinical presentation
- (a) Symptoms include headache, visual changes, and tinnitus.
- (b) This is a slow growing, but locally aggressive tumor.

Radiology
- (a) Hypo- or isointense on T1-weighted MRI and hyperintense on T2-weighted MRI. Destructive lobulated mass with calcifications and variable enhancement.
- (b) Chondrosarcomas are difficult to distinguish from chordomas on imaging.
- (c) Chondrosarcomas typically arise from the petroclival synchondrosis and often involve the petrous apex.

Treatment
- (a) Craniofacial resection or endoscopic resection.
- (b) Tumor has a better prognosis than chordoma.
- (c) Common approaches are transsphenoidal, transclival, or transpterygoid.

Metastases

Epidemiology
    (a) 1% of all sellar and parasellar tumors.
    (b) Breast and lung cancers more commonly metastasize to this area.
    (c) The posterior lobe of the pituitary is more likely to be affected by metastatic lesions. This is due to blood supply which comes directly from the carotid artery.

Clinical presentation
    (a) Symptoms include diabetes insipidous which is likely due to the predilection for the posterior lobe, visual changes, headache, and hypopituitarism.

Radiology
    (a) Hypo or isointense on T1-weighted images and varying hyperintensity on T2. These lesions are difficult to differentiate from pituitary adenoma.

Treatment
    (a) Biopsy is required to confirm diagnosis. Excisional biopsy is a reasonable option for those lesions causing mass effect.
    (b) Palliative treatment with radiation is often the appropriate therapy.

Esthesioblastoma

Origin/Epidemiology
    (a) Arises from the olfactory epithelium.
    (b) Age range for diagnosis is 12-70, with a mean age around 40.

Clinical presentation
    (a) Symptoms include nasal obstruction, epistaxis, unilateral nasal discharge, and headache.
    (b) Metastases is uncommon, however cervical lymphadenopathy is seen in 10% to 15% of patients.

Treatment
    (a) Surgical resection with postoperative radiation is treatment of choice. Controversy still exist regarding appropriate surgical between endoscopic and open craniofacial resection. If cervical metastasis is present then neck dissection is included in the treatment protocol.
    (b) Common approaches are transnasal and anterior cranial fossa.

Encephalocele/CSF leak (Figure 29-5)

Origin/Epidemiology
    (a) Etiology includes trauma, spontaneous, tumor, and congenital.
    (b) Common locations for leak include cribriform plate, fovea ethmoidalis, sphenoid, and temporal bone.

Clinical presentation
    (a) Intermittent clear rhinorrhea.
    (b) Preoperative evaluation should include history and physical including nasal endoscopy.
    (c) Assessment should include size of bony defect, degree of dural disruption, intracranial pressure, meningoencephalocele formation, and site of defect.
    (d) Spontaneous leaks are most often caused by increased intracranial pressure (ICP), also known as benign intracranial hypertension (BIH) or pseudotumor cerebri.
    (e) Normal intracranial opening pressure is between 10 and 15 cm H_2O, however, elevated pressures are typically around 25-27 cm H_2O.
    (f) BIH presents with headache, pulsatile tinnitus, balance problems, and visual changes.
    (g) Most patients with BIH are women and obese.

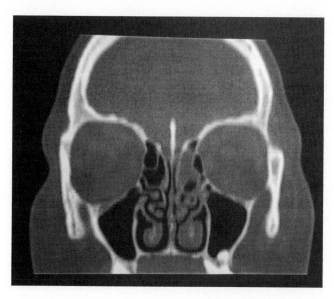

Figure 29-5 Arrow pointing to lateral lamella; site of encephalocele.

   (h) The most common site for spontaneous leaks and encephaloceles associated with elevated ICP is the lateral sphenoid recess, which historically has been referred to as Sternberg canal.

   (i) Endoscopic sinus surgery and neurologic surgery are the two most common procedures leading to iatrogenic CSF leaks.

   (j) Particular vulnerable areas of injury include the thin lateral lamella of the cribriform plate and the posterior wall of the frontal sinus.

   (k) Congenital encephaloceles are most commonly found adjacent to the vertical attachment of the middle turbinate.

   (l) Diagnostic evaluation should include beta 2 transferrin and imaging studies including CT and MRI.

Radiology

   (a) CT scan performed to look for bony defects. CT scans can localize active leaks when intrathecal contrast is used, referred to as a CT cisternogram. This test is not useful for intermittent leaks.

   (b) Radiolabelled cisternogram used intrathecal injection of a radioactive marker which if positive is detected on pledgets placed in the nasal cavity. This technique is better for intermittent leaks as the pledgets are in place for several hours. This is rarely used because of the invasiveness of using radioactive markers and the high false positive rate.

   (c) MRI is useful for detecting encephaloceles. It is also helpful in detecting empty sella which is seen with elevated ICP.

   (d) Low dose intrathecal fluorescein can be used to detect and localize leaks. This technique is most commonly performed in the operating room. This allows dissection as needed and confirmation of a watertight seal after reconstruction.

Treatment

   (a) In general, the defect is exposed in a 360 degree manner, sinus mucosa is stripped to prevent mucocele, if an encephalocele is present it is reduced using bipolar cautery, and an appropriate multi-layer closure is performed.

Reconstruction

(a) Multilayered Reconstruction include: Inlay and onlay grafts.
(b) Inlay grafts are placed between the dural matter and skull base.
(c) Onlay grafts are placed extracranially.
(d) Inlay, as known as underlay, grafts include abdominal fat, acellular dermis, and fascia lata.
(e) Onlay, as known as overlay, grafts include avascular graft, pedicled vascular flap such as nasoseptal flaps, turbinate flaps, and regional flaps.
(f) Vascularized flaps have a lower leak rate than free grafts.
(g) Small defects less than 1 cm in diameter can be repaired with any multilayer reconstruction, and results in greater than 90% success rate.
(h) Vascularized flaps have multiple benefits including ease of use, low donor site morbidity, low complication rate, and accelerated healing process.
(i) Examples of vascularized tissue flaps include nasoseptal flap, inferior turbinate flap (anterior or posterior pedicle), middle turbinate flap, and pericranial flap.
(j) Current opinion is that the nasoseptal flap is the workhorse for skull base reconstruction.
(k) Vascularized flaps have taken the postoperative CSF leak rates down to approximately 5%.

Nasoseptal Flap

(a) A vertical incision is made parallel to the anterior segment of the inferior turbinate. However, the anterior extent may be adjusted to accommodate the size and shape of the defect.
(b) Two parallel incisions are then made superiorly and inferiorly. Superiorly the incision begins at the superior or inferior edge of a widened sphenoid ostium and carried in a sagittal plane 1 to 2 cm below the superior edge of the nasal septum. Inferiorly the incision is carried medially along the posterior choana, down the free edge of the nasal septum, and anteriorly along the maxillary crest.
(c) The flap is then elevated creating a mucoperichondrial flap, which once mobilized can be placed in the nasopharynx or maxillary antrostomy.
(d) This flap is supplied by the sphenopalatine artery and its posterior septal branch.
(e) Figure 29-6.

Rescue Nasoseptal Flap

(a) This flap can be created if there is a possible, but not likely risk of an intra-operative CSF leak.
(b) The advantage of a rescue nasoseptal flap is decreased donor morbidity and decreased duration of dissection.
(c) The disadvantage of this flap is its constant need for retraction and its impedance in exposing the floor of the sphenoid.
(d) The superior incision is only extended 1/3 to ½ anteriorly. The superior and posterior flap is elevated using a dissecting instrument, starting with the superior edge. The contralateral sphenoid is then widely opened and a posterior septectomy is performed.

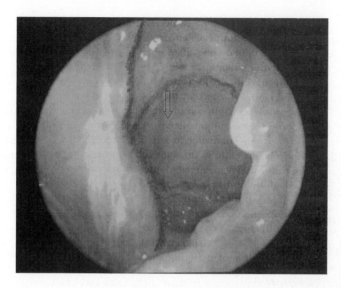

Figure 29-6 Arrow. NSF: Nasoseptal flap; Left NSF located on planum and posterior wall of sphenoid sinus.

Inferior Turbinate Flap

(a) For both techniques the mucosa is dissected off the bone inferiorly and superiorly leaving either an anterior or posterior pedicled base.

(b) Anteriorly pedicled inferior turbinate flap: blood supply is the turbinate branch of sphenopalatine artery, anterior ethmoid artery, and lateral nasal artery.

(c) Anterior flap is used for defects in the anterior cranial fossa.

(d) Posteriorly pedicled inferior turbinate flap: blood supply is the inferior turbinate artery.

(e) Posterior flap is used for clival defects.

Middle Turbinate Flap

(a) This flap can be used for sellar, tuberculum, and fovea ethmoidalis repair.

(b) A vertical incision is made at the anterior aspect of the vertical portion of the middle turbinate. The mucosa is dissected of the bone which is carried posteriorly and allows the flap to open like a book.

(c) The flap is supplied by the posterior lateral nasal artery.

Pericranial Flap

(a) Indication includes a large anterior skull base defect.

(b) This flap is traditionally harvested using a bicoronal incision, however, an endoscopic approach using a small glabellar incision has been described.

(c) Endoscopic harvesting of the pericranial flap is performed using two endoscopes, very similar to an endoscopic brow lift approach.

(d) A horizontal incision is then made at the glabella and an osteotomy is performed. The flap is then retrieved from the supraorbital region and placed intranasally.

(e) Blood supply for this flap is the supratrochlear artery.

Gasket Seal Closure

(a) This technique is used for defects > 1cm. It includes: soft tissue graft (fascia lata), rigid material (Medpore, Vomer, Titanium plate), vascularized flap (nasoseptal flap, middle turbinate flap), and duraSeal.

(b) Intrathecal fluorescein can be used to help detect intra-operative CSF leaks and confirm watertight reconstructions as the end of the case.

(c) This is an off label use of fluorescein, but has been documented as a safe drug based on multiple studies.

(d) There is several serious but rarely occurring complications from this medication including seizure, chemical meningitis, transient radicular neuropathy, and transient paraparesis and hemiparesis.

Complications of Endoscopic Skull Base Surgery

(a) Postoperative CSF leak is the most common complication after endoscopic skull base surgery.

(b) Appropriate multilayer reconstruction based on defect size and location will decrease the risk of postoperative leak.

(c) Tension pneumocephalus is less common after the endoscopic approach in comparison to an open approach.

(d) Signs and symptoms of tension pneumocephalus include rapid neurologic decline consistent of confusion and loss of consciousness.

(e) Perioperative bleeding typically begins intraoperatively and ranges from venous bleeding to carotid injury.

(f) Hemostatic techniques include warm irrigation, gelfoam with thrombin packing, floseal, cautery, and aneurysm clipping.

(g) Carotid injury is rare and should be treated with immediate packing of the nasal cavity and lowering of blood pressure. A piece of meshed muscle taken from the neck or thigh can be placed over the injured carotid after which the nasal cavity is tightly repacked.

(h) Immediate after control of bleeding, the patient should be taken to interventional radiology for angiogram and stenting/embolization.

(i) Cerebrovascular accident can be due to accidental injury to the circulation, venous infarct due to drastic changes in CSF pressure, or embolic phenomena.

(j) Infectious complications are rare and typically are due to a local infection from postoperative crust which is a breeding ground for bacterial overgrowth.

(k) Minor complications may include sinusitis, vestibular burns, anosmia, and synechiae.

Comparison Between the Microscopic and Endoscopic Approach

(a) There are distinct advantages to the microscopic approach including: neurosurgeon familiarity with equipment, namely the microscope, ability to have a three dimensional view, constant safe trajectory to the sella, and less operative time.

(b) Disadvantages to the microscopic approach include narrowed field of view with restricted view of key structures such as carotid protuberance, opticocarotid recess, sellar floor, cavernous sinus wall, and optic chiasm.

(c) The endoscopic approach provides several advantages including panoramic views of the sphenoid which allows for identification of key landmarks. A greater portion of the tumor resection can be visualized directly. With the use of a 0, 30, and 45 degree endoscope post resection evaluation can be completed which increases the chance for gross total resection.

(d) Disadvantages to the endoscopic approach include neurosurgeon unfamiliarity with the endoscope, increased operating room time on the part of the otolaryngologist, and possible trauma to the nasal mucosa.

Bibliography

Anand VK, Schwartz TH. *Practical Endoscopic Skull Base Surgery*. San Diego, CA: Plural Publishing; 2007.

Cavallo LM, Cappabianca P, Messina A, et al. The extended endoscopic endonasal approach to the clivus and cranio-vertebral junction: anatomical study. *Childs Nerv Syst*. 2007;23(6):665-671. Epub 2007 Apr 6.

Hadad G, Bassagasteguy L, Carrau RL, Mataza JC, Kassam A, Snyderman CH, Mintz A. A novel reconstructive technique after endoscopic expanded endonasal approaches: vascular pedicle nasoseptal flap. *Laryngoscope*. 2006 Oct;116(10):1882-1886.

Inoue T, Rhoton AL Jr, Theele D, Barry ME. Surgical approaches to the cavernous sinus: a microsurgical study. *Neurosurgery*. 1990;26(6):903-932.

Kennedy DW, Hwang PH. *Rhinology: Diseases of the Nose, Sinus, and Skull Base*. New York, NY: Thieme; 2012.

Questions

1. Which component of the multilayer skull base reconstruction has been heralded as the workhorse of skull base reconstruction and has led to a significant decline in postoperative CSF leaks?

   A. Fascia lata graft

   B. Abdominal fat graft

   C. Nasoseptal flap

   D. Inferior turbinate flap

2. What are radiographic findings seen in empty sella syndrome?

   A. T2-weighted hyperintense lesion within the sella on MRI

   B. Absent pituitary gland on MRI

   C. Hyperintense lesion on T1- and T2-weighted MRI

   D. Rim-enhancing lesion within the sella

3. What is considered normal intracranial pressure?

   A. 5-9 cm H_2O

   B. 10-15 cm H_2O

   C. 16-20 cm H_2O

   D. 21-25 cm H_2O

4. Which is not a technique used for hemostasis during skull base surgery?
   A. Gelfoam
   B. Warm saline irrigation
   C. Strip of muscle
   D. Dextran

5. What is the blood supply to the nasoseptal flap?
   A. Supratrochlear artery
   B. Sphenopalatine artery
   C. Nasociliary artery
   D. Posterior lateral nasal artery

Chapter 30
Salivary Gland Diseases

Anatomy

Parotid Gland

    A. Lateral aspect of face.
    B. Anterior border is the masseter muscle.
    C. Superior border is the zygomatic arch.
    D. Posterior border is the tragal cartilage and sternocleidomastoid muscle.
    E. Inferior tail of parotid is between the ramus of the mandible and sternocleidomastoid muscle, overlying the digastric muscle.
    F. Deep border is the prestyloid compartment of the parapharyngeal space.
    G. Superficial and deep lobes of the parotid are divided by the facial nerve.
    H. Eighty percent of the parotid parenchyma is the superficial lobe.
    I. Parotid is overlying the posterior aspect of mandible.
    J. Covered by parotidomasseteric fascia.
       i. Attaches to the root of zygoma.
      ii. Thin fascia separates from tragal and conchal cartilage by blunt dissection.
     iii. Thick fascia attaches to the mastoid process.
     iv. Thick fascia at the anterior and inferior tip of the parotid separating the parotid from the submandibular gland.

K. Arterial anatomy.
    i. External carotid artery courses medial to the parotid gland dividing into the maxillary artery and the superficial temporal artery.
    ii. The superficial temporal artery gives off the transverse facial artery.
L. Venous anatomy.
    i. The maxillary and superficial temporal veins form the retromandibular vein.
    ii. Retromandibular vein joins the external jugular vein via the posterior facial vein.
    iii. Retromandibular vein can give off an anterior facial vein that joins the internal jugular vein that is just deep to the marginal mandibularis branch of the facial nerve.
M. Stensen duct.
    i. Traverses over the masseter muscle.
    ii. Duct punctum exits the oral mucosa adjacent to the second upper molar.
N. Great auricular nerve.
    i. Arises from C2 and C3 cervical nerve branches.
    ii. Divides into anterior and posterior branches.
    iii. The posterior branch can frequently be saved, reducing auricular numbness.
O. Facial nerve.
    i. Extratemporal segment exits the skull base through the stylomastoid foramen posterolateral to the styloid process and anteromedial to the mastoid process.
    ii. The facial nerve branches as it enters the parotid forming the *pes anserinus*.
    iii. The upper divisions include the temporal-facial branches.
    iv. The lower divisions include the cervico-facial divisions.
    v. Numerous branching patterns are possible.
    vi. Facial nerve trunk and divisions more superficial in children younger than 2 years.
P. Anatomic landmarks to identify the facial nerve.
    i. Tympano-mastoid suture line.
    ii. Posterior belly of the digastric muscle.
    iii. Tragal pointer.
    iv. Stylomastoid artery.
    v. Retrograde identification by tracing one of the facial nerve branches.
Q. Autonomic nerve supply.
    i. Glossopharyngeal nerve (cranial nerve [CN] IX) supplies parasympathetic innervation.
    ii. Superior cervical ganglion supplies sympathetic innervation.
R. Parapharyngeal space.
    i. Inverted pyramid with the base at the petrous bone of the skull base; medial boundary is the lateral pharyngeal wall; the lateral boundary is the medial pterygoid muscle; the posterior boundary is the carotid sheath and vertebral bodies; the anterior boundary is the pterygomandibular raphe.
    ii. Deep parotid tumors can extend into the prestyloid compartment.
    iii. Poststyloid compartment contains the carotid sheath structures.

Submandibular Gland

A. Superior margin is the mandible and the inferior margin is the anterior and posterior bellies of the digastric muscle forming the submandibular triangle.

    B. Arterial anatomy.
        i. Facial artery courses deep to the posterior belly of the digastric muscle.
        ii. Facial vein lies lateral to the gland.
        iii. Wharton ducts open in the floor of the mouth and cross deep to the lingual nerve.
    C. Neural anatomy.
        i. The facial nerve via the chorda tympani nerve provides secretomotor innervation to the submandibular and sublingual glands.
        ii. The lingual nerve, a sensory nerve, traverses the floor of mouth and during submandibular gland surgery attaches to the deep superior surface of the submandibular gland via the submandibular ganglion.
        iii. The hypoglossal nerve provides motor function to the tongue and is medial to the digastric muscle and the submandibular gland.
    D. Lymph nodes of the submandibular gland are periglandular unlike the parotid where there are (about 20) intraglandular as well as periglandular.

Sublingual and Minor Salivary Glands

    A. The sublingual glands are paired, located opposite the lingual frenulum, superior to the mylohyoid muscle, and drain individually in the floor of mouth via Rivinus ducts or via the submandibular duct via the Bartholin duct.
    B. Mucoceles of the sublingual glands are called ranulas.
    C. Minor salivary glands are located throughout the upper airway, but are concentrated in the oral cavity, especially the palate, and number 600 to 1000.

Imaging

Neoplasms

Imaging studies in small, mobile, superficial parotid lesions are elective. Ultrasound to distinguish solid from cystic mass and ultrasound for fine-needle aspiration (FNA) guidance.

    A. Ultrasound.
        i. Cost-effective, available in office setting, no radiation exposure (especially important in the pediatric population).
        ii. Color Doppler ultrasound may suggest malignancy because of the increased nodular vascularity.
        iii. Loss of fatty hilum, round lymph nodes, and abnormal peripheral vascularity can suggest malignancy.
        iv. Less information than computed tomography (CT) and magnetic resonance (MR) in deep lobe lesions, retromandibular lesions, and extraparotid extension.
        v. Useful for obtaining image-guided biopsies when needed.
    B. Magnetic resonance imaging (MRI) is the best study for lesions suspect for neoplasm (noninflammatory).
        i. Fat (the parotid gland has a high fat content) is hyperintense (bright) on unenhanced T1-weighted images.
        ii. Almost all neoplasms are visualized as hypointense (dark) on T1 images.

     iii. T1 images can determine invasion of bone, that is, skull base extension.

     iv. Tissue with abundant water content is hypointense (dark) on T1 images and hyperintense on unenhanced T2-weighted images.

     v. Less cellular differentiated masses (benign and low-grade malignancy) tend to be hyperintense on T2 unenhanced images as they may have more water content than their malignant counterpart which are more likely hypointense.

     vi. Cellular benign mixed tumors are hypointense on T1; hyperintense on T2.

     vii. Warthin tumors are isointense/hyperintense on T1 (cysts containing cholesterol); variable/hetergenous intensity on T2.

     viii. Gadolinium-enhanced images can be hyperintense with inflammatory lesions or neoplasms and can help distinguish a purely cystic from solid tumor.

     ix. Distinguishing between benign and malignant lesions by MRI is *not* reliable but malignancy can be suspected with irregular margins or extraglandular infiltration of tumor.

     x. MR imaging in the setting of possible recurrent neoplasm after prior treatment is complemented by positron emission tomography (PET) scan and FNA.

C. Noncontrast CT scan reliably detects submandibular and parotid sialoliths.

     i. Most neoplasms have a similar appearance on CT; contrast allows discerning between a purely cystic lesion, lipoma, and a neoplasm.

     ii. MR is superior to CT in determining the extent of soft tissue disease.

     iii. Early cortical involvement of the mandible or skull base is better determined by CT; MR is better at determining bone marrow and intracranial involvement.

     iv. CT-guided FNA can be diagnostic in nonpalpable lesions.

D. Nuclear scintigraphy.

     i. Tc-99m pertechnetate is rarely used but may help in diagnosing Warthin tumor.

E. PET fluorodeoxyglucose (PET-FDG) for initial evaluation is not reliable, not anatomic, and expensive. Pleomorphic adenoma and Warthin tumors are FDG-avid, while many malignant cancers are low grade so can't reliably distinguish between adenoma and carcinoma.

F. Parapharyngeal tumors.

     i. Deep lobe parotid tumors and ectopic salivary gland tumors in the prestyloid space.

     ii. Poststyloid space lesions are usually schwannomas and paragangliomas.

G. Inflammatory lesions.

     i. Ultrasound or unenhanced CT for calculi, but, plain radiographs are also used.

     ii. Sialography is contraindicated in the acute setting of sialadenitis, but is useful in evaluating for stones, ductal strictures, penetrating trauma, and inflammatory disorders.

     iii. MR sialography can image the salivary ducts and does not require cannulation of the duct.

H. Systemic diseases.

     i. Ultrasound or CT may identify calcifications in Sjögren disease or sarcoidosis.

     ii. Sialography or MR sialography may help stage Sjögren disease.

     iii. MR is most sensitive in determining a mucosa-associated lymphoid tissue (MALT) lymphoma in the Sjögren patient.

     iv. Bilateral parotid cysts can be identified with imaging and may suggest an HIV-positive patient.

Physiology and Related Topics

    A. Embryology
- i. Parotid glands develop in the seventh embryonic week near the eventual duct orifice near the angle of the stomodeum.
- ii. The parotid anlage grows posterior and the facial nerve grows anterior.
- iii. A true capsule is not formed.
- iv. Salivary secretion starts after birth.
- v. Intraparotid lymph nodes form within the pseudocapsule of the parotid but lymph nodes do not form within other salivary glands.

    B. Physiology—autonomic nervous system
- i. Flow of saliva is regulated by the autonomic nervous system.
- ii. Parasympathetic cholinergic stimulation is dominant and uses mostly the neurotransmitter acetylcholine to activate phospholipase C which activates second messenger Ca^{2+}. Its functions include fluid formation, and transport activity in the acinar and ductal cells.
- iii. Sympathetic beta-adrenergic neurotransmitter is predominantly norepinephrine using G-protein–activated second messenger, cyclic adenosine monophosphate (cAMP). Its functions include exostosis and protein metabolism.
- iv. In the acinar cell Na^+, Cl^-, and HCO_3^- are secreted into the acinar lumen after the parasympathetic neurotransmitter attaches to the parasympathetic M3 muscarinic receptor.
- v. Water is drawn into the acinar lumen by the osmotic gradient of NaCl.
- vi. Water impermeable ductal cells in the ductal lumen reabsorb NaCl and secrete $KHCO_3$, (and a small amount of protein) making saliva less isotonic and more alkaline.

    C. Physiology—sialochemistry
- i. Saliva is 99.5% water and the remainder proteins and electrolytes.
- ii. Humans secrete about a liter of saliva per day.
- iii. Saliva becomes more viscous in the following order; parotid, submandibular gland, sublingual gland, minor salivary gland.
- iv. Ca^{2+} concentration is twice as high in the submandibular gland.
- v. Parotid gland secretion is proteinaceous, watery, and serous and is the predominant saliva that is stimulated.
- vi. Gustatory and olfactory stimulation induce predominantly parotid secretion.
- vii. Submandibular gland secretion has a higher mucin content and a higher basal flow rate and is the predominant unstimulated saliva.
- viii. Alpha-amylase is the most abundant protein with 40% of the body amylase produced by salivary glands.
- ix. Salivary osmolality increases during stimulation (NaCl is not reabsorbed as much).

    D. Physiology—sialometry
- i. Flow of saliva can be measured by volumetric techniques or with dynamic radionucleotide scintigraphy using Tc-99m pertechnetate.
- ii. Normal values are difficult to establish because of variability of the flow rates in healthy individuals.
- iii. No substantial age-related effect on stimulated salivary flow.
- iv. Decreased basal salivary flow with age.
- v. Unilateral salivary gland resection does not usually result in subjective xerostomia.

E. Physiology—salivary gland function
   i. Amylase starts the digestion of starch.
   ii. Saliva lubricates the food bolus with mucous glycoproteins assisting with speech, mastication, swallowing, and taste.
   iii. Saliva buffers with bicarbonate (HCO_3^-).
   iv. Antimicrobial proteins include secretory immunoglobulin A, mucins, lysozyme, histamine, lactoferrin, and amylase.
   v. Salivary proteins have a dental protective function preventing dental plaque formation and promoting remineralization.
   vi. Excretory function includes viruses (HIV) and inorganic elements (lead).
   vii. Oral epidermal growth factor is reduced with loss of salivary gland function and impedes oral wound healing.
F. Pathologic states
   i. Cystic fibrosis results in abnormal chloride regulation with failure of reabsorption of NaCl in the ductal cells resulting in more viscous saliva with decreased flow rates and sludging of saliva.
   ii. Prescription and nonprescription drugs are the most common sources of xerostomia, in particular anticholinergic medications (antihistamines and antidepressants).
   iii. Aging results in loss of acinar cells, and decreased salivary flow combined with other systemic disease and medications leads to xerostomia.

Histology and Related Topics

A. Parotid gland
   i. Acinar cells are pyramidal shape with a basal nucleus and secretory granules at the apex.
   ii. The serous cells of the parotid are interposed by myoepithelial cells that have a contractile function.
   iii. Acinar duct leads to the intercalated duct, the intralobular striated duct, and the excretory duct.
   iv. The intercalated and striated ducts can modify the salivary composition.
   v. Adipose cells in the parotid parenchyma increase with aging.
B. Submandibular gland—predominantly serous with 10% mucous cells often surrounded by serous cells in a demilune pattern
C. Sublingual glands and minor salivary glands
   i. Mucous acinar cells with an even higher percent of mucous acini in minor salivary glands, which are unencapsulated.
   ii. Ebner glands are serous minor salivary glands located posteriorly on the tongue.
D. Ultrastructure
   i. Secretory granules are prominent on the apical (facing the acinar lumen) aspect of the acinar cell.
   ii. Protein production occurs mostly in acinar cells, starts in the mitochondria and endoplasmic reticulum of the acinar cell, with further posttranslational protein modification in the Golgi complex and storage in the secretory granules.
   iii. Water permeable acinar cells are highly polarized and the apical and basolateral membranes are separated by tight junctions.
   iv. The extracellular matrix separates the acinar cells from the interstitium.

      v. Myoepithelial cells are located between connective tissue and acinar basal membranes (as well as intercalated duct cells) and contain both smooth muscle and epithelial cells and are rich in adenosine triphosphate (ATP).

  E. Adenomatoid hyperplasia
      i. Idiopathic asymptomatic nodule generally on the hard palate.
      ii. Biopsy reveals normal minor salivary gland with excision being curative.

  F. Sialadenosis
      i. Painless enlargement of the salivary glands.
      ii. Enlarged acinar cells.
      iii. Myoepithelial atrophy and degenerative changes in neural elements.

  G. Oncocytic metaplasia
      i. Mitochondria are enlarged and more numerous.
      ii. Idiopathic and associated with aging and most common in the parotid.

  H. Sebaceous metaplasia
      i. Sebaceous cells found in normal salivary glands, most commonly parotid.
      ii. Fordyce granules: sebaceous cells in the oral mucosa.
      iii. Metaplasia occurs with sebaceous cells replacing cells of the intercalated or striated duct.

  I. Necrotizing sialometaplasia (unilateral or midline ulcer on the posterior hard palate or at the junction of the hard and soft palates).
      i. Exuberant squamous metaplasia.
      ii. Inflammatory response in minor salivary glands.
      iii. Can be misinterpreted as a malignant process.

  J. Accessory and heterotopic salivary gland tissue (SGT)
      i. Accessory SGT: ectopic salivary gland tissue with a duct system, most commonly located anterior to the main parotid gland.
      ii. Accessory SGT: drains into the main parotid duct.
      iii. Accessory SGT: adjacent to the buccal branch of the facial nerve.
      iv. Heterotopic SGT: has acini in an abnormal location without a duct system.
      v. Heterotopic SGT: most commonly in cervical lymph nodes with rare examples in the middle ear, thyroid, and pituitary.

  K. Amyloidosis
      i. Rarely reported in salivary glands.
      ii. Positive Congo red staining (apple-green birefringence on polarized view).
      iii. Painless salivary gland enlargement.

  L. Lipomatosis
      i. Tumor-like accumulation of intraparenchymal fat tissue.
      ii. Fibrous capsule, discreet mass.
      iii. Associated with aging, diabetes, alcoholism, and malnutrition.

  M. Cheilitis glandularis
      i. Nodular swollen lower lip of adult males.
      ii. Can express saliva
      iii. Nonspecific histologic finding, hyperplasia, fibrosis, and ectasia.

Sialadenitis

  A. Acute suppurative sialadenitis.
      i. Elderly, debilitated, and postsurgical (abdominal and hip) patients most commonly involves the parotid gland.

    ii. Parotid is less mucinous and has less antimicrobial activity than submandibular gland.

    iii. Sialoliths more commonly involve the submandibular gland.

    iv. Etiology: salivary stasis.

        a. *Staphylococcus aureus* is most common pathogen (monitor for MRSA).

        b. *Streptococcus viridans* anaerobes.

    v. Parotitis presents with typically unilateral painful gland swelling and purulence from Stensen duct.

    vi. Ultrasound or CT may identify stone or abscess; sialography is contraindicated as it results in more inflammation.

    vii. Treatment: Usually beta-lactamase and anaerobic sensitive antibiotics, (unless case is mild), hydration, posterior to anterior massage, and sialagogues.

    viii. Parotid abscess can be difficult to diagnose clinically with anaerobic infections.

    ix. Drainage of abscess involves elevation of facial flap and radial incisions in the parotid parenchyma in the direction of the facial nerve.

B. Chronic sialadenitis.

    i. Sialolithiasis may result in scarred, stenotic ducts, and sialectasia leading to diminished secretory function of the gland.

    ii. Rx: Antibiotics, hydration, sialogogues—50% improve.

    iii. Removal of sialolith can return gland function, obviate gland removal.

    iv. Kuttner tumor—heavy lymphoid infiltrate in submandibular gland, may mimick neoplasm.

C. Mumps.

    i. "Epidemic" parotitis, paramyxovirus, prevent with measles, mumps, and rubella (MMR) vaccine.

    ii. Peak age 4 to 6 years.

    iii. Most common viral infection, mostly bilateral parotid involved, also fevers, malaise, orchitis, encephalitis, or sensorineural hearing loss.

    iv. Dx: clinical, serologic; Rx: supportive.

D. HIV.

    i. Parotid enlargement from lymphoid hyperplasia, infection, lymphoma.

    ii. May be presenting sign of HIV.

    iii. Lymphoepithelial cysts only in parotid but not in other salivary glands because of the incorporation of lymph nodes in parotid embryology.

    iv. May develop a sicca syndrome similar to Sjögren syndrome—diffuse infiltrative lymphocytosis syndrome (DILS).

    v. Dx: HIV+ serology, associated cervical adenopathy, and nasopharyngeal lymphoid hypertrophy.

    vi. Deforming bilateral cysts can form, cyst unlikely malignant, Rx: anti-retroviral meds and in select patients sclerotherapy; surgery rarely recommended.

    vii. Solid mass—40% risk of malignancy.

E. Granulomatous diseases.

    i. Tuberculosis increasing secondary to HIV and immigrant population.

        a. Primary is through intraglandular lymph nodes, mostly parotid.

        b. Secondary; after infection of lungs with hematogenous spread.

        c. *Dx*: Purified protein derivative (PPD), FNA–acid-fast bacilli, culture, Langhans giant cells.

    ii. Atypical mycobacteria—children 16 to 36 months.
        a. Violaceous hue of skin, sinus tracts
        b. Chest x-ray (CXR) negative, PPD nonreactive
        c. Dx: serology
        d. Rx: incision and curettage, surgical excision of gland
    iii. Actinomycosis—gram-positive anaerobic actinomyces, sulfur granules.
        a. Risk factors—poor oral hygiene, impaired immunity
        b. Sinus tracts, multiloculated abscesses
        c. Rx: Penicillin G IV × 6 weeks, then PO erythromycin or clindamycin
    iv. Cat scratch disease—*Bartonella henselae,* rickettsial pathogen.
        a. Associated with lymphatics of parotid
        b. Dx: serology and polymerase chain reaction (PCR), lymphadenopathy, positive Warthin-Starry stain reaction, pathologic features
        c. Rx: observation, azithromycin
    v. Toxoplasmosis—*Toxoplasmosis gondii,* protozoan parasite, increased incidence with HIV epidemic, under cooked meats, and cat feces.
        a. Dx: culture, acute and convalescent titers.
        b. Rx: pyrimethamine and sulfadiazine, plus folinic acid.
    vi. Sarcoidosis: systemic, unknown etiology, noncaseating granulomas.
        a. Heerfordt disease/syndrome—acute parotitis, uveitis, polyneuritis (facial nerve palsy).
        b. Rx: steroids.
F. Sjögren syndrome—autoimmune disease, destruction acinar, and ductal cells.
    i. Xerophthalmia, xerostomia—primary.
    ii. With collagen vascular disease (rheumatoid arthritis)—secondary.
    iii. More common in women, immune-mediated disease, alleles HLA-B8, HLADr3 genetic predisposition.
    iv. Parotid hypertrophy.
    v. Dx: (+) anti-Ro (SS-A) and anti-La (SS-B) serologies, minor salivary gland biopsy can demonstrate increased lymphocyte infiltration.
    vi. Higher rate of non-Hodgkin lymphoma from prolonged stimulation of autoreactive B cells.
    vii. Histology—benign lymphoepithelial lesion with proliferation of epimyoepithelial islands.
    viii. Rx: oral hygiene, salivary substitutes, pilocarpine, and cevimeline.
G. Sialolithiasis.
    i. Sialoliths—exact etiology unknown. Typically cause pain and swelling with meals. Tend to enlarge over time.
    ii. Sialolith imaging includes plain and dental (submental vertex) x-rays, sialography (determines strictures, dilations, and filling defects), ultrasound (can detect stones and ductal dilation), noncontrast CT, scintigraphy (secretory function), and MR sialography.
    iii. Intraoral sialolithotomy—incise floor of mouth mucosa, removes stone, heals by secondary intention or suturing of duct.
    iv. Transoral proximal Wharton duct stone excision—gland sparing.
    v. Incision of Stensen duct can lead to duct stenosis.
    vi. Submandibular sialoliths often in the duct, parotid often in the parenchyma.

    H. Sialendoscopy for diagnosis of salivary gland swelling without obvious cause (occult sialolith, stricture, or kink) and removal of select small sialoliths.
       i. Stones larger than 5 mm are not able to be removed with a basket.
      ii. Wharton duct is more difficult to cannulate than Stensen duct.
    I. Extracorporeal lithotripsy—not FDA approved in United States. Compressive shock waves brought to focus through acoustic lenses results in stone fragmentation. Residual stone fragments can be removed by sialendoscopy.
    J. Intracorporeal lithotripsy delivers laser energy through a fiberoptic cable.

Pediatric Salivary Gland Disease

    A. Hyposalivation—dehydration, radiotherapy (XRT) for malignancy, anticholinergic drugs
    B. Parotitis
       i. Neonatal suppurative parotitis—preterm, male neonates. *Staphylococcus aureus* most common
      ii. Recurrent parotitis of childhood—more common in boys, age 3 to 10, recurs weekly or monthly, no pus from duct, imaging shows ectasia of ducts, Rx: antibiotic for *Staphylococcus aureus,* dilation of Stensen duct, and sialendoscopy.
      iii. Viral—mumps (paramyxovirus), HIV, cytomegalovirus.
      iv. Bacterial—uncommon.
    C. Congenital cysts
       i. Parotid dermoid: an isolated midline cystic structure
      ii. Dermoid floor of mouth: midline, unlike a ranula
      iii. Branchial: associated with frequent infections, less than 5% of branchial anomalies are first branchial cleft abnormalities, present from the external auditory canal to the angle of the mandible, Type I has a tract to the membranous external auditory canal, Type II without tract to external auditory canal; Rx: complete surgical resection
      iv. Polycystic parotid gland has multiple cysts, primitive or mature ducts, remnant acini
    D. Acquired cysts
       i. Ranula—extravasation, not a true cyst; blue translucent swelling, simple type in sublingual space; plunging type posterior to mylohyoid, extending into the neck, Rx: complete resection of sublingual gland
      ii. Mucocele—pseudocyst, lower lip most common location
    E. Neoplasms—vascular neoplasm most common salivary neoplasms of children (20%)
       i. Hemangiomas present at birth usually involute between age 2 and 5 (50% by 5 years, 70% by 7 years).
         a. Most commons salivary gland neoplasm in children.
         b. 80% single lesion, 20% multiple lesions.
         c. Surgery only if impending complications, otherwise can remove postinvolution sparing facial nerve.
         d. Rx with propranolol.
      ii. Lymphangiomas mostly present in the first year of life, rarely involute; Rx— surgery: can be difficult with involvement of nerves and deep tissue planes, OK-432 sclerosing agent.
      iii. Most common benign solid neoplasms: pleomorphic adenoma.
      iv. Fifty percent of solid salivary gland neoplasms malignant (higher rate than in adults), most common malignancy is mucoepidermoid carcinoma.

     F. Sialorrhea
        i. Children with cognitive and physical disabilities, metal poisoning.
        ii. Conservative Rx—glycopyrrolate, scopolamine, Botox.
        iii. Surgery—bilateral parotid duct ligation (risks: sialadenitis and fistulization) and submandibular gland excision.
     G. Recurrent aspiration of saliva from ptyalism/sialorrhea.
        i. Tracheotomy often unsuccessful in prevention.
        ii. Laryngotracheal separation is successful; reversible in select patients.

Benign Tumors and Cysts

     A. Benign mixed tumor
        i. Most common salivary gland neoplasm in adults and children.
        ii. About 85% present in the parotid, most of these in the tail of parotid.
        iii. Can extend into the prestyloid parapharyngeal space, presenting as an oropharyngeal mass—transoral resection leads to higher recurrence.
        iv. Ultrasound is inexpensive imaging technique. MR is superior to CT.
        v. FNA accurate in diagnosis.
        vi. Incomplete fibrous capsule.
        vii. Histology—biphasic-benign epithelial cells and stromal cells.
        viii. Hypercellular (epithelial rich) firmer tumors are usually present at an earlier stage; hypocellular myxoid tumors are more generally at an advanced stage and more prone to rupture.
        ix. Informed consent should include transient and permanent facial nerve dysfunction, ear numbness, gustatory sweating (Frey syndrome), sialocele, hematoma, and recurrence.
        x. Facial nerve dysfunction and Frey syndrome less frequent for partial superficial parotidectomy with nerve dissection compared to complete superficial or total parotidectomy. No higher recurrence.
        xi. Extracapsular dissection is an alternative technique that does not dissect the facial nerve; only for select tumors in expert hands.
        xii. Enucleation results in unacceptably high recurrence rate.
        xiii. Recurrence with facial nerve dissection procedures is 1% to 4%.
        xiv. Recurrences are usually multinodular.
        xv. Definitive treatment for recurrence involves resection of all gross tumor and postoperative radiation therapy.
        xvi. Surgery for recurrent mixed tumors: high rate of temporary facial nerve injury.
     B. Myoepithelioma—1% of salivary gland neoplasms, most present in the parotid
     C. Warthin tumor—papillary cystadenoma lymphomatosum
        i. Almost exclusively in the parotid.
        ii. Second most common benign neoplasm of the parotid.
        iii. Slow growing mass, occasionally can become inflamed and painful.
        iv. Up to 20% are multifocal, 5% are bilateral.
        v. Associated with smoking, but no clonal population by PCR, so not considered a true neoplasm.
        vi. Technetium TC-99m pertechnetate uptake is due to oncocytic cell component.
        vii. Histology—oncocytic epithelium, papillary architecture, lymphoid stroma, and cystic spaces.
        viii. Treatment—complete resection or observation.

    D. Basal cell adenoma
       i. About 5% occur in the parotid, 2% to 5% of salivary gland tumors.
       ii. Can mimic solid subtype adenoid cystic carcinoma.
    E. Canalicular adenoma—usually in upper lip, slow growing, asymptomatic
    F. Oncocytoma
       i. About 1% of salivary gland neoplasms.
       ii. Oncocytes—epithelial cells with accumulations of mitochondria.
       iii. Oncocytic metaplasia—transformation of acinar and ductal cells to oncocytes—associated with aging.
       iv. Oncocytosis—proliferation of oncocytes in salivary glands.
       v. Minor salivary gland oncocytomas can be locally invasive.
    G. Lipomas—CT and MRI have characteristic appearance.
    H. Acquired cysts of the salivary glands
       i. About 5% to 10% of salivary gland diseases are different types of cysts.
       ii. True cysts have an epithelial lining—retention cysts.
       iii. Pseudocysts are common in minor salivary glands—mucocele—most common, often from biting the lip.
       iv. Glands of Blandin and Nuhn—mucoceles of anterior lingual salivary glands.
       v. Benign lymphoepithelial cysts in non-HIV patients form from epithelial ductal inclusions in lymph nodes that then become cystic.
    I. Sialadenosis
       i. Noninflammatory, nonneoplastic, mostly symmetric salivary hypertrophy.
       ii. Etiology, endocrine (diabetes mellitus, adrenal disorders), dystrophic—metabolic (alcoholism, malnutrition) and neurogenic (anticholinergic medications).
       iii. Normal acinar cells are 30 to 40 μm in diameter, whereas in sialadenosis the diameters are 50 to 70 μm.
       iv. Sialadenosis from a peripheral autonomic neuropathy.
       v. FNA or gland biopsy may be diagnostic.
       vi. Idiopathic: diagnosis of exclusion.
       vii. Rx: Correction of underlying systemic problem.

Malignant Tumors

    A. Incidence: 1 to 2 per 100,000 with no causative relationship with smoking and/or alcohol. Radiation exposure may be a causative factor.
    B. Embryology similar to benign tumors.
       i. Reserve cell theory—salivary gland neoplasms derived from stem cells.
       ii. Multicellular theory—all cells in the salivary unit are capable of replication.
    C. General consideration.
       i. One-half present as a painless mass; growth rates variable.
       ii. Facial nerve dysfunction, adenopathy, trismus, and numbness uncommon.
       iii. Imaging can, but generally does not distinguish from benign lesions.
       iv. T1: 0 to 2 cm, T2: 2 to 4 cm, T3 > 4 cm, T4: gross invasion (mandible, facial nerve, ear canal).
    D. Treatment—complete surgical excision.
       i. Ratio of malignant to benign tumors: sublingual > minor > submandibular > parotid.
       ii. If the facial nerve is functioning, nerve preservation is feasible if plane of dissection between nerve and tumor can be achieved.

    iii. If the facial nerve is grossly involved with tumor and sacrificed, immediate nerve grafting should be performed.

    iv. Submandibular gland mass: FNA to determine neoplasm or inflammatory mass and if malignant submandibular triangle dissection with complete surgical removal; neck dissection for high-grade tumors or positive cervical lymphadenopathy.

    v. Malignancy of the sublingual gland is rare; complete resection recommended.

    vi. Minor salivary gland resection depends on the location in the upper respiratory tract. Most common location is on the hard palate.

    vii. Comprehensive neck dissection, levels I to V, is appropriate for N+ disease (20%-30% occult metastases to level 5 for parotid lesions). Elective neck dissection can be considered in the N0 neck with high-grade histology, high-grade histologic subtype, T3 and T4 disease, extraglandular extension, and facial nerve dysfunction (submandibular site more aggressive site than parotid for metastasis).

    viii. Mastoidectomy may be required if the main trunk of the facial nerve is resected in order to achieve a negative proximal nerve margin.

    ix. Preoperative imaging is important.

    x. Postoperative radiotherapy is indicated with close surgical margins, extraglandular extension, facial nerve preservation with close margins, perineural invasion, metastatic lymphadenopathy, high-grade tumors, recurrent low-grade tumors; all represent risk for recurrence.

    xi. Neutron beam XRT for recurrent and gross residual disease improves local control over photons but not overall survival.

    xii. Intensity-modulated radiation therapy (IMRT) distributes high doses to the intended target, limiting doses to critical normal structures.

    xiii. Overall rate of distant metastasis is about 25%.

    xiv. Chemotherapy presently not effective; reserved for palliation.

    xv. Molecular-targeted Rx so far not effective.

    xvi. Vascular endothelial growth factor (VEGF), p53 c-erbB markers—poor prognosis.

E. Mucoepidermoid carcinoma (MEC).

    i. Most common malignant tumor of the salivary glands in adults and children.

    ii. Low-grade histology—glandular and microcystic structures, associated with translocation mutation t(11;19).

    iii. Intermediate-grade histology—more epidermoid cells.

    iv. High-grade histology—solid sheets tumor, +Ki-67, Her2/neu-poor prognosis.

    v. Adenopathy associated with increasing histologic grade.

    vi. Surgical Rx: Complete surgical resection.

    vii. Radiotherapy: High-grade tumor, positive margins, positive cervical adenopathy.

F. Adenoid cystic carcinoma.

    i. About 10% of malignant salivary gland neoplasms.

    ii. Second most common malignant neoplasm.

    iii. Most common malignant tumor of minor salivary, submandibular, and sublingual salivary glands.

    iv. Palate most common site in the oral cavity.

    v. Propensity for perineural invasion and distant metastases (lung most common).

    vi. Lymphatic metastasis not common except for submandibular origin.

    vii. T1-weighted fat-suppressed MRI helps determine perineural tumor spread.

    viii. Cribriform type—Swiss cheese pattern—best prognosis.

    ix. Tubular pattern—low-grade tumor.

     x. Solid pattern—high-grade tumor.

     xi. Delayed local and distant spread—survival does not stabilize at 5 years.

     xii. Rx: Complete surgical resection and postoperative radiation therapy for almost all.

     xiii. Most common mode of failure is distant metastasis.

G. Acinic cell carcinoma.

     i. Most common in the parotid, occasionally bilateral, most low-grade tumors; plus proliferation marker *Ki-67*-high grade

     ii. Multiple subtypes do not have prognostic significance

     iii. Treatment: complete surgical resection

     iv. Recurrence more likely local than regional

H. Epithelial-myoepithelial carcinoma.

     i. Mostly in parotid, locoregionally aggressive

     ii. Low mortality

I. Salivary duct carcinoma.

     i. High-grade tumor with resemblance to mammary ductal carcinoma

     ii. Can present de novo or in setting of carcinoma ex-pleomorphic adenoma

     iii. Early regional metastasis

     iv. Rx: complete resection, postoperative radiation therapy

J. Polymorphous low-grade adenocarcinoma.

     i. Second most common salivary malignant tumor in oral cavity (usually hard palate).

     ii. Rarely in parotid.

     iii. Overall good prognosis; rarely metastasizes to the neck.

     iv. Can have perineural spread.

K. Adenocarcinoma, not otherwise specified (NOS).

     i. Shrinking category that used to include salivary duct carcinoma, epithelial-myo-epithelial carcinoma, and others.

L. Carcinoma ex-pleomorphic adenoma.

     i. Most common malignant mixed tumor.

     ii. Up to 10% of salivary gland malignancies.

     iii. Arises from long-standing mixed tumor.

     iv. Presents as a rapid growth of tumor in a long-standing salivary mass.

     v. Comprised of epithelial-derived carcinoma arising with mixed tumor.

     vi. Rx: complete resection, postoperative radiation therapy.

     vii. Poor long-term survival.

     viii. Carcinoma sarcoma—metastasis must display both malignant epithelial and malignant mesenchymal components—fulminant natural history.

     ix. Metastasizing pleomorphic adenoma—rare entity—behaves with unequivocally malignant features but with benign histologic features.

M. Lymphoma.

     i. Parotid is most common salivary gland involved. Sjögren patients are at higher risk.

     ii. Extranodal (primary lymphoma) arises from lymphocytes within the parotid.

     iii. Most common extranodal lymphoma is MALT lymphoma.

     iv. MALT lymphomas are marginal zone B-cell lymphomas.

     v. The central feature of MALT lymphoma is the lymphoepithelial lesion.

     vi. MALT lymphomas often localized disease-favorable prognosis.

     vii. Localized Rx for MALT lymphoma includes resection and/or radiation.

     viii. Nodal or secondary lymphoma is occasionally seen with systemic non-Hodgkin lymphoma.

     ix. Rx for secondary lymphoma is systemic.

Metastasis to Major Salivary Glands

    A. Squamous cell carcinoma (most common) and melanoma comprise the overwhelming number of neoplasms that metastasize to the parotid.
        i. Others include Merkel cell, eccrine, and sebaceous carcinoma.
        ii. Can occur by direct invasion; lymphatic metastasis from a nonsalivary gland primary; and hematogenous spread from a distant primary.
    B. Basal cell carcinoma.
        i. Most involve parotid by direct invasion.
    C. Cutaneous squamous cell carcinoma.
        i. About 5% of cutaneous squamous cell carcinomas metastasize to the parotid or neck.
        ii. Usually within 1 year of the index cancer.
        iii. Histologic factors will not distinguish between the rare primary salivary gland squamous cell carcinoma.
        iv. Risk factors: Diameter > 2 cm, thickness > 4 mm, local recurrence, perineural invasion, preauricular skin, or external ear index lesion.
        v. Superficial parotidectomy should be considered in the treatment of selected preauricular squamous cell cancers.
        vi. Parotid metastasis from skin primary is associated with 25% rate of clinical neck metastasis and 35% rate of occult neck metastasis.
        vii. Metastasis from a cutaneous primary posterior to the external auditory canal is unlikely to involve the parotid.
        viii. Radiation therapy is used with surgery for metastasis to the parotid.
        ix. Neck and parotid metastasis has worse prognosis than parotid metastasis.
    D. Melanoma
        i. Most parotid melanoma arises from a head and neck cutaneous primary.
        ii. Regional metastatic rates correlate with tumor thickness; < 5% in tumors < 1 mm, 20% from tumors between 1 and 4 mm, and up to 50% for tumors > 4 mm.
        iii. Sentinel node biopsy appropriate for T2, T3, T4, and N0; use lymphoscintigraphy and handheld gamma probe, blue dye injected intradermally.
        iv. Melanoma with unexpected drainage patterns.
        v. A high rate of patients with parotid metastasis will have neck metastasis.
        vi. Metastasis to the parotid poor prognosis.

Radiation-Induced Xerostomia

    A. Impacts 40,000 patients annually in the United States.
    B. Impaired mastication and speech and leads to dental caries.
    C. Acinar cell loss with relative sparing of ductal cells.
    D. Irreversible radiation damage begins at 25 Gy.
    E. Can also occur with radioiodine treatment (dose related).

Palliative Therapy

    A. Frequent water drinking, oral sialogogues, oral wash, salivary substitutes
    B. Pilocarpine, cevimeline—side effects often result in cessation of treatment
    C. Amifostine-radioprotector—acts intracellularly to scavenge and bind oxygen-free radicals and assist in DNA repair after radiation exposure

    D. Palifermin—epithelial proliferation
    E. For radioactive iodine induced sialadenitis, stenosis and mucous plugs–interventional sialendoscopy

Submandibular Salivary Gland Transfer

    A. Gland released and repositioned in the submental space.
    B. Retrograde blood flow to the transferred gland must be assured.
    C. Submandibular gland is shielded from radiation therapy; less xerostomia.

Parotid Gland Surgery

    A. Parotidectomy
       i. FNA to help determine presence or absence of neoplasm, benign versus malignant neoplasm, and less reliably specific type of tumor.
      ii. Ultrasound guidance improves diagnostic accuracy.
     iii. About 90% accurate; false positives for malignant tumors uncommon.
     iv. Preservation of the posterior branch of the greater auricular nerve results in less numbness of auricle.
      v. Landmarks: tympanomastoid suture line, posterior belly of the digastric muscle, tragal pointer, stylomastoid artery.
     vi. Once the main trunk of the facial nerve is identified dissection can proceed with care to protect the nerve from injury.
    vii. Retrograde facial nerve dissection is useful for recurrent tumors with significant scarring in the area of the main trunk of the facial nerve.
   viii. Abdominal fat, AlloDerm, SMAS flap, sternocleidomastoid transposition flap, or free tissue transfer may improve defect.
     ix. Frey syndrome (gustatory sweating)—abnormal neural connection between parasympathetic cholinergic nerve fibers of the parotid with severed sympathetic receptors innervating sweat glands.
      x. Frey syndrome can be treated with botulinum toxin.
     xi. Sialocele will usually resolve within 1 month.
    xii. Deep lobe parotid tissue—20% of volume dissected after superficial lobe removed, imaging helpful.
   xiii. Most deep lobe and parapharyngeal space tumors can be removed by a transcervical approach, mandibulotomy is occasionally needed; methods to preserve the inferior alveolar nerve are preferred.
   xiv. Parapharyngeal tumors can present as a mass pushing the tonsil fossa medially in the oral cavity; should generally not be removed by a transoral approach.
    xv. Accessory parotid tissue is located anterior to the parotid gland; slightly higher incidence of malignancy compared to the parotid. Usually in close proximity to the zygomatic and buccal branches of the facial nerve.
   xvi. Recurrent multifocal mixed tumor may require resection of skin with flap reconstruction.
  xvii. Incision for submandibular gland resection is via an upper neck crease with care to preserve the marginal mandibular branch of the facial nerve.
 xviii. The hypoglossal nerve is medial to the digastric muscle.

        xix. Caudal retraction of the submandibular gland and anterior retraction of the mylo-hyoid muscle expose the lingual nerve superiorly.

        xx. Small sublingual tumors may be removed via a transoral approach, transferring Wharton duct if possible or resecting the submandibular gland if this is not possible.

        xxi. Larger sublingual tumors may require en-bloc resection of floor of mouth.

        xxii. Minor salivary gland tumors usually present as a submucosal mass. Imaging is necessary; endoscopy may be necessary for pharyngo-laryngo-tracheal lesions.

Clinical Guidelines

Approach to Evaluation for Salivary Gland Disease

A. History

    i. Age and gender

    ii. Salivary glands involved (onset, duration, progression)

    iii. Presence/absence of pain (character, intensity and duration)

    iv. Presence/absence of cranial nerve deficit (facial/trigeminal)

    v. Presence/absence of salivary discharge

    vi. Presence/absence of other symptoms

        a. Xerostomia and xerophthalmia

        b. Malocclusion, dental caries, trismus

        c. Otalgia

        d. Fever, unintentional weight loss

        e. Neck swelling/lymphadenopathy

        f. Thorough review of systems

    vii. Social history: Smoking/alcohol exposure, international travel, infectious exposure, and sexual history

    viii. Family history

        a. Autoimmune disorders

        b. Head and neck neoplasms

        c. Leukemia/lymphoma

        d. Genetic disorders/syndromes

B. Physical examination

    i. Vital signs (systemic signs of disease)

    ii. Complete head and neck examination

        a. Unilateral/one gland versus bilateral/multiglandular

        b. Careful examination of salivary ducts and orifices

        c. Careful examination of eyes and lacrimal glands and ducts

        d. Cranial nerve examination

        e. Neck examination for lymphadenopathy (unilateral versus bilateral)

    iii. Comprehensive body examination (lung, cardiovascular, skin changes/rashes/lesions, musculoskeletal/joints)

C. Imaging studies

    i. CXR: hilar lymphadenopathy, parenchymal infiltrate, lung lesions

    ii. Sialography (rarely used; largely replaced by sialendoscopy): evaluate ductal system

      iii. Ultrasound: no radiation, inexpensive, able to do in-office setting

      iv. CT: radiation exposure, quick, relatively inexpensive (compared to MRI)

      v. MRI: no radiation; improved soft-tissue imaging; can be used in lieu of sialendoscopy/sialography

D. Laboratory studies

    i. Order selectively and **not** as an all-inclusive panel (don't use "shotgun approach"); useful for the diagnosis of systemic disorders.

    ii. Particularly helpful in the diagnosis or exclusion of infectious, granulomatous, metabolic, autoimmune, hormonal, and other systemic disorders.

      a. Complete blood count.

      b. Erythrocyte sedimentation rate (ESR)

      c. Serum calcium and angiotension-converting enzyme elevation (sarcoidosis)

      d. Autoantibodies-rheumatoid factor (RF), antinuclear antibodies (ANA), anti-SSA and anti-SSB (Sjögren syndrome)

      e. Thyroid-stimulating hormone (hypothyroidism)

      f. Complete metabolic panel (hepatic or renal dysfunction)

      g. Human immunodeficiency virus test

      h. Nutritional or vitamin deficiencies

E. Sialendoscopy

    i. Diagnostic sialendoscopy may be utilized for visualization and inspection of the ductal system.

    ii. Inspection may reveal sialoliths, ductal stenosis, or salivary mucosal lesions such as polyps or sialodochitis.

    iii. Diagnose and potentially treat disorder/issues.

      a. Stricture

      b. Stenosis

      c. Sialolithiasis

      d. Inflammatory debris/mucous plugs

F. Fine needle aspiration biopsy (FNAB)

    i. Cytopathology results of FNAB must be carefully correlated with physical examination and other investigations in order to maximize the benefit of this diagnostic information.

    ii. Accurate method for the diagnosis of both neoplasms and nonneoplastic salivary gland swelling/disorders.

      a. Benign versus malignant neoplasm

      b. Lymphoma

      c. Chronic sialadenitis

      d. Sialadenosis

    iii. Beneficial in characterizing acute and chronic infections.

    iv. Special stains and cultures of aspirates.

      a. Tuberculosis

      b. Cat-scratch disease

      c. Actinomycosis

      d. Bacterial sialadenitis

      e. Radiation sialadenitis

    v. Limitation of FNAB.

      a. Inadequate tissue sampling

      b. Expertise of the cytopathologist

G. Diagnostic gland biopsy
   i. Lower lip biopsy of minor salivary glands is simple and valuable method of tissue sampling for inflammatory disorder (Sjögren syndrome).
   ii. Rarely, an incisional biopsy of the parotid gland is warranted in order to render a definitive diagnosis.
      a. Diffuse/generalized process
      b. Amyloidosis
      c. Sarcoidosis
      d. Sjögren syndrome
      e. Lymphoma

Classification of Salivary Gland Disorders

A. Nonneoplastic salivary gland disorders and dysfunction
   i. Inflammatory disorders and dysfunction
      a. Acute sialadenitis
         1. Sialolithiasis
         2. Viral (cytomegalovirus, coxsackie virus A and B, influenza, echovirus, and lymphocytic choriomeningitis virus)
         3. Bacterial (adult and neonatal suppurative, recurrent parotitis of childhood)—in difficult cases/aseptic cultures rule out tuberculosis
         4. Radiation-induced
      b. Chronic sialadenitis
         1. Obstructive
            • Primary infection with secondary obstruction
            • Primary obstruction with secondary infection
         2. Granulomatous disease
            • Sarcoidosis
            • Wegener granulomatosis
            • Tuberculosis
            • Cat-scratch disease
            • Actinomycosis
         3. Autoimmune (Sjögren syndrome)
         4. HIV-associated cystic sialadenitis
   ii. Noninflammatory disorders and dysfunction
      a. Acute
         1. Trauma
         2. Necrotizing sialometaplasia
         3. Pneumoparotitis
      b. Chronic
         1. Aging
         2. Sialadenosis
            • Endocrine disorders
               (a) Diabetes mellitus
               (b) Hypothyroidism
               (c) Acromegaly
               (d) Menopause
               (e) Pregnancy and lactation

- Nutritional disorders
  - (a) Alcoholism
  - (b) Obesity
  - (c) Nutritional/vitamin deficiency states
- Behavioral
  - (a) Anorexia
  - (b) Bulimia
- Medications
  - (a) Iodine
  - (b) Drugs affecting the adrenergic and cholinergic autonomic nervous system
  3. Amyloidosis
  4. Idiopathic
  B. Neoplastic salivary gland disease
    i. Benign
      a. Pleomorphic adenoma
      b. Warthin tumor
      c. Oncocytoma
    ii. Malignant
      a. Mucoepidermoid carcinoma
      b. Adenoid cystic carcinoma
      c. Adenocarcinoma
      d. Acinic cell carcinoma
      e. Squamous cell carcinoma
      f. Melanoma (metastatic to intraparotid lymph nodes and parotid gland)

Bibliography

Berg EE, Moore CE. Office-based sclerotherapy for benign parotid lymphoepithelial cysts in the HIV-positive patient. *Laryngoscope.* 2009;119:868-870.

Iro H, Zenk J, Escudier MP, et al. Outcome of minimally invasive management of salivary calculi in 4,691 patients. *Laryngoscope.* 2009;119:263-268.

Prendes BL, Orloff LA, Eisele DW. Therapeutic sialendoscopy for the management of radioiodine sialadenitis. *Arch Otolaryngol Head Neck Surg.* 2012;138(1):15-19.

Seikaly H, Jha N, Harris JP, et al. Long-term outcomes of submandibular gland transfer for prevention of postradiation xerostomia. *Arch Otolaryngol Head Neck Surg.* 2004;130:956-961.

Thackray A, Lucas R. Tumors of the major salivary glands. *Atlas of Tumor Pathology, Series 2, Fascicle 10.* Washington, DC: Armed Forces Institute of Pathology; 1974:107-117.

Questions

1. Which nerve supplies parasympathetic nerve fibers to the submandibular gland?

   A. Hypoglossal nerve

   B. Facial nerve

   C. Lingual nerve

   D. Mylohyoid nerve

   E. Vidian nerve.

2. What is the most common malignant tumor of the parotid gland?
   A. Mucoepidermoid carcinoma
   B. Acinic cell carcinoma
   C. Adenoid cystic carcinoma
   D. Lymphoma
   E. Salivary ductal carcinoma

3. What is the most common salivary gland neoplasm in children?
   A. Hemangioma
   B. Pleomorphic adenoma
   C. Mucoepidermoid carcinoma
   D. Lymphoma
   E. Adenoid cystic carcinoma

4. Which salivary gland tumor is strongly associated with tobacco exposure?
   A. Polymorphous low-grade adenocarcinoma
   B. Adenoid cystic carcinoma
   C. Pleomorphic adenoma
   D. Carcinoma ex-pleomorphic adenoma
   E. Warthin tumor

5. A 46-year-old woman, who received 150 mCi of Iodine-131 following total thyroidectomy for papillary thyroid carcinoma, presents with intermittent painful swelling of the parotid glands bilaterally. Patient is afebrile without white blood count elevation. There is decreased salivary production from Stenson duct with gland massage. Noncontrast CT scan shows diffuse parotid swelling. In addition to conservative measures (warm compresses, sialogogues, gland massage), the patient should also receive a/an
   A. 2-week course of oral clindamycin
   B. 4-6 week course of intravenous vancomycin
   C. sialendoscopy
   D. minor salivary gland lip biopsy
   E. MRI with gadolinium

Chapter 31
The Oral Cavity, Pharynx, and Esophagus

Normal Anatomy

Boundaries and Subunits

Oral Cavity

- Boundaries: vermilion border to junction of hard and soft palate and circumvallate papillae (linea terminalis).

Subunits: include lip, buccal mucosa, upper and lower alveolar ridges, retromolar trigones, oral tongue (anterior to circumvallate papillae), hard palate, and floor of mouth.

Oropharynx

- Boundaries: from junction of hard and soft palate and circumvallate papillae to vallecu-lae (plane of hyoid bone).

Subunits: include soft palate and uvula, base of tongue, pharyngoepiglottic and glossoepi-glottic folds, palatine arch (including tonsillar fossae, palatine tonsils, and pillars), valleculae, and lateral and posterior oropharyngeal walls.

Hypopharynx

- Boundaries: from level of hyoid bone (pharyngoepiglottic folds) to level of inferior bor-der of cricoid cartilage.

Subunits: include pyriform (piriform) sinus (laryngopharyngeal sulcus) which is bordered by aryepiglottic folds medially and thyroid cartilage anteriorly with its apex at the level of the cri-coid cartilage, posterior and lateral pharyngeal walls (lateral merges with lateral wall of pyriform sinus), and postcricoid region, which is inferior to the arytenoids, extends to inferior margin of cricoid cartilage, and is contiguous with medial walls of pyriform sinuses.

Esophagus

- Boundaries: from cricoid cartilage to cardia of stomach.

Subunits: include upper esophageal sphincter, body (cervical—thoracic—intra-abdominal), and lower esophageal sphincter.

Dimensions: incisors to cricopharyngeal sphincter is approximately 16 cm, to stomach 38 to 40 cm (in adults).

Anatomy of the Oral Cavity

Salivary Ducts

A. Parotid (Stenson): orifice is lateral to second molars.

B. Submaxillary (Wharton): orifice is in midline floor of mouth adjacent to lingual frenulum.

C. Sublingual (Rivinus): multiple orifices draining into floor of mouth or into submaxillary duct.

Teeth

- Deciduous teeth: 20

Adult: 32, which are numbered superiorly right to left (1-17), inferiorly left to right (17-32)

Tongue

Surface anatomy

A. Papillae: over the anterior 2/3 of the tongue including filiform (no taste function), fungiform (diffuse), and foliate (lateral tongue). The circumvallate papillae are large and lie in a V-shape at the junction of the anterior and posterior portions of the tongue.

B. Sulcus terminalis: a grove at the anterior margin of the circumvallate papillae.

C. Foramen cecum: a pit at the junction of the sulcus terminalis from which the embryologic thyroid begins its descent (etiology of thyroglossal duct cyst).

D. Frenulum: anterior fold of mucous membrane attaches the anterior inferior aspect of the tongue to the floor mouth and gingiva. Wharton ducts open on either side of the frenulum. May be congenitally short (tongue tied).

E. Lingual tonsil: lymphoid tissue extending over the base of the tongue (considered to be in oropharynx). Size varies among individuals. Blood supply from lingual artery and vein.

F. Valleculae: depressions on either side of the midline glossoepiglottic fold extending to the level of the hyoid bone. (Considered to be in oropharynx.)

Muscles

A. Extrinsic muscles of the tongue (cranial nerve XII): include the geniglossus, hyoglossus, styloglossus, and palatoglossus.

B. Intrinsic muscles (cranial nerve XII): include superior and inferior longitudinal, vertical, and transverse.

C. Fibrous septae—(septum linguae): defines midline and contains a triangular fat pad that is visualized on axial CT scan.

Sensory innervation: anterior different from posterior

A. Anterior 2/3 (oral tongue): sensations of touch, pain, temperature transmitted via lingual nerve (V3). Taste sensation is transmitted via lingual nerve to chorda tympani.

Taste:

Papillae ⟶ Afferent fibers ⟶ lingual nerve ⟶ chorda tympani ⟶
geniculate ganglion ⟶ intermediary nerve ⟶ nucleus solitarius

B. Posterior 1/3 (tongue base): touch and gag (visceral afferent) sensation is transmitted via cranial nerve IX to nucleus solitanius.

Taste: Circumvallate papillae and mucosa of epiglottis and valleculae ⟶ nucleus solitarius of the pons via cranial nerve IX.

Vascular supply

A. Lingual artery: second branch external carotid

B. Lingual vein: travels with hypoglossal nerve (veins of Ranine) (place hypoglossal nerve at risk during attempts to control bleeding)

Lymphatic drainage
  A. Anterior tongue: central drains to ipsilateral and contralateral nodes, tip to submental nodes, and marginal (lateral) to ipsilateral nodes. Skip nodes may be encountered in level 4.
  B. Posterior tongue drains to both ipsilateral and contralateral deep cervical nodes (jugulodigastric).
  C. Hard palate: forms the anterior 2/3 of the palate and consists of the palatine process of the maxilla and horizontal plates of the palatine bones. Covered with stratified squamous epithelium attached firmly to underlining bone.
  D. Foramina of the palate. → *Descending palatine artery + nerve*
       i. Greater palatine foramen: conveys descending palatine branch of V2 to innervate palate as well as descending palatine artery (third division of maxillary artery). Depression palpable 1 cm medial to second molar.
       ii. Accessory palatine foramen: posterior to greater palatine foramen, conveys lesser descending palatine artery to soft palate.
       iii. Incisural foramen: lies in midline of anterior palate, transmits incisural artery to anterior septum.
  E. Blood supply To palate.

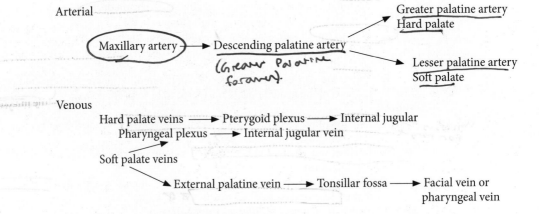

Arterial

Maxillary artery → Descending palatine artery → Greater palatine artery / Hard palate
                   (Greater Palatine foramen) → Lesser palatine artery / Soft palate

Venous

Hard palate veins → Pterygoid plexus → Internal jugular
Pharyngeal plexus → Internal jugular vein
Soft palate veins → External palatine vein → Tonsillar fossa → Facial vein or pharyngeal vein

Saliva (See also Chapter 30)
  A. Total of 1500 mL/day. When unstimulated, two-thirds is secreted by submaxillary glands, when stimulated, 2/3 by parotid glands. Reduced by radiotherapy, medications (primarily anticholinergics).
  B. Is 99.5% water with only 0.5% organic/inorganic solids. Electrolyte composition is sodium 10 mEq/L, potassium 26 mEq/L, chlorine 10 mEq/L, and bicarbonate 30 mEq/L. pH is 6.2:7.4.
  C. Organic component: includes glycoprotein and amylase (Circulating amylase of salivary origin can be distinguished from that of pancreatic origin).

Muscles of mastication
  A. Masseter, temporal, lateral pterygoid, medial pterygoid
  B. Blood supply: branches of maxillary artery
  C. Nerve supply: V3 (motor branch)

Anatomy of the Pharynx
Soft Palate
- Muscles
  (a) Palatoglossus (anterior pillar): approximates palate to tongue and narrows oropharyngeal opening.
  (b) Palatopharyngeus (posterior pillar): raises larynx and pharynx, closing oropharyngeal aperture.
  (c) Musculus uvulae: shortens uvula.
  (d) Levator veli palatini: raises soft palate to contact posterior pharyngeal wall.
  (e) Tensor veli palatini: pulls soft palate laterally to give rigidity and firmness to palate. Muscle originates in part on the eustachian tube cartilage, so contraction opens tube.
- Motor innervation
  (a) V3 motor division ⟶ pharyngeal plexus ⟶ tensor veli palatini
  (b) X ⟶ pharyngeal plexus ⟶ remainder of palatal muscles
- Sensory innervation: Cranial nerves V2, IX, X
- Blood supply: (see above)

Minor Salivary Glands
Palatine Tonsils
- Embryology: the lateral extension of the second pharyngeal pouch is absorbed and the dorsal remnants persist to become epithelium of palatine tonsil. The tonsillar pillars originate from the second and third branchial arches. The tonsillar crypts are first noted during the 12th week of gestation and the capsule during the 20th week.
- Anatomy: Lymphoid tissue with germinal centers containing 6 to 20 epithelial lined crypts. Capsule over deep surface is separated from the superior constrictor by thin areolar tissue. Lymphoid tissue of the palatine tonsil is contiguous with that of the lingual tonsil.
- The plicae triangularis is a variable fold consisting of lymphaic tissue and connective tissue, lies between tongue and palatoglossus, dorsal to glossopalatine arch.
- Gerlach tonsil: lymphoid tissue within lip of fossa of Rosenmueller—involves Eustachian tube.
- Arterial blood supply to the palatine tonsil.
  (a) Facial ⟶ Tonsillar branch ⟶ tonsil (main branch)
  (b) Facial ⟶ Ascending palatine ⟶ tonsil
  (c) Lingual ⟶ Dorsal lingual ⟶ tonsil
  (d) Ascending pharyngeal ⟶ tonsil
  (e) Maxillary ⟶ Lesser descending palatine ⟶ tonsil
- Venous blood supply.
  (a) Lingual vein
  (b) Pharyngeal vein
- Immunology.
  (a) B lymphocytes proliferate in germinal centers.
  (b) Immunoglobulins (IgG, A, M, D), compliment component, interferron, lysozymes, and cytokines accumulate in tonsil tissue.
  (c) The role of the tonsil remains controversial and to date there is no proven immunologic effect from tonsillectomy.
- Microbiologic environment of the adult mouth.
  (a) Staphylococci (first oral microbe in neonate; from skin contamination)

(b) Nonhemolytic streptococci
(c) Lactobacilli
(d) *Actinomyces*
(e) *Leptothrix*
(f) *Neisseria*
(g) *Bacteroides*
(h) Spirochetes
(i) Micrococci
(j) Viruses
  ○ Myxovirus
  ○ Adenovirus
  ○ Picornavirus
  ○ Coronaviruses
  ○ Human papilloma virus (HPV)

Oropharyngeal Walls

- Passavant ridge: visible constriction of superior end of superior constrictor where fibers of the palatopharyngeal constrictor interdigitate. Visualized endoscopically during approximation of palate to posterior pharyngeal wall and during elevation of the pharynx during swallowing.
- Lateral pharyngeal bands: are rests of lymphoid tissue just behind posterior pillars.
- Muscles.
- Pharyngeal constrictors.
  (a) Superior constrictor: originates on the medial pterygoid plate, mandible, and base of tongue and inserts on median raphe.
  (b) Middle constrictor: originates on the hyoid bone and stylohyoid ligament.
  (c) Inferior constrictor: origin is on the oblique line of thyroid cartilage.
- Pharyngeal and laryngeal elevators (shorten pharynx) and origins.
  (a) Salpingopharyngeus: temporal bone and eustachian tube
  (b) Stylopharyngeus: styloid process
  (c) Stylohyoid: styloid process
- Upper esophageal sphincter: the cricopharyngeus muscle is the most inferior portion of inferior constrictor, and is separated from it by a triangular dehiscence termed Killian dehiscence (through which a Zenker diverticulum can form). Other dehiscences include the traiangular Laimer-Haeckerman space between the posterior cricopharyngeus and the esophageal musculature, and the Killian-Jamieson space, a lateral dehiscence inferior to the cricopharyngeus through which branches of the inferior thyroid artery pass. During rest, the muscle is in tonic contraction and relaxes during swallowing. The sphincter is actively dilated by laryngeal elevation during deglutition.

Physiology of Normal Swallowing

Overview

The laryngopharynx functions as a "time-share" for respiration and deglutition. The most basic function of larynx is airway protection. Some herbivores and infants are able to breathe and swallow simultaneously, whereas adults must interrupt respiration (usually during expiration) to swallow. During deglutition the formed bolus must be moved completely through the pharynx while the glottis is closed. Defective deglutition results in either inadequate nutrition, aspiration due to failure to protect the airway, or both. The normal swallow is best understood by dividing into three phases:

A. The oral phase prepares the food for delivery to the pharynx (some authors term this the oral preparatory phase). Components include:
   i. Mastication
   ii. Addition and mixing of saliva
   iii. Control of bolus: tongue, lips, buccinator, palate
   iv. Selection and verification of safety of bolus (volume, taste, fish bones, etc)

The oral phase is under voluntary control, and ends when the bolus is pressed against the faucial arches to precipitate the involuntary pharyngeal phase. Pressure-sensitive receptors on anterior tonsillar pillar (IX, X) trigger the involuntary pharyngeal swallow.

B. The pharyngeal phase of the swallow moves the bolus quickly (in less than one second) past the closed glottis and through upper esophageal sphincter into the esophagus. The components of the pharyngeal phase are:
   i. Nasopharyngeal closure with palate elevation (levator, tensor vs palatini) and contraction of superior constrictor (Passavant ridge)
   ii. Cessation of respiration (usually during expiration)
   iii. Glottic closure: with approximation of true vocal cords, false vocal cords and arytenoids to epiglottis (in order).
   iv. Bolus propulsion: via tongue base protrusion ("tongue driving force") and contraction of the pharyngeal constrictor muscles.
   v. Laryngeal elevation and pharyngeal shortening: results in protection of laryngeal vestibule, epiglottic rotation, and active dilatation of cricopharyngeal sphincter.
   vi. Epiglottic rotation: active due to laryngeal elevation, passive due to pressure of bolus.
   vii. UES dilatation: relaxation of cricopharyngeus muscle, active dilatation due to laryngeal elevation, and pressure of bolus. Subatmospheric pressure can be measured at UES ahead of bolus.

C. The *esophageal phase* conveys bolus to the stomach in an average of 3 to 6 seconds with primary peristalsis and relaxation of LES.

D. Nerves of Swallowing
   i. Sensory receptors: found on soft palate, tongue base, tonsillar pillars, posterior pharyngeal wall.
   ii. Central ganglions: V—gasserian, IX—inferior (Andersch) and superior (petrosal) ganglions, X—inferior (jugular) and superior (nodose) ganglions
   iii. Efferent pathways: (List)
      a. V: Teeth, jaw, masticators, buccinator
      b. V, X: Palate
      c. VII: Lips, facial musculature
      d. IX: Pharynx
      e. X: Pharynx, larynx, esophagus
      f. XII: Tongue

Anatomy of the Esophagus

40 cm in length in adult

Muscles

A. No serosa.
B. Outer longitudinal layer.
C. Inner circular layer.
D. Upper 5 cm skeletal muscle.
E. Lower ½ smooth muscle.
F. Upper-mid portion is overlap of striated and smooth muscle.
G. Innervation: myenteric plexus of Auerbach within muscle layers (parasympathetic ganglion cells).
H. Vagus nerves rotate clockwise when viewed from above: left moves to anterior surface, R moves to posterior surface.

Bolus transit: upper one third is striated muscle and has most rapid peristalsis—less than 1-second transit. Lower two-thirds smooth muscle, approximately 3-second transit. Gravity plays only minor role in normal swallowing, so position changes minimal. Overdistension of esophagus leads to spasm.

Peristalsis

A. Primary: physiologic propulsive wave of sequential constriction and shortening.
B. Secondary: nonphysiologic retrograde peristalsis
C. Tertiary: nonphysiologic segmental constriction without propulsion

Submucosa: Contains connective tissue, blood and lymphatic vessels, and parasympathetic ganglion cells and fibers: myenteric plexus of Meissner.
Mucosa: Contains muscularis mucosae, the lamina propria, and stratified squamous epithelium with minimal secretory function and poor absorption.

Lower Esophageal sphincter (LES)

A. Closure prevents reflux of gastric contents into esophagus.
B. Is not a true anatomic structure, but an active zone of high pressure extending 1 to 2 cm above and below diaphragm that relaxes during passage of the peristaltic wave.
C. The Angle of His is the oblique angle of entry of the esophagus into the stomach. It is absent in infants, predisposing them to reflux—2/3 of 4-month-old infants reflux.
D. LES function is controlled by parasympathetic tone (acetylcholine) and gastrin.
E. The diaphragmatic crura surrounding hiatus create a sling which assists in sphincteric function. This effect is lost with a hiatus hernia.

Disorders of the Oral Cavity, Pharynx, and Esophagus_____

Disorders of the Oral Cavity

Dental Developmental Abnormalities

A. Anodontia (partial or complete): is the hereditary absence of teeth.
B. Dilaceration: the tooth root, as a result of trauma, fails to develop normally, resulting in an angular malformation of the root. The condition is associated with rickets and cretinism.
C. Supernumerary teeth.

    D. Enamel hypoplasia.

    E. Enamel discoloration: may be due to antibiotic exposure (tetracycline) prior to eruption.

Periapical Disease

    A. Granuloma (asymptomatic)

    B. Alveolar abscess (due to caries involving root canal)

       i. May lead to sinusitis, osteomyelitis, Ludwig angina, or bacteremia.

    C. Radicular cyst

Inflammation of Oral Mucosa: Stomatitis is the general term for any inflammatory disorder of the oral mucosa. It can be associated with the following diseases:

    A. Gingivitis

    B. Periodontitis (pyorrhea)

    C. Periodontitis: is chronic degenerative destruction of the periodontal tissue. Papillon-Lefevre syndrome is periodontitis, hyperkeratosis of the soles of the feet and palms of the hands, and calcification of the dura.

    D. Acute necrotizing ulcerative gingivitis (ANUG, Vincent angina, trench mouth) is due to synergistic mixed anaerobic infection including *Borrelia vincentii* (fusiform bacillus). Symptoms are a fetid odor to the breath, excessive salivation, and bleeding gingiva. Treatment is oral hygiene and penicillin.

    E. Herpetic gingivostomatitis and herpes labialis are usually due to herpes simplex. Herpes labialis is the most common viral infection of the mouth. Shingles due to herpes zoster is rare.

    F. Herpangina (group A coxsackievirus): is a vesicular eruption of the soft palate, usually associated with fever and coryza.

    G. Noma: is an acute necrotizing gingivitis that rapidly spreads into adjacent soft tissue. It is most commonly seen in third world countries, with the highest incidence in children. *Borrelia* and other anaerobic fusiform bacilli are always present.

    H. Bacterial stomatitis (Streptococci, Staphylocci, Gonococci).

    I. Thrush (*Candida albicans*): often seen in presence of immunocompromise, xerostomia, or in patients using inhaled steroids. Topical or systemic anti-fungal therapy may be used for treatment.

    J. Actinomycosis: (filiform bacillis): Forms abscesses with masses of bacteria that resemble "sulfur granules".

    K. Blastomycosis.

    L. Histoplasmosis *(Histoplasm capsylatum)*.

    M. Pyogenic granuloma: when forms on gingival termed "epulis".

    N. Mucositis: commonly encountered as a result of chemotherapy or radiation therapy.

Noninfectious Lesions

    A. Sutton disease (recurrent aphthous ulcers [RAU]): forms multiple, large deep ulcers that can cause extensive scarring of the oral cavity.

    B. Erythema multiforme: "iris like" lesions that may involve the oral cavity, conjunctiva, and skin. Often preceded by upper respiratory infection (URI).

    C. Pemphigus vulgaris (intraepidermoid bullae)

    D. Pemphigoid (subepidermoid bullae): differentiation from pemphigus requires histologic examination with staining for basement membrane.

    E. Lichen planus: is a reticular branching pattern of leukoplakia with most common site on buccal mucosa. Advanced cases termed erosive lichen planus with a 10% to 15% chance of progression to squamous cell carcinoma. Treatment is topical steroids.

  F. Systematic lupus erythematosus.

  G. Bechet disease: oral ulcerations, conjunctivitis, iritis, and urethretis.

Oral Mucosal Manifestations of Systematic Processes

  A. Pernicious anemia: is caused by a lack of vitamin B_{12}. The tongue may show lobulations of its surface or, in advanced cases, be shiny, smooth, and red. Oral mucosa may exhibit an irregular erythema.

  B. Iron deficiency anemia: oral mucosa is ash gray (may be associated with Plummer-Vinson syndrome). Tongue is smooth and devoid of papillae.

  C. Thalassemia (mediterranean anemia): oral mucosa has diffuse pallor and cyanosis.

  D. Polycythemia: oral mucosa is bright blue-red with gingival bleeding.

  E. Osler-Weber-Rendu disease (hereditary hemorrhagic telangiectasia): forms spider-like blood vessels or angiomatous-appearing lesions on the oral mucosa, tongue, and nasal mucosa and is associated with recurrent epistaxis. The gastrointestinal tract may be involved and transfusion may be required.

  F. Sturge-Weber syndrome: port-wine stain of the face, oral cavity, or tongue associated with vascular malformations of the meninges and cerebral cortex.

  G. Thrombocytopenic purpura: purpura due to marked decrease in platelets from a variety of causes. Initial manifestations are often oral petechiae and ecchymosis.

  H. Menopausal gingivostomatitis (senile atrophy): is dry oral mucosa with a burning sensation, diffuse erythema, shiny mucosa, and occasionally fissuring in the melobuccal fold. Pathophysiology unknown and treatment is symptomatic.

  I. Nutritional pathology (deficiency).

    i. Riboflavin: atrophic glossitis, angular cheilitis, gingivostomatitis

    ii. Pyridoxine: angular cheilitis

    iii. Nicotinic acid: angular cheilitis

    iv. Vitamin C: gingivitis and "bleeding gums"

  J. Kaposi sarcoma: often presents as violaceous macules on the oral mucosa. Uncommon except in association with AIDS where it is considered an AIDS-defining condition.

Pigmentation Changes of the Oral Cavity

  A. Melanosis: physiologic pigmentation, often seen as dark patches of the oral mucosa.

  B. Amalgam tattoo: inadvertent tattoo of gingiva from dental amalgam introduced through a mucosal laceration.

  C. Peutz-Jeghers syndrome: melanotic macules periorally

  D. Bismuth: black

  E. Lead: blue-gray line (Burton line) that follows margin of gingiva

  F. Mercury: gray/violet

  G. Silver: violet/blue/gray

  H. Addison disease: brown

  I. Hemochromatosis: bronze

  J. Xanthomatous disease: yellow/gray

  K. Kaposi sarcoma: violaceous macules

Common Childhood Diseases with Oral Cavity Manifestations

  A. Measles (rubeola): Koplik spots (pale round spots on erythematous base) seen on buccal and lingual mucosa

  B. Chicken pox (varicella): vesicles

  C. Scarlet fever: strawberry tongue

  D. Congenital heart disease: gingivitis, cyanotic gums

  E. Kawasaki disease: strawberry tongue

i. **Leukoplakia (white plaque)**: Descriptive term for a white hyperkeratoic lesion that may or may not be associated with dysplastic change on histologic examination. It occurs most frequently on the lip (vermilion) and then in descending order of frequency on the buccal mucosa, mandibular gingiva, tongue, floor of mouth, hard palate, maxillary gingiva, lip mucosa, and soft palate. Less than 10% of *isolated* (see nodular variant below) leukoplakia will demonstrate carcinoma or severe dysplasia on biopsy.

ii. **Erythroplakia (red plaque)**: is a granular erythematous area, often encountered in association with leukoplakia (nodular leukoplakia). 50% will demonstrate severe dysplasia or carcinoma *in situ* on biopsy.

iii. **Nodular leukoplakia**: (mixed white and red plaques). Greater malignant potential, similar to erythroplakia in risk of malignancy. May be seen in association with frank invasive cancer.

iv. **Median rhomboid glossitis**: is a smooth reddish area of the midline of the tongue devoid of papillae. It sometimes has a corresponding lesion along the hard palate. It may be associated with candida overgrowth.

v. **Fordyce granules**: are painless, pinpoint yellow nodules that occur bilaterally on the posterior buccal mucosa. These represent enlarged ectopic sebaceous glands.

vi. **Macroglossia**: can be due to several causes.
 a. Hemangioma
 b. Lymphangioma
 c. Myxedema
 d. Acromegaly
 e. Amyloidosis
 f. Benign cysts
 g. Pierre Robin (actually relative macroglossia due to micrognathia)
 h. Tertiary syphilis
 i. Von Gierke disease (glycogen storage disease Type I)
 j. Hurler syndrome (mucopolysaccharidosis)
 k. Down syndrome
 l. Infection, that is, actinomycosis

Tumors of the Mandible (Excluding Carcinoma)

A. **Mandibular tori**: are benign bony exostoses commonly seen on lingual or buccal aspect of anterior mandible.

B. **Odontogenic fibroma**: presents as a circumscribed radiolucency with smooth borders, occurring around the crown of unerupted teeth in children, adolescents and young adults. Radiographically it resembles a dentigerous cyst. Treatment is excision and nearly always curative.

C. **Ameloblastoma**: is a neoplasm of enamel origin that presents in the third and fourth decade. The most common site is the mandible, especially the molar region. Tumors are slow growing and painless, expanding surrounding bone. Treatment is excision.

D. **Cementomas**: are a broad class of lesions that form cementum (bone-like connective tissue that covers tooth root). Tumors usually arise at the tip of tooth roots in young adults. The radiographic appearance can vary from radiolucent to densely radiopaque, depending on the lesion. Treatment is simple enucleation.

E. **Odonotoma**: is a tumor composed of ameloblasts (enamel) and odontoblasts (dentin). It appears as irregular radiopaque mass, often between tooth roots and is associated with unerupted teeth. Simple enucleation is sufficient.

F. Adenoameloblastoma: is a well-encapsulated follicular cyst, occurring most commonly in the anterior maxilla of adolescent girls in association with impacted teeth. A rare malignant variant exists. Treatment is excision.

G. Ameloblastic fibroma: is a slow-growing, painless lesion seen in the molar area of the mandible in adolescents and children. It contains both epithelial and mesenchymal tissue and is radiographically similar to an ameloblastoma.

H. Ameloblastic sarcoma: malignant fast-growing, painful, and aggressive variant of ameloblastic fibroma. Occurs most commonly in young adults. Treatment is surgical excision. Recurrence is common.

I. Ewing sarcoma: rapidly growing tumor with local pain and swelling. It is most common between ages 10 and 25 years. The mandible is the most common site in head and neck. Treatment is radiation and chemotherapy. Survival is about 50%.

J. Osteogenic sarcoma: rapidly growing, aggressive malignant tumor of bone. It occurs primarily in adolescents and young adults. Survival of mandibular variant better than long bone. Combined therapy often utilized.

Odontogenic Cysts

A. Radicular cyst: is the most common cyst, called a "periapical cyst" when it involves the tooth root. Secondary to dental infection and is usually asymptomatic. It presents as a radiolucent area on x-ray, and treatment is extraction or root canal therapy.

B. Dentigerous (follicular) cyst: is a development abnormality caused by a defect in enamel formation. It is always associated with an unerupted tooth crown, and most common in the mandibular third molar or maxillary cuspid. Ameloblastoma formation occurs in the cyst wall.

C. Odontogenic keratocyst: mimicks dentigerous cysts if associated with a tooth root. Diagnosis is based on histology, and treatment is excision. Curettage and partial excision result in a high rate of recurrence.

Other Oral Cavity Lesions

A. Hairy tongue: hyperplasia of filiform papillae. It may be black, blue, brown or white depending on microflora and nicotine staining, and is often associated with candida overgrowth.

B. Epulis: nonspecific term for tumor or tumor like masses of the gingiva, often a pyogenic granuloma. Common in pregnancy. Congenital epulis is rare and resembles a granular cell myoblastoma. A giant cell epulis (giant cell reparative granuloma) is more common and histologic examination demonstrates reticular and fibrous connective tissue with numerous giant cells. Radiographs show cuffing or sclerotic margins of bone.

C. Ranula: mucocele of the sublingual gland that presents in the floor of the mouth. *Plunging ranula* penetrates the mylohyoid muscle and presents as a soft submental neck mass. Excision should include the entire sublingual gland in order to prevent recurrence, with care taken to protect the submandibular duct and the lingual nerve.

D. Torus palatini: benign excessive bone growth in midline of palate that continues to enlarge beyond puberty. Occasionally it must be removed in order to prevent denture irritation.

Disorders of the Oropharynx

Soft Palate

A. Cleft palate: is due to failure of fusion, and associated with a characteristic voice change and nasal regurgitation of liquids. A submucous cleft may be present. Eustachian tube disorder is due to failure of tensor veli palatini to open ET on swallowing.

   B. Congenital elongation of the uvula.
   C. Squamous Papillomas.
   D. Aphthous ulcers.
   E. Leukoplakia, erythroplakia, squamous cell cancer.
   F. Minor salivary gland tumors.
   G. Quincke disease: Swelling of the uvula often in association with acute bacterial tonsillitis. Uvular swelling can also occur with trauma, (heroic snoring, burn from hot food or beverage).
   H. Angioneurotic edema: can occur as familial (C1 esterase deficiency), allergic, or due to ACE inhibitor. ACE inhibitor induced angioedema is more common in those of African descent and can occur at any time following initiation of therapy. Severe swelling may be preceded by sentinel swelling. Tracheotomy may be required.

Palatine Tonsils: Differential Diagnosis of Tonsillar Mass
   A. Acute tonsillitis
   B. Tonsillolith
   C. Peritonsillar abscess
   D. Mononucleosis
   E. Parapharyngeal space mass
   F. Lymphoma
   G. Squamous cell cancer (SCC)

SCC may be either standard variant (found in smokers/drinkers) or HPV-related (HPV 16 and 18, high levels of P16, often found in nonsmokers, different biological behavior and response to treatment).

Acute tonsillitis
   A. Etiology
      i. Group A beta-hemolytic streptococci (GABHS)
      ii. Haemophilus influenza
      iii. *Streptococcus pneumoniae*
      iv. Staphylococci (with dehydration, antibiotics)
      v. Tuberculosis (immunocompromised)
   B. Differential diagnosis
      i. Infectious mononucleosis
      ii. Malignancy (lymphoma, leukemia, carcinoma)
      iii. Diphtheria
      iv. Scarlet fever
      v. Vincent angina
      vi. Leukemia
      vii. Agranulocytosis
      viii. Pemphigus

Acute peritonsillar abscess
   A. Pus located deep to tonsil capsule between tonsil and superior constrictor muscle
   B. Presents with deviation of the tonsil and uvula toward the midline, swelling of soft palate, often with trismus
   C. Complications of peritonsillar abscess
      i. Parapharyngeal abscess (due to rupture through superior constrictor)
      ii. Venous thrombosis, phlebitis, bacteremia, endocarditis
      iii. Arterial involvement to include thrombosis, hemorrhage, pseudoaneurysm
      iv. Mediastinitis
      v. Brain Abscess

      vi. Airway Obstruction

     vii. Aspiration pneumonia

    viii. Nephritis (due to streptococcal antigen)

     ix. Peritonitis

      x. Dehydration

Tonsillectomy

  A. Procedure referred to by Celsius in De Medicina (10AD)

  B. First documented surgery by Cague of Rheims (1757)

  C. Indications of tonsillectomy:

      i. Recurrent infections: 3 per year for 3 years, 5 per year for 2 years, 7 or more in 1 year, or greater than 2 weeks of school or work missed in 1 year.

     ii. Hypertrophy causing upper airway obstruction (sleep disordered breathing or frank sleep apnea)

    iii. Peritonsillar abscess

    iv. Suspicion of malignancy, either unilateral enlarged or search for unknown primary

     v. Hypertrophy causing deglutition problems

    vi. Recurrent tonsillitis causing febrile seizures

    vii. Diptheria carrier

   viii. Treatment of early stage cancer (often performed with robotic assistance (TORS)

    ix. Morbidity: postoperative hemorrhage 2% to 4%

     x. Mortality 1 in 25,000 (hemorrhage, airway obstruction, anesthesia)

Disorders of the Tongue Base

  A. Lingual tonsillar hypertrophy

  B. Lingual tonsillitis

  C. Lingual thyroid (failure of the descent)

  D. Benign vallecular cysts

  E. Neoplasms

      i. Squamous cell cancer

     ii. Lymphoma

    iii. Minor salivary gland tumors (usually malignant)

    iv. Lingual thyroid (due to failure of descent)

Disorders of the Oropharyngeal Walls

  A. Inflammation of the lateral pharyngeal bands

  B. Cobblestoning: of posterior wall (inflammation of lymphoid rests)

  C. Trauma (child falling with stick in mouth)

  D. Squamous cell cancer

  E. Eagle syndrome (pain due to elongated styloid process)

Diseases of the Hypopharynx

  A. Inflammation (associated with supraglottis)

  B. Angioneurotic edema (often associated with ACE-inhibitor usage)

  C. Osteophyte

  D. Aberrant carotid artery

  E. Carotid aneurysm

  F. Parapharyngeal space mass

  G. Hypopharyngeal carcinoma

Dysphagia

May be oral, pharyngeal, or esophageal. Common in elderly or debilitated. Associated with shortened survival in elderly patients with dementia.

Evaluation

- History
  - (a) Underlying disease, onset and progression
  - (b) Weight loss, odynophagia, dietary changes and consistencies, coughing with meals
  - (c) Recurrent pneumonia, aspiration
  - (d) Voice change, "mucus"
  - (e) Oral control, failure of swallowing initiation
  - (f) Location of sensation of food sticking
  - (g) Odynophagia, substernal chest pain, heartburn
- Complete head and neck examination
- Radiographic studies
  - (a) Esophagram: evaluates esophagus
  - (b) Modified barium swallow (3-phase swallow, "cookie" swallow): evaluates pharyngeal function.
    - ○ Radiographic findings: pharyngeal dilatation, penetration or aspiration into trachea, into larynx, stenosis, obstruction, disorders of peristalsis, persistent cricopharyngeal bar
    - ○ Fiberoptic examination of swallowing (FEES) with or without sensory testing (at same time as physical examination)
    - ○ Esophagoscopy sedated transoral or unsedated transnasal route (TNE)
- Pathologic entities
  - (a) Anatomic defects: such as cleft palate, tumor, head and neck surgery, stenosis.
  - (b) Timing: Neurologic defects such as stroke or head injury, alterations in level of consciousness, injury to brain stem, cerebellum, long tracts, or peripheral cranial nerves: either sensory or motor.
  - (c) Motor: Muscle weakness due to weight loss and sarcopenia (frailty), primary myopathy, peripheral neuropathy—cranial nerve or injury to myoneural plexis, or central injury to brain stem or cerebellum. Disorders of peristalsis.

Diseases Associated With Dysphagia

- Inflammatory lesions of the pharynx associated with viral infections
- Vincent angina
- Thrush (*Candida*)
- Tonsillitis (peritonsillar abscess and lingual tonsillitis)
- Retropharyngeal abscess
- Plummer-Vinson syndrome
- Polio and post-polio syndrome
- Parkinson disease
- Stroke
- Pseudobulbar palsy
- Cerebrovascular accident
- Acute myelogenous leukemia
- Multiple sclerosis
- Myasthenia gravis

- Polyneuritis
- Dermatomyositis
- Myotonia congenita or dystrophica
- Muscular dystrophy
- Primary muscular tumors
- Primary muscular invasion due to tumor
- Zenker diverticulum
- Squamous cell carcinoma of esophagus
- Adenocarcinoma of esophagus
- Tongue, pharyngeal, or laryngeal carcinoma
- Thyroid mass
- Achalasia
- Chagas disease
- Scleroderma
- Raynaud phenomenon
- Esophageal webs
- Esophageal spasm
- Psychologic illness
- Schatzki ring (lower esophageal)
- Burns
- Dysphagia lusoria
- Leiomyoma (benign)

Specific Neuromuscular Disorders of Swallowing (sensory, motor, or central coordination)

Usually more than one etiology is present.

A. Tongue base weakness: inanition, neuromuscular disease, stroke, brain stem disorder, poor bolus propulsion with residue in vallecula and over tongue base on MBS or FEES. Treatment is chin tuck to close vallecula, tongue base strengthening exercises, and liquid rinse during meals.

B. Oral dysfunction: tumor or surgery, stroke, (especially brain stem), and other neuromuscular disorder. Poor oral control, oral residue, and failure to initiate swallow. Treatment is tongue strengthening exercises, and articulation exercises.

C. Pharyngeal sensory loss: associated with stroke, gastroesophageal reflux, aging, or surgical injury. Retained pharyngeal secretions on MBS or FEES, with decreased sensation on sensory testing. Silent (without coughing) penetration of laryngeal vestibule, and aspiration, typically worse with thin liquids. Treatment is thickening of liquids to provide more time for pharyngeal response.

D. Vocal cord paralysis: suspected with voice change and aspiration of thin liquids. Treatment is vocal cord medialization.

E. Vocal cord weakness: associated with aging, general debilitation, and Parkinson disease. It is manifested by failure of glottic closure, vocal cord bowing, and weak, breathy voice. Treatment is vocal cord adduction exercises and vocal cord augmentation.

F. Failure of laryngeal elevation: associated with neuromuscular disorders, generalized debilitation, and stroke (especially brain stem). MBS and FEES demonstrate tongue base and pyriform sinus residue and failure of cricopharyngeal opening. Treatment is laryngeal elevation exercises, Mendelson maneuver (hold larynx as high as possible for as long as possible with each swallow), EMG biofeedback, and transcutaneous electric stimulation of suprahyoid muscles.

G. Generalized pharyngeal weakness: associated with stroke and a variety of general and neuromuscular diseases. It is manifested by moderate to severe residue with failure to clear completely on subsequent swallows, secondary penetration/aspiration, often worse with solids than with liquids. Treatment is multiple consecutive swallows, small bites, and liquid wash between bites.

H. Failure of UES opening: associated with failure of laryngeal elevation, gastro-esophageal reflux, neuromuscular disease, and Zenker diverticulum. It is manifested by a cricopharyngeal "bar" or a pharyngeal diverticulum seen on radiographic examination, pharyngeal residue, or regurgitation following a swallow. (Pharyngeal bar may be present in up to 30% of asymptomatic elderly). Treatment depends on diagnosis and may be addressed by either strengthening of active UES opening or reduction of sphincteric closure (chemodenervation or cricopharyngeal myotomy).

I. Disorders of peristalsis: reduced, (atony) excessive, (spasm) or disordered (secondary or tertiary).

Diseases of the Esophagus

Inflammatory Disease
A. Gastroesophageal reflux with esophagitis.
B. Barrett esophagitis: metaplasia of squamous epithelium to columnar mucosa.
C. Infections: Candidiasis—common in HIV. Treat with antifungal, including topical or systemic.

Diverticuli
A. Zenker diverticulum: occurs in Killian dehiscence inferior to fibers of the inferior constrictor and superior to cricopharyngeus. Associated with failure of UES opening due incomplete cricopharyngeal muscle relaxation, muscle fibrosis, or failure of active dilatation due to inadequate laryngeal elevation. Symptoms include regurgitation of undigested food, dysphagia and weight loss, aspiration and cough. Treatment is cricopharyngeal myotomy, with or without excision, suspension, or inversion of sac) or endoscopic diverticulotomy with either laser or stapler.
B. Epiphrenic diverticulum: occurs just superior to cardioesphogeal junction, usually on the right side. Symptoms are minimal, and constitutes13% of all esophageal diverticula.
C. Traction diverticulum: are usually midesophageal, typically on left side, and often due to traction of adjacent inflammatory process (usually tuberculosis).

Hiatal Hernia (HH)
Hiatal hernia is defined as a portion of stomach passing up through the esophageal hiatus of the diaphragm. HH may be either *sliding* (most common) in which the esophagogastric junction (EGJ) herniates into the thorax, or *paraesophageal* in which the EGJ is below the diaphragm while the fundus of the stomach bulges around it and through the diaphragm into the chest cavity. Associated conditions for sliding HH include:
A. Increased intra-abdominal pressure due to pregnancy, obesity, tight clothing, ascites, constipation.
B. Age: the incidence is 30% in the older population.
C. Weakness of esophageal hiatus: results in incompetence of the LES.
D. Kyphoscoliosis.
E. Sandifer syndrome: is abnormal contortions of the neck associated with unrecognized hiatus hernia in children.
F. Saint triad: is gallbladder disease, colonic diverticular disease, and hiatus hernia.

Motility Disorders

Diagnosis made with contrast barium study and manometry. Radiographic findings include: tertiary contractions trapping barium in segments, retrograde displacement of barium ("intraesophageal reflux"), spontaneous waves not preceded by a swallow, or three to five repetitive waves following a single swallow. Following are some common pathologic causes of motility disorders:

- Polymyositis: muscle weakness secondary to inflammatory and degenerative changes in *striated muscle*. Proximal muscle weakness (hip and shoulder) is most common presenting symptom. When associated with skin rashes, it is termed *dermatomyositis*. Involves the striated muscle of the hypopharynx and upper esophagus. Peristalsis is diminished and poorly coordinated, and the esophagus may be dilated. Manometric evaluation demonstrates decreased UES pressure and reduced peristaltic waves. Hiatus hernia and reflux are absent.
- Scleroderma (Progressive systemic sclerosis): involves smooth muscle with a marked decrease in lower esophageal sphincter pressure, associated reflux, and esophagitis. May have Raynaud phenomenon. 60% have significant dysphagia and up to 40% of patients develop a stricture secondary to reflux. Normal peristalsis may be seen in the upper esophagus, with aperistalsis, dilation, and gastroesophageal reflux distally. Barium may distend the esophagus in the supine position with free passage in the upright position.
- Achalasia: disorder of esophageal motility characterized by aperistalsis, esophageal dilatation, and failure of LES relaxation. Barium swallow demonstrates failure of peristalsis, dilatation, and an air-fluid level in the upright position.
  - (a) Primary achalasia: due to idiopathic degeneration of the ganglion cells of Auerbach plexis.
  - (b) Secondary achalasia: due to carcinoma, CVA, Chagas disease, postvagotomy syndrome, or diabetes mellitus.

Other Motility Disorders of the Esophagus

- A. Esophageal spasm: simultaneous, repetitive, nonperistaltic and often powerful contractions of the esophagus.
- B. Presbyesophagus: associated with age and manifested by incoordination of sphincter function, reduced peristalsis, and frequent tertiary contractions.
- C. Ganglion degeneration: associated with achalasia, Chagas disease, and seen in the elderly.
- D. Motility disorder due to irritant such as gastroesophageal reflux or corrosive injury.
- E. Neuromuscular disorder due to diabetes, alcoholism, ALS, or other dysautonomia.
- F. Spasm may be described as "curling", "tertiary contractions", "corkscrew esophagus", or "rosary bead esophagus".
- G. Cricopharyngeal achalasia: is failure of UES dilatation—see discussion above.
  - i. Lower esophageal ring (Shatzki ring): concentric ring that occurs at the esophagogastric junction (EGJ). It is encountered in 6% to 14% of barium studies, but only one third are symptomatic. Symptoms are rare unless the lumen is less than 13 mm. Dysphagia is intermittent and primarily to solid food. Heartburn is rare and manometry is normal. Is best seen in barium studies done in recumbent position or EGD. Often not seen on rigid esophagoscopy. A Shatzki ring involves only mucosa, whereas peptic stricture due to reflux involves both mucosa and muscle layers.

     ii. Esophageal Webs: dysphagia develops slowly, are asymmetric (as opposed to rings and strictures). Usually on anterior wall, often associated with Plummer-Vinson syndrome (Patterson-Kelly, sideropenic dysphagia).

     iii. Plummer-Vinson syndrome: Most common in females (F:M 10:1) typically of Scandinavian descent. Syndrome is associated with iron deficiency anemia, upper esophageal web, hypothyroidism, glossitis, cheilitis, and gastritis. Dysphagia may be present even in the absence of a web. Anemia may precede other features. There is an increased risk of postcricoid carcinoma (15% in one study). Diagnosis is by barium swallow (which may show abnormalities in esophageal propulsion and/or a web). Check CBC, serum iron, ferritin levels. Treatment is with iron replacement and dilatation of the web. Etiology is unclear—possible relationship to GERD.

Esophageal Trauma

- Boerhaave syndrome: a linear tear 1 to 4 cm in length through all three layers of the esophagus due to sudden increase in esophageal pressure, usually due to vomiting. Rare, 90% occur on left, encountered in males more commonly (5:1). Presents with severe knife-like epigastric pain radiating to left shoulder, may not have significant hematemesis. Develop respiratory difficulty, subcutaneous emphysema, and shock. CXR demonstrates initially widened mediastinum, then left pleural effusion or hydro-pneumothorax. Tear may be difficult to differentiate from myocardial infarction, pulmonary embolus, or perforated ulcer. Treatment is thoracotomy and repair.
- Mallory-Weiss Syndrome: tear of gastroesophageal junction or cardia of stomach due to forceful vomiting. Is most commonly encountered in alcoholics, (usually men older than 40) and presents with massive hematemesis.
- Esophageal foreign bodies: most common location is at site of physiologic or pathologic narrowing, such as cricopharyngeus, scar from prior burn or surgery, or at site of peptic stricture. Use of barium studies and flexible endoscopy is controversial. Appropriate instrumentation and experience in esophagoscopy necessary to assure optimal outcome. Button batteries lead to particularly severe injury due to leakage of alkaline contents.
- Iatrogenic perforation: most commonly occur at sites of narrowing. Clinical picture is sore throat, neck and chest pain following procedure, often with tachycardia out of proportion to fever. Fever and subcutaneous emphysema develop later. Chest radiograph and CT required if clinical suspicion present. Antibiotics, fluid resuscitation, and early surgical exploration with repair are required to assure optimal outcome.
- Esophageal compression: may be either anatomic or pathologic.
  - (a) Anatomic: include cricopharyngeus (UES), aorta, left mainstem bronchus, and diaphragm (LES)
  - (b) Pathologic: include enlarged thyroid or thymus, osteophyte of cervical spine, mediastinal mass, cardiac enlargement or aortic aneurysm, or massive enlargement of the liver

Gastroesophageal Reflux Disease (GERD)

- Symptoms: may be typical (substernal chest pain, waterbrash) or atypical (laryngeal symptoms of hoarseness, voice change, sore throat, globus, or cough).
- Diagnosis: is often made by history, laryngeal examination, 24-hour pH-metry, esophageal biopsy, or response to empiric therapy. Barium swallow may demonstrate esophagitis, stricture, etc. Occasionally reflux may be seen, but absence of reflux of barium does not rule out GERD. Bernstein test (reproduces symptoms by instillation

of acid into esophagus) primarily of historical interest. Esophagoscopy (transoral or transnasal [TNE]) may be required for diagnosis. Up to 50% of selected patients with GERD symptoms may have esophageal abnormalities on TNE examination.

- Complications: may be esophageal (ulceration, stricture, Barrett esophagitis, carcinoma), laryngeal (chronic laryngitis, vocal process granulomata, ulceration, or subglottic edema), or pulmonary (asthma). Role of GERD in sinusitis, pediatric otitis media, and laryngeal cancer remains controversial.
- Barrett esophagitis: Lower esophagus lined with (columnar) gastric epithelium instead squamous epithelium. Barretts divided into short (< 3 cm) and long segment (> 3 cm). Increasing incidence noted in recent decades. Progressess to cancer of the esophagus at the rate of 1% to 2% per year. Barrett ulcer is deep peptic ulceration in an area of Barrett esophagitis.
- Treatment of gastroesophageal and gastropharyngeal reflux: includes elevation head of bed, dietary changes, avoidance of caffeine and nicotine and antiacids. Many patients respond to H2 blockers, but proton pump inhibitors now commonly used for both diagnosis and therapy. Carcinoma of the esophagus: accounts for 4% of cancer deaths with a male preponderance of 5:1. It is increasing in incidence, and is associated with alcohol and tobacco usage, Barrett esophagitis, or prior burn, scar, or stricture. Cancers arising in the upper third are usually squamous cell carcinoma, whereas those in the distal 2/3 likely to be adenocarcinoma. In decreasing order, most common are distal 1/3 (40%-50%), next is middle 1/3 (30%-40%), and less than 1/3 arise in upper 1/3. Other malignant neoplasms include sarcomas such as liomyosarcoma or fibrosarcoma. Benign tumors of the esophagus are rare and include leiomyoma, fibroma, or lipoma.

Congenital Lesions

- Congenital diaphragmatic hernias: posterior termed pleuroperitoneal (Bochdalek) whereas anterior is retrosternal (Morgagni). Treatment is surgical.
- Tracheoesophageal fistulae: occur in 1 in 3,000 births and are associated with polyhydramnios (16%), cardiac abnormalities, vestibular abnormalities imperforate anus, and genital-urinary abnormalities. These may be of various types: the most common (85%) is a distal TEF with upper esophageal atresia. Less common are blind upper and lower esophageal pouches without a connection to the trachea (8%) and a true H-type fistula (4%). In less than 1%, the proximal esophagus opens into the trachea. Infants present with drooling and feeding difficulties, coughing, abdominal distention, vomiting, and cyanosis. Radiographs demonstrate marked air filling the stomach and proximal intestine and often right upper lobe pneumonia (aspiration). Passage of an NG tube that meets obstruction 9-13 cm from the nares suggests the diagnosis. A chest radiograph with the catheter in place can demonstrate position of pouch as well air in stomach and intestine. Sixty to eighty percent survive, however if cardiac or genital-urinary abnormalities present, survival drops to 22%. Barium study is diagnostic.
- Dysphagia lusoria (Bayford syndrome): is symptomatic compression of the esophagus by anomalous location of the right subclavian artery. Instead of arising from the innominate artery, the anomalous right subclavian originates from the descending aortal distal to the left subclavian and passes posterior to the esophagus to get to the arm. It is associated with a nonrecurrent right recurrent laryngeal nerve and aneurysms of the aorta and the aberrant right subclavian artery. Dysphagia is intermittent but can lead to weight loss. Barium swallow will show posterior compression, CT diagnostic. Treatment is ligation and division with anastomosis of distal subclavian artery to carotid.

- Esophageal burns: have become more rare since improvements in public awareness and packaging. Alkalis (lye) are more likely to cause deep burns than acids. Concentrated acids, however, are associated with gastric rupture. Oral burns are not present in 8% to 20% of those with esophageal burns. Esophagoscopy for diagnosis within 24 hours. If no burn is found, follow up with a barium swallow in two weeks. If a burn is identified, do not advance beyond burn. Treat with antibiotics and steroids (2-3 weeks). Nasogastric intubation is controversial—can function as a lumen-finder. Pathologic sequence of burns is as follows:
  - (a) 0-24 hours: dusky cyanotic edematous mucosa
  - (b) 2-5 days: gray-white coat of coagulated protein fibroblasts appear
  - (c) 4-7 days: slough with demarcation of burn depth. Esophageal wall is weakest from days 5 through 8
  - (d) 8-12 days: appearance of collagen
  - (e) 6 weeks: scar formation and evident stricture

Bibliography

Carrau RL, Murry T. *Comprehensive Management of Swallowing Disorders*. San Diego, CA: Singular Publishing Group, Inc;1999.

Hollingshead WH. *Textbook of Anatomy*. 3rd ed. New York, NY: Harper & Row; 1974.

Mitchell SL, Teno JM, Kiely DK, et al. The clinical course of advanced dementia. *N Engl J Med*. 2009:361:1529-1538.

Ney DM, Weiss, JM, Kind AJ, Robbins J. Senescent swallowing; impact, strategies, and interventions. *Nutr Clin Pract*. 2009;24:395.

Postma GN, Cohen JT, Belafsky PC, et al. Transnasal esophagoscopy: revisited (over 700 consecutive cases). *Laryngoscope*. 2005:115:321-323.

Vieth M, Schubert B, Lang-Schwarz K, Stolte M. Frequency of Barrett's neoplasia after initial endoscopy with biopsy: a long-term histopathological follow-up study. *Endoscopy*. 2006;38:1201-1205.

Questions

1. A 38-year-old asymptomatic woman is undergoing right thyroid lobectomy. During the procedure the right recurrent laryngeal nerve cannot be identified. Review of the CT scan is likely to demonstrate:

   A. aberrant take-off of right subclavian artery, which passes behind the esophagus

   B. anterior displacement of the nerve by an unexpectedly enlarged parathyroid gland

   C. congenital laryngeal rotation with hypertrophy of Galen anastomosis

   D. right-sided porencephaly with congenital absence of right vagus nerve

2. An 88-year-old woman complains of burning mouth. Examination reveals "shiny" tongue. The most likely diagnosis is

   A. xerostomia due to medications

   B. senile atrophy

   C. malabsorption syndrome with essential nutrient deficiency

   D. congenital absence of filiform papillae

3. During esophagoscopy in a 75-kg adult a mass was encountered at 40 cm from the incisors. It appeared to be a malignancy and was biopsied. The most likely diagnosis is

A. squamous cell carcinoma

B. adenocarcinoma

C. malignant paraganglioma

D. metastatic renal cell carcinoma

4. A 46-year-old woman is found to have anesthesia of her left hard palate. Sensation in her cheek and upper lip are normal. A CT scan demonstrates a mass in her ipsilateral posterior nasal cavity. Of the following, which is the most likely site of nerve involvement?

A. Incisural foramen

B. Foramen rotundum

C. Descending palatine canal

D. Glossopharyngeal nerve

5. A 45-year-old man is referred for "hard tumors" of his mandible. Examination reveals bilateral multiple prominent bony-hard protuberances on his anterior-medial mandible just below the gum line. The most likely diagnosis is

A. ostegenic carcinoma

B. ameleoblastoma

C. Ewing sarcoma

D. mandibular exostoses

Chapter 32
Neck Spaces and Fascial Planes

The advent of advanced imaging and powerful antimicrobial therapy has allowed more deep neck space infections to be managed with medical therapy alone. However, detailed knowledge of the neck spaces and fascial planes is mandatory in order to predict patterns of spread and the possible effects on surrounding structures. In addition, detailed knowledge is required should surgical intervention prove necessary. The goal of surgery for deep neck space infections is to stop the progression of disease while preserving normal vital structures. With the rise of resistant organisms such as methicillin-resistant staphylococcus aureus (MRSA), surgery will continue to remain a critical component in the management of deep neck space infections.

Anatomy

Triangles of the Neck (Figure 32-1)
Anterior Cervical Triangle
    A. Boundaries:
        i. Superior: mandible
        ii. Anterior: midline
        iii. Posterior: sternocleidomastoid
    B. Subordinate triangles:
        i. Submaxillary (digastric) triangle
            a. Superior: mandible
            b. Anterior: anterior belly of digastric
            c. Posterior: posterior belly of digastric
        ii. Carotid triangle
            a. Superior: posterior belly of digastric
            b. Anterior: superior belly of omohyoid
            c. Posterior: sternocleidomastoid
        iii. Muscular triangle
            a. Superior: superior belly of omohyoid
            b. Anterior: midline
            c. Posterior: sternocleidomastoid
        iv. Submental (suprahyoid) triangle
            a. Superior: symphysis of mandible
            b. Inferior: hyoid bone
            c. Lateral: anterior belly of digastric

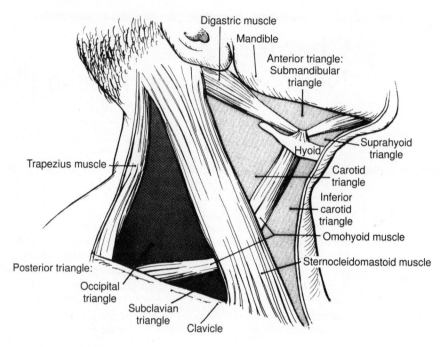

Figure 32-1 Triangles of the neck.

Posterior Cervical Triangle
    A. Boundaries:
        i. Anterior: sternocleidomastoid
        ii. Posterior: trapezius
        iii. Inferior: clavicle
    B. Subordinate triangles:
        i. Occipital triangle:
            a. Anterior: sternocleidomastoid
            b. Posterior: trapezius
            c. Inferior: omohyoid
        ii. Subclavian triangle:
            a. Superior: omohyoid
            b. Inferior: clavicle
            c. Anterior: sternocleidomastoid

Fascial Planes of the Neck (Figure 32-2)
Superficial Cervical Fascia
    A. Envelopes:
        i. Platysma
        ii. Muscles of facial expression
    B. Boundaries:
        i. Superior: zygomatic process
        ii. Inferior: clavicle

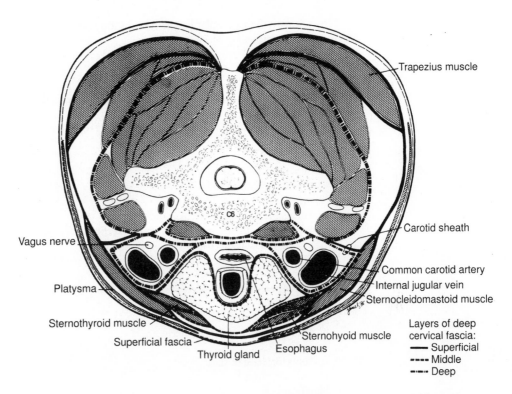

Figure 32-2 Fascial planes of the neck. (*Adapted with permission from Paonessa DF, Goldstein JC: Anatomy and physiology of head and neck infections (with emphasis on the fascia of the face and neck),* Otolaryngol Clin North Am. *1976 Oct;9(3):561-580.)*

   C. Significance:
      i. Main plane of resistance to deep neck spread of cellulitis
      ii. Allows mobility of skin over deep neck structures
      iii. Easily separated when raising neck flaps from deep cervical fascia in the subplatysmal potential space (adipose, sensory nerves, blood vessels)

Deep Cervical Fascia
   A. **Superficial layer (investing fascia)**
      i. Envelopes:
         a. Trapezius, sternocleidomastoid, strap muscles
         b. Submandibular and parotid glands
         c. Muscles of mastication: masseter, pterygoids, temporalis
      ii. Boundaries:
         a. Superior: mandible and zygoma
         b. Inferior: clavicle, acromion, spine of scapula
         c. Anterior: hyoid bone
         d. Posterior: mastoid process, superior nuchal line of cervical vertebrae
      iii. Significance:
         a. Outlines masticator space superiorly

      b. Forms stylomandibular ligament posteriorly (separates parapharyngeal and submandibular spaces)

      c. Splits anteroinferiorly to form suprasternal space of Burns

B. **Middle Layer (visceral fascia)**

   i. Envelopes:

      a. Muscular division: strap muscles (sternohyoid, sternothyroid, thyrohyoid, omohyoid)

      b. Visceral division: pharynx, larynx, trachea, esophagus, thyroid, parathyroid, buccinators, constrictor muscles of pharynx

   ii. Boundaries:

      a. Superior: base of skull

      b. Inferior: mediastinum

   iii. Significance:

      a. Forms pretracheal fascia over the trachea

      b. Forms buccopharyngeal fascia which overlies pharyngeal wall (anterior border of retropharyngeal space)

      c. Buccopharyngeal fascia forms midline raphe (posterior midline) and pterygo-mandibular raphe (lateral pharynx)

C. **Deep Layer (prevertebral fascia)**

   i. Envelopes:

      a. Paraspinous muscles

      b. Cervical vertebrae

   ii. Boundaries:

      a. Superior: base of skull

      b. Inferior: chest

   iii. Significance:

      a. The deep layer of the deep cervical fascia comprises two layers.

      b. The *prevertebral layer* attaches to the transverse processes laterally and covers the vertebral bodies, paraspinous and scalene muscles. Extends from the base of skull to the coccyx.

      c. The *alar layer* lies between the prevertebral layer and the visceral layer of the middle fascia and covers the cervical sympathetic trunk. Extends from the base of skull to the mediastinum.

      d. The *danger space* is the space between the alar and prevertebral layers of the deep cervical fascia.

D. **Carotid Sheath Fascia (Figure 32-3)**

   i. Envelopes:

      a. Common carotid artery

      b. Internal jugular vein

      c. Vagus nerve

   ii. Boundaries:

      a. Superior: base of skull

      b. Inferior: thorax

   iii. Significance:

      a. Comprised of all three layers of the deep cervical fascia

      b. Potential avenue for rapid spread of infection called the "The Lincoln Highway of the Neck"

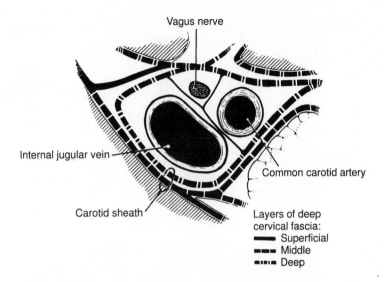

Figure 32-3 Fascial layers of the carotid sheath.

Neck Spaces (Table 32-1)

Parapharyngeal Space

A. Boundaries:
  i. Superior: base of skull (middle cranial fossa)
  ii. Inferior: hyoid bone
  iii. Anterior: pterygomandibular raphe
  iv. Posterior: prevertebral fascia
  v. Medial: pharyngobasilar fascia (superiorly), superior constrictor
  vi. Lateral: deep lobe of parotid gland, mandible, medial pterygoid

B. Contents: styloid process divides into a prestyloid and poststyloid compartment. The poststyloid compartment is where the major vessels and cranial nerves reside.
  i. Prestyloid compartment: muscular (anterior to styloid process)
    a. Fat
    b. Lymph nodes
    c. Internal maxillary artery
    d. Inferior alveolar, lingual, auriculotemporal nerves
    e. Medial and lateral pterygoid muscles
    f. Deep lobe parotid tissue
  ii. Poststyloid compartment
    a. Carotid artery
    b. Internal jugular vein
    c. Sympathetic chain
    d. Cranial nerves IX, X, XI, XII

Pterygopalatine (Pterygomaxillary) Fossa

A. Boundaries:
  i. Superior: sphenoid body, palatine bone (orbital process)
  ii. Anterior: posterior wall of maxillary antrum

Table 32-1 Major Deep Neck Spaces and Contents

Neck Space	Boundaries	Contents	Communicating Spaces
Peritonsillar	• Medial: palatine tonsil • Lateral: superior constrictor muscle	• Loose connective tissue • Tonsillar branches of the lingual, facial, ascending pharyngeal vessels	• Parapharyngeal
Parapharyngeal	• Superior: base of middle fossa • Inferior: hyoid bone • Anterior: pterygomandibular raphe • Posterior: prevertebral fascia • Medial: superior constrictor • Lateral: deep lobe parotid, medial pterygoid	Prestyloid • Fat • Lymph nodes • Int. max. artery • Auricolotemporal, • Lingual, inferior alveolar n. • Pterygoid muscles • Deep lobe parotid Poststyloid • Carotid • Internal jugular • Superior sympathetic • CN IX, X, X, XII	• Perotonsillar • Submandibular • Visceral • Retropharyngeal • Carotid • Masticator • Parotid
Infratemporal fossa	• Superior: sphenoid and temporal skull, fossa medial to zygomatic arch • Anterior: infraorbital fissure, maxilla • Lateral: ramus and coronoid of mandible • Medial: lateral pterygoid plate with tensor and levator palatine muscles	• Pterygoid muscles • Temporalis tendon • Int. max. artery • Pterygoid venous plexus • Mandibular nerve (V3) with otic ganglion	• Temporal fossa • Pterygomaxillary fossa
Pterygomaxillary fossa	• Superior: sphenoid body, palatine bone • Anterior: posterior wall or maxillary antrum • Posterior: pterygoid process, greater wing of sphenoid • Medial: palatine bone • Lateral: temporalis muscle via ptery-gomaxillary fossa	• Maxillary nerve (V2) • Sphenopalatine ganglion • Int. max. artery	• Infratemporal fossa • Parapharyngeal space • Masticator space • Temporal fossa
Temporal fossa	• Superior: temporal line of skull • Inferior: zygomatic arch • Lateral: temporalis fascia • Medial: pterion skull	• Temporalis muscle • Temporal fat pad	• Infratemporal fossa • Pterygomaxillary fossa
Parotid	• Medial: parapharyngeal space • Lateral: parotid fascia	• Parotid gland • Facial nerve • External carotid artery • Posterior facial vein	• Parapharyngeal • Temporal fossa • Masticator

(continued)

Table 32-1 (*continued*) **Major Deep Neck Spaces and Contents**

Neck Space	Boundaries	Contents	Communicating Spaces
Masticator	• Medial: fascia medial to pterygoid muscles • Lateral: fascia overlying masseter	• Masseter muscle • Pterygoid muscles • Ramus and posterior body of mandible • Inferior alveolar nerve • Int. max. artery	• Parotid • Pterygomaxillary • Parapharyngeal
Submandibular	• Superior: floor of mouth • Inferior: digastric muscle • Anterior: mylohyoid and anterior belly digastric muscle • Posterior: posterior belly of digastric and stylomandibular ligament • Medial: hyoglossus and mylohyoid • Lateral: skin, platysma, mandible	• Sublingual and submandibular glands • Wharton duct • Lingual nerve • Lymph nodes • Facial artery and vein • Marginal branch of VII	• Parapharyngeal • Visceral space
Visceral	• Superior: hyoid bone • Inferior: mediastinum • Anterior: superficial layer of deep cervical fascia • Posterior: retropharyngeal space; prevertebral fascia • Lateral: parapharyngeal space	• Pharynx • Esophagus • Larynx • Trachea • Thyroid gland	• Submandibular • Parapharyngeal • Retropharyngeal
Carotid sheath	• Anterior: sternocleidomastoid muscle • Posterior: prevertebral space • Medial: visceral space • Lateral: sternocleidomastoid muscle	• Carotid artery • Int. jugular vein • Vagus nerve • Ansa cervicalis nerve	• Visceral space • Prevertebral • Parapharyngeal
Retropharyngeal	• Superior: base of skull • Inferior: superior mediastinum • Anterior: pharynx, esophagus • Posterior: alar fascia • Medial: midline raphe of superior constrictor • Lateral: carotid sheath	• Lymph nodes • Connective tissue	• Carotid sheath • Superior mediastinum • Parapharyngeal space • Danger space
Danger	• Superior: Base of skull • Inferior: diaphragm • Anterior: alar fascia of deep layer of deep cervical fascia • Posterior: prevertebral fascia of the deep layer of the deep cervical fascia.	• Loose areolar tissue	• Retropharyngeal • Prevertebral • Mediastinum
Prevertebral	• Superior: base of skull • Inferior: coccyx • Anterior: prevertebral fascia • Posterior: vertebral bodies • Lateral: transverse process of vertebrae	• Dense areolar tissue • Paraspinous, prevertebral, scalene muscles • Vetebral artery and vein • Brachial plexus • Phrenic nerve	• Danger space

      iii. Posterior: pterygoid process, greater wing of sphenoid

      iv. Medial: palatine bone, nasal mucoperiosteum

      v. Lateral: temporalis muscle via pterygomaxillary fissure

  B. Contents:

      i. Maxillary nerve (V2)

      ii. Sphenopalatine ganglion

      iii. Internal maxillary artery

Masticator Space

  A. Boundaries:

      i. Lateral: fascia over masseter muscle (superficial layer of deep cervical fascia)

      ii. Medial: fascia medial to pterygoid muscles (superficial layer of deep cervical fascia)

  B. Contents:

      i. Masseter muscle

      ii. Lateral and medial pterygoid muscles

      iii. Ramus and posterior body of mandible

      iv. Temporalis muscle tendon

      v. Inferior alveolar nerve (V3)

      vi. Internal maxillary artery

Temporal Fossa

  A. Boundaries:

      i. Superior: temporal lines on lateral surface of skull (attachment of temporalis muscle)

      ii. Inferior: zygomatic arch

      iii. Lateral: temporalis fascia

      iv. Medial: skull including pterion

  B. Contents:

      i. Temporalis muscle

      ii. Temporal fat pad

Infratemporal Fossa

  A. Boundaries

      i. Medial: lateral pterygoid plate with tensor and levator palatini muscles, superior constrictor

      ii. Lateral: mandibular ramus , coronoid process

      iii. Anterior: infratemporal surface of maxilla; inferior orbital fissure

      iv. Superior: infratemporal crest bone (sphenoid and temporal bones) medially, space deep to zygomatic arch laterally

  B. Contents:

      i. Medial and lateral pterygoid muscles

      ii. Insertion of temporalis on coronoid process

      iii. Internal maxillary artery and branches

      iv. Pterygoid venous plexus

      v. V3 with otic ganglion and chorda tympani

      vi. Posterior superior branch of V3

Parotid Space

  A. Boundaries:

      i. Medial: parapharyngeal space

      ii. Lateral: parotid fascia (superficial layer of deep cervical fascia)

B. Contents:
   i. Parotid gland
   ii. Facial nerve
   iii. External carotid artery and branches
   iv. Posterior facial vein

Peritonsillar Space
   A. Boundaries:
      i. Medial: Palatine tonsil
      ii. Lateral: Superior constrictor muscle
   B. Contents:
      i. Loose connective tissue
      ii. Tonsillar branches of lingual, facial, ascending pharyngeal vessels

Submandibular (Submaxillary) Space (Figure 32-4)
   A. Boundaries:
      i. Superior: floor of mouth mucosa
      ii. Inferior: digastric
      iii. Anterior: mylohoid and anterior belly of digastric
      iv. Posterior: posterior belly of digastric and stylomandibular ligament
      v. Medial: hyoglossus and mylohyoid
      vi. Lateral: skin, platysma, mandible
   B. Contents: the mylohyoid line divides the submandibular space into a sublingual (infections anterior to second molar) and submaxillary (infections of second and third molars) compartments.
      i. Sublingual (supramylohyoid) space:
         a. Sublingual gland
         b. Wharton duct
         c. Lingual nerve

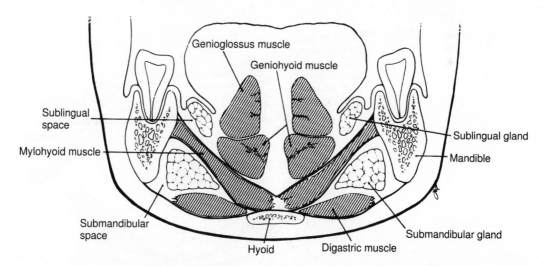

Figure 32-4 Division of the submandibular space into supramylohyoid and inframylohyoid spaces by mylohyoid muscle. (*Adapted with permission from Hollinshead WH, ed:* Anatomy for Surgeons, Head and Neck. *3rd edition. Philadelphia, PA: Harper & Row; 1982.*)

      ii. Submaxillary (inframylohyoid) space:
         a. Submandibular gland
         b. Lymph nodes
         c. Hypoglossal nerve (anterior)
         d. Facial vein and artery
         e. Marginal branch of facial nerve

Carotid Sheath Space (See Figure 32-3)
  A. Boundaries:
     i. Anterior: sternocleidomastoid
     ii. Posterior: prevertebral space
     iii. Medial: visceral space
     iv. Lateral: sternocleidomastoid
  B. Contents:
     i. Carotid artery
     ii. Internal jugular vein
     iii. X nerve
     iv. Ansa cervicalis

Visceral Space (Pretracheal Space) (Figure 32-5)
  A. Boundaries:
     i. Superior: hyoid bone
     ii. Inferior: mediastinum (T4 level/ arch of aorta)
     iii. Anterior: superficial layer of deep cervical fascia
     iv. Posterior: retropharyngeal space; prevertebral fascia
     v. Lateral: parapharyngeal space; carotid fascia
  B. Contents:
     i. Pharynx
     ii. Esophagus

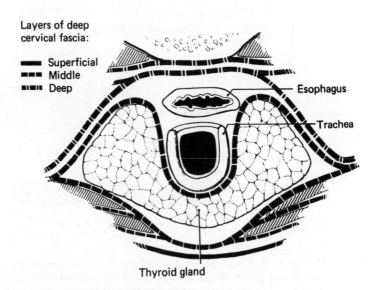

Figure 32-5 Fascial layers surrounding the visceral space.

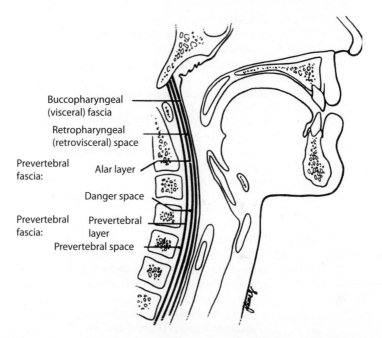

Buccopharyngeal (visceral) fascia

Retropharyngeal (retrovisceral) space

Prevertebral fascia:

Alar layer

Danger space

Prevertebral fascia:

Prevertebral layer

Prevertebral space

Figure 32-6 Fascial layers of the retrovisceral space. (*Adapted with permission from Hollinshead WH, ed: Anatomy for Surgeons, Head and Neck. 3rd edition. Philadelphia, PA: Harper & Row; 1982.*)

iii. Larynx
iv. Trachea
v. Thyroid gland

Retropharyngeal (Retrovisceral) Space (Figure 32-6)
  A. Boundaries:
    i. Superior: base of skull
    ii. Inferior: superior mediastinum; tracheal bifurcation (T4); middle layer of deep cervical fascia fuses with alar layer of deep cervical fascia.
    iii. Anterior: pharynx and esophagus (middle layer of deep cervical fascia-buccopharyngeal fascia).
    iv. Posterior: alar fascia
    v. Medial: Midline raphe of superior constrictor muscle (results in unilateral abscess in this space)
    vi. Lateral: carotid sheath
  B. Contents:
    i. Retropharyngeal lymph nodes (pediatric infections of sinuses or nasopharynx)
    ii. Connective tissue

Danger Space (See Figure 32-6)
  A. Boundaries:
    i. Superior: base of skull
    ii. Inferior: diaphragm
    iii. Anterior: alar fascia of deep layer of deep cervical fascia
    iv. Posterior: prevertebral fascia of deep layer of deep cervical fascia

B. Contents:
    i. Loose areolar tissue (Danger spaced named due to potential for rapid spread of infection through this space.)

Prevertebral Space (See Figure 32-6)

A. Boundaries
    i. Superior: base of skull
    ii. Inferior: coccyx
    iii. Anterior: prevertebral fascia (results in midline abscess in this space)
    iv. Posterior: vertebral bodies
    v. Lateral: transverse process of vertebrae
B. Contents
    i. Dense areolar tissue
    ii. Muscle: paraspinous, prevertebral, scalene
    iii. Vetebral artery and vein
    iv. Brachial plexus and phrenic nerve

Deep Neck Space Infections

A. **Etiology (Figure 32-7)**
    i. Dental infections (most common adult)
    ii. Acute pharyngitis of Waldeyer ring (most common pediatric)
    iii. Cervical lymphadentitis (must rule out associated cancer in adult)
    iv. Acute rhinosinusitis (retropharyngeal lymphadenitis)
    v. Acute mastoiditis (Bezold abscess)
    vi. Iatrogenic (oral surgery; intubation or endoscopic trauma)
    vii. Sialadenitis
    viii. Foreign body
    ix. Penetrating cervicofacial trauma (includes IV drug injection)
    x. Cellulitis
    xi. Congenital cysts (thyroglossal duct; branchial cleft)
    xii. Acquired cysts (laryngoceles; saccular cysts)
B. Microbiology
    i. Mixed aerobic and anaerobic polymicrobial oropharyngeal flora (most common)
    ii. Streptococcus viridians
    iii. *Strepococcus pyogenes* (group A beta-hemolytic strep)
    iv. Peptostreptococcus
    v. Staphylococcus epidermidis
    vi. Staphylococcus aureus
    vii. Methicillin-resistant staphylococcus aureus (MRSA) (the most common isolate in community acquired deep neck infections in children younger than 2 years)
    viii. Bacteroides
    ix. Fusobacterium
    x. *Neisseria, Pseudomonas, Escherichia, Haemophilus* (occasional)
    xi. Actinomyces (gram-positive oropharyngeal saprophyte; necrotic granulomas with "sulfur granules")
    xii. Mycobacteria (tuberculous and nontuberculous; necrotizing cervical caseating granulomas; Pott abscess of vertebral body with spread to prevertebral space; acid fast bacterium; cough, fever, sweats, weight loss).
    xiii. Bartonella henselae (cat scratch disease; large tender cervical lymph nodes, fever, fatigue)

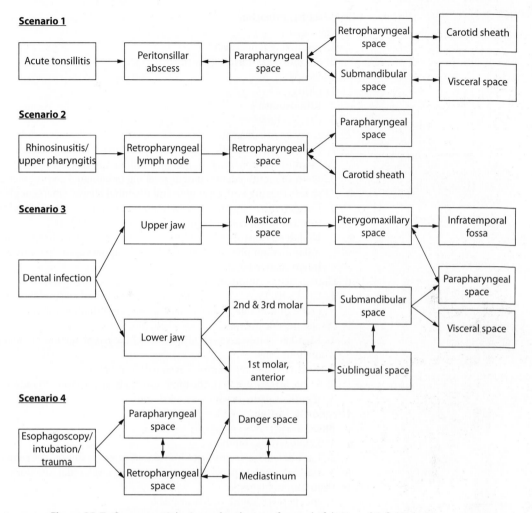

Figure 32-7 Common etiologies and pathways of spread of deep neck infections.

C. **Clinical Evaluation**
  i. **History**
    a. Inflammatory symptoms: pain, fever, swelling, redness.
    b. Localizing symptoms: dysphagia/ odynophagia/drooling (retropharyngeal abscess), "hot potato voice," trismus (peritonsillar abscess), hoarseness, dyspnea, ear pain, neck swelling, otalgia.
    c. Recent infection: dental, sinusitis, otitis.
    d. Recent trauma: IV drug use.
    e. Recent surgery: dental, intubation, endoscopy.
    f. Past medical history: antibiotic allergies.
    g. Immunodeficiency (diabetes; HIV; autoimmune disorder; collagen-vascular disease; hematologic malignancy; recent chemotherapy or steroid) causes increased risk of atypical pathogens and rapidly progressive symptoms.

ii. **Physical Examination**
   a. Palpation:
      1. Localizing tenderness
      2. Crepitus (gas-forming organism)
   b. Otoscopy:
      1. Otitis
      2. Rhinosinusitis
      3. Foreign body
   c. Oral cavity and pharynx
      1. Poor dentition (tooth infection; possible anaerobic organisms)
      2. Trismus (parapharyngeal, pterygomaxillary, masticator spaces)
      3. Floor of mouth edema/ tongue swelling (sublingual and submandibular spaces causing Ludwig angina and potential airway emergency)
      4. Purulent discharge from Wharton or Stenson duct (parotid and sublingual/ submandibular spaces; bimanual palpation for stones)
      5. Unilateral tonsil swelling with deviation of uvula (peritonsillar abscess if inflammation present; think tonsil or parapharyngeal space tumor if no inflammation)
   d. Cranial nerve examination
      1. CN II, III, IV, V, VI can cause reduced vision and eye mobility via retrograde flow of infection through valveless ophthalmic veins.
   e. Awake flexible fiberoptic airway evaluation
      1. Mandatory if hoarseness, dyspnea, stridor, dysphagia/odynophagia without obvious cause.
      2. Normal oximetry common even with critical airway.
      3. Stable airway needs verification prior to transportation to radiology suite.
      4. Identifies patients who may need intubation.

iii. **Diagnostic Testing**
   a. Blood tests
      1. Leukocytosis common
      2. Lack of leukocytosis (virus; immunodeficiency; tumor; congenital cyst)
      3. Basic electrolyte panel (glucose; hydration level; renal function)
   b. Plain film radiography
      1. Inexpensive, rapid, widely available
      2. Jaw films (Panorex): lucency at dental root (odontogenic abscess); salivary stones
      3. Lateral neck films: air-fluid level; > 5 mm thickening (child) or > 7 mm thickening (adult) at C2 (retropharyngeal infection); arytenoid or epiglottic thickening (thumbprint sign) (supraglottitis)
      4. Chest films (dyspnea; tachycardia; cough): widened mediastinum (mediastinitis); lower lobe infiltrate (aspiration pneumonia)
   c. Computed tomography with IV contrast
      1. Best overall visualization of neck spaces and structures.
      2. Determines neck spaces requiring drainage, which can be misidentified in 70% of cases based on physical examination alone.
      3. Difficult to differentiate between abscess (pus) or phlegmon (edema). No pus is found on 25% of neck explorations.
      4. Can differentiate between contained (within node) and noncontained (neck spaces) abscess.

5. Metastatic adenopathy (from oropharyngeal primary) needs to be ruled out since this can mimic neck abscess on CT in adult patient.

6. IV contrast contraindications: allergy, renal failure.

d. Magnetic resonance imaging

1. Helpful in select cases (intracranial communication or complication; infection of vertebral bodies)

2. Not recommended if airway or swallowing issues

3. MR angiography helpful if thrombi or pseudoaneurysm of major vessel suspected

e. Ultrasonography

1. Advantages: noninvasive; no radiation; allows fine needle aspiration; pediatric patients

2. Limitations: deeper abscesses; obese patients

D. **Treatment**

i. **Airway Management**

a. Loss of airway main source of mortality from deep neck infection.

b. Airway most at risk with infection of:

1. Submandibular space

2. Parapharyngeal space

3. Retropharyngeal space

c. Fiberoptic exam evaluates at-risk airway

d. First-line therapy:

1. Oxygenated face tent with cool humidity

2. Intravenous steroids

3. Epinephrine nebulizers

4. ICU observation if stable and airway > 50 % normal caliber

e. Tracheotomy

1. Worsening stridor, dyspnea, or obstruction with < 50% of normal airway diameter

2. Awake flexible intubation possible if glottis large enough to pass adult flexible bronchoscope (6 mm)

3. Awake tracheotomy if patient not easily intubatable

4. Elective tracheotomy if prolonged (> 48 h) airway edema anticipated. Elective tracheotomy is associated with reduced hospital days and costs compared to prolonged intubation.

ii. **Fluid Resuscitation**

a. Dehydration common due to dysphagia (peritonsillar, retropharyngeal).

b. Dehydration may be cause of sialadenitis.

c. Signs of dehydration:

1. Tachycardia

2. Dry, pasty mucous membranes

3. Decreased skin turgor

d. Initial resuscitation: 1 to 2 L of isotonic IV fluids.

iii. **Intravenous Antibiotic Therapy (Table 32-2)**

a. Broad-spectrum empiric therapy indicated at diagnosis (should not be delayed for culture).

b. Clindamycin first-line therapy of choice for children < 2 years due to increasing rates of MRSA.

Table 32-2 **Recommended Antibiotic Therapy for Deep Neck Infections**

Community-acquired infection (gram-positive cocci; gram-negative rods; anaerobes)

- Ampicillin-sulbactam 1.5-3.0 g IV every 6 h *or*
- Clindamycin (*if PCN allergy*) 600-900 mg IV every 8 h
- Moxifloxacin (*if Eikenella suspected*) 400 mg QD

Immunocompromised/Nosocomial infection

Pseudomonal and gram-negatives

- Ticarcillin-clavulanate 3g IV every 6 h *or*
- Pipercillin-tazobactam 3g IV every 6 h *or*
- Imipenem-cilastin 500 mg IV every 6 h *or*
- Ciprofloxacin (*if PCN allergy*) 400 mg IV every 12 h
- Levafloxacin (*if PCN allergy*) 750 mg IV every 24 h

Methicillin-resistant *Staphylococcus aureus* (MRSA)

- Clindamycin 600-900 mg every 8 h *and* vancomycin 1 g IV every 12 h
- Trimethoprim-Sulfamethoxazole 10 mg/kg/day divided every 8 h (*if clindamycin resistant*), *and* vancomycin 1 g IV every 12 h

Necrotizing fasciitis **(mixed gram-positive and expanded anaerobes)**

- Ceftriaxone 2 g IV every 8 h *and* clindamycin 600-900 mg every 8 h *and* metronidazole 500 mg IV every 6 h

Actinomycoses

- Penicillin G 10-20 million units divided every 6 h per day for 4 weeks *then*
- Penicillin V oral 2-4 g divided every 6 h per day for 4-6 mo *or*
- Clindamycin IV and PO if PCN allergy

    c. Fluids from aspiration/ drainage should be sent for culture and sensitivity monitoring.

    d. Clindamycin-resistance is currently present in 5% to 10% of community-acquired MRSA infections.

    e. May delay need for surgical drainage in stable patient:

        1. Contained abscess (intranodal) or phlegmon.

        2. Most pediatric cases.

        3. Abscess size < 2.5 cm contained within single neck space.

        4. Patient kept NPO if surgery is considered.

        5. Repeat imaging and/or surgical intervention indicated if no improvement after 48 to 72 hours of therapy.

        6. If improved, continue IV 24 hours beyond symptom resolution followed by 2 weeks of PO therapy.

  iv. **Surgical Management**

    a. Indications for surgical exploration:

        1. Air-fluid level in neck or gas-forming organism

        2. Abscess present in fascial spaces of neck

        3. Threatened airway compromise from abscess or phlegmon

        4. Failure to respond to 48 to 72 hours of IV antibiotics

    b. Goals of surgical exploration:

        1. Drainage of abscess

        2. Fluid sampling for culture and sensitivity

3. Irrigation of involved neck space
4. Establishment of external drainage pathway to prevent recurrence.
5. Removal of infectious source (dental extraction; foreign body removal)

c. Needle aspiration
1. Lymph nodes containing small abscesses
2. Congenital cysts (with delayed excision after infection subsides)
3. Peritonsillar abscess (adolescent/adult)
4. CT image-guided techniques possible for deep neck spaces

d. Transoral incision and drainage
1. Peritonsillar abscess
   - Adolescent/adult.
   - Performed if not adequately drained by needle aspiration.
   - Premedicate with IV fluids, antibiotics, steroids, and pain medication.
   - Topical anesthetic spray followed by 2 to 3 cc of lidocaine injection over lateral soft palate.
   - Incision on lateral soft palate 5 to 10 mm behind anterior tonsillar pillar.
   - Irrigation of incision with sterile saline.
   - Oral antibiotics for 10 days.
   - Recurrent abscess possible in 16% adults and 7% of children.
2. Alveolus
   - Remove infected tooth (teeth)
3. Buccal space
   - Incision of buccal mucosa
   - Blunt spreading of buccinator muscle parallel to facial nerve
4. Masticator space
   - Incision through mucosa lateral to retromolar trigone
   - Blunt dissection to masseter
5. Pterygomaxillary space
   - Alveobuccal sulcus above third maxillary molar with tunnel dissected posteriorly, superiorly, and medially around maxillary tuberosity into pterygomaxillary fossa
   - Alternative route: through posterior wall of maxillary sinus through Caldwell-Luc or transnasal endoscopic approach)
6. Retropharyngeal space
   - Difficult to access through the neck
   - Access with tonsil gag
   - Determine location of abscess with needle aspiration
   - Incision made over abscess with blunt dissection into pocket
   - Avoid lateral dissection (carotid) or pulsatile areas (retropharyngeal carotid)

e. Tonsillectomy (Peritonsillar abscess)
1. Indications for delayed tonsillectomy:
   - Recurrent peritonsillar abscess
   - Recurrent/chronic tonsillitis
   - Tonsillar hypertrophy with obstructive symptoms
2. Indications for acute "quinsy" tonsillectomy:
   - Recurrent peritonsillar abscess.
   - Massive tonsils causing acute airway obstruction.
   - Patient already under general anesthesia due to comfort issues or poor exposure.

  f. Transcervical incision and drainage
   1. Three surgical approaches (choice depends on involved spaces)
    • Modified blair (parotid) incision
     (a) Parotid space
     (b) Temporal and infratemporal fossa
     (c) Submandibular and parapharyngeal spaces (with extension of neck incision)
    • Horizontal lateral neck incision upper neck (2 cm below mandible body)
     (a) Masticator space (lower border of mandible and staying along lateral surface)
     (b) Submandibular space (between posterior belly of digastric and mandible body)
     (c) Sublingual space (lateral to anterior digastric belly with blunt spreads through mylohoid muscle)
     (d) Parapharyngeal space/Pterygomaxillary space (anterior traction of submandibular gland with blunt dissection superior and medial to posterior belly of digastrics along medial surface of mandible angle)
    • Horizontal lateral neck incision mid-neck (level 3 at cricoid cartilage)
     (a) Retropharyngeal/danger/prevertebral spaces.
     (b) Dissection medial to carotid sheath (retracted laterally) and lateral to strap muscles (retracted medially).
     (c) Deep cervical fascia and paraspinous muscles identified.
     (d) Blunt dissection superior (skull base) to inferior (mediastinum).
   2. Surgical technique
    • Divide superficial cervical fascia and superficial layer of deep fascia.
    • Blunt dissection with hemostat and Kittner sponge into involved space.
    • Overdissection puts normal structures at risk and provides path for infection to spread.
    • Avoid finger dissection if suspect IV drug use (broken needles).
    • Culture inflammatory drainage or pus.
    • Copious irrigation of wound.
    • External drainage with Penrose or rubber band drain.
    • Loose closure of wound.
E. **Selected complications of deep neck infections**
 i. **Ludwig angina**
  a. Severe infection of the sublingual and submental spaces.
  b. High mortality from asphyxia.
  c. Most commonly dental origin.
  d. Rapid spread through fascial planes (not lymphatics).
  e. Swelling causes posterior tongue displacement and airway obstruction.
  f. Erect, drooling patient, with edema of tongue and floor of mouth; woody, indurated neck.
  g. Airway management is first priority (tracheotomy versus awake fiberoptic intubation).
  h. Wide drainage of bilateral submandibular and sublingual spaces.
  i. IV antibiotic therapy with anaerobic coverage.
 ii. **Cavernous sinus thrombosis**
  a. Life-threatening condition with mortality rate of 30% to 40%
  b. Upper dentition common source of infection

    c. Retrograde spread via valveless ophthalmic veins to cavernous sinus

    d. Symptoms: fever, lethargy, orbital pain

    e. Signs: proptosis, reduced extraocular mobility, dilated pupil, reduced pupillary light reflex

iii. **Lemierre syndrome**

    a. Potentially fatal if not recognized.

    b. Thrombophlebitis of the internal jugular (IJ) vein.

    c. Most common organism: Fusobacterium necrophorum (anaerobic, gram-negative bacillus).

    d. Bacterium spreads to IJ from tonsillar veins where endotoxin causes platelet aggregation.

    e. Associated with pharyngitis, spiking "picket fence" fevers, lethargy, lateral neck tenderness, septic emboli (nodular chest infiltrates and/or septic arthritis).

    f. Tobey-Ayer Test: compression of the thrombosed IJ during spinal tap does not increase CSF pressure as opposed to the contralateral side.

    g. CT with IV contrast can demonstrate filling defect in IJ vein.

    h. Intravenous beta-lactamase resistant antibiotics indicated for 2 to 3 weeks.

    i. Heparin anticoagulation can be considered.

    j. Vein ligation and excision indicated if clinical deterioration occurs.

iv. **Carotid artery pseudoaneurysm or rupture**

    a. Associated with infection of retropharyngeal or parapharyngeal space.

    b. Mortality rate of 20% to 40%

    c. Frequency of bleed: internal carotid artery (49%); common carotid artery (9%); external carotid artery (4%); miscellaneous (14%).

    d. Possible signs: pulsatile neck mass, Horner syndrome, palsies of CN IX-XII, expanding hematoma, neck ecchymosis, sentinel bright red bleed from nose or mouth, hemorrhagic shock

    e. Diagnosis: MRA or angiography.

    f. Treatment: Urgent ligation or stenting of carotid artery.

v. **Mediastinitis**

    a. Associated with infections of the retropharyngeal (most common; superior mediastinum) and danger spaces (posterior mediastinum to diaphragm).

    b. Mortality rate as high as 30% to 40%

    c. Possible signs: diffuse neck edema, dyspnea, pleuritic chest pain, tachycardia, hypoxia.

    d. CXR: mediastinal widening, pleural effusion.

    e. Improved survival with combined cervical and thoracic drainage (81%) versus cervical drainage alone (53%).

vi. **Necrotizing Fasciitis**

    a. Mortality of 20% to 30% (highest with mediastinal extension).

    b. More common in older or immunocompromised patients.

    c. Dental infection most common cause; mixed aerobic and anaerobic flora.

    d. Signs: diffuse spreading erythematous pitting edema of neck with "orange-peel" appearance; subcutaneous crepitus.

    e. Neck CT shows tissue gas in 50% of cases.

    f. Treatment: critical care support; broad-spectrum antibiotics, surgical exploration; hyperbaric oxygen.

    g. Surgery: debridement to bleeding tissue.

Bibliography

Alexander D, Leonard J, Trail M. Vascular complications of deep neck abscesses. *Laryngoscope.* 1968;78:361.

Brook I. The increased risk of community-acquired methicillin-resistant Staphylococcus aureus in neck infections in young children. *Curr Infect Dis Rep.* 2012;14:119-120.

Brook I. Microbiology and management of peritonsillar, retropharyngeal, and parapharyngeal abscesses. *J Oral Maxillofac Surg.* 2004;62:1545-1550.

Cheng J, Elden L. Children with deep space neck infections: our experience with 178 children. *Otolaryngol Head Neck Surg.* 2013;148:1037-1042.

Corsten MJ, Shamji FM, Odell PF, et al. Optimal treatment of descending necrotizing mediastinitis. *Thorax.* 1997;52:702-708.

Crespo AN, Chone CT, Fonseca AS, et al. Clinical versus computed tomography evaluation in the diagnosis and management of deep neck infection. *Sao Paulo Med J.* 2004;122:259-263.

Elliott M, Yong S, Beckenham T. Carotid artery occlusion in association with a retropharyngeal abscess. *Int J Pediatr Otorhinolaryngol.* 2005;70:359-363.

Golpe R, Marin B, Alonso M. Lemierre's syndrome (necrobacillosis). *Postgrad Med J.* 1999;75:141-144.

Kluka EA. Emerging dilemmas with methicillin-resistant *Staphylococcus aureus* infections in children. *Curr Opin Otolaryngol Head Neck Surg.* 2011;19:462-466.

Plaza Mayor G, Martinez-San Millan J, Martinez-Vidal A. Is conservative treatment of deep neck space infections appropriate? *Head Neck.* 2001;23:126-133.

Potter JK, Herford AS, Ellis 3rd E. Tracheotomy versus endotracheal intubation for airway management in deep neck space infections. *J Oral Maxillofac Surg.* 2002;60:349-354.

Smith 2nd JL, Hsu JM, Chang J. Predicting deep neck space abscess using computed tomography. *Am J Otolaryngol.* 2006;27:244-247.

Tung-Yiu W, Jehn-Shyun H, Ching-Hung C, et al. Cervical necrotizing fasciitis of odontogenic origin: a report of 11 cases. *J Oral Maxillofac Surg.* 2000;58:1347-1352.

Questions

1. The prestyloid parapharyngeal space contains all of the following *except*
   A. fat
   B. lymph nodes
   C. glossopharyngeal nerve
   D. deep lobe of parotid
   E. medial and lateral pterygoid muscles

2. Masticator space infections can spread directly to all the following spaces *except*
   A. parotid space
   B. parapharyngeal space
   C. pterygomaxillary space
   D. retropharyngeal space
   E. buccal space

3. An 18-month-old child presents with fever, dysphagia, drooling, and neck tenderness. The most likely organism is
   A. Pneumococcus

    B. MRSA

    C. Moraxella catarrhalis

    D. Haemophilus influenzae

    E. Peptostreptocossus

4. A patient presents with fever, dysphagia, and odynophagia. Transoral examination is within normal limits. Pulse oximetry is 100%. The most appropriate next step in management is

    A. modified barium swallow

    B. PO antibiotic therapy

    C. antifungal therapy for likely esophageal thrush

    D. fiberoptic laryngoscopy

    E. reflux management

5. An emergency room physician calls you concerning a 48-year-old man with poor dentition, unilateral neck swelling, sore throat, odynophagia, and asymmetric tonsils. The neck CT shows a large level II lymph node with rim enhancement just deep to the skin. The next most appropriate step includes

    A. surgical I&D of the neck abscess

    B. transoral I&D of presumed peritonsillar abscess

    C. repeat oral antibiotics with follow-up in 2 to 3 weeks

    D. dental referral for likely odontogenic infection

    E. full head and neck examination with FRNA of neck mass for cytopathology

Chapter 33
Thyroid and Parathyroid Glands

"The extirpation of the thyroid gland for goiter typifies perhaps better than any operation the supreme triumph of the surgeon's art."

—Halsted, 1920

Anatomy and Embryology

Background

A. Anatomy
   i. The thyroid is composed of two lateral lobes connected by an isthmus, which rests at the level of the second to fourth tracheal cartilages.
   ii. Each thyroid lobe measures approximately 4 cm high, 1.5 cm wide, and 2 cm deep.
   iii. A pyramidal lobe, a remnant of descent of the thyroid is present in up to 40% of patients.

B. Embryology
   i. The thyroid's medial anlage arises as a ventral diverticulum from the endoderm of the first and second pharyngeal pouches at the foramen cecum.
   ii. The diverticulum forms at 4-week gestation and descends from the base of the tongue to its adult pretracheal position in the route of the neck through a midline anterior path, assuming its final adult position by 7-week gestation.
   iii. Parafollicular C cells arising from the neural crest of the fourth pharyngeal pouch as ultimobranchial bodies migrate and infiltrate the forming lateral thyroid lobes.
   iv. If thyroid migration is completely arrested, a lingual thyroid results without normal tissue in the orthotopic site.
   v. If the inferior most portion of the thyroglossal duct tract is maintained, a pyramidal lobe is formed. If a remnant of thyroid tissue is left along the thyroglossal duct tract, it develops into a cyst, enlarges, and presents in the adult as a midline neck mass, frequently in close association with the hyoid bone.

C. Lymphatics
   i. An extensive regional intra- and periglandular lymphatic network exists. The isthmus and medial thyroid lobes drain initially to Delphian, pretracheal, and superior mediastinal nodes, while the lateral thyroid drains initially to the internal jugular chain. The inferior pole drains initially to paratracheal, peri-recurrent laryngeal nerve (RLN) nodes.

D. Fascia
  i. The cervical viscera—including trachea, larynx, and thyroid—are ensheathed by the middle layer (visceral) of the deep cervical fascia.

It is important to distinguish between the true thyroid capsule and the areolar tissue present in the interval between the true thyroid capsule and the undersurface of the strap muscles (ie, the perithyroid sheath). The true thyroid capsule is tightly adherent to the thyroid parenchyma and continuous with fibrous septa that divide the gland's parenchyma into lobules. As the strap muscles are elevated off the ventral surface of the thyroid, the thin areolar tissue of the perithyroid sheath is encountered as thin cobweb-like tissue that is typically easily lysed and occasionally associated with small bridging vessels extending from the undersurface of the strap muscles to the true thyroid capsule. As dissection extends around the posterolateral lobe of the thyroid during thyroidectomy, separation of the layers of the perithyroid sheath allows recognition of the superior parathyroid, which is usually closely associated with the posterolateral thyroid capsule of the superior pole. It is posterior to the plane of the recurrent nerve when viewed in a sagittal orientation.

Ligament of Berry

- The thyroid elevates with the larynx and trachea with deglutition.
- The thyroid is attached to the laryngotracheal complex through anterior and posterior suspensory ligaments.
- The anterior suspensory ligament arises from the anterior aspect of the first several tracheal rings and inserts on the undersurface of the thyroid isthmus.
- The posterior suspensory ligament of the thyroid (ligament of Berry) is a condensation of the thyroid capsule, it is well vascularized, deriving a branch of the inferior thyroid artery.
- The RLN can actually penetrate the thyroid gland within the ligament of Berry in a significant percentage of patients.

Recurrent and Superior Laryngeal Nerves

- The cervical branches of the vagus nerve that are of concern during thyroid surgery include the superior laryngeal nerve (SLN), both internal and external branches, as well as the RLN (Figure 33-1).
- The SLN's internal branch supplies sensation (general visceral afferents) to the lower pharynx, supraglottic larynx, and base of tongue as well as special visceral afferents to epiglottic taste buds.
- The SLN's external branch provides motor innervation (branchial efferents) to the cricothyroid muscle and inferior constrictor.
- The RLN provides motor innervation (branchial efferents) to the inferior constrictor and all intrinsic laryngeal muscles except the cricothyroid muscle.
- The RLN supplies sensation (general visceral afferents) to the larynx (vocal cords and below), upper esophagus, and trachea as well as parasympathetic innervation to the lower pharynx, larynx, trachea, and upper esophagus.
- A right nonrecurrent RLN occurs in approximately 0.5% to 1% of cases.
- The right RLN enters the neck base at the thoracic inlet more laterally than does the left recurrent. The right RLN ascends the neck, traveling from lateral to medial, crossing the inferior thyroid artery.
- The left RLN emerges from underneath the aortic arch and enters the thoracic inlet on the left in a more paratracheal position and extends upward in or near the tracheoesophageal groove, ultimately crossing the distal branches of the inferior thyroid artery.

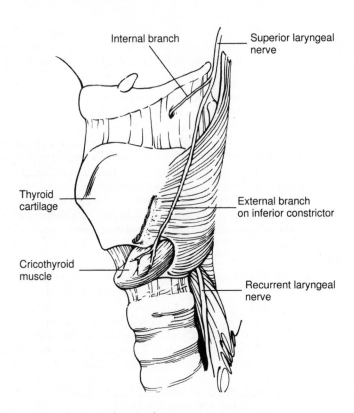

Figure 33-1 Recurrent and superior laryngeal nerves.

Typically, for the last centimeter or so, the RLN, prior to laryngeal entry, travels close to the lateral border of the trachea.

- In approximately one-third of cases, the RLN branches prior to its laryngeal entry point (Figure 33-2).
- The SLN arises from the upper vagus nerve and descends medial to the carotid sheath. It divides into internal and external branches about 2 to 3 cm above the superior pole of the thyroid.
- The internal branch travels medially to the carotid system, entering the posterior aspect of the thyrohyoid membrane, providing sensation to the ipsilateral supraglottis.
- The external branch descends to the region of the superior pole and extends medially along the inferior constrictor muscle to enter the cricothyroid muscle. As the external branch slopes downward on the inferior constrictor musculature, it has a close association with the superior pole pedicle.
- Typically, the external branch diverges from the superior pole vascular pedicle 1 cm or more above the superior aspect of the thyroid superior pole.
- In 20% of cases, the external branch is closely associated with the superior thyroid vascular pedicle at the level of the capsule of the superior pole, placing it at risk during ligation of the superior pole vessels. Also in approximately 20% of cases the external branch travels subfasically on the inferior constrictor as it descends making it difficult to visualize, though still identifiable through neural stimulation.

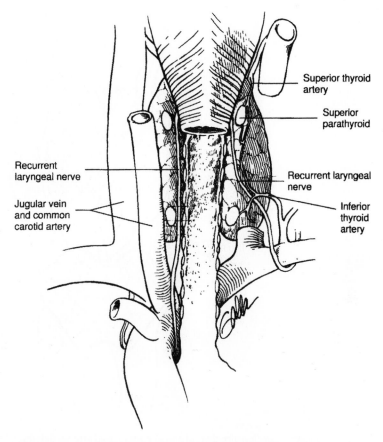

Figure 33-2 Posterior view of thyroid showing superior and inferior thyroid arteries and their relationship to the RLNs.

Vasculature

- The arterial supply to the thyroid is from the superior thyroid artery, a branch of the external carotid artery, and the inferior thyroid artery, a branch of the thyrocervical trunk.
- The thyroid ima artery is a separate unpaired inferior vessel which may rise from the innominate artery, carotid artery, or aortic arch directly and is present in 1.5% to 12% of cases.
- The thyroid veins include the superior, middle, and inferior thyroid veins (Figure 33-3). The superior thyroid vein derives as a branch of the internal jugular vein and travels with the superior thyroid artery in the superior pole vascular pedicle. The middle thyroid vein travels without arterial complement and drains into the internal jugular vein. The inferior thyroid vein also travels without arterial complement, extending from the inferior pole to the internal jugular or brachiocephalic vein.

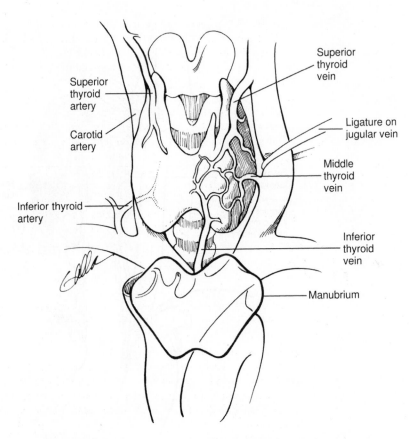

Figure 33-3 Superior thyroid and inferior thyroid arteries (left figure) and superior, middle, and inferior thyroid veins (right figure).

Hormones

The thyroid is composed of follicles that selectively absorb and store iodine from the blood for production of thyroid hormones (TH). The follicles are composed of a single layer of thyroid epithelial cells, which secrete thyroid hormone (triiodothyronine) (T_3) and thyroxine (T_4)

    A. T_3
        i. Several times more physiologically potent than T_4.
       ii. Ten percent of thyroid gland's production of TH.
      iii. Half-life is 1 day, so reassessment of thyroid function tests after dose change of exogenous T_3 is performed after 1 to 2 weeks.
      iv. Eighty percent of circulating T_3 is created from conversion of T_4 in the periphery.
       v. Exogenous T_3 (levotriiodothyronine) is available as liothyronine.
    B. T_4
        i. Strongly correlates with thyroid-stimulating hormone (TSH) level and is believed to play a predominant role in TSH negative feedback.

      ii. About 90% of the thyroid gland's production of TH.

      iii. Half-life is 6 to 7 days; therefore, with change in exogenous T_4 dose, thyroid function tests are reassessed after 5 to 6 weeks.

      iv. Exogenous T_4 is available as levothyroxine.

  C. Both T_4 and T_3

      i. Stimulate calorigenesis, potentiate epinephrine, lower cholesterol levels, and have roles in normal growth and development.

      ii. Iodine is actively transported into the thyroid follicular cell and is oxidized to thyroglobulin-bound tyrosine residues. Four such iodinizations result in the formation of T_4; removal of one residue results in the formation of T_3.

      iii. Subsequently stored bound to thyroglobulin in colloid. The stored hormone is, upon release, taken up from colloid, cleaved off thyroglobulin, and released into the circulation.

      iv. Predominately protein bound (mainly to thyroid-binding globulin), with less than 1% representing free (ie, unbound) hormone.

Thyroid Function Tests

Thyroid hormone (TH) production and secretion is regulated by the pituitary's TSH. The two thyroid hormones are T_4 and T_3. As TH decreases, TSH increases in an effort to stimulate the thyroid to maintain the preexisting set point. Increased TSH levels stimulate gland size and vascularity. As TH increases, TSH release is suppressed.

  A. TSH assays (third-generation ultrasensitive assays capable of detecting 0.01 mU/L) are the sole test necessary to sensitively diagnose hypo- or hyperthyroidism.

  B. TSH measurements are now used not only to monitor replacement therapy but also to measure suppressive therapy both for thyroid nodules and postoperatively for thyroid carcinoma.

  C. If TSH is high and T_4 is normal, subclinical hypothyroidism is diagnosed. Such a pattern is typically seen in early Hashimoto thyroiditis.

  D. If TSH is low and T_4 and T_3 are normal, subclinical hyperthyroidism is diagnosed. Such a pattern is often seen in multinodular goiter, as the patient develops progressive hyperfunctional regions within the thyroid and grades toward frank hyperthyroidism.

  E. Total T_4 and total T_3 laboratory tests measure total amount of protein-bound and free hormone.

  F. There can be significant fluctuation in these total measures depending upon changes in thyroid-binding globulin level.

  G. It is the T_3 resin uptake test that allows for correction of total T_4 level for fluctuation in thyroid-binding globulin. T_3 resin uptake measures the binding capacity of existing thyroid-binding globulin. The more available binding sites on native thyroid-binding globulin, the less resin uptake of radiotagged T_3.

  H. Thus, in states of thyroid-binding globulin excess, T_3 resin uptake is low.

      i. High levels of thyroid-binding globulin occur in pregnancy or with use of birth control pills.

      ii. Low thyroid-binding globulin levels can occur in hypoproteinemic states in acromegaly, and with androgen and anabolic steroids (Table 33-1).

TABLE 33-1 **Patterns Of Thyroid Function Tests**

	Euthyroid	*Hyperthyroid*	*Hypothyroid*	*States of High TBG*	*States of Low TBG*
TSH	Normal	↓	↑	Normal	Normal
Total T_4	Normal	↑	↓	↑	↓
T_3 resin uptake (or THBR)	Normal	↑	↓	↓	↑
Free T_4 index	Normal	↑	↓	Normal	Normal

TBG, thyroid-binding globulin; TSH, thyroid-stimulating hormone; T_4, thyroxine; T_3, triiodothyronine.

Benign Thyroid Disease

Hypothyroidism

- Hypothyroidism is the functional state characterized by increased TSH and decreased TH.
- Hypothyroidism has a variety of causes and can present with a multitude of symptoms (Table 33-2).
- Treatment for hypothyroidism is typically started at a low dose to avoid abrupt correction, especially in elderly patients or in patients with coronary artery disease.
- Typically, T_4 is started at 0.05 mg PO per day and is slowly increased, titrated to thyroid function levels.

Myxedema refers to nonpitting edema secondary to increased glycosaminoglycans in tissue in severe hypothyroidism.

Hyperthyroidism

- *Hyperthyroidism* refers to the physiologic state of increased TH biosynthesis and secretion.

TABLE 33-2 **Hypothyroidism**

Differential Diagnosis	*Clinical Manifestations*
1. Primary gland failure (common)	Fatigue, slowed mentation, change in memory, depression, cold intolerance, hoarseness, brittle hair, dry skin, thick tongue, weight gain, constipation/ileus, menstrual disturbance, bradycardia, nonpitting edema, hyporeflexia, psychosis, hyponatremia, hypoglycemia, coma. In infants, mental retardation/cretinism.
A. Hashimoto thyroiditis	
B. Iodine deficiency	
C. Associated with thyroiditis (lymphocytic/postpartum, subacute)	
D. Radiation-induced (I^{131} or external beam)	
E. Postsurgical	
F. Drugs (lithium, iodine)	
G. Hereditary metabolic defects in hormonogenesis	
2. Central hypothyroidism (rare)	

TABLE 33-3 **Hyperthyroidism**	
Differential Diagnosis	*Clinical Manifestations*
1. Graves disease	Weight loss, fatigue, nervousness, tremor, palpitations, increased appetite, heat intolerance, muscle weakness, diarrhea, sweating, menstrual disturbance
2. Toxic nodule/multinodular goiter	
3. Thyroiditis	
4. Exogenous hyperthyroidism/struma ovarian/functional thyroid cancer	
5. Thyrotropin, thyrotropin-like secreting tumor (pituitary, trophoblastic, other)	

- Hyperthyroidism can occur as a result of several pathologic entities and presents with characteristic symptoms (Table 33-3).
- By far, Graves disease and toxic nodular goiter account for most hyperthyroidism. Hyperthyroidism referable to thyroiditis is self-limiting.

Thyrotoxicosis refers to the clinical syndrome of TH excess.

Graves Disease
- A. Accounts for 60% of clinical hyperthyroidism.
- B. Autoimmune disease resulting from immunoglobulin, autoantibody binding to the TSH receptor, which results in TSH-like activity.
- C. More common in females, presents in the third to fourth decades.
- D. Physical examination shows a diffusely enlarged thyroid. Increased metabolic activity is reflected by increased blood flow; thus a thyroid bruit can often be heard.
- E. Histologically shows scattered lymphocytic infiltration.
- F. Patients may have an infiltrative ophthalmopathy with exophthalmos. Although considered a part of Graves disease, the ophthalmopathy typically follows an independent course relative to the thyroid.
- G. Patients may also exhibit an infiltrative dermopathy, resulting in localized myxedema (eg, pretibial) and, rarely, thyroid acropachy, characterized by digital clubbing and edema of the hands and feet.
- H. Iodine-123 (I^{123}) scanning shows a diffuse increased gland uptake.
- I. Treatments include radioactive iodine ablation, antithyroid drugs, or surgery; treatment in United States, except in children and young adults, usually involves radioactive iodine initially.

Hyperthyroidism can also arise from a toxic nodular goiter. In these cases, unlike Graves disease, the hyperfunctional tissue is restricted to one or more regions within the thyroid gland, which is enlarged in a nodular pattern.

Toxic Multinodular Goiter
- A. Develops from preexisting nontoxic nodular goiter.
- B. Occurs more frequently in endemic goiter, occurring in iodine-deficient regions, and presents more commonly in females.
- C. No eye or skin findings that characterize Graves disease.
- D. Progressive nodule formation and evolution of hyperfunctional regions, which elaborate excess TH, resulting in suppression of TSH. This TSH suppression results in the adjacent normal gland becoming less active on I^{123} scans, with hyperfunctional areas being hot.

E. At this stage the hyperfunctional region is not autonomous and a suppression I^{123} shows no uptake. This prehyperthyroid pattern of suppressed TSH but normal T_4 and T_3 is referred to as subclinical hyperthyroidism.

F. The development of overt hyperthyroidism in such patients with exogenous iodine administration (eg, iodine CT contrast) is referred to as the Jod-Basedow phenomenon.

G. With time, the hyperfunctional regions become truly autonomous, continuing to secrete TH despite significant TSH suppression. When true autonomy occurs, I^{123} scanning shows focal hot regions with complete absence of adjacent normal gland. Suppression scanning at this time shows ongoing focal uptake, demonstrating autonomy despite TSH suppression.

Uninodular Toxic Goiter

A. Hyperthyroidism typically does not occur until the nodule is 3 cm or larger.

B. Such nodules are usually characterized by enhanced T_3 production relative to T_4.

C. Unlike Graves disease, low rate of spontaneous remission after antithyroid drug therapy is withdrawn in toxic nodular goiter.

D. Treatment is either surgery or radioactive iodine, antithyroid medications are considered only as a pretreatment prior to more definitive surgical or radioablative treatment.

E. Surgery quickly and definitively corrects hyperthyroidism and is associated with low morbidity.

Treatment of Hyperthyroidism

When medical treatment is initially offered for hyperthyroidism, treatment is usually initiated with antithyroid drugs in order to render the patient euthyroid. Radioiodine ablation represents a more definitive modality. Radioiodine ablation involves the oral administration of I^{131}. Areas of increased uptake are preferentially injured through beta-radiation. It is contraindicated in women who are pregnant or lactating.

Antithyroid Medication

A. Propylthiouracil (PTU) and methimazole:
   i. Block iodine organification and TH synthesis , PTU also blocks peripheral conversion of T_4-T_3.
   ii. PTU is given q3d; methimazole qd.
   iii. Administration over 6 to 8 weeks before rendering a patient euthyroid.
   iv. Side effects include rash, fever, lupus-like reaction, and bone marrow suppression (0.3%-0.4% of cases), which is reversible if detected early. PTU has recently been associated with liver failure especially in children and so methimazole is considered the first-line therapy for hyperthyroidism.
   v. Contraindicated in pregnancy and lactation.

B. Iodides:
   i. Potassium iodide and Lugol solution inhibit organification and prevent TH release.
   ii. Given preoperatively to decrease thyroid gland vascularity.
   iii. Antithyroid effect is transient, with escape within 2 weeks, and is termed the Wolff-Chaikoff effect.
   iv. Prolonged high-dose iodides, especially in the setting of toxic nodular goiter, can result in hyperthyroidism.

C. Beta-adrenergic blockers
   i. Examples include propranolol or nadolol.
   ii. Block peripheral TH effects (do not alter TH production).

   iii. Useful in symptomatic control while other treatments are initiated and also in transient forms of hyperthyroidism associated with thyroiditis (see later).
   iv. Contraindicated in patients with asthma, chronic obstructive pulmonary disease (COPD), cardiac failure, insulin-dependent diabetes, bradyarrhythmias, and those taking monoamine oxidase inhibitors.
 D. Advantages in the treatment of hyperthyroidism:
   i. Quick onset of action
   ii. May facilitate remission with ongoing euthyroid status after discontinuation of the medicine
 E. Disadvantages
   i. Risk of agranulocytosis
   ii. High rate of hyperthyroid relapse (74% of patients relapsed if followed over a period of 5 years)
   iii. Liver failure with PTU

Radioactive Iodine Ablation

 A. Represents definitive treatment and has low but significant long-term side effects in terms of risk of developing malignancy and no teratogenic effects (conception must be delayed more than 6 months after radioactive iodine treatment).
 B. *Disadvantages*: Up to 80% of patients with Graves disease and up to 50% of those with toxic nodules treated with radioactive iodine ultimately become hypothyroid.
 C. Less rapid normalization of TH levels than surgery (typically 6-8 weeks).
 D. Some reluctance to treat young patients with radioablation given the potential for long-term development of second malignancies.

Surgery for Hyperthyroidism

 A. Correction of the hyperthyroid state faster than radioactive iodine and without the risks of antithyroid drugs.
 B. Surgery is especially suited for toxic nodules, where one discrete region of the thyroid may be resected with preservation of contralateral normal tissue.
 C. Many studies show that when properly done, surgery poses a lower risk of hypothyroidism than radioactive iodine ablation.
 D. Surgery for Graves is considered when there is: (1) failure or significant side effects after medical treatment, (2) need for rapid return to euthyroidism, (3) massive goiter, (4) a wish to avoid radioactive iodine, (5) concern regarding RAI and eye disease or, (6) Graves with nodules.
 E. Preoperative endocrinologic management is essential in order to return the patient to the euthyroid state so as to avoid perioperative thyroid storm. Euthyroidism is obtained typically by antithyroid drugs used for 6 weeks prior to surgery with or without beta-adrenergic blockers.
 F. When the patient is euthyroid, some consider a 2-week course of preoperative iodide (super saturated potassium iodide [SSKI] or Lugol solution), which is believed to decrease vascularity and gland friability, although the efficacy of such treatment is controversial.
 G. The goal of surgery for hyperthyroidism is to remove the hyperfunctional tissue typically for Graves diseases as a total thyroidectomy. It is difficult to preserve sufficient thyroid tissue to render the patient euthyroid and so total thyroidectomy is preferred. Implicit in the surgical philosophy is that it is preferable to render the patient hypothyroid rather than to provide inadequate resection with recurrent hyperthyroidism.

    H. Surgical treatment for Graves disease:
- i. The standard surgery for Graves disease is total thyroidectomy with resection of any existing pyramidal lobe.
- ii. Alternatives include total lobectomy on one side and contralateral subtotal resection or bilateral subtotal thyroidectomy.
- iii. When remnants are left during surgery for Graves disease, they generally range from 4 to 8 g.
- iv. Complication rates of bilateral subtotal thyroidectomy for Graves disease in expert hands show an average of 0.4% permanent hypoparathyroidism and 1.2% permanent vocal cord paralysis.
- v. The rate of postoperative recurrent hyperthyroidism after bilateral subtotal thyroidectomy for Graves disease in expert hands is about 6% and is proportional to the size of the remnant left, the iodine content of the diet, and the degree of lymphocytic infiltration of the gland.

    I. Surgical treatment for toxic nodule(s):
- i. Resection of the involved portion of the gland, (lobectomy).
- ii. In toxic multinodular goiter it is best to consider both scintillographic and sonographic information in constructing a rational surgical plan for toxic multinodular goiter as hot regions of the gland may not correspond to the areas of gross nodularity.

Thyroiditis

Hashimoto Thyroiditis

- A. Most common form of thyroiditis and most common single thyroid disease.
- B. Autoimmune disease, increased thyroid peroxidase antibodies in 70% to 90% of patients.
- C. More common in females in third to fifth decade of life.
- D. Usually patients are euthyroid at presentation, but hypothyroid symptoms may occur at presentation in up to 20%. Hypothyroidism may develop with time and results from progressive loss of follicular cells.
- E. Presents as painless, firm, symmetric goiter, although regional pain has been reported; typically both lobes are enlarged.
- F. Histologically, there is lymphocytic infiltration with germinal center formation, follicular acinar atrophy, Hürthle cell metaplasia, and fibrosis.
- G. Iodine[123] scanning typically contributes little information to the workup.
- H. If patient is hypothyroid, treatment with TH resolves symptoms and usually decreases the size of the goiter.
- I. Surgery is only considered if the goiter is large, symptomatic, or refractive to TH.
- J. The development of any discrete palpable abnormality that is not part of the diffuse goiter process despite a preexisting diagnosis of thyroiditis should be evaluated with fine-needle aspiration (FNA).
- K. Rarer fibrous variants of Hashimoto form a massive, firm goiter.
- L. A rare complication of Hashimoto is development into thyroid lymphoma. A rapidly enlarging mass within a Hashimoto gland should raise concern regarding lymphoma and warrants FNA or biopsy.

Subacute Granulomatous Thyroiditis

- A. Also known as deQuervain thyroiditis, most common cause of painful thyroid.
- B. Viral in etiology, presents with enlarged, painful thyroid, often after upper respiratory tract infection, fever and malaise are common.

    C. Pain in the perithyroid region typically radiates up the neck to the angle of the jaw and ear. The pain and enlargement may only involve a portion of the gland and later migrate to the opposite side.

    D. About 50% of patients with subacute granulomatous thyroiditis (SGT) present with hyperthyroidism with an elevated TH and sedimentation rate. Pain in the hyperthyroid phase typically resolves in 3 to 6 weeks.

    E. I^{123} scanning typically shows less than 2% uptake, this low uptake distinguishes the transient hyperthyroidism of SGT from that of Graves disease or toxic multinodular goiter.

    F. About 50% of patients will enter a hypothyroid phase lasting several months. Most patients ultimately revert to euthyroidism; only 5% will develop permanent hypothyroidism.

    G. Self-limiting disease, treat as needed with nonsteroidal anti-inflammatory drugs (NSAIDs) such as aspirin, and rarely steroids.

Lymphocytic Thyroiditis

    A. Also termed silent, painless, or postpartum thyroiditis.

    B. Etiology unknown, but believed to be an autoimmune process.

    C. Painless with course similar to subacute thyroiditis.

    D. Occurs sporadically but is common in postpartum females; it may occur in up to 5% of such women.

    E. Presents as painless, symmetric thyroid enlargement and reversible hyperthyroidism.

    F. Thyrotoxicosis is self-limiting, no treatment needed.

Acute Suppurative Thyroiditis

    A. Rare thyroid infection with abscess formation.

    B. Most often bacterial (commonly due to *Staphylococcus, Streptococcus,* or *Enterobacter*) but can be fungal or even parasitic.

    C. Typically presents in the setting of an upper respiratory tract infection (URTI).

    D. Treatment is with incision and drainage and parenteral antibiotics.

    E. Children may demonstrate left pyriform sinus fistulae, so after acute treatment, evaluation for this condition is reasonable, including barium swallow, CT, or endoscopy.

Riedel Struma

    A. Rare inflammatory process of unknown etiology; thyroid equivalent to sclerosing cholangitis or retroperitoneal fibrosis.

    B. Large, nontender goiter with a woody consistency fixed to surrounding structures.

    C. Clinical course characterized by progressive regional symptoms, include dysphagia, tracheal compression, and possibly RLN paralysis.

    D. Patient's present euthyroid but can progress to hypothyroidism.

    E. Histologically, extensive fibrotic process, the hallmark of which is extrathyroidal extension of fibrosis into surrounding neck structures.

    F. Treatment may require a biopsy, often in the form of isthmectomy, which may be sufficient to relieve symptoms of tracheal and esophageal pressure. Aggressive surgery is usually avoided because of the loss of surgical planes due to extensive extrathyroidal fibrosis.

Euthyroid goiter (nontoxic diffuse and multinodular goiter)

    A. Thyroid enlargement without significant functional derangement may occur with diffuse enlargement (nontoxic diffuse goiter) or through multinodular formation (multinodular goiter).

B. Goiter development can be sporadic or associated with iodine deficiency, inherited metabolic defects, or exposure to goitrogenic agents.

C. Thyroid function tests are normal for nontoxic diffuse goiter. For multinodular goiter, thyroid function tests may show a normal T_4 and T_3, with TSH low normal (subclinical hyperthyroidism) as some of the nodules slowly grade toward autonomy.

D. Goiter may be stable over a period of years or can slowly grow. Nodules within multinodular goiter may also undergo rapid, painful enlargement secondary to hemorrhage. Such a rapid increase in size may be associated with pain and an increase in regional symptoms, including airway distress.

E. Several studies suggest that from 15% to 45% of patients with large cervical goiters or substernal goiters may be asymptomatic. Of note, patients may be asymptomatic and yet have radiographic evidence of tracheal compression and evidence of airway obstruction on flow volume studies.

F. When patients with goiter are symptomatic, they may present with chronic cough, nocturnal dyspnea, choking, and difficulty breathing in different neck positions or in recumbency. Several surgical series show that approximately 20% of patients with cervical and retrosternal goiters present with acute airway distress, with up to 10% requiring intubation.

G. Surgical consideration should be given to all patients who are symptomatic, all patients with significant radiographic evidence of airway obstruction, and all patients with substernal goiter should be offered surgery.

H. Other surgical indications include significant cosmetic issue and all substernal goiters, as the substernal tissue represents abnormal tissue, which is unavailable for routine physical examination, monitoring, or FNA.

I. The physical examination of such patients should include evaluation of respiratory status, tracheal deviation, and substernal extension. The development of venous engorgement or subjective respiratory discomfort with the arms extended over the head (Pemberton sign) can suggest obstruction of the thoracic inlet from a large or substernal goiter.

J. All patients should have vocal cord mobility assessed.

K. All patients should have a TSH test to rule out subclinical hyperthyroidism.

L. Ultrasound should be performed even when multiple nodules are present. It is recommended that nodules measuring 1.0 to 1.5 cm, those with suspicious sonographic appearance such as microcalcification and intranodular hypervascularity should be aspirated as should isofunctioning or nonfunctioning nodules, especially those with suspicious sonographic features.

M. If there is significant concern regarding tracheal deviation, compression or substernal extension an axial CT scan should be performed.

N. Thyroxin suppression can reduce goiter size and has been found to be more helpful in diffuse than in multinodular goiter. The reduction in goiter size is, however, unpredictable. Goiter growth typically resumes after T_4 discontinuation.

O. During the surgery for goiter, nerve identification is of course necessary as in all cases of thyroidectomy. It may be necessary to use a superior approach with identification of the nerve at the laryngeal entry point after superior pole dissection and then retrograde dissection of the nerve.

P. Multiple surgical series suggest that sternotomy for large cervical and substernal goiters is rarely needed. The surgery necessary for cervical and substernal goiter ranges from lobectomy to total thyroidectomy. Subtotal thyroidectomy, may rarely be appropriate depending on intraoperative parathyroid findings in order to preserve parathyroid tissue. The incidence of carcinoma (usually small intrathyroidal papillary carcinomas) in such multinodular goiters is approximately 7.5%.

Management Of Thyroid Nodules

A. Thyroid nodules are common. They occur in 4% to 7% of the adult population. Approximately 1 in 20 new nodules can be expected to harbor carcinoma. The incidence of thyroid cancer is increasing both throughout the world and in the United States, mostly secondary to earlier detection. An estimated 62,980 new cases of thyroid cancer are expected in the United States in 2014. The majority, 47,790 new cases, are in women with 15,190 new cases expected in men. Disease-specific death from thyroid cancer has not changed significantly, with 1890 thyroid-specific deaths anticipated in 2014 in the United States.

B. Ninety-five percent of thyroid nodules are colloid nodules, adenomas, thyroid cysts, focal thyroiditis, or cancer. Less likely entities are also possible (Table 33-4). A colloid or adenomatous nodule is a nodule within a gland affected by multinodular goiter. It represents a focal hyperplastic disturbance in thyroid architecture and is generally not a true clonal neoplasm.

C. True follicular adenomas are monoclonal tumors arising from follicular epithelium and can be autonomous or nonautonomous. It is unknown whether some follicular adenomas have the capability of evolving to follicular carcinoma.

D. *Risk of malignancy*: The history and physical examination should provide us with a clinical setting within which we interpret the FNA (Table 33-5). Patients who are less

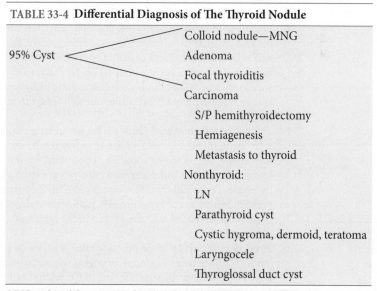

TABLE 33-4 **Differential Diagnosis of The Thyroid Nodule**

95% Cyst
- Colloid nodule—MNG
- Adenoma
- Focal thyroiditis
- Carcinoma
  - S/P hemithyroidectomy
  - Hemiagenesis
  - Metastasis to thyroid
- Nonthyroid:
- LN
- Parathyroid cyst
- Cystic hygroma, dermoid, teratoma
- Laryngocele
- Thyroglossal duct cyst

MNG, multinodular goiter; LN, lymph node; S/P, status post.

TABLE 33-5 **Degree Of Clinical Concern For Carcinoma in a Thyroid Nodule Based on History and Physical Examination**

Less Concern	More Concern
Chronic stable examination	Age < 20 > 60 years
Evidence of a functional disorder (eg, Hashimoto toxic nodule)	Males
	Rapid growth, pain
Multinodular gland without dominant nodule	History of radiation therapy
	Family history of thyroid carcinoma
	Hard, fixed lesion
	Lymphadenopathy
	Vocal cord paralysis
	Size > 4 cm
	Aerodigestive tract compromise (eg, stridor, dysphagia)

than 20 years of age have a higher risk of carcinoma. In patients who are above 60 years of age, nodular disease is more common and malignant disease, if ultimately found, has a considerably worse prognosis. A history of exposure to ionizing radiation is a risk factor for the development of benign and malignant thyroid nodularity, with palpable nodularity being present in up to 17% to 30% of patients exposed. Approximately 1.8% to 10.0% of those exposed to low-dose radiation will eventually develop thyroid carcinoma. Some studies suggest that patients with palpable thyroid lesions with a history of radiation therapy may have a 30% to 50% risk of malignancy, though other studies suggest a lower incidence of malignancy.

E. Low-dose radiation therapy (eg, 200-500 rads), has been given in the past for adenoidal and tonsillar hypertrophy, thymic enlargement, facial acne, and tinea of the head and neck. Such treatment ended in approximately 1955 in the United States. Nodules may develop with a latency of up to 20-30 years, requiring ongoing vigilance. Exposure to nuclear fallout, high-dose therapeutic radiation as for Hodgkin disease, or scatter exposure from breast radiation also seems to increase the risk of thyroid nodular disease.

F. The risk of follicular malignancy is higher in larger nodules. Also, lesions greater than 4 cm are at increased risk for false-negative results during FNA. Generally the firmer the nodule, the more one should be concerned for carcinoma (see elastography). Lymphadenopathy and vocal cord paralysis are strong correlates of malignancy. Family history of medullary carcinoma is certainly important to elicit but is infrequently present. Symptoms of rapid growth, pain, or aerodigestive tract compromise may occur with advanced malignancy but more commonly are associated with benign disease.

G. *Physical examination of the thyroid gland*: It is best to orient toward the thyroid through adjacent cartilaginous laryngeal reference points. Once the thyroid cartilage notch is identified, the anterior ring of the cricoid can be easily found. One thumbbreadth below the cricoid, the isthmus can be palpated on the underlying upper cervical trachea. When identifying the isthmus in the midline or the bilateral thyroid lobes laterally, it is useful to have the patient swallow in order to have the thyroid roll upward underneath the thumb. With such an examination, nodules of 1 cm or greater can be routinely detected. It is important to determine the firmness of the thyroid nodule and its mobility or fixation to the adjacent laryngotracheal complex. All patients with thyroid lesions should have a vocal cord examination to assess vocal cord motion. It should be strongly emphasized that voice and swallowing can be normal in the setting of complete unilateral vocal cord paralysis.

Workup: Laboratory Evaluation

A. Sensitive TSH assay.
B. Excellent screening test to definitively diagnose euthyroidism, hyperthyroidism, or hypothyroidism and is recommended in the initial evaluation of patients with a thyroid nodule.
C. Thyroid peroxidase (TPO) antibodies are helpful if the diagnosis of Hashimoto thyroiditis is suspected.
D. Thyroglobulin
   i. Secreted by both normal and to some degree by malignant thyroid tissue.
   ii. The assay is interfered with by antithyroglobulin antibodies that occur in approximately 15% to 25% of patients.
   iii. Extensive overlap in thyroglobulin levels exists between benign thyroid conditions and thyroid carcinoma.
   iv. Thyroglobulin measures are not useful in the workup of the thyroid nodule
E. Calcitonin, because of the rarity of medullary carcinoma of the thyroid, is not thought to be a reasonable routine screening test in patients with a solitary nodule.
F. Radionuclide scanning (with technetium 99m or I^{123}):
   i. Has been used in the past for the workup of thyroid nodularity.
   ii. Ninety-five percent of all nodules are typically found to be cold; only 10% to 15% of cold nodules are malignant.
   iii. Thyroid scanning does not make it possible to separate nodules into benign and malignant categories.

Ultrasonography

It is recommended that thyroid sonography should be performed in all patients with one or more suspected thyroid nodules. Ultrasonography does not distinguish benign from malignant lesions, but it can provide an accurate baseline. A sonogram can identify the number, size, and shape of cervical nodes surrounding and distant from the thyroid. Concerning ultrasound features of lymph nodes suggestive for malignancy include microcalcifications, irregular borders, hypervascularity, and loss of the lymph node hilum. Sonography may also be useful in screening the thyroid for small lesions in patients presenting with metastatic thyroid cancer and for the evaluation of the thyroid in patients with a history of head and neck radiation.

Fine-Needle Aspiration

A. Fine-needle aspiration (FNA) via ultrasound guidance is strongly recommended as the diagnostic procedure of choice for the evaluation of thyroid nodules (Table 33-6). Effectiveness of FNA is, in turn, related to the skill of both aspirator and cytopathologist. FNA has significantly decreased the number of patients being sent to surgery by 20% to 50%, and has significantly increased the yield of carcinoma found in surgical specimens by 10%-15% (Table 33-7).

TABLE 33-6 Algorithm for The Evaluation of Thyroid Nodules

1. Patients found to have thyroid nodules greater than 1-1.5 cm should undergo a complete history, physical examination, and measurement of serum TSH.

2. If low TSH, then I^{123} or Tc^{99} scanning, if uniform increased uptake or "hot" then evaluate and treat for hyperthyroidism.

3. Normal or elevated TSH, proceed with ultrasound (U/S).

4. If no nodule is seen sonographically and TSH is high then evaluate and treat hypothyroidism; if TSH is normal then no further workup.

5. If U/S shows a posterior nodule, a nodule greater than 1-1.5 cm, or a nodule greater than 50% cystic then U/S guided FNA should be performed.

6. FNA results:

   A. Nondiagnostic/inadequate: repeat U/S-guided FNA in 3 months, if inadequate again, then close follow-up or surgery.

   B. Malignant: surgery

   C. Indeterminate: If suspect carinoma then surgery; if suspect neoplasia then consier I^{123}, hot nodules are followed, cold nodules should proceed to surgery.

   D. Benign: It is recommended that nodules found to be benign on FNA and are easily palpable be followed clinically at 6-18 month intervals. Benign nodules not easily palpated should be followed with U/S at the same follow-up intervals. If there is evidence of benign nodule growth repeat FNA with U/S guidance is recommended.

7. Cysts less than 4 cm can be aspirated and potentially suppressed, with surgery reserved for recurrent cyst formation. Cysts larger than 4 cm should be resected.

Data from Cooper DS, Doherty GM, Haugen BR, et al. Management guidelines for patients with thyroid nodules and differentiated thyroid cancer. *Thyroid*. 2006 Feb;16(2):109-142.

TABLE 33-7 Guidelines for The Role of FNA Biopsy

1. Recommendations

   A. FNA is the procedure of choice in evaluation of thyroid nodules.

   B. Repeated nondiagnostic aspirates of cystic nodules need close observation or surgical excision. Surgery is highly recommended if the nondiagnostic nodule is solid.

   C. Surgery is recommended for all aspirates categorized as malignant.

   D. Nodules found to be benign on cytology do not require further diagnostic studies or treatment.

   E. Readings suspicious for papillary carcinoma or Hürthle cell neoplasm, should be treated with either lobectomy or total thyroidectomy. There is no need for radionuclide scanning.

Data from Cooper DS, Doherty GM, Haugen BR, et al. Management guidelines for patients with thyroid nodules and differentiated thyroid cancer. *Thyroid*. 2006 Feb;16(2):109-142.

B. In the past thyroid FNA cytopathologic categories include (1) malignant, (2) suspicious/indeterminate, (3) benign, and (4) nondiagnostic.

C. In an attempt to establish a standardized diagnostic terminology/classification system and morphologic criteria for reporting thyroid, FNA, a six-tiered diagnostic classification system based on a probabilistic approach, was initiated (the Bethesda classification) and is increasing in use (Table 33-8).

D. When FNA is read as malignant, the chance of malignancy is very high, with a false-positive rate of only 1%. Medullary carcinoma of the thyroid can have a variety of histologic and cytologic forms. Once medullary carcinoma is suspected, calcitonin immunohistochemistry can confirm the FNA diagnosis. Anaplastic carcinoma is often easily identified based on the degree of anaplasia. Lymphoma can be suggested by FNA, but additional tissue with open biopsy is often required to confirm the diagnosis.

E. The main difficulty with FNA in the identification of malignancy is the differentiation of follicular adenoma from follicular carcinoma. This diagnosis hinges on a histologic finding of pericapsular vascular invasion. In order to definitively differentiate follicular adenoma from follicular carcinoma, histologic evaluation of the entire capsule is necessary. This goal cannot be obtained with FNA. The FNA of follicular adenomas is graded as to several cytopathologic features ranging from macrofollicular to microfollicular. The least worrisome finding on FNA of a follicular lesion is described as a macrofollicular lesion, or as a colloid adenomatous nodule. With a lesion that is read as microfollicular with little colloid and little follicular sheeting, the risk of carcinoma ranges from 5% to 15% and increases with the nodule's size.

F. Hürthle cells are large polygonal follicular cells with granular cytoplasm. A Hürthle cell-predominant aspirate may indicate an underlying Hürthle cell adenoma or Hürthle cell carcinoma. Hürthle cells can also be present as metaplastic cells in a variety of thyroid disorders, including multinodular goiter and Hashimoto thyroiditis. Because of the risk of an underlying Hürthle cell carcinoma, patients with FNAs described as Hürthle cell-predominant are recommended to have surgery.

TABLE 33-8 **The Bethesda System for Reporting Thyroid Cytopathology: Implied Risk of Malignancy and Recommended Clinical Management**

Diagnostic Category	Risk of Malignancy (%)	Usual Management[a]
Nondiagnostic or unsatisfactory	1-4	Repeat FNA with ultrasound guidance
Benign	0-3	Clinical follow-up
Atypia of undetermined significance or follicular lesion of undetermined significance	~ 5-15[b]	Repeat FNA
Follicular neoplasm or suspicious for a follicular neoplasm	15-30	Surgical lobectomy
Suspicious for malignancy	60-75	Near-total thyroidectomy or surgical lobectomy[c]
Malignant	97-99	Near-total thyroidectomy[c]

[a] Actual management may depend on other factors (eg, clinical and sonographic) besides the FNA interpretation.

[b] Estimate extrapolated from histopathologic data from patients with "repeated atypicals."

[c] In the case of "suspicious for metastatic tumor" or a "malignant" interpretation indicating metastatic tumor rather than a primary thyroid malignancy, surgery may not be indicated.

Modified with permission from Ali Sz and Cibas ES: *The Bethesda System for Reporting Thyroid Cytopathology definitions, criteria, and explanatory notes.* Springer, 2010.

Nondiagnostic aspirates occur in about 15% of cases, with about 3% of these ultimately showing malignancy. Such aspirates should be repeated, 3 months from the last attempt.

G. FNA false-negative rate ranges from 1% to 6%. False negatives occur with greater frequency in small lesions less than 1 cm or large lesions greater than 3 cm as well as in cystic lesions.

H. Options for management of patients with FNAs reported as benign include (1) following the patient with repetitive examinations and sonograms; (2) administering suppressive therapy; and, rarely, (3) surgery. Lesions founds to be malignant and suspicious lesions (microfollicular, Hürthle cell-predominant) are resected.

I. Cysts account for about 20% of all thyroid nodules. The identification of a thyroid nodule as a cyst is not necessarily equivalent to a benign diagnosis. Papillary carcinomas can present with cystic metastasis with or without hemorrhage. In general, the color of cyst fluid is not helpful in diagnosis (except that parathyroid tumors may have clear fluid), but hemorrhagic fluid and a quick recurrence of the cyst are potentially suggestive of cystic papillary carcinoma. The technique of repetitive FNA cyst drainage plus or minus suppressive therapy is generally ineffective when cysts are greater than 3 to 4 cm in diameter. Surgery is recommended in these cases. The risk of carcinoma in a cyst that has persisted after aspiration attempts ranges from 10% to 30%.

J. Efforts to personalize care for patients with indeterminate nodules have explored the potential of molecular testing. Many molecular markers have been proposed, but only a small minority have been robust to modify clinical decision-making and impact care. Diagnostic testing using a gene expression classifier (GEC) measures the expression of 167 gene transcripts from aspirated material from thyroid nodules. The material is classified as either benign or suspicious based on a priori results to maximize sensitivity and negative predictive value. Another strategy utilizes tested markers to rule in cancer based on markers including the BRAF mutation that should not be present in benign aspirates. Molecular testing of FNA biopsies, especially for BRAF, but also a combination of markers including BRAF, RAS, RET/PTC, and PAX8/PPAR gamma, can improve accuracy of the preoperative FNA diagnosis from cytology.

Elastography

Recently, the newly developed US elastography (USE) has been applied to study the hardness/elasticity of nodules and to differentiate malignant from benign lesions especially in indeterminate nodules on cytology.

USE is a newly developed diagnostic tool that evaluates the degree of distortion of US beam under the application of an external force and is based upon the principle that the softer parts of tissues deform easier than the harder parts under compression, thus allowing a semi-quantitative determination of tissue elasticity. Preliminary data obtained in a limited number of patients suggested that USE might be useful in the differential diagnosis of nodules with indeterminate cytology.

Well-Differentiated Thyroid Carcinoma (WDTC)

Papillary Carcinoma of the Thyroid

A. *Histopathology*: Papillary carcinoma is characterized histologically by the formation of papillae and unique nuclear features. The nuclei of the neoplastic epithelium are large, with nuclear margins folded or grooved and with prominent nucleoli giving a "Orphan Annie eye" appearance. Lesions with any papillary component, even if follicular features predominate, are believed to follow a course consistent with papillary carcinoma. Unfavorable histologic forms of papillary carcinoma include diffuse sclerosing, tall-cell and columnar cell variants.

B. *Clinical behavior and spread*: Papillary carcinoma is strongly lymphotropic, with early spread through intrathyroidal lymphatics as well as to regional cervical lymphatic beds. Papillary carcinoma nodal metastases can often undergo cystic formation and may be dark red or black in color.

C. It is now understood that the multiple foci of papillary carcinoma often seen within the thyroid gland represent true multifocality rather than intraglandular lymphatic spread.

D. At presentation, approximately 30% of patients harbor clinically evident cervical nodal disease (up to 60% of pediatric patients) with a rate of distant metastasis at presentation of approximately 3%. The high prevalence of microscopic disease in regional neck nodal basins and in the contralateral thyroid lobe is in stark contrast to the low clinical recurrence in the neck (< 9%) and in the contralateral lobe (< 5%).

E. Most studies suggest that the presence of microscopic cervical lymph node metastasis has no significant prognostic implications. There is some evidence to suggest that the presence of cervical lymph node metastasis may increase the subsequent rate of nodal recurrence, particularly with macroscopic nodal disease.

F. *Etiology and demographics*: The majority of papillary carcinomas arise spontaneously. Low-dose radiation exposure is thought to have an inductive role in some patients with papillary carcinoma.

   i. The mitogen-activated protein kinase (MAPK) pathway is central to malignant transformation. In 70% of all cases alteration in this pathway is found. Papillary thyroid cancer (PTC) is associated with mutually exclusive alterations to MAPK pathway effectors. Ras, RET, and *BRAF* are part of a linear signaling pathway. A RET oncogene rearrangement has been identified in 10% to 30% of patients with papillary carcinoma. The *BRAF* (T1799A) somatic mutation encodes the constitutively active kinase B-Raf (Val600Glu). This mutation is found almost exclusively in PTC, accounting for approximately 50% of all cases. The presence of a BRAF mutation appears to be a negative prognosticator. These tumors show higher frequency of extrathyroidal invasion and a predisposition to neck lymph node and distant metastasis. PTCs with *BRAF* mutations also have a higher recurrence rate, and the metastatic recurrences have diminished radioiodine avidity. Detection of somatic mutations in FNA specimens of PTC with the *BRAF* (T1799A) mutation can be performed with good sensitivity and specificity.

Follicular Carcinoma

A. *Histopathology*: Follicular carcinoma is the well-differentiated thyroid malignancy, with follicular differentiation lacking features typical of papillary carcinoma. Follicular carcinoma, typically seen as small follicular arrays or solid sheets of cells, has significant morphologic overlap with the benign follicular adenoma. Pericapsular vascular invasion is the most reliable indication of malignancy. The degree of invasiveness, a strong prognostic correlate, varies. Lesions may be widely invasive or "minimally" invasive.

B. *Clinical behavior and spread*: Follicular carcinoma is less likely present with nodal metastasis than papillary carcinoma, but it has a higher rate of distant metastasis at presentation. Reports of distant metastasis vary and are estimated at 16% overall. Follicular carcinoma is typically unifocal lesion. The incidence of contralateral disease for follicular carcinoma approaches zero.

    C. *Etiology and demographics*: Follicular carcinoma occurs more commonly in females than in males and in an older age group than papillary carcinoma, with the median age in the sixth decade. Little is known regarding the etiology. There is however an increased incidence of follicular thyroid carcinoma (FTC) in regions of iodine-deficient endemic goiter felt to be associated with chronic TSH elevation.

    D. Prognosis for follicular carcinoma relates to a number of patient and tumor characteristics—mainly the degree of invasiveness, the presence of metastatic disease, and age at presentation.

    E. Hürthle cell carcinoma is considered a subtype of follicular carcinoma. It is also known as follicular carcinoma, oxyphilic type. It is believed to follow a more aggressive course than follicular carcinoma overall, especially with respect to distant metastasis. Metastasis usually occurs hematogenously, but lymph node metastasis is also not uncommon. Radioactive iodine uptake is typically poor, with greater reliance being placed on surgery. The overall mortality rate is 30% to 70%.

Prognostic Risk Grouping for WDTC

    A. The identification of key prognostic variables makes it possible to segregate patients with WDTC into a large low-risk group and a small high-risk group. Mortality in the low-risk group is approximately 1% to 2%, while in the high-risk group it is approximately 40% to 50%. Segregation of patients into high- and low-risk groups permits appropriately aggressive treatment in the high-risk group with avoidance of excess treatment and its complications in patients in low-risk category.

    B. The key elements of existing prognostic schema for WDTC include:

        i. *Age*: Typically, for females below age 50 and for males below age 40 prognosis is improved.

        ii. *Degree of invasiveness/extrathyroidal extension*: Increased invasiveness increases the risk of local, regional, and distant recurrence and decreases survival.

        iii. *Metastasis*: The presence of distant metastasis increases mortality.

        iv. *Sex*: Males generally have a poorer prognosis than females.

        v. *Size*: Lesions larger than 5 cm have a worse prognosis and lesions smaller than 1.5 cm have a better prognosis. There is controversy as to the exact cutoff, some describing decreased prognosis with lesions greater than 4 cm.

    C. *The two best-known prognostic schema* Hay scheme for papillary carcinoma is summarized by the mnemonic AGES—for age, gender, extent, and size. Cady prognostic schema is for papillary carcinoma and follicular carcinoma and is summarized by the mnemonic AMES—for age, metastasis, extent, and size.

Guidelines for Preoperative Staging of WDTC

    A. It is recommended that patients with malignant cytologic findings on FNA, being treated with thyroidectomy, undergo preoperative neck ultrasound for evaluation of the contralateral lobe and cervical lymph nodes. CT scanning of the neck can be considered.

Extent of Thyroidectomy

In 1987, Hay provided excellent data suggesting that the extent of thyroidectomy should be tailored to the patient's prognostic risk grouping. He found that survival was equivalent for low-risk-group patients with unilateral or bilateral surgery. Survival in the high-risk group was improved with the offering of bilateral thyroid surgery over unilateral thyroid surgery. However, total thyroidectomy offered no survival benefit above near-total thyroidectomy.

Specific Guidelines for Appropriate Operative Management of WDTC

  A. Recommendations:
   i. Total thyroidectomy is indicated in patients with greater than 1 cm cancers diagnosed on preoperative cytology. In addition, those with suspicious cytology with bilateral nodular, who prefer to undergo bilateral thyroidectomy to avoid the possibility of requiring a future surgery on the contralateral lobe should also undergo total thyroidectomy.
   ii. The majority of patients with thyroid cancer should have a total or near-total thyroidectomy initially.
   iii. Lobectomy alone may be sufficient only for small, low-risk, isolated, intrathyroidal papillary carcinomas without cervical nodal disease.
  B. Level VI neck dissection may be considered for patients with advanced stage papillary thyroid carcinoma.
  C. Near-total or total thyroidectomy without central node dissection may be appropriate for follicular cancer.
  D. In patients with biopsy-proven metastatic cervical lymphadenopathy a lateral neck compartmental lymph node dissection should be performed.

Surgical Treatment of the Neck for WDTC

In all cases, systematic evaluation of the central neck nodal beds should be performed (including Delphian, perithyroid, pretracheal, RLN, upper mediastinal, and perithymic regions), with resection of grossly enlarged lymph nodes. If nodal disease is evident in the lateral neck, a selective neck dissection sparing all structures encompassing levels 2-4, ± 5 depending on imaging findings, rather than "berry picking" is recommended. Such a systematic neck dissection seems to decrease subsequent nodal recurrence and the need for complicated reoperation, but has an unclear impact on survival.

The management of the central neck in a patient without clinical disease evidence by either radiologic means or physical examination remains a controversial contemporary topic. Proponents of a prophylactic or elective central node dissection argue that the routine removal of the central nodal beds will remove a potential recurrence source and the potential re-operative morbidity associated with it, permit accurate long-term surveillance, and improve staging accuracy to intensify treatment with radioactive iodine. Opponents of routine prophylactic central node dissection would argue that subclinical metastases are of uncertain importance. There is no clear literature evidence in terms of lowering recurrence or mortality rates, and there is morbidity associated with the intensification of the procedure. Although in expert, high volume centers, the rates of recurrent laryngeal nerve injury are not reported to be higher, there is a higher rate of hypoparathyroidism with routine elective central neck dissection. Furthermore, when increased surgery is performed to remove lymph nodes, there is the potential to upstage patients and intensify with radioactive iodine that may not have been given to a lower stage patient. The high rate of micrometastatic disease that is known to be present will become evident when sought through more extensive surgery.

Invasive Disease

When disease is focally adherent to a functioning RLN, it should be dissected off, removing gross disease and preserving the functioning nerve. An infiltrated RLN is resected if preoperative paralysis is present or if gross disease cannot be removed from the nerve. Extracapsular disease involving the strap muscles is usually easily managed with resection of the involved musculature. Disease invasive to the larynx and trachea is managed with resection of gross disease, with preservation of vital structures when possible. Near-total excision with postoperative adjuvant treatment is equivalent with respect to survival to more radical resection.

Postoperative Follow-up for WDTC

A. TH, usually T_4, is given to suppress TSH to 0.1-0.3 mU/L or lower in high-risk patients. I^{131} can be given post-thyroidectomy based on the patient's risk grouping and likelihood of harboring metastatic disease. Typically, high-risk patients with papillary carcinoma and most patients with follicular carcinoma are considered for treatment.

B. I^{131} is given in ablative doses ranging from 30 to 100 mCi if patients have undergone less than total thyroidectomy and greater than 2% uptake on regional neck scanning. Such treatment completes thyroid ablation, rendering the patient hypothyroid. It is recommended that the minimum radioactivity necessary for ablation be used. Thereafter, with a TSH greater than 30 mU/L, whole body scanning can be performed. Patients should undergo thyroid hormone withdrawal by stopping use of levothyroxine (with or without switching to levotriiodothyronine) for a number of weeks prior to whole body scanning. Metastatic well-differentiated thyroid carcinoma cells require increased TSH levels to drive them to take up sufficient I^{131} scanning doses to reveal their presence on whole body scanning. If disease is identified on such whole body scans, therapeutic doses of I^{131} (100-150 mCi) are given.

C. External beam radiation (typically using from 50-60 Gy) has been employed to palliate extensive central neck disease, prolong local control, and improve quality of life in inoperable cases or where gross disease persists postoperatively. It has also been used to palliate bony and central nervous system (CNS) metastasis.

D. Thyroglobulin is produced by normal and, to some degree, malignant thyroid tissue and can serve as a marker of well-differentiated thyroid cancer. Thyroglobulin is usually elevated after total thyroid ablation in patients with known metastatic disease and, along with whole body scanning, can be used to assess the status of metastatic disease. If thyroglobulin is low (< 2 ng/mL on T_4 suppression) or unmeasurable after total thyroid ablation and whole body scanning is negative, patients rarely harbor clinically significant metastatic disease.

E. Cervical ultrasound (U/S) performed at 6 and 12 months and then annually for 3 to 5 years is recommended to evaluate the thyroid bed and central and lateral cervical nodal compartments for disease recurrence or metastasis.

F. PET/CT scanning may be performed and useful on patients with WDTC who have a negative I^{131} scan who have thyroglobulin > 10 ng/mL.

Medullary Carcinoma of the Thyroid

A. *Histopathology*: This lesion arises from parafollicular C cells (not thyroid follicular cells). Calcitonin is secreted by normal parafollicular C cells, and calcitonin elevation occurs in C-cell hyperplasia and all forms of medullary carcinoma of the thyroid (MTC). This tumor marker has proven extremely useful in establishing a diagnosis in asymptomatic relatives of hereditary cases and in postoperative screening for recurrent disease. RET oncogene point missense germ-line mutations have been identified in patients with inherited MTC.

B. *Clinical behavior and spread*: There is no significant effective therapy available for medullary carcinoma of the thyroid other than surgery. Surgical recommendation is for total thyroidectomy and central neck dissection for all cases of medullary carcinoma. Medullary carcinoma of the thyroid has a strong tendency toward paratracheal and lateral neck nodal involvement. Therefore all patients with medullary carcinoma of the thyroid should have, at time of surgery, thorough central neck dissection emphasizing the paratracheal regions. Given the high incidence of microscopic lateral neck disease, all patients with palpable medullary carcinoma of the thyroid should have ipsilateral level II to V neck dissections with a consideration for bilateral dissection. MTC tends to recur locally and may metastasize hematogenously to lung, liver, or bone. For all types of MTC, the 5-year survival rate is between 78% and 91%; the 10-year survival rate is between 61% and 75%.

C. *Etiology and demographics*: MTC represents approximately 5% to 10% of all thyroid cancers. Approximately 75% of medullary carcinoma occurs as a sporadic neoplasm, typically presenting in the fourth decade as a unifocal lesion without associated endocrinopathy. Hereditary MTC accounts for the remaining 25%, occurring in a younger age group with multifocal thyroid lesions (Table 33-9). All three forms of hereditary MTC are inherited as autosomal dominant traits and are associated with multifocal MTC. All are preceded by multifocal C-cell hyperplasia.

Lymphoma

A. *Histopathology*: Primary thyroid lymphomas are typically of the non-Hodgkin type. Primary thyroid Hodgkin disease is extremely rare.

B. *Clinical behavior and spread*: They are highly curable malignancy if diagnosed promptly and managed correctly. Treatment is based on the lymphoma subtype and the extent of disease and is similar to the treatment of non-Hodgkin lymphoma (NHL) at other sites. Treatment is radiation therapy and chemotherapy. Surgery is mainly restricted to biopsy.

C. *Etiology and demographics*: Thyroid lymphomas constitute only 3% of all NHLs and approximately 5% of all thyroid neoplasms. Thyroid lymphoma usually occurs in women in the sixth decade of life, presenting typically as a rapidly enlarging firm, painless mass. Patients may present with evidence of RLN paralysis, dysphagia, and regional adenopathy. Often, there is a history of preexisting hypothyroidism (30%-40% of cases). The incidence of primary thyroid lymphomas in patients with Hashimoto thyroiditis is markedly increased.

Anaplastic Carcinoma

A. *Histopathology*: Anaplastic thyroid cancer (ATC) is believed to occur from a terminal dedifferentiation of previously undetected long-standing differentiated thyroid carcinoma. About 25% of undifferentiated thyroid cancers have *BRAF* mutations, and this proportion is probably higher in tumors with documented evidence of progression from a pre-existing well-differentiated PTC.

B. *Clinical behavior and spread*: Patients present with a rapidly growing neck mass. Patients present with large, widely invasive primaries often fixed to the laryngotracheal complex, vocal cord paralysis, cervical adenopathy, and, frequently, distant metastasis. Patients may present with hoarseness, weight loss, bone pain, weakness, and cough. There is often a history of preexisting goiter that has been stable for years.

C. Surgical treatment is generally limited to debulking or isthmusectomy, for biopsy, often combined with tracheotomy. It is important to obtain sufficient biopsy material to rule out lymphoma, which is readily treatable. Aggressive surgery directed toward the thyroid or laryngotracheal complex is, in general, not warranted. Treatment

TABLE 33-9 Subtypes Of Medullary Thyroid Carcinoma (MTC)

	Mode of Transmission	Family History	Age at Presentation (Decade)	Likelihood of Regional LN Involvement	Subtypes of MTC		
					Pheochromocytoma	Hyperparathyroidism	Mucosal Neuromata Marfanoid Habitus
Sporadic	—	Negative	Fourth	High	No	No	No
MEN IIa	Autosomal dominant	Positive or negative	Third	High if Dx with mass / Low if Dx with screen	Yes	Yes	No
MEN IIb	Autosomal dominant	Usually negative	First or second	High	Yes	No	Yes
FMTC	Autosomal dominant	Positive or negative	Fourth	Low	No	No	No

LN, lymph node; MEN, multiple endocrine neoplasia; FMTC, familial nonmutiple endocrine neoplasia medullary carcinoma of the thyroid (now FMTC is considered a nonpenetrant form of MEN 2A).

recommendations generally include hyperfractionated external beam radiation combined with chemotherapy.

D. *Etiology and demographics*: Anaplastic carcinoma represents less than 5% of thyroid cancers and occurs in an older age group. The Anaplastic carcinoma is one of the most lethal human malignancies with an average survival of about 6 months. ATC does not concentrate iodine.

Thyroidectomy: Surgical Anatomy

A. A collar-type thyroid incision is made, typically 1 or 2 finger breadths above the sternal notch in a curvilinear fashion, within a normal skin crease. A subplatysmal skin flap is raised superiorly up to the level of the thyroid notch.

B. Strap muscles are identified in the midline, and the sternohyoid (more medial) and sternohyoid (more lateral) are elevated in one layer off the ventral surface of the thyroid lobe.

C. Through primarily blunt dissection, the lobe is dissected and mobilized. As this is done, the thyroid gland is retracted medially, and the strap muscles are retracted laterally. The middle thyroid vein should be ligated, providing lateral exposure of the mid lobe (Figure 33-4).

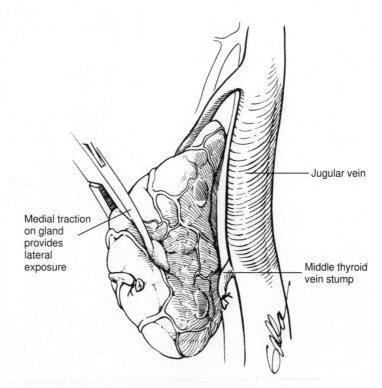

Jugular vein

Medial traction on gland provides lateral exposure

Middle thyroid vein stump

Figure 33-4 Middle thyroid vein division provides for greater lateral exposure.

D. The inferior pole is dissected with an eye toward identifying the inferior parathyroid, which is typically located within 1 cm inferior or posterior to the thyroid's inferior pole. The inferior parathyroid is often within the uppermost thyrothymic horn (upper thymus).

E. The RLN can be identified through the lateral approach at the midpolar level just below the ligament of Berry and its laryngeal entry point or medial to the tubercle of Zuckerkandl. The RLN is identified as a white, wave-like structure with characteristic vascular stripe. Extralaryngeal branching can occur in about one-third of patients above the crossing point of the RLN and inferior thyroid artery. On the right, the RLN angles more laterally than on the left. Nerve stimulation can be used to facilitate nerve identification. The laryngeal entry point is indicated by the inferior cornu of the thyroid cartilage. The possibility of a nonrecurrent RLN on the right should be kept in mind. Goitrous enlargement of the thyroid gland can significantly distort RLN position, as can peri-RLN nodal paratracheal disease.

F. The RLN should be identified visually in all cases and confirmed electrically through neural monitoring.

G. The distal branches of the inferior and superior thyroid arteries should always be taken as close to the thyroid as possible in order to optimize parathyroid preservation (Figure 33-5). If the parathyroid has turned black as a result of its dissection or has a

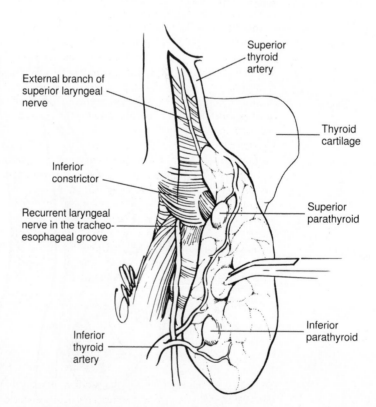

Figure 33-5 Laterally, the inferior thyroid artery and superiorly, the superior thyroid artery are followed to identify inferior and superior parathyroid glands.

questionable vascular pedicle, it can be biopsied, confirmed as parathyroid, and then minced and placed into several muscular pockets in the sternocleidomastoid muscle (SCM).

H. Downward and lateral retraction of the superior pole allows dissection in the interval between the thyroid cartilage medially and the superior pole laterally (cricothyroid space). The superior polar vessels are then ligated at the level of the thyroid capsule. The external branch of the SLN can be, in approximately 20% of cases, closely related to the superior pole vessels at the level of the thyroid capsule and is, therefore, vulnerable to injury.

I. In those cases where a portion of the lobe is left in place in order to preserve parathyroid tissue, it is the posterolateral portion of the thyroid lobe that should be left in situ.

Surgical Complications

A. RLN paralysis rates vary because many studies do not involve postoperative laryngeal examination, which is essential for determination of accurate postoperative paralysis rates. Many reports reveal rates of 6% to 7%, with some reports as high as 23%. The incidence of RLN paralysis increases with bilateral surgery, revision surgery, surgery for malignancy, surgery for substernal goiter, and in patients brought back to surgery for bleeding. The authors believe that the RLN should be clearly identified and dissected along its entire course at thyroidectomy and that identification should be made both visually and through neural electric stimulation. Such stimulation is safe and allows the surgeon to identify a neurapraxic nerve injury and potentially postpone contralateral thyroid surgery. Temporary RLN paralysis generally resolves within 6 months. Bilateral RLN paralysis may result in a nearly normal voice but also respiratory insufficiency with postoperative stridor. SLN external branch paralysis occurs in 0.4% to 3% of cases and results in reduction of cricothyroid vocal cord tensing with loss of high vocal registers. The affected cord will be lower and bowed, with laryngeal rotation.

B. Hypoparathyroidism can result in perioral and digital paresthesias. Progressive neuromuscular irritability results in spontaneous carpopedal spasm, abdominal cramps, laryngeal stridor, mental status changes, QT prolongation on the electrocardiogram, and ultimately tetanic contractions. Chvostek sign is the development of facial twitching with light tapping over the facial nerve. This sign must be assessed preoperatively, as approximately 5% of the normal population has a positive Chvostek sign in the setting of eucalcemia. Trousseau sign is induced carpal spasm through tourniquet-induced ischemia. Treatment for hypocalcemia is usually begun when the calcium level falls below 7.5 mg/dL or in the symptomatic patient. Temporary hypoparathyroidism, defined as being of less than 6 months duration, occurs in from 17% to 40% of patients after total thyroidectomy. Permanent hypoparathyroidism after total thyroidectomy in the community occurs in approximately 10% of patients.

Parathyroid Glands

A. The parathyroid glands' hormonal product, parathyroid hormone (PTH), maintains calcium levels through increased calcium absorption in the gut, mobilization of calcium in bone, inhibition of renal calcium excretion, and stimulation of renal hydroxylase to maintain vitamin D levels.

B. Total calcium levels vary with protein fluctuation, but ionized calcium is maintained within strict ranges. In patients with normal albumin, total serum calcium can be followed. If the albumin level is abnormal, total serum calcium levels can be corrected (total serum calcium levels fall by 0.8 mg/dL for every 1 g/dL fall in albumin) or the ionized calcium can be followed.

C. Adenomatous or hyperplastic change to the parathyroid glands can increase PTH levels and produce hypercalcemia.

    i. *Adenoma* implies a single enlarged gland, typically in the context of three other normal glands. Adenomas have been found to be benign clonal neoplasms. Such glands are hypercellular, consisting of chief and oncocytic cells, with decreased intra- and intercellular fat.

    ii. *Hyperplasia* implies that all four glands are involved in the neoplastic change, though the gross enlargement of the glands may be quite asymmetric. Histologically, in hyperplasia there is an increased number of chief and oncocytic cells in multiple parathyroid glands.

D. Primary hyperparathyroidism (HPT), which occurs in approximately 1 out of 500 females and 1 out of every 2000 males, can be spontaneous, familial, or associated with multiple endocrine neoplasia (MEN) syndromes; HPT is usually mediated by a single gland's adenomatous change (approximately 85%), but it can be caused by four-gland hyperplasia in approximately 5% to 15% of cases. Four-gland hyperplasia can be sporadic or can occur in familial HPT or in MEN I (Werner) and MEN IIa (Sipple) syndromes.

    i. Double adenomas account for 2% to 3% of cases and are more common in elderly patients.

    ii. Parathyroid carcinoma occurs rarely and accounts for approximately 1% of cases of HPT. One should suspect parathyroid carcinoma if calcium and, especially, PTH levels are significantly elevated. In cases of parathyroid carcinoma, preoperative examination may be notable for a perithyroid mass. Such findings do not occur in benign HPT.

    iii. Secondary HPT represents a hyperplastic response of parathyroid tissue, typically to renal failure.

    iv. When this parathyroid response becomes autonomous, persisting after correction of the primary metabolic derangement (typically renal transplant) with increased PTH levels despite normalization of calcium, it is termed tertiary HPT.

    v. Elevated calcium and decreased phosphorus with elevated PTH help establish the diagnosis of HPT, elevated calcium levels can be caused by many other entities (Table 33-10).

E. *Benign familial hypocalciuric hypercalcemia (BFHH)*: Like HPT, BFHH is associated with high calcium and PTH levels. It is an autosomal dominant inherited disease characterized by excess renal calcium reabsorption, leading to high serum calcium and low urine calcium levels which are stable throughout life. Surgery is not indicated.

F. While chronically elevated calcium levels in the past have been detected through "painful bones, kidney stones, abdominal groans, psychic moans, and fatigue overtones," the majority of primary HPT today is detected in asymptomatic or mildly symptomatic patients on routine laboratory screening panels (Table 33-11).

G. Symptomatic hypercalcemia warrants surgical treatment. In addition, typically patients with significantly elevated calcium levels greater than 1 mg/dL above the upper limit of normal are also offered surgery. Surgery is also offered for young patients under 50 years of age because of the potential for development of symptoms

TABLE 33-10 **Differential Diagnosis of Hypercalcemia**

Primary hyperparathyroidism

Secondary hyperparathyroidism

Tertiary hyperparathyroidism

Pseudohyperparathyroidism

Sarcoid

Granulomatous disease (tuberculosis, berylliosis, eosinophilic granuloma)

Milk-alkali syndrome

Benign familial hypocalciuric hypercalcemia

Malignancy (breast, lung, multiple myeloma)

Pheochromocytoma

Vitamin D intoxication

Excess calcium intake

Lithium and thiazide diuretics

Hyperthyroidism

Adrenal insufficiency

Immobilization

Paget disease

Factitious hypercalcemia (tourniquet effect)

if followed nonsurgically. Also, surgery is offered to all patients who desire it or who have had a previous episode of life-threatening hypercalcemia. Controversy exists for patients over 50 years of age who are asymptomatic. In such patients, if there is evidence of significant bone or renal dysfunction, surgery is recommended. If creatinine clearance in this patient group is decreased by 30% for age without other obvious cause, urinary calcium is greater than 400 mg/dL, or bone density is less than two standard deviations below the mean corrected for age, gender, and race, surgery is recommended.

Localization Studies

A. *Preoperative localization studies*: If unilateral, guided or minimal access is planned, localization studies should be considered. Most agree that localization studies are warranted in revision cases (Figure 33-6).

   i. Parathyroid scintigraphy is the best imaging modality for preoperative localization of parathyroid adenomas. Sestamibi scanning, initially introduced as a cardiac scan, has been found to be an excellent study for preoperative localization in HPT. Technetium 99m methoxyisobutyl isonitrile (Tc^{99}MIBI) is initially taken up by both thyroid and parathyroids. The thyroid uptake is, over time, washed out, yet sestamibi is retained by adenomatous parathyroid glands. The uptake and retention of sestamibi is thought to be related to cellular mitochondrial content. Two hour washout scans reveal the enlarged parathyroids. This scan seems to be one of

TABLE 33-11 Manifestations of Chronic Hypercalcemia

Weight loss

Polyuria–polydipsia

Malaise

Fatigue

Confusion

Depression

Memory changes

Hypertension

Renal dysfunction (ranging from nephrolithiasis to nephrocalcinosis)

Duodenal and peptic ulcers

Constipation

Pruritus

Pancreatitis

Arthritis

Gout

Bone pain, cysts, demineralization, fracture

Band keratitis, palpebral fissure calcium deposition

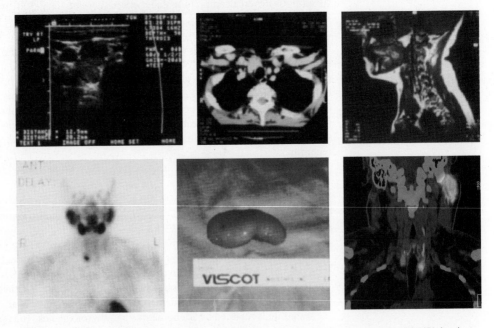

Figure 33-6 Parathyroid localization tests: parathyroid adenoma seen on sonogram, CT, MRI, (top), and planar sestamibi scanning, fuset SPECT/CT and gross pathology of parathyroid adenoma (bottom).

the most sensitive tests available for HPT, with sensitivity in the literature ranging from 70% to 100%. Single proton emission computerized tomography (SPECT) scanning for primary hyperparathyroidism increases the accuracy of routine sestamibi scanning by about 2% to 3% by providing a three-dimensional picture rather than a planar (PA) view.

ii. Hybrid SPECT/CT combines the three-dimensional functional information of SPECT with the anatomic information of CT, further improving preoperative localization.

iii. Sonography is relatively inexpensive, with sensitivities in the literature ranging from 22% to 82%. Sonography is, however, extremely operator-dependent, and is poor in evaluating lesions behind the larynx and trachea or in the mediastinum.

iv. CT scanning has been found to be less sensitive than magnetic resonance imaging (MRI) but 4D CT has been shown to be helpful by identifying typical contrast perfusion characteristics of abnormal parathyroid glands.

v. MRI is expensive, with sensitivities ranging from 50% to 80%.

Surgical Theory for Hyperparathyroidism

A. Although a single adenoma is more likely, hyperplasia must always be kept in mind when creating the surgical plan. Unilateral exploration augmented by preoperative localization studies should allow shorter operative times, a decrease in postsurgical complications, and resultant cost savings.

B. At this time there seems to be a general trend toward unilateral surgery and minimally invasive approaches with increased reliance on preoperative localization testing and intraoperative PTH assays. Given the short half-life of PTH, approximately 10 minutes after resection of an adenoma, the PTH falls to within normal limits. Once sufficient PTH fall occurs, the surgery can be successfully halted.

C. Four-gland hyperplasia. Surgical strategies include three and one half-gland subtotal resection to four-gland resection with autotransplantation to the forearm. In general, the aggressiveness of the surgical approach should relate to the clinical severity of the subtype of four-gland hyperplasia.

Parathyroid: Surgical Anatomy

A. Parathyroid glands have been described as flat-bean or leaf-like shaped yellow-tan, caramel, or mahogany in color and thus may be distinguished from the brighter, less distinct yellow fat with which the parathyroids are typically closely associated. They can be observed as discrete bodies gliding within the more amorphous fat surrounding them as this fat is gently manipulated (the gliding sign).

B. The vast majority of humans have four parathyroid glands, but approximately 5% of patients will have more than four glands.

C. Mirror-image symmetry occurs for the upper parathyroids as well as for the lower parathyroids. Finding a left gland can then assist in finding the corresponding right gland.

Superior Parathyroid: Surgical Anatomy

A. The superior parathyroid derives from the fourth branchial pouch and is associated with the lateral thyroid anlage/C-cell complex.

B. As such, the superior parathyroid tracks closely with the posterolateral aspect of the bilateral thyroid lobes.

C. The final adult position of the superior parathyroid is less variable than that of the inferior parathyroid because of its shorter embryologic migratory path.

D. The superior parathyroid typically occurs at the level of the cricothyroid articulation of the larynx, approximately 1 cm above the intersection of the RLN and inferior thyroid artery. It is closely related to the posterolateral aspect of the superior thyroid pole, often resting on the thyroid capsule in this location. The superior parathyroid is located at a plane deep (dorsal) to the plane of the RLN in the neck. And may lie quite deep in the neck and tends toward a retrolaryngeal and retroesophageal location.

Inferior Parathyroid: Surgical Anatomy

A. The inferior parathyroids derive from the third branchial pouch and migrate with the thymus anlage. The inferior parathyroid has a more varying adult position.

B. The inferior parathyroid is found in close association with the inferior pole of the thyroid, often on the posterolateral aspect of the capsule of the inferior pole or within 1 to 2 cm. It is often closely associated with the thickened fat of the thyrothymic horn (ie, thyrothymic ligament).

C. The inferior parathyroid is generally located superficial (ventral) to the RLN.

Guided Parathyroid Surgery

A. Patients first undergo a preoperative localization scan with double-phase sestamibi, SPECT, or fused SPECT/CT imaging.

B. Only those with a positive scan are candidates for minimally invasive guided surgery. Patients should understand that localization does not occur or if the adenoma is not readily found a formal exploration may be necessary.

C. Delayed imaging is acquired 2 hours after injection and an ink mark is placed on the skin over the aberrant parathyroid.

D. Patients are then brought to the operating room. A horizontal incision is then made in a skin area abutting the mark and either using the localization scan alone or in conjunction with a handheld gamma probe may be used as a guide to the surgeon to the area of highest radioactivity levels. Blunt dissection is performed until the adenoma is identified and resected. Resected tissue may be sent for frozen pathology to confirm and/or rapid PTH levels may also be obtained postresection.

Parathyroid Exploration

A. The overriding technical principle in parathyroid exploration is meticulous dissection in a bloodless field to avoid blood staining of tissues. Loupe magnification is helpful. The surgeons should have a low threshold to identify the RLN, depending on the depth of the needed dissection. Intraoperative PTH drop can be extremely helpful in determining when exploration can be successfully halted as long as strict criteria for its use are met.

B. The first step in parathyroid exploration involves a full exploration of all normal parathyroid gland locations.

C. In the case of "missing glands"
   i. If the inferior gland is missing, then the thyrothymic horn is exposed/resected and the region greater than 1 cm lateral to the inferior pole and medial to the inferior pole adjacent to the trachea is dissected.
   ii. If this search is unrewarding, then frank ectopic inferior gland locations are explored, including the lower thymus.

iii. An undescended ectopic gland is then considered; therefore the carotid sheath is opened and explored from hyoid to thoracic inlet.

iv. Consideration should also be given to a subcapsular or intrathyroidal inferior parathyroid.

v. If the superior gland is missing, the extended normal locations for the superior gland should be explored, including the posterolateral aspect of the upper half of the thyroid lobe and retrolaryngeal, retroesophageal regions.

vi. If this search is unrewarding, then the superior gland can be searched for more inferiorly in the para- and retroesophageal region, extending from the hyoid down to the posterior mediastinum.

vii. If the above search is unrewarding and has revealed only four normal-appearing glands, one should consider a fifth gland. Such a fifth-gland adenoma is typically found in the thymus; therefore more aggressive thymic exploration and resection are warranted.

viii. One should avoid empiric thyroidectomy and never remove a normal thyroid gland.

Complications of Parathyroid Surgery

In experienced surgical hands, persistent hypercalcemia occurs postoperatively in less than 5% of patients with primary HPT caused by adenoma. A higher failure rate of approximately 10% to 50% exists when HPT is caused by hyperplasia, some forms of inherited HPT (eg, MEN I), or secondary HPT.

A. Reasons for failure (ie, persistent or recurrent hypercalcemia) in surgery for HPT include failure to find the adenomatous gland in a normal cervical location, failure to find a second adenoma, failure to recognize four-gland hyperplasia, failure to identify a supernumerary gland (ie, fifth gland), regrowth of adenoma from the unresected stump of a resected adenoma, unrecognized parathyroid carcinoma, or incorrect diagnosis (eg, BFHH).

B. The most common ectopic locations for parathyroid adenomas include retroesophageal, retrotracheal, anterior mediastinal, intrathyroidal, carotid sheath, and hyoid/angle of mandible. Hypoparathyroidism can occur after surgery for HPT.

C. Permanent hypoparathyroidism occurs after surgery for adenoma in approximately 5% of cases overall.

D. Permanent hypoparathyroidism occurs after surgery for hyperplasia or secondary HPT in about 10% to 30% of cases.

Bibliography

Alexander EK, Schorr M, Klopper J, Kim, et al. Multicenter clinical experience with the Afirma Gene Expression Classifier. *J Clin Endocrinol Metab.* 2014; 99(1):119-125.

Mazzaferri EL, Young RL. Papillary thyroid carcinoma: a ten-year follow-up report on the impact of treatment in 576 patients. *Am J Med.* 1981;70:511-518.

Randolph G, Kamani D. The importance of preoperative laryngoscopy in patients undergoing thyroidectomy: voice, vocal cord function, and the preoperative detection of invasive thyroid malignancy. *Surgery.* 2006;139(3):357-362.

Randolph G. *Surgery of the Thyroid and Parathyroid Glands.* 2nd ed. Philadelphia, PA: Elsevier Saunders; 2013.

Randolph GW, Henning D, The International Neural Monitoring Study Group. Electrophysiologic recurrent laryngeal nerve monitoring during thyroid and parathyroid surgery: international standards guideline statement. *Laryngoscope.* 2011;121:S1-S16.

Questions

1. Generally most thyroid nodules are biopsied if they
   A. are > 1 cm
   B. are < 1 cm
   C. are between 1 and 2 mm or larger
   D. are palpated and felt to be benign
   E. cause cosmetic deformity

2. Most parathyroid glands
   A. are vascularized by the superior thyroid artery
   B. are in the mediastinum
   C. are close to or on the thyroid gland
   D. are often found to be adenomatous at thyroid surgery
   E. are removed and autotransplanted at surgery

3. Papillary thyroid cancer
   A. prognosis is worse in the young adult
   B. is associated with frequent nodal metastasis at presentation
   C. is associated with capsular invasion
   D. is typically associated with C-cell hyperplasia
   E. cannot occur in the pyramidal lobe

4. Medullary cancers
   A. may be associated with RET oncogene mutation
   B. are always inherited
   C. result in decrease of calcitonin and carcinoembryonic antigen (CEA)
   D. never spread to liver or lung
   E. are always associated with parathyroid disease

5. Graves disease
   A. is associated with focal increased uptake in the thyroid
   B. can be managed with surgery
   C. cannot usually be treated with radioactive iodine
   D. is always associated with eye disease
   E. generally can be operated on without preoperative medical management

Chapter 34
Cysts and Tumors of the Jaw

Introduction

Pathologic lesions of the jaws necessitate a wide differential diagnosis. A thorough clinical history and physical examination aid in diagnosis, though in most situations, radiographs and histopathological analysis are necessary to determine proper treatment. Many are asymptomatic and found on routine dental radiograph screening. All jaw cysts, except periapical cysts, are generally associated with vital teeth, unless coincidental disease of adjacent teeth is present. Tooth vitality can be assessed by ice testing or electrical pulse testing. Needle aspiration prior to open incisional biopsy of a radiolucent lesion is important to exclude diagnosis of arteriovenous malformation and, although not always reliable, can give insight into cystic versus solid masses. Aspiration of a solid tumor would usually yield a dry tap. Radiographs play a critical role in management of such lesions of the jaws as they may appear radiolucent ("radiographically cystic"), radiopaque, or sometimes contain characteristics of both (Figures 34-1 and 34-2). Computed tomography (CT) scans can be helpful when lesions are large, neurologic changes are present, or malignancy is suspected. Pertinent clinical, histopathologic, and radiographic features as well as treatment and prognosis will be reviewed for these lesions.

Cysts of the Jaw

A true cyst contains an epithelial lining.

Odontogenic

Inflammatory
  A. Periapical cyst (radicular cyst)
      i. Clinical features
          a. Overall most common odontogenic cyst of the jaws.
          b. Associated with *nonvital* tooth or trauma, not always symptomatic.
          c. Necrotic dental pulp creates inflammatory response at apex leading to granuloma formation or fistula to the gingiva or through cheek/jaw skin.
      ii. Radiographic features: radiolucent, single lesion, well-demarcated, unilocular, surrounding apex of tooth
      iii. Histopathologic features: polymorphonuclear leukocytes (PMNs) intermixed with inflammatory exudate, cellular debris, necrotic material, bacterial colonies

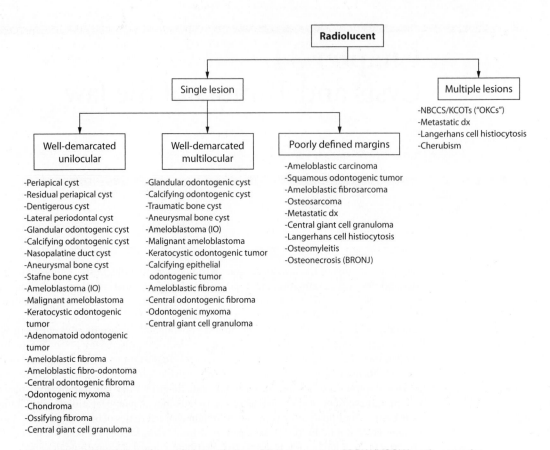

Figure 34-1 Clinical algorithm: radiolucent lesions. (IO: intraosseous; ARONJ/MRONJ: antiresporptive osteonecrosis of the jaw/medication-related osteonecrosis of the jaw; NBCCS: nevoid basal cell carcinoma syndrome; KCOTs: keratocystic odontogenic tumors, previously known as odontogenic keratocysts "OKCs")

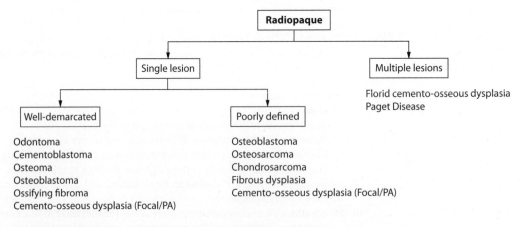

Figure 34-2 Clinical algorithm: radiopaque lesions. (PA: periapical)

      iv. Treatment: removal of underlying inflammatory process through endodontic treatment (root canal) or tooth extraction with enucleation and curettage; antibiotics and drainage of any soft tissue abscess (if occurs)

      v. Prognosis: excellent

B. Residual periapical cyst

      i. Clinical features

        a. At the site of previous tooth extraction

        b. Remnant of process that led to tooth loss versus insufficient curettage during tooth extraction versus continuation of epithelial rest inflammatory response after tooth extraction

        c. Generally asymptomatic

      ii. Radiographic features: radiolucent, single lesion, well-demarcated, unilocular

      iii. Histopathologic features: same as periapical cyst

      iv. Treatment: enucleation and curettage

      v. Prognosis: excellent

Developmental

A. Dentigerous cyst

      i. Clinical features

        a. Second most common odontogenic cyst of the jaws (after periapical cyst).

        b. Most common between ages of 10 and 30 years.

        c. Associated with the crown of *unerupted tooth.*

        d. Most commonly arises from mandibular third molar or maxillary canines, although can occur at any *unerupted* tooth.

        e. May grow extensively, associated with painless expansion of bone.

        f. 18G needle aspiration can yield *straw-colored fluid.*

      ii. Radiographic features: radiolucent, single lesion, well-demarcated, unilocular, associated with crown of *unerupted tooth*

      iii. Histopathologic features: fibrous capsule surrounded by inflammatory infiltrate

      iv. Treatment: extraction of affected tooth with enucleation and curettage; if larger cyst, may consider two-stage approach with prolonged decompression with drain prior to formal treatment

      v. Prognosis: excellent, very low recurrence rate

B. Eruption cyst

      i. Clinical features

        a. Occurs during tooth eruption process in children younger than 10 years.

        b. *Bluish* cyst appears under the gingiva, can sometimes be painful.

      ii. Radiographic features: not typically necessary but can confirm presence of erupting tooth; diagnosis usually made clinically

      iii. Histopathologic features: surface oral epithelium with underlying inflammatory infiltrate

      iv. Treatment: usually not needed, resolves when tooth erupts through it; if fails to occur, then simple excision

      v. Prognosis: excellent

C. Lateral periodontal cyst

      i. Clinical features:

        a. Asymptomatic, *only found on radiograph.*

        b. Occurs in people aged 40 to 70 years; rarely in younger than 30 years.

        c. About 80% occur in mandibular premolar/canine/lateral incisor area.

    ii. Radiographic features: radiolucent, single lesion, well-demarcated, unilocular, lateral to roots of vital teeth, usually less than 1 cm in size

    iii. Histopathologic features: thin epithelial lining with foci of glycogen-rich clear cells

    iv. Treatment: enucleation with preservation of tooth

    v. Prognosis: excellent

D. Glandular odontogenic cyst

    i. Clinical features

        a. Occurs in middle aged adults; rarely in younger than 20 years.

        b. About 80% occur in mandible, generally anterior.

        c. Small cysts can be asymptomatic, but larger ones can expand to produce pain/paresthesias.

    ii. Radiographic features: radiolucent, single lesion, well-demarcated, unilocular or multilocular

    iii. Histopathologic features: lined with stratified squamous epithelium with small microcysts and clusters of mucous cells present

    iv. Treatment: generally, enucleation and curettage, consideration of enbloc resection

    v. Prognosis: variable recurrence rates reported, but some greater than 30% as there is potential for locally aggressive behavior

E. Calcifying odontogenic cyst (Gorlin cyst)

    i. Clinical features

        a. Variable clinical behavior

        b. Variable age, infant to elderly

        c. Variable location, intraosseous versus extraosseous

    ii. Radiographic features: radiolucent, single lesion, well-demarcated, unilocular or multilocular; irregular calcifications can be present

    iii. Histopathologic features: cystic lining with eosinophilic *ghost cells*

    iv. Treatment: enucleation and curettage for intraosseous; excision for extraosseus

    v. Prognosis: good

Nonodontogenic Cysts

A. Nasopalatine duct cyst/incisive canal cyst

    i. Clinical features

        a. Overall, most common *nonodontogenic* cyst

        b. Forms during fusion of primary and secondary palate

        c. Most common in 30 to 60 years of age, rare in less than 10 year of age despite being of embryological origin

        d. Male predominance

    ii. Radiographic features: *heart-shaped* radiolucent lesion, single lesion, well-demarcated, unilocular, above roots of central incisors

    iii. Histopathologic features: variable depending on proportion of respiratory (nasal) epithelium and squamous (oral) epithelium

    iv. Treatment: enucleation

    v. Prognosis: excellent

B. Nasolabial cyst

    i. Clinical features

        a. Soft tissue cyst, occurs between ala and lip from trapped epithelium during embryologic fusion; remnants of nasolacrimal duct

        b. Female predominance, 30 to 50 years of age

        c. Generally asymptomatic

      ii. Radiographic features: due to origin in soft tissues, *no* radiographic changes usually present; generally, no changes are present, however can sometimes saucerize adjacent bone of maxilla

      iii. Histopathologic features: ciliated pseudostratified columnar epithelium with goblet cells (respiratory epithelium)

      iv. Treatment: surgical excision

      v. Prognosis: excellent

Pseudocysts

Cystic appearance, but *do not* have a true epithelial lining.

A. Traumatic bone cyst
    i. Clinical features
      a. Does *not* necessarily have traumatic history.
      b. Most common between ages 10 and 20 years.
      c. Male predominance.
      d. Affects mandible more than maxilla.
      e. 18G needle aspiration yields nothing or scant blood.
    ii. Radiographic features: radiolucent, single lesion, well-demarcated, multilocular; can scallop roots of adjacent teeth
    iii. Histopathologic features: thin, vascular, connective tissue membrane with *no* epithelial lining
    iv. Treatment: surgical exploration of cyst alone will often induce healing process
    v. Prognosis: excellent

B. Aneurysmal bone cyst
    i. Clinical features
      a. Affects mandible more than maxilla.
      b. Rapid swelling of jaw can occur.
      c. 18G needle aspiration can yield blood.
    ii. Radiographic features: radiolucent, single lesion, well-demarcated, unilocular or multilocular; can have "soap bubble" appearance
    iii. Histopathologic features: blood-filled space surrounded by connective tissue; *no* epithelial lining
    iv. Treatment: generally curettage, possible sclerotherapy; resection in severe cases
    v. Prognosis: excellent

C. Stafne bone cyst
    i. Clinical features
      a. Asymptomatic, *radiographic finding*
      b. Thought to be developmental, may occur due to submandibular gland developing close to lingual surface leading to thinner bone formation
      c. Inferior to mandibular canal where inferior alveolar nerve runs in posterior mandible
      d. Most commonly unilateral
      e. Strong male predominance
    ii. Radiographic features: radiolucent, single lesion, well-demarcated, unilocular
    iii. Histopathologic features: biopsy not needed
    iv. Treatment: none required
    v. Prognosis: excellent as no treatment needed

Tumors of the Jaws

Odontogenic Tumors

- About 94% to 97% of odontogenic tumors are benign.

Epithelial

Ameloblastoma

A. Benign locally aggressive neoplasm
B. Three variants: solid or multicystic (92%) greater than unicystic (6%) greater than peripheral (2%)
C. Solid or multicystic (intraosseous)
   i. Clinical features
     a. Generally occurs after 20 years of age
     b. About 85% occur in the mandible, most commonly in molar/ramus region
     c. Slow, painless expansion of jaw
   ii. Radiographic features
     a. Radiolucent, single lesion, well-demarcated, unilocular or multilocular
     b. Resorption of tooth roots, cortical bone expansion
   iii. Histopathologic features
     a. The epithelium demonstrates peripheral columnar cells exhibiting reversed polarization; *piano key* appearance.
     b. Multiple subtypes: Follicular, plexiform, acanthomatous, granular cell, desmoplastic, basal cell variant.
   iv. Treatment
     a. Optimal method has been controversial.
     b. Most favor resection with 1 cm past radiographic extent of tumor.
   v. Prognosis: Good with regular clinical and radiographic surveillance.
D. Unicystic (intraosseous)
   i. Clinical features
     a. Majority occur in the mandible, generally molar/ramus region.
     b. Painless swelling of the jaws.
   ii. Radiographic features: radiolucent, single lesion, well-demarcated unilocular or multilocular
   iii. Histopathologic features:
     a. Subtypes: luminal unicystic, intraluminal unicystic, mural unicystic
   iv. Treatment: varies on subtype
     a. Luminal/intraluminal: resection with clear margins
     b. Mural: resection with clear margins
   v. Prognosis: Good overall, but there is 10% to 20% recurrence rate
E. Peripheral (extraosseous)
   i. Clinical features
     a. Middle age adult
     b. Sessile or pedunculated gingival mass, not ulcerated, usually posterior location
   ii. Radiographic features: limited utility since extraosseous
   iii. Histopathologic features: ameoloblastic epithelium below the lamina propria
   iv. Treatment: surgical excision
   v. Prognosis: recurrence rate 15% to 20%

Malignant Ameloblastoma and Ameloblastic Carcinoma

A. Difference between these is best described under *histopathologic features* below.
   i. Clinical features
      a. Presence of metastasis can be spaced out by time from treatment of initial ameloblastoma.
      b. Sites of metastasis: lung and cervical lymph nodes.
   ii. Radiographic features
      a. Malignant ameloblastoma: radiolucent, single lesion, well-demarcated, unilocular or multilocular
      b. Ameloblastic carcinoma: radiolucent, single lesion, poorly defined margins
   iii. Histopathologic features: Malignant ameloblastoma has no cytologic changes from benign ameloblastoma other than the fact that it is metastatic; ameloblastic carcinoma has malignant cytologic changes in both the primary and the metastatic sites
   iv. Treatment: depends on stage
   v. Prognosis: poor

Keratocystic Odontogenic Tumor

A. Formerly known as odontogenic keratocyst (OKC).
B. Reclassified by World Health Organization (WHO) in 2005; this was based on histologic and genetic studies.
   i. Clinical features
      a. Majority involve the posterior body and ramus of mandible.
      b. 18G needle aspiration can yield a *white/yellow, cheese-like material.*
      c. If multiple, need to be worked up for nevoid basal cell carcinoma syndrome (NBCCS, Gorlin syndrome).
      d. Autosomal dominant.
      e. Multiple basal cell carcinomas, multiple keratocystic odontogenic tumors (KCOTs)/"OKCs," skin cysts, palmar/plantar pits, calcified falx cerebri, increased head circumference, rib/vertebral malformations, hypertelorism (mild), and spina bifida.
   ii. Radiographic features: radiolucent, single lesion, well-demarcated, unilocular or multilocular
   iii. Histopathologic features: parakeratinized or orthokeratinized epithelial lining, with hyperchromatic palisaded basal cell layer
   iv. Treatment: controlled decompression with intraoral drain (if large to reduce size), enucleation and curettage with extraction of involved teeth, +/− peripheral ossectomy
   v. Prognosis: locally aggressive behavior, up to 30% recurrence rate (peripheral budding)

Adenomatoid Odontogenic Tumor

A. Clinical features
   i. Most commonly occurs in those below 20 years of age.
   ii. Female predominance.
   iii. Majority occur in the anterior maxilla.
   iv. Slow growing, relatively asymptomatic.
B. Radiographic features
   i. Radiolucent, single lesion, well-demarcated, unilocular
   ii. May contain small calcifications which helps differentiate from dentigerous cyst
C. Histopathologic features: variable duct-like structures within fibrous stroma

    D. Treatment: enucleation

    E. Prognosis: excellent

Calcifying Epithelial Odontogenic Tumor (Pindborg)

    A. Clinical features

        i. Generally occurs between 30 and 50 years of age

        ii. More common in mandible than maxilla

        iii. Painless, slowly progressive swelling

    B. Radiographic features: radiolucent, single lesion, well-demarcated, multilocular

    C. Histopathologic features: large areas of amyloid-like extracellular material, forming concentric rings known as "Liesegang ring" calcifications (Congo red staining)

    D. Treatment: resection with small margin of normal bone

    E. Prognosis: good

Squamous Odontogenic Tumor

    A. Clinical features

        i. Variable age

        ii. Variable location

    B. Radiographic features: radiolucent, single, poorly defined margins

    C. Histopathologic features: patches of squamous epithelium in fibrous stroma

    D. Treatment: conservative local excision or curettage

    E. Prognosis: excellent

Mixed Epithelial and Ectomesenchymal

Ameloblastic Fibroma

    A. Clinical features

        i. Generally occurs in younger than 30 years

        ii. Male predominance

        iii. Most common in posterior mandible

    B. Radiographic features: radiolucent, single lesion, well-demarcated, unilocular or multilocular

    C. Histopathologic features: odontogenic epithelium in mesenchymal stroma

    D. Treatment

        i. *Initial*: enucleation and curettage

        ii. *Recurrence*: en bloc resection

    E. Prognosis: good, but close surveillance needed, up to 18% recur

Ameloblastic Fibro-odontoma

    A. Clinical features

        i. Most common in children

        ii. Posterior mandible

    B. Radiographic features: radiolucent, single lesion, well-demarcated; unilocular with flecks of calcification

    C. Histopathologic features: cords of odontogenic epithelium in loose connective tissue resembling dental papilla

    D. Treatment: enucleation with conservative curettage

    E. Prognosis: excellent

Ameloblastic Fibrosarcoma (Malignant)

    A. Clinical features

        i. Generally occurs in young adults

        ii. Majority occur in mandible

        iii. Pain, swelling, rapid growth

    B. Radiographic features: radiolucent, single lesion, poorly defined margins

    C. Histopathologic features: odontogenic epithelium intermixed in mesenchymal stroma with pleomorphic cells

    D. Treatment: radical resection

    E. Prognosis: poor

Odontoma

    A. Clinical features

        i. Commonly occurs during 10 to 30 years of age

        ii. Asymptomatic, found on routine dental radiographic screening

    B. Radiographic features: radiopaque, single lesion, well-demarcated. Two types:

        i. Compound-appears as small tooth-like structures

        ii. Complex-enamel and dentin, no resemblance to tooth

    C. Histopathologic features: irregular tooth-like structures in an enamel matrix

    D. Treatment: enucleation

    E. Prognosis: excellent

Ectomesenchymal

Odontogenic Fibroma (Central, Intraosseous)

    A. Clinical features

        i. More common after the age of 40 years

        ii. Most commonly located in posterior mandible, anterior maxilla

        iii. Generally asymptomatic, may cause bony expansion or loose teeth

    B. Radiographic features: radiolucent, single lesion, well-demarcated, unilocular (when small) or multilocular (when large)

    C. Histopathologic features: fibroblasts in collagen matrix

    D. Treatment: enucleation and curettage

    E. Prognosis: good

Odontogenic Fibroma (Peripheral, Extraosseous)

    A. Clinical features

        i. Can occur at variable ages

        ii. Slow growing gingival mass with normal overlying mucosa

    B. Radiographic features: none, extraosseous

    C. Histopathologic features: same as central

    D. Treatment: surgical excision

    E. Prognosis: excellent

Odontogenic Myxoma

    A. Clinical features

        i. More commonly occurs in mandible

        ii. Painless expansion of bone (when large)

    B. Radiographic features: radiolucent, single, well-demarcated, unilocular or multilocular, "soap bubble" pattern; appears similar to ameloblastoma

    C. Histopathologic features: stellate cells in loose myxoid stroma

    D. Treatment: resection as often locally aggressive

    E. Prognosis: good, but close follow-up needed as average recurrence rate is about 25%

Cementoblastoma

    A. Clinical features

        i. Majority occur in molar/premolar region of mandible

        ii. Most common in those younger than 30 years

    B. Radiographic features: radiopaque, single lesion, well-demarcated, associated with root

    C. Histopathologic features: cementoblasts

    D. Treatment: extraction of tooth with attached mass

    E. Prognosis: excellent

Nonodontogenic Tumors
Primary Tumors
Osteoma
    A. Clinical features
      i. Young adults
      ii. Asymptomatic, slowly growing
      iii. Usually found at angle of mandible
      iv. Gardner syndrome
        a. Autosomal dominant (chromosome 5).
        b. Colonic polyposis, multiple osteomas of the jaws, skin fibromas, impacted teeth.
        c. Close surveillance with colonoscopy is needed as there is a high rate of malignant transformation of colonic polyps.
    B. Radiographic features: radiopaque, single lesion, well-demarcated; can have multiple lesions in Gardner syndrome
    C. Histopathologic features: normal appearing bone (either cancellous or compact)
    D. Treatment: observation or surgical excision (if symptomatic)
    E. Prognosis: excellent
Osteoblastoma
    A. Clinical features
      i. Commonly painful
      ii. Majority occur under age of 30 years
    B. Radiographic features: radiopaque, single lesion, well-demarcated or poorly defined
    C. Histopathologic features: irregular bony trabecular pattern
    D. Treatment: enucleation and curettage
    E. Prognosis: good
Osteosarcoma
    A. Clinical features
      i. Most common between ages 10 and 20 years
      ii. Equal incidence in both mandible and maxilla
      iii. Swelling, pain, loosening of teeth
    B. Radiographic features
      i. Radiolucent, single lesion, poorly defined margins or radiopaque, single lesion, poorly defined
      ii. *Sunburst* appearance
      iii. Widening of periodontal ligament around teeth
    C. Histopathologic features: osteoblastic, chondroblastic, or fibroblastic depending on the amount of osteoid, cartilage, or collagen produced
    D. Treatment: radical resection usually with pre- and postoperative chemotherapy
    E. Prognosis: fair
Chondroma
    A. Clinical features:
      i. Most common between ages 30 and 50 years
      ii. Most commonly located in anterior maxilla or condyle
      iii. Painless, slow growing

    B. Radiographic features: radiolucent, single lesion, well-demarcated, unilocular with central area of radiopacity
    C. Histopathologic features: mature hyaline cartilage
    D. Treatment: resection
    E. Prognosis: good

Chondrosarcoma

    A. Clinical features:
        i. Occurs in older adults
        ii. More common in maxilla than mandible
        iii. Painless swelling
    B. Radiographic features: radiopaque, single lesion, poorly defined
    C. Histopathologic features: three grades exist
        i. Grade 1, similar to chondroma
        ii. Grade 2, increased cellularity
        iii. Grade 3, increased cellularity with spindle cell proliferation
    D. Treatment: radical resection; tends to be less responsive to radiation or chemotherapy.
    E. Prognosis: dependent on histologic grade

Metastatic Disease

    A. Clinical features
        i. Older adults may be initial presentation of primary malignancy.
        ii. Breast most common, then lung, then prostate.
        iii. May present with pain, paresthesias, or nonhealing extraction sites.
    B. Radiographic features: radiolucent, generally multiple (although can have single lesion, poorly defined margins)
    C. Histopathologic features: consistent with primary malignancy
    D. Treatment and prognosis: depends on primary malignancy

Fibro-Osseus Lesions

Fibrous Dysplasia

    A. Clinical features
        i. Generally asymptomatic
        ii. May cease or "burn out" after puberty
        iii. Two subtypes
            a. Monostotic, 80%
            b. Polyostotic
        iv. *McCune-Albright syndrome*: polyostotic fibrous dysplasia, café au lait skin lesions, endocrinopathies such as precocious puberty, pituitary or thyroid abnormalities
    B. Radiographic features: radiopaque, single lesion, poorly defined; "ground glass" appearance
    C. Histopathologic features: irregular bony trabeculations in fibrous stroma
    D. Treatment: observation or surgical excision; dependent on size, location, symptom severity
    E. Prognosis: variable, depending on location and extent of disease

Ossifying Fibroma

    A. Clinical features
        i. Most common between ages 20 and 40 years
        ii. Female predominance
        iii. More common in premolar/molar region of mandible
        iv. Painless swelling

B. Radiographic features: radiolucent or radiopaque (can be mixed), well-demarcated unilocular
C. Histopathologic features: woven bone and cementum-like material surrounded by fibrous connective tissue
D. Treatment: enucleation
E. Prognosis: good

Cemento-osseous Dysplasia

A. Clinical features
   i. Strong female predominance
   ii. More common in African Americans
   iii. Middle age
   iv. Three subtypes
      a. Focal: posterior mandible
      b. Periapical: anterior mandible, around tooth root
      c. Florid: diffuse involvement
B. Radiographic features: radiopaque, single lesion, well demarcated or poorly defined; extent depends on subtype as florid can have mulltiple lesions
C. Histopathologic features: spicules of bone and cementum intermixed within connective tissue
D. Treatment: generally, none needed
E. Prognosis: good

Central Giant Cell Granuloma

A. Clinical features
   i. Majority occur in those younger than 30 years.
   ii. Majority occur in the mandible.
   iii. Can cross midline in anterior maxilla.
B. Radiographic features: radiolucent, single lesion, well-demarcated, unilocular or multilocular lesions or ill defined
C. Histopathologic features: multinucleated giant cells in loose cellular stroma
D. Treatment
   i. Closely resembles brown tumor and hyperparathyroidism should be ruled out in all cases
   ii. *Medical:* intralesional steroids, calcitonin, interferon
   iii. *Surgical:* aggressive curettage (usually treated surgically)
E. Prognosis: good

Manifistations of Systemic Conditions

Langerhans Cell Histiocytosis

A. Clinical features
   i. Most common in children
   ii. Males more than females
   iii. Dull pain common
B. Radiographic features: radiolucent, single or multiple lesions, poorly defined; teeth appear to be "floating in air"
C. Histopathologic features: Histiocytes intermixed with plasma cells, lymphocytes, giant cells
D. Treatment: radiation or chemotherapy
E. Prognosis: poor

Cherubism
  A. Clinical features:
     i. Autosomal dominant
     ii. Most common during 2 to 5 years of age, can enlarge with growth and become stable by puberty
     iii. Painless, bilateral cheek swelling due to expansion of posterior mandible
  B. Radiographic features: radiolucent, multiple lesions, upper and lower jaws
  C. Histopathologic features: vascular fibrous tissue containing giant cells
  D. Treatment: observation versus surgical excision depending on symptom severity
  E. Prognosis: variable

Paget Disease
  A. Clinical features
     i. Male predominance
     ii. More common in Caucasians than African Americans
     iii. Usually occurs after 50 years of age
     iv. Chronic, slowly progressive
     v. Can have cranial neuropathies if foramina are involved
  B. Radiographic features: radiopaque, multiple lesions; "cotton-wool" appearance
  C. Histopathologic features: uncontrolled osteoblastic and osteoclastic activity
  D. Treatment: bisphosphonates, calcitonin (slows bone turnover)
  E. Prognosis: chronic disease, rarely causes death

Osteonecrosis

Osteomyelitis
  A. Clinical features
     i. More common in mandible than maxilla
     ii. Fever, leukocytosis, swelling, lympadenopathy
  B. Radiographic features: radiolucent, single, poorly defined margins
  C. Histopathologic features: necrotic bone, surrounding inflammation
  D. Treatment: Intravenous antibiotic and surgical debridement
  E. Prognosis: variable

Osteoradionecrosis
  A. Clinical features:
     i. Complication from head and neck radiation, leaving bone hypocellular and hypoxic
     ii. Can be very painful
  B. Radiographic features: radiolucent, single, poorly defined margins
  C. Treatment
     i. If mild, good oral hygiene, hyperbaric oxygen therapy, debridement as needed
     ii. If severe, may require surgical resection with vascularized flap reconstruction
  D. Prognosis: variable, dependant on severity

Antiresorptive Osteonecrosis of the Jaw (ARONJ) or Medication-related Osteonecrosis of the Jaw (MRONJ)
  A. Clinical features
     i. Occurs in patients undergoing dental procedures after receiving PO/IV bisphosphonate therapy, or other antiresorptive (ie, RANK ligand inhibitor, denosumab) or antiangiogenic medications; *previously termed, bisphosphonate-related osteonecrosis of the jaw (BRONJ).*

  ii. No history of radiation therapy

  iii. Can be very painful

 B. Radiographic features: radiolucent, single, poorly defined margins

 C. Treatment: variable, can range from good oral hygiene, debridement, to surgical resection and reconstruction

 D. Prognosis: variable, dependent on severity

Bibliography

Avelar RL, Antunes AA, Carvalho RW, Bezerra PG, Oliveira Neto PJ, Andrade ES. Odontogenic cysts: a clinicopathological study of 507 cases. *J Oral Sci.* 2009;51:581-586.

Carlson E. Odontogenic cysts and tumors. In: Miloro M, Ghali G, Larsen P, et al, eds. *Peterson's Principles of Oral and Maxillofacial Surgery.* 2nd ed. Hamilton (Canada): BC Decker; 2004:575-596.

Curran AE, Damm DD, Drummond JF. Pathologically significant pericoronal lesions in adults: histopathologic evaluation. *J Oral Maxillofac Surg.* 2002;60:613-617; discussion 618.

Jing W, Xuan M, Lin Y, et al. Odontogenic tumours: a retrospective study of 1642 cases in a Chinese population. *Int J Oral Maxillofac Surg.* 2007;36:20-25.

Luo HY, Li TJ. Odontogenic tumors: a study of 1309 cases in a Chinese population. *Oral Oncol.* 2009;45:706-711.

Neville BW, Damm DD, Allen CM, Bouquot JE. *Oral and Maxillofacial Pathology.* 2nd ed. Philadelphia, PA: WB Saunders; 2002.

Ochsenius G, Escobar E, Godoy L, Penafiel C. Odontogenic cysts: analysis of 2,944 cases in Chile. *Med Oral Patol Oral Cir Bucal.* 2007;12:E85-91.

Osterne RL, Matos Brito RG, Negreiros Nunes Alves AP, Cavalcante RB, Sousa FB. Odontogenic tumors: a 5-year retrospective study in a Brazilian population and analysis of 3406 cases reported in the literature. *Oral Surg Oral Med Oral Pathol Oral Radiol Endod.* 2011;111:474-481.

Pogrel MA. Benign nonodontogenic lesions of the jaws. In: Miloro M, Ghali G, Larsen P, et al, eds. *Peterson's Principles of Oral and Maxillofacial Surgery.* 2nd ed. Hamilton, (Canada): BC Decker; 2004:597-616.

Prockt AP, Schebela CR, Maito FD, Sant'Ana-Filho M, Rados PV. Odontogenic cysts: analysis of 680 cases in Brazil. *Head Neck Pathol.* 2008;2:150-156.

Ruggiero SL, Dodson TB, Fantasia J, Goodday R, Aghaloo T, Mehrotra B, Ryan F. Medication-related osteonecrosis of the jaw—2014 update. *American Association of Oral and Maxillofacial Surgeons, Position Paper.* 2014:1-26.

Questions

1. Which of the following is the most likely diagnosis to require *no* treatment?

 A. Keratocystic odontogenic tumor

 B. Ameloblastoma

 C. Eruption cyst

 D. Osteomyelitis

 E. Periapical cyst

2. Which of the following lesions is radiopaque?

 A. Aneurysmal bone cyst

 B. Odontogenic myxoma

C. Stafne bone cyst

D. Ossifying fibroma

E. Nasopalatine duct cyst

3. Which of the following radiolucent lesions is classically associated with the crown of an unerupted third molar?

A. Lateral periodontal cyst

B. Calcifying odontogenic cyst

C. Ameloblastoma

D. Dentigerous cyst

E. Glandular odontogenic cyst

4. Which of the following lesions has epithelium consisting of columnar cells with reversed polarization in a "piano key" appearance?

A. Cementoblastoma

B. Ossifying fibroma

C. Cemento-osseous dysplasia

D. Fibrous dysplasia

E. Ameloblastoma

5. The presence of a nonvital tooth is a requirement for the diagnosis of

A. dentigerous cyst

B. glandular odontogenic cyst

C. calcifying odontogenic cyst

D. periapical cyst

E. lateral periodontal cyst

Chapter 35
Carotid Body Tumors and Vascular Anomalies

Carotid Body Tumors and Other Tumors of the Poststyloid Parapharyngeal Space

Carotid Body Tumors

Presentation and Natural History

- Also known as glomus caroticum
- Benign neuroendocrine tumor arising from carotid body paraganglia
- Normal function of carotid body is as a chemoreceptor for changes in blood oxygen, carbon dioxide, and hydrogen ion concentration
- Two cell types:
- Chief cells (Type I)—neural crest derived and are the cells capable of releasing neurotransmitters
- Sustentacular cells (Type II)—supporting cells similar to glia
- Arranged in "zellballen" configuration (tumor nests surrounded by fibrovascular stroma)
- Most common paraganglioma of the head and neck (45%-60%)
- Sporadic
- Typically present in fifth and sixth decades
- Unusual in children
- No gender predilection
- Rarely bilateral (5%)
- Familial
- Related to mutations in succinate dehydrogenase genes
- Present at a younger age than sporadic cases
- Less likely to be malignant
- Increased incidence of bilaterality (30%) and other paraganglia including pheochromocytoma
- Hyperplastic
  - (a) Described in populations living at higher altitudes
  - (b) Thought to be due to chronic hypoxia
  - (c) More commonly in women (may be related to anemia from menses)
- Physical examination
  - (a) Most common presentation is neck mass (deep mass high in the neck)
  - (b) Tethered vertically but mobile horizontally (Fontaine sign)

(c) May be pulsatile or have a bruit
- Slow growing and often overlooked for years by patients
- May encase carotid or invade artery and surrounding structures
- Shamblin classification
    (a) I—small tumor easily separated from carotid
    (b) II—tumor partially encircles carotid and is difficult to separate
    (c) III—tumor completely encircles carotid and is densely adherent
- Malignancy is rare (5%-10%)
    (a) Pain is the most predictive feature, along with young age and rapid enlargement.
    (b) No histologic criteria of malignancy for primary tumor.
    (c) Malignancy is defined as the presence of regional or distant metastases; local invasion or destructive behavior does not establish malignancy.
- Rarely functional (1%-3%)
    (a) If history of hypertension or flushing consider workup for catecholamine byproducts (best screening test is plasma free metanephrines, second best is 24-hour urine fractionated metanephrines).
    (b) Symptoms may also be due to another, synchronous tumor (eg, pheochromocytoma).

Diagnosis and Management
- Contrast-enhanced computed tomography (CT) or magnetic resonance imaging (MRI):
    (a) Best, first imaging study
    (b) Demonstrates relationship to carotid and can help differentiate between other potential tumors in that area (eg, schwannoma)
    (c) Hypervascular mass typically splaying internal and external carotid
        ○ If mass pushes both vessels anteromedially a vagal tumor should be considered.
        ○ If mass pushes vessels laterally a sympathetic tumor should be considered.
        ○ However, both tumors can mimic carotid body tumors on CT or MRI.
        ○ If the tumor is located above the bifurcation, even if it splays the carotids, an entity other than a carotid body tumor should be expected.
    (d) MRI appearance described as "salt and pepper."
    (e) Halo between carotid and tumor suggests a good plane of separation.
- Angiography:
    (a) Classic finding is "lyre sign," splaying of internal and external carotid by vascular mass.
    (b) Most useful if preoperative embolization planned; however, preoperative embolization has not been shown to reduce intraoperative blood loss and is usually not necessary.
- If carotid sacrifice is a possibility (eg, Shamblin III), angiography or CT/MR angiography is often used to evaluate circle of Willis and collateral blood flow.
- Fine-needle aspiration (FNA) to be avoided, core-needle or open biopsy to be condemned.
- Surgical resection:
    (a) Preferred modality for small tumors in healthy patients.
    (b) Transcervical approach begins with level II to III selective neck dissection to improve exposure and sample lymph nodes.
    (c) Cranial nerves identified and preserved; it is imperative that the connections between the vagus and hypoglossal are not separated as this can lead to dysfunction of both nerves.

(d) Dissection is in avascular plane between carotid and tumor; classic teaching is to resect in subadventitial plane but this is usually not necessary and weakens the arterial wall.

(e) The external carotid is sometimes sacrificed to improve mobilization of the tumor.

(f) Vascular surgery should be available for carotid replacement as decision to resect the carotid made intraoperatively.

(g) Complications of surgery
   ○ Cranial nerves (CNs) X and XII most commonly injured but incidence should be low for most tumors
   ○ First bite syndrome—intense parotid pain on initiating eating due to injury of cervical sympathetics; usually worst in the morning and tends to improve with time
   ○ Baroreflex failure—tachycardia and blood pressure lability due to loss of carotid sinus reflex mediated by Hering nerve (branch of CN IX); more significant for patients with bilateral surgery

- Radiation therapy:
  (a) An option for unresectable cases, poor operative candidates, or by patient preference.
  (b) Tumors typically do not regress but remain radiologically stable.
  (c) Postoperative radiotherapy (RT) should be considered for metastatic cases.

- Observation:
  (a) Appropriate for small tumors based on patient preference or for poor surgical candidates
  (b) Yearly CT or MRI to monitor the growth

Vagal Paragangliomas

Presentation and Natural History

- Also known as glomus vagale.
- Represent 5% to 9% of head and neck paragangliomas.
- Histopathology same as for carotid body tumors.
- Have a higher incidence of malignancy than carotid body tumors (16%).
- Typically arise from the inferior (nodose) ganglion but can arise from middle or superior ganglion.
- Can extend to skull base or intracranially.
- Preoperative weakness of CN X occurs in one-third of patients.

Diagnosis and Management

- Contrast-enhanced CT or MRI
  (a) Vascular tumor typically displacing carotids anteromedially without splaying.
  (b) Vagal tumors tend to separate the jugular vein from the carotid sheath, whereas sympathetic tumors typically do not.
  (c) Can splay carotids and mimic a carotid body tumor.
- Surgical resection
- Essentially guarantees vagal paralysis.
- Used for aggressive tumors invading the skull base and for patients with preexisting vagal paralysis.
- Cervical approach used for lower tumors and lateral skull base approach for higher tumors.
- If diagnosis of vagal paraganglioma made intraoperatively when carotid body tumor is suspected, it is reasonable to abort procedure and either give radiation or observe the patient.

- Radiation therapy or observation
- Preferred for patients with small tumors and no preexisting vagal weakness
- Otherwise same as for carotid body tumors

Schwannomas

Presentation and Natural History

- Encapsulated tumor composed of Schwann cells.
- Derived from neural crest cells
- Normally produce myelin for extracranial nerves
- Tumors also called neurilemomas or neurinomas
- Two histologic patterns:
  - (a) Antoni A—more cellular and organized, palisading Schwann cells arranged in Verocay bodies
  - (b) Antoni B—random arrangement within loose stroma
- Genetics
- Approximately 90% sporadic
- No gender predilection
- Associated with alterations in neurofibromatosis type 2 (NF-2) gene and can rarely be associated with the NF-2 syndrome.
- Presentation similar to carotid body tumors.
- Most schwannomas of the head and neck occur in the parapharyngeal space.
- Schwannomas are the second most common tumor of the parapharyngeal space.
- Sympathetic chain and CN X most common, but can also involve IX, XI, XII, and cervical or brachial plexus.

Diagnosis and Management

- Nerve weakness
- Can occur in nerve of origin (eg, Horner for a sympathetic chain tumor)
- However, not diagnostic of the nerve of origin as nerve weakness may be due to compression or invasion by a tumor arising from another local structure (eg, carotid body tumor causing Horner syndrome)
- Contrast-enhanced CT or MRI
- Tumors will demonstrate enhancement during venous phase, but do not show as intense enhancement as paragangliomas and do not demonstrate flow voids on MRI.
- Sympathetic tumors may displace carotids laterally or mimic carotid body tumor.
- Vagal tumors are as above for vagal paragangliomas.
- Surgical resection
- Preferred modality and usually curative.
- Most tumors can be enucleated with preservation of nerve.
- Substantial incidence of postoperative nerve weakness which is greatly increased in setting of preoperative nerve weakness.

Vascular Anomalies

Hemangioma

Presentation and Natural History

- True vascular tumor.
- Two types: congenital and infantile.

- Congenital hemangioma is the rare tumor present at birth.
- Two types: rapidly involuting and noninvoluting
- Glucose transporter-1 (GLUT1) negative
- Infantile hemangioma is the most common vascular anomaly in head and neck.
- Presents after birth, usually as a distinct, bright red mass.
- Firm and rubbery (unlike compressible vascular malformations).
- Diagnosis typically made clinically.
- GLUT1 positive; stain used to confirm diagnosis if in question.
- Three anatomic locations:
  - (a) Superficial: bright red, cobblestoned, cutaneous, or mucosal mass
  - (b) Deep: no cutaneous/mucosal component, bluish hue of overlying skin
  - (c) Compound: superficial and deep components
- Three phases of growth, which occur independent of the growth of the patient:
  - (a) Proliferative—first 9 to 12 months of life
    - ○ Can have two periods of rapid proliferation
      - – One to 3 months, usually 80% of growth occurs
      - – Five to 6 months
  - (b) Involution—variable course of regression over many years
    - ○ Graying of lesion, "herald spot," is usually the first indication of involution.
  - (c) Involuted—almost all involuted by 9 years of age; classic teaching is 50% involuted by 5 years, 70% by 7 years and 90% by 9 years
    - ○ Three distributions:
      - – Focal—classic solitary mass
      - – Multifocal—multiple masses
        - ◊ When more than five cutaneous masses present, must rule out liver and gastrointestinal (GI) involvement with abdominal ultrasound (US)
      - – Segmental distribution—multiple cervicofacial subunits or large areas of upper aerodigestive tract
        - ◊ Usually follows trigeminal territory (V1, 2, and/or 3).
        - ◊ Two-thirds of children with V3 ("beard") distribution will have synchronous subglottic hemangioma—must evaluate airway.
        - ◊ PHACES syndrome—anomalies of
          - * *P*osterior cranial fossa
          - * Segmental *H*emangiomas
          - * Intracranial or cervical *A*rteries
          - * *C*ardiac (heart and aorta)
          - * *E*ye
          - * *S*ternum
        - ◊ Subglottic hemangioma
        - ◊ Must be ruled out as a source of stridor in any infant with a cutaneous hemangioma
        - ◊ Typically a bluish or reddish, compressible mass in the posterior left subglottis
        - ◊ Parotid hemangioma
        - ◊ Most common parotid tumor of infancy
        - ◊ Deep, firm mass within substance of gland

Diagnosis and Management
- Diagnosis usually made clinically and biopsy not necessary.
- Ultrasound can be helpful in differentiating from arteriovenous malformation (AVM) if in question.

- Subglottic hemangiomas may show asymmetric narrowing of subglottis on neck x-ray and typically require rigid endoscopy for full assessment.
- Classically, observation is advised in most cases of cutaneous hemangiomas although trend is for earlier intervention prior to rapid growth phases to prevent scarring and cosmetic deformities.
- Intervention imperative for:
- Symptomatic—for example, bleeding, ulcerated, massive and resulting in chronic heart failure (CHF) or Kasabach-Merritt phenomenon (consumptive coagulopathy)
- Critical anatomic locations—eyelids, lips, ears, airway
- Inconspicuous hemangiomas can be managed with observation and reassurance.
- Medical management:
- Intralesional steroid injections.
- Systemic steroids or chemotherapy (alpha-interferon, vincristine) have significant side effects but are used for symptomatic or critically located tumors.
- Most recently propranolol has shown success in causing regression of hemangiomas and may become a first-line therapy, pending further experience and data from specialized centers.
- Laser therapy:
- Flash lamp pulsed-dye laser (585 nm) effective for superficial lesions (no deep component).
- Nd:YAG has deeper penetration and can be used for superficial and deep lesions.
- Laser therapy also used to manage ulcerated lesions, promote resurfacing, and for postregression telangiectasia.
- Scar may still require surgical excision after regression of lesion.
- Surgical therapy:
- Used for localized lesions or postregression remnants
- Subglottic hemangiomas—no consensus on management:
- Rarely observation for nonobstructing lesions.
- Medical therapy.
  (a) Steroid injections and dilation for small lesions
  (b) Systemic or combined therapy for larger lesions
  (c) Beta blockers (propranolol) may become first-line therapy
- Endoscopic CO_2 or KTP laser ablation or excision effective, but should be avoided in circumferential lesions because of high risk of subglottic stenosis.
- Open removal with airway reconstruction if necessary.
- Regardless of approach, preservation of mucosa is key to prevent subglottic stenosis.
- Tracheotomy usually is not required and should be avoided unless absolutely necessary; tracheotomy is detrimental during key speech and language milestones of childhood.

Vascular Malformations

Presentation and Natural History

- Not considered as tumors
- Tend to grow with the patient
- Categorized by blood flow: slow flow and fast flow
- Slow flow: capillary, venous, and lymphatic
- Capillary (venular)
  (a) Telangiectasias, nevus flammeus (port wine stain), spider angioma
  (b) Sturge-Weber syndrome (port wine stain of face with ipsilateral intracranial angiomas/AVMs)

- Venous
  (a) Usually diagnosed early in life with finding of a soft, compressible mass.
  (b) Continue to grow with patient throughout life, by both expansion and proliferation.
  (c) Incidence is 1:10,000, usually sporadic.
  (d) Superficial lesions have bluish coloration to overlying skin or mucosa.
  (e) Deep lesions associated with muscle groups.
  (f) Can present later in life with continued growth or pain and rapid expansion secondary to clot formation.
- Lymphatic
  (a) Usually diagnosed in childhood when noticed at birth or when expand secondary to local infection (eg, upper respiratory infection [URI] or otitis media).
    ○ Noncompressible lesions, usually deep with normal overlying skin.
    ○ Mucosal lesions often have overlying vesicles.
  (b) Most common site in body is the cervicofacial region; diffuse lesions can involve the upper aerodigestive tract.
  (c) Large upper aerodigestive tract lesions may be diagnosed on prenatal ultrasound and require emergency airway management or ex utero intrapartum treatment (EXIT) procedure during delivery.
  (d) *Main classification*: macrocystic and microcystic
    ○ Macrocystic is easier to treat and have a better prognosis.
    ○ Some small, posterior triangle, macrocystic lymphatic malformations regress spontaneously within the first year of life.
  (e) Orbital lymphatic malformations can have associated intracranial vascular anomalies that must be ruled out.
    ○ Fast flow: arteriovenous malformations (AVMs) and arteriovenous fistulas (AVFs)
    ○ AVMs
      – Form from a nidus of abnormal capillary beds.
      – Lesions usually present as a vascular blush that expands as the patient grows.
      – Lesions can be pulsatile to palpation and have a bruit.
      – Advanced lesions can have local tissue and bone destruction, bleeding, and pain.
      – Often misdiagnosed as hemangioma in infancy until regression does not occur, with considerable additional morbidity.
      – Can present much later in life (eg, fourth-fifth decade), with evidence of a posttraumatic etiology.
      – Most diagnosed in infancy or childhood and grow intermittently secondary to environmental stimuli.
      – Recent evidence of hormonal receptors in AVMs; indeed, hormonal changes such as puberty and pregnancy appear to stimulate growth.
    ○ AVFs
      – Posttraumatic
      – Defined by single arteriovenous connection, rather than a nidus of multiple connections

Diagnosis and Management
- Slow-flow vascular malformations.
- Ultrasound is most useful for diagnosis.
  (a) Venous malformations will have phleboliths and slow blood flow on Doppler.

(b) Determination between macrocystic and microcystic can be made for lymphatic malformations.
- MRI is helpful for delineating extent of lesions and relationship to surrounding structures.
- Conservative management with elevation of head of bed is used to discourage swelling and expansion; warm compresses and nonsteroidal anti-inflammatory drugs (NSAIDs) are used for thrombosis of venous malformations.
- Sclerotherapy to stimulate inflammation and fibrosis, ultimately decreasing expansion and shrinking lesion.
  (a) Most are delivered via radiologic guidance.
  (b) Procedure of choice for macrocystic lymphatic malformations.
  (c) Ethanol, sodium tetradecyl sulfate, bleomycin, glues, and polymers.
  (d) OK-432, inactivated *Streptococcus pyogenese*, is the subject of several clinical trials and has been shown to be 80% to 90% effective for macrocystic lymphatic malformations but less so for microcystic lymphatic malformations.
  (e) Must ensure sclerosant is not systemically absorbed, especially for high-drainage venous malformations.
  (f) Complications include overlying skin necrosis, scarring, and neuropathy.
- Laser therapy
  (a) KTP and Nd:YAG lasers are first-line therapy for skin and mucosal venous malformations.
  (b) Pulsed-dye lasers are also useful for capillary malformations.
  (c) Interstitial Nd:YAG can be used for deeper venous malformations.
- Surgery
  (a) Can be challenging, but best option for "cure."
  (b) More effective than sclerotherapy for microcystic lymphatic malformations.
  (c) Preoperative sclerotherapy to decrease intraoperative blood loss should be considered for venous malformations.
  (d) Must ensure complete excision to prevent recurrence.
  (e) Postoperative scarring and fibrosis can be significant, especially for lymphatic malformations.
- AVMs
  (a) Doppler US will demonstrate rapid blood flow, and MRI will usually show flow voids.
  (b) CT angiogram is useful for operative planning.
  (c) Treatment is difficult and multidisciplinary.
    ○ Embolization of nidus with alcohol or polymers.
    ○ Surgical resection following embolization.
      – Small, easily resectable lesions
      – Life-threatening, destructive lesions; often requires massive resection with adjacent or free tissue transfer
    ○ Recurrence is common.
- AVFs
  (a) Angiography or CT angiography demonstrates single arteriovenous connection.
  (b) Embolization only for deep, inconspicuous lesions.
  (c) Surgical resection in highly visible lesions (eg, lip) to eliminate residual scar and return of normal function.
    ○ Consider preoperative embolization to decrease intraoperative blood loss.
    ○ If no embolization, it is useful to identify and clip feeding artery early in resection.

Bibliography

Boedeker CC, Neumann HP, Offergeld C, et al. Clinical features of paraganglioma syndromes. *Skull Base*. 2009;19:17-25.

Buckmiller LM, Richter GT, Suen JY. Diagnosis and management of hemangiomas and vascular malformations of the head and neck. *Oral Dis*. 2010;16:405-418.

Colen TY, Mihm FG, Mason TP, Roberson JB. Catecholamine-secrting paragangliomas: recent progress in diagnosis and perioperative management. *Skull Base*. 2009;19:377-385.

Jalisi S, Netterville JL. Rehabilitation after cranial base surgery. *Otolaryngol Clin North Am*. 2009;42:49-56.

Netterville JL, Jackson CG, Miller FR, Wanamaker JR, Glasscock ME. Vagal paraganglioma: a review of 46 patients treated during a 20-year period. *Arch Otolaryngol Head Neck Surg*. 1998;124:1133-1140.

Questions

1. A patient presents with a lateral neck mass demonstrating a 'lyre sign' on CT angiogram. The most likely diagnosis is
   A. vagal paraganglioma
   B. carotid body tumor
   C. vagal schwannoma
   D. sympathetic schwannoma
   E. glomus jugulare

2. A child with PHACES syndrome would have all of the following findings **except**
   A. choanal atresia
   B. segmental hemangiomas
   C. eye abnormalities
   D. intracranial or cervical artery abnormalities
   E. cardiac defects

3. An infant presents to your office with 3 weeks of increasing stridor but no cyanosis or apneic episodes. A large red lesion is noted on his right cheek, extending to the oral commissure. The next appropriate step would be
   A. intralesional dexamethasone injection in the office
   B. oral propranolol and reevaluation in 2 days
   C. airway endoscopy
   D. contrast-enhanced CT
   E. biopsy with staining for GLUT1

4. Which of the following is the most common vascular tumor of the head and neck?
   A. carotid body tumor
   B. jugular paraganglioma
   C. infantile hemangioma
   D. vascular malformation

5. Histologic findings in carotid body tumors include all of the following **except**
   A. physaliferous cells.
   B. Zellballen configuration.
   C. sustentacular cells.
   D. chief cells.
   E. all of the above findings are seen in carotid body tumors.

Chapter 36
TNM Classification in Otolaryngology—Head and Neck Surgery

Introduction

The TNM system describes a cancerous tumor's involvement at the primary site (T), as well as spread to regional lymph nodes (N) and distant metastasis (M).

Objectives of Staging System

The TNM staging system was created to describe cancer in a uniform fashion and provide physicians a common language to discuss the disease. This allows for a better understanding of prognosis and accurate patient counseling. Treatment protocols can be devised based on treatment results of similar tumors. Finally, it is useful for stratifying cancers for clinical research and for measuring outcomes to various treatment options.

History

The American Joint Committee on Cancer (AJCC) was formed in 1959, unifying previous classification systems and providing a foundation for our current staging system. Since then, the AJCC has continued to update a stage classification system for all anatomic sites and subsites. The most recent revision was published in 2010.

Definitions of TNM Categories

T describes the extent of the primary tumor. There are seven categories: TX (primary tumor cannot be assessed), T0 (no evidence of primary tumor) T*is* (tumor in situ), T1, T2, T3, and T4. Within the head and neck size of the tumor generally defines the T stage. Notable exceptions include vocal fold mobility in larynx cancer. Depth of invasion is not included in the staging system as it relates to primary tumor size. Modifiers "a" (less severe) and "b" (more severe) can be used within some T categories to further describe the tumor.

N describes spread of the cancer to regional lymph nodes in five categories: NX (regional lymph nodes cannot be assessed) N0, N1, N2, and N3. This is basically described by size of the lymph nodes and is modified by location of the involved nodes. Evaluation of surgically excised lymph nodes by a pathologist can further affect N stage.

M describes the presence of distant metastasis, either as MX, M0, or M1. A patient with a metastasis beyond the regional lymph nodes has M1 disease. M0 describes no evidence of metastasis after an appropriate evaluation. MX designates that a metastatic workup has not been completed, but the likelihood of metastasis is low.

Prefix modifiers are also used to further describe the staging. The "c" prefix refers to staging based on clinical examination. The "p" prefix refers to staging based on pathological examination after surgical resection.

The current staging system, including sites and subsites, are summarized in the following tables (detailed descriptions can be found in the updated AJCC manual). These are divided into four categories:

A. Lips, oral cavity, pharynx, and larynx (Tables 36-1 to 36-7)
B. Nasal cavity and paranasal sinuses (Tables 36-8 and 36-9)
C. Major salivary glands (Table 36-10)
D. Thyroid gland (Table 36-11)

Nodal staging (Table 36-12) and stage groupings (Tables 36-13 and 36-14) are shown in subsequent tables.

Table 36-1 Lips and Oral Cavity[a]

T1	< 2 cm
T2	> 2 cm and < 4 cm
T3	> 4 cm
T4a	Moderately advanced local disease (lip). Invades through bone, inferior alveolar nerve, floor of mouth or skin (oral cavity). Invades adjacent structures only, such as bone, extrinsic tongue muscles, and skin
T4b	Very advanced local disease. Tumor invades masticator space, pterygoid plates, skull base, or encases internal carotid artery

[a]Includes oral tongue, buccal mucosa, hard palate, alveolar ridge, retromolar trigone, floor of mouth, and lips

Table 36-2 Nasopharynx

T1	Confined to nasopharynx
T2	Extends to oropharynx, or nasal cavity, or parapharyngeal extension
T3	Invades bony structures or paranasal sinsuses
T4	Intracranial extension, involves cranial nerves, hypopharynx, orbit, or extends into infratemporal fossa or masticator space

Table 36-3 Oropharynx a

T1	< 2 cm
T2	> 2 cm and < 4 cm
T3	> 4 cm
T4a	Moderately advanced local disease. Invades larynx, extrinsic tongue muscles, medial pterygoid, hard palate, or mandible
T4b	Very advanced local disease. Invades lateral pterygoid muscle, pterygoid plates, lateral nasopharynx, skull base, or encases carotid artery

Table 36-4 Hypopharynx a

T1	< 2 cm and limited to one subsite
T2	> 2 cm, < 4 cm, or invades adjacent subsite of hypopharynx or adjacent site
T3	> 4 cm or fixed hemilarynx
T4a	Moderately advanced local disease. Invades cartilage, hyoid bone, thyroid gland, or central compartment soft tissue, including strap muscles
T4b	Very advanced local disease. Invades prevertebral fascia, encases carotid artery, or involves mediastinum

a Includes piriform sinus, pharyngeal wall, and postcricoid area

Table 36-5 Supraglottic Larynx a

T1	Limited to one subsite
T2	Spreads to adjacent subsite within supraglottic larynx or outside of supraglottic larynx
T3	Vocal cord fixation, or invades adjacent structures (postcricoid area, preepiglottic tissue, paraglottic space, minor thyroid cartilage invasion)
T4a	Moderately advanced local disease. Invades thyroid cartilage or beyond larynx
T4b	Very advanced local disease. Invades prevertebral fascia, encases carotid artery, or involves mediastinum

a Includes lingual and laryngeal and infrahyoid epiglottis, false cords, arytenoids, and aryepiglottic folds

Table 36-6 Glottic Larynx

T1	Limited to vocal cord(s)
T2	Extends to supra or subglottis and/or impaired mobility
T3	Limited to larynx with vocal cord fixation
T4a	Moderately advanced local disease. Tumor extends beyond outer cortex of thyroid cartilage and/or invades tissue beyond larynx

Table 36-7 **Subglottic Larynx**

T1	Limited to subglottis
T2	Extends to vocal cord(s) with normal or impaired mobility
T3	Extends to vocal cord(s) with fixation
T4a	Moderately advanced local disease. Invades cartilage or extends beyond larynx
T4b	Very advanced local disease. Invades prevertebral fascia, encases carotid artery, or involves mediastinum

Table 36-8 **Nasal Cavity and Ethmoid Sinuses**

T1	Limited to one subsite, with or without bony invasion
T2	Invades two subsites in a single region or extending to adjacent region
T3	Extends to medial wall, floor of orbit, maxillary sinus, palate, or cribriform plate
T4a	Moderately advanced local disease. Invades anterior orbit, skin, pterygoid plates, frontal or sphenoid sinus, and extends minimally into anterior cranial fossa
T4b	Very advanced local disease. Invades orbital apex, dura, brain, middle cranial fossa, cranial nerve (CN) other than V2, nasopharynx, and clivus

Table 36-9 **Maxillary Sinus**

T1	Limited to mucosa
T2	Invades infrastructure
T3	Invades subcutaneous tissue, posterior wall, orbital floor, ethmoids
T4a	Moderately advanced local disease. Invades anterior orbit, skin, pterygoid plates, frontal or sphenoid sinus, and cribriform plate
T4b	Very advanced local disease. Invades orbital apex, dura, brain, middle cranial fossa, CN other than V2, nasopharynx, and clivus

Table 36-10 **Major Salivary Glands**[a]

T1	< 2 cm
T2	> 2 cm and < 4 cm
T3	> 4 cm or extraparenchymal extension
T4a	Moderately advanced local disease. Invades skin, mandible, ear canal, and facial nerve
T4b	Very advanced local disease. Invades skull base, pterygoid plates, or encases carotid artery

[a]Includes: parotid, submandibular, and sublingual

Table 36-11 Thyroid

T1	< 2 cm
T1a	< 1 cm
T1b	> 1 cm but < 2 cm
T2	> 2 cm or < 4 cm
T3	> 4 cm or minimal extrathyroid extension (eg, sternothyroid muscle)
T4a	Moderately advanced local disease. Extends beyond thyroid capsule to invades subcutaneous soft tissue, larynx, trachea, esophagus, or recurrent laryngeal nerve
T4b	Very advanced local disease. Invades prevertebral fascia, encases carotid or mediastinal vessels

Note: Nodal status is either N0 for no regional lymph node metastasis or N1a for pretracheal/paratracheal lymph nodes and N1b for other cervical or mediastinal lymph node.

Table 36-12 Staging for Regional Lymph Nodes

N0	No nodes
N1	Ipsilateral < 3 cm
N2a	Ipsilateral > 3 cm and < 6 cm
N2b	Ipsilateral multiple < 6 cm
N2c	Bilateral or contralateral < 6 cm
N3	> 6 cm

Table 36-13 Stage Groupings (Except Thyroid)[a]

Stage I	TI	N0	M0
Stage II	T2	N0	M0
Stage III	T3	N0	M0
	T1-3	N1	M0
Stage IV	T4	N0	M0
	Any T	N2	M0
	Any T	N3	M0
	Any T	Any N	M1
Nasopharynx			
Stage I	TI	N0	M0
Stage II	T2	N0	M0
Stage III	T3	N0	M0
	T1-3	N1	M0
	T1-3	N2	M0
Stage IV	T4	N0	M0
	Any T	N3	M0
	Any T	Any N	M1

[a]Lips, oral cavity, pharynx, larynx, nose, sinuses, salivary glands (except nasopharynx)

Table 36-14 **Thyroid Stage Grouping**

Papillary or follicular thyroid cancer			
Under 45 years			
Stage I	Any T	Any N	M0
Stage II	Any T	Any N	M1
45 years and older			
Stage I	TI	N0	M0
Stage II	T2	N0	M0
Stage III	T3	N0	M0
	T1-3	N1a	M0
Stage IV	T4	N0	M0
	Any T	N1b	M0
	Any T	Any N	M1
Medullary thyroid cancer			
Stage I	TI	N0	M0
Stage II	T2	N0	M0
	T3	N0	M0
Stage III	T1-3	N1a	M0
Stage IV	T4	N0	M0
	Any T	N1b	M0
	Any T	Any N	M1
Anaplastic thyroid cancer			
Stage IV	All anaplastic thyroid cancer is Stage IV		

Bibliography

American Joint Committee on Cancer. *Cancer Staging Manual.* 7th ed. New York, NY: Springer-Verlag; 2010.

Questions

1. A 65-year-old patient with hoarseness is noted to have a 1-cm lesion on the left vocal cord, extending toward the anterior commissure. The vocal cord is mobile and no neck masses are noted on examination or imaging. A computed tomography (CT) chest is unremarkable. Biopsy reveals squamous cell carcinoma. Which answer best describes the TNM staging?
   A. T1N0M0
   B. T1N1M0

C. T2N0M0

D. TXN0M0

E. Unable to determine based on the information provided

2. A 70-year-old former smoker presented with hoarseness and dysphagia for 3 months. Laryngoscopy shows a tumor of the right false vocal cord extending to true vocal cord and medial wall of pyriform sinus on the same side. The vocal cord is mobile and there is no contralateral spread. CT neck reveals a right larynx mass with extension into the paraglottic space and a 1.8-cm lymph node on the right at level III. Biopsy confirms squamous cell carcinoma. Chest and brain imaging are negative. Which answer best describes the TNM staging?

A. T1N0M0

B. T1N1M0

C. T2N1M0

D. T2N2M0

E. T3N1M0

3. A 49-year-old woman is evaluated for a left-sided thyroid mass. On ultrasound, it measures 16 mm × 14 mm and no enlarged lymph nodes are identified. A chest x-ray (CXR) is negative and needle aspiration confirms papillary thyroid cancer. Which answer best describes the TNM staging?

A. T1aN0M0

B. T1bN0M0

C. T2N0M0

D. T3N0M0

E. T4N0M0

4. A 75-year-old smoker is seen for an ulcerative mass of the right oral tongue and floor of mouth. It measures 3.5 cm in greatest diameter and invades through cortical bone of the mandible. There are multiple right-only cervical lymph nodes, the largest of which is 2 cm. A positron emission tomography (PET) scan shows no evidence of distant disease. A biopsy shows squamous cell carcinoma. Which answer best describes the TNM staging?

A. T3N1M0

B. T3N2aM0

C. T3N2bM0

D. T4N2aM0

E. T4N2bM0

5. A 25-year-old man is evaluated for a right parotid mass. It measures 3 cm in greatest dimension. Imaging shows no evidence of spread to regional lymph nodes or beyond. At surgery, the tumor is noted not to extend beyond the parotid parenchyma. Final histology reveals adenoid cystic carcinoma. Which answer best describes the TNM staging?

A. T1N0M0

B. T1N1M0

C. T2N0M0

D. T2N1M0

E. T3N0M0

Chapter 37
Malignant Melanoma of the Head and Neck

Essentials of Otolaryngology- Head and Neck Surgery

Incidence

- 76,100 estimated new cases of malignant melanoma in the United States in 2014.
- 9,710 estimated deaths from melanoma in the United States in 2014.
- 20% to 30% of melanomas are located in the head and neck region.
- Alarming increases in incidence (5% per year) and mortality (2% per year).
- Highest incidence in areas with high sun-exposure and populations with fair skin (eg, Australia).

Risk Factors

- Sun-exposure
  - (a) Frequent, intermittent exposure to intense sunlight appears to be the highest risk factor.
  - (b) Ultraviolet light causes a photochemical reaction in DNA, leading to the formation of pyrimidine (thymine and cytosine) dimers.
  - (c) Ultraviolet B (290-310 nm).
    - More potent cause of DNA damage
  - (d) Ultraviolet A (320-400 nm).
    - More abundant in natural sunlight than UVB
    - Can also cause oxidative DNA damage
  - (e) Visible light may also contribute to the pathogenesis.
  - (f) Sunblock is protective.
    - Most products protect against UVB
    - SPF rating considers UVB only
    - Newer compounds (avobenzone, benzophenones) block UVA
- Tanning beds
  - (a) Produce mostly UVA radiation, but some models increase UVB fraction.
  - (b) Recent evidence supports an increased risk of malignant melanoma with frequent use.
- Fair skin (Fitzpatrick type I), blond or red hair
- Family history of melanoma

674

- Freckling of the upper back
- History of 3 or more blistering sunburns before the age of 20 years
- History of 3 or more years at an outdoor job as a teenager
- Presence of actinic keratoses

Hereditary Syndromes

- Familial Melanoma/dysplastic nevus syndrome
  - (a) Multiple atypical moles
  - (b) Lifetime risk of melanoma approaches 100%
  - (c) Genetic defect = CDKN2A gene at chromosome 9p21, which encodes p16(INK4a) and p14ARF
- Xeroderma pigmentosa
  - (a) Autosomal recessive
  - (b) 1000-fold increased risk of skin cancer, often before the age of 10
  - (c) Early onset freckling (before 2 years of age)
  - (d) Caused by a heterogeneous group of defects in the nucleotide excision repair pathway → cannot appropriately repair the constant DNA damage (specifically, thymine dimers) caused by UV exposure

Molecular Biology of Sporadic Melanoma

- Ras-Raf-Mek-Erk pathway
  - (a) Important pathway in regulation of cell proliferation.
  - (b) Activating NRas mutations are the most common Ras family mutations.
  - (c) Activating BRAF mutations are found in 50% to 70% of cutaneous melanomas.
  - (d) Several **BRAF inhibitors** and **MEK inhibitors** approved by the Food and Drug Administration (FDA) to treat malignant melanomas with activating mutations in BRAF.
- PI3K/PTEN
  - (a) Activation of this pathway associated with cell proliferation and malignant transformation.
  - (b) Most commonly observed events → activating mutations in PI3K, loss or silencing of PTEN, or amplification of AKT.
  - (c) Several drugs affecting this pathway, including PI3K and AKT inhibitors, are currently being studied.
- c-kit
  - (a) Tyrosine kinase receptor for stem cell factor.
  - (b) Activating mutations and amplifications cause constitutive activation of growth and proliferation pathways.
  - (c) More commonly found in melanoma unrelated to sun-exposure, namely acral or mucosal melanoma.
  - (d) Imatinib: A combined Abelson murine leukemia viral oncogene (ABL), c-kit, platelet-derived growth factor receptor (PDGFR) inhibitor, very successful in treating GI stromal tumors, and chronic myelogenous leukemias. Imatinib or other kit inhibitors may have activity in melanomas with activating c-kit mutations (more common in acral lentiginous and mucosal melanomas).

Premalignant Lesions

Up to 80% of malignant melanomas may arise in a preexisting lesion.

- Congenital nevi
  - (a) Has characteristics of benign nevus (mole), but present at birth
  - (b) May or may not develop coarse surface hairs ("congenital hairy nevus")
  - (c) Occurs in 1% to 2% of newborns
  - (d) May be part of a rare syndrome, neurocutaneous melanosis, where patients also develop melanotic neoplasms of the central nervous system
  - (e) Large or "giant" nevi (> 20 cm) have approximately 10% lifetime risk of conversion to melanoma
- Dysplastic nevus/atypical mole
  - (a) Generally larger than normal moles, with irregular/indistinct borders
  - (b) Often heterogeneous coloration
  - (c) Controversy over malignant potential exists
  - (d) Dysplastic nevi should be followed closely or removed if there is a high suspicion for melanoma, or if malignant characteristics of the lesion evolve
- Lentigo maligna (Hutchinson melanotic freckle)
  - (a) Melanoma *in situ*.
  - (b) Preinvasive phase (radial growth only) of *lentigo maligna melanoma* (vertical growth, as well).
  - (c) Large, thin, flat, irregular pigmented lesion.
  - (d) Frequently on the face and neck, areas of sun-damaged skin.
  - (e) Rate of progression is generally low, but reports vary between 2% and 33%.

Melanoma Subtypes

- Lentigo maligna melanoma
  - (a) Least common, 5% to 10% of all cases.
  - (b) Prolonged radial growth (years to decades).
  - (c) Lentigo maligna becomes lentigo maligna melanoma once it invades into the papillary dermis.
- Superficial spreading
  - (a) Most common, 75% of cases.
  - (b) Initial radial growth phase, with progression to vertical growth phase (often with ulceration or bleeding).
  - (c) Cells are very uniform in appearance.
  - (d) Smaller lesions generally have good prognosis due to lack of vertical growth.
- Nodular
  - (a) 10% to 15% of all cases.
  - (b) No radial growth phase: rapid vertical growth.
  - (c) Commonly ulcerated.
  - (d) Small lesions are often thick and have a poor prognosis.
- Acral lentiginous
  - (a) Found predominantly on the soles, palms, beneath the nail plate.
  - (b) Sun exposure does not seem to be a risk factor.
  - (c) Approximately 10% of cases overall, but most common among African Americans, Latin Americans, Native Americans, and Japanese.
- Desmoplastic
  - (a) Rare variant of melanoma, but most common site is head and neck.
  - (b) Appearance is variable, and often amelanotic.

(c) Histology: spindle-shaped tumor cells among a fibrous stroma, may show neuron-like differentiation.

(d) High affinity for perineural spread, and low rate of lymphatic metastasis.

- Mucosal Melanoma
  (a) < 1% of melanomas, but ~10% of all head and neck melanomas.
  (b) See the end of this chapter for a brief review of mucosal melanoma.

Differential Diagnosis

Benign lesions

- Sebhorreic keratosis
  (a) Light brown lesions, "stuck-on" appearance
- Pigmented actinic keratosis
- Benign melanocytic lesions
  (a) Mongolian spot: congenital patch of melanocytes, completely benign
  (b) Blue nevus
    ○ A rest of melanocytes; rare lesion, but more common in Asian patients. There are rare cases of melanoma arising from blue nevi.
    ○ Two variants exist:
      – Common blue nevus: common in head and neck
      – Cellular blue nevus: atypical lesions, can be difficult to differentiate from melanoma
  (c) Melanocytic nevus
    ○ Hamartomatous lesion composed of melanocytes
    ○ Spitz nevus
      – Childhood lesion composed of large or spindle-shaped melanocytes. Can have a phase of rapid growth, but it is benign. Can be difficult to differentiate from childhood melanoma.
      – Reports exist describing metastases from atypical spitz nevi, but it is debated whether these are Spitz nevi or malignant melanomas
  (d) Nevus of Ota: melanocytic hamartoma in the V2/V3 distribution
  (e) Nevus of Ito: similar to nevus of Ota, except occurring in shoulder region
- Lentigo maligna
- Atypical (dysplastic) nevus

Malignant lesions

- Basal cell carcinoma
- Keratoacanthoma
  (a) Low-grade malignancy that resembles well-differentiated squamous cell carcinoma
- Squamous cell carcinoma
- Sebaceous carcinoma
- Merkel cell carcinoma
  (a) Neuroendocrine carcinoma of the skin

Histologic Appearance of Malignant Melanoma

- Malignant melanoma is often characterized by:
  (a) Enlarged cells with cytologic atypia
  (b) Large, pleomorphic, hyperchromic nuclei

    (c) Prominent nucleoli

    (d) "Pagetoid" growth (upward, out of the basal layer) is commonly observed; this can also occur in melanocytic nevi, however more extensive lateral spread and cytological atypia favor the diagnosis of melanoma.

    (e) Presence of melanin on hematoxylin and eosin (H&E) stain or with the aid of Fontana stain

- However, melanomas can be "amelanotic."
- The histologic pattern and differentiation of melanoma can vary greatly.
- Melanoma has been called a "great mimicker," and belongs in the differential diagnosis of any undifferentiated tumor.
- Common immunohistochemical markers:

    (a) HMB-45, S-100, Melan-A, and Vimentin.

    (b) Cytokeratin is usually negative.

- **Depth of invasion** and **number of mitoses** have an important impact on prognosis.

Evaluation

History and Physical Examination

- Thorough history to determine risk of melanoma (see risk factors).
- Common characteristics of malignant melanoma (ABCDE checklist):

    (a) **A**symmetry, **B**order irregularities, **C**olor variegation, **D**iameter > 6 mm or recent increase in size, **E**volution - changes in size, color, texture, etc.

- A thorough physical examination of the head and neck is always warranted, but there are several important considerations specific to malignant melanoma.

    (a) **Location** has a significant impact on prognosis.

    (b) Generally, head and neck melanoma has a worse prognosis than other sites.

    (c) Specific subsites of the head and neck carry a worse prognosis.

       ◦ (worst) scalp > ear > cheek > neck (improved)

    (d) Note signs of aggressive/advanced disease:

       ◦ Ulceration

       ◦ Nodularity

       ◦ Satellite lesions

    (e) Thorough examination of the draining lymph node basin is required.

       ◦ Include parotid lymph nodes, especially for anterior scalp, temple, or cheek melanomas

       ◦ occipital nodes, especially for retroauricular or posterior scalp lesions.

Imaging

- Stage I or II disease: **chest X-Ray** is often obtained, and is the only imaging study necessary unless suspicion for distant metastasis exists based on clinical examination or laboratory findings.
- **CT with IV contrast** of the head and neck is used to evaluate the extent of local-regional disease. Therefore, obtain in any patient with thick lesions, evidence of local invasion, or evidence on clinical examination for regional metastasis.
- Metastatic imaging work-up includes:

    (a) CT chest, abdomen, pelvis with IV contrast.

    (b) MRI of the brain.

    (c) Recently, PET and PET-CT have been shown to be highly sensitive for the detection of systemic metastasis, and may replace whole-body CT scan.

- **Consider** metastatic screening in the following patients:
    - (a) Patients with thick melanomas (> 4 mm), satellitosis, ulceration, or recurrent lesions
- Metastatic evaluation is **required** in the following patients:
    - (a) Patients with regional metastases (stage III)
    - (b) Patients with signs or symptoms of metastatic disease on examination or laboratory evaluation
    - (c) Patients with known systemic disease (stage IV)

Other

- Baseline CBC, basic chemistry panel, total protein, albumin
- Elevated alkaline phosphatase may signify metastatic disease to bone or liver
- Elevated ALT/AST may signify metastatic disease to the liver
- Elevated lactate dehydrogenase (LDH) is nonspecific, but may signify the presence of metastasis. It is also a useful marker to follow for the development of metastatic disease during follow-up. Recommended in any patient at risk for systemic disease.

Biopsy

- All lesions suspicious for malignant melanoma should undergo biopsy by a method that will give a definitive diagnosis and provide information on depth of invasion.
- Shave and needle biopsies of the primary tumor should not be performed.
- **Excisional biopsy**
    - (a) Acceptable if lesion is very small
    - (b) Excise with 1 to 2-mm margins → wide excision of margins necessary if pathologic review yields malignant melanoma
    - (c) Excision of large lesions may disrupt lymphatic drainage, altering results on lymphoscintigraphy
- **Incisional** or **punch biopsies** through the thickest portion of tumor is recommended.
    - (a) Allows adequate assessment of depth of invasion.
    - (b) Does not disrupt border of tumor in order to determine appropriate margins for wide local excision.
    - (c) Does not affect lymphatic drainage of the lesion if lymphoscintigraphy is planned.

Staging

- The most important prognostic factors in malignant melanoma are depth of invasion, ulceration, mitotic index, satellitosis, degree of lymph node involvement, and distant metastasis.
- A description of Clark levels, and Breslow thickness (Table 37-1) are presented here as these are commonly referenced, however the current standard of evaluation and prognostication are the recent guidelines proposed in the staging system developed by the American Joint Council on Cancer (AJCC) (Table 37-2).
- Note that AJCC staging includes clinical and pathologic staging. Pathologic staging incorporates pathologic information about the regional lymph nodes after lymph node biopsy/neck dissection, subdividing stage III disease into the categories shown. Only pathologic stage is presented here, as sentinel lymph node biopsy has become routine for medium thickness melanomas at most centers.

Treatment

Surgery
Primary Lesion

- A diagnosis of malignant melanoma requires wide local excision of the primary lesion, unless systemic metastases are present and palliative resection is unwarranted.

Table 37-1 **Definitions of Clark Levels and Breslow Thickness for Malignant Melanoma**

Clark Levels	Level of Invasion
Level I	Epidermis only (*carcinoma in situ*)
Level II	Papillary dermis (not to papillary-reticular interface)
Level III	Fills/expands papillary dermis to reticular interface
Level IV	Reticular dermis
Level V	Subcutaneous tissue
Breslow Thickness	
Stage I	≤ 0.75 mm
Stage II	0.76-1.50 mm
Stage III	1.51-4.0 mm
Stage IV	≥ 4.1 mm

Margins
- General guidelines:
    - (a) **1-cm** margin for tumors <1 mm thick
    - (b) **Consider >1 cm** margin for lesion with 1 to 2-mm thickness.
    - (c) **2-cm** margin for tumors > 2 mm thick, or ulcerated
- Appropriate margins for melanoma have been debated for decades, and recommendations of 1 to 2 cm are often not feasible due to functional and cosmetic considerations in the head and neck.
- Depth of resection varies based on the region of the head and neck involved. Some important considerations:
    - (a) **Scalp lesions:** resected to the calvarial periosteum; the outer table of the cranium can be included if lesion is thick and encroaches upon the periosteum.
    - (b) **Auricular lesions** often require partial or total auriculectomy depending on the size of the tumor and presence or absence of satellitosis.
    - (c) Lesions that involve the **ear canal** may require lateral temporal bone resection.
    - (d) **Facial lesions** are often resected down to the level of the facial mimetic muscles, unless lesion is thicker and requires resection of muscle or even facial bone.
    - (e) **Lesions overlying the parotid gland** resected down to parotid-masseteric fascia, unless thickness requires that a superficial parotidectomy be included in resection.

Cervical Lymph Nodes
- **Therapeutic neck dissection**
    - (a) Patients with evidence of lymphatic metastasis on clinical examination or imaging require a neck dissection to remove gross disease.
    - (b) Anterior scalp, temple, ear, or facial melanomas with evidence of regional disease require a **superficial parotidectomy** as well. Chin and neck melanomas do not require parotidectomy.
    - (c) For posterior scalp, posterior ear, or retroauricular melanomas with evidence of regional disease, the **postauricular and suboccipital nodes** must be included in the neck dissection.

Table 37-1 TNM Staging for Malignant Melanoma

T Classification	Thickness (mm)	Ulceration Status/Mitoses
T1	≤1.0	a: w/o ulceration and mitoses <1/mm² b: with ulceration or mitoses ≥1/mm²
T2	1-2 mm	a: w/o ulceration and mitoses <1/mm² b: with ulceration or mitoses ≥1/mm²
T3	2-4 mm	a: w/o ulceration and mitoses <1/mm² b: with ulceration or mitoses ≥1/mm²
T4	>4 mm	a: w/o ulceration and mitoses <1/mm² b: with ulceration or mitoses ≥1/mm²

N Classification	No. of Metastatic Nodes	Nodal Metastatic Mass
N1	1 node	a: micrometastasis* b: macrometastasis**
N2	2-3 node	a: micrometastasis* b: macrometastasis** c: in transit met(s)/satellite(s) without metastatic nodes
N3	4 or more metastatic nodes, matted nodes, or in transit met(s)/satellite(s) with metastatic node(s)	

*Micrometastases are diagnosed after sentinel lymph node biopsy and completion lymphadenectomy (if performed).
**Macrometastases are defined as clinically detectable nodal metastases confirmed by therapeutic lymphadenectomy or when nodal metastasis exhibits gross extracapsular extension.

M Classification	Site	Serum LDH
M1a	Distant skin, subcutaneous, or nodal mets	Normal
M1b	Lung metastases	Normal
M1c	All other visceral metastases Any distant metastasis	Normal Elevated

Reproduced with permission of Edge S, Byrd DR, Compton CC, et al: *AJCC Cancer Staging Manual*, 7th edition. Chicago, IL: Springer Science and Business Media LLC; 2010.

Anatomic Stage/Prognostic Groups

Clinical Staging*				Pathologic Staging**			
Stage 0	Tis	N0	M0	0	Tis	N0	M0
Stage IA	T1a	N0	M0	IA	T1a	N0	M0
Stage IB	T1b	N0	M0	IB	T1b	N0	M0
	T2a	N0	M0		T2a	N0	M0
Stage IIA	T2b	N0	M0	IIA	T2b	N0	M0
	T3a	N0	M0		T3a	N0	M0
Stage IIB	T3b	N0	M0	IIB	T3b	N0	M0
	T4a	N0	M0		T4a	N0	M0
Stage IIC	T4b	N0	M0	IIC	T4b	N0	M0
Stage III	Any T	≥N1	M0	IIIA	T1-4a	N1a	M0
					T1-4a	N2a	M0
				IIIB	T1-4b	N1a	M0
					T1-4b	N2a	M0
					T1-4a	N1b	M0
					T1-4a	N2b	M0
					T1-4a	N2c	M0
				IIIC	T1-4b	N1b	M0
					T1-4b	N2b	M0
					T1-4b	N2c	M0
					any T	N3	M0
Stage IV	Any T	Any N	M1	IV	Any T	Any N	M1

* Clinical staging includes microstaging of the primary melanoma and clinical/radiologic evaluation for metastases. By convention, it should be used after complete excision of the primary melanoma with clinical assessment for regional and distant metastases.
** Pathologic staging includes microstaging of the primary melanoma and pathologic information about the regional lymph nodes after partial or complete lymphadenectomy. Pathologic Stage 0 or Stage IA patients are the exception; they do not require pathologic evaluation of their lymph nodes.

- **Elective neck dissection / Sentinel lymph node biopsy**
  - (a) Elective neck dissection has been largely replaced by sentinel lymph node biopsy, with neck dissection reserved for cases with positive sentinel lymph nodes.
  - (b) Sentinel lymph node biopsy is recommended for patients with T2 or T3 tumors (depth 1-4 mm) and no evidence on clinical examination of lymph node metastasis ("N0 neck")
  - (c) Also indicated for lesions extending to Clark levels IV or V, lesions with an increased mitotic index (> $1/mm^2$), or ulceration, regardless of the thickness of the lesion.
  - (d) The parotid lymph nodes and neck levels IB, II, III, and IV are at risk when primary lesions involve the anterior scalp (anterior to a vertical line drawn superiorly from the external auditory canal), temple, facial lesions, and ear.
  - (e) Posterior scalp (posterior to a vertical line drawn superiorly from the external auditory canal) and retroauricular lesions drain to the posterolateral neck—levels II, III, IV, and V—along with the retroauricular and suboccipital lymph nodes.
- Technical aspects of sentinel lymph node biopsy
  - (a) **Lymphoscintigraphy**, or lymphatic mapping, is performed 1 to 24 hours prior to sentinel node biopsy.
  - (b) Dermal layer of the bed of primary lesion (or region of recent resection if excisional biopsy was performed) is injected with Technecium-99-labeled sulfur colloid .
  - (c) Two-dimensional nuclear imaging, or three-dimensional SPECT/CT is performed to map the lymph nodes draining the site of the lesion.
  - (d) **Sentinel lymph node biopsy** is then performed.
    - ○ If lymphoscintigraphy was performed just before surgery, no additional Tc-99-labelled sulfur colloid is injected.
    - ○ If lymphoscintigraphy was performed the day before, additional tracer is injected 1 hour before surgery.
    - ○ Isosulfan blue can be injected into the primary site at the time of surgery as an adjunctive method to identify sentinel nodes.
    - ○ A hand-held gamma probe is used to identify the sentinel lymph node.
    - ○ The sentinel node, ideally identified with the guidance of the lymphatic map, the gamma probe, and visualized with uptake of isosulfan blue, is removed.
    - ○ If localization is to parotid region, superficial parotidectomy may be necessary.
    - ○ Additional nodes (usually ~ 3-4 lymph nodes) are removed until the reading from the gamma probe in the surgical bed is reduced to 10% of the highest reading from the resected lymph nodes.
    - ○ Sentinel lymph nodes undergo standard sectioning with H&E staining, as well as additional sectioning with IHC evaluation using HMB-45, S-100, and Melan-A.
  - (e) Sentinel lymph nodes positive for metastatic melanoma necessitates complete neck dissection, including a parotidectomy or removal of the postauricular/suboccipital nodes if the location of primary disease places these regions at risk of metastasis.

Reconstruction
- Choose from "reconstructive ladder" (secondary intention-→ primary closure → skin graft → regional flap → free flap) depending on location and size of defect.
- DO NOT perform a complex reconstruction (ie, regional or free flap) until the margin status has been defined on the final pathologic report.
- If necessary, place a dressing or skin graft over large/complex wounds and return to the OR for reconstruction after margins have been deemed negative.
- May also perform neck dissection at the time of reconstruction if the sentinel lymph node biopsy results are deemed positive.

External Beam Radiation

- Used to improve local-regional control in the following settings:
  - (a) Postoperative radiation following resection/neck dissection of palpable lymphatic disease
  - (b) Radiation to regional lymph nodes for patients with T2b-T4, N0 disease who cannot undergo sentinel lymph node biopsy or neck dissection
  - (c) Radiation to regional recurrence in patients who have previously undergone neck dissection
  - (d) Radiation to primary site in patients at high risk of local failure (eg, T4 lesions, desmoplastic melanoma, etc.)
- Hypofractionated treatment schedule (6 Gy fractions up to a total dose of 30 Gy) is most effective.

Chemotherapy

- Systemic therapy is used in two settings:
  - (a) For patients at high risk for the development of distant metastasis (ie, Stage III or recurrent disease)
  - (b) Patients with known distant metastases (ie, Stage IV disease)
- Available therapies:
  - (a) **Dacarbazine** and derivatives
    - ○ Alkylating agent, FDA approved for the treatment of advanced melanoma → 10% to 20% response rate
- **Interferon α-2b**
  - (a) Cytokine normally produced by lymphocytes
  - (b) FDA approved for treating malignant melanoma
  - (c) Mechanism of action not well understood- modulates immune response to cancer cells
- **IL-2**
  - (a) Biologic modifier similar to INFα-2b
- **Ipilimumab** – a monoclonal antibody that blocks cytotoxic T lymphocyte antigen-4 (CTLA-4), approved to treat unresectable or metastatic melanoma. CTLA-4 is found on the surface of T-cells, and when activated leads to down regulation of T-cell activity. Inhibition of CTLA-4 promotes the T-cell response to tumor cell antigens.
- **MAP kinase (Ras-Raf-MEK-ERK) pathway inhibitors**
  - (a) **Vemurafenib**: small molecule selective inhibitor of BRAF which is approved to treat unresectable or metastatic melanoma with activating mutations in BRAF (eg, BRAF V600E mutations).
  - (b) **Dabrafenib**: BRAF inhibitor used to treat patients with tumors containing activating BRAF mutations.
  - (c) **Trametinib:** a MEK inhibitor, approved to treat patients with tumors containing BRAF mutations.
  - (d) Dabrafenib and Trametinib have been approved as single agents and in combination.
- Exploratory Strategies
  - (a) **Tumor vaccines** have been well-studied in malignant melanoma, but results have not shown a benefit, to date.
  - (b) **Tumor-induced lymphocyte therapy**
    - ○ Patients' lymphocytes are extracted and cultured in the presence of melanoma antigens.
    - ○ These "activated" lymphocytes are reintroduced into the patient after chemotherapeutic lymphodepletion.

(c) **Lambrolizumab**: promising investigational drug that targets the programmed death receptor-1 (PD-1). Many tumors express PD-L1, the ligand for PD-1. Activated PD-1 on T-Cells leads to suppression, a mechanism to evade the immune response. PD-1 and PD-L1 inhibitors disrupt this mechanism of immunosuppression, and enhance the immune response.

See Figure 37-1.

Management Algorithm

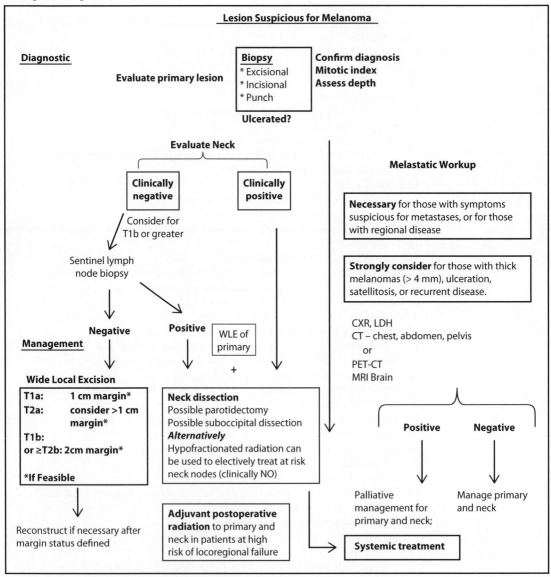

Figure 37-1 Management Algorithm.

Follow-Up

- Recommendations vary, but typical follow-up schedules are every 3 to 6 months for 4 years, and annually thereafter.
- Periodic LDH and CXR recommended.
- Frequency of examination, laboratory testing, and radiologic examinations should increase for more advanced stage.

Other Considerations in Head and Neck Melanoma

Desmoplastic Melanoma

- Often nonpigmented, initially benign-appearing.
- Rare, spindle-cell variant with a propensity for perineural spread.
- These lesions can be purely desmoplastic in nature, or can have elements of both desmoplastic and conventional melanoma features (mixed desmoplastic).
- Pure desmoplastic melanomas metastasize to regional lymph nodes very infrequently and therefore sentinel lymph node biopsy is not recommended.
- Considerations for sentinel lymph node biopsy for mixed desmoplastic lesions are the same as for conventional cutaneous melanoma.
- Excision with wide margins (2 cm if feasible) with adjuvant radiotherapy is recommended for all melanomas with desmoplastic features.

Mucosal Melanoma

- Rare variant of melanoma, but most common site is in the head and neck.
- Most common sites: nasal > paranasal sinuses > oral cavity > nasopharynx.
- Prognosis: (best) Nasal > oral cavity > paranasal sinuses (worst).
- Disease can be indolent with vague symptoms, thus patients often present with an advanced stage of disease.
- Often amelanotic.
- Depth of invasion has not been shown to be a predictor of prognosis.
- Treatment:
  (a) Surgical resection
  (b) Therapeutic neck dissection for clinically positive lymph nodes
  (c) Elective neck dissection not recommended
  (d) Radiation at high dose (> 54 Gy) and standard fractionation can improve local-regional control
- Many patients succumb to distant metastasis.

Unknown Primary Melanoma

- Melanoma identified in cervical lymph nodes or parotid nodes with no evidence or history of a primary lesion.
- Thorough history and physical examination necessary to identify potential primary lesion, and metastatic workup indicated.
- Theorized that primary lesions can spontaneously regress.
- Treat with surgical resection/neck dissection and postoperative hypofractionated radiation (ie, treat as a Stage III melanoma).

Bibliography

American Joint Committee on Cancer (AJCC). Melanoma of the skin. In: Edge SB, Byrd DR, Compton CC, eds. *AJCC Cancer Staging Manual.* 7th ed. New York, NY: Springer; 2010.

Anderson TD, Weber RS, Guerry D, et al: Desmoplastic neurotropic melanoma of the head and neck: the role of radiation therapy. *Head Neck.* 2002;24:1068-1071.

Ballo MT, Ross MI, Cormier JN, et al: Combined-modality therapy for patients with regional nodal metastases from melanoma. *Int J Radiat Oncol Biol Phys.* 2006;64:106-113.

Gomez-Rivera F, Santillan A, McMurphey AB, et al. Sentinel node biopsy in patients with cutaneous melanoma of the head and neck: recurrence and survival study. *Head Neck.* 2008;30:1284-1294.

Moreno MA, Roberts DB, Kupferman ME, et al. Mucosal melanoma of the nose and paranasal sinuses, a contemporary experience from the M.D. Anderson Cancer Center. *Cancer.* 2010;116:2215-2223.

Morton DL, Thompson JF, Cochran AJ, et al (MSLT Group). Final trial report of sentinel-node biopsy versus nodal observation in melanoma. *N Engl J Med.* 2014;370(7):599-609.

Saranga-Perry V, Ambe C, Zager JS, et al. Recent developments in the medical and surgical treatment of melanoma. *CA Cancer J Clin.* 2014;64(3):171-185.

Questions

1. Which of the following is *not* a risk factor for the development of head and neck melanoma?

   A. Fitzpatrick type I skin type

   B. Ultraviolet A exposure from tanning booths

   C. Presence of multiple nevi on the cheeks

   D. Four blistering sunburns in the teenage years

2. Which of the following drugs does not modulate the immune response to melanoma?

   A. Vemurafenib

   B. Ipilimumab

   C. IL-2

   D. Lambrolizumab

3. What is the proper margin, if feasible, for a nonulcerated lesion with 1.25 mm depth of invasion?

   A. 0.5 cm

   B. 1 cm

   C. 1.5 cm

   D. 2 cm

4. You are planning to resect an ulcerated malignant melanoma that has 2.1 mm depth of invasion from the left anterior parietal scalp of a 40-year-old male patient. He has no cervical or parotid lymphadenopathy and no suspicious nodes on imaging. What is the most appropriate next step in management?

   A. Wide local excision with 2-cm margin

   B. Wide local excision with 1-cm margin, elective neck dissection

   C. Wide local excision with 2-cm margin, with sentinel lymph node biopsy

   D. Wide local excision with 2-cm margin, radiation therapy to the draining lymph node basin, including the parotid gland

5. A patient presents with a large, left auricular melanoma with three palpable lymph nodes in the left neck. Which of the following is not an appropriate test for distant metastasis?

A. LDH

B. Brain MRI

C. Full body PET-CT

D. Evaluation for V600E activation mutation in BRAF

Chapter 38
Tumors of the Larynx

Laryngeal Cancer

- Second most common malignancy of upper aerodigestive tract (Table 38-1)
- Represents 1% to 5% of all malignancies
- Squamous cell carcinoma (SCCA) represents 85% to 95% of laryngeal malignancies
- M:F ratio 4:1
- Risk factors
  - (a) Tobacco
    - ○ Risk does not decrease to baseline despite cessation for years
  - (b) Alcohol
  - (c) Prior head and neck SCCA
  - (d) History of recurrent respiratory papillomatosis
  - (e) Environmental factors reported in literature such as exposure to wood dust, paint, etc.
- Clinical Presentation
  - (a) Hoarseness
  - (b) Dysphagia
  - (c) Odynophagia
  - (d) Referred otalgia
  - (e) Dyspnea
  - (f) Stridor
  - (g) Aspiration
  - (h) Hemoptysis
  - (i) Weight loss
  - (j) Globus sensation
  - (k) Sore throat greater than 2 weeks

Clinical Evaluation

- History
  - (a) Pertinent risk factors
  - (b) Duration of symptoms

Table 38-1 **Differential Diagnosis of Laryngeal Mass**

Nonneoplastic Lesions	*Primary Laryngeal Malignancies*
Mucus retention cyst	Epithelial
Laryngocele	Squamous cell carcinoma
Vocal fold polyp	Verrucous
Vocal process granuloma	Spindle cell
Keratosis	Adenoid
Hyperplasia—squamous cell	Basaloid
Hyperplasia—pseudoepitheliomatous	Clear cell
Amyloidosis	Adenosquamous
Infectious—tuberculosis (TB), *Candida*	Giant cell
Inflammatory—Wegener, relapsing	Lymphoepithelial
Polychondritis	Malignant salivary gland tumors
Benign neoplasms	*Neuroendocrine tumors*
Papilloma	Carcinoid
Pleomorphic adenoma	Small cell carcinoma
Oncocytic papillary cystadenoma	Malignant paraganglioma
Lipoma	*Malignant soft tissue tumors/sarcomas*
Neurofibroma	Malignant bone/cartilage tumors
Leiomyoma	Chondrosarcoma
Paraganglioma	Osteosarcoma
Chondroma	Lymphoma
Giant cell tumor	Extramedullary plasmacytoma
Premalignant lesions	
Squamous cell dysplasia	
Carcinoma in situ	

Adapted with permission from Flint PW, Haughey BH, Lund VJ, et al: *Cummings Otolaryngology Head and Neck Surgery.* 5th ed. St. Louis, Mo: Mosby Elsevier; 2010.

    (c) Comorbidities
    (d) History of prior cancers
    (e) Dysphagia, malnutrition, dehydration, weight loss
    (f) Dyspnea, stridor
- Physical examination
    (a) Comprehensive head/neck examination
    (b) Voice characteristics
    (c) Neck examination for lymphadenopathy
    (d) Dental evaluation

  (e) Flexible laryngoscopy
  (f) Videostroboscopy
- Diagnostic tests/studies
  (a) Pathologic diagnosis
    ○ Endoscopy with biopsy
    ○ Fine-needle aspiration (FNA) of palpable neck node
  (b) Imaging
    ○ Computed tomography (CT) or magnetic resonance imaging (MRI) of neck
      – Extent of disease
      – Spread of tumor to pre-epiglottic, paraglottic, posterior cricoid areas
      – MRI more sensitive for cartilage invasion
    ○ CT chest
      – Exclude pulmonary metastasis
      – Isolated pulmonary nodule more likely to be second primary than metastatic laryngeal cancer
    ○ Laboratory studies
      – Electrocardiography (ECG) for preoperative clearance
      – Prealbumin and albumin for nutritional status
      – Complete blood count (CBC), electrolyte panel, liver function tests

Laryngeal Anatomy and Boundaries

- Supraglottis
  (a) Third and fourth branchial arch derivative with no midline fusion
  (b) Blood supply: superior laryngeal arteries
  (c) Bilateral lymphatic drainage
  (d) Superior surface of epiglottis to lateral margin of ventricle at junction of false vocal fold with true vocal fold
  (e) *Quadrangular membrane*: fiberoelastic membrane; extends from epiglottis to arytenoids and corniculate cartilage
  (f) *Subsites*: suprahyoid epiglottis, infrahyoid epiglottis, aryepiglottic folds, arytenoids, ventricle, false vocal folds
- Glottis
  (a) Sixth branchial arch derivative
  (b) Blood supply: inferior laryngeal arteries
  (c) Extends 1 cm below apex of ventricle
  (d) *Conus elasticus*: fibroelastic membrane; extends from cricoid cartilage to vocal ligament; limits spread of cancer laterally
  (e) *Broyles' tendon*: insertion of vocalis tendon to thyroid cartilage, potential area for tumor spread to thyroid cartilage (absence of perichondrium in this area)
  (f) *Subsites*: true vocal folds (including anterior/posterior commissure)
- Subglottis
  (a) Sixth branchial arch derivate
  (b) Blood supply: inferior laryngeal arteries
  (c) Extends from glottis to inferior border of cricoid cartilage
  (d) *Subsites*: none
- Preepiglottic space (Figure 38-1)
  (a) Anterior to epiglottis

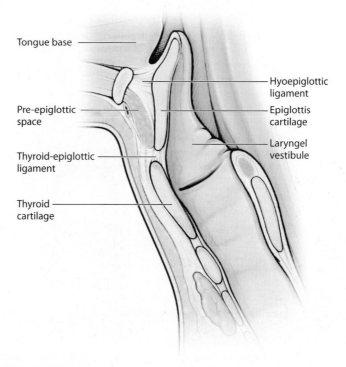

Figure 38-1 Sagittal view of larynx.

   (b) Extends from hyoepiglottic ligament/vallecula to thyroid cartilage/thyroepiglottic ligament; bounded anteriorly by thyroid membrane
   (c) Contains fibrofatty tissue
   (d) Contiguous with paraglottic space
- Paraglottic space (Figure 38-2)
   (a) Space outside conus elasticus and quadrangular membrane
   (b) Contains fibrofatty tissue
   (c) May allow for submucosal, transglottic spread of tumor
- Reinke space
   (a) Superficial lamina propria of true vocal fold

Premalignant Laryngeal Lesions

- Spectrum from hyperplasia → atypia → dysplasia (mild/moderate/severe) → carcinoma in situ (CIS)
- *Mild dysplasia*: cellular abnormalities; limited to basal one-third of epithelium
- *Moderate dysplasia*: cellular abnormalities; up to two-thirds of epithelium thickness
- *Severe dysplasia*: cellular atypia; greater than two-thirds of epithelium thickness
- *CIS*: intraepithelial neoplasm; no basement membrane or stromal invasion

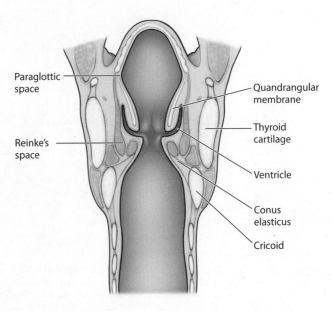

Figure 38-2 Coronal sagittal view of larynx.

- Interval to malignant transformation variable (3-10 years)
    (a) Mild/moderate dysplasia: 7% to 11% lesions undergo malignant transformation.
    (b) Severe dysplasia: 18% lesions undergo malignant transformation, older studies state 30%.
    (c) Clinically, severe dysplasia and CIS behave similarly.
- Biopsy is gold standard of diagnosis
    (a) Techniques include incisional biopsy, excisional biopsy, or microflap excision
- Treatment – early lesions
    (a) Endoscopic excision ± CO_2 laser as needed
        ○ Repeat surgery as needed for local control
    (b) Radiation
        ○ Effective alternative – very elderly, frail, and multifocal lesions
    (c) Both surgery and radiation have excellent local control with early lesions
    (d) Requires close, life-long follow-up to detect recurrent and second primary lesions

Laryngeal Squamous Cell Carcinoma

- Histology
    (a) Normal tissue
        ○ Supraglottis: ciliated pseudostratified columnar epithelium
        ○ Glottis: stratified squamous epithelium
        ○ Subglottis: ciliated pseudostratified columnar epithelium

    (b) Squamous cell cancer
- Well-differentiated: keratinization, intercellular bridges, pleomorphic nuclei
- Moderately differentiated: less keratinization, more atypical nuclei
- Poorly differentiated: minimal keratinization, minimal intercellular bridges, numerous atypical nuclei

- Staging
  - (a) Supraglottic
    - T1: limited to one subsite.
    - T2: more than one subsite of supraglottic larynx or spreads outside of supraglottic larynx, without vocal fold fixation.
    - T3: vocal fold fixation or invasion of adjacent structures (postcricoid, pre-epiglottic space, paraglottic space, inner cortex of thyroid cartilage).
    - T4a: (moderately advanced) invades thyroid cartilage or beyond larynx.
    - T4b: (very advanced) invades prevertebral fascia, encases carotid artery, or invades mediastinum.
    - Usually presents with mild odynophagia, dysphagia, and referred otalgia (via Arnold nerve).
    - Most common subsite is epiglottis.
    - Tumor spreads typically to base of tongue or pre-epiglottic space.
    - 25% to 50% have cervical nodal metastases at time of presentation.
      - Incidence based on T stage: T1 (10%), T2 (29%), T3 (38%), T5 (57%).
      - Incidence of occult nodal metastasis increases based on T stage: T1 (0%), T2 (20%), T3 (25%), T4 (40%).
      - Typically spreads to level II-IV of neck (levels I and V rarely involved and only when there is disease in other levels).
      - Risk of contralateral neck involvement increased if tumor centrally located.
  - (b) Glottic SCCA
    - T1: limited to vocal folds with normal vocal fold movement
      - T1a: one vocal fold
      - T1b: bilateral vocal folds
    - T2: extends to subglottis or supraglottis, or impaired vocal fold mobility
    - T3: vocal fold fixation or invasion of adjacent structures (paraglottic space, inner cortex of thyroid cartilage)
    - T4a: (moderately advanced) invades thyroid cartilage or beyond larynx
    - T4b: (very advanced) invades prevertebral fascia, encases carotid artery, or invades mediastinum
    - Most common site of laryngeal cancer with most cancers in anterior two-thirds of true vocal folds (TVF)
    - Typical symptoms include hoarseness and globus sensation
    - Incidence of cervical metastasis low and based on T stage: T1/T2 (<5%), T3/T4 (20%-25%)
    - Cervical metastasis typically unilateral and in levels II, III, IV, and VI
    - Transglottic lesions extend into subglottis/supraglottis and have higher rates of nodal metastasis and cartilage invasion
      - Occurs when tumors extend through anterior commissure
      - Can also become transglottic by spread through paraglottic space or spreading along arytenoid cartilage posterior to ventricle
  - (c) Subglottic SCCA
    - T1: limited to subglottis

- T2: involves vocal folds with normal or impaired mobility
- T3: involves vocal folds with fixation
- T4a: (moderately advanced) invades cricoid or thyroid cartilage or beyond larynx
- T4b: (very advanced) invades prevertebral fascia, encases carotid artery, or invades mediastinum
- Rare, aggressive, and poorly differentiated
- Can present with airway obstruction, stridor, or dyspnea
- Incidence of cervical metastasis low (one study detected disease in 33% of level VI nodes)
- May also present with metastasis to superior mediastinum (associated with stomal recurrence after treatment with total laryngectomy)
(d) Distant metastasis
- Most common hematogenous spread to lungs > liver > skeletal system
- Most common lymphatic spread to mediastinum
- Increased risk with advanced stage, neck disease, locoregional recurrence, or primary site with supraglottis/subglottis greater than glottis
- Treatment of early laryngeal cancer (Stage I/II)
  (a) Mainly treated with single modality – radiation or surgery
  - Treatment individualized to patient depending mainly on stage and subsite
  - External beam radiation
    - Radiation field depends on subsite
    - *Advantages*: useful in nonoperative candidates, avoids up-front tracheotomy in certain patients
    - *Disadvantages*: mucositis, laryngeal edema, dysphagia, Xerostomia, risk of chondronecrosis, increased difficulty in detecting recurrence
    - Usually involves 6-week course of treatment (total 60-70 Gy)
    - Local control rates 90% to 98% with T1 or certain T2 lesions
  - Based on subsite involved, different surgical procedures can be used
    - Endoscopic resection with or without laser
    - Local control rates of 95% for T1 and 80% for T2 lesions
    - Open procedures now less often used (historic interest)
  (b) Supraglottic SCCA
  - Supraglottic laryngectomy
    - *Indications*: T1 or T2 with normal vocal fold mobility, tumor limited to supraglottis 2 to 5 mm from anterior commissure.
    - *Contraindications*: vocal fold fixation, interarytenoid involvement, poor pulmonary status, thyroid cartilage invasion.
    - *Advantages*: minimal effect on voice, possibility of avoiding irradiation, appropriate pathologic staging.
    - *Disadvantages*: applicable to select patients, may require initial tracheotomy, requirement for postoperative swallowing therapy (almost all patients have dysphagia and aspirate postoperatively).
    - Can be endoscopic or open.
    - Postoperative radiation is indicated for positive margins, perineural spread, extracapsular spread, greater than or equal to two positive lymph nodes.
  - External beam radiation
    - Nonsurgical option especially for patients with poor pulmonary status and other comorbidities

- Management of neck
  - Because of incidence of occult neck disease, neck should be incorporated into radiation field or patient should undergo selective neck dissection for N0 neck.
  - Both sides of neck should be treated especially for midline lesions.
- (c) Glottic SCCA
  - Endoscopic laser excision or microlaryngeal surgery
    - *Advantages*: possibility of avoiding irradiation, similar local control as radiation.
    - *Disadvantages*: poorer voice outcomes compared to radiation.
    - Endoscopic procedures have largely replaced open procedures such as vertical partial laryngectomy and hemilaryngectomy.
      ◊ Avoidance of tracheotomy and improved dysphagia outcomes
    - *Indications*: T1 or T2 lesions with limited involvement of contralateral vocal fold, limited infraglottic extension, limited involvement of arytenoids.
      ◊ Preservation of arytenoid complex results in decreased postoperative dysphagia and improved vocal outcomes
    - *Contraindications*: vocal fold fixation or bilateral vocal fold impaired motion, interarytenoid involvement, poor pulmonary status, difficult exposure endoscopically.
    - Postoperative radiation may be needed for positive margins.
  - External beam radiation
    - Excellent local control for T1 size lesions and good voice outcomes
    - High failure rate of up to 30% with T2 lesions that have impaired mobility of TVF
  - Involvement of anterior commissure
    - Lower locoregional control rates
    - Surgically best addressed with open procedure such as supracricoid partial laryngectomy with preservation of cricoid and one arytenoid joint, defect closed with approximation of base of tongue to laryngeal remnant
  - Management of neck
    - Low incidence of occult neck disease
    - Neck does not need to be treated in clinically N0 cases
- Treatment of advance laryngeal cancers (Stage III/IV)
  - (a) Concurrent chemoradiation for most T3 and early T4 lesions
  - (b) Partial laryngectomy or endoscopic partial laryngectomy for selected cases
  - (c) Total laryngectomy with adjuvant CRT for advanced T4 lesions if stridor or aspiration present
  - (d) Traditional treatment had been total laryngectomy with postoperative radiation
  - (e) Laryngeal preservation protocols developed due to morbidity of procedure (physical appearance and impaired communication)
  - (f) Treatment considerations include patient's comorbidities or preferences, physician's expertise, and access to resources
  - (g) Landmark studies
    - VA laryngeal study (1991)
      - Compared induction chemotherapy (cisplatin/5-FU) with definitive radiation versus total laryngectomy and postoperative radiation
      - Patients with poor response to chemotherapy underwent total laryngectomy and postoperative radiation

- No difference in survival between the two groups (68% 2-year survival for both groups)
- 64% laryngeal preservation in induction chemotherapy group
- Pattern of recurrence differed between the two groups with the nonsurgical group having more locoregional recurrence and surgical group have more incidence of distal disease
- Patients with T4 cancers were more likely to need salvage laryngectomy
- Patients with fixed vocal folds and gross cartilage invasion also did worse with nonsurgical treatment
  - ○ RTOG 91-11 study (2003)
    - Compared nonsurgical treatments with induction chemotherapy (cisplatin/5-FU) with radiation, concurrent chemoradiation (cisplatin), and radiation alone
    - Included patients with stage III or IV disease (T2, T3, and low-volume T4)
    - Comparable incidence of toxic effects namely mucositis, nausea/vomiting, neutropenia with induction chemotherapy followed by radiation and concurrent chemoradiation
    - Laryngectomy-free survival and locoregional control better in concurrent chemoradiation group: 88% at 2 years
    - Study often criticized for not having surgical arm
  - ○ 10-year follow-up study
    - Concurrent group had improved locoregional control and laryngeal preservation compared with induction and radiotherapy alone groups
    - Laryngectomy-free survival improved in both induction and concurrent group (both superior to radiotherapy alone group)
- (h) Laryngeal preservation surgery
  - ○ Supracricoid laryngectomy can be considered in select T2-T4 patients
  - ○ Defect reconstructed with cricohyoidopexy (CHP) or cricohyoidoepiglottopexy (CHEP) if epiglottis is spared
  - ○ *Indications*: good pulmonary function, limited thyroid cartilage or epiglottic involvement
  - ○ *Contraindications*: involvement of both arytenoid joints, infraglottic extension to cricoid cartilage, invasion of hyoid bone or posterior arytenoid mucosa
- (i) Primary treatment strategy for patients with advanced laryngeal cancer who are not candidates for laryngeal preservation surgery is chemoradiation with cisplatin
  - ○ Applies to most patients with T3 laryngeal cancer
  - ○ Success of chemoradiation treatment depends on adherence to protocol as efficacy of radiation dramatically decreases with treatment breaks
- (j) Total laryngectomy with adjuvant radiation recommended for most patients with T4 disease, cartilage invasion, or inability to tolerate chemoradiation
- (k) Management of neck
  - ○ Elective treatment of neck in clinical N0
    - Glottic T3
    - T4 lesions
    - Especially with transglottic involvement
    - Radiation or neck dissection with levels II to IV and VI
  - ○ Clinical neck disease
    - Comprehensive neck dissection or definitive radiation is recommended regardless of site or T stage

- Planned neck dissection not necessary if complete response to chemoradiation (risk of isolated neck recurrence 0%-11%)
- Postoperative adjuvant therapy
  - (a) Postoperative concurrent chemoradiation
    - Radiation Therapy Oncology Group (RTOG) and EORTC studies in 2004
    - High-risk patients with all sites of head and neck SCCA
      - Defined as positive margins, extracapsular extension, perineural disease in EORTC study
      - Defined as positive margins, two or more positive lymph nodes, extracapsular extension in RTOG trial
      - Both studies showed improved locoregional control with significantly higher toxicities
      - EORTC showed survival benefit
  - (b) Subglottic laryngeal cancer
    - Usually presents at advanced stage
    - Treatment of choice is total laryngectomy with adjuvant therapy
    - Paratracheal lymph nodes need to be treated due to risk of peristomal recurrence (radiation and surgical resection)
  - (c) Voice rehabilitation after total laryngectomy
    - Tracheoesophageal prosthesis most reliable technique
    - Esophageal speech
      - Difficult to learn
      - Requires trapping, swallowing, and expulsion of air to create voice via vibration of pharyngoesophageal mucosa
    - Electrolarynx
      - Considered too mechanical by many patients
- Major complications of treatment
  - (a) Surgery
    - *Pharyngocutaneous fistula*
      - Increased incidence if history of radiation therapy
      - Treatment: local wound care, debridement, possible flap closure
    - *Stomal stenosis*
      - May be secondary to stomal recurrence
      - May require patient to wear appliance such as laryngectomy tube
    - Dysphagia secondary to pharyngeal stenosis
  - (b) Chemoradiation
    - *Esophageal stenosis*: usually secondary to scarring or high-intensity radiotherapy
    - *Nonfunctional larynx*
      - Can result from severe local side effects after chemoradiation
      - May require tracheotomy, g-tube, or total laryngectomy
    - *Chondritis*: increased risk with biopsy post-chemoradiation treatment
- Follow-Up
  - (a) National Comprehensive Cancer Network (NCCN) recommendations
    - First year after treatment: 1 to 3 months
    - Second year after treatment: 2 to 4 months
    - Third through fifth year after treatment: 4 to 6 months
    - Every 6 to 12 months thereafter

- (b) Important to detect recurrences and second primary tumors
- (c) Thyroid function test every 6 to 12 months (20%-65% incidence of hypothyroidism depending on treatment modality)
- Treatment of recurrent or metastatic SCCA
  - (a) Recurrences can be salvaged approximately 50% of the time.
  - (b) Signs of local recurrence:
    - ○ Increased edema or impairment of vocal fold mobility
    - ○ Mass lesion
    - ○ Ulceration
  - (c) Symptoms include increased pain, worsening dysphonia, worsening dysphagia.
  - (d) Positron emission tomography (PET)/CT helpful in assessing tumor response following treatment and in differentiating between scar and fibrosis from residual tumor.
    - ○ Recommend timing after therapy is 10 to 12 weeks
    - ○ Associated with higher false-positive rate if performed sooner after treatment
  - (e) Most suspected recurrences require biopsy confirmation.
  - (f) Treatment modalities for recurrence:
    - ○ Surgery
      - – Based on site and size of recurrence
      - – May require partial or total laryngectomy
      - – Neck dissection for clinically N0 neck has no survival advantage but may show improvement in locoregional control
    - ○ Reirradiation with or without concurrent chemotherapy limited by greater risk of side effects
    - ○ Cetuximab
      - – Monoclonal antibody against epidermal growth factor receptor (EGFR) which is overexpressed in cancer cells
      - – FDA approved for monotherapy in recurrent or metastatic head and neck cancer
      - – May be used in platinum refractory treatment and concomitantly for locoregionally advanced disease without metastases
      - – May prolong life and improve locoregional control
    - ○ Palliative care if cancer is incurable

Variants of Laryngeal Squamous Cell Carcinoma

- Verrucous carcinoma:
  - (a) 1% to 2% of laryngeal cancers.
  - (b) Characterized by exophytic growth of well-differentiated keratinizing epithelium.
  - (c) On histology, margins of tumor are pushing rather than infiltrative.
  - (d) Does not metastasize unless it has foci of conventional SCCA.
  - (e) Treatment is wide local surgical excision unless patient is poor candidate.
  - (f) No need for nodal dissection.
  - (g) Radiation therapy generally not required.
- Additional variants of squamous cell carcinoma in the larynx have been reported.
  - (a) Poorly characterized mainly in case series.
  - (b) Treatment largely unchanged.
  - (c) Includes spindle cell carcinoma.

- Nonsquamous cell malignancies of the larynx include adenocarcinoma, adenoid cystic carcinoma, neuroendocrine tumors, mucoepidermoid carcinoma, sarcomas (including chondrosarcoma), and rare metastatic lesions.

Practical Clinical Guidelines

- Early laryngeal cancer may be treated with surgical interventions such as endoscopic CO_2 laser resection or primary radiation therapy.
- Advanced laryngeal cancer may require multi-modality therapy including surgical interventions such as partial or total laryngectomy as well adjuvant therapy such as postoperative chemoradiation.
- Initial evaluation includes identification of primary subsite of lesion and clinical evidence of cervical nodal metastasis.
- Imaging should evaluate for distant metastases and is invaluable in determining tumor extent, invasion into critical structures, and feasibility of organ preservation surgical procedures.
- Endoscopy with biopsy should be considered for aid in tumor mapping, tissue diagnosis, and staging.

Bibliography

Armstrong WB, Volkes DE, Maisel RH. Malignant tumors of the larynx. In: Flint PW, Haughey BH, Lund VJ, et al, eds. *Cummings Otolaryngology Head and Neck Surgery.* 5th ed. St. Louis, MO: Mosby Elsevier; 2010:1482-1511.

Hartl DM. Evidence-based practice: management of glottic cancer. *Otolaryngol Clin North Am.* 2012;45(5):1143-1161.

Jenckel F, Knecht R. State of the art in the treatment of laryngeal cancer. *Anticancer Res.* 2013;33(11):4701-4710.

National Comprehensive Cancer Network. Clinical Practice Guidelines in Oncology. *Head Neck Cancers.* Version 1.2014.

Sinha P, Okuyemi O, Haughey BH. Early laryngeal cancer. Loehn BC, Kunduk M, McWhorter AJ. Advanced laryngeal cancer. In: Johnson JT, Rosen CA, eds. *Bailey's Head and Neck Surgery – Otolaryngology.* 5th ed. Baltimore, MD: Lippincott Williams & Wilkins; 2014:1940-1977.

Questions

1. A 55-year-old patient presents with history of hoarseness for 6 months and on examination is found to have an ulcerative lesion extending from the right true vocal fold across the anterior commissure to the left vocal fold. He is recommended to obtain a CT scan to assess possible spread of disease to the thyroid cartilage. What structure facilitates this process?

   A. Conus elasticus

   B. Quadrangular membrane

   C. Broyle ligament

   D. Ventricle

   E. Vocal ligament

2. A 78-year-old man presents with history of laryngeal cancer limited to the true vocal folds. He has had multiple prior resections endoscopically with his last one being about 5 years ago. He reports recently starting smoking again after undergoing a cervical spine fusion procedure. On examination, he has a suspicious lesion at the anterior commissure, which was biopsied and noted to be CIS. He is very interested in preserving his voice. What is the best treatment?

   A. Observation and vocal cord stripping if he has progression

   B. Radiation

   C. Endoscopic surgery

   D. Total laryngectomy

   E. Laryngofissure with excision of lesion and keel placement

3. A 45-year-old man presents with 5-month history of worsening odynophagia and otalgia. He is noted on physical examination to have an ulcerated mass over the lingual epiglottis extending to the false vocal fold on the right. He is also noted to have some decreased mobility of his right vocal fold. He is noted to have bilateral enlarged lymph nodes with largest being 2.5 cm in size. What is the clinical stage for this patient?

   A. T3N2c

   B. T3N1

   C. T2N1

   D. T3N2b

   E. T2N2c

4. A 67-year-old man presents with odynophagia and otalgia for 4 months. He is noted to have a 2-cm exophytic, ulcerating mass on the right false vocal fold. He has no evidence of enlarged lymph nodes on CT scan and on biopsy is reported to have verrucous carcinoma. What is the best treatment?

   A. Observation

   B. Radiation

   C. Supraglottic laryngectomy with bilateral neck dissection

   D. Total laryngectomy

   E. Wide local excision

5. A 27-year-old man presents with history of hoarseness and a whitish lesion that was biopsied and noted to be severe dysplasia. What is the rate of malignant transformation?

   A. 10%

   B. 20%

   C. 40%

   D. 50%

   E. 60%

Chapter 39
Carcinoma of the Oral Cavity, Pharynx, and Esophagus

According to the World Cancer Research Fund International, in 2012 there were 529,000 cases of cancer of the oral cavity and pharynx accounting for 3.7% of all cancers and 456,000 cases of cancer of the esophagus accounting for 3.7% of all cancers. The American Cancer Society estimates that in 2014 there will be 42,440 cases of cancer of the oral cavity and pharynx with 8390 deaths and 18,170 cases of esophageal cancer with 15,450 deaths in the United States. These cancers are at least 2.5 times more common in men than in women.

- Ninety percent of malignant neoplasms arising within the oral cavity and pharynx are squamous cell carcinomas (SCCAs).
- Variants arising from minor salivary glands distributed throughout the oral cavity are the second most common.

Etiology

- Tobacco is the major risk factor for head and neck cancer. The combined use of tobacco and alcohol has a multiplicative rather than an additive effect resulting in a 15-fold increased risk for developing these cancers.
- Human papilloma virus particularly for oropharyngeal carcinoma.
- Epstein-Barr virus (EBV) in the development of nasopharyngeal carcinoma.
- Gastroesophageal reflux disease has been implicated in the development of hypopharyngeal esophageal carcinomas.
- Genetic: (uncommon) Li-Fraumeni syndrome and Fanconi anemia.

Anatomy

Traditionally, the oral cavity and pharynx have been grouped together for epidemiologic study and ease of categorization. However, the carcinomas of the oral cavity and pharynx differ greatly in anatomic, biologic, and pathologic features. Furthermore, the pharynx is subdivided into three distinct regions: the oropharynx, hypopharynx, and nasopharynx (Figure 39-1).

Oral Cavity

The oral cavity extends from the cutaneous-vermilion junction of the lips to the anterior tonsillar pillars. The posterior border of the oral cavity also includes the circumvallate papillae inferiorly and the junction of the hard and soft palate superiorly.

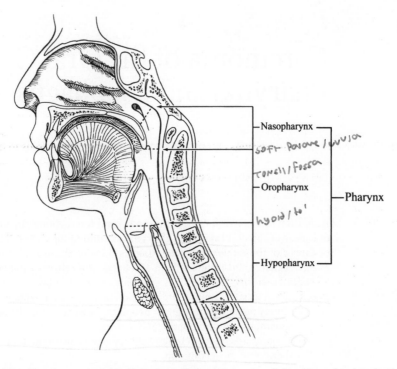

Figure 39-1 The pharynx is divided into three distinct anatomic subsites. The soft palate, hyoid bone, and cricoid cartilage serve to demarcate each region.

Subsites within the oral cavity include
- Lips
- Oral tongue, anterior two-thirds
- Floor of mouth
- Buccal mucosa
- Gingiva (alveolar ridge), upper and lower
- Retromolar trigone (RMT)
- Hard palate

Oropharynx

The oropharynx begins at the anterior tonsillar pillars and extends posteriorly to include the soft palate, tonsillar fossa, posterior pharyngeal wall, and base of tongue. The oropharynx extends vertically from the inferior surface of the soft palate at the junction with the hard palate superiorly to the plane of the superior surface of the hyoid bone. The oropharynx is divided into four anatomic subsites:
- A. Base of tongue
- B. Soft palate and uvula
- C. Tonsil/tonsillar fossa
- D. Pharyngeal wall (lateral and posterior)

Hypopharynx

The hypopharynx begins superiorly at the superior border of the hyoid and extends inferiorly to the lower border of the cricoid cartilage. It includes three subsites:

    A. Pyriform sinuses (or fossa), left and right
    B. Posterior hypopharyngeal wall
    C. Postcricoid region

The postcricoid area extends from the arytenoid cartilages to the inferior aspect of the cricoid and connects the two pyriform sinuses, thus forming the anterior wall of the hypopharynx. Each pyriform sinus extends from the pharyngoepiglottic folds to the upper end of the cervical esophagus and is bounded laterally by the thyroid cartilage and medially by the surface of the aryepiglottic fold and the arytenoid and cricoid cartilages.

Nasopharynx

The nasopharynx is the superior portion of the pharynx between the choanae of the nasal cavity and free edge of the soft palate inferiorly. The nasopharynx is divided into three subsites:

    A. Lateral walls (including the fossa of Rosenmüller and eustachian tube orifice)
    B. Vault or roof
    C. Posterior wall

TNM Staging

The tumor (T), lymph node (N), metastasis (M) or TNM system is a clinical staging schema based on the extent of disease as determined by physical examination and imaging prior to initial treatment. TNM staging provides a useful estimation of prognosis, aids in treatment selection, and permits the assessment of treatment outcomes. The American Joint Committee for Cancer (AJCC) coordinates and periodically updates the criteria for assessment and staging.

TNM Staging for Oral Cavity, Oropharynx, Hypopharynx
Primary Tumor (T)

- Tx: primary tumor cannot be assessed.
- T0: no evidence of primary tumor.
- Tis: carcinoma in situ.
- T1: tumor < 2 cm in greatest dimension.
- T2: tumor > 2 but not > 4 cm in greatest dimension.
- T3: tumor > 4 cm in greatest dimension.
- T3 (hypopharynx) tumor > 4 cm or with fixation of the larynx.
- T4 (lip): tumor invades adjacent structures (eg, through cortical bone, inferior alveolar nerve, floor of mouth, skin of face).
- T4 (oral cavity): tumor invades adjacent structures (eg, through cortical bone, into deep (extrinsic) muscles of tongue, maxillary sinus, skin. Superficial erosion alone of bone/tooth socket by gingival primary is not sufficient to classify as T4.

◻ T4 (oropharynx): tumor invades adjacent structures (eg, pterygoid muscles, mandible, hard palate, deep muscle of tongue, larynx).

◻ T4 (hypopharynx): tumor invades adjacent structures (eg, thyroid/cricoid cartilage, carotid artery, soft tissues of neck, prevertebral fascia/muscles, thyroid and/or esophagus).

Regional Lymph Nodes (N) for Oral Cavity, Oropharynx, and Hypopharynx

- Nx: regional lymph nodes cannot be assessed.
- N0: no regional lymph node metastasis.
- N1: metastasis in a single ipsilateral node measuring < 3 cm.
- N2a: metastasis in a single ipsilateral node, < 3 cm but not > 6 cm in greatest dimension.
- N2b: metastasis in multiple ipsilateral nodes, none > 6 cm in greatest dimension.
- N2c: metastases in bilateral or contralateral nodes, none > 6 cm in greatest dimension.
- N3: metastasis in a node > 6 cm in greatest dimension.

Distant Metastasis (M) for Oral Cavity, Oropharynx, Hypopharynx

- Mx: distant metastasis cannot be assessed.
- M0: no distant metastasis.
- M1: distant metastasis.

TNM Staging for Nasopharynx

Primary Tumor (T)

- Tx: primary tumor cannot be assessed.
- T0: no evidence of primary tumor.
- Tis: carcinoma in situ.
- T1: tumor confined to the nasopharynx.
- T2: tumor extends to soft tissues of the oropharynx and/or nasal fossa:
  - (a) T2a: without parapharyngeal extension
  - (b) T2b: with parapharyngeal extension
- T3: tumor invades bony structures and/or paranasal sinuses.
- T4: tumor with intracranial extension and/or involvement of cranial nerves, infratemporal fossa, hypopharynx or orbit.

Regional Lymph Nodes (N)

- Nx: regional lymph nodes cannot be assessed.
- N0: no regional lymph nodes metastasis.
- N1: unilateral lymph node metastasis < 6 cm in greatest dimension above the supraclavicular fossa.
- N2: bilateral metastasis in lymph nodes < 6 cm in greatest dimension above the supraclavicular fossa.
- N3a: metastasis in a lymph node > 6 cm in dimension.
- N3b: metastasis in a lymph node with extension to the supraclavicular fossa.

Distant Metastasis (M) for Nasopharynx

- Mx: distant metastasis cannot be assessed.
- M0: no distant metastasis.
- M1: distant metastasis.

See Figure 39.2.

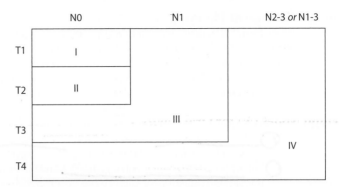

Figure 39-2 TNM staging for the oral cavity, oropharynx, and nasopharynx. Roman numerals indicate stage.

Evaluation and Treatment of Carcinoma of the Oral Cavity and Pharynx: General Considerations

Signs and Symptoms

- Early signs and symptoms may include a nodule, or ulcerative lesion of the lip or mucosa, odynophagia, dysphagia, otalgia, eustachian tube dysfunction or hoarseness lasting more than 2 weeks duration.
- Lymphadenopathy, cranial nerve dysfunction, nasal obstruction, severe dysphagia, unintentional weight loss, hemoptysis, and respiratory distress are observed in more advanced disease.

Diagnostic Studies

- The diagnosis is confirmed by histologic evaluation of a tissue biopsy from the primary site and/or cytologic evaluation of a fine-needle aspirate from an enlarged lymph node.

Imaging Studies

- A computed tomography (CT) scan or magnetic resonance imaging (MRI) with contrast of the soft tissue of the neck provides important clinical staging information about the size and location of the primary tumor and involvement of surrounding anatomical structures as well as lymph node involvement.
- For most patients, CT is adequate and more cost effective. MRI is preferred with nasopharyngeal, sinonasal, and skull base tumors.
- A chest x-ray or chest CT scan is important screening tests for the presence of distant metastases or a primary lung cancer.
- Panorex or dental x-rays should be considered if the patient might require radiation therapy.
- PET18-fluorodeoxyglucose positron emission tomography (FDG-PET) provides a sensitive whole body survey for sites of metabolically active tissue such as tumor and distinguishes it from normal tissues. It is helpful in delineating regional nodal and distant metastases. This should be done for patients who have a high risk for metastases (eg, stage III-IV disease)
- Some authors recommend FGD-PET for assessing response to treatment. This is best done 3 to 4 months after the end of radiation for 97% to 100% accuracy in predictive value.

Multidisciplinary Treatment Planning

Optimal care of patients with oral and pharyngeal cancer occurs within a multidisciplinary, collaborative setting between experts in the fields of head and neck surgery, radiation and medical oncology, radiology, and pathology. The management of aesthetic and functional outcomes requires close coordination of reconstructive surgeons, speech pathologists, dentists, oral surgeons, physical therapists, and maxillofacial prosthodontists.

General Principles of Treatment

- Early-stage (stage I-II) carcinoma of the oral cavity and pharynx (excluding nasopharynx) can be treated with radiation therapy or surgery.
- For advanced-stage tumors (stage III-IV), treatment with a combination of chemotherapy and radiation, or surgery and postoperative radiation results in improved rates of locoregional control and overall survival compared to single modality therapy.
- Radiation therapy with or without chemotherapy is the standard treatment for nasopharyngeal carcinoma.
- Traditionally, surgery with postoperative radiation has been the mainstay of therapy for advanced-stage SCCA of the head and neck.
- The development of trans-oral robotic surgery has allowed improved access and visibility to expand the indications for surgical removal of small and intermediate volume cancers arising from the posterior oral cavity, oropharynx, larynx and hypopharynx.
- Chemotherapy and radiation for both definitive therapy and organ preservation has gained popularity as well. This is particularly true for advanced-stage carcinomas of the oropharynx and hypopharynx where preservation of organ function is critical for speech and swallowing.
- Several clinical trials have demonstrated the effectiveness of combined chemoradiation regimens in achieving excellent locoregional control, disease-free survival, and reduction in the rate of distant metastases.
- Induction chemotherapy with cisplatin and fluorouracil alone or in combination with docetaxel in locally advanced SCCA of the head and neck has been investigated: long-term results of the TAX 324 randomized phase 3 trial. However, there is no evidence that this induction approach provides better survival compared to concomitant chemoradiation.
- Postoperative, combined chemoradiotherapy has been shown to result in improved locoregional control, disease-free survival, and improved overall survival in patients with positive resection margins from the primary tumor, extracapsular extension of tumor within one or more lymph nodes or multiple positive lymph nodes.
- The addition of chemotherapy to radiation results in significant treatment-related toxicities that may not be well tolerated in patients with poor performance status and multiple medical comorbidities.
- The use of biologic agents to block the epidermal growth factor receptor (EGFR) present on the cell surface of epidermal cancer cells also has a role. Cetuximab, a monoclonal antibody against the ligand-binding site of EGFR, has been shown to significantly improve locoregional control and survival in patients with advanced-stage disease when combined with radiation therapy.
- Intensity-modulated radiotherapy (IMRT) utilizes multiple beams of variable radiation intensity to deliver escalated dose to the tumor while decreasing doses to nearby organs at risk.
- The decision of an appropriate treatment regimen must take into consideration the extent and location of the tumor, clinical stage at diagnosis, and the overall medical condition of the patient.

Management of the N0 Neck

The incidence of occult cervical metastasis is significant for patients with oral and pharyngeal squamous cell carcinoma. While the rate depends on the primary site and its size, there is little debate that most patients are at high risk for regional failure.

Several treatment options are advocated for managing N0 neck disease:

- Expectant management.
- Elective cervical lymphadenectomy.
- Elective radiotherapy to the neck.
- With expectant management, the "wait and watch" policy may result in diminished regional control and overall survival and salvage rates for delayed regional metastasis may be lower.
- Many advocate elective neck dissection over radiation therapy in patients if the incidence of occult metastasis is greater than 15% to 20%.
- While occult metastasis can be managed with similar results, histopathologic examination of the neck dissection specimen provides important prognostic data, such as the number of lymph nodes involved and the presence of extracapsular spread (ECS). Adjuvant therapy can then be given to these high-risk patients.
- If no metastasis is present, if micrometastasis is present, or if a single node without ECS is present, the patient can be spared radiation therapy.

Second Primary Malignancy in Head and Neck Squamous Cell Carcinoma

- The incidence of second primary tumors is approximately 5% to 10%.
- A synchronous second primary tumor is found simultaneously with the initial head and neck cancer, while a metachronous tumor develops after treatment.
- Approximately 50% of second primaries arise within the head and neck, while the lung is the next most common site (20%).

Molecular Biology of Head and Neck Squamous Cell Carcinoma

- Slaughter first elucidated the concept of "field cancerization." Chronic exposure to tobacco, alcohol, or other carcinogens produces alterations of the normal squamous mucosa of the entire upper aerodigestive tract resulting in dysplastic epithelial changes from which cancers can arise.
- Phenotypic changes such as dysplasia or cancer have been correlated to changes at the molecular level.
- Genetic alterations are the result of inactivation of tumor suppressor genes (eg, p53, retinoblastoma, p16) or activation of proto-oncogenes to oncogenes (eg, RET, EGFR, RAS).
- The accumulation of several mutations ultimately results in the progression from normal mucosa to dysplasia to carcinoma.

Distant Metastasis

- Distant metastasis (DM) develops in 15% of patients with head and neck cancer.
- The incidence of distant metastases at the time of presentation is estimated to be 5% to 7%.
- There is a clear correlation between distant metastasis and the following factors: higher nodal stage, the number of lymphatic metastases, advanced T stage, and the hypopharynx as primary tumor site.
- Patients with ECS, multiple positive lymph nodes, and locoregional recurrence have a significantly higher risk for developing DM.
- Screening for the presence of distant metastasis may include plain chest x-ray, chest CT scan, or PET/CT scan depending on the presumed risk as noted above.
- For an isolated pulmonary metastasis, resection may be indicated.

Follow-up

- Most patients with head and neck cancer die as a result of local or regional failure. Therefore, after definitive treatment, regular follow-up examinations are important. When recurrence is identified early, salvage therapy may be effective.
- Recurrences usually present in the first 2 years after treatment, so a head and neck examination should be performed every 4 to 6 weeks during the first year and every 3 months during the second year.
- During years 3 to 5 follow-up should continue at 4- to 6-month intervals.
- Because the incidence of developing a second primary cancer remains constant at about 4% to 5% per year, routine tumor surveillance visits should be performed every 6 to 12 months for life.
- If the patient should become symptomatic at any time between visits, the surgeon should perform a thorough examination and order any ancillary tests and procedures that might be necessary.
- Pain is a sensitive indicator for tumor recurrence and should serve as a "warning sign" for the head and neck oncologist.

Carcinoma of the Oral Cavity

Carcinoma of the Lip

- Most common site for cancer of the oral cavity with incidence 1.8 per 100,000.
- Greater than 95% SCCA. Remainder are minor salivary gland carcinomas or basal cell carcinomas (BCCs).
- 95% lower lip, 5% upper lip.
- BCC is more common on the upper lip than lower lip, but SCCA is still the most common cancer of the upper lip.
- Age at time of diagnosis: 50% patients between 50 and 69 years.
- Male predilection: 20:1-35:1 for lower lip, but 5:1 for upper lip.
- Risk factors: sunlight exposure, lack of pigmented layer, tobacco smoking.
- Diagnosed early because of prominent location.
- Symptoms of lip cancer:
  Early: blistering, crusting, ulceration, or leukoplakia
  Late: mandibular invasion, involvement of mental nerve
- Regional metastasis occurs in approximately 10% of patients, usually later in the course of disease as compared to other oral cavity sites.
- Lymphatic drainage is primarily to submental, submandibular nodes.
- Bilateral metastasis is a concern for lesions near the midline.

Treatment of Lip Cancer

- Goals of treatment in order of importance. (1) Complete eradication of tumor (2) Maintain or restore oral competence (3) Achieve acceptable cosmesis
- Small (T1, T2) lesions treated with either radiation or surgery only.
- Large (T3, T4) lesions usually require combined modality therapy.
- Neck dissection performed for clinically apparent lymphadenopathy.
- Extent of resection determines reconstruction.
- Proper alignment of vermilion border is critical with closure in four layers.
- Reconstruction (lower lip) is based on the size of the defect.
- Less than one-fourth to one-third: primary closure, facilitated by V-shaped excision.
- One-fourth to one-half: bilateral advancement flaps or "lip-switch" flaps: Abbe, when close to oral commissure; Estlander, when involving the oral commissure.

- One-half to two-thirds: Karapandzic flap.
- Two-thirds to total: local flap reconstruction (Bernard-Burrow or Gillies fan flap) or free tissue transfer.
- Postoperative radiation therapy is indicated in high-risk patients with locally advanced disease (T3-T4), perineural invasion at the primary site, positive margins, multiple lymphatic metastases or extracapsular spread (ECS).
- Primary radiation is an option for patients unsuitable for or unwilling to undergo resection.
- Local and regional control greater than 90% in patients without cervical lymph node involvement.
- Carcinoma of the upper lip or oral commissure has 10% to 20% lower survival.
- 5-year rates of survival. Overall: 91%
  (a) Stage I-II greater than 90% with surgery or radiation
  (b) Stage III-IV 30% to 70%
- Recurrent disease, mandibular invasion, and lymph node involvement result carry a poor prognosis.

Carcinoma of the Oral Tongue

- Includes the mobile portion of the tongue anterior to the circumvallate papillae.
- Second most common tumor of the oral cavity (30%).
- Most often arises along the lateral borders of the tongue.
- Risk factors: tobacco, alcohol, immunosuppression, and possibly poor oral hygiene.
- Depth of tumor invasion greater than 2-4 mm correlated with higher rates of regional metastasis, recurrence, and mortality.
- Perineural invasion at the primary site is another indicator of recurrence and increased mortality.
- The incidence of SCCA of the tongue in young patients has increased in the United States, from 4% in 1971 to 18% in 1993. In this young population, no clinical features or risk factors (age, substance abuse) have been clearly identified and an increased genetic susceptibility to carcinogenesis has been postulated.
- Thorough oral cavity examination by dentists, oral surgeons, otolaryngologists, and primary care physicians especially in patients with risk factors is critical for early detection.
- Erythroplakia (red, inflammatory lesion) is the most common presentation of early SCCA.
- Late symptoms include tongue fixation, decreased tongue sensation, alteration in speech and swallowing, and cervical lymphadenopathy.
- Screening methods include vital staining, spectral analysis, ViziLite (chemiluminescence), and brush biopsies.
- Most lesions are amenable to biopsy in the office for tissue diagnosis.
- Regional metastases occur with primary nodal drainage to levels I-III (Figure 39-3).
- Incidence of nodal metastases depends on size of primary tumor and depth of invasion with 25% to 33% clinically detectable and 20% to 25% occult.
- Risk of bilateral cervical lymph node metastases with midline dorsum or ventral surface of tongue.
- Treatment requires management of the primary with partial glossectomy for early T1-T2 lesions and reconstruction by primary closure, secondary intention, or skin graft.
- External beam radiation with or without brachytherapy may be used in patients with T1-T2 lesions that are not suitable for or refuse surgery.
- Near-total or total glossectomy may be necessary for extensive local disease.

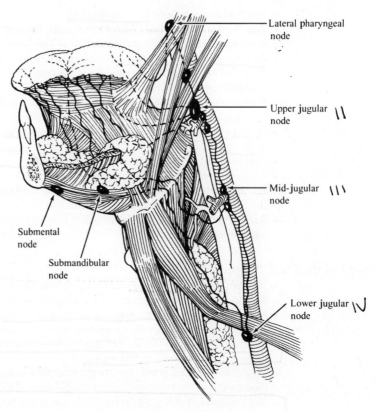

Lateral pharyngeal node

Upper jugular node \\

Mid-jugular node \\\

Submental node

Submandibular node

Lower jugular node \J

Figure 39-3 Lymphatic drainage of the oral tongue and oropharynx.

- Even with flap reconstruction, there is significant morbidity associated with deglutition and maintenance of an adequate airway. Aspiration may be a chronic problem; thus laryngectomy may be necessary.
- In select patients, total glossectomy may be possible without total laryngectomy.
- Chemoradiation may be considered for T4 tongue cancers. However, bone involvement usually requires surgical resection.

Management of Mandibular Invasion
- Tumors extending superficially to the gingiva should be resected with periosteum as the deep margin.
- Tumors involving periosteum require at least a marginal mandibulectomy which may include a horizontal cuff of alveolar ridge or sagittal resection of the inner or outer cortex.
- Patients with an edentulous mandible are more likely to require a segmental mandibulectomy because of decreased bone stock and increased risk for fracture.
- Segmental mandibulectomy is indicated for direct bone invasion.

Management of the Neck
- Upper jugular nodes (73%), submandibular nodes (18%), the middle jugular nodes (18%), and the submental nodes (9%) are the most frequent sites of metastasis for SCCA of the oral tongue.

- Elective treatment of the neck with either surgery or radiation is recommended for primary tumors with greater than 2 to 4 mm depth of invasion.
- Selective neck dissection should include at least levels I-III (supraomohyoid neck dissection).
- Bilateral neck dissections should be performed for midline dorsum or ventral tongue cancers.
- Observation may be considered for those patients with less than 2-mm depth of invasion or carcinoma in situ.
- Elective neck dissection results in better outcomes than observation.
- Survival following salvage treatment for regional metastasis is only 35% to 40%.
- Sentinel lymph node biopsy has been demonstrated to be feasible and accurate for staging the regional lymphatics in patients with T1-T2, N0 oral cavity cancers.

Treatment Outcomes
- 5-year locoregional control rates of 91%
- 5-year survival rates
  (a) Stage I, II: 60% to 75%
  (b) Stage III, IV: 25% to 40%.
- Impact of ECS on survival: 5-year disease-specific and overall survival rates for patients with pathologically negative necks (pN−) were 88% and 75%; for pN+/ECS− patients, 65% and 50%; and for pN+/ECS+ patients, 48% and 30%.

Carcinoma of the Floor of the Mouth

- Floor of the mouth (FOM) extends from the lingual aspect of the alveolar ridge to the ventral surface of the tongue.
- The mylohyoid and hyoglossus muscles provide the muscular support for the FOM.
- The orifices of the submandibular duct (Wharton duct) open in the FOM on either side of the lingual frenulum.
- FOM is the third most common site for oral cavity tumor.
- Small lesions isolated to the FOM may be relatively asymptomatic while more extensive lesions may invade the mandible or extend to the root of the tongue.
- Invasion of lingual or mental nerves results in decreased tongue mobility, alterations in speech and swallowing, and decreased sensation over the tongue, lip, or skin of the cheek.
- Tumor may track along the submandibular duct or obstruct its orifice resulting in distension of the submandibular gland.
- Cervical metastasis is most frequently seen in the submandibular (64%), upper jugular (43%), and the submental nodes (7%).
- Bilateral metastasis is not uncommon given the midline location of the tumor.

FOM SCC Treatment
- Management of the primary tumor, mandible involvement, and cervical lymphatics is similar to that described for oral tongue cancer noted earlier.

Treatment Outcomes
- Locoregional control: Recurrence at the primary site (41%) is twice as common as failure in the neck (18.5%).
- 5-year survival rates for patients with cancer of the FOM:
  (a) Stage I = 64%-80%
  (b) Stage II = 61%-84%
  (c) Stage III = 28%-68%
  (d) Stage IV = 6%-36%

Carcinoma of the Retromolar Trigone

- The RMT is a triangulated region of gingiva overlying the ascending ramus of the mandible.
- The RMT represents a watershed area, near the buccal mucosa, tonsillar fossa, glossopharyngeal sulcus, lateral floor of mouth, tongue base, soft palate, and, deeply, the masticator space.
- The true incidence of RMT carcinoma is difficult to determine since tumors often involve both the retromolar trigone and adjacent sites making it difficult to ascertain the tumor's epicenter.
- A thin layer of mucosa and underlying soft tissue overlies the mandible, and bony involvement may develop early.
- Involvement of the inferior alveolar nerve (V3) may occur early due to close proximity to the mandibular foramen.
- At presentation, regional metastases are common: 10% to 20%.
- Lymphatic drainage is predominantly to the upper jugular lymph nodes (level II).

Treatment

- For stage I or II tumors, surgery and radiation are equally effective.
- Management of early disease involving extensive superficial lesions that involve the soft palate but do not invade bone, radiotherapy may be a better treatment option, since palatal resection can result in poor speech and swallowing outcomes.
- Management of advanced-stage lesions often requires a combination of surgery and radiation.
- Marginal mandibulectomy sometimes possible if only periosteum is involved.
- The majority of advanced tumors with bony invasion require composite resection. The approach may be transcervical after raising the soft tissue flap over the bone or translabial (lip splitting incision) with a lateral mandibulotomy.
- Reconstructive options for small (< 5 cm) defects of the lateral mandible include the use of a mandibular reconstruction bar to span the bony defect and a soft tissue flap such as pectoralis major myocutaneous flap or radial forearm free flap.
- Reconstruction of larger mandibular defects greater than 5 cm usually require a composite flap such as a fibula osteocutaneous free flap.
- Obturators may be necessary if the resection involves a significant portion of the palate.
- Unilateral elective neck dissection (levels I-III) or therapeutic neck dissection should be performed in those patients with an increased risk of nodal disease.

Treatment Outcomes

- Improved locoregional control and disease-free survival with surgery and radiotherapy versus radiotherapy alone.
- 5-year locoregional control (surgery + radiotherapy)
  - (a) Stages I-III = 87%
  - (b) Stage IV = 62%
  - (c) Overall = 71% C
- 5-year cause-specific survival (surgery + radiotherapy)
  - (a) Stages I-III = 83%
  - (b) Stage IV = 61%
  - (c) Overall = 69%

Carcinoma of the Alveolar Ridge Gingival Mucosa

- 10% of all malignancies in the oral cavity.
- Most commonly arise in edentulous areas or at the free margin of the gingiva of the lower alveolar ridge.

- Approximately 40% of patients will have invasion of the mandible or maxilla at the time of diagnosis.
- Superficial bone invasion does not constitute a T4 tumor stage.
- Open tooth sockets or small defects in the edentulous mandibular ridge provide ready access for tumor invasion into bone.
- Cancers of the upper alveolar ridge may extend through bone into the nasal cavity or maxillary sinus.
- Lymphatic drainage for alveolar ridge cancers is most often to level I (submandibular and submental) and level II (upper deep jugular nodes). Regional metastases are clinically detectable in 25% to 30% while occult metastases occur in15%.
- Management of small cancers of the alveolar ridge can be resected transorally.
- Partial maxillectomy may be required for lesions of the upper alveolar ridge or mandibulectomy for those of the lower alveolar ridge is often required, since invasion of mandible or maxilla is not uncommon.
- Management of mandibular invasion requires reconstructive options similar to that described for floor of mouth cancer earlier.
- Small defects of the maxillary alveolar ridge may be closed with a local rotational flap from the palate, skin grafting, or healing by secondary intention.
- Larger defects involving the maxillary sinus can be reconstructed with an obturator or dental prosthesis, temporalis muscle flap, or free tissue transfer.
- Therapeutic, comprehensive treatment of the neck is indicated in all patients who have clinically positive neck disease.
- Early-stage primary cancers with clinically N0 necks may be observed; however, in patients with advanced T stage, radiologic or histologic evidence of mandibular invasion, and/or decreased tumor differentiation, elective treatment of the neck is recommended.
- Adjuvant radiotherapy is recommended for patients with extensive nodal disease, perineural invasion, lymphovascular invasion, or inadequate margins of resection.
- Radiation therapy as primary modality is not recommended because of the close proximity of tumor to the underlying bone unless the patient is an unsuitable operative candidate.

Treatment Outcomes
- Local and regional control: 70% to 80% with 5-year survival rates: 50% to 65%.
- The presence of mandibular cortical invasion decreases 5-year survival from 85% to 68%.
- Cervical metastases also decrease 5-year survival (86% vs 59%).

Carcinoma of the Hard Palate

- The hard palate extends from the lingual surface of the maxillary alveolar ridge to the posterior edge of the palatine bone.
- Only half of all tumors are SCCAs with minor salivary gland tumors also common.
- Necrotizing sialometaplasia is a benign mucosal inflammatory lesion that can be mistaken for malignancy in the hard palate.
- Most carcinomas manifest as a granular superficial ulceration of the hard palate with the mucoperiosteum providing a barrier to tumor spread.
- With more advanced lesions, tumor may extend through the periosteum of bone into adjacent regions of the oral cavity, such as the paranasal sinuses and floor of the nose.
- The incisive foramen anteriorly and the greater and lesser palatine foramina posteriorly serve as potential sites for tumor extension into the nasal cavity and skull base respectively.

- 10% to 25% of patients present with cervical nodal metastases.
- Lymph node basins include the retropharyngeal, upper jugular, and submandibular.
- Preoperative imaging should be performed to assess the lateral pharyngeal nodes, since these are difficult to evaluate on clinical examination.
- Careful assessment of the trigeminal nerve is crucial, and perineural invasion to the gasserian ganglion should be evaluated with MRI.
- Although radiation can be used to treat carcinomas of this site, surgery is preferred.
- Radiation is more commonly reserved for adjuvant treatment. Management of the primary by wide local excision is performed to obtain surgical margins.
- Infrastructure maxillectomy may be necessary for tumors' partially eroding bone.
- For extensive involvement of the adjacent bony and soft tissue structures, a total maxillectomy, with or without orbital exenteration, or resection of cheek skin may be required.
- Management of the neck with elective treatment of the neck is generally not performed because of the low rate of occult metastases.
- Reconstruction of small and/or superficial defects of the hard palate may be done with a local palatal flap or a regional temporalis muscle flap.
- For reconstruction of larger hard palate or infrastructure maxillectomy defects, an obturator with or without a skin graft is a common method of reconstruction.
- The obturator is fabricated from a synthetic polymer and provides oronasal separation, which can yield normal speech and swallowing function.
- Use of an obturator provides the advantage of direct visualization of the surrounding primary site for tumor surveillance.
- A disadvantage is that it may leak air or food and require multiple adjustments to maintain a proper fit.
- Composite defects may require reconstruction with free tissue transfer to reconstruct bone and soft tissue defects. The fibula, scapular or iliac crest free flaps are more commonly used.
- Radiotherapy can be selected for primary or adjuvant management of palate cancer.
- Postoperative radiotherapy is often recommended in advanced disease or in cancers with adverse pathologic features mentioned previously to decrease local and regional recurrence.

Treatment Outcomes

- Local recurrence rate are 53% while regional recurrence rate are 30%.
- 5-year survival: 44% to 75%.

Carcinoma of the Buccal Mucosa

- The buccal mucosa comprises the inner lining of the lips and cheeks.
- In the United States, less than 10% of all oral cavity cancer occurs at this site.
- A high incidence of cancer at this site in India is attributed at least in part to the prevalent practice of chewing "pan," a combination of betel nut, lime, and tobacco.
- SCCA more often arises from preexisting leukoplakia at this site compared to other locations in the oral cavity.
- Verrucous carcinoma, a more indolent variant of SCCA, has a predilection for the buccal mucosa.
- The buccinator muscle and buccal fat pad are easily invaded and provide little or no barrier to tumor spread.
- Invasion of the mandible, hard palate, maxillary sinus, cheek skin, or pterygoid muscles may occur with advanced disease.

- Tumor thickness (> 6 mm) correlates with increased morbidity and mortality.
- Regional metastases are most common in the buccinator, submental, and submandibular lymph nodes.
- While management of the primary with radiation alone can be used for early stage cancers, surgical resection is the preferred method of treatment for the primary tumor.
- Small, early stage lesions can be resected transorally while more extensive lesions may require marginal or segmental mandibulectomy, resection of cheek skin, or partial palatal resection.
- Management of the N0 neck with elective supraomohyoid neck dissection is recommended most often though external beam radiation may be used.
- Reconstructive options for early-stage lesions may be by secondary intention or closure with skin grafts or mucosal advancement flaps.
- A regional flap (eg, pectoralis major, temporalis muscle) or free tissue transfer (eg, radial forearm, fibula, scapula) may be necessary for more extensive defects.
- The use of adjuvant therapy in the form or radiation or chemoradiation is recommended for those patients with advanced stage and/or adverse pathologic features mentioned earlier.

Treatment Outcomes

- Locoregional recurrence ranges from 43% to 80%.
- 5-year survival
  - (a) Stage I = 78%
  - (b) Stage II = 66%
  - (c) Stage III = 62%
  - (d) Stage IV = 50%

Carcinoma of the Oropharynx

- The subsites of the oropharynx include the palatine tonsils and tonsillar pillars, base of tongue, soft palate, and posterior pharyngeal wall.
- Squamous cell carcinoma accounts for approximately 90% of all carcinomas of the oropharynx.
- Lymphoid tissue is abundantly present in the oropharynx as part of Waldeyer ring. Therefore, the next most common malignancy encountered is lymphoma, primarily of the palatine tonsils and base of the tongue.
- In addition to these tissues, minor salivary glands are present in the oropharynx and can undergo malignant transformation resulting in various forms of salivary gland carcinoma (eg, adenoid cystic carcinoma, mucoepidermoid carcinoma).
- The incidence of a second primary tumor is significant.
- Chronic tobacco and alcohol use are the major etiologic factors.
- More recent studies have shown a relationship between human papillomavirus, especially subtype 16 (HPV-16), and oropharyngeal carcinoma arising in patients without other risk factors.
- Approximately 60% of cancers of the tonsil and tongue base are HPV-16 positive.
- HPV positive cancers are on the rise primarily in Caucasian males with a history of multiple sexual partners.
- Cancers arising within the oropharynx can become quite large before the patient becomes symptomatic. Therefore, these tumors tend to present at an advanced stage.
- A careful assessment of larynx and nasopharynx is needed to assess for local tumor extension to these sites.

- Cervical lymph node metastasis is present in greater than 50% of all patients and is often the initial presenting sign.
- Lymph nodes along the jugular chain are most commonly involved (levels II-IV).
- The retropharyngeal nodes are potential sites of lymph node metastasis and must be taken into consideration during treatment planning.
- It may be difficult to distinguish between direct spread into the neck from the primary tumor and extensive nodal involvement with extracapsular extension.
- Metastatic cervical lymph nodes from oropharyngeal sites may present as cystic in nature and can be mistaken for branchial anomalies.
- Early-stage cancers of the oropharynx are effectively treated with surgery or radiation as single modality therapy.
- Hyperfractionation delivery of external beam radiation therapy (XRT) and concurrent "boost" radiotherapy may improve local and regional control. If surgery is the preferred method of treatment, transoral robotic surgery is used in many centers.
- Treatment of advanced-stage oropharyngeal carcinoma has undergone a paradigm shift over the past 10 to 15 years. Traditionally, surgery with pre- or postoperative radiation therapy has been the standard for treatment for advanced-stage carcinoma of the oropharynx. However, organ preservation strategies with combinations of chemotherapy and radiation have proven efficacious and are now commonly used for treatment of oropharyngeal cancer.

Carcinoma of the Soft Palate

- Comprises less than 2% of all mucosal head and neck cancers.
- Occurs most frequently on the oral surface of the soft palate. Therefore, these tumors are readily visible and symptomatic earlier than other oropharyngeal sites.
- Increased incidence of additional primary tumors with second primary tumor ~ 13% and metachronous tumor ~ 26%.
- Cancer may appear as an area of leukoplakia, erythroplakia, or raised lesion.
- Extension of primary tumor to tonsil, tonsillar pillars, nasopharynx, or hard palate.
- Cervical metastasis is clinically present in up to 50% of patients.
- For the soft palate, tumor thickness (> 3 mm) has correlated with regional metastasis and survival.
- For even small midline lesions of the soft palate, the propensity for regional metastasis is great (> 40%).
- The rate of bilateral cervical metastases ranges from 5% to 15%.
- Lymphatic drainage is to the upper jugular nodes (level II).
- Small primary tumors can be treated surgically by a transoral approach or by radiation therapy.
- Recently, the use of robotic devices has been advocated to aid the transoral surgical approach.
- Larger primary tumors are more commonly treated with radiation or chemoradiation in an attempt at tissue preservation to prevent velopharyngeal insufficiency.
- Because of the increased risk for bilateral cervical lymph node metastases, treatment of both necks with neck dissection and/or external beam radiation should be performed depending on tumor staging.
- Reconstruction of the soft palate is difficult from a functional standpoint.
- No reconstruction or reconstruction with local flaps can be done for small defects.
- Larger defects are best reconstructed by free tissue transfer with thin, pliable soft tissue such as a radial forearm flap.

Treatment Outcomes

- Locoregional control for
  - (a) Stage I-II = 75%-90%
  - (b) Stage III = 75%
  - (c) Stage IV = 35%
- 5-year overall survival:
  - (a) Stage I-II = 70%-80%
  - (b) Stage III = 64%
  - (c) Stage IV = 20%-40%

Carcinoma of the Tonsil and Tonsillar Pillars

- Most common site for carcinoma of the oropharynx
- Asymptomatic during early stages while later symptoms include dysphagia, odynophagia, otalgia, neck mass, and/or trismus.
- Invasion of adjacent structures is common including soft palate, retromolar trigone, tongue base, mandible, and pterygoid muscles.
- Clinically positive lymphadenopathy ranges from 66% to 76%.
- Lymphatic drainage is primarily to levels II-IV and the retropharyngeal lymph nodes.
- Rate of contralateral lymph node metastases reportedly as high as 22%.
- Radiation or combined chemoradiation is generally the treatment modality of choice.
- Surgical resection is useful for salvage or for patients with extensive bony invasion.
- Exposure of the tumor is the main challenge to surgical resection. Access to the tonsil and lateral oropharynx is facilitated with use of robotics leading to increased use of transoral excision for early stage cancers. Treatment of the neck with concurrent or staged neck dissection is done.
- Resection of more advanced disease requires anterior mandibulotomy with mandibular swing. These approaches are useful for tonsil and tongue base cancers without bony invasion.
- Composite resection, the en bloc resection of posterior mandible and primary tumor is utilized for large tumors involving multiple subsites with mandibular invasion.
- Neck dissection may be performed before radiation or chemoradiation in patients with N1-N3 disease.
- Neck dissection may be performed post-treatment for patients with N2 or greater disease and/or clinically detectable residual disease.
- Some controversy exists over the need for neck dissection in patients with N1 disease following treatment with radiation or chemoradiation assuming no clinically detectable disease remains.
- Reconstructive options for small defects include primary closure or healing by secondary intention.
- Regional pedicled flaps provide excellent soft tissue bulk and adequate skin for closure of large mucosal defects involving the lateral oropharynx and tongue base.
- The pectoralis major remains as one of the workhorse flaps for oropharyngeal reconstruction.
- Other pedicled flaps include latissimus dorsi and trapezius muscle.
- Free tissue transfer with radial forearm or anterolateral thigh flap is useful for larger soft tissue defects of the lateral oropharynx and tongue base.
- Composite defects may be reconstructed with fibula or scapular osteocutaneous flaps.

Treatment Outcomes

- Locoregional control:
  - (a) Stage I-II = 75%-90%

   (b) Stage III = 50%
   (c) Stage IV = 20%
- 5-year overall survival:
   (a) Stage I-II = 80%
   (b) Stage III = 50%
   (c) Stage IV = 20%-50%

Carcinoma of the Base of Tongue

- Anatomically, it is the region of the tongue posterior to the circumvallate papillae including the vallecula.
- Less common than carcinoma of the oral tongue.
- More aggressive than cancer of the oral tongue.
- Lingual tonsil tissue at base of tongue may give rise to lymphoma in addition to squamous cell carcinoma.
- The most common presenting signs are referred otalgia and odynophagia.
- Visualization of the tongue base is difficult making early detection difficult.
- Palpation of the tongue base is an important part of the evaluation for accurate diagnosis and to assess the extent of tumor.
- Tumor may invade the adjacent structures of the larynx, tonsil, soft palate, and hypopharynx.
- The rate of lymphatic metastases is high regardless of T stage with more than 60% of patients having clinically detectable cervical lymph node metastases at the time of presentation.
- The rate of bilateral cervical metastases approaches 20% due to extensive and bilateral lymphatic drainage of the tongue base.
- Neck zones II-IV are the most common site for lymph node metastases.
- Management of tongue base cancer is similar to other cancers of the oropharynx. It is treated primarily with radiation therapy or chemoradiation.
- In general, surgery is used for small primary tumors or for salvage following radiation or chemoradiation.
- There are several surgical approaches to the tongue base depending on the size and location of the primary cancer.
- Mandibular swing or composite resection as discussed in the section on "Carcinoma of the tonsil and tonsillar pillar."
- Median mandibuloglossotomy involves division of the mandible at the symphysis and the tongue along the medial raphe to access small tumors isolated to the mid-portion of the tongue base. Lateral exposure is limited.
- Suprahyoid pharyngotomy approaches the tongue base through a neck incision by entering the pharynx immediately above the hyoid bone. This is useful for smaller neoplasms of the tongue base without extension to other sites.
- "Blind entry" into the pharynx risks the possibility of entering into tumor.
- Transoral laser resection may be performed for small, superficial lesions in selected patients.
- Laryngectomy may be necessary to prevent chronic aspiration in patients undergoing total glossectomy.
- Options for reconstruction of the tongue base are similar to other sites in the oropharynx noted above. For total glossectomy defects, a flap with significant bulk is useful such as pedicled pectoralis major or anterolateral thigh free flap.

Treatment Outcomes

- Locoregional control:
  - (a) Stage I-II = 75%-90%
  - (b) Stage III = 50%
  - (c) Stage IV = 20%
- 5-year overall survival:
  - (a) Stage I-II = 85%
  - (b) Stage III-IV = 20%-50%
- The incidence of distant metastases in oropharyngeal cancer is approximately 15% to 20%.
- Large tumors with extensive nodal disease should be followed carefully for local and regional recurrence and also for signs of distant failure.
- CT scan of the chest or PET/CT scan may be useful in the initial evaluation of patients believed to be at increased risk for distant metastases.

Carcinoma of the Hypopharynx

- Anatomically, the hypopharynx extends from the level of the hyoid bone to the lower level of the cricoid cartilage and is in immediate approximation to the larynx.
- Hypopharynx subsites include the pyriform sinus, posterior hypopharyngeal wall and postcricoid region
- Greater than 90% of hypopharyngeal cancer is squamous cell carcinoma.
- Risk factors are chronic tobacco and alcohol use and gastroesophageal reflux disease.
- Plummer-Vinson syndrome is associated with hypopharyngeal cancer. This disorder affects women between the ages of 30 and 50 years and consists of a combination of iron deficiency anemia, dysphagia, mucosal webs, weight loss, angular stomatitis, and atrophic glossitis.
- In the United States, pyriform sinus carcinoma predominates (accounting for 60%-70% of cases), while in Europe, postcricoid carcinomas predominate.
- The most common symptoms are odynophagia, referred otalgia, dysphagia, hoarseness, and/or a neck mass that present late in the disease.
- The rich lymphatic network in the submucosal tissue surrounding the hypopharynx allows early spread to regional lymph nodes and direct extension into adjacent soft tissues.
- 60% to 75% of patients with hypopharyngeal carcinoma have palpable cervical metastases at presentation.
- Carcinoma of the medial wall of the hypopharynx may behave differently and have a greater propensity for contralateral metastasis than lesions of the lateral wall.
- Extension of tumor into the larynx is common for cancer arising along the medial pyriform wall.
- Posterior cricoid cancers may invade into the cricoarytenoid muscles and cartilage of the larynx.
- Lateral hypopharyngeal cancers may extend superiorly to the oropharynx and nasopharynx, inferiorly to involve the esophagus or deep into the prevertebral fascia.
- Lesions that involve more than one subsite within the hypopharynx have significant increase in mortality.
- A characteristic feature of hypopharyngeal cancer is its tendency for submucosal spread which must be taken into consideration during surgical resection in order to obtain a negative margin.

- Management of hypopharyngeal carcinoma remains both challenging and controversial with treatment selection depending on stage, subsite, performance status of the patient, and institutional preference.
- Radiation therapy is advocated as a primary modality of treatment for T1 and selected T2 lesions, and may provide a better functional (organ preserving) result.
- Radiation therapy may be used to treat bilateral cervical nodal basins as well as retropharyngeal nodes with diminished morbidity.
- Neck dissection prior to radiation may be considered in certain patients with extensive but resectable cervical metastasis.
- Postoperative adjuvant radiation therapy plays a crucial role following surgery for advanced-stage carcinomas of the hypopharynx, improving local and regional control, and increasing survival.
- Indications for postoperative radiation include multiple levels or bulky nodal disease, cartilage invasion, ECS, positive surgical margins.
- The role of concurrent chemotherapy and radiation therapy in the treatment of hypopharyngeal SCCA remains unclear. (1) The European Organization for Research and Treatment of Cancer (EORTC) Head and Neck Cooperative Group showed results comparable to surgery and post-operative XRT, but the 5-year survival rate was only 35%.
- Selected tumors of the posterior hypopharyngeal wall can be resected with laryngeal preservation if there is no fixation to the prevertebral fascia.
- These can be approached via transhyoid or median labiomandibular glossotomy.
- Postcricoid tumors usually present at an advanced stage and therefore require total laryngopharyngectomy or if involving the cervical esophagus, they require laryngopharyngoesophagectomy.
- Pyriform sinus may be treated by extended partial laryngopharyngectomy which was first described by Ogura and may be indicated for selected T1 and T2 carcinomas. Supracricoid hemilaryngopharyngectomy which preserves cricoid integrity and the contralateral arytenoid and vocal cord. Oncologic results are comparable when adjuvant radiation therapy was used.
- Total laryngopharyngectomy, however, is often required for complete oncologic resection.
- Steiner and colleagues have demonstrated the effectiveness of transoral CO_2 laser microsurgery as an organ-preserving approach for cancers of the hypopharynx (and also oropharynx). The goal of this approach is to perform an oncologic resection with preservation of uninvolved tissues.
- With transoral resection, elective or therapeutic neck dissection is also performed and surgery is followed by postoperative external beam radiation therapy.
- Reconstructive options include primary closure for patients undergoing partial laryngopharyngectomy or total laryngectomy with partial pharyngectomy.
- Pectoralis major myocutaneous flap is useful for partial laryngopharyngectomy defects when remaining mucosa is insufficient for primary closure.
- Tubed pectoralis major flap can be utilized for total laryngopharyngectomy defects but overall tissue bulk and stenosis at the anastomotic sites are problematic.
- Radial forearm and anterolateral thigh flaps have been used for partial pharyngectomy defects. Tubed radial forearm, rectus, or other fasciocutaneous flaps have been described for closure of total laryngopharyngectomy defects.
- Free jejunal autograft can also be used for reconstruction following total laryngopharyngectomy.

- Gastric pull-up is indicated when total laryngopharyngectomy with esophagectomy is performed.
- Price et al noted a high incidence (20%) of occult, synchronous esophageal carcinoma.

Treatment Outcomes

- Local and regional control:
  (a) Pyriform sinus = 58%-71%
  (b) Pharyngeal wall: T1 = 91%; T2 = 73%; T3 = 61%; T4 = 37%
  (c) Postcricoid carcinoma: less than 60%.
- 5-year survival rates:
  (a) Pyriform sinus: 20%-50%
  (b) Pharyngeal wall: 21%
  (c) Postcricoid carcinoma: 35%
- Distant metastasis occur in about 20% of patients with hypopharyngeal carcinoma.

Carcinoma of the Nasopharynx

World Health Organization (WHO) Classification

- Type I: keratinizing SCCA is similar to other epidermoid carcinoma of the head and neck
- Type II: non-keratinizing SCCA
- Type III: undifferentiated carcinomas are historically known as lymphoepithelioma or Schmincke tumors. These poorly differentiated tumors are infiltrated by nonmalignant T-cell lymphocytes. This is the most common form of carcinoma of the nasopharynx (NPC).
- Distribution in North America: Type I = 25% Type II = 12% Type III = 63%
- Histological classification of NPC:
  (a) Keratinizing SCCA (WHO type I)
  (b) Nonkeratinizing carcinoma differentiated (WHO type II)
  (c) Undifferentiated (WHO type III)
- Endemic NPC (WHO type II or III) is found predominantly in the southern provinces of China, Southeast Asia, certain Mediterranean populations, and among the Aleut Native Americans.
- Risk factors include EBV, genetic predisposition (HLA class I and II haplotypes), environmental factors (food-preserving nitrosamines frequently used in Cantonese salted fish).
- The incidence of NPC among Chinese born in North America is significantly lower than among native-born Chinese but still greater than the risk for Caucasians, emphasizing a synergistic role of environmental factors.
- Sporadic NPC, (WHO type I) is related to tobacco and alcohol exposure with a peak incidence in the fifth and sixth decades of life However, 20% of NPC develop in patients under the age of 30.
- Younger patients tend to have undifferentiated (WHO III) tumors.
- EBV plays a major role in the pathogenesis of NPC. EBV is a double-stranded DNA virus that is part of the human herpesvirus family. It establishes persistent, chronic infection, usually in B lymphocytes. Six nuclear proteins (EBNAs) and three membrane proteins (LMPs) are believed to mediate EBV-related carcinogenesis.

- EBV antibodies are acquired earlier in life in tropical rather than in industrialized countries, but by adulthood 90% to 95% of populations have demonstrable EBV antibodies.
- EBV is detected in virtually all patients with NPC, and EBV-encoded RNA is present in virtually all NPC tumor cells.
- EBV serology may be useful in regions where NPC is prevalent.
- IgA antibodies to viral capsid or to the early antigen complex are present in high titers compared to those in matched controls.
- Prospective serologic screening detected occult NPC and anticipated recurrences after therapy.
- Molecular cytogenetic studies have confirmed that EBV infection is an early, possibly initiating event in the development of nasopharyngeal carcinoma.
- Clonal EBV DNA was present in premalignant lesions, suggesting that NPC arises from a single EBV-infected cell.
- B-cell lymphocytes should serve as the only reservoir of EBV and persistent infection within epithelial cells strongly suggests premalignancy or NPC.
- Nasopharyngeal brush biopsy or swab has been advocated for screening and early diagnosis by using polymerase chain reaction (PCR) to detect the EBV genome within nasopharyngeal epithelia. Further studies will be needed to confirm the accuracy and efficacy of this approach.
- Early symptoms are rare.
- The development of a neck mass (usually level II or V), aural fullness, and nasal dysfunction are more common symptoms.
- Cranial neuropathies (especially cranial nerves III-VI) are common and indicate orbital and/or skull base invasion. Further extension may involve cranial nerve XII at the hypoglossal foramen or the cervical sympathetic chain, resulting in Horner syndrome.
- Cervical lymph node metastases to jugulodigastric, posterior cervical, and/or retropharyngeal lymphadenopathy are frequently present at the time of diagnosis
- Spread to the parotid nodes can occur through the lymphatics of the eustachian tube. Low cervical metastases (to the lower jugular or supraclavicular chains) are uniformly associated with poor prognosis.
- Approximately 87% of patients present with palpable nodal disease and 20% have bilateral metastases.
- Concurrent administration of chemotherapy with radiation therapy has been shown to improve overall survival rates in a phase III study performed in the United States. This approach in an Asian population has shown similar results to the US data.
- Surgical resection of NPC is technically difficult due to the architecture and inaccessibility of the anterosuperior skull base and the retropharyngeal lymphatics.
- Surgery is reserved for highly selected patients in cases of radiation failure or tumor recurrence. Several approaches have been advocated including an infratemporal fossa approach, described by Fisch, a combined transpalatal, transmaxillary, transcervical approach, and an extended osteoplastic maxillotomy or "maxillary swing."
- Persistent postradiation lymphadenopathy is treated with radical or modified radical neck dissection.
- CT is useful for identifying paranasopharyngeal extension of tumor and skull base invasion.
- MRI is used to assess the extent of soft tissue involvement, perineural invasion, and retropharyngeal and cervical lymph node involvement.

- PET scanning may be useful to assess for distant metastases or to detect persistent or recurrent cancer following treatment.
- Radiation therapy or chemoradiation is the primary treatment modalities for nasopharyngeal carcinoma. When properly delivered, external beam therapy can spare adjacent tissues and limit morbidity to the pituitary, eyes, ears, and frontal and temporal lobes. Improved imaging with CT and MRI has permitted better dosimetry and treatment outcomes.
- Re-irradiation (with external beam and brachytherapy) may play a role in the treatment of certain recurrent NPCs, especially using conformal intensity-modulated therapy.
- When delivered through a traditional intra-cavitary approach, brachytherapy offered little advantage over external beam therapy. A transnasal interstitial implant was developed to deliver a more effective tumoricidal dose.
- Wei and colleagues have advocated a transpalatal approach for the placement of gold grain, the preferred radiation source.

Treatment Outcomes

- Local and regional control Radiation: 60%
- Radiation with concurrent chemotherapy: 70% to 80%
- 5-year survival radiation 36% to 58%, radiation with concurrent chemotherapy 70% to 80%
- 10-year survival: The risk of recurrence continues after 5 years; 10% to 40%.
- Nasopharynx is the subsite within the head and neck that has the highest rate of distant metastases.
- Distant metastases are present or develop in 25% to 30% of patients. Whereas local and regional failure previously accounted for most morbidity and mortality, distant metastasis now is a frequent mode of failure and death.

Carcinoma of the Esophagus

- The majority (> 90%) of esophageal cancer is SCCA or adenocarcinoma.
- Greater than 75% of adenocarcinomas occur in the distal esophagus.
- Squamous cell carcinoma is more evenly distributed throughout the esophagus.
- The most common site for primary esophageal cancer is the lower third of the esophagus followed by the middle third and rarely the cervical esophagus.
- Carcinoma involving the cervical esophagus most commonly results from extension of hypopharyngeal cancer inferiorly into the cervical esophagus.
- The cervical esophagus extends from the lower border of the cricoid cartilage to the thoracic inlet.
- Risk factors for squamous cell carcinoma include tobacco and alcohol use, achalasia, caustic injury, Plummer-Vinson syndrome, history of head and neck cancer, history of radiation therapy to the mediastinum, low socioeconomic status, and nonepidermolytic palmoplantar keratoderma (tylosis).
- Risk factors for adenocarcinoma include Barrett esophagus, acid reflux, tobacco use, and history of radiotherapy to the mediastinum.
- Barrett esophagus is characterized by metaplasia of the normal squamous mucosa of the distal esophagus to a villiform, columnar epithelium similar to the epithelial lining of the stomach which may progress to dysplasia and eventually adenocarcinoma.
- The annual rate of malignant transformation of Barrett esophagus is 0.5%.
- Common symptoms of esophageal carcinoma include dysphagia, odynophagia, and weight loss. Hoarseness may occur if there is recurrent laryngeal nerve invasion or direct tumor involvement of the larynx.

- Barium esophagogram, CT scan with contrast of neck, chest, abdomen, and pelvis, and PET scan are useful imaging studies to assess regional lymphadenopathy and detect distant metastases.
- Flexible or rigid endoscopy is performed to assess extent and location of lesion and to obtain tissue for histopathologic diagnosis.
- Cancer involving the cervical esophagus may extend to involve the larynx and trachea.
- Tracheoesophageal fistula may result from invasion of cancer through the posterior wall of the trachea.
- Distal esophageal cancer may extend inferiorly to involve the esophagogastric junction.
- At the time of diagnosis, more than 50% of patients have metastases or an unresectable primary tumor.
- Early-stage disease is treated surgically with a transthoracic or transhiatal approach for partial or total esophagectomy.
- Transcervical approach for upper cervical esophagus or inferior extension from hypopharynx.
- Laryngectomy with or without partial tracheal resection may be necessary for upper cervical esophageal cancer.
- Endoscopically placed stents may be deployed for palliative treatment of dysphagia in advanced-stage disease.
- Primary radiotherapy may be used as an alternative treatment in patients with medical comorbidities that prevents surgical resection.
- No improvement in survival has been demonstrated with preoperative radiation therapy.
- Postoperative radiotherapy improves local disease control.
- Preoperative chemotherapy may result in a reduction in primary tumor size as well as treat regional and distant metastases, but no survival benefit has been demonstrated.
- Postoperative chemotherapy may also treat regional and distant metastases but results in increased toxicity, morbidity and no improvement in survival.
- Combined chemoradiation (CRT) leads to increased toxicity but better tumor response with combined therapy. When utilized preoperatively in patients with locally advanced disease, the reduction in tumor size may allow for complete surgical resection. CRT offers no clear survival benefit when used preoperatively.
- Useful as primary treatment modality in patients with unresectable disease.
- Reconstructive options include gastric transposition (pull-up) utilized in patients undergoing total esophagectomy. Cervical esophagectomy or total laryngopharyngectomy is best repaired with free tissue transfer including free jejunal flap or tubed radial forearm free flap.
- Pedicled, tubed pectoralis major flap is possible but difficult due to excessive tissue bulk.

Treatment Outcomes
- The overall 5-year survival rate for esophageal cancer is approximately 14%.
- 5-year overall survival rates
  (a) Stage I = 50-80%
  (b) Stage IIA = 30%-40%
  (c) Stage IIB = 10%-30%
  (d) Stage III = 10%-15%
  (e) Stage IV = 0%
- There are several independent predictors of poor prognosis such as decrease in weight equal to 10% of body mass, dysphagia, lymphatic micrometastases, advanced age, and large primary tumor.

Bibliography

Al-Sarraf M, Le Blanc M, Giri PG, et al. Chemoradiotherapy versus radiotherapy in patients with advanced nasopharyngeal cancer: phase III randomized inter-group study 0099. *J Clin Oncolm.* 1998;16:1310-1317.

Bernier J, Domenge C, Ozsahin M, et al. Postoperative irradiation with or without concomitant chemotherapy for head and neck cancer. *N Engl J Med.* 2004;350:1945-1962.

Bhayani MK, Holsinger FC, Lai SY. A shifting paradigm for patients with head and neck cancer: transoral robotic surgery (TORS). *Oncology (Williston Park).* 2010; 24:1010-1015 (Review).

Bonner JA, Harari PM, Giralt J, et al. Radiotherapy plus cetuximab for locoregionally advanced head and neck cancer: 5-year survival data from a phase 3 randomised trial, and relation between cetuximab-induced rash and survival. *Lancet Oncol.* 2010;11(1):21-28.

Enzinger PC, Mayer RJ. Esophageal cancer. *N Engl J Med.* 2003;349:2241-2252. http://www.cancer.org/research/cancerfactsstatistics/cancerfactsfigures2014/. http://www.wcrf.org/cancer_statistics/world_cancer_statistics.php. World Cancer Research Fund International.

Lorch JH, Golou-beva O, Haddad RI, et al. TAX 324 Study Group. *Lancet Oncol.* 2011;12:153-159.

Wei WI, Sham J. Nasopharyngeal carcinoma. *Lancet.* 2005;365:2041-2054.

Yao M, Graham MM, Hoffman HT, et al. The role of post-radiation therapy FDG PET in prediction of necessity for post radiation therapy neck dissection in locally advanced head and neck squamous cell carcinoma. *Int J Radiat Oncol Biol Phys.* 2004;59:1001-1010.

Questions

1. Elective neck dissection for T2N0M0 cancer of the floor of mouth should include neck levels
   A. unilateral levels I, II, III
   B. bilateral levels II, III, IV
   C. bilateral level I
   D. unilateral levels II, III, IV
   E. bilateral levels I, II, III

2. Common risk factors for cancer of the tongue base include tobacco, alcohol, and
   A. human papilloma virus 11 and 18
   B. Epstein-Bar virus
   C. ingestion of smoked fish
   D. Plummer-Vinson syndrome
   E. human papilloma virus 16

3. In the surgical treatment of oral cavity cancer, which of the following lesions require bilateral elective neck dissection?
   A. T2 anterior tongue
   B. T2 midline lip
   C. T2 lateral tongue
   D. T3 buccal mucosa
   E. T1 hard palate

4. The appropriate surgical treatment for T2 N1M0 cancer of the left base of tongue includes
   A. transoral excision of the primary and left neck dissection levels I-III
   B. transoral excision of the primary alone
   C. transoral excision of the primary and bilateral neck dissections levels II-IV
   D. transoral excision of the primary and bilateral neck dissections levels I-V
   E. transoral excision of the primary and left neck dissection levels I-V

5. Risk factors for hypopharyngeal carcinoma include
   A. smoking
   B. alcohol
   C. gastroesophageal reflux disease
   D. Plummer-Vinson syndrome
   E. all of the above

Chapter 40
The Role of Chemotherapy for Head and Neck Cancer

Chemotherapy as a Single Modality

- Chemotherapy has come to be recognized as a vital part of treatment of the locally advanced head and neck cancer patient. The goals of chemotherapy are outlined in Table 40-1.

What had been clear since the 1970s were the high rates of response to induction chemotherapy with single agents such as methotrexate, bleomycin, cisplatin, and 5-Fluorouracil (5-FU).

- Table 40-2 lists the most commonly used chemotherapeutic and biologic agents for head and neck cancer.
  In the 1980s, with the introduction of the combination of cisplatin and 5-FU, rates of complete remission approached 25% while overall response rates approached 45%. Treatment was always followed by definitive local therapy with either radiation therapy or surgery as responses were always thought to be transient. The combination was also noted to be effective in the treatment of distant metastatic disease.
- The cisplatin/5-FU combination soon became established as the standard regimen for the treatment of locally advanced and metastatic head and neck squamous cell carcinomas. However, for patients with previously treated disease, the rate of response to systemic chemotherapy was substantially diminished to disappointing rates of 5% to 15%. Nonetheless, this dramatic sensitivity to chemotherapy in previously untreated disease suggested that this treatment modality might decrease distant metastatic disease, improve locoregional control, permit organ preservation, and boost overall survival.
- A number of trials were conducted during the 1970s and 1980s to test adjuvant chemotherapy for head and neck cancer. Meta-analysis showed an insignificant overall improvement in cancer mortality of 0.5%. Neither single agent nor combination chemotherapy produced a significant reduction of cancer deaths. The mortality rate from chemotherapy in nine series averaged 6.5%. These disappointing results have led to the abandonment of adjuvant chemotherapy following definitive treatment for locally advanced head and neck squamous cell carcinomas, with the prominent exception of the nasopharyngeal subsite.

Table 40-1 **Potential Goals of Chemotherapy**

1. Act as a radiosensitizer and improve locoregional control
2. Treat micrometastatic disease and improve overall survival
3. Organ preservation
4. Palliate metastatic disease
5. Debulk large tumors to make surgery feasible

Chemotherapy Combined With Radiation Therapy

- The goal of concurrent chemotherapy with radiation is to increase locoregional control and prevent distant metastases. A number of single agents have been studied since the late 1960s, including bleomycin, methotrexate, hydroxyurea, mitomycin-C, 5-FU, and cisplatin.
- Most studies failed to report an improvement in overall survival, although a number of agents conferred an increase response rate to radiation therapy. Chemotherapy also was complicated by systemic toxicity from the agent used. Methotrexate conferred significant mucosal and cutaneous toxicity, bleomycin produced significant mucositis and skin toxicity, 5-FU potentiated mucositis, and mitomycin-C produced pulmonary toxicity.
- It was ultimately cisplatin that produced a significant enough benefit in terms of overall survival to warrant its use in spite of its nephro-, oto-, and neurotoxicity. Common side effects of the most commonly used drugs are listed in Table 40-3.
- Based on several studies, chemoradiation has now become a standard of care for locally advanced head and neck cancer, although there is recognition that chemoradiation results in higher acute toxicity rates and greater long term end organ dysfunction.
- The addition of another agent or agents in combination with cisplatin (eg, 5-FU or taxanes) concomitant with radiation therapy has not added to the clinical complete response rate but increased local side effects, especially mucositis. Thus, platinum agents alone (cisplatin or carboplatin) appear to be the chemotherapeutic drug of choice for concurrent chemotherapy with radiation therapy in patients with head and neck cancers. At the present time, cisplatin given alone on a 3-week schedule is most widely used in the United States, while weekly carboplatin is increasingly being used with concurrent radiation after triplet induction therapy.

Table 40-2 **Commonly Used Chemotherapeutic and Biological Agents in Head and Neck Cancer**

1. 5-Fluoruracil (5-FU)
2. Cisplatin
3. Carboplatin
4. Docetaxel
5. Paclitaxel
6. Cetuximab

Table 40-3 **Single-Agent Drug Therapy**

Drug	N + V	Mucositis	Bone marrow	Alopecia	Kidney	Nerve	Vesicant	Other
			Toxicity (1-4+)					
5-FU	1+	3+	2+	1+	—	—	—	
Cisplatin	4+	—	3+	2+	4+	3+	—	Ototoxicity 3+
Carboplatin	3+	—	4+	2+	—	3+	—	
Paclitaxel	4+	—	4+	4+	—	3+	—	
Docetaxel	4+	—	4+	4+	—	2+	—	
Cetuximab	1+	—	—	—	—	—	—	Rash 3+

Based on several studies, chemoradiation has now become a standard of care for locally advanced head and neck cancer, although there is recognition that chemoradiation results in higher acute toxicity rates and greater long.

Experience With Cisplatin-Based Regimen

- The concept of concurrent chemoradiation with systemic chemotherapy has been most successful in the treatment of nasopharyngeal carcinoma, which represents a unique subsite of the head and neck region. Nasopharyngeal carcinoma is often EBV (Epstein-Barr virus) driven and has a propensity to metastasize.
- Nonetheless, systemic chemotherapy for nasopharyngeal cancer still remains controversial and has not been fully accepted outside of the United States.

Chemoradiation for Laryngeal Preservation

- The RTOG 9111 study specifically compared neoadjuvant chemotherapy followed by radiation with concurrent chemoradiation and radiation therapy alone. All three groups had equivalent survival, but locoregional control was significantly better in the concurrent chemoradiation group. Other studies have also established the superiority of concurrent chemoradiation therapy for locally advanced head and neck cancer, and it has become an established standard of care for such patients.

Induction Chemotherapy Followed by Chemoradiation Therapy

- The advent of the taxanes changed the role of neoadjuvant chemotherapy in the treatment of locally advanced head and neck cancer but has not established a firm role for systemic neoadjuvant chemotherapy.
- The clinical activity of single agent docetaxel and single agent paclitaxel has been established in several Phase II studies.
- Based on these studies, TAX 324 was conducted. Five hundred and one patients (all of whom had stage III or IV disease with no distant metastases and tumors considered to be nonresectable or were candidates for organ preservation) were randomly assigned to receive either TPF (docetaxel, cisplatin, 5-FU) or PF (cisplatin, 5-FU) induction chemotherapy, followed by chemoradiotherapy with weekly carboplatin therapy and radiotherapy for 5 days per week. The primary end point was overall survival.
- The authors concluded that induction chemotherapy with the addition of docetaxel (TPF) significantly improved progression-free and overall survival in patients with nonresectable squamous cell carcinoma of the head and neck.

- In the randomized phase III DeCIDE trial, patients with N2/N3 locally advanced squamous cell carcinoma of the head and neck were assigned to two cycles of induction chemotherapy—docetaxel, cisplatin, and fluorouracil (TPF)—followed by concurrent chemoradiation, or to chemoradiation alone. Compared with their counterparts who did not get induction chemotherapy, those who did showed trends toward better recurrence-free survival and distant failure–free survival. However, overall survival was statistically indistinguishable.
- The randomized phase III PARADIGM trial also compared chemoradiation alone versus TPF induction chemotherapy followed by chemoradiation in patients with locally advanced stage III or IV squamous cell carcinoma of the head and neck. The 3-year survival and progression free survival rates were similar in each arm.
- Due to the conflicting results of these studies, induction chemotherapy still remains controversial for locally advanced head and neck cancer.

Intra-Arterial Cisplatin Chemoradiation Therapy

- Capitalizing on the cis-diamine dichloroplatium (DDP)-neutralizing agent sodium thiosulfate and its pharmacokinetic properties, enormous concentrations of cisplatin can be infused directly into large head and neck tumors through a targeted IA approach. In a Phase I study, it was determined that cisplatin could be safely administered to patients with advanced and recurrent head and neck cancer at a dose intensity of 150 mg/m^2 per week.
- Rasch et al presented data from their randomized Phase III study comparing intravenous to intra-arterial chemotherapy and confirmed the equivalence of intra-arterial chemotherapy to intravenous therapy.
- Damascelli et al capitalized on the intra-arterial approach and a novel albumin bound taxane, abraxane, to conduct a Phase I study. Eighteen patients (78%) had a clinical and radiologic objective response (complete, 26%; partial, 52%). The toxicities encountered were hematologic (8.6%) and neurologic (8.6%). Two catheter-related complications occurred: one reversible brachiofacial paralysis and one asymptomatic occlusion of the external carotid artery.

Postoperative Chemoradiation Therapy

- The use of chemotherapy combined with radiation therapy (concomitant chemoradiation) following surgery also has proven to be successful. As the final conclusion of two trials differed slightly, and in order to better define risk, a combined analysis of prognostic factors and outcome from the two trials was performed. This analysis demonstrated that patients in both trials with extracapsular nodal spread of tumor and/or positive resection margins benefited from the addition of cisplatin to postoperative radiotherapy. For those with multiple involved regional nodes without extracapsular spread, there was no survival advantage.

Biologic Therapies

- The most recent advent to head and neck cancer chemotherapy has been the biologic agents. Cetuximab has been the most studied agent. A humanized monoclonal antibody, it specifically blocks the epidermal growth factor receptor, present in over 90% of head and neck cancers. Other monoclonal agents available against this receptor include panitumumab.

- Bonner et al randomized patients with stage III or IV head and neck cancer to receive either radiation alone or radiation therapy with weekly cetuximab. Median survival for patients treated with cetuximab was 49 months, compared with 29.3 months for patients who received radiation therapy alone. With the exception of acneiform rash and infusion reactions, the incidence of grade 3 or greater toxic effects, including mucositis, did not differ significantly between the two groups.
- Vermorken et al reported the results of single agent cetuximab in the treatment of platinum refractory head and neck cancer. Disease control rate (complete response/partial response/stable disease) was 46%, and median time to progression (TTP) was 70 days.
- Subsequently, Vermorken et al studied the addition of cetuximab to chemotherapy in untreated recurrent or metastatic head and neck cancer in a Phase III randomized study. Adding cetuximab to platinum-based chemotherapy with fluorouracil (platinum-fluorouracil) prolonged the median survival. The authors concluded that cetuximab could be safely added to standard chemotherapy for metastatic head and neck squamous cell carcinoma and provide significant benefit.
- However, no benefit in survival was seen when cetuximab or panitumumab was added to chemoradiation for primary treatment of locally advanced head and neck cancer. These results have curbed the enthusiasm of incorporating cytotoxic chemotherapy together with anti-EGFR therapy.
- The future direction of chemotherapy will test questions such as whether or not cetuximab and radiation is equivalent to chemoradiation (RTOG 1016), will risk stratify and guide therapy based on factors such HPV status, and will incorporate other biological therapies, including small molecule tyrosine kinase inhibitors in novel combinations.

Bibliography

Bonner JA, Harari PM, Giralt J, et al. Radiotherapy plus cetuximab for squamous-cell carcinoma of the head and neck. *N Engl J Med.*2006;354(6):567-578.

Cohen E, Karrison T, Kocherginsky M, et al. DeCIDE: A phase III randomized trial of docetaxel (D), cisplatin (P), 5-fluorouracil (F) (TPF) induction chemotherapy (IC) in patients with N2/N3 locally advanced squamous cell carcinoma of the head and neck (SCCHN). Paper presented at: 2012 ASCO Annual Meeting, 2012.

Damascelli B, Patelli GL, Lanocita R et al. A Novel Intraarterial Chemotherapy Using Paclitaxel in Albumin Nanoparticles to Treat Advanced Squamous Cell Carcinoma of the Tongue: Preliminary Findings. American Journal of Roentgenology.2003;181(1):253–260

Giralt J, Fortin A, Mesia R, et al. A phase II, randomized trial (CONCERT-1) of chemoradiotherapy (CRT) with or without panitumumab (pmab) in patients (pts) with unresected, locally advanced squamous cell carcinoma of the head and neck (LASCCHN). 2012 ASCO Annual Meeting.

Posner MR, Hershock DM, Blajman CR, et al. Cisplatin and fluorouracil alone or with docetaxel in head and neck cancer. *N Engl J Med.* 2007;357(17):1705-1715.

Rasch CRN, Hauptmann M, Schornagel J, et al. Intra-arterial versus intravenous chemoradiation for advanced head and neck cancer: Results of a randomized phase 3 trial. Cancer.2010;116:2159–2165.

Vermorken JB, Remenar E, van Herpen C, et al. Cisplatin, fluorouracil, and docetaxel in unresectable head and neck cancer. *N Engl J Med.* 2007;357(17):1695-1704.

Questions

1. Chemotherapy can do all of the following except:
    A. act as a radiosensitizer
    B. palliate metastatic disease
    C. cure head and neck cancer single handedly
    D. debulk large tumors
    E. help preserve an organ

2. All of the following are drugs used to treat head and neck cancer except:
    A. cisplatin
    B. carboplatin
    C. cetuximab
    D. doxorubicin
    E. docetaxel

3. Side effects of cisplatin include all of the following except:
    A. nephrotoxicity
    B. ototoxicity
    C. neurotoxicity
    D. nausea and vomiting
    E. cardiomyopathy

4. All of the following are high risk features that merit post-operative chemoradiation except:
    A. positive margins
    B. multiple positive nodes
    C. extracapsular spread

5. Successful uses of chemotherapy include all of the following except:
    A. post-surgical chemoradiation in patients with high-risk features
    B. induction chemotherapy followed by chemoradiation
    C. primary chemoradiation
    D. adjuvant chemotherapy given postradiation
    E. single agent therapy in the metastatic disease setting

Notes

The authors are grateful to Ms. Kissindra Moore who has diligently prepared the manuscript for publication.

Chapter 41
Radiation Therapy for Head and Neck Cancer

Background

- Radiation induced double strand breaks within DNA kill tumor cells.
- Normal tissues have a greater ability to repair radiation induced damage as compared to tumor cells.
- This difference is exploited in radiation oncology.
- Radiation is usually given in small daily fractions, given 5 days a week over 6 to 7 weeks
- This allows for maximal normal tissue healing.

Radiation Dose

- The unit of radiation is Gray (Gy) and 1 Gy is equal to 1 joule (J) of energy absorbed per kilogram of matter.
- Daily doses of radiation are usually in the range of 1.8 to 2.0 Gy/day.
- Total radiation doses depend on tumor type and histology, but in general:
  (a) > 50 Gy/25 fractions (fx) is used to sterilize microscopic disease such as in the clinically negative neck at risk for lymphatic nodal spread.
  (b) 60 Gy/30 fx is used in the postoperative setting to control microscopic residual disease within the postoperative bed and is also used for intermediate-risk areas, such as lymph node levels with involved nodal disease.
  (c) 66 Gy/33 fx is used for close or positive margins.
  (d) 70 Gy/35 fx is used to control gross tumor with curative intent.
- The relationship between the daily dose and the total dose is not linear, for example, thirty-five 2-Gy fractions of irradiation leads to a total of 70 Gy, but this is biologically very different than receiving ten 7-Gy fractions of irradiation.
- The relationship is linear quadratic and given by the formula:

$$\text{Biologic equivalent dose (BED)} = nd(1 + d/(\alpha/\beta))$$

Where n = number of fractions, dose-dose per fraction, α and β represents the linear and quadratic components of cell killing, respectively. α/β is given a value of 10 for most tumors.

- The ability to simultaneously dose different portions of the tumor based on risk now exists.

(a) For example, using IMRT in nasopharyangeal cancer, one can give gross tumor 2.12 Gy per fraction, while giving the entire nasopharynx and high-risk nodal areas (retropharyngeal nodes, levels II-III, V) 1.8 Gy per fraction, while giving the uninvolved low-neck 1.64 Gy per day in 33 daily fractions.

(b) This provides a total dose of 69.92 Gy to the primary tumor and gross lymph nodes, 59.4 Gy to high-risk areas, and 54.12 Gy to low-risk areas.

Altered Fractionation Schemes

- Investigators have examined effects of changes in the radiation dose fractionation scheme, above the generally accepted 5 fractions per week of 1.8 to 2.0 Gy.
- This has come in various forms including: six fractions per week, or dosing to certain portions of the target volume at doses > 2.0 Gy per day (eg, 2.2 Gy/day), or giving an additional fraction of irradiation during the last few weeks of treatment.
- The exact differences and the relative advantages and disadvantages of the various approaches is beyond the scope of this text.
- Invariably these techniques have demonstrated improved local control rates particularly in patients with locally advanced disease.
- The combination of accelerated fractionation, in combination with systemic chemotherapy, however, does not seem to add any therapeutic benefit although it does add toxicity.
- Thus the use of altered fractionation in today's clinical practice is largely limited to cases of locally advanced tumors in patients who can't tolerate systemic therapy.

Radiation Therapy Techniques

Three-Dimensional Conformal Radiation Therapy (3D-CRT)

- Refers to CT-based radiation planning.
- The tumor and critical avoidance structures, such as the brain stem or parotid glands, are contoured on axial CT images.
- Radiation therapy is planned, usually with 2 to 6 beams, with the goals of treating the tumor and avoiding critical structures.
- If a critical structure is adjacent to the tumor, it may be impossible to deliver the desired dose to the tumor without overdosing the critical structure. In this situation, either tumor underdosing or acceptance of the risk of treating to full dose is required.

Intensity-Modulated Radiation Therapy (IMRT)

- IMRT is a significant advance over 3D-CRT and is now used standardly for treatment of most head and neck tumors.
- IMRT uses many beams or arcs and requires the use of computer-based planning to create sophisticated radiation plans in which small leaves move in and out of each radiation field to block critical structures.
- Essentially this makes it possible to curve the delivered radiation dose around critical structures such as the parotid gland or spinal cord in order to deliver dose to targets.

Image-Guided Radiation Therapy (IGRT)

- IGRT refers to the incorporation of three-dimensional imaging prior to radiation delivery.
- Prior to each treatment, an imaging study is performed to confirm alignment of the target volume.
- This consists of either orthogonal diagnostic quality x-rays or a limited volume CT scan.
- IGRT improves the likelihood that treatment is delivered accurately and thus reduces the risk of "marginal miss."
- IGRT can also reduce the margin of normal tissue used to account for potential setup error and thus can reduce the amount of normal tissue exposed to the treatment dose.

The Role of Radiation in Head and Neck Cancers

- Radiation therapy plays a critical role in the management of head and neck cancers.
- It plays a dual role and can be used as curative intent treatment alone or with combined chemotherapy.
- Additionally, it can also be used postoperatively for patients with an elevated risk of recurrence based on final pathologic findings.
- It also allows for organ and functional preservation approaches.
- At some institutions, radiation is used preoperatively before planned surgical resection, although this is not a common practice.

The Role of Radiation Therapy in Specific Disease Sites

Larynx Cancer

- Radiation therapy is often used for early stage larynx carcinoma, T1-2N0
- In these settings narrow field irradiation, consisting of a 5 to 6 cm square field extending from the hyoid bone down to the cricoid is often used.
- Given there is no coverage of elective lymph nodes, and no chemotherapy, this treatment is generally well tolerated.
- Randomized trials have demonstrated a benefit to using doses of greater than 2 Gy per fraction, and a common fractionation scheme is 63 Gy in 2.25 Gy fractions for T1N0 tumors, and 65.25 Gy in 2.25 Gy fractions for T2N0 tumors.
- Larynx preservation has emerged as an option for patients with locally advanced laryngeal tumors, with either T3-T4 disease or positive nodes.
- Concurrent chemoradiation has shown the best rates of larynx preservation, with an 88% rate of larynx preservation at 2 years in RTOG 91-11.
- Patients with extensive cartilage invasion have often been offered surgery, as the control rates induction chemotherapy and radiation in the VA larynx trial in such patients was < 50%.
- Survival is equivalent for patients receiving laryngectomy or larynx preservation so long as early surgical salvage is considered for patients with residual or recurrent disease.

Hypopharynx Cancer

- Similarly to larynx cancer, trials of larynx preservation therapy for hypopharynx cancer have been attempted and also found to be successful, although the rate of success is lower than in larynx cancer.
- Concurrent chemoradiation is the preferred approach when attempting larynx preservation in patients with hypopharyngeal cancer.

Nasopharynx Cancer

- Nasopharynx cancers are generally felt to be unresectable, have high rates of subclinical nodal involvement, and are usually managed nonoperatively.
- Patients have a high rate of level II, V, and retropharyngeal nodal involvement, and these areas should be covered in all patients.
- Patients have a propensity to along the base of skull, and thus, a detailed cranial nerve examination is important in all patients.
- PET/CT and MRI studies are useful parts of the staging process.
- For T1N0 tumors radiation alone can be considered.
- For T2N0 or more advanced disease cisplatin-based chemoradiation is the treatment of choice.
- Three cycles of adjuvant chemotherapy are typically given following this chemoradiation, although the necessity of this is a source of controversy.
- Current studies are examining whether Epstein-Barr virus titers can better predict who would benefit from adjuvant therapy.

Oral Cavity Tumors

- Oral cavity cancers are generally managed surgically, with consideration of radiation as an adjuvant therapy based on the final pathologic results.
- For small early stage (T1-2N0), well-lateralized tumors of the buccal mucosa, retromolar trigone, hard palate, and gingiva, radiation therapy to the primary site and ipsilateral neck can be considered.
- For larger lesions or node positive tumors in these locations, we have generally advocated treatment of both necks.
- For tongue cancers and floor of mouth tumors we have generally considered radiation therapy to both necks in patients that warrant irradiation.
- See the section Postoperative Radiation Therapy.

Oropharynx Cancer

- The incidence of oropharyngeal carcinoma is increasing.
- This is likely due to an increase in human papillomavirus (HPV)-associated tumors, with estimates that currently around 70% of all newly diagnosed tumors are associated with HPV.
- Data demonstrates that HPV-associated tumors carry a favorable prognosis.
- In the RTOG 0129 study, HPV-associated tumors had a 3-year overall survival of 82.4% versus a 3-year overall survival of 57.1%.
- It should be noted that HPV associated tumors in smokers with a greater than 10-pack-year history of smoking have a worse prognosis than nonsmokers.
- Current trials are aimed and potentially deescalating therapy for HPV associated tumors.

- Patients with early staged tumors undergoing radiation can be treated with radiation alone.
- Advanced disease is usually treated with concurrent chemoradiation.
- Patients with small, well-lateralized tumors with no or minimal nodal disease can be considered for ipsilateral only irradiation.

Salivary Gland Tumors

- Salivary gland tumors are managed surgically, with adjuvant irradiation based on the results of final pathology.
- Radiation should be considered in patients with high-grade tumors, node positive tumors, in cases with close or positive margins, perineural invasion, and in patients with recurrent tumors.
- In the particular instance of adenoid cystic carcinomas, adjuvant irradiation should always be given.
    (a) In this situation, consideration should be given to radiate the pathway of any named nerves involved with perineural invasion to their location at the base of skull.
    (b) For example, in an adenoid cystic carcinoma of the parotid, irradiation would be given to the path of the 7th cranial nerve to the base of skull, in order to decrease the rate of relapse due tracking of tumor cells along the nerve.

Postoperative Radiation Therapy

- Radiation therapy is often offered to patients postoperatively depending on the final pathologic results.
- Potential indications for irradiation include
    (a) Close (< 5 mm) or positive margins
    (b) Extracapsular extension of lymph nodes
    (c) Multiple nodes positive
    (d) T3-T4 primary tumors
    (e) Perineural invasion
    (f) Lymphovascular invasion
- In the case of positive margins or extracapsular extension of lymph nodes chemotherapy (preferably with cisplatin) concurrently with irradiation should be considered.
- The timing of radiation in the postoperative setting matters, and data has shown the ideal time period from the date of surgery until the completion of irradiation is 11 weeks.
- This implies that radiation, which is usually 6.0 to 6.5 weeks in length, should optimally start 4 to 5 weeks post surgery.

Reirradiation

- Failures arising in an irradiated field are difficult to manage.
- The ideal treatment in this situation is surgical resection.
- Often, however, if surgery is not possible, and a repeat course of irradiation therapy is the only potentially curative option.

- Reirradiation is potentially curative for a minority of patients. In highly selected patient populations it is associated with a 2-year survival of approximately 10% to 30%.
- Reirradiation therapy has a potentially high likelihood of toxicity and patient selection is paramount.
- The time interval between the initial course of irradiation and the consideration of re-irradiation is of critical importance.
- Recurrences that occur < 1 year after the initial course of irradiation are likely somewhat radiation resistant, and likely are the poorest candidates for re-irradiation.
- The ideal patient is one who has a new primary cancer in an area that was previously irradiated many years ago.
- Effort must be made to limit overlap and in the case of reirradiation we have typically only treated gross tumor alone with no elective irradiation.
- We have also typically reirradiated in conjunction with radiosensitizing chemotherapy.
- The dose used in the reirradiation setting varies by institution, but our approach has been to use 60 Gy, which is considerably lower than one would use in the upfront setting.
- Consideration should be given to hyperfractionated irradiation when performing reirradiation, that is, breaking of the daily dose of irradiation into two fractions given 6 hours apart.
  (a) This has been shown to lead to less late toxic effects.
  (b) A commonly used regiment with this approach is 1.2 Gy given twice daily to a total dose of 60 Gy.
  (c) The downside of this approach is the logistical issues of requiring a patient to come to the radiation center twice daily.
- One can also consider reirradiation in the adjunct setting. This was tested in a randomized trial and shown to lead to an improvement in locoregional control and disease-free survival, although no overall survival benefit was noted. Toxicity was significant with nearly 40% of patients having Grade 3-4 late toxicity at 2 years.

Neck Dissection Following Definitive Chemoradiation

- The practice of elective neck dissection for patients undergoing chemoradiation has generally fallen out of favor due to high rates of neck dissection which showed no residual tumor.
- Prospective study has supported our current approach of performing a 12-week post-therapy PET/CT scan and observing patients with PET-negative disease.

Bibliography

Ang KK, et al. *Human papillomavirus and survival of patients with oropharyngeal cancer.* (1533-4406 (Electronic)).

Ang KK, et al. *Randomized trial addressing risk features and time factors of surgery plus radiotherapy in advanced head-and-neck cancer.* (0360-3016 (Print)).

Bernier J, et al. *Defining risk levels in locally advanced head and neck cancers: a comparative analysis of concurrent postoperative radiation plus chemotherapy trials of the EORTC (#22931) and RTOG (# 9501).* (1043-3074 (Print)).

Forastiere AA, et al. *Concurrent chemotherapy and radiotherapy for organ preservation in advanced laryngeal cancer.* (1533-4406 (Electronic)).

Induction chemotherapy plus radiation compared with surgery plus radiation in patients with advanced laryngeal cancer. The Department of Veterans Affairs Laryngeal Cancer Study Group. (0028-4793 (Print)).

Janot F, et al. *Randomized trial of postoperative reirradiation combined with chemotherapy after salvage surgery compared with salvage surgery alone in head and neck carcinoma.* (1527-7755 (Electronic)).

Questions

1. Patients found to have extracapsular extension following surgical resection should be treated with
   A. concurrent cisplatin
   B. concurrent cetuximab
   C. accelerated radiation alone
   D. observation

2. The dose of irradiation traditionally used for gross disease is
   A. 50 Gy
   B. 60 Gy
   C. 70 Gy
   D. 80 Gy

3. Radiation therapy is usually given in daily doses of
   A. 1 Gy/day
   B. 1.5 Gy/day
   C. 2 Gy/day
   D. 2.5 Gy/day

4. Which is true in general about larynx preservation?
   A. Rates of larynx preservation are generally < 50%.
   B. Larynx preservation allows a substantial percentage of patients to preserve their larynx, however, this comes at the cost of inferior survival.
   C. Induction chemotherapy followed by radiation offers the best chance of larynx preservation.
   D. The rate of larynx preservation in patients with gross penetration through the thyroid cartilage is less than 50%.

5. Studies have demonstrated that surgery and postoperative radiation should be completed in what time period for optimal results?
   A. 6 weeks
   B. 11 weeks
   C. 13 weeks
   D. 15 weeks

Chapter 42
Tumor Biology of Head and Neck Cancer

Recent advances in analyses of expression and alterations of genes and proteins has made it obvious that these tools will be critical for estimating prognosis and determining appropriate therapy for head and neck cancers. A recent effort, The Cancer Genome Atlas (TCGA), supported by the National Cancer Institute (NCI) has provided detailed information about common gene defects and expression patterns, as well as protein expression patterns found in head and neck squamous cell carcinoma (HNSCC). Although similar data is emerging for some salivary cancer types and molecular analyses of thyroid cancers are rapidly evolving, we will limit discussion here to HNSCC.

HPV-associated HNSCC should be considered a different disease from tobacco-associated or sporadic HNSCC that arises in nonsmokers. Clinically, HPV-positive (HPV(+)) HNSCC have much better survival than HPV-negative (HPV(−)), occur in a younger cohort with different risk factors, and have a distinct set of molecular defects driving the tumor. Because of these differences, HPV(−) and HPV(+) HNSCC will be presented separately.

HPV-Negative HNSCC

The etiology of HNSCC not associated with HPV is primarily driven by tobacco use. Tobacco carcinogens are thought to drive genetic changes that result in cancer. Common or distinct genetic events observed in HPV(−) HNSCC are categorized below. **Percentages listed are amongst HPV(−) HNSCC.**

    A. *Tumor suppressors* (inactivating events)
        i. P53: proliferation, apoptosis, genome maintenance
            a. Mutation: 80%
        ii. CDKN2A (p16INK4a): proliferation
            a. Mutation: 25%
            b. Deletion: 32%
            c. Methylation: 32%
        iii. FAT1: migration, proliferation
            a. Mutation: 25%
            b. Deletions: 7%
        iv. NOTCH1: differentiation
            a. Mutation: 20%
        v. CASP8: apoptosis
            a. Mutation 10% (linked with HRAS activation)

vi. Let-7c miRNA: differentiation
    a. Copy number loss: 35%
B. *Oncogenes* (activating events)
    i. PIK3CA: proliferation, survival
        a. Mutation: 19%
        b. Amplification: 20% (large amplicon 3q26-ter, not clear if PIK3CA is the target)
    ii. 11q13: amplification of multiple genes- 32%
        a. CCND1(cyclin D1): proliferation
        b. EMS1 (cortactin): migration, invasion, proliferation
        c. FADD: apoptosis (role as oncogene questionable)
    iii. EGFR: proliferation, survival
        a. Amplification: 12%
    iv. FGFR1: proliferation, survival
        a. Amplification: 12%
    v. HRAS: proliferation, migration, survival
        a. Mutation: 5% (linked with CASP8 mutations)

The most commonly amplified and deleted chromosomal regions and involved genes are
A. *Commonly amplified regions*
    i. 11q13: 32%
        a. Genes in amplicon: cyclin D1, EMS1 (cortactin), FADD
    ii. 3q26-ter: 20%
        a. Genes in amplicon: PIK3CA, p63, h-TERC, SOX2, others
    iii. 8q24: 14%
        a. Genes in amplicon: POU5F1B (functional isoform OCT4)
    iv. 7p11: 12%
        a. Genes in amplicon: EGFR
    v. 8p11: 12%
        a. Genes in amplicon: FGFR1
B. *Commonly deleted regions*
    i. 9p21: 32%
        a. Genes in deleted region: CDKN2A

Major Biological Pathways Altered in HPV(−) HNSCC and Genetic Alterations Driving These Pathways

Common names of genes are given m=mutation, a=amplification, d=deletion
    For amplification/deletions, chromosomal region is listed (eg, d:9p21 = deletion of chromosomal region 9p21)
A. Proliferation/Cell cycle: p53 (m), CDKN2A (p16^{INK4a}, m, d:9p21) , CCND1 (cyclin D1, a:11q13), EMS1 (cortactin, a:11q13), EGFR (a:7p21), FGFR (a:8p11), FAT1 (m), PIK3CA (m, a:3q26-ter), HRAS (m)
B. Survival/Apoptosis: p53 (m), PIK3CA (m, a:3q26-ter), HRAS (m), EGFR (a:7p11), FGFR1 (a:8p11), CASP8 (m)
C. Differentiation: NOTCH (m), p63 (a:3q26-ter),
D. Migration: EMS1 (a:11q13), HRAS (m), FAT1 (m)

HPV(+)

HPV-associated HNSCC are epidemiologically, biologically, and clinically different compared to HPV-negative head and neck cancers. Molecular differences distinguishing HPV(+) form

HPV(-) HNSCC, include distinct gene expression profiles and significantly fewer somatic mutations and chromosomal abnormalities in HPV-positive HNSCC. Since major HPV oncoproteins E6 and E7 inactivate p53 and Rb, respectively, HPV(+) HNSCCs almost always harbor wild-type p53 and express high levels of CDKN2A, which encodes p16^{INK4a}—the Rb upstream regulator. Irrespective of HPV status, head and neck squamous cancers demonstrate losses of 3p and 8p and gains of 3q and 8q chromosomal regions, suggesting commonalities of molecular pathogenesis.

Genetic events found in HPV(+) HNSCC are listed below.
A. *Tumor suppressors* (inactivating events)
    i. NOTCH1: differentiation
      a. Mutation: 17%
    ii. TRAF3: immunity
      a. Focal deletions and point mutations: 20%
    iii. let-7c miRNA: differentiation
      a. Copy number loss: 17%
B. *Oncogenes* (activating events)
    i. PIK3CA: proliferation, survival
      a. Mutation: 37%
      b. Amplification: 27% (large amplicon at 3q, not clear if PIK3CA is the target)
    ii. E2F1: proliferation, survival
      a. Focal amplifications: 19%
    iii. FGFR3: angiogenesis, cell migration
      a. Activating FGFR3-TACC3 fusion: 6%

The most commonly amplified and deleted chromosomal regions and involved genes are
A. *Commonly amplified regions*
    i. 3q: 27%; genes in amplicon (possible targets): PIK3CA, p63, h-TERC, SOX2, others
    ii. 8q: 17%
B. *Commonly deleted regions*
    i. 3p: 11%

Major Biological Pathways Altered in HPV(+) HNSCC and Genetic Alterations Driving these Pathways

Names of genes are given; m=mutation, a=amplification, d=deletion, f=fusion.
A. Proliferation/cell cycle: p53(inactivated by HPV E6), Rb (inactivated by HPV E7), PIK3CA (m, a:3q26-ter), E2F1 (focal a)
B. Survival/apoptosis: PIK3CA (m, a:3q26-ter), FGFR3 (FGFR3-TACC3 f)
C. Immunity: TRAF3 (focal d and m)
D. Differentiation: NOTCH1 (m), p63 (a:3q26-ter)

Differences Between HPV(+) and HPV(−) HNSCC Protein Expression and Activation; RPPA

Using reverse phase protein array (RPPA), our group evaluated expression of 137 total and phosphorylated proteins in 29 HPV(+) and 12 HPV(−) prospectively collected HNSCCs. 33 proteins and 8 phosphoproteins were expressed in tumors in HPV-dependent manner. Four major pathways that distinguish HPV(+) from HPV(−) HNSCCs include: (1) DNA repair, (2) cell cycle, (3) apoptosis, and (4) PI3K/AKT/mTOR.

A. DNA repair is the largest functional category of differentially expressed proteins (12 of 41 differentially expressed proteins (29%), including PARP1, BRCA2, PCNA, and XRCC1) with total protein levels significantly upregulated in HPV(+) as compared to HPV(−) tumors.

B. Cell cycle: Due to HPV E7-dependent downregulation of Rb, which in turn unleashes transcriptional activity of E2F1, HPV(+) tumors express lower levels of Rb and higher levels of S and G2/M cyclins E1 and B1. In contrast, HPV(−) HNSCC expresses higher levels of cyclin D1 and corresponding higher levels of phospho-Rb.

C. Increased markers of **apoptosis,** including cleavage of caspases 3 and 7, were found in HPV(+) tumors.

D. PI3K/AKT/mTOR: Mutant PIK3CA in HPV(+) tumors preferentially activates the mTOR, but not AKT pathway. Direct Akt targets, including phospho-Raf, phospho-GSK3β and phospho-TSC2, were expressed at relatively lower levels in HPV(+) tumors.

Brief Mechanistic Description for Major Players in HPV(+) and HPV(−) HNSCC

- **P53** is one of the two major tumor suppressors in human cancer, and p53 function must be altered by some means in all or nearly all cancers. P53 functions in response to abnormal proliferative signals, DNA damage, viral infection and other cellular stresses resulting in cell cycle arrest or death. HPV(-) HNSCC inactivate p53 through mutation in the vast majority of cases, while tumors driven by HPV express the E6 viral oncoprotein to degrade and inactivate p53. P53 inhibits **survival** and **proliferation** and is an effector of **DNA damage response**.

- **Retinoblastoma (Rb)** is the other major tumor suppressor in human cancer, and like p53 its function is universally, or nearly universally inhibited in tumors. Unlike p53 there are few mutations in Rb in HNSCC; however, Rb is inhibited in nearly all HPV(−) HNSCC by loss of CDKN2A (p16) or amplification of CCND1 (cyclin D1). HPV(+) tumors inactivate Rb through expression of the vial oncoprotein, E7. Rb is a major regulator of **cell cycle and proliferation**.

- **CDKN2A (p16^{INK4a})** binds and inhibits cyclin-dependent kinase 4 and 6 (CDK4/CDK6) preventing their phosphorylation and inhibition of Rb. Loss of p16INK4a allows CDK4 or CDK6 (see below) to inactivate Rb, which promotes **proliferation**. Of interest and clinical utility, p16 is highly expressed in HPV(+) HNSCC due to Rb inactivation by HPV E7.

- **CCND1 (cyclin D1)** binds to CDK4 or CDK6 activating them to phosphorylate and inactivate Rb. Cyclin D1 family member, cyclin D2, is also amplified in a small percentage of HNSCC (3%). Overexpression of cyclin D1 inhibits Rb, which promotes **proliferation**.

- **E2F1** is a transcription factor that is inhibited by Rb, which tethers it preventing its entry into the nucleus. In the nucleus, E2F1 is a transcription factor that transcribes many genes to **promote proliferation**. E2F1 is amplified in 19% of HPV(+) tumors.

- **HPV16 E6 oncoprotein** in combination with a cellular protein, E6-associated protein, ubiquitinates p53 resulting in its degradation, therefore **inhibiting apoptosis and promoting uncontrolled proliferation**.

- **HPV16 E7 oncoprotein** inactivates Rb via direct binding, ubiquitination, and protesome-dependent degradation, resulting in release and activation of transcriptional factor E2F driving expression of S-phase genes, **deregulating cell cycle and promoting cellular replication**.
- **FAT1** is a protocadherin that inhibits WNT signaling by inhibiting b-catenin. Mutations in FAT1 allow b-catenin signaling which promotes **proliferation and migration** and has a role in stem cell maintenance.
- **NOTCH1** is a transmembrane receptor that signals after binding of ligands Delta-like-1 and Jagged-1. For signaling, NOTCH is cleaved by γ-secretase releasing a portion of the Notch intracellular domain that translocates to the nucleus. NOTCH1 can function as an oncogene or tumor suppressor depending on cell context. In HNSCC, mutations are inactivating suggesting that NOTCH1 acts as a tumor suppressor. Notch signaling plays a role in cellular **differentiation.**
- **EGFR** (epidermal growth factor receptor) is a receptor tyrosine kinase activated by binding to epidermal growth factor or other ligands. EGFR family members include HER2 that is amplified in a small percentage of HNSCC (3%). Signaling through EGFR promotes **survival and proliferation**.
- **FGFR1** (fibroblast growth factor receptor 1) is a receptor tyrosine kinase activated by binding to its ligands, fibroblast growth factors. Signaling through FGFR1 promotes **survival and proliferation**.
- **FGFR3** (fibroblast growth factor receptor 3) is a receptor tyrosine kinase that plays an important role in the regulation of **cell proliferation and apoptosis**.
- **PIK3CA** is the catalytic subunit of the phosphoinositide 3-kinase that converts phosphatidylinositol 4,5 bi-phosphate (PIP2) to phosphatidylinositol 3,4,5 tri-phosphate (PIP3). PTEN is a tumor suppressor that catalyzes the opposite conversion of PIP3 to PIP2 and is lost in a low percent of HNSCC. Activation of PIK3CA results in PI3K signaling through AKT, mTOR and other targets to promote **proliferation and survival**.
- **HRAS** is an oncogene activated by binding to GTP stimulated by upstream signaling from receptor tyrosine kinases and other receptors. Ras is inactivated by hydrolysis of GTP to GDP and mutations prevent this inactivation. HRAS signals through PI3K, RAF and MAPK, and RALGDS to promote **proliferation and survival**.
- **TRAF3** is a member of the TNF receptor associated factor (TRAF) protein family. The protein has an important role in activating type I interferon response against DNA viruses; it also negatively regulates the alternative NF-kB pathway. Inactivation of TRAF3 exclusively in HPV(+) HNSCC most likely represents a mechanism for escape of **both innate and acquired anti-viral responses**.
- **Let-7c microRNA (miRNA)** is a candidate tumor suppressor that controls cell **proliferation and differentiation**.

Questions

1. Which one of the following is not a tumor suppressor gene?
   A. p53
   B. FAT1
   C. NOTCH1
   D. EGFR

2. Which type of HNSCC has better survival?
   A. HPV+
   B. HPV−

3. Which type of HNSCC has more somatic mutations and chromosomal abnormalities?
   A. HPV+
   B. HPV−

4. Which one of the following is not an oncogene?
   A. FGFR1
   B. HRAS
   C. TRAF3
   D. PIK3CA

5. Loss of which chromosome arm is common in HNSCC?
   A. 3p
   B. 3q
   C. 8q
   D. 10p

Chapter 43
Skull Base Surgery

Introduction

Advances in surgical technique as well as strategies to deliver adjuvant radiation therapy in the last few decades have drastically improved outcomes in patients with malignant tumors invading the skull base. Tumors of the upper aerodigestive tract and neck involving the intracranial space can now be addressed with the combined expertise of head and neck surgeons and neurological surgeons.

Approaches

Procedures are classified as anterior, middle and posterior according to the cranial fossa to which the surgery is directed. In addition lesions of the midline such as the region of the sella turcica and clivus require a central approach. Far lateral approaches are utilized for access to the region of the brain stem and medulla (Figure 43-1). Expanded endonasal approaches to sinonasal malignancies involving the skull base have also been described for select anterior skull base malignancies.

Anatomy

Anterior Skull Base

The anterior skull base is defined as the bony partition between the frontal lobes in the anterior cranial fossa and the midline and paramedian facial structures including nasal cavity and eyes.

The gyri of the frontal lobes overlie most of the anterior cranial fossa, the ocular gyri and gyrus rectus lie lateral to the midline. The floor of the anterior cranial fossa is composed of ethmoid, sphenoid, and frontal bones. Anteriorly it forms the crista galli and cribiform plate of the ethmoid bone and covers the upper nasal cavity. The crista galli defines the midline of the anterior skull base. Posteriorly it forms the planum sphenoidale. Laterally the frontal bone and lesser wing of the sphenoid form the roof or the orbit and the optic canal; blending medially into the anterior clinoid process. The cribiform plate is the thinnest portion of the ethmoid bone and transmits the first cranial nerve to the olfactory fossa through multiple foramina.

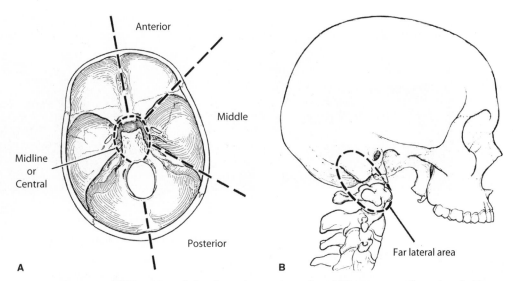

Figure 43-1 (A) Diagram outlining the various regions of cranial base surgery. (*Reproduced with permission from Donald PJ: Surgery of the Skull Base. Philadelphia, PA: Lippincott-Raven; 1998.*) (B) The far lateral approach.

Infratemporal Fossa

The infratemporal fossa is located inferiorly to the temporal fossa. The temporalis muscle is located in the temporal fossa and inserts into the coronoid process and down the mandibular ramus. Distally the temporalis muscle traverses deep to the zygomatic arch forming the lateral wall of the infratemporal fossa. The roof of the infratemporal fossa is the floor of the middle cranial fossa.

The boundaries of the infratemporal fossa include the maxillary sinus anteriorly, the parotid gland posteriorly, the ascending ramus of the mandible and the temporalis muscle laterally, the zygomatic arch and the greater wing of the sphenoid superiorly as well as the pterygoid fascia medially. It includes the parapharyngeal space containing the internal carotid artery, internal jugular vein, CN VI to XII and the masticator space that contains the maxillary and mandibular branches of the trigeminal nerve, the internal maxillary artery, the pterygoid venous plexus and the pterygoid muscles. The infratemporal fossa is connected to the middle cranial fossa via multiple foramina (ie, carotid canal, jugular foramen, foramen spinosum, foramen ovale, foramen lacerum).

Middle Cranial Fossa

The middle cranial fossa contains the temporal lobe of the brain. The anterior wall of this fossa is penetrated medially by the superior orbital fissure and the optic canal. The floor of the middle cranial fossa is composed of temporal bone and to a small extent the lesser wing of the sphenoid. Both petrous pyramids of the temporal bone meet in the middle where they articulate with the sphenoid bone that is aerated by the sphenoid sinus and indented superiorly by the sella turcica.

The Gasserian ganglion situated in Meckel Cave and the mandibular branch (V3) of the trigeminal nerve exiting through the foramen ovale are the key anatomical structure of the middle fossa. Meckel cave and the trigeminal ganglion are located medially near the apex of the petrous bone. Along the anterior border of the petrous bone are also the Glasscock and Kawase triangles.

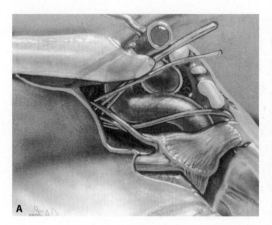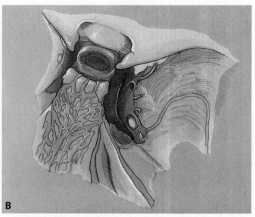

Figure 43-2 (A) The cavernous sinus showing the cranial nerves and the ICA. (B) The venous connections to the cavernous sinus.

The boundaries of Glasscock triangle form a line from the foramen spinosum to the facial nerve hiatus laterally, the greater superficial petrosal medially and the V3 anteriorly. Kawase triangle is made by the greater superficial petrosal nerve laterally, the petrous ridge medially, and the arcuate eminence at the base. The petrous carotid artery is found beneath the greater superficial petrosal nerve. V3 travels inferiorly to the infratemporal fossa. The foramen rotundum is also medially located and carries V2 to the pterygopalatine fossa. Foramen spinosum houses the middle meningeal artery. The internal carotid artery runs under the Gasserian ganglion and is separated from it by a thin plate of bone.

The cavernous sinus receives the internal carotid artery as it ascends the foramen lacerum. It is located laterally to the sphenoid sinus and contains the third, fought and sixth cranial nerves, the former two in a double fold of dura in its lateral wall and the latter in a sparse adventitia of the lateral wall of the ICA (Figure 43-2). In addition numerous extracranial veins and dural venous sinuses connect in the cavernous sinus including the superior and inferior petrosal sinuses posteriorly and the sphenoparietal sinus anteriorly. The cavernous sinus connects to the contralateral sinus via the circular sinus around the pituitary and the basilar plexus across the clivus.

Temporal Bone/Petrous Apex

The temporal bone has four parts: mastoid, squamosa, tympanic, and petrous. The petrous apex is shaped like a pyramid and is located between the middle and posterior fossae. The petrous apex forms three surfaces, anterior (temporal), posterior (posterior fossa), and inferior (occipital).

Anterior Surface

The anterior superior surface forms the middle fossa floor. The arcuate eminence is the bulge along the superior surface overlying the superior semicircular canal. The facial hiatus transmits the greater superficial petrosal nerve and exits anterolaterally to the arcuate eminence.

Posterior Surface

The posterior surface of the petrous apex is the anterolateral wall of the posterior cranial fossa. It extends medially from the posterior semicircular canal and the endolymphatic sac to the petroclinoid ligament and the canal for the abducens nerve (Dorello canal). It is bounded superiorly and inferiorly by the superior and inferior petrosal sinuses. The internal auditory (IAC) canal lies midway across its surface. The lateral portion of the IAC is divided into a superior and an inferior portion by a horizontal ridge called the transverse or falciform crest. The facial nerve and superior vestibular nerve are superior to this crest while the cochlear nerve and inferior vestibular nerve are inferior to this crest. The facial nerve is located anterior to the superior vestibular nerve and is separated by a vertical ridge of bone called Bill bar. The endolymphatic duct lies on the posteroinferior face of the temporal bone. The vestibular aqueduct enters the temporal bone lateral to the operculum and travels to the inferior surface of the vestibule.

Inferior Surface

The inferior surface is bounded by the jugular bulb and the inferior petrosal sinus. It contains the carotid canal situated anterior to the jugular foramen and medial to the styloid process. It proceeds superiorly to the petrous apex and turns 90 degrees anteromedially. The digastric ridge runs sagittally medial to the mastoid tip and intersects with the stylomastoid foramen. The styloid process is anterior to the stylomastoid foramen. The jugular foramen is medial to the styloid process. The jugular bulb lies in the lateral compartment. The mastoid compartment contains cranial nerves nine, ten and eleven. The cochlear aqueduct enters medially between the jugular fossa and the carotid canal. The spine of the sphenoid is anterior to the vertical segment of the carotid canal. The cartilaginous portion of the Eustachian tube begins medial to the spine of the sphenoid. The hypoglossal canal is medial and inferior to the jugular foramen.

Clinical Investigation

History and Physical Examination

Timing, progression and quality of symptoms should be evaluated. Any aggravating or alleviating factors should be noted. For patients that have had previous treatment past operative and pathology reports, laboratory tests and records of previous examinations should be reviewed. The most common symptoms associated with base of skull neoplasms are anosmia, blindness or diplopia when the orbit or cavernous sinus is invaded, facial numbness when the trigeminal nerve is involved and dysphagia or hoarseness with involvement of the jugular foramen. Facial pain usually indicates a locally advanced malignancy with perineural spread. Trismus is an important symptom as it is common in sinus malignancies with posterior extension or pharyngeal carcinomas with involvement of the pterygoid region. Rare presenting symptoms seen mostly in locally advanced disease include headache and clear rhinorrhea (CSF leak).

Physical examination should be performed in a systematic fashion as outlined below.

- Face/Scalp skin: examined for any premalignant or malignant lesions. Any scars of previous skin excisions should be noted and discussed with the patient.
- Eyes: The symmetry of the orbits should be compared and any proptosis or differences in scleral show should be noted. Ectropion can be found in cases of facial nerve paralysis. The conjunctiva should be evaluated for erythema or irritation. Pupil size and reactivity as well as visual field testing are important. Extraocular mobility should be evaluated in 9 directions (up, down, right, left, and diagonally right up, right down, left up, left down). Spontaneous nystagmus should be evaluated by having the patient wear Frenzel lenses while gaze nystagmus is elicited by having the patient follow the examiners finger performing a "cross" type movement. Positional nystagmus is provoked by the Dix-Hallpike maneuver.
- Ears: The skin of the pinna and the external auditory canal should be evaluated as well as the postauricular skin. The tympanic membrane should be evaluated with pneumatic otoscopy and microscopic otoscopy when evaluation with handheld otoscope is suspicious. Tuning fork evaluation is an essential part of the otologic examination.

- Nasal cavity/Nasopharynx: Anterior rhinoscopy with or without decongestion will reveal abnormalities of the septum, turbinates, and nasal mucosa. When pathology is noted rigid endoscopy provides a better visualization of the paranasal sinus meatus to evaluate extent of disease. The nasopharynx should be evaluated endoscopically with focus on the Eustachian tubes, Fossa of Rosenmuller, posterior and lateral pharyngeal wall and palate mucosa and mobility.
- Oral cavity/Oropharynx: Carefully evaluate oral mucosa, teeth, and tongue. Tongue should be evaluated for movement, atrophy or fasciculations. In the case of hypoglossal nerve dysfunction the tongue will deviate toward the lesion. The drainage from the parotid and submandibular ducts should be evaluated while massaging the corresponding salivary glands. The oropharynx begins at the boundary of the hard and soft palate superiorly and the circumvallate papillae inferiorly. The mucosa of the palatine tonsils, the lingual tonsils, the soft palate and the lateral and posterior pharyngeal walls should be evaluated carefully with direct visualization, mirror examination and/or fiberoptic endoscopy. The movement of the palate as well as presence of a gag reflex should be noted. The base of tongue and tonsils should be palpated and any symmetry noted.
- Larynx: Evaluation of vocal cord mobility and laryngeal sensation is important in evaluation of skull base lesions. Videostroboscopy can provide detailed information related to anatomy and function when needed.
- Neck: Careful palpation should be performed. Mobility, location, and size should be noted. Vertically fixed masses raise suspicion for carotid body tumor.
- Cranial nerves: A full cranial nerve examination is imperative in all skull base cases.

Radiography

- CT/MRI scan: Complementary and essential in every case, should be obtained in axial, coronal and sagittal planes. Fine cut CT scan has advantage of detecting bone erosion. MRI with Gadolinium based IV-contrast with fat-suppression software is employed to differentiate fat from tumor tissue. MRI can narrow down the differential diagnosis for lesions of the cerebellopontine angle and the petrous apex (Table 43-1).
- Angiogram: Useful for hypervascular lesions such as glomus tumors, carotid body tumors or juvenile angiofibromas. Also useful in cases of suspected carotid artery invasion. Balloon test occlusion is useful in assessing cerebral perfusion through the noninvolved internal carotid artery. This helps determine if carotid bypass will be needed in cases where sacrifice of the internal carotid artery is expected.
- PET CT: Positron emission tomography is most useful in detecting recurrence or distant metastatic disease.

Table 43-1 MRI Findings of Cerebellopontine Angle and Petrous Apex Lesions

Tumor	T_1	T_1-Gad	T_2
Vestibular schwannoma	Iso or mildly hypointense	Marked enhancement	Moderately Hyperintense
Meningioma	Iso or mildly hypointense	Marked enhancement	Hypo to hyperintense
Cholesteatoma (epidemoid)	Hypointense (variable)	No enhancement	Hyperintense
Arachnoid cyst	Hypointense	No enhancement	Hyperintense
Lipoma	Hyperintense	No enhancement	Intermediate
Cholesterol granuloma	Hyperintense	No enhancement	Hyperintense

Preparation

While some tumors of this region (ie, angiofibromas, acoustic neuromas, meningiomas and paragangliomas) can sometimes be diagnosed by radiographic imaging, others will require a pathological diagnosis. In the case of deep tumors were fine needle aspiration may not be feasible, diagnosis should be pursued through an endoscopic skull base approach. Due to the complexity of anatomy and surgical planning in this area tissue diagnosis before embarking on "en-bloc" resection is paramount as resection often involves sacrifice of critical neurovascular structures. Unresectability criteria include invasion of the brain stem, involvement of both internal carotid arteries, involvement of both cavernous sinuses, invasion of brain parenchyma that if resected will lead to poor quality of life and invasion of the spinal cord. Invasion of the optic chiasm would lead to bilateral blindness and is a relative contraindication. Patient factors such as distant metastasis, multiple comorbidities, and lack of consent should also be taken into account. In addition patients with chemo or radio responsive tumors, that is lymphoma, should not undergo surgical resection.

Extensive surgery of the skull base can entail placement of a tracheostomy, lumbar drain, temporary tarsorrhaphy or gold weight in eyelids, anesthetic vascular monitoring and installation of scalp electrodes to monitor brain activity if carotid artery clamping is anticipated.

Anterior Skull Base

Malignancies of the Anterior Skull Base

A. Epithelial
    i. Squamous cell carcinoma of sinonasal origin
    ii. Minor salivary gland malignancies
        a. *Adenoid Cystic carcinoma*
        b. *Mucoepidermoid carcinoma*
        c. *Adenocarcinoma*
    iii. Neuroendocrine carcinoma
    iv. Mucosal melanoma
    v. Olfactory neuroblastoma
    vi. Sinonasal undifferentiated carcinoma
B. Nonepithelial
    i. Chordoma
    ii. Chondrosarcoma
    iii. Osteogenic sarcoma
    iv. Soft tissue sarcoma
        a. *Fibrosarcoma*
        b. *Malignant fibrous histiocytoma*
        c. *Hemangiopericytoma*
        d. *Angiosarcoma*
        e. *Kaposi Sarcoma*
        f. *Rhabdomyosarcoma*
    v. Lymphoproliferative
        a. *Lymphoma*
        b. *Polymorphic reticulosis*
        c. *Plasmacytoma*
C. Metastatic

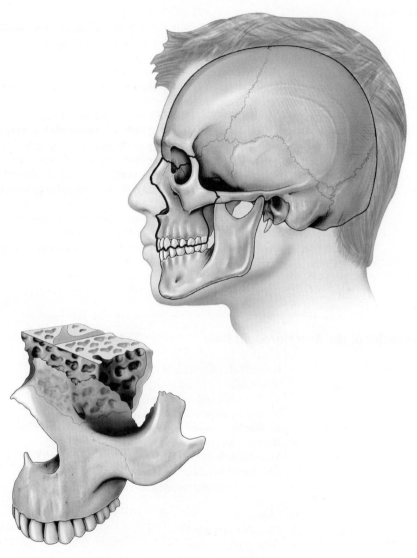

Figure 43-3 Anterior craniofacial resection with sparing of the orbit.

Craniofacial Resection (Figure 43-3)

A. Lateral rhinotomy incision or midface degloving.
B. Medial maxillary ostectomy with registering of fixation plates first.
C. Can extend to total maxillectomy if tumor is extensive.
D. Ethmoidectomy and medial maxillectomy.
E. If tumor invades to the posterior maxillary wall, remove.
F. If pterygomaxillary space invaded drill pterygoid plates and remove soft tissue with adequate margin.

G. Drill out anterior wall and floor of sphenoid sinus.
H. Small portions of the lateral sphenoid wall and the medial cavernous sinus can be removed with care not to disrupt the ICA.
I. Palatal muscles can be removed if involved.
J. The Eustachian tubes are removed if the lateral wall of the nasopharynx is involved.
K. At the completion of the extracranial portion margins are checked. Only the anterior cranial floor should have residual tumor.
L. Bicoronal flap raised with preservation of the pericranium.
M. Posterior scalp is raised to give appropriate length to pericranial flap.
N. Two parallel incisions are made in the calvarial periosteum on either side of the frontal skull to the origin of the temporalis muscle. Incisions are connected across the vertex posterior to the scalp incision. The flap is elevated down to the supraorbital rims.
O. The pericranial flap is pedicled on the supraorbital and supratrochlear vessels.
P. Neurosurgeon performs a low small craniotomy to extirpate intracranial extent of tumor.
Q. Tumor invading dura or brain should be cleared by a margin of 5 mm.
R. The neurosurgeon delineates the circumference of tumor penetrating the anterior fossa floor and clears areas involved with a margin of 5 to 10 mm.
S. Multiple frozen sections are obtained to ensure clear margins.
T. The dura is repaired with temporalis fascia, fascia lata, lyophilized dura, or bovine pericardium grafts.
U. The pericranial flap is placed under the dural reconstruction and wedged between the healthy dura and beyond the posterior extremity of the defect and the residual anterior fossa floor at this site.
V. A dacryocystorhinostomy can be considered with placement of sialastic stent through the lacrimal pucta if the duct has been severed.
W. Free microvascular flaps are reserved for cases requiring a total maxillectomy, facial skin or an extensive resection of the infratemporal fossa resulting in a large cavity.
X. Orbital exenteration is usually indicated with gross invasion of the periorbital fat, extraocular muscles, or optic nerve.
Y. Orbital exenteration: periorbita is incised over the superior and lateral orbital rims. Dissection continues along the roof of the orbit and lateral walls until the superior orbital fissure (SOF) and the optic foramen are exposed. Lidocaine is injected around these structures to prevent autonomic-induced cardiac arrhythmias. The neurovascular structures of the SOF are carefully ligated and divided. The optic nerve and ophthalmic artery are also ligated and divided. The extraocular muscles are transected at the orbital apex. The medial and inferior orbital wall should be removed en bloc in patients with sinonasal carcinoma.

Expanded Endonasal Endoscopic Approach to Anterior Skull Base

-   Benefits include the avoidance of large transfacial and scalp incisions, better visualization through magnification and angled scopes as well as avoidance of brain retraction.
-   Can be combined with small craniotomy approach in some cases.
-   Recent case series have quoted a 5-year survival of up to 60%, in endoscopic management of sinonasal malignancies, which is comparable to that achieved with the traditional craniofacial approach.
-   Randomized controlled trials comparing both open and endoscopic techniques, however, are still not available due to the difficulty in designing a trial with these two surgical arms due to ethical and logistical reasons.

- Drawbacks include limited lateral exposure, problems with hemostasis, and high incidence of CSF leak.
- Ideal for small midline lesions.
- Contraindications include:
  (a) Orbital involvement
  (b) Involvement of far lateral maxillary sinus
  (c) Dural involvement lateral to the orbit
  (d) Invasion of brain parenchyma
  (e) Cavernous sinus or carotid involvement
  (f) Lesion lateral to the cavernous carotid or superolateral to the optic nerve
- In sinonasal malignancies the site of origin of the tumor should be removed en bloc with adequate margins.
- Water tight closure of the skull base defect is paramount.
- Hadad-Bassagasteguy flap (pedicled nasoseptal mucosal flap) has been shown to reduce incidence of CSF leak.
- Procedure:
  (a) Nasoseptal flap harvested and tucked in nasopharynx.
  (b) Tumor is debulked endonasally to visualize margins, origin and site of skull base involvement.
  (c) Maxillary sinus antrostomies, ethmoidectomy, and sphenoidotomy performed for identification of landmarks of the nasal cavity and visualization of the optic and carotid canals.
  (d) May resect posterior wall of frontal sinus, medial wall of orbits, roof of sphenoid and septum if needed for adequate margins.
  (e) A Draf III procedure is performed to remove the floor of the frontal sinus.
  (f) The nasal septum is transected below the tumor to the sphenoid rostrum.
  (g) The anterior and posterior ethmoid arteries are ligated and divided at skull base.
  (h) The anterior skull base is drilled thin and elevated, it is removed from the crista galli to the planum sphenoidale and from the medial orbital wall to the contralateral medial orbital wall.
  (i) The dura is cauterized and opened around tumor with adequate margin.
  (j) Cortical blood vessels are elevated and olfactory roots are transected.
  (k) Margins are confirmed through multiple frozen sections.
  (l) Closure of dural defect done in multilayered fashion. Can use dural graft matrix in the subdural space followed by fascia graft followed by nasoseptal flap. This is later secured in place using fibrin glue followed by gelfoam or fat.
  (m) Reconstruction is buttressed with nasal packing, the use of nasal trumpets can reduce the risk of pneumocephalus while preserving nasal airway. In certain cases tracheotomy can also be used to divert the flow of air and prevent pneumocephalus.

Surgery of the Infratemporal Fossa

    A. Three approaches described by Fisch et al.
      i. Type A: access to the temporal bone
      ii. Indications
        a. Glomus Tumors
        b. Salivary gland cancers
        c. Squamous cell carcinoma

   d. Cholesteatoma
   e. Neurinoma
   f. Meningioma
   g. Rhabdomyosarcoma, teratoma, myxoma
  iii. Type B: access to the clivus
  iv. Indications
   a. Chordoma
   b. Chondroma
   c. Squamous cell carcinoma
   d. Dermoid/epidermoid cysts
   e. Meningioma, craniopharyngioma, plasmacytoma, arachnoid cyst, and cranio-pharyngeal fistulae
  v. Type C: access to the parasellar region and nasopharynx
  vi. Indications
   a. Salvage surgery for squamous cell carcinoma
   b. Adenoid cystic carcinoma around Eustachian tube
   c. Advanced juvenile nasopharyngeal angiofibroma
 B. Approach to intratemporal fossa:
  i. C-shaped incision from the temporal region extending 4 cm postauricularly then down into the neck.
  ii. A periosteal flap pedicled on the EAC anteriorly is created.
  iii. EAC is transected at the bony cartilaginous junction deep to the periosteal flap.
  iv. The lateral EAC is everted and closed.
  v. The periosteal flap is rotated anteriorly and sutured to the closed EAC.
  vi. The neck dissection is performed and cranial nerves IX, X, XI, XII, internal carotid artery and internal jugular vein are exposed.
  vii. The facial nerve is identified at the stylomastoid foramen.
  viii. A mastoidectomy removing the mastoid tip, entire bony auditory canal, medial canal skin, tympanic membrane and middle ear contents is performed.
  ix. The facial nerve is translocated anteriorly at the stylomastoid foramen.
  x. The mandibular condyle is mobilized and the glenoid fossa is exposed.
  xi. The internal carotid artery is dissected from the neck to the skull base to its position below the cochlea.
  xii. The posterior and middle fossa dura can be opened to expose the cranial cavity when intracranial extension is present.
  xiii. Can sacrifice the labyrinth and/or cochlea to access the internal carotid artery, the petrous apex, the clivus or the anterior brain stem.
  xiv. Several techniques can be applied for reconstruction including recontouring with allogenic tissue matrix, temporalis muscle-fascia flap or microvascular free flap.
  xv. A layered closure is performed and a pressure dressing applied for 24 hours.

Surgery of the Middle Cranial Fossa

 A. **Tumors of the Middle Cranial Fossa:**
  i. Chordoma
  ii. Chondrosarcoma
  iii. Meningioma
  iv. Trigeminal schwanomma

     v. Osteosarcoma

    vi. Cholesteatoma

   vii. Cholesterol granuloma

  viii. Squamous cell carcinoma

    ix. Lymphoma

B. **Approach to Middle Cranial Fossa:**

  i. Combines infratemporal fossa approach with a small, low, middle fossa craniotomy.

    a. Incision begins near the midline of the calvarium, 2 cm behind the hairline. It is carried inferiorly in front of the ear for parotid, sinus and neck lesions or behind the ear for lesions of the temporal bone or clivus.

    b. The flap is elevated forward to the level of the lateral orbital rim and angle of the mandible.

    c. The external auditory canal (EAC) is severed across the bony cartilaginous junction.

    d. The temporal branch of the facial nerve is protected by elevating a patch of temporal fascia deep to the branch during the skin elevation.

    e. The ICA and internal jugular vein are identified in the neck to obtain proximal vascular control.

    f. The temporalis muscle is elevated through and incision made in the pericranium about 2 cm outside the periphery of its origin. The muscle is elevated to its insertion in the coronoid process of the mandible.

    g. The arch of the zygoma and the condyle of the mandible are removed (Figure 43-4)

    h. Under magnification, the tympanomeatal flap is raised and the middle ear is entered anteriorly, exposing the opening of the Eustachian tube.

    i. Using a small cutting burr, cuts are made within the tympanic annulus at 2 o'clock and 7 o'clock. The superior cut is directed superiorly into the middle ear, across the tensor tympani canal anterior to the cochleariform process into the superior part of the protympanum. The inferior cut is made across the hypotympanum into the mouth of the Eustachian tube.

    j. The external canal is then drilled down to the level of the dura into the squamosal part of the temporal bone superiorly and inferiorly through the thickness of the external canal into the glenoid fossa.

    k. The cut through the glenoid fossa is only about 2 mm deep and is directed toward the foramen spinosum where the middle meningeal artery is ligated.

    l. Neurosurgery performs small craniotomy through greater wing of the sphenoid and squamous temporal bone connecting the cut in the external auditory canal posteriorly to the pterygoid plates anteriorly.

    m. When bone flap is removed a greenstick fracture occurs so that the protympanum is fractured across and the internal carotid artery is exposed as it enters the posterior wall of the bony Eustachian tube.

    n. The internal carotid artery can be dissected from the fibrous ring at the opening of the carotid canal through the vertical and horizontal portions all the way to the cavernous sinus if involved with tumor.

    o. The tumor is removed en bloc and frozen sections are checked to ensure margins are negative.

    p. The carotid artery may be grafted if sacrifice necessary to clear margins versus leaving microscopic disease on the carotid adventitia.

    q. The Eustachian tube is removed subcranially to expose the nasopharynx. If involved the entire Eustachian tube and the clivus can be excised.

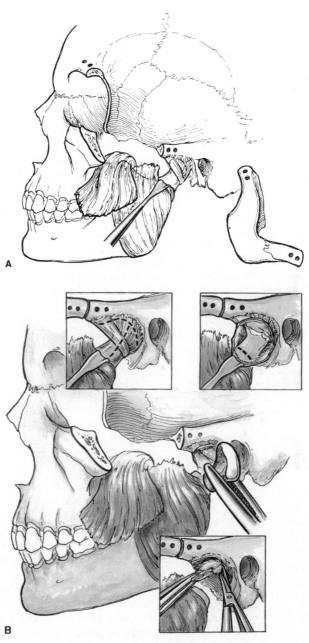

Figure 43-4 (A) Bony excision complete. (B) Condylectomy: Lateral aspect of the temporomandibular joint capsule is opened and connected to the mandibular neck. The condylar neck is transected and the condyle removed. The meniscus and attached soft tissue are removed. (*Reproduced with permission from Donald PJ:* Surgery of the Skull Base. *Philadelphia, PA: Lippincott-Raven; 1998.*)

  r. Dura is closed with fascia grafts and nasopharynx is separated from cranial cavity with either a pedicled temporalis muscle flap or a rectus abdominis free flap.

  s. Finally the craniotomy bone flap and zygomatic arch are plated into position.

The Far Lateral Approach

A. Appropriate for tumors originating from clivus, upper posterior neck or extending posteroinferiorly from the temporal bone.

B. Incision is a question mark beginning high in the occiput and coursing around the postauricular area descending to the upper neck.

C. Trapezius, splenius capitis, semispinalis capitis, and longissimus capitis are separated from the basioocciput exposing the cervical spine.

D. The bone of the spinous processes of the cervical spine is carefully drilled with care not to injure the vertebral artery.

E. Usually the vertebral artery can be taken safely if invaded by tumor.

F. If vertebral artery sacrifice is anticipated, a preoperative balloon occlusion test should be performed to establish the safety of sacrificing the artery.

G. If not sacrificed the artery is mobilized to the foramen magnum and the atlanto-occipital joint is exposed.

H. The lateral mass of the atlas is drilled away with care not to injure the occipital emissary vein and the hypoglossal canal.

I. Occipital craniotomy is performed.

J. Can extend resection up to the temporal bone with a mastoidectomy to expose the jugular bulb.

K. Neurosurgeon can perform an occipital-spinal fusion if concern for spinal instability.

L. A fascial graft can be used for dural closure if necessary.

M. The occipital bone graft is replaced and the muscles are reapproximated before closure.

Tumors of the Temporal Bone

- Glomus tumors are the most common lesions in this area.
  - (a) Glomus tumors are paragangliomas that arise from paraganglionic tissue derived from the migration of neural crest cells during embryonic development.
  - (b) May present with hearing loss, pulsatile tinnitus, vertigo, cranial nerve neuropathies (V, VI, VII, IX, X, XI and XII) aural pain or neck mass.
  - (c) Physical examination includes a full neurologic examination and otomicroscopic evaluation.
  - (d) 1% of paragangliomas display physiologically significant catecholamine secretion. Presence of tachycardia, arrhythmias, flushing or liable hypertension should prompt analysis of 24 hour urine specimen for vanillylmendelic acid, metanephrine and normetanephrine levels.
  - (e) Audiogram is required part of initial evaluation.
  - (f) CT scan, arteriography, MRI with gadolinium and MRA are useful to evaluate bone invasion, vascularity and soft tissue extension respectively.
  - (g) Two major classifications:
    - ○ Fisch classification
      - – Class A: limited to mesotypanum

    – Class B: limited to hypotympanum, mesotympanum and mastoid
    – Class C: involvement of infralabyrinthine components and extending to petrous apex
       ◊ Type C1 - limited involvement of the vertical portion of the carotid canal
       ◊ Type C2 - invading the vertical portion of the carotid canal
       ◊ Type C3 - invasion of the horizontal portion of the carotid canal
    – Class D: intracranial extension
       ◊ Type D1 - intracranial extension less than 2 cm in diameter
       ◊ Type D2 - intracranial extension greater than 2 cm in diameter
  ◦ Glasscock-Jackson classification
    – Glomus tympanicum:
       ◊ Small mass limited to the promontory filling the middle ear.
       ◊ Tumor completely filling middle ear space
       ◊ Tumor filling middle ear extending into mastoid
       ◊ Tumor filling middle extending into mastoid or through tympanic membrane to fill external auditory canal
    – Glomus jugulare:
       ◊ Involving jugular bulb, middle ear and mastoid
       ◊ Extending under internal auditory canal
       ◊ Extending into petrous apex, may have intracranial extension
       ◊ Extending beyond petrous apex into clivus or infratemporal fossa, may have intracranial extension

- Other tumors of the temporal bone
  - (a) EAC
    - ◦ Benign
      - Pleomorphic adenoma
      - Ceruminous adenoma
        - ◊ Malignant
          - * Squamous cell carcinoma
          - * Basal cell carcinoma
          - * Sarcoma
          - * Melanoma
          - * Lymphoma
          - * Adenocarcinoma
          - * Adenoid cystic carcinoma
          - * Ceruminous adenocarcinoma
  - (b) Middle ear and mastoid
    - ◦ Benign
      - Paraganglioma
      - Myxoma
      - Lipoma
      - Hemangioma
      - Schwannoma
      - Neurofibroma
      - Ostema
      - Chondroblastoma
      - Giant cell tumor
      - Meningioma
      - Teratoma

- ○ Malignant
  - – Squamous cell carcinoma
  - – Basal cell carcinoma
  - – Adenocarcinoma
  - – Carcinoid tumor
  - – Rhabdomyosarcoma
  - – Malignant paraganglioma
  - – Malignant schwanomma
  - – Hemangiopericytoma
  - – Osteosarcoma
  - – Chondrosarcoma
  - – Malignant germ cell tumor
- Staging of SCC of the temporal bone determines surgical approach
  - (a) T1 – Limited to EAC, no bone erosion – Lateral temporal bone resection
  - (b) T2 – Limited bony EAC erosion – Lateral temporal bone resection
  - (c) T3 – Full thickness EAC erosion with limited < 5 mm soft tissue involvement or middle ear involvement or facial paresis – Subtemporal temporal bone resection
  - (d) T4 – Erosion of cochlea, petrous apex, medial wall of middle ear, carotid canal, jugular foramen dura, and > 5 mm soft tissue involvement – total temporal bone resection
- Lateral temporal bone resection
  - (a) C shaped preauricular incision curved into a cervical neck crease
  - (b) In ear canal incision is made in the cartilaginous EAC encompassing the lesion.
  - (c) Auriculectomy or partial auriculectomy may be required.
  - (d) Stepped incision is made through the fascia, muscle, and periosteum.
  - (e) Flap elevated anteriorly to the root of the zygoma.
  - (f) Elevation of the soft tissues over the mastoid done in a subperiosteal plane.
  - (g) Ear canal is sectioned at the bony cartilageous junction and closed in multiple layers.
  - (h) The temporalis muscle and the temporoparietal fascia can be preserved and reflected forward to be used later in reconstruction.
  - (i) Mastoidectomy with skeletonization of the facial nerve, tegmen, sigmoid sinus and bony ear canal is performed.
  - (j) Extended facial recess approach is performed and dissection continues into glenoid fossa anteriorly. The incudostapedial joint is sectioned and the incus is removed.
  - (k) The tensor tympani is sectioned.
  - (l) The stylomastoid foramen is decompressed and the digastric muscle is exposed.
  - (m) A chisel is used to lightly cantilever the mobilized specimen.
  - (n) Parotidectomy and supraomohyoid neck dissection is performed for staging in a majority of patients.
  - (o) A rotational flap or rectus free flap may be required for closure if auriculectomy performed.
- Subtemporal bone temporal bone resection removed the temporal bone lateral to the petrous apex including the otic capsule and includes mobilization of the petrous carotid artery and an infratemporal fossa dissection.
- Total temporal bone resection includes resection of the petrous apex with or without resection of the petrous carotid artery. It involves an extensive infratemporal fossa dissection with mobilization or resection of the petrous carotid artery and middle and posterior fossa craniotomy.

Tumors of the Internal Auditory Canal and the Cerebellopontine Angle

- 90% of tumors at the cerebellopontine angle are acoustic schwanommas.
- 10% are either meningiomas, arachnoid cysts, cholesteatomas, facial neuromas or metastatic lesions.
- Acoustic neuromas are benign tumors of the superior and inferior vestibular nerves that originate at the junction of the Schwann cells and astrocytes typically in the internal auditory canal. Their growth rate is 1 to 4 mm per year on average.
- 95% occur in a sporadic fashion while 5% are associated with neurofibromatosis type 2 or familial acoustic neuroma.
- Up to 1/3 of acoustic neuromas remain stable in size when monitored over time.
- Hearing loss with gradual progression is the most common presenting symptom but 20% of patients can present with sudden-onset sensorineural hearing loss.
- Tinnitus is present in up to 70% of patients presenting with an acoustic tumor.
- Facial nerve deficits are observed in 10% of patients.

Approaches to the Internal Auditory Canal and Cerebellopontine Angle

- **Three approaches have been described:**
  (a) Translabyrinthine approach
    ○ Advantages
      − Minimized cerebellar retraction and potential subsequent atrophy
      − Less postoperative headaches
      − Visualize facial nerve prior to tumor dissection
    ○ Disadvantages
      − Up to 21% incidence of CSF fistula
      − Loss of residual hearing
      − Longer exposure time
  (b) Retrosigmoid approach
    ○ Advantages
      − Quicker approach
      − 50% hearing preservation in tumors less than 2 cm
    ○ Disadvantages
      − Twenty-three percent incidence of postoperative headache.
      − Requires cerebellar retraction with possible subsequent atrophy.
      − 7% to 21% incidence of CSF fistula.
      − In larger tumors, dissection precedes identification of the facial nerve.
  (c) Middle cranial fossa approach
    ○ Advantages
      − 50% to 75% chance of hearing preservation
      − Minimal risk of CSF fistula
    ○ Disadvantages
      − Slight increased risk to facial nerve if tumor originates on inferior vestibular nerve
      − Requires some temporal lobe retraction which could pose additional risks in the elderly

Translabyrinthine Approach

This approach was first introduced in 1904 by Panse but did not become a standard approach until its reintroduction by William House.

Technique

A. curved postauricular incision is made 3 cm behind the postauricular crease.
B. A complete mastoidectomy is performed.

C. The sigmoid sinus is skeletonized and only a very thin wafer of bone is left covering the sinus (Bill island).

D. Dura is exposed anterior and 2 cm posterior to the sinus allowing compression of the sinus for improved exposure.

E. A complete labyrinthectomy is performed.

F. The internal auditory canal is skeletonized 180°.

G. All bone covering the dura from the sigmoid sinus to the porus acousticus is removed as well as the bone covering the middle fossa dura.

H. The jugular bulb is skeletonized.

I. The intralabyrinthine segment of the facial nerve is identified together with the vertical crest (Bill bar) which separates the facial nerve from the superior vestibular nerve in the lateral most aspect of the IAC.

J. The dura over the IAC and posterior fossa is incised.

K. The superior vestibular nerve together with the tumor is reflected off of the facial nerve.

L. Tumor debulking proceeds with bipolar cautery, CO_2 laser, or Cavitron ultrasonic surgical aspirator (CUSA) together with microdissection.

M. The epitympanum is filled with temporalis fascia and open air cell tracts are occluded with bone wax.

N. Mastoid cavity is packed with abdominal fat.

O. Three layer closure of incision.

Transotic Approach

The transotic approach as described by Fisch is a modification of the translabyrinthine approach. It adds additional exposure anterior to the IAC and decreases the risk of a post-operative CSF fistula. In addition to the steps of a translabyrinthine approach, the following components are added:

Technique

A. A 4-cm-by-4 cm craniotomy is performed immediately posterior to the sigmoid sinus.

B. A dural flap is created and retracted.

C. Arachnoid is incised and CSF is drained from the cisterna magna.

D. The cerebellum is covered with a cottonoid and retracted posteriorly with a flat blade retractor.

E. The CPA is now visualized.

F. At this point, tumor can be excised, vestibular nerve sectioned, or the trigeminal, facial, or vestibular nerve can be decompressed.

G. Tumor is debulked with bipolar cautery, Cavitron ultrasonic aspirator, or CO_2 laser.

H. Once adequate exposure of the posterior face of the petrous bone and operculum is exposed, the dura overlying the IAC is incised and elevated.

I. The IAC is skeletonized from posterosuperiorly.

J. The operculum is an important landmark, which identified the entry point of the endolymphatic duct.

K. Remaining anteromedial to the endolymphatic duct while approaching the IAC decreases the risk of entry into the labyrinth with resultant deafness.

L. In general, up to 7 mm of bone can be removed safely from the medial aspect of the IAC.

M. Once the facial nerve is identified, the remainder of the tumor is peeled off of the nerve and excised.
N. All exposed air cells are occluded with bone wax.
O. Fascia is placed over the IAC.
P. The dural flap over the CPA is closed.
Q. The craniotomy defect is filled with bone chips or a cranioplasty is performed, with hydroxylapatite cement and the wound closed.

Retrolabyrinthine Approach

Originally described by Hitselberger and Pulec in 1972 for section of the fifth nerve, use of this approach has been expanded. Presently its use is limited to vestibular nerve sections and management of hemifacial spasm by microvascular decompression. There are minimal advantages to this approach and a significant disadvantage of limited visualization.

Technique

A. A postauricular incision is made and a layered flap created.
B. A cortical mastoidectomy is performed.
C. The dura is skeletonized along posterior fossa and superiorly along the middle fossa dura.
D. The facial nerve, labyrinth, and incus are identified.
E. The sigmoid sinus is decorticated and retrosigmoid air cells are removed to expose the retrosigmoid dura.
F. A dural flap is made parallel to the sigmoid sinus (behind the endolymphatic sac) up to the level of the superior petrosal sinus.
G. The cerebellum is retracted and the arachnoid incised, exposing the seventh to eighth nerve complex.
H. The vestibular nerve is sectioned or a nerve decompression performed.
I. The tumor is removed or the nerve sectioned.
J. The wound is closed with silk sutures on the dura; abdominal fat may be used to obliterate the surgical defect prior to layered closure.

Approaches to the Petrous Apex

Evaluation of the patient with pathology at the petrous apex must include consideration of lesions involving the clivus, pituitary, nasopharynx, sphenoid, temporal bone, and meninges.

Lesions of the Petrous Apex

- Cholesteatoma
  (a) Arise from the foramen lacerum from the epithelial elements congenitally included in Sessel pocket of the cephalic flexure of the embryo.
  (b) Ninety-four percent of cases present with hearing loss.
- Mucocele
- Metastatic tumor
- Mesenchymal tumor (chondroma)
- Osteomyelitis, including malignant external otitis and mastoiditis
- Clival tumor (chordoma)
- Glomus tumor
- Nasopharyngeal tumors

- Meningioma
- Neurinoma (trigeminal or acoustic)
- Aneurysm of the ICA
- Cholesterol granuloma
- Histiocytosis X

Symptoms

- Cranial neuropathy
  - (a) Nerves III, IV, V, VI, VII, and VIII
  - (b) Jugular foramen syndrome of nerves IX, X, and XI
  - (c) Hypoglossal foramen XII
- Headache (often retro-orbital or vertex)
- Tinnitus, hearing loss
- Eustachian tube dysfunction; serious effusion
- Meningitis
- Gradenigo syndrome (otorrhea, lateral rectus palsy, trigeminal pain)

Goals of Surgical Management

A. Provide exposure or permit easy access for exteriorization.
B. Preserve residual hearing.
C. Preserve facial function.
D. Preserve the ICA.
E. Protect the brain stem.
F. Prevent CSF leakage.

Approaches

A. Infracochlear
B. Supralabyrinthine
C. Retrolabyrinthine
D. Middle cranial fossa
E. Trans-sphenoid
F. Partial labyrinthectomy
G. Transcochlear
H. Infratemporal fossa

The Transcochlear Approach

This approach provides access to the skull base medial to the porus acusticus and anterior to the petrous apex and brain stem.

Technique

A. An extended postauricular incision is made.
B. A cortical mastoidectomy is performed.
C. The facial nerve is skeletonized from the stylomastoid foramen to the geniculate ganglion.
D. Bone covering the posterior fossa dura, sigmoid sinus, and middle fossa dura is removed.
E. A labyrinthectomy is performed.
F. The chordae tympani and greater superficial petrosal nerves are divided and the facial nerve is mobilized posteriorly.

G. The stapes and incus are removed and the cochlea is drilled out.
H. The dissection is bounded by the carotid artery anteriorly, the superior petrosal sinus above, the jugular bulb below, and the sigmoid sinus posteriorly; the medial extent is the petrous apex just below Meckel cave.
I. Following tumor removal, the wound may be filled with harvested fat and closed in layers.

Surgery for Vertigo

Only in persistent incapacitating vertigo which has failed medical management surgical intervention considered.
A. Ménière disease
  i. Symptoms, signs, medical treatment
    a. Fluctuating hearing loss.
    b. Episodic vertigo.
    c. Tinnitus.
    d. Aural pressure.
    e. Fifteen percent to 30% bilateral.
    f. Medical management includes low-salt diet (< 2000 mg/d), diuretics, stress reduction, vestibular rehabilitation therapy.
    g. Other possible medical therapies include corticosteroids, (both systemic and intratympanic) and Meniett therapy (micropressure therapy).
    h. Differential diagnosis includes autoimmune inner ear disease, tertiary syphilis, vestibular schwannoma, perilymphatic fistula, basilar migraine.
  ii. Surgical options
    a. Endolymphatic shunt or sac decompression 60% to 75% success rate drops to 50% at 5 years; 1% to 3% hearing loss.
    b. Intratympanic gentamycin (3/4 cc gentamycin 40 mg/mL mixed with 1/4 cc of bicarbonate 0.6M); 85% to 90% success rate. Limit use to unilateral disease. Two to six treatments up to 20% incidence of SNHL.
    c. Labyrinthectomy used in patients with unilateral disease with nonserviceable hearing in the affected ear; 85% success rate.
    d. Vestibular neurectomy used in patients with unilateral disease and serviceable hearing bilaterally; 90% success rate; 10% incidence of SNHL.
B. Benign paroxysmal positional vertigo
  i. Signs, symptoms, medical treatment
    a. Vertigo induced by head motion and lasts for less than 1 minute. Resolves over weeks to months. Frequently recurrent.
    b. Halpike demonstrating rotatory nystagmus with 5 to 10 seconds latency and 10 to 30 seconds duration is pathognomonic.
    c. Vertigo is secondary to posterior semicircular canal debris.
    d. Canalith repositioning maneuver is effective 74% to 91% of the time.
  ii. Surgical options
    a. *Singular neurectomy:* 90% success rate with 25% risk of complete or partial hearing loss
    b. *Posterior semicircular canal occlusion:* 90% success rate with 20% risk of hearing loss
C. Perilymphatic fistula

      i. Signs, symptoms, medical treatment
         a. SNHL.
         b. Vertigo.
         c. Symptoms exacerbated with Valsalva or loud noises.
         d. Site of leak around stapes footplate and round window.
         e. Treat initially with bed rest and stool softeners.
      ii. Surgical options
         a. Exploratory tympanotomy and closure of fistula by denuding surrounding mucosa and sealing small pieces of fascia.
    D. Unilateral labyrinthine injury (trauma, vascular, viral, tumor)
      i. Signs, symptoms, medical treatment
         a. Manage with vestibular rehabilitation therapy
      ii. Surgical options
         a. Labyrinthectomy
         b. Vestibular neurectomy via retrosigmoid, middle cranial fossa, or translabyrinthine approaches, 85% success rate
    E. Superior canal dehiscence syndrome
      i. Signs, symptoms, medical treatment
         a. Vertigo and oscillopsia in response to Valsalva or loud noises
         b. Chronic disequilibrium or positional vertigo
         c. Autophone
         d. Possible mild conductive hearing loss
      ii. Surgical options
         a. Plug superior semicircular canal via middle cranial fossa approach
      iii. Resurface superior semicircular canal via the middle cranial fossa approach

Complications and Outcomes

Most series quote a complication rate of approximately 50% in complicated skull base surgical resections. One of the most common complications is cerebrospinal fluid leak that can lead to tension pneumocephalus and meningitis. CSF leaks commonly resolve spontaneously but should be repaired if not resolved in 7 to 10 days. Although the efficacy of prophylactic antibiotics for CSF leak is still in question the practice of continuing perioperative antibiotics until resolution is commonplace. The likelihood of this complication is diminished with the use of vascularized free flap reconstruction of the skull base. Wound complications including wound dehiscence, infection, craniotomy bone flap loss and free flap failure are also common.

Functional and cosmetic results can be enhanced by the use of therapeutic devices and prosthetics. Orthognathic retraining and the use of an active rehabilitation mandibular exercise program, for example, can often address trismus.

Mortality after resection of tumors of the skull base has been reported mostly in the context of vascular sacrifice of the carotid artery. This complication has been known to occur despite pre-operative balloon occlusion tests. Fortunately a majority of lesions can be resected utilizing the aforementioned approaches without requiring vascular sacrifice, decreasing the risk of vascular complications. Myocardial infarction, pulmonary embolism, and cerebral edema make up the remainder of the commonest causes of perioperative death and occur mostly in the elderly with multiple medical comorbidities.

Current data support the use of surgical resection of skull base lesions, followed by radiation therapy for high-risk pathology, dural invasion, or positive margins on final pathology.

When employing this techniques multiple institutions report an average of approximately 50% overall survival at 5 years. Emphasizing that although there have been significant improvements in the field new modalities of therapy for high-risk tumors should continue to be pursued to improve on these results.

Bibliography

Almeida JR, Su SY, Koutourousiou M, et al. Endonasal endoscopic surgery for squamous cell carcinoma or the sinonasal cavities and skull base: oncologic outcomes based on treatment strategy and tumor etiology. *Head Neck Surg.* 2014; accepted article.

Bentz BG, Bilsky MH, Shah JP, Kraus DH. Anterior skull base surgery for malignant tumors: a multivariate analysis of 27 years of experience. *Head Neck.* 2003:25(7):515-520.

Hanna EY, DeMonte F. *Comprehensive Management of Skull Base Tumors.* New York, NY: Informa Healthcare USA, Inc; 2008: 256-257.

Har-El G. Anterior craniofacial resection without facial skin incisions – A review. *Otolaryngol Head Neck Surg.* 2004;130(6):780-787.

Oldring D, Fisch U. Glomus tumors of the temporal region: surgical therapy. *Am J Otol.* 1979;1(1):7-18.

Questions

1. Which of the following is a contraindication to an extended endoscopic approach to anterior skull base tumors?
   A. Extension through lateral maxillary sinus wall
   B. Involvement of the cavernous sinus
   C. Orbital involvement
   D. Tumor extension superolateral to orbital nerve
   E. Dural involvement
   F. A, B, C and D are correct

2. Which of the following cerebellopontine angle lesions has the characteristic MRI finding of high signal intensity on both T1 and T2 weighted images?
   A. Lipoma
   B. Cholesterol granuloma
   C. Arachnoid cyst
   D. Cholesterol granuloma
   E. Vestibular schwannoma
   F. Meningioma

3. Which one of the following is a "relative contraindication" to surgery of the skull base?
   A. Invasion of both cavernous sinuses
   B. Invasion of the optic chiasm
   C. Invasion of bilateral carotid arteries
   D. Invasion of the spinal cord
   E. Invasion of the brain stem

4. This approach is ideal for small intracanalicular tumors where hearing preservation is a priority:
   A. middle fossa approach
   B. retrosigmoid approach
   C. translabyrinthine approach
   D. retrolabyrinthine approach

5. The most important factor in 5-year survival in the resection of skull base malignancies is
   A. a watertight dural seal
   B. the presence of tumor-free margins at the end of resection
   C. the postoperative use of irradiation therapy
   D. the use of free flap reconstruction
   E. the use of laser in the resection of the tumor

Part 5
Laryngology

Chapter 44
The Larynx

Anatomy

The larynx is a valve between the upper aerodigestive tract and the lower airway. The vocal folds are a dynamic valve controlling this opening.

Laryngeal Cartilages

A. *Hyoid bone* is the most rostral component.
   i. U-shaped bone
   ii. Suspended from the mandible and base of the skull by ligaments
   iii. Provides stability to the larynx and pharynx
   iv. Site of attachment for cervical strap muscles and the geniohyoid muscle
B. *Thyroid cartilage* is the largest component of the laryngeal skeleton.
   i. Shield-shaped structure, formed of two ala, fused anteriorly, and opened posteriorly.
   ii. Forms the protuberance known as Adam's apple, larger in males.
   iii. Provides anterior support and protection for the larynx.
   iv. Posteriorly, each ala has superior and inferior cornuae.
   v. Thyrohyoid ligament connects the superior cornuae to the hyoid bone.
   vi. Inferior cornuae articulates with the cricoid cartilage.

C. *Cricoid cartilage* is the strongest of the laryngeal cartilages.
   i. The only complete rigid ring in the airway
   ii. Shaped like a signet ring: the flat portion is posterior
D. Epiglottic cartilage is leaf shaped.
   i. Attached to the inside of the thyroid cartilage anteriorly and projects posteriorly above the glottis.
   ii. The petiole is the point of attachment to the thyroid cartilage.
E. *Arytenoid cartilages* are the chief moving parts of the larynx.
   i. Muscles that open and close the glottis act by moving the arytenoids
   ii. Pear shaped, with broad bases that articulate with shallow ball and socket joints on the posterior superior surface of the cricoid
   iii. Vocal process:
       a. Anterior projection of each arytenoid
       b. Site of attachment for thyroarytenoid muscle
   iv. Muscular process:
       a. Lateral projection of arytenoid adjacent to piriform sinus
       b. Site of insertion of the lateral and posterior cricoarytenoid muscles
   v. The interarytenoid muscle connects the medial surfaces of these cartilages.
F. *Sesamoid cartilages*: Small cartilages above the arytenoid in the aryepiglottic fold.
   i. Corniculate cartilages (also called cartilages of Santorini)
   ii. Cuneiform cartilages (also called cartilages of Wrisberg)
   iii. Triticeous cartilage (not always present)—small elastic cartilage in thyrohyoid ligament; sometimes mistaken for a foreign body on soft tissue x-ray films

Laryngeal Joints

A. *Cricoarytenoid joint*:
   i. Motion is primarily rotational, about a variable axis, with little gliding motion.
   ii. Synovial joint
   iii. Arytenoid rotates externally to move vocal process upward and outward.
   iv. Arytenoid rotates internally to move the vocal process medially and inferiorly.
B. *Cricothyroid joints*:
   i. Primary motion is like a visor, or bucket handle, with minimal sliding.

Extrinsic Ligaments

A. *Thyrohyoid membrane*:
   i. Connects thyroid cartilage and hyoid bone
   ii. Pierced on each side by superior laryngeal vessels and internal branch of superior laryngeal nerve
B. *Median thyrohyoid ligament*: thickened median portion of the thyrohyoid membrane
C. *Thyrohyoid ligament*: thickened lateral edge on each side of the thyrohyoid membrane
D. *Cricothyroid membrane*: connects the anterior surfaces of cricoid and thyroid
   i. Relatively avascular
   ii. May be pierced for emergency tracheotomy (cricothyrotomy)
E. *Cricotracheal ligament*:
   i. Attaches the cricoid cartilage to the first tracheal ring
F. *Thyroepiglottic ligament*:
   i. From anterior epiglottis anteriorly to thyroid cartilage
G. *Hyoepiglottic ligament*:
   i. Connects the posterior surface of the hyoid bone and the lingual side of the epiglottis

Intrinsic Ligaments and Membranes

    A. *Quadrangular membrane*:
       i. Horizontal extent: from epiglottis to the arytenoids and corniculate cartilages
      ii. Extends inferiorly to the false vocal fold
     iii. Forms upper part of the elastic membrane (the fibrous framework of the larynx)
    B. *Conus elasticus*:
       i. Also known as cricovocal membrane or triangular membrane
      ii. Inferior attachment: superior border of the cricoid cartilage inferiorly
     iii. Superior anterior attachment: deep surface of apex of the thyroid cartilage
     iv. Superior posterior attachment: vocal process of the arytenoid cartilage
      v. Forms lower portion of elastic membrane (below the ventricle)
    C. *Median cricothyroid ligament*:
       i. A thickening of the anterior conus elasticus
    D. *Vocal ligament*: the free upper edge of the conus elasticus
       i. Inserts onto the anterior thyroid cartilage as Broyle ligament.
      ii. Anterior and posterior macula flavae are condensations at each end of vocal ligament.
     iii. Flavae are believed to manufacture subepithelial connective substances.

Extrinsic Laryngeal Muscles

Connect the larynx to other structures.
    A. *Depressor muscles (and innervation)*: Sternohyoid (C2, C3), thyrohyoid (C1), and omohyoid (C2, C3).
    B. *Elevator muscles (and innervation)*: Geniohyoid (C1), digastric (anterior belly V; posterior belly VII), mylohyoid (V), and stylohyoid (VII).
    C. *Pharyngeal constrictor muscles*: Paired, with insertion on posterior midline raphe (innervated by pharyngeal plexus):
       i. *Superior constrictor*: does not attach to the larynx
      ii. *Middle constrictor*: arises from hyoid and stylohyoid ligament
     iii. *Inferior constrictor*: arises from oblique line on thyroid cartilage
    D. *Cricopharyngeus*: Continuous muscle that surrounds the esophageal inlet and attaches to each side of the cricoid cartilage. It is the upper esophageal sphincter.

Intrinsic Laryngeal Muscles

    A. Innervation: recurrent laryngeal nerve, except for the cricothyroid muscle, which is supplied by the external branch of the superior laryngeal nerve
    B. *Thryroarytenoid muscle*:
       i. Origin: anterior interior surface of thyroid cartilage.
      ii. Insertion: vocal process and anterior surface of the arytenoid.
     iii. *Medial* (vocalis muscle): controls length, tension, and stiffness.
     iv. *External*: adducts vocal fold. Small portion inserts on quadrangular membrane as thyroepiglottic muscle which narrows the laryngeal inlet.
    C. *Lateral cricoarytenoid muscle*:
       i. Origin: lateral cricoid arch
      ii. Insertion: muscular process of arytenoid cartilage
     iii. Action: pulls the muscular process forward, which rotates the arytenoid so that the vocal process moves inward and down.
    D. *Interarytenoid muscle*:
       i. The only unpaired muscle in the larynx.
      ii. Connects the two arytenoid cartilages.

        iii. Oblique fibers constrict the laryngeal inlet.

        iv. Transverse fibers assist in closing the posterior glottis.

E. *Aryepiglottic muscle*: small muscle in free edge of the aryepiglottic fold

F. *Posterior cricoarytenoid muscle*:

     i. Origin: posterior cricoid lamina

    ii. Insertion: muscular process of the arytenoid cartilage

   iii. Two compartments: medial (transverse) and lateral (oblique)

   iv. Action: the only abductor of the larynx

      a. Pulls muscular process down and back to rotate arytenoid so that vocal process moves up and out

      b. Co-contracts with adductor muscles during phonation

G. *Cricothyroid muscle*:

     i. Origin: anterior arch of the cricoid cartilage

    ii. Insertion: thyroid cartilage

   iii. Action:

      a. Closes the cricothyroid space and increases the distance between the anterior commissure and the posterior cricoid

      b. Increases length and tension in the vocal fold

Compartments of Laryngeal Lumen

A. *Vestibule*: from the inlet of the larynx to the edges of the false vocal folds

     i. Anterior boundary: posterior surface of the epiglottis

    ii. Posterior boundary: interarytenoid area

   iii. Lateral boundary: false vocal folds

B. *Ventricle (ventricle of Morgagni)*: a deep recess between the false and true vocal folds

     i. Saccule is a conical pouch that ascends from the anterior part of the ventricle.

    ii. Numerous minor salivary glands open into the ventricle.

C. *Glottis (rima glottidis)*: The space between the free margins of the true vocal cords

     i. Pentagonal when the vocal folds are abducted widely

    ii. Narrows to a slit during phonation

      a. Closes completely during swallow, Valsalva, and cough

D. *Pyriform fossa*: a pharyngeal recess within the thyroid lamina but lateral to paraglottic space

Divisions of the Larynx

A. *Supraglottis*: from the tip of the epiglottis to the beginning of squamous epithelium at the junction between the lateral wall and the floor of the ventricle

B. *Glottis*: the true vocal folds and the posterior commissure

     i. Membranous vocal fold: from anterior commissure to vocal process of arytenoid

      a. Composed of soft tissues: vocal ligament, muscle, and the vocal cover

      b. From anterior commissure to the vocal process of the arytenoid cartilage

      c. These structures vibrate to produce the voice

    ii. Cartilaginous vocal fold: arytenoid cartilages

   iii. Posterior commissure: mucosa and the interarytenoid muscle

C. *Subglottis*: from undersurface of the true vocal folds to the inferior cricoid edge

Spaces in the Larynx

A. *Paraglottic space*: between thyroid ala, conus elasticus, and quadrangular membrane

B. *Preepiglottic space*: bounded by the vallecula, thyroid cartilage, thyrohyoid membrane, and epiglottis

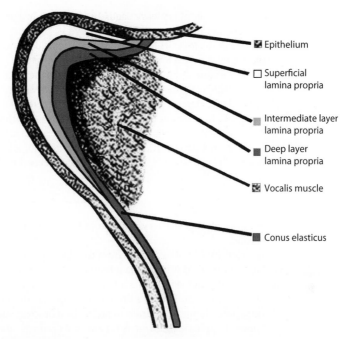

Figure 44-1 Illustration of membranous vocal fold.

Laryngeal Mucosa

    A. Stratified squamous epithelium over vocal folds and upper vestibule
    B. Ciliated columnar epithelium elsewhere
    C. Mucosa of vibratory edge of vocal fold is specialized for phonatory vibration, with an organized submucosal structure that allows the epithelium to vibrate freely over the underlying vocal ligament.
    D. Three layers in the lamina propria (Figures 44-1)
        i. *Superficial*: very loose fibrous tissue and hyaluronic acid
        ii. *Middle layer*: denser, with more elastic fibers
        iii. *Deep*: cross-linked collagen, progressively denser toward the vocal ligament

Nerve Supply

Two branches of the vagus nerve
    A. *Superior laryngeal nerve* (SLN)
        i. Exits vagus at nodose ganglion and divides into two branches
            a. Internal (sensory) branch pierces thyrohyoid membrane and carries afferent sensation from the larynx at and above the glottis.
            b. The external (motor) branch supplies cricothyroid muscle.
    B. *Recurrent laryngeal nerve* (RLN)
        i. Motor innervation to all ipsilateral intrinsic laryngeal muscles except cricothyroid.
        ii. Interarytenoid muscle receives bilateral innervation.
        iii. Motor nucleus is the nucleus ambiguous.
        iv. Sensory fibers from the subglottis and trachea to nucleus solitaries.
        v. Longer course left side: Fibers descend into chest with vagus nerve, and then loop around the ligamentum arteriosum to ascend in tracheoesophageal groove.

vi. Right RLN fibers leave vagus and loop upward around the subclavian artery to ascend in tracheoesophageal groove.

vii. On both sides, RLN enters larynx near cricothyroid joint.

viii. Extralaryngeal branching may be encountered.

ix. Embryonic branchial arch system causes the circuitous routes of the RLNs.

    a. RLN is the nerve of the sixth segmental arch.

    b. Left artery of sixth arch as the ductus arteriosus (ligamentum arteriosum).

    c. Right artery of the sixth arch disappears, so that right RLN loops around the fourth arch, which becomes the subclavian artery.

    d. Nonrecurrent RLN is associated with anomalous retroesophageal subclavian.

C. *Nerve of Galen*: (ramus communicans) connects the SLN and RLN.

Blood Supply and Lymphatic Drainage

A. Superior laryngeal artery arises from the superior thyroid artery, a branch of external carotid.

B. Inferior thyroid artery arises from the thyrocervical trunk.

C. Superior thyroid vein drains into internal jugular vein.

D. Inferior thyroid vein drains into the innominate vein.

E. Supraglottic lymphatics drain to upper jugular lymph nodes, some crossover.

F. Infraglottic lymphatics drain to pretracheal or lower jugular nodes with some crossover.

G. Glottic lymphatic drainage is very sparse drainage, and only ipsilateral.

Embryology

A. Fourth week of embryologic development: Respiratory diverticulum appears as a thickening on the ventral wall of the foregut, just caudal to the fourth branchial arch.

B. Diverticulum elongates to form the larynx, trachea, and lungs.

C. The laryngeal cartilages arise from the fourth and sixth branchial arches.

D. The cricothyroid muscle is derived from the fourth arch and is supplied by the superior laryngeal nerve.

E. All other intrinsic laryngeal muscles are from the sixth arch, supplied by the recurrent laryngeal nerve. The laryngeal lumen becomes obliterated by mesenchyme during the sixth week, but begins to recanalize during the 10th week.

Development

A. At birth, the larynx is at the level of the second or third vertebra and epiglottis is in contact with the soft palate. This creates two separate channels in the aerodigestive tract: one for food and the other for swallowing. This arrangement is characteristic of mammals.

B. After birth, the larynx gradually descends in the neck due to expansion of the cranial cavity.

C. By 4 to 6 months, the epiglottis is no longer in contact with the soft palate.

    i. One common cavity in the pharynx

    ii. Increased risk of aspiration during swallow

D. By the age of 6 to 8 years, the larynx descends to the level of the fifth cervical vertebrae. The pharyngeal space is a good resonating chamber for phonation and versatile organ for articulation.

E. During adolescence in males, the larynx doubles in anterior-posterior diameter and undergoes a second descent, resulting in a deeper voice than that of females.
F. During adolescence in both males and females, the subepithelial connective tissue of the vocal fold edge differentiates into a layered structure.
G. Ossification:
    i. *Hyoid bone*: Begins shortly after birth in six centers, complete by 2 years of age.
    ii. Thyroid cartilage: Begins at puberty, at inferior margin, progressing cranially.
    iii. Cricoid cartilage begins in young adulthood in the posterior superior area and progresses caudally.
    iv. Arytenoid cartilages calcify in the third decade.

Physiology

Protection of the Lower Airway: Primary and Phylogenetically Oldest Function

A. To prevent aspiration during swallowing
    i. Larynx moves up and forward, out of path of ingested bolus.
    ii. Epiglottis moves down and back, diverts bolus away from the midline.
    iii. Aryepiglottic folds contract to constrict laryngeal inlet.
    iv. Both true and false vocal folds close tightly. True vocal fold closure is the most important barrier to aspiration.
B. *Cough*: to clear foreign matter from the lower airway, the larynx
    i. Opens widely during inspiratory phase
    ii. Closes tightly during compressive phase
    iii. Opens widely during expulsive phase
C. Variation of glottic resistance according to respiratory demand
    i. Glottis opens during inspiration, wider with deep breathing or panting.
    ii. Glottis gradually closes during exhalation. Degree of closure determines the rate of passive exhalation.
D. *Valsalva maneuver*: Larynx closes tightly with inflated lungs
    i. Stabilizes thorax for muscular actions (eg, heavy lifting)
    ii. Increases intra-abdominal pressure for defecation, vomiting, and childbirth

Reflexes

A. Reflex closure in response to tactile or chemical stimulus.
B. Laryngospasm with strong stimulus or reduced threshold (anesthesia, hyperoxia).
C. Arrhythmia, bradycardia, and occasionally cardiac arrest may result from stimulating the larynx, as with intubation. This could be an exaggeration of responses that alter heart rate in response to respiratory cycle. These responses can be blocked with atropine.
D. Sudden infant death may be due to hyperactive laryngeal reflex.

Phonation

Adducted vocal folds vibrate passively, powered by exhaled air.
A. Mechanism:
    i. Exhaled air increases subglottic pressure to push vocal folds apart.
    ii. Airflow through glottis creates negative pressure, pulling vocal folds back together (Bernoulli effect).
    iii. Myoelastic forces also pull the vocal folds back together.
    iv. Cycle begins again as glottis closes.

B. Requirements for normal phonation:
   i. Appropriate vocal fold approximation
      a. Too loose → breathiness
      b. Too tight→ strained voice
   ii. Adequate expiratory force
   iii. Control of length and tension
   iv. Intact layer structure of lamina propria for mucosal mobility
   v. Adequate vocal fold bulk—(vocalis muscle may become atrophic with aging, neuropathy, or disuse)
   vi. Resonance of vocal tract
C. *Acoustics*: The voice is not a sinusoidal wave, but a complex waveform that can be described as a summation of various frequencies.
   i. If frequencies are harmonic, the voice quality is pleasing and clear.
   ii. Increase in nonharmonic frequencies produces a rough voice.
D. *Resonance*: The cavities of the supraglottis, hypopharynx, oropharynx, and nasopharynx modulate the sound signal by acting as resonance chambers that filter sound and selectively amplify certain frequencies.
E. *Articulation*: The palate, tongue, teeth, pharynx, and lips shape vocal sound into vowels and create consonants.

Clinical Evaluation of Hoarseness

A. Define what the patient means
   i. Change in sound of the voice
   ii. Increased effort of speaking
   iii. Vocal fatigue
B. Establish time course
   i. Onset: gradual or sudden
   ii. Duration: acute or chronic
   iii. Stable, progressing, or improving
C. Medical history to assess causes, contributing factors
   i. Trauma, intubation surgery
   ii. Systemic illnesses
   iii. Gastro-esophageal reflux symptoms
   iv. Allergy, rhinitis
   v. Neurological problems
   vi. Medications
   vii. Substance use (tobacco, alcohol, psychotropic drugs)
D. Voice history
   i. Previous voice problems—recurrent laryngitis
   ii. Professional or occupational demands on voice
   iii. Vocal training
   iv. Vocal abuse: shouting, speaking over noise
E. Perceptually assess the voice
   i. Quantify hoarseness:
      a. GRBAS Rating Scale each parameter rated on a scale of 0-3
         1. Grade (severity)
         2. Roughness
         3. Breathiness

        4. Aesthenia (weakness)

        5. Strain

    b. Maximum phonation time (MPT), the maximum length of time a patient can vocalize after taking a deep breath

        1. 10 seconds or less is abnormal

        2. 5 seconds or less is disabling

F. Examine the larynx endoscopically—indirect mirror examination generally inadequate.

    i. Video recording provides visual record and allows playback for detailed assessment

    a. Flexible endoscopy

        1. Generally well tolerated

        2. Allows assessment during connected speech and other tasks

        3. Distal chip images are clearer than fiberoptic

        4. In general, insufficient light for good stroboscopy

    b. Rigid endoscopy

        1. Transoral: 90 or 70 degree Hopkins rod telescope

        2. Allows brighter light, clearer image

        3. Cannot view during connected speech

        4. Tolerance limited by gag reflex

    c. Stroboscopy

        1. Light flashing near fundamental frequency of voice

        2. Simulates slow motion vibration

        3. Demonstrates pliability of vocal folds

        4. Detects adynamic segments and submucosal lesions

        5. Detects asymmetric vibration

        6. May differentiate between dysplasia and invasive carcinoma

        7. Light flashing at fundamental frequency results in still view in one phase

        8. If vibration is irregular, stroboscopy is not feasible

    d. High speed video

        1. Provides true slow motion

        2. Good for irregular vibration

        3. Can detect abnormalities of onset, as in spasmodic dysphonia

        4. Requires so much light that the endoscope could burn tissue

        5. Expensive, not practical for most clinicians

G. Objective measures of voice: no accepted standards analogous to audiology and not generally used clinically

    i. Phonetogram: Determines frequency and loudness range

    ii. Digital acoustic analysis: Various measures of periodicity and signal to noise

    iii. Electroglottography – monitors electrical impedance across the neck to document changes in glottal closure during phonation

    iv. Aerodynamic measures : Document airflow and pressure during phonation

H. Quality of life measures

Common Causes of Hoarseness

Acute Laryngitis

Common Causes

A. Infectious: Laryngeal inflammation usually results from coughing, not direct infection. Forceful closure can result in interarytenoid edema.

        i. Bacterial: Moraxella catarrhalis, Haemophilus influenza, Streptococcus pneumonia, Staphylococcus aureus

        ii. Viral: Parainfluenza, Influenza, Herpes Simplex Virus

        iii. Fungal: Candida albicans

  B. Noxious chemicals.

  C. Angioedema.

  D. Vocal trauma: shouting and loud talking require tight closure.

  E. Allergy.

  F. Irritants.

Diagnosis

  A. History of sudden onset of hoarseness.

  B. History of inciting factor (voice abuse, upper respiratory infection [URI], reflux symptoms).

  C. Acid reflux may not manifest symptoms of gastroesophageal reflux disease (GERD), such as heartburn, etc.

  D. No dyspnea (this suggests another diagnosis).

  E. Reflux should be strongly suspected if hoarseness occurs after a patient has gone to bed soon after a large meal, or after drinking alcohol. A foul taste in the mouth on awakening is another sign of nocturnal reflux.

Physical Examination

  A. *Routine head and neck examination*: seeks signs of URI, sinusitis, and tonsillitis.

  B. Voice may be rough, weak, or breathy and increased adductor effort is required to speak.

  C. Laryngeal examination: rule out other causes of hoarseness:

        i. Assure normal vocal fold motion

        ii. No lesions on vocal fold

        iii. Look for interarytenoid edema, which may limit glottic closure

Natural History

  A. Generally resolves spontaneously over 1 to 2 weeks.

  B. May evolve into chronic laryngitis.

  C. Laryngitis precipitated by one factor may be prolonged by other factors, such as pre-existing gastroesophageal reflux or poor vocal habits.

Treatment: Symptomatic and Supportive

  A. Vocal hygiene—absolute silence not required.

  B. Hydration.

  C. Decongestant for nasal obstruction.

  D. Cough suppression.

  E. Mucolytic.

  F. Avoid drying antihistamines.

  G. H_2 blockers or proton pump inhibitors (PPIs) if acid reflux detected or suspected.

  H. Steroids only for urgent need to use voice (performance, etc). Steroids mask symptoms, therefore performers should be monitored closely to detect injury due to overuse.

  I. If infectious treatment can be targeted to most likely organism or culture, biopsy could be performed to help direct treatment.

Chronic Laryngitis

  A. Laryngeal inflammation can become self-perpetuating.

        i. Interarytenoid edema increases the effort that is required to close the glottis.

        ii. This increased force on arytenoids exacerbates edema.

    iii. Edema is perceived as "something in the throat."

    iv. Patient makes frequent efforts to clear the throat, which perpetuates edema.

Common Causes

A. Infectious

    i. Bacterial: Klebsiella pneumonia

    ii. Mycobacterial: Mycobacterium tuberculosis, Mycobacterium leprae

    iii. Spirochete: Treponema pallidum

    iv. Fungal: Candida albicans, Blastomyces dermatitidis, Histoplasma capsulatum, Coccidiodes immitis, Cryptococcus neoformans

B. Allergy

C. Laryngopharyngeal reflux

D. Smoking

E. Radiation

F. Vocal abuse

G. Environmental irritants

Diagnosis

A. May require biopsy to provide diagnosis and exclude carcinoma and many of these can be mimickers.

Treatment

A. Culture directed antimicrobial for offending organism.

B. Consider more aggressive treatment for cause such as Nissen fundoplication for LPR, immunotherapy for allergies, change of occupation for environmental allergens and persistent vocal abusers.

Laryngopharyngeal Reflux

A. *Symptoms*: globus, dysphonia, dysphagia, chronic cough, throat clearing and mucous, only 25% to 35% have heartburn

B. *Pathophysiology*: upper esophageal sphincter dysfunction, worse with physical exertion and increase intra-abdominal pressure

C. *Diagnosis*:

    i. Clinical symptoms with resolution with maximal medication management

    ii. Endoscopy

        a. Vocal folds edema, thick mucous, pseudosulcus (subglottic swelling which resembles sulcus), interarytenoid swelling, diffuse edema and erythema

    iii. 24-hour dual sensor pH probe (gold standard)

        a. Improved results with impedance measuring

    iv. Pharyngeal pH monitoring (Restech probe)

        a. Placed into the nares under topical anesthesia and probe is located around superior aspect of oropharynx

        b. Can measure both acidic liquid and gaseous vapor

        c. Normalized values provide reference for diagnosis

        d. Better predictive value over proximal pH monitoring for extraesophageal symptoms and response to surgical treatment

D. *Treatment*

    i. Maximal medication regimen

        a. BID Proton Pump Inhibitor taken 30 minutes prior to breakfast and dinner

        b. Can add H2 blocker at nighttime

    ii. Diet modification

    iii. Behavioral modification

     iv. Esophagoscopy
     v. Surgical management
       a. Fundoplication

Vocal Nodules: Calluses on the Vocal Folds

A. Cause: vocal abuse:
    i. Phonating too loudly, too much, or with improper vocal technique
    ii. Occasionally severe coughing leads to nodules

B. Epidemiology:
    i. Frequently occur in young children and cheerleaders, not common in adult males.
    ii. Nodules are an occupational hazard for singers and grade school teachers.
    iii. In singers, small nodules may be protective, with no impact on the voice.

C. Diagnosis:
    i. History
      a. Voice is chronically raspy and there may be frequent bouts of laryngitis.
      b. Singers may report reduced vocal range or require longer warm-up before singing.
      c. History of voice use is important to identify contributing factors.
    ii. Physical
      a. Laryngoscopy reveals opposing, usually symmetric swelling or masses of the middle portion of the membranous vocal fold.
      b. Experienced examiner can confidently rule out malignancy as a consideration.
      c. Soft and edematous in early stages, firm and cornified when mature.
      d. Significant asymmetry suggests another pathology (polyp or cyst).

D. Treatment
    i. Voice restriction or rest can often result in temporary improvement.
    ii. The cornerstone of treatment is voice therapy. If vocal habits are corrected, nodules nearly always resolve. This process may require weeks or months.
    iii. Occasionally, early surgical removal may be recommended.
    iv. If underlying vocal problem is not corrected, recurrence after surgery is likely.
    v. Surgery can result in permanent vocal impairment due to scarring.
    vi. Surgery for symptomatic lesions persisting after adequate voice therapy.
      a. Nodules may be too large or firm to regress.
      b. Lesion may be a polyp or cyst rather than a nodule.
    vii. Treatment decisions should be based on vocal function, not appearance.

Vocal Fold Polyp: Sessile or Pedunculated Soft tissue Mass Membranous Vocal Fold

A. *Histology*: out-pouching of mucosa, distended by edema and loose stroma
B. *Etiology*: unknown, sometimes due to resolving hematoma
C. *Primary symptom*: hoarseness
    i. Bleeding into polyp can cause sudden enlargement.
D. Diagnosis:
    i. *History*: chronic hoarseness, recurring bouts of laryngitis are common; large polyps may cause dyspnea
    ii. *Physical examination*: smooth soft tissue mass, usually pale
E. Treatment:
    i. *Surgery*: excision via direct microlaryngoscopy
    ii. *Voice therapy*: polyps do not regress, but voice may improve

Contact Ulcer and Granuloma

A. Laryngeal ulcers and granulomas typically appear on the vocal process of the arytenoid cartilage, but may occasionally be seen on the free edge of the vocal fold.

B. *Causes*: Vocal abuse, throat clearing, intubation, and gastroesophageal reflux.

C. Diagnosis:
   i. *History*: Symptoms are very similar to chronic laryngitis. May include:
      a. Foreign body sensation and/or hoarseness
      b. Frequent throat clearing
      c. History of intubation
      d. Acid reflux symptoms
      e. Heavy voice use, vocally demanding occupation
   ii. Physical examination
      a. Large granuloma seen easily with mirror.
      b. Detection of ulcers may require rigid telescope or chip camera.
      c. Flexible endoscopy detects abusive laryngeal posture during speech.

D. Treatment:
   i. Control of acid reflux:
      a. Lifestyle and diet changes PPIs
      b. May require 6 months or more for resolution
      c. Effective even in patients without symptoms of GERD
   ii. Vocal hygiene instruction.
   iii. Voice therapy if vocal abuse detected.
   iv. Botulinum toxin injection of the thyroarytenoid muscle should be considered in refractory cases or as adjunct to surgical removal.
   v. *Surgical removal*: Only for symptomatic lesions which do not respond to medical therapy, or when a tumor or other pathology is suspected.
      a. Recurrence rate very high
      b. Recurrent lesions often more recalcitrant than original lesions

Vocal Cysts and Sulci: Subtle Lesions That Can Significantly Impair Voice

A. *Etiology*: possibly congenital, or acquired by vocal trauma

B. *Pathophysiology*: vocal impairment due to the mass lesion and/or deficiency of lamina propria
   i. *Cysts*: epithelial lined spaces; may be mucus retention or epidermoid
   ii. *Sulci*: depression in mucosa of vocal fold edge. Two types:
      a. Epithelial lined pocket (could be a ruptured cyst)
      b. Area of deficient lamina propria (also known as sulcus vergeture)
   iii. Pseudocysts:
      a. Submucosal collections of scar or connective tissue
      b. Not encapsulated by epithelium
      c. Probably the result of chronic trauma

C. *Presentation*: chronic hoarseness

D. Diagnosis:
   i. Cysts or sulci may be seen on routine office endoscopy, but are often occult.
   ii. Laryngeal stroboscopy can reveal submucosal masses or restriction of the mucosal wave.
   iii. Often the diagnosis is only apparent with direct microlaryngoscopy.

E. Treatment:
   i. *Cysts*: direct laryngoscopy and microsurgical excision:

       a. Hoarseness may persist or be worse, due to scarring or persistent deficiency.

       b. Patients must be counseled about this risk and surgery must be carefully considered.

     ii. *Sulci*: Unreliable outcome of surgery. Approaches include excision, collagen or steroid injection, mucosa "slicing" technique, or mucosal elevation with submucosal grafting.

Epithelial Hyperplasia

A. Keratosis and leukoplakia are premalignant epithelial lesions of laryngeal mucosa.

B. *Etiology*: Smoking, vocal abuse, chronic laryngitis, GERD, and vitamin deficiencies.

C. *Presentation*: hoarseness.

D. *Physical examination*: Thickened, white or reddish patches.

     i. *Stroboscopy*: Lesions usually impair glottal closure, but restriction of mucosal wave suggests possible invasive cancer.

E. *Diagnosis*: Requires biopsy. However, a trial of conservative measures may be indicated if malignancy is not strongly suspected.

F. Treatment:

     i. *Conservative*: cessation of smoking, antireflux therapy, and voice therapy

     ii. Direct microlaryngoscopy with excisional biopsy or microflap excision of lesion

     iii. Periodic follow-up to detect recurrence, or possible new lesions

G. *Complications*: Excision can cause scarring with chronic hoarseness.

Laryngocele: Dilation of the Appendix of the Ventricle, Filled With Air or Fluid

A. Types

     i. *Internal laryngocele*: totally within the thyroid cartilage framework

     ii. *External laryngocele*: extends through the thyrohyoid membrane

     iii. *Combined lesion*: dilation spanning both areas

B. Etiology:

     i. Increased intrapharyngeal pressure (glass blowers and wind instrument players)

     ii. Idiopathic

C. Presentation:

     i. Hoarseness.

     ii. External laryngocele presents as swelling in the neck that may increase in size with "puffing" maneuver.

D. Diagnosis:

     i. Physical examination may show enlargement of the false vocal fold or entire supraglottis.

     ii. Definitive diagnosis is by computed tomography (CT) or magnetic resonance imaging (MRI).

     iii. Direct laryngoscopy is required to rule out an obstructing tumor.

E. Treatment:

     i. Endoscopic marsupialization or excision for internal laryngoceles

     ii. External approach for external or recurrent laryngoceles

Laryngeal Papillomatosis: Benign Warty Tumor Caused by Human Papilloma Virus

A. Primary site of involvement is the larynx, but aggressive papilloma may involve trachea or even distal bronchi. Papilloma may also involve pharynx or tonsils.

B. Epidemiology:

      i. Juvenile onset

        a. Maternal transmission from mothers with genital warts. (Cesarean section does not reduce the incidence of transmission.)

        b. Risk factors are first-born child, young mother, and vaginal delivery.

      ii. Adult onset

        a. Most likely sexual transmission

C. *Presentation*:

      i. Children: usually present with stridor and dyspnea due to difficulty diagnosing hoarseness

      ii. Adults: present with early sign of hoarseness and later sign is stridor and dyspnea

D. Diagnosis:

      i. Can usually be strongly suspected with office examination.

      ii. Definitive diagnosis requires laryngoscopy and biopsy.

E. Treatment:

      i. Suspension microlaryngoscopy and excision are usually required. Microdebrider or CO_2 laser is most commonly used, but microsurgical instruments are also used, particularly for smaller single site lesions.

      ii. Office-based endoscopic procedures with local anesthesia can be used in some adults. Most commonly performed with KTP laser.

      iii. Other approaches include cryotherapy, photodynamic therapy, or injection of antiviral agents (cidofovir).

      iv. Airway management can be critical with obstructing lesions and requires close communication with the anesthesiologist.

      v. Recurrence is common. Repeated surgery can lead to permanent scarring and webbing.

      vi. Single site lesions are less prone to recurrence. Pediatric papillomatosis has been reported to regress at puberty.

      vii. Malignant transformation may occur, particularly with subtypes 6 and 11.

      viii. Tracheotomy should be avoided, as there is concern that it has been associated with subglottic and tracheal spread of lesions. However, it has also been noted that urgent tracheotomy is more likely in cases with aggressive disease, and so the association may not be causative.

Chondroma: Slowly Growing Tumor

A. Presentation:

      i. Hoarseness, dyspnea, dysphagia, and globus sensation.

      ii. More common in men than women.

      iii. Most frequent site is posterior plate of the cricoid cartilage, followed by the thyroid, arytenoid, and epiglottis.

B. *Diagnosis*: Submucosal mass may be seen on mirror examination or office endoscopy, but is often only apparent on CT scanning.

C. *Treatment*: Surgical excision.

      i. Thyrotomy for anterior tumors.

      ii. Lateral approach for other areas.

      iii. Recurrence is common.

Rare Benign Tumors

A. Neurofibroma, arising from Schwann cells, most often in aryepiglottic fold

B. Granular cell myoblastoma, usually in posterior vocal fold

      C. Adenoma

      D. Lipoma

Neurologic Disorders

Laryngeal Paresis

A. *Symptoms*: dysphonia, vocal fatigue, diplophonia, odynophonia, decreased projection, decreased range

B. *Pathophysiology*: Partial denervation leading to weakening of the muscles

C. *Diagnosis*:
    i. Laryngoscopy – unilateral or bilateral hypomobility or bowing (exaggerated with repetitive phonation), may have concomitant muscle tension dysphonia
    ii. Laryngeal EMG
        a. Can help differentiate cause of bowing
        b. Findings are similar to peripheral nerve injury (decreased recruitment, large or polyphasic motor units, fibrillation potentials, complex repetitive discharges)

D. *Treatment*:
    i. Observation
    ii. Voice therapy
    iii. Augmentation with either injection or thyroplasty

Laryngeal Paralysis

A. Presentation
    i. Symptoms vary greatly.
    ii. Unilateral paralysis
        a. *No symptoms*: immobile vocal fold noted during routine examination
        b. Most often, hoarseness and breathy due to inadequate glottal closure during phonation
        c. Occasionally, aspiration during swallowing
    iii. Bilateral paralysis
        a. Weak or normal voice
        b. Stridor to respiratory distress

B. Etiology
    i. *Cancer*: lung, thyroid, esophagus, and other
    ii. *Surgery*: thyroidectomy, cervical spine, intrathoracic
        a. Thyroidectomy is most common cause of bilateral laryngeal paralysis.
    iii. *Cardiovascular*: aortic aneurysm, cardiac hypertrophy, etc
    iv. *Inflammatory*: collagen vascular disorders, sarcoidosis, Lyme disease, and syphilis
    v. Central lesions: Arnold-Chiari malformation, multiple sclerosis, etc
        a. Isolated laryngeal paralysis due to other central lesions (such as stroke) is rare, as other cranial nerves are usually affected.
        b. *Idiopathic*: in about 20% of cases.

C. Pathophysiology
    i. Position of paralyzed vocal fold may be lateral immediately after injury, and shifts to paramedian position over a few months.
    ii. Paramedian vocal fold position determined by residual or regenerated innervation.

        a. Nerve injuries regenerate to varying degrees and partial injuries common.

        b. Regenerated or repaired nerve does not restore motion, but can restore muscular tone.

        c. Regenerating RLN preferentially reinnervates adductor muscles, so there is inadequate posterior cricoarytenoid muscle (PCA) force to abduct; so vocal fold lies in paramedian position.

    iii. If vocal fold is completely denervated (central or high vagus nerve injury), it is flaccid and lies in lateral, cadaveric position.

D. Diagnosis

    i. Differentiate neural paralysis from mechanical fixation.

        a. Electromyography (EMG) may can help to determine nerve injury and identify the stage of reinnervation if present.

            1. Absence of EMG activity or synkinetic activity predicts poor recovery.

        b. Direct laryngoscopy with palpation of the vocal process to assess for mobility.

    ii. It is very important to detect and treat the underlying cause.

E. Treatment

    i. For unilateral paralysis, goal is to improve glottal closure.

        a. Voice therapy

        b. Injection laryngoplasty:

            1. Via direct laryngoscopy, under local or general anesthesia, or in the office, through the mouth, or through the neck.

            2. The ideal substance would be well tolerated and permanent. Currently, no injectable substance is ideal for the treatment of laryngeal paralysis.

- Teflon injection was the most widespread treatment through the 1970s, but is no longer used as granulomas eventually developed in many patients.
- Gelfoam is a temporary, off-label treatment, effective for 8 to 10 weeks. Indicated when recovery is expected within a short time.
- Cadaveric micronized dermis, requires preparation prior to use, needs over injection. Lasts 2 to 4 month to 1 year, has FDA approval.
- Hyaluronic acid gels, lasts 6 to 9 months, requires no preparation.
- Calcium hydroxylapatite, lasts greater than 1 year, the carrier gel carboxymethylcellulose lasts 2 to 3 months, requires no preparation
- Autologous fat, harvested by liposuction or excision. Unpredictable survival—sometimes dissipates within a short time, but may survive for years.
- Type I thyroplasty (permanent medialization laryngoplasty):

        c. Vocal fold medialized by permanent implant placed in paraglottic space, via a window in thyroid cartilage.

            1. Usually performed under local anesthesia, so that results can be monitored during the procedure.

            2. Ishiki originally described carving the implant from a silastic block. Other options are prefabricated implants or strips of Gortex.

            3. Complications:

- Postoperative airway obstruction due to edema.
- Late extrusion of implant.
- Failure to achieve adequate voice, usually because implant is too high or too anterior. Also, implant may be effective intraoperatively, but prove to be too small after resolution of operative edema or subsequent muscle atrophy.

- Medialization laryngoplasty is not effective for patients with flaccid paralysis and a large, posterior gap, or with vocal processes on different levels.
  d. *Arytenoid adduction:* Mimics the action of the lateral cricoarytenoid muscle.
  1. *Indications:* large glottal gap, vocal processes on different levels, aspiration.
  2. It may be performed in combination with injection or thyroplasty.
  3. Muscular process is exposed by transecting the attachments of the inferior constrictor muscles to the thyroid ala, and reflecting the pyriform fossa mucosa.
  4. Suture through muscular process is passed through anterior thyroid cartilage, and traction applied to rotate arytenoid internally.
  5. *Laryngeal reinnervation:* Most commonly, a branch of the ansa cervicalis is anastomosed to the distal recurrent laryngeal nerve. An alternate approach is to use a neuromuscular pedicle. Reinnervation by either technique is reported to restore bulk and tone to the reinnervated muscles, but not functional motion. It is less effective in patients over the age of 51.
  ii. Treatment for bilateral laryngeal paralysis
  a. Improves airway, with minimal impact on voice.
  1. Tracheotomy is the gold standard. Speech is still possible with digital occlusion of the tracheotomy tube or use of a Passy-Muir valve.
  2. Arytenoidectomy:
     - External or endoscopic
     - Total, medial, or subtotal
  3. Endoscopic cordotomy, cordectomy, or suture lateralization.
  4. Arytenoid abduction by external approach.
  5. Reinnervation does not restore abductor function.
  6. Laryngeal "pacing" with an implantable stimulator is still experimental.

Spasmodic Dysphonia: Focal Dystonia of the Larynx

A. *Pathophysiology:* Intermittent involuntary spasms of intrinsic laryngeal muscles during speech.
B. *Etiology:* Unknown.
C. Presentation:
  i. Adductor form:
  a. Most frequent form
  b. Strained and strangled voice with frequent voice breaks
  c. Breaks commonly occur at onset of words beginning with vowels (eg, "—eggs")
  ii. Abductor form:
  a. About 1 in 10 patients with spasmodic dysphonia (SD)
  b. Whispering or breathy voice
  c. Voice breaks between plosive consonants and vowels (eg, "pu—pp—y")
D. *Diagnosis:* Based on the perceptual assessment and laryngeal examination to rule out anatomic pathology. A recent research conference at National Institute on Deafness and Other Communication Disorders (NIDCD) established diagnostic criteria.
  i. Patient perceives increased effort in speaking.
  ii. Difficulty fluctuates over time and/or between tasks.
  iii. Symptoms have lasted more than 3 months.
  iv. One or more of these vocal tasks are normal: laugh, cry, shout, whisper, sing, or yawn.

       v. Laryngeal examination shows normal laryngeal anatomy and normal function for nonspeech tasks.

E. Treatment modalities:

    i. Speech therapy alone has very limited efficacy.

    ii. Recurrent laryngeal nerve transection was the first effective treatment.

       a. However symptoms often recur within 3 years.

       b. Many patients have unacceptable breathiness.

    iii. Botulinum toxin injection of the thryoarytenoid muscle is currently the most widely used treatment for adductor SD.

       a. Very small amounts of toxin are injected on one or both sides of the larynx, to weaken, but not paralyze the muscle.

       b. Injection can be percutaneous, usually with EMG guidance, or through the mouth, with endoscopic guidance.

       c. The effective dose varies between patients and must be established by trial and error and titration.

       d. Botulinum toxin is less often effective for abductor SD, and requires injection into the posterior cricoarytenoid muscle.

    iv. Surgical treatment:

       a. The "Berke" procedure transects adductor branches of the RLNs and reinnervates with branches of the ansa cervicalis.

       b. Medialization thyroplasty improves glottal closure in patients with abductor SD.

       c. Lateralization thyroplasty has been reported effective for adductor SD.

Dysphagia With Severe Aspiration

A. Loss of protective laryngeal function. Even when oral feeding is withheld, aspiration of secretions can result in life-threatening pneumonia.

B. *Etiology*: Brain stem or cranial nerve deficits.

C. *Treatment*: Numerous surgical techniques have been proposed as treatment, and none is ideal.

    i. Tracheotomy. Cuffed tube does not prevent aspiration, but allows for suctioning and may decrease amount of material reaching lungs.

    ii. Surgical separation of the larynx and trachea and creation of a tracheostoma.

    iii. Epiglottic flap to arytenoids.

    iv. Lindeman tracheoesophageal diversion procedure with proximal trachea to esophagus anastomosis and creation of a distal permanent tracheostoma.

    v. Suturing vocal folds together via a laryngofissure. Theoretically reversible procedure.

    vi. Total laryngectomy.

Laryngeal Infections

Candidiasis

A. *Risk factors*: powdered inhaled steroids for asthma or chronic obstructive pulmonary disease (COPD), acid reflux, immune compromise, and antibiotic therapy

B. Diagnosis:

    i. History of progressive hoarseness, cough, and/or globus sensation.

    ii. Examination of larynx shows white patches on bright red mucosa.

    iii. May appear to be leukoplakia.

C. Treatment:

    i. Systemic antifungal treatment. Topical and swallowed nystatin is ineffective.

    ii. Withhold steroid.

    iii. Biopsy necessary for persistent lesions to rule out carcinoma.

Epiglottitis: Infectious Inflammation and Edema of the Supraglottis

A. *Pathophysiology*: The swollen epiglottis acts as a ball valve, with rapidly progressive dyspnea. If untreated, death can occur within a few hours.

B. *Etiology*: Usually *Haemophilus influenzae*, although it may be caused by other bacteria or viruses. The occurrence of epiglottitis has decreased steadily in the United States since the *H influenzae* type B vaccine became a routine childhood immunization in the late 1980s.

C. *Presentation*: Sore throat, dysphagia and drooling, fever, stridor, dyspnea, (relieved somewhat by leaning forward.), "hot potato" voice.

D. Diagnosis:

    i. Primarily based on history.

    ii. Point tenderness at the hyoid level in midline is a characteristic sign.

    iii. Examination should be careful and gentle to avoid stimulating a gag, which can precipitate sudden upper airway obstruction. Do not use a tongue blade. Flexible endoscopy can usually be used in adults.

    iv. Imaging should not delay treatment when diagnosis is strongly suspected.

        a. In doubtful cases, with mild dyspnea, a lateral soft tissue demonstrates the swollen epiglottis.

        b. A CT scan may demonstrate the rare occurrence of an abscess of the epiglottis. However, when the diagnosis is strongly suspected, treatment should not be delayed to obtain imaging.

        c. Any patient who is sent for imaging for suspected epiglottitis should be continuously attended by a physician capable of emergency airway management.

    v. Blood cultures are more likely than mucosal cultures to document the pathogen, but securing the airway has a higher priority than obtaining cultures.

E. Treatment:

    i. Establish airway in the operating room, under controlled conditions, with tracheotomy or orotracheal intubation.

    ii. Selected adults who present more than 8 hours after onset without severe stridor may be managed without intubation or tracheotomy, but only with close monitoring.

    iii. Intravenous antibiotics and possibly steroids.

Croup (Acute Laryngotracheobronchitis)

A. Croup primarily occurs in children between the ages of 1 and 3 years.

B. *Cause*: Virus, parainfluenza types 1 to 4, *H influenzae*, streptococci, staphylococci, or pneumococci are often cultured.

C. Symptoms:

    i. Congestion and barking cough, with hoarseness, progressing to stridor.

    ii. With increasing obstruction, suprasternal retractions and accessory muscle use.

    iii. Agitation and an increased pulse are signs of hypercarbia.

    iv. Circumoral pallor and cyanosis are late signs.

D. Diagnosis:

    i. History

    ii. *Imaging*: "steeple" sign on soft tissue anteroposterior (AP) image (subglottic narrowing due to edema)

E. *Treatment*: Depends on severity.

i. Cool mist inhalation may result in quick resolution.

ii. Steroids.

iii. Hospitalization for persistent and significant distress.

iv. Humidified oxygen, intermittent racemic epinephrine.

v. Antibiotics if indicated by fever and/or culture.

vi. Airway intervention if obstruction is severe (severe croup may actually be bacterial tracheitis).

vii. Recurrent croup is an indication for operative endoscopy, due to possible anomaly such as subglottic stenosis, cyst, laryngeal cleft, or hemangioma.

Bacterial Tracheitis

A. It is a rare but serious complication of viral and laryngotracheal bronchitis.

B. *Etiology*: *Staphylococcus, Streptococcus,* and/or *Streptococcus pneumoniae*

C. *Symptoms*: High fever, stridor, and symptoms of severe croup

D. Management:

i. Bronchoscopy reveals purulent tracheitis, with obstruction due to edema and sloughed necrotic mucosa and mucus casts.

ii. Debris must be removed, and repeated bronchosocopy is often required.

iii. Intravenous antibiotics are administered on the basis of culture results.

iv. High incidence of progression to pneumonia.

Less Common Laryngeal Infections

Laryngeal Tuberculosis

A. Almost always secondary to activate pulmonary tuberculosis.

B. Gross appearance may mimic laryngeal cancer.

C. Most common site is the posterior larynx, followed by the laryngeal surface of the epiglottis.

Syphilis

A. Very rare.

B. The larynx is never affected in the primary stage of the disease.

C. Lesions may mimic laryngeal cancer.

D. Diagnosis is based on serologic tests.

Scleroma

A. Caused by *Klebsiella rhinoscleromatis*, rare in the United States, but endemic in humid climates in Africa, Middle East, Asia, Eastern Europe, Central and South America.

B. Three stages cataharral, granulomatous, and sclerotic.

C. Treatment:

i. Oral tetracycline and steroids

ii. May require endoscopic excision, and/or tracheotomy

Glanders

A. Caused by *Burkholderia mallei* (formerly *Pseudomonas mallei*)

B. Multiple granulomatous abscesses throughout the body

Leprosy

A. *Etiology*: *Mycobacterium leprae*, or Hansen bacillus

B. Involves larynx in 10% of the cases

C. Treatment:

i. DDS (diaminodiphenylsulfone; dapsone) for 1 to 4 years

ii. Corticosteroids

iii. Tracheotomy for obstruction

Diphtheria
  A. *Etiology*: *Corynebacterium diphtheriae*.
     i. Rare in United States due to immunization.
  B. Symptoms
     i. Onset is insidious, beginning with hoarse, croupy.
  C. Diagnosis
     i. Characteristic signs are grayish-white membrane in the throat and "wet mouse" smell.
     ii. Attempts to remove membrane causes bleeding.
  D. Death is by airway obstruction.
  E. *Treatment*: Secure airway and administer antitoxin and penicillin.
Mycotic Infections
  A. *Blastomycosis*:
     i. *Etiology*: *Blastomyces dermatitidis*.
     ii. *Epidemiology*: Endemic in the Southwestern United States
     iii. *Pathophysiology*:
        a. Mainly a disease of the skin and lungs.
        b. Primary involvement of the larynx does occur, with diffuse nodular infiltration of the larynx, vocal cord fixation, ulcer, and stenosis.
     iv. *Diagnosis*: Isolating the yeast forms on culture.
     v. *Treatment*: Intravenous amphotericin B. Less severe infection may be treated with ketoconazole or itraconazole.
  B. *Histoplasmosis*
     i. *Etiology*: Caused by *Histoplasma capsulatum*
     ii. *Epidemiology*: Endemic to the Ohio, Mississippi, and Missouri River valleys. It is usually associated with pulmonary histoplasmosis.
  C. *Treatment*: Amphotericin B.

Systemic Diseases Affecting the Larynx

Sarcoidosis

  A. This is a systemic granulomatous disease that usually affects the lungs. Laryngeal involvement is not common. Granulomatous masses can cause hoarseness while mediastinal adenopathy or neural involvement can cause laryngeal paralysis or paresis.
  B. *Presentation*: cough, hoarseness, globus sensation, occasionally dyspnea.
  C. *Diagnosis*: Granulomas are seen as pale submucosal supraglottic masses, usually on epiglottis, but sometimes on aryepiglottic folds, false vocal folds, subglottis, and occasionally the true vocal fold.
     i. Diagnosis requires biopsy, showing noncaseating granulomas.
     ii. Fungal infections and other granulomatous diseases must be excluded.
  D. *Treatment*:
     i. Systemic steroids, chronic therapy.
     ii. Intralesional steroid injection, repeated as necessary.
     iii. Large lesions may require excision, debulking, or even tracheotomy.
     iv. Consider rheumatology or pulmonology referral

Rheumatoid Arthritis

A. Rheumatoid arthritis can cause inflammatory fixation of the cricoarytenoid joint and/or inflammatory nodules (Bamboo nodules) on the vocal fold. Other causes of inflammatory joint fixation include other collagen vascular diseases, gout, Crohn disease, ankylosing spondylitis, and trauma. Gonorrhea, tuberculosis, and syphilis are rare causes of cricoarytenoid arthritis.

B. *Presentation*: Hoarseness, pain, globus, referred otalgia. Bilateral arthritis causes stridor and dyspnea.

C. *Diagnosis*:
   i. May have history of rheumatoid arthritis.
   ii. Physical examination shows immobile arytenoid with erythema and edema in arthritis. Nodules may appear similar to common vocal nodules, but usually unilateral and erythematous.
   iii. Serology: Elevated erythrocyte sedimentation rate, rheumatoid factor, decreased complement levels, abnormal lupus panel.
   iv. High-resolution CT scan can show erosion of joint and soft tissue swelling.

D. *Treatment*:
   i. Medical: steroids, immunomodulators, nonsteroidal anti-inflammatory medications.
   ii. Tracheotomy may be required to relieve airway obstruction. May be removed if stridor resolves with treatment.
   iii. Nodules can be excised with microsurgery or injected with steroids, but may recur.

Systemic Lupus Erythematosis

A. This is an autoimmune connective tissue that affects many organ systems, including the myocardium, kidneys, lungs, and central nervous system (CNS). Laryngeal involvement is rare.

B. *Presentation*: Skin rash is very common presentation, typically in the malar areas following sun-exposure, and many patients have oral ulcers. Laryngeal involvement causes hoarseness by several mechanisms and may cause stridor.

C. *Diagnosis*:
   i. Established diagnosis of systemic lupus erythematosus (SLE) and hoarseness.
   ii. Physical examination shows edema, paralysis, erythematous asymmetric vocal nodules, or joint arthritis.

D. *Treament*: Primarily steroids.

Wegener Granulomatosis

A. This is an autoimmune vasculitis that primarily affects the lungs and kidneys. In up to 25% of cases, the larynx is affected, with exophytic granulation tissue that often progresses to subglottic stenosis.

B. *Presentation*: Cough, hoarseness, stridor. Many have prior diagnosis of Wegener.

C. Diagnosis:
   i. Biopsy shows necrotizing granulomas and capillary thrombosis.
   ii. Antinuclear antibody (ANA) may be positive, but antineutrophil cytoplasmic antibody (C-ANCA) is more sensitive.

D. Treatment:
   i. *Medical*: Steroids and cytotoxic drugs.
   ii. *Surgical*: Stenosis can be excised but often recurs. Tracheotomy is often required.

Relapsing Polychondritis

A. This causes chronic multisystem inflammation of cartilage.
B. *Presentation*:
    i. Commonly begins with painful swelling and erythema of auricles.
    ii. About half develop stridor due to progressive cartilage destruction.
C. *Diagnosis*: Primarily based on history and physical examination. Biopsy is nonspecific, but may exclude other etiologies.
D. *Treatment*:
    i. Steroids, dapsone, azathioprine, cyclophosphamide, cyclosporine, penicillimine, plasma exchange.
    ii. Surgical reconstruction is ineffective. Airway disease can progress to death from pneumonia or obstructive respiratory failure.

Pemphigus and Pemphigoid

A. These are autoimmune diseases that produce blistering of skin and/or mucosa:
    i. *Pemphigus*: Destruction of desmogleins and disrupts connections between epithelial cells, causing intraepithelial blistering.
    ii. *Pemphigoid*: Destruction of basement membrane causes subepithelial blisters.
B. *Presentation*: Mouth and throat pain and hoarseness. Both disorders usually begin with mouth ulcers that can spread as far caudal as the larynx, but do not involve the subglottis or trachea.
C. *Diagnosis*:
    i. Biopsy with immunoflourescent stain may demonstrate the antibodies causing the lesions, but histology often shows only nonspecific necrosis particularly in the center of ulcerated lesions.
    ii. Serology is sometimes helpful.
D. *Treatment*: Dapsone, steroids, and azathiaprine
E. *Prognosis*:
    i. Mortality as high as 15%.
    ii. Scarring may obstruct the airway.

Amyloidosis

A. It is the accumulation of abnormal fibrillar substance within tissues, either primary or secondary to multiple myeloma. It can attack any organ.
B. Death from disseminated amyloidosis is usually from renal or cardiac failure.
C. However, amyloid that involves the larynx is usually localized to that area alone.
D. *Presentation*: Hoarseness, stridor, globus, and dysphagia.
E. *Diagnosis*: Laryngeal examination shows waxy lesions that may be gray or orange, typically on the epiglottis, but sometimes glottic or subglottic.
F. *Biopsy*: Histology stained with hematoxylin and eosin (H&E) is nonspecific. Specimens should be processed with Congo red stain and viewed under polarized light to show apple green birefringence.
G. *Treatment*:
    i. Endoscopic excision or open surgery to remove or debulk symptomatic lesions.
    ii. Total removal often impossible with frequent recurrence.
    iii. Tracheotomy may be required.

Laryngeal Trauma

A. Blunt trauma to the larynx can cause laryngeal fractures without significant external signs.

B. *Pathophysiology*:

    i. Laryngeal fractures are not common, since the larynx is protected posteriorly by the spine, and anteriorly, the chin and sternum provide some shielding.

    ii. Laryngeal fractures usually result from a direct anterior blow with the head extended.

    iii. Such trauma can also injure the cervical spine. Another cause of laryngeal fracture is strangulation, with a crushing injury.

C. *Presentation*:

    i. Increasing airway obstruction with dyspnea and stridor. However, patient may be in an asymptomatic interval.

    ii. Nearly half of patients who sustain a laryngeal fracture asphyxiate at the scene of the accident.

    iii. In other cases, airway obstruction develops after a fairly asymptomatic interval, and can be suddenly fatal.

    iv. Dysphonia or aphonia.

    v. Cough and hemoptysis.

    vi. Dysphagia and odynophagia.

D. *Physical signs*:

    i. Loss of neck contour due to flattening of thyroid cartilage

    ii. Neck hematoma

    iii. Subcutaneous emphysema

    iv. Crepitus over the laryngeal framework

E. *Management*: determined by stability of the airway.

    i. Acute airway distress

        a. Proceed directly to operating room for tracheotomy with local anesthesia, followed by direct laryngoscopy under general anesthesia to assess the injury.

        b. Be prepared to perform emergency tracheotomy en route should the airway be suddenly lost.

        c. Orotracheal intubation is not recommended, as laryngeal distortion makes this difficult, and the tube may create a false passage.

    ii. Stable airway:

        a. Flexible laryngoscopy to assess vocal fold motion and look for lacerations and exposed cartilage.

        b. If fiberoptic examination is normal, manage conservatively with observation, humidification, and steroids.

        c. If fiberoptic examination shows hematoma, swelling, decreased motion, or other distortion, perform CT scan. If CT shows displaced fracture, proceed to surgical repair. Otherwise, conservative management with steroids, humidified air, and observation.

        d. If examination shows lacerations or exposed cartilage, proceed directly to operating room for urgent tracheotomy under local, followed by direct laryngoscopy under general anesthesia.

    iii. *Surgical repair*:

        a. If mucosal laceration a midline thyrotomy is used to expose laryngeal mucosa. All lacerations should be carefully sutured. Local flaps or free mucosal grafts may be used to close defects.

b. If an arytenoid cartilage is completely avulsed and displaced, it is better to remove it than attempt to reposition it.
c. Laryngeal cartilage fractures should be reduced and immobilized. The use of plates has made this easier.
d. Laryngeal stents may be used to add stability, but can stimulate granulation tissue. Should be considered in severely comminuted fracture to provide stability.

Laryngeal and Tracheal Stenosis

A. *Etiology*: Usually results from trauma due to intubation or external injury. May also be caused by systemic disease or be idiopathic. Frequently associated with acid reflux.
B. *Presentation*: Symptoms and treatment vary with location, severity, and etiology. Supraglottic stenosis is much less common than glottic or subglottic.
C. *Presentation*: Progressive stridor and dyspnea, with or without hoarseness.
D. Diagnosis:
   i. Prior history of intubation or trauma
   ii. Office endoscopy to evaluate supraglottic and glottic airway and vocal fold motion
   iii. CT scan to evaluate subglottic and tracheal airway, and cricoarytenoid joints
   iv. Direct laryngoscopy and bronchoscopy to determine extent of lesion and palpate immobile vocal folds
E. *Treatment*:
   i. Supraglottic stenosis
      a. Endoscopic excision of scar may be effective but often stenosis recurs.
      b. External excision, essentially supraglottic laryngectomy, can be effective.
   ii. Glottic stenosis
      a. If obstructive symptoms are present nearly always involves fixation of the vocal folds due to posterior scarring, anterior stenosis usually affects voice more than respiration.
      b. Treatment must consider resulting vocal function.
      c. If vocal fold mobility cannot be restored, then the airway can only be restored by static enlargement of the airway, which impairs the voice. This would include arytenoidectomy or cordotomy. Sometimes a tracheotomy is the best option.
   iii. Subglottic stenosis
      a. Can be managed by endoscopic excision if the scar is thin and not circumferential, and the cricoid support is intact.
      b. Can perform with or without radial incision and balloon dilation or rigid dilation
      c. Reconstructive surgery can be considered with either laryngotracheoplasty, or cricotracheal resection.
   iv. Tracheal stenosis
      a. Definitively treated by resection and end-to-end anastomosis
      b. Can be managed with balloon dilation if thin band or poor surgical candidate
   v. Airway stenosis that involves multiple sites or that occurs in patients with complex medical conditions is very difficult to treat. An option for reconstructive surgery is a T-tube, to stent the airway.
   vi. Expanding endotracheal stents are not advised, due to complications of granulation and potential erosion into the mediastinum.

Congenital Anomalies

Laryngomalacia

A. It is the most common cause of neonatal stridor.

B. *Pathophysiology*: Supraglottis is flaccid, and epiglottis or interarytenoid tissue collapse during inspiration to obstruct the airway.

C. *Etiology*: Unknown, probably neurologic or structural immaturity.

D. *Classification*:
   i. Type 1, foreshortened or tight aryepiglottic folds
   ii. Type 2, redundant tissue in the supraglottic
   iii. Type 3, posterior epiglottic collapse due to underlying neuromuscular disorders

E. *Presentation*:
   i. Stridor is noted soon after birth.
   ii. Breathing better in prone position, worse when prone than when supine.
   iii. However because of the current "Back to Sleep" initiative to prevent sudden infant death syndrome, parents often do not place child in supine position.

F. *Diagnosis*:
   i. Flexible endoscopy in the office: Epiglottis is classically described as "omega" shaped and falls backward during inspiration. Shortened aryepiglottic folds tethering epiglottis posteriorly. Redundant arytenoid mucosa can prolapse into glottic airway with inspiration. Vocal fold mobility is normal.
   ii. Operative endoscopy is indicated if other anomalies are suspected or if stridor is very severe, with cyanosis.

G. *Treatment*:
   i. Usually observation and assurance that this will resolve by 12 to 16 months.
   ii. Proton pump inhibitor treatment can help temporize symptoms to avoid surgical procedure.
   iii. Endoscopic supraglottoplasty for severe stridor or failure to thrive.
   iv. Tracheotomy may be required.

Laryngeal Paralysis

A. It is the second most common cause of newborn stridor. Most commonly unilateral but may be bilateral.
   i. *Causes*: idiopathic, birth trauma, cardiomegaly, Arnold-Chiari malformation, ligation of persistent ductus arteriosis
   ii. *Presentation*: weak cry, inspiratory stridor, and/or feeding difficulties
   iii. *Diagnosis*
      a. Fiberoptic endoscopy
      b. Imaging to rule out cardiac and neurologic causes
      c. Barium swallow advisable to detect aspiration
   iv. *Treatment*
      a. Observation for hoarseness and mild stridor.
      b. Tracheotomy for severe stridor (usually bilateral paralysis).
      c. Swallowing team consultation for feeding issues—pneumoencephalography (PEG) if severe issues.
      d. Definitive laryngeal surgery deferred pending potential recovery and growth.
      e. Laryngeal reinnervation
         1. Effective for decreasing synkinetic inspiratory stridor, which can occur later in life.
         2. Provides bulk and tone of cord to allow for close to normal voice production.

Hemangioma

A. It is the vascular lesion that causes airway obstruction.
B. *Presentation*:
    i. Progressive inspiratory stridor with onset soon after birth
    ii. Sometimes progressive episodes of croup
    iii. Voice usually normal
    iv. Skin hemangioma in 50% of cases, increased incidence with beard distribution
C. *Diagnosis*:
    i. Direct laryngoscopy and bronchoscopy show compressible erythematous most often involving the anterior subglottis.
    ii. Do not biopsy.
    iii. Extent can be assessed with imaging.
D. *Treatment*:
    i. Observation: Natural history is expansion for several months followed by involution.
    ii. Systemic steroids and racemic epinephrine for acute stridor.
    iii. Systemic propranolol can result in dramatic involution.
    iv. CO_2 laser excision, external excision, or tracheotomy if obstruction does not respond to propranolol.

Laryngeal Web or Atresia

A. A congenital band over part (web) or all (atresia) of the glottis
B. *Presentation*:
    i. Laryngeal atresia presents with complete obstruction at birth, unless a distal T-E fistula provides some connection from trachea to outer air. Other anomalies are usually present and mortality is quite high. Death may follow if not promptly recognized and treated.
    ii. Webs usually involve anterior larynx. Small web may be asymptomatic, larger webs cause weak or hoarse cry.
C. *Diagnosis*: endoscopic examination
D. *Treatment*:
    i. Tracheotomy for relief of airway obstruction.
    ii. Web is best corrected when child is larger and anatomy is more distinct.
    iii. Successful division of web may not improve the voice.

Congenital Laryngeal Cysts

A. Supraglottic or subglottic.
B. Diagnosis and treatment are accomplished by endoscopy with rupture or marsupialization of the cyst.
C. Recurrence is infrequent, but subsequent endoscopy is required to monitor for such an occurrence.

Congenital Subglottic Stenosis

A. Congenital, or secondary to intubation
B. *Presentation*: stridor and respiratory failure, usually after attempts to extubate
C. *Diagnosis*: bronchoscopy
D. *Treatment*: tracheotomy, balloon dilation, cricoid split, or laryngotracheal reconstruction

Laryngeal Clefts

A. Laryngeal cleft is a rare anomaly caused by incomplete fusion of the laryngotracheal septum.

B. *Presentation*: cyanosis with feeding, stridor, recurrent pneumonia. Severity due to extent of cleft.

C. *Classification*: Benjamin Parsons
  i. Type 1 – interarytenoid region
  ii. Type 2 – partial involvement of cricoid
  iii. Type 3 – extension through cricoid cartilage
  iv. Type 4 – extension into posterior wall of trachea

D. *Diagnosis*: Direct laryngoscopy and bronchoscopy.

E. *Treatment*: Some can be observed and will eventually improve, others require repair by endoscopic or open repair.

Cri-Du-Chat Syndrome

A. This is named because of the abnormal cry.

B. It is caused by partial deletion of a no. 5, group B chromosome.

C. There are multiple other accompanying anomalies including mental retardation, facial abnormalities, hypotonia, and strabismus.

Foreign Bodies in the Larynx and Tracheobronchial Tree

A. Choking on food causes about 3000 deaths per year in the United States, predominantly between the ages of 1 and 3.

B. In infants less than 1 year of age, suffocation from foreign body aspiration is the leading cause of accidental death.

C. The most common foods causing fatal aspiration are hot dogs, grapes, and peanuts.

D. Smaller objects do not cause complete airway obstruction.

E. *Presentation*: Foreign bodies that do not cause obstruction present with wheezing or chronic cough.
  i. Often the initial aspiration event is not observed.
  ii. An observed choking event may be followed by an asymptomatic interval.
  iii. Recurrent pneumonia is a late manifestation.

F. *Diagnosis*:
  i. Physical examination
  ii. Tracheal foreign body—biphasic stridor, may have audible slap or palpable thud
  iii. Bronchial—expiratory wheeze, decreased breath sounds on involved side
  iv. Chest radiograph
    a. Only radiopaque foreign bodies are visible.
    b. Fluoroscopy or inspiratory and expiratory films show atelectasis on inspiration, hyperinflation on expiration on the side of the foreign body.
    c. Obstructive emphysema and consolidation may be seen.

G. *Treatment*:
  i. Removal by rigid ventilation bronchoscope.
    a. Bronchoscopy indicated whenever diagnosis is suspected. All signs and symptoms need not be present. Performing a negative endoscopy is much better than neglecting an occult foreign body.
    b. Removal requires teamwork and communication, with all equipment available, assembled, and working.

          c. Telescopes and optical forceps greatly facilitate removal.

          d. General anesthesia is required, with spontaneous ventilation, may be supplemented by topical anesthesia.

          e. Steroids are recommended to reduce edema.

    H. *Complications*:

        i. Edema, bronchitis, pneumonia, ulceration, granulation tissue.

        ii. Pneumothorax, pneumomediastinum.

        iii. Vegetable matter may swell and become impacted.

        iv. Total obstruction, as foreign body becomes lodged in larynx during removal. This may be managed by pushing foreign body back into bronchus.

Tracheotomy

    A. It is done to form a temporary opening in the trachea. Tracheostomy, in which the trachea is brought to the skin and sewed in place, provides a permanent opening.

    B. Indications

        i. Airway obstruction at or above the level of the larynx

        ii. Inability to clear secretions

        iii. Need for prolonged mechanical ventilation

        iv. Pulmonary insufficiency that benefits from reduction of upper airway resistance and dead space

        v. Severe obstructive sleep apnea

    C. Signs of airway obstruction

        i. It is best to intervene early rather than wait for late signs of upper airway obstruction.

          a. Early signs

            1. Retractions (suprasternal, supraclavicular, intercostal)

            2. Inspiratory stridor

          b. Later signs

            1. Agitation and/or altered consciousness

            2. Rising pulse and respiratory rate, paradoxical pulse

          c. Danger signs

            1. Pallor or cyanosis late danger signs

            2. Fatigue and exhaustion

    D. Postoperative care

        i. Secure tube tightly, preferably with direct sutures, to prevent accidental dislodgement.

        ii. Chest x-ray films (AP and lateral) determine the length and position of the tracheotomy tube and detect pneumomediastinum or pneumothorax.

        iii. Do not change external tube for 3 to 4 days, to prevent reentry into false passage.

        iv. Frequent suctioning and removal and cleaning of inner cannula.

    E. Complications

        i. *Immediate*: bleeding, pneumothorax, pneumomediastinum, subcutaneous emphysema, dislodged or obstructed tube, false passage with tube outside trachea, postobstructive pulmonary edema, apnea due to loss of hypoxic drive, tube too short or inappropriate shape (especially in morbidly obese patients)

        ii. *Delayed*: granulation tissue, stomal infection, subglottic or tracheal stenosis, tracheomalacia, tracheoesophageal fistula, displacement of tube, tracheoinnominate fistula, persisting tracheocutaneous fistula after decannulation

Swallowing and Management of Dysphagia

Stages of Swallowing

      A. Voluntary
         i. Oral Preparatory - Prepares food for swallowing
            a. Lip closure, tensions from labial and buccal musculature (CN VII)
            b. Rotary jaw motion (CN VII)
            c. Lateral tongue rolling (CN XII)
            d. Anterior bulging of soft palate seals oral cavity and widens nasal airway (CN IX and X)
         ii. *Oral*: Food moves from oral cavity to pharynx
            a. Posterior propulsion of food by tongue along hard palate (CN XII)
            b. Triggers pharyngeal swallow by glossopharyngeal nerve (CN IX)
               1. Delayed trigger by superior laryngeal nerve at laryngeal inlet
            c. Prolonged with age and increased velocity
      B. Involuntary
         i. Pharyngeal
            a. Airway protection with laryngeal elevation and closure (CN XI and XII)
            b. Velopharyngeal closure preventing nasopharyngeal regurgitation (CN IX and X)
            c. Pharyngeal contraction (CN IX)
            d. Cricopharyngeal/UES opening (CN X)
               1. Muscle is under tonic contracted to prevent air ingestion with inhalation and reflux from esophagus
         ii. Esophageal
            a. Peristalsis
               1. Upper 1/3 of mixed voluntary muscles
               2. Lower 2/3 involuntary

Dysphagia

      A. *Signs and symptoms*: coughing, choking, recurrent pneumonia, malnutrition, dehydration, weight loss, regurgitation, globus sensation, food impaction
      B. *Diagnosis*:
         i. Patient assessment
            a. Patient questionnaire indicating the severity of dysphagia and effect on quality of life
            b. EAT 10 validated questionnaire, numerous other quality of life tools
            c. Used for research purposes and to tract patient's progress with treatment
         ii. Bedside evaluation
            a. Screening tool used to assess whether patient needs further testing or is cleared for oral intake
            b. Uses trial with water and various consistencies monitoring outcomes of oxygen saturation or coughing to pass or fail patient
            c. None are valid or reliable
         iii. Manometry
            a. Probes with graded pressure sensors placed in office and patient observed with numerous swallows
            b. Useful to show function of UES, LES, and coordination of peristalsis
            c. Performed in the office with minimal anesthesia

    iv. Functional Endoscopic Examination of Swallowing (FEES)
- a. Visualization of pharynx before and after swallow
- b. Uses different consistencies with or without food coloring
- c. Good for detection of penetration, aspiration, pooling, retained secretions, effectiveness of cough
- d. Examination
  1. Start with pharyngeal squeeze (high pitched strained phonation in rising crescendo)
  2. Start with water/ice chips and progress to puree then crackers
  3. Pre-swallow
     - Secretion level: assess amount and location of secretion prior to swallow
     - Can indicate patients who are at high risk for aspiration due to open glottis during bolus formation and transit
  4. Post swallow
     - Assess whether food contents have penetrated larynx or if the patient aspirated the contents.
     - Location of residue (velleculae, pharyngeal wall, pyriform)
     - Can be used in conjunction with compensatory maneuvers to test for benefit
     - Limitation is that one cannot visualize oral phase, events during swallow or upper esophageal sphincter function

    v. Functional Endoscopic Exam of Swallowing and Sensory Testing (FEESST)
- a. FEES with additional sensory testing
- b. Test laryngeal adduction reflex, which is triggered by particulate matter in the larynx
- c. Can use light touch with endoscope, presence of residue without patient attempt to clear or air puffs
- d. Adjunct to MBS or FEES in neurologically impaired patients
- e. Useful in patients who are bedridden and incapacitated who cannot undergo MBS

    vi. Videofluroscopy
- a. Barium swallow (Esophagram)
  1. Large amount of barium with one swallow
  2. Evaluates anatomy of UES, esophagus, and LES
  3. Assess for motility problems, cricopharyngeal function and LES function

    vii. Modified barium swallow
- a. Smaller sips of barium with different consistencies used
- b. Assess all phases of swallowing and allows for visualization of structural movement
- c. Can be used to evaluate compensatory mechanisms for effectiveness
- d. Can also be used to visualize UES and diagnose cricopharyngeal dysfunction

C. *Causes and Treatment*
- i. Oropharyngeal dysphagia
  - a. Cause: neurological impairment (Parkinson, stroke, ALS, Bell palsy, Myasthenia Gravis, Oculopharyngeal Muscular Dystrophy), structural impairment (radiation, post-surgical defects or scarring, xerostomia, mucositis, inflammatory lesions)
  - b. Diagnosis:
    1. MBS or FEES

    c. Treatment
       1. Diet modification
       2. Direct compensatory measures – involve a swallow
- Supraglottic swallow - inhale and hold breath then place bolus in swallow position; Swallow while holding breath and cough after swallow before inhaling
  - (a) Use in vocal fold paresis, paralysis, laryngeal sensory deficits
  - (b) Voluntary airway closure technique
- Effortful swallow - Squeeze hard with all muscles
  - (a) Helps propel bolus into oropharynx
  - (b) Careful in patients with oropharyngeal weakness or poor vocal fold closure
- Mendelsohn maneuver - Dry swallows while feeling thyroid prominence, lift and hold for several seconds
  - (a) Opens UES through extending duration of laryngeal elevation
  - (b) Patients with poor laryngeal excursion or elevation or poor coordination
- Head tilt – Tilt head to side of a paralyzed vocal fold prior to swallow
  - (a) Directs food away from open glottis and collapses pharynx on affected side to prevent aspiration.

       3. Indirect compensatory measures – does not involve a swallow
- Lingual strengthening
  - (a) Improves handling of bolus and transmission
- Shaker head lift
  - (a) Supine position with head lifts while shoulders on floor or bed
  - (b) Strengthen muscles contributing to UES opening (geniohyoid, thyrohyoid, digastric)
  - (c) Decrease hypopharyngeal bolus pressure into UES
  - (d) Decreased residue
- Expiratory Muscle Strength Training
  - (a) Strength gains in suprahyoid muscles
  - (b) Increase hyolaryngeal movement

       4. Stimulation
- Electrical stimulation
  - (a) Percutaneous – hook wire electrodes to target muscles
  - (b) Transcutaneous – stimulated sensory fibers in skins and target muscles
- Thermal tactile
  - (a) Rubbing anterior tonsillar pillars with cold
  - (b) Increases sensitivity minimizing pharyngeal delay

ii. Diffuse idiopathic skeletal hyperostosis
    a. Most common location C5-6
    b. Pathophysiology: causes mechanical obstruction and can produce inflammation, which can cause associated neck and back stiffness and pain
    c. Symptoms: Solid food dysphagia due to mechanical obstruction and aspiration of retained secretions post swallow
    d. Diagnosis: MBS or endoscopy
    e. Treatment: conservative management with NSAIDS and rarely surgical excision

   iii. Schatzki Ring
- a. Symptoms: intermittent dysphagia to solids, do not start until diameter < 13 mm
- b. Pathophysiology: lower esophageal mucosal ring above GE junction possibly related to GERD as a decrease has been seen with acid suppression
- c. Diagnosis: esophagram or endoscopy
- d. Treatment: dilation

   iv. Achalasia
- a. Symptoms: regurgitation of food, chest pain, cough, dysphagia to solids and liquids, heartburn,
- b. Pathophysiology:
  1. Esophageal motility disorder due to dysfunction of inhibitory neurons of myenteric plexus
  2. Can also be caused by Chagas disease and malignancy
- c. Diagnosis:
  1. Esophageal manometry
     - High resting LES pressure and failure to relax
     - Aperistalsis from lack of triggering from LES relaxation
  2. Esophagram – Bird's beak appearance of LES with dilated esophagus
- d. Treatment:
  1. Endoscopic dilation and Botox to LES
  2. Heller myotomy with or without fundoplication 70% to 90% success rate

   v. Diffuse esophageal spasm
- a. Symptoms: dysphagia, regurgitation, heartburn
- b. Pathophysiology: neuroinhibitory dysfunction with normal peristaltic contractions with high amplitude contraction of esophageal smooth muscle
- c. Diagnosis:
  1. Manometry shows normal swallows with abnormal pressure waves
  2. Esophagram – corkscrew appearance
- d. Treatment:
  1. Smooth muscles relaxants such as anticholinergics and calcium channel blockers
  2. Botox injections

   vi. Zenker diverticulum
- a. Symptoms: dysphagia, regurgitation, halitosis, neck swelling, aspiration, gurgling after eating, dysphonia
- b. Pathophysiology: pseudodiverticulum at Killian triangle between inferior constrictor and cricopharyngeus
  1. Discoordination between UES and pharyngeal contraction causing increased intraesophageal pressure
  2. More frequently in men, 7th-8th decade, and left side
  3. Possible relationship to reflux
- c. Diagnosis – Barium swallow
- d. Treatment
  1. Diverticulopexy – open procedure with suturing intact diverticulum superiorly to prevertebral fascia to prevent entrance of food
  2. Imbrication – purse string around lumen with inversion of sac
  3. Diverticulectomy with cricopharyngeal myotomy

- Risks include mediastinitis, RLN injury, pneumonia, hematoma, infection, pharyngocutaneous leak,
- Decreased recurrence with CP myotomy and compared to endoscopic procedures
- Requires Nasogastric tube for 2 to 5 days post op
- Can use canal suture or staple to repair pharyngeal defect

4. Endoscopic
   - Requires exposure to perform procedure with a bivalve laryngoscope, which is difficult to place in patients with prominent teeth, cervical kyphosis, retrognathia, TMJ
   - 5% conversion rate to open
   - Can use electrocautery, CO_2 laser, KTP laser, stapler
     (a) Stapler must be modified as tip does not contain staples
     (b) May require 2 for diverticulum greater than 6 cm
     (c) Can perform only myotomy for small diverticulum
   - Small leak rate
   - 5% recurrence rate
   - Can consider feeding post-operative day 0/1

vii. Killian Jamieson diverticulum is between inferior cricopharyngeus and esophagus

viii. Cricopharyngeal dysfunction
   a. Symptoms: dysphagia to solids > liquids, globus sensation, food sticking
   b. Pathophysiology: hypertrophy of muscle, inability to relax muscle due to neuromuscular disorder (muscular dystrophy, stroke, Parkinson, vagus nerve palsy), fibrosis from radiation
   c. Diagnosis:
      1. Esophagram or Video Oropharyngeal Swallow Study
         - Will show Cricopharyngeal bar
         - Can help identify poor surgical candidates
           (a) Impaired pharyngeal strength
           (b) Impaired hyolaryngeal elevation
             ○ Manometry – tonic contraction of cricopharyngeus without relaxation
   d. Treatment
      1. Dietary modification to soften food
      2. Dilation
         - Increase success in patients with fibrosis and stenosis
      3. Botox
         - Can inject in office or in operating room.
         - Can last 5 to 6 months.
         - 73% of Botox failures improved with myotomy therefore cannot be used to predict surgical improvement.
         - Risk of intralaryngeal muscle diffusion and vocal fold paralysis.
         - Doses of 50-100 Units split into 3 to 4 injection sites.
      4. Endoscopic myotomy
         - Performed with bivalve endoscope
         - Similar to management of Zenker diverticulum exposure is most important part of surgery
         - Most commonly use CO_2 laser
         - Incise through mucosa and cricopharyngeus

- Leaves buccopharyngeal fascia and areolar tissue intact, which prevents pharyngeal leak
  5. Open myotomy
     - Similar approach to Zenker's
     - Can place bougie prior to surgery to provide cutting surface
     - Remove portion of muscle to prevent rehealing

Care of the Professional Voice

A. Definition
   i. Person whose career depends on speaking or singing skill
   ii. Vocal quality and endurance are critically important to vocal performers
B. Presentation of the professional voice user
   i. Healthy check-up: establish baseline and check for potential problems
   ii. Chronic voice change
   iii. Acute change in voice
   iv. Urgent need to perform
   v. Factors influencing motivation of performer to seek care
      a. Date and importance of next performance
      b. Severity and acuity – may use OTC meds for mild problems
      c. Singing versus speaking
      d. Medical Insurance—lack of inhibits
C. New patient healthy voice visit
   i. Vocal history:
      a. Professional status and voice goals
      b. Performance commitments
      c. Working environment
   ii. Medical history.
   iii. Training: Show choir director versus classically trained vocal pedagogist.
   iv. Vocal range: is it appropriate? Singing outside range is abusive.
      a. Male: Bass, Baritone, Tenor
      b. Female: Alto, Mezzo-soprano, Soprano
   v. Useful terms in discussing singing problems:
      a. Vocal registers
         1. Chest voice, head voice, falsetto
      b. Passaggio
         1. Least stable portion of range
         2. Where chest and head voice overlap
         3. Yodeling is vacillation between chest and head or falsetto
         4. Classical voice training smoothes transition between registers
      c. Tessitura: the portion of range where voice is most brilliant
      d. Singers Formant or "Ring"—Resonance that allows singers to be heard over the orchestra
   vi. Lifestyle issues in performers:
      a. Late nights
      b. Meals and noisy parties after performance
      c. Extroverted personalities
      d. May use alternative Rx's

vii. Baseline examination—including stroboscopy—performers may have asymptomatic nodules or other lesions, which could be "red herrings" if there is a subsequent voice disorder

viii. Voice Recording

ix. Instruction in voice hygiene

D. Assessment for voice change

   i. Professional voice users have the same pathologies as nonprofessional voice patients, but

      a. Vocal performance places stress on the larynx

      b. Changes in vocal quality have greater impact

         1. normal pitch drop with menopause can be devastating for singer

         2. Laryngeal atrophy with age weakens the voice

E. Voice abuse

   i. Excessive performance

   ii. Faulty technique

   iii. Poor audio feedback during performance

F. Common faults in singing technique

   i. Tension: jaw, neck, tongue, chest

   ii. Breathiness

   iii. Poor resonance

   iv. Hard glottal attack

   v. Singing outside range

Vocal Emergency: Sudden Voice Change Just Before Performance

A. To perform or not to perform?

   i. Can it be done without damage? (Risk to future career?)

      a. Status of vocal folds—hemorrhage or tear is absolute contraindication

      b. Severity of illness

      c. Demands of performance

      d. How will it sound?

      e. Skill and training

      f. Bad performance worse for reputation than canceling

      g. How important is the performance?

      h. Financial concerns

Management of Acute Laryngitis for a Performance

A. Examination to rule out contraindication to performance.

B. Voice rest.

C. Hydration.

D. Mucolytics.

E. Cough suppression:

   i. No scopolamine or antihistamine

F. Reflux management.

G. Manage concurrent rhinitis.

   i. Decongestant

   ii. Antibiotics?

H. Steroids to reduce vocal fold edema-oral just as effective as parenteral.

I. Topical oxymetazoline rarely needed for vocal fold edema.

J. These are all short-term measures for an important limited performance that cannot or should not be canceled.

K. Ideal management of laryngitis includes voice rest, as continued performance perpetuates the problem.

Bibliography

Blitzer A, Crumley RL, Dailey SH, et al. Recommendations of the neurolaryngology study group on laryngeal electromyography. *Otolaryngol Head Neck Surg.* 2009;140(6):782-793.

Fitch WT, Giedd J. Morphology and development of the human vocal tract: a study using magnetic resonance imaging. *J Acoust Soc Am.* 1999;106(3 Pt 1):1511-1522.

Hirano M. Phonosurgical anatomy of the larynx. In: Ford CN, Bless DM, eds. *Phonosurgery.* New York, NY: Raven Press; 1991.

Laitman JT, Reidenber JS. Advances in understanding the relationship between the skull base and larynx with comments on the origins of speech. *Hum Evol.* 1998;3:99.

Ludlow CL, Adler CH, Berke GS, et al. Research priorities in spasmodic dysphonia. *Otolaryngol Head Neck Surg.* 2008;139(4):495-505.

Paniello RC, Edgar JD, PhD, Kallogieri D, Piccirillo JF. Medialization vs. reinnervation for unilateral vocal fold paralysis: a multicenter randomized clinical trial. *Laryngoscope.* 2011;121(10):2172-2179.

Sans V, de la Roque ED, Berge J, et al. Propranolol for severe infantile hemangiomas: follow-up report. *Pediatrics.* 2009;124(3):423-431.

Woodson G. Arytenoid abduction: indications and limitations. *Ann Otol Rhinol Laryngol.* 2010;119(11):742-748.

Woodson GE. Spontaneous laryngeal reinnervation after recurrent laryngeal or vagus nerve injury. *Ann Otol, Rhinol Laryngol.* 2007;116(1):57-65.

Questions

1. The superior laryngeal nerve supplies which of the following muscles?

    A. Vocalis

    B. Cricothyroid

    C. Cricopharyngeus

    D. Lateral cricoarytenoid

    E. Superior pharyngeal constrictor

2. The medial wall of the paraglottic space is the

    A. thyroid ala

    B. conus elasticus

    C. aryepiglottic fold

    D. Broyle ligament

    E. thyrohyoid membrane

3. A patient with adductor spasmodic dysphonia will have the most difficulty with which of the following words?
   A. Mama
   B. Puppy
   C. Elephant
   D. Rainbow
   E. Candle

4. The arytenoid adduction procedure mimics the action of which muscle?
   A. Cricothyroid
   B. Interarytenoid
   C. Thyroarytenoid
   D. Lateral cricoarytenoid
   E. Posterior cricoarytenoid

5. Laryngeal stroboscopy is most useful in the diagnosis of
   A. spasmodic dysphonia
   B. laryngeal paralysis
   C. epiglottitis
   D. vocal fold sulcus
   E. laryngopharyngeal reflux

Chapter 45
Embryology of Clefts and Pouches

Correlation Between Age and Size of Embryo	
Weeks	*Millimeters*
2.5	1.5
3.5	2.5
4	5
5	8
6	12
7	17
8	23
10	40
12	56
16	112
5-10 mo	160-350

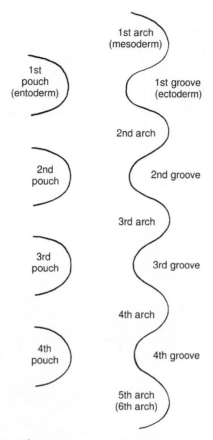

Figure 45-1 Pouches and grooves.

Development of the Branchial Arches

The first 8 weeks constitute the period of greatest embryonic development of the head and neck. There are five arches that are named either pharyngeal or branchial. Between these arches are the grooves or clefts externally and the pouches internally. Each pouch has a ventral or dorsal wing. The derivatives of the arches are usually of mesoderm origin. The groove is lined by ectoderm, and the pouch is lined by entoderm (Figure 45-1).

Each arch has an artery, nerve, and cartilage bar. These nerves are anterior to their respective arteries, except in the fifth arch where the nerve is posterior to the artery. (Embryologically, the arch after the fourth is called the fifth or sixth arch depending on the theory one follows. For simplicity in this synopsis, it is referred to as the fifth arch.) Caudal to all the arches lies the 12th nerve. The sternocleidomastoid muscles are derived from the cervical somites posterior and inferior to the above arches.

There are two ventral and two dorsal aortas in early embryonic life. The two ventral aortas fuse completely, whereas the two dorsal ones only fuse caudally (Figure 45-2A). During the course of embryonic development, the first and second arch arteries degenerate. The second arch artery has an upper branch that passes through a mass of mesoderm, which later chondrifies and ossifies as the stapes. This stapedial artery usually degenerates during late fetal life but

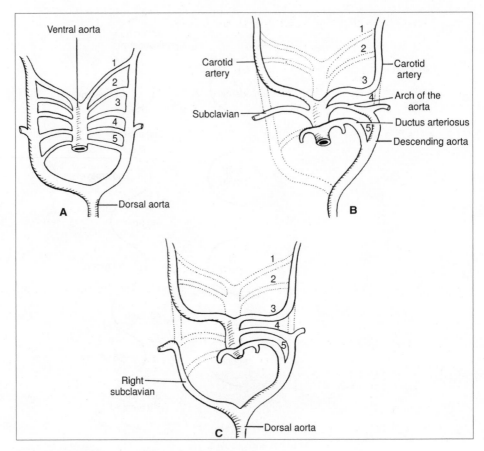

Figure 45-2 Development of the embryonic arteries.

occasionally persists in the adult. The third arch artery is the precursor of the carotid artery in both left and right sides. The left fourth arch artery becomes the arch of the aorta. The right fourth arch artery becomes the proximal subclavian. The rest of the right subclavian and the left subclavian are derivatives of the seventh segmental arteries. The left fifth arch artery becomes the pulmonary artery and ductus arteriosus. The right fifth arch artery becomes the pulmonary artery with degeneration of the rest of this arch vessel (Figure 45-2B).

Should the right fourth arch artery degenerate and the right subclavian arise from the dorsal aorta instead, as shown in Figure 45-2C, the right subclavian becomes posterior to the esophagus, thus causing a constriction of the esophagus without any effect on the trachea (dysphagia lusoria). The innominate artery arises ventrally. Hence when it arises too far from the left, an anterior compression of the trachea results (anomalous innominate).

The fifth arch nerve is posterior and caudal to the artery. As the connection on the right side between the fifth arch artery (pulmonary) and the dorsal aorta degenerates, the nerve (recurrent laryngeal nerve) loops around the fourth arch artery, which subsequently becomes the subclavian. On the left side, the nerve loops around the ductus arteriosus and the aorta. Table 45-1 lists the branchial arches and their derivatives.

Table 45-1 **Branchial Arches and Their Derivatives**

Arch	Ganglion or Nerve	Derivatives
First (mandibular)	Semilunar ganglion V$_3$	Mandible
		Head, neck, manubrium of malleus
		Body and short process of incus
		Anterior malleal ligament
		Sphenomandibular ligament
		Tensor tympani
		Mastication muscles, mylohyoid
		Anterior belly of digastric muscle
		Tensor palati muscle
Second (hyoid)	Geniculate ganglion VII	Manubrium of malleus
		Long process of incus
		All of stapes superstructure except footplate and annular ligament (vestibular portion)
		Stapedial artery
		Styloid process
		Stylohyoid ligament
		Lesser cornu of hyoid
		Part of body of hyoid
		Stapedius muscle
		Facial muscles
		Buccinator, posterior belly of digastric muscle
		Styloid muscle
		Part of pyramidal eminence
		Lower part of facial canal
Third	IX	Greater cornu of hyoid and rest of hyoid
		Stylopharyngeus muscle, superior and middle constrictors; common and internal carotid arteries
Fourth	Superior laryngeal nerve	Thyroid cartilage, cuneiform, inferior pharyngeal constrictor, cricopharyngeus, cricothyroid muscles, aorta on the left, proximal subclavian on the right
Fifth[a]	Recurrent laryngeal nerve	Cricoid, arytenoids, corniculate, trachea, intrinsic laryngeal muscles, inferior constrictor muscle, ductus arteriosus

[a] Often called the *sixth arch* from the standpoint of evolution and comparative anatomy.

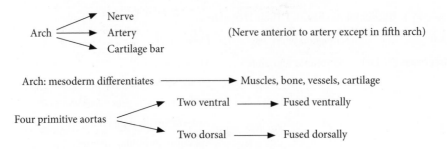

Derivatives of the Pouches

A. Each pouch has a ventral and a dorsal wing. The fourth pouch has an additional accessory wing. The entodermal lining of the pouches proliferates into glandular organs.

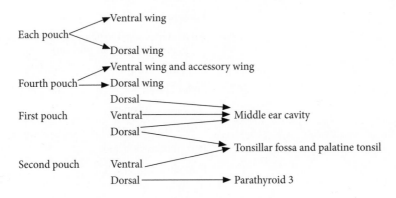

B. During embryonic development the thymus descends caudally, pulling with it parathyroid 3. Consequently, parathyroid 3 is inferior to parathyroid 4 in the adult.

C. The ultimobranchial body becomes infiltrated by cells of neural crest origin, giving rise to the interfollicular cells of the thyroid gland. These cells secrete thyrocalcitonin.

D. As these "out-pocketing" pouches develop into glandular elements, their connections with the pharyngeal lumen, referred to as pharyngobranchial ducts, become obliterated. Should obliteration fail to occur, a branchial sinus (cyst) is said to have resulted.

E. The second pharyngobranchial duct (between the second and third arches) is believed to open into the tonsillar fossa, the third pharyngobranchial duct opens into the pyriform sinus, and the fourth opens into the lower part of the pyriform sinus or larynx. An alternative school of thought believes that branchial sinuses and cysts are not remnants of patent pharyngobranchial ducts but, rather, are remnants of the cervical sinus of His.

F. The cutaneous openings of branchial sinuses, if present, are always anterior to the anterior border of the sternocleidomastoid muscle. The tract always lies deep to the platysma muscle, which is derived from the second arch (Figure 45-3).

   i. Course of a second arch branchial cyst

      a. Deep to second arch derivatives and superficial to third arch derivatives

      b. Superficial to the 12th nerve and anterior to the sternocleidomastoid

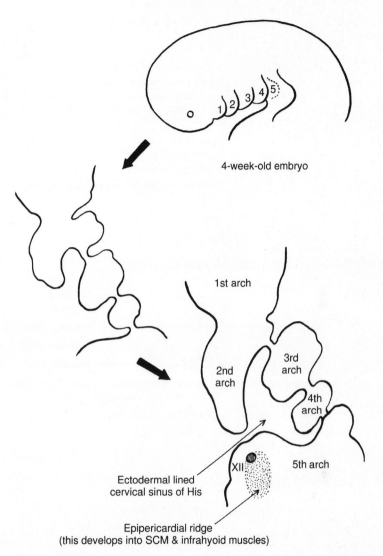

4-week-old embryo

1st arch

2nd arch

3rd arch

4th arch

5th arch

XII

Ectodermal lined cervical sinus of His

Epipericardial ridge
(this develops into SCM & infrahyoid muscles)

Figure 45-3 Pharyngobranchial ducts.

    c. In close relation with the carotid sheath but superficial to it

    d. Superficial to the ninth nerve, pierces middle constrictor, deep to stylohyoid ligament, opens into tonsillar fossa

  ii. Course of a third arch branchial cyst

    a. Again, subplatysmal and opens externally anterior to the sternocleidomastoid muscle

    b. Superficial to the 12th nerve, deep to the internal carotid artery and the ninth nerve

    c. Pierces the thyrohyoid membrane above the internal branch of the superior laryngeal nerve and opens into the pyriform fossa

iii. Course of a fourth arch branchial cyst
    a. Right
       1. The tract lies low in the neck beneath the platysma and anterior to the sternocleidomastoid muscle.
       2. It loops around the subclavian and deep to it, deep to the carotid, lateral to the 12th nerve, inferior to the superior laryngeal nerve; opens into the lower part of the pyriform sinus or into the larynx.
    b. Left
       1. Because the fourth arch vessel is the adult aorta, the cyst may be intrathoracic, medial to the ligamentum arteriosus and the arch of the aorta.
       2. It is lateral to the 12th nerve, inferior to the superior laryngeal nerve.
       3. It opens into the lower pyriform sinus or into the larynx.

Arches

First Arch (Mandibular Arch), Meckel Cartilage

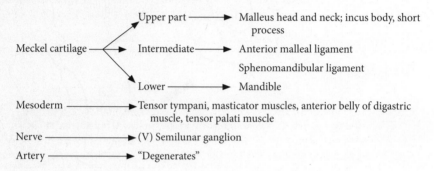

Meckel cartilage →
- Upper part → Malleus head and neck; incus body, short process
- Intermediate → Anterior malleal ligament / Sphenomandibular ligament
- Lower → Mandible

Mesoderm → Tensor tympani, masticator muscles, anterior belly of digastric muscle, tensor palati muscle

Nerve → (V) Semilunar ganglion

Artery → "Degenerates"

Second Arch (Hyoid Arch)

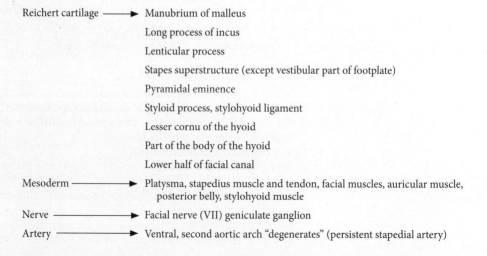

Reichert cartilage →
- Manubrium of malleus
- Long process of incus
- Lenticular process
- Stapes superstructure (except vestibular part of footplate)
- Pyramidal eminence
- Styloid process, stylohyoid ligament
- Lesser cornu of the hyoid
- Part of the body of the hyoid
- Lower half of facial canal

Mesoderm → Platysma, stapedius muscle and tendon, facial muscles, auricular muscle, posterior belly, stylohyoid muscle

Nerve → Facial nerve (VII) geniculate ganglion

Artery → Ventral, second aortic arch "degenerates" (persistent stapedial artery)

Third Arch

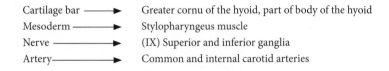

Cartilage bar ⟶ Greater cornu of the hyoid, part of body of the hyoid
Mesoderm ⟶ Stylopharyngeus muscle
Nerve ⟶ (IX) Superior and inferior ganglia
Artery ⟶ Common and internal carotid arteries

Fourth Arch

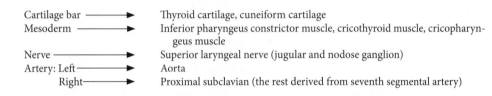

Cartilage bar ⟶ Thyroid cartilage, cuneiform cartilage
Mesoderm ⟶ Inferior pharyngeus constrictor muscle, cricothyroid muscle, cricopharyngeus muscle
Nerve ⟶ Superior laryngeal nerve (jugular and nodose ganglion)
Artery: Left ⟶ Aorta
Right ⟶ Proximal subclavian (the rest derived from seventh segmental artery)

Fifth Arch

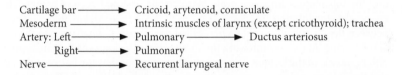

Cartilage bar ⟶ Cricoid, arytenoid, corniculate
Mesoderm ⟶ Intrinsic muscles of larynx (except cricothyroid); trachea
Artery: Left ⟶ Pulmonary ⟶ Ductus arteriosus
Right ⟶ Pulmonary
Nerve ⟶ Recurrent laryngeal nerve

Embryology of the Thyroid Gland

In a 4-week-old embryo, a ventral (thyroid) diverticulum of endodermal origin can be identified between the first and second arches on the floor of the pharynx. It also is situated between the tuberculum impar and the copula. (The tuberculum impar together with the lingual swellings becomes the anterior two-thirds of the tongue, and the copula is the precursor of the posterior one-third of the tongue.) The ventral diverticulum develops into the thyroid gland. During development it descends caudally within the mesodermal tissues. At 4.5 weeks the connection between the thyroid diverticulum and the floor of the pharynx begins to disappear. By the 6th week it should be obliterated and atrophied. Should it persist through the time of birth or thereafter, a thyroglossal duct cyst is present. This tract travels either superficial to, through, or just deep to the hyoid and reaches the foramen cecum (Figure 45-4).

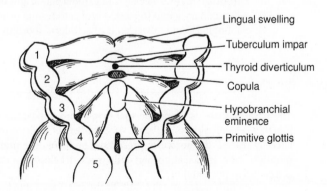

Figure 45-4 Four-week-old embryo.

Table 45-2 **Embryonic Development of the Tongue**

Age (Weeks)	Structure
4	Tuberculum impar, lingual swellings, copula
7	Voluntary muscles, nerve XII, papillae, tonsillar tissues
8-20	Circumvallate papillae
11	Filiform and fungiform papillae

Embryology of the Tongue

The tongue is derived from ectodermal origin (anterior two-thirds) and entodermal origin (posteriorly). At the fourth week, two lingual swellings are noted at the first arch, and a swelling, the tuberculum impar, appears between the first and second arches. These three prominences develop into the anterior two-thirds of the tongue. Meanwhile, another swelling is noted between the second and third arches, called the copula. It develops into the posterior one-third of the tongue. At the seventh week the somites from the high cervical areas differentiate into voluntary muscle of the tongue. The circumvallate papillae develop between the 8th and 20th weeks and the filiform and fungiform papillae develop at the 11th week (Table 45-2).

Embryology of Tonsils and Adenoids

A. Palatine tonsil (8 weeks) develops from the second pouch (ventral or dorsal).
B. Lingual tonsil (6.5 weeks) develops between the second and third arch ventrally.
C. Adenoids (16 weeks) develop as a subepithelial infiltration of lymphocytes.

Embryology of Salivary Glands

A. Parotid gland (5.5 weeks) is of ectodermal origin derived from the first pouch.
B. Submaxillary gland (6 weeks) is of ectodermal origin derived from the first pouch.
C. Sublingual gland (8 weeks) is of ectodermal origin derived from the first pouch.

Embryology of the Nose

The nasal placode is of ectodermal origin and appears between the middle of the third and fourth weeks of gestation (Figure 45-5A). It is of interest to note that at this stage the eyes are laterally placed, the auricular precursors lie below the mandibular process, and the primitive mouth is wide. Hence abnormal embryonic development at this stage may result in these characteristics in postnatal life.

At the fifth week, the placodes become depressed below the surface and appear as invaginated pits. The nasal pit extends backward into the oral cavity but is separated from it by the

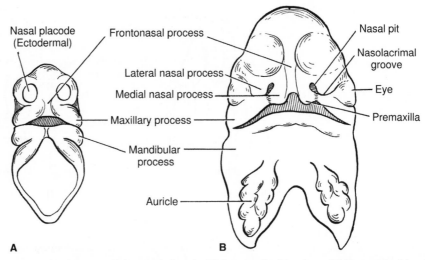

Figure 45-5 Development of the nasal placode. (A) Four-week-old embryo; (B) Five-week-old embryo.

bucconasal membrane (Figure 45-5B). This membrane ruptures at the seventh to eighth week of gestation to form the posterior nares. Failure in this step of development results in choanal atresia. The nasal pit extends backward as well as upward toward the forebrain area. Epithelium around the forebrain thickens to become specialized olfactory sensory cells.

Anteriorly, the maxillary process fuses with the lateral and medial nasal processes to form the anterior nares. The fusion between the maxillary process and the lateral nasal process also creates a groove called the nasolacrimal groove. The epithelium over the groove is subsequently buried, and, when the epithelium is resorbed, the nasolacrimal duct is formed, opening into the anterior aspect of the inferior meatus. The duct is fully developed at birth.

The frontonasal process (mesoderm) is the precursor of the nasal septum (Figure 45-6). The primitive palate (premaxilla) located anteriorly is also a derivative of the frontonasal process (mesoderm). Posteriorly (Figure 45-7), the septum lies directly over the oral cavity until the ninth week, at which time the palatal shelves of the maxilla grow medially to fuse with each other and with the septum to form the secondary palate. The hard palate is formed by the eighth to ninth week (Figure 45-8), and the soft palate and the uvula are completed by the 11th to 12th week.

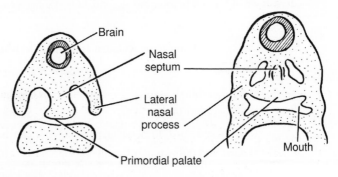

Figure 45-6 Development of the nasal septum (see text).

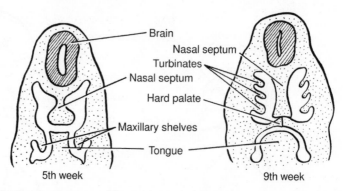

Figure 45-7 Further development of the nasal septum (see text).

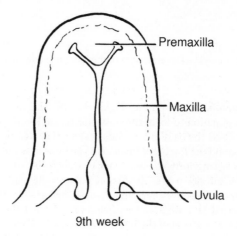

9th week

Figure 45-8 Parts of the palate.

From the 8th week to the 24th week of embryonic life, the nostrils are occupied by an epithelial plug. Failure to resorb this epithelium results in atresia or stenosis of the anterior nares.

Along the lateral wall of the nasal precursor, the maxilloturbinal is the first to appear, followed by the development of five ethmoturbinals and one nasoturbinal. Table 45-3 gives the derivatives of each embryonic anlage, and Table 45-4 gives a timetable of their development.

Table 45-3 Embryonic Anlagen and Their Derivatives

Anlagen	*Derivatives*
Maxilloturbinal	Inferior concha
First ethmoturbinal	Middle concha
Second and third ethmoturbinals	Superior concha
Fourth and fifth ethmoturbinals	Supreme concha
Nasoturbinal	Agger nasi area

Table 45-4 **Timetable of Nasal Development**

Structures	Time of Development (Week)
Inferior concha formed	7
Middle concha formed	7
Uncinate process formed	7
Superior concha formed	8
Cartilage laid down	10
Vomer formed and calcified	12
Ethmoid bone calcified	20
Cribriform plate calcified	28
Perpendicular plate, crista galli calcified	After birth

Embryology of the Larynx

Figure 45-9 depicts the embryonic development of the larynx between the 8th and 28th weeks of fetal life.

The entire respiratory system is an outgrowth of the primitive pharynx. At 3.5 weeks, a groove called the laryngotracheal groove develops in the embryo at the ventral aspect of the foregut. This groove is just posterior to the hypobranchial eminence and is located closer to the fourth arch than to the third arch. During embryonic development, when a single tubal structure is to later become two tubal structures, the original tube is first obliterated by a proliferation of lining epithelium, then as resorption of the epithelium takes place, the second tube is formed and the first tube is recannulized. Hence any malformation involves both tubes. This process of growth accounts for the fact that more than 90% of tracheoesophageal fistulas are associated with esophageal atresia. During development the mesenchyme of the foregut grows medially from the sides, "pinching off" this groove to create a separate opening. With further maturation, two separate tubes, the esophagus and the laryngotracheal apparatus, are formed.

This laryngotracheal opening is the primitive laryngeal aditus and lies between the fourth and fifth arches. The sagittal slit opening is altered to become a T-shaped opening by the growth of three tissue masses. The first is the hypobranchial eminence, which appears during the third week. This mesodermal structure gives rise to the furcula, which later develops into the epiglottis. The second and third growths are two arytenoid masses, which appear during the fifth week. Later, each arytenoid swelling shows two additional swellings that eventually mature into the cuneiform and corniculate cartilages.

As these masses grow between the fifth and seventh weeks, the laryngeal lumen is obliterated. At the ninth week the oval shape lumen is reestablished. Failure to recannulize may result in atresia or stenosis of the larynx. The true and false cords are formed between the 8th and 10th weeks. The ventricles are formed at the 12th week.

The two arytenoid masses are separated by an "interarytenoid notch," which later becomes obliterated. Failure of this obliteration to occur results in a posterior cleft up to the cricoid cartilage, and opening into the esophagus. This is a culprit of severe aspiration in the newborn.

Table 45-5 outlines the muscular and cartilaginous development of the larynx.

The laryngeal muscles are derivatives from the mesoderm of the fourth and fifth arches and hence are innervated by the 10th nerve. The infant larynx is situated at a level between the

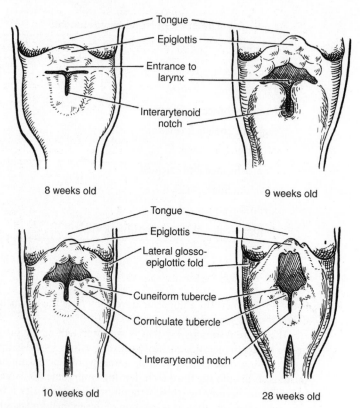

Figure 45-9 Development of the fetal larynx.

Table 45-5 **Laryngeal Muscular and Cartilaginous Development With Embryonic Age**

Development	*Age (weeks)*
Muscular	
Inferior pharyngeal constrictor and cricothyroid muscles formed	4
Interarytenoid and postcricoarytenoid muscles formed	5.5
Lateral cricoarytenoid muscle formed	6
Cartilaginous	
Development of epiglottis (hypobranchial eminence)	3
Thyroid cartilage (fourth arch) and cricoid cartilage (fifth arch) appear	5
Chondrification of these two cartilages begins	7
Development and chondrification of arytenoid (fifth arch) and corniculate (fifth arch) (vocal process is the last to develop)	12
Chondrification of the epiglottis	20
Development of the cuneiform cartilage (fourth arch)	28

Table 45-6 **Development of Paranasal Sinuses**

Sinus	Characteristics	Age
Maxillary	Arises as a prolongation of the ethmoid infundibulum	12 wk
	Pneumatizes	At birth
	Reaches stable size	18 y
Frontal	Arises from the upper anterior area of the middle meatus	Starts at late fetal life or even after birth
	Pneumatizes	After 1 y
	Full size	20 y
Sphenoid	Arises from the epithelial outgrowth of the upper posterior region of the nasal cavity in close relation with the sphenoid bone	Starts at third fetal month
	Pneumatizes	During childhood
	Full size	15 y
Ethmoid	Arises from the evagination of the nasal mucosa into the lateral ethmoid mass	Sixth fetal month
	Pneumatization completed	7 y
	Full size	12 y

second and third cervical vertebrae. In the adult it lies opposite the body of the fifth cervical vertebra.

Table 45-6 outlines the development of the paranasal sinuses.

Ossification of Laryngeal Skeleton

Hyoid → Ossification from six centers → Starts at birth; completed by 2 years

Thyroid → Starts at 20-23 years; starts at inferior margin

        Extends posteriorly at each ala

        Superior margin never ossified

Cricoid → Starts at 25-30 years

        Incomplete

        Starts at inferior margin

Arytenoids → Starts at 25-30 years

Middle Ear Cleft

Embryology of the ear and congenital deformities (Tables 45-7A and B)

Table 45-7a **Embyrology of the Ear**

Week	External ear	Middle ear	Inner ear	Facial nerve
3-5	Ectoderm—first branchial groove Endoderm—first branchial pouch	Second branchial pouch—middle ear space, second mesenchymal arch—stapes arch	Neuroectoderm + ectoderm—otic placode evolves to otic pit, vesicle, and endolymphatic duct and sac; ventral—vestibule; dorsal—cochlea, acoustic ganglion; superior—vestibular; inferior—cochlear, otic capsule from mesenchyme tissue	Primoridal facial–acoustic—sensory fibers: chordae tympani nerve, nervus intermedius, geniculate ganglion, greater superficial petrosal nerve
6-9	First to second arch form hillocks of His First arch 1 tragus 2 helical crus 3 helix Second arch 4 antihelix 5 antitragus 6 loblule	Malleus and incus—single mesenchymal mass, mesenchymal stapes footplate; Meckel's cartilage—head and neck of malleus, body and short process of incus; Reichert cartilage—manubrium of malleus, long process of incus, stapes arch	Semicircular canals, macula divides: upper—utricle, lower—saccule; cochlea—2.5 turns wk 6-8.5	VII and VIII separate, extends to facial muscles, fallopian canal evolves as sulcus ninth wk. and fuses with Reichert cartilage
10-14	Hillocks fuse—auricle	Stapes arch formed, four mucosal pouches formed: anterior—anterior pouch of von Trolch; medius—petrous and epitympanium; superior—posterior pouch of von Trolch, mastoid; posterior—oval and round window niche, sinus tympani	Vestibular end organs formed, otolithic membrane, macula, cochlea tectorial membrane, scala tympani, fissula ante fenestram, fossula post fenestram	Extensive facial branching, location anterior in relation to external ear
15-20	Auricle recognizable, tympanic ring formed	Ossicles adult size, ossification begins	Membranous labyrinth complete without end organs, ossification begins at 14 sites	Located anterior and superficial, migration posterior
21-28	(External auditory canal) EAC epithelial core reabsorbs, complete 28th wk	Drum formed 28th wk; ectoderm—squamous; mesoderm—fibrous; entoderm—mucosal	Ossification complete 23rd wk; last to ossify fissula ante fenestrum, fossula post fenestrum; cochlea structures formed	Fallopian canal closes and ossifies

Table 45-7a **Continued**

Week	External ear	Middle ear	Inner ear	Facial nerve
30-Birth	Auricle and ear canal continued to grow to age 9 y	Middle ear air space formed; tympanic ring ossifies by age 3; eustachian tube grows 17-36 mm	Membranous and bony labyrinth adult size; endolymphatic sac grows until adulthood	Facial nerve lateral until mastoid tip formed at age 3; 25% fallopian canals dehiscent

Grade	Microtia	Atresia
I	Slight deformity of pinna	EAC normal—atretic, ossicles—deformed or fixed, abnormal course of facial nerve
II	Deformed cartilage framework of pinna	Atresia, absent tympanic bone, small middle ear space, deformed ossicles, facial nerve anterior and lateral
III	Soft tissue remnant of pinna	Middle and inner ear deformities
IV	Anotia	Severe inner ear deformities: Scheibe—collapse e of cochlear duct, deformed organ of corti; Michel aplasia—absent inner ear

Congenital deformities incidence: microtia 0.13-6 per 1000 live births; atresia 1.2-5.5 per 1000 births; ossicular abnormalities 2% of patients having stapes surgery; bilateral deformities 10%; congenital hearing loss: sensorineural 85%; conductive 15% with external deformities in 50%.
Common syndromes associated with conductive hearing loss: mandibulofacial dysostosis (Treacher Collins); hemifacial microsomia; oculoauricular vertebral dysplasia (Goldenhar); craniofacial dysostosis (Crouzon disease).
Data from Sataloff RT. *Embryology and Anomalies of the Facial Nerve and Their Surgical Implications.* New York, NY: Raven Press; 1991.

Table 45-7b **Microtia–Atresia**

External ear deformities

Preauricular pits and sinuses:

Etiology: failure of complete closure first and second branchial arch hillock

Incidence: white 0.18%, black 1.49%

Pathology: epithelial-lined tract, may be associated with chronic inflammation, may extend to tragus or scaphoid fossa

Management: observation unless infected; excision of complete fistula tract

Auricular deformities:

Microtia grade I-IV often associated with atresis grade I-IV; protruding ear–cupped ear–deep conchal bowl; helical and antihelical rim deformities

Management: dependent on severity of deformity; otoplasty—reconstruction

Evaluation congenital hearing loss and deformities:

Audiology: birth—otoacoustic emissions (OAE); brainstem-evoked response audiometry (BERA); play audiometry at the age of 18 mo

Expected hearing loss:

Atresia: 60-70 dB conductive loss

Stapes fixation: 50-65 dB conductive loss; presence of a carhart notch may suggest abnormal course of facial nerve

Table 45-7b *Continued*

Ossicular abnormalities: 25-50 dB conductive loss

Facial nerve impinging on stapes: 20-35 dB conductive loss

Radiology: conductive hearing loss—compute d tomography (CT) thin 0.6 mm sections, axial and coronal views prior to surgery

Sensorineural hearing loss—early childhood CT 0.6 mm, MR I < 1 mm of the cochlea and labyrinth, axial and coronal

Management

Amplification: 6 mo of age hearing aids, sound stimulation

Cochlear implant: age 1-2 y with profound sensorineural hearing loss

Bone anchored hearing device considered for nonsurgical patients—age 6 y

Surgical reconstruction: external and middle ear

Reconstruction of pinna prior to EAC and middle ear; age 5-8 y, depending on size of opposite ear. Four stages:

1. Bury carved rib cartilage skeleton of pinna. 2. Construct lobule. 3. Elevate helical rim and graft postauricular sulcus. 4. Construct conchal bowl and tragus, may be combined with atresia surgery.

Atresia, middle ear reconstruction: indications—conductive hearing loss > 30 dB, bone conduction < 20 dB, aerated and accessible middle ear space. reconstruction 70% tympanoplasty—ea r canal, drum, and ossicular chain, stapes and oval window 17%, 60% have additional ossicular abnormalities, facial nerve covers the oval window 13% requiring fenestration of the horizontal canal.

Alternative treatment: bone anchored auricular prosthesis and hearing aid; no treatment with normal or aidable opposite ear.

Bibliography

Anson BJ, Donaldson JA. *The Ear: Developmental Anatomy and Surgical Anatomy of the Temporal Bone.* 3rd ed. Philadelphia, PA: WB Sanders Company; 1981:23-57.

Isaacson G, ed. Congenital anomalies of the head and neck. *Otolaryngol Clin North Am.* 2007;40:1-8.

Jahrsdoerfer R. Congenital malformations of the ear. *Ann Otolaryngol.* 1980;89:348-353.

Lambert PR. Congenital aural atresia. In: Bailey, ed. *Head & Neck Surgery–Otolaryngology.* Philadelphia, PA: Lippincott–Raven; 1998:1997-2010.

Sataloff RT. *Embryology and Anomalies of the Facial Nerve and Their Surgical Implications.* New York, NY: Raven Press; 1990.

Questions

1. The ultimobranchial body is responsible for cells that produce
   A. insulin
   B. parathyroid hormone
   C. thyrocalcitonin
   D. amylase
   E. thyroxine

2. What is the precursor to the nasal septum?
   A. Medial nasal process
   B. Lateral nasal process
   C. Frontonasal process
   D. Maxillary process
   E. Ethmoturbinal

3. The anterior two-thirds of the tongue is derived from
   A. endoderm
   B. ectoderm
   C. mesoderm
   D. neural crest cells
   E. thyroid cells

4. Which nerve is associated with the fourth branchial arch?
   A. Hypoglossal nerve
   B. Facial nerve
   C. Glossopharyngeal nerve
   D. Superior laryngeal nerve
   E. Trigeminal nerve

5. Cutaneous openings of branchial arch sinus tracts are always anterior to
   A. hyoid bone
   B. submandibular gland
   C. sternocleidomastoid muscle
   D. angle of the mandible
   E. recurrent laryngeal nerve

Chapter 46
Cleft Lip and Palate

Overview/Introduction

- Cleft lip with or without cleft palate is the most common congenital malformation of the head and neck occurring in 1:1000 live births.
- Each patient should be evaluated for congenital anomalies, developmental delay, neurologic disorders, and psychosocial concerns.
- A multidisciplinary team is recommended to ensure that every aspect of care is appropriately coordinated among providers.
- A fundamental understanding by the surgeon of each step of care is warranted.

Anatomy

- Lip (Figure 46-1)
  - (a) Primary muscle: orbicularis oris (innervated by CN VII)—creates a sphincter around the mouth
  - (b) Primary blood supply: superior labial artery—runs deep to the orbicularis oris muscle
  - (c) Vermillion border (white roll): mucoepithelial junction between the cutaneous lip and mucosal lip— a 1 mm discrepancy in re-approximation is easily visible
  - (d) Dry lip: portion of mucosal lip exposed to air
  - (e) Wet lip: separated from dry lip by the wet-dry junction
  - (f) Philtral ridges: paramedian columns formed at embryonic fusion plane between maxillary and frontonasal prominences—elevation of the vermillion at the junction with the philtrum forms the peak of cupid's bow
  - (g) Philtral dimple: midline dimple above central portion of cupid's bow formed by decussation of muscles to contralateral philtral column and attachment of orbicularis oris to dermis
- Palate
  - (a) Primary palate: anterior to the incisive foramen
  - (b) Secondary palate: posterior to the incisive foramen
    - Hard palate: posterior to incisive foramen but anterior to levator veli palatini muscle
    - Soft palate: posterior to hard palate, comprised of levator veli palatini, tensor veli palatini, musculus uvula

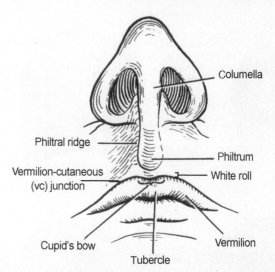

Figure 46-1 Anatomy of the lip. (*Reproduced with permission from Lee KJ, ed.* Essential Otolaryngology. *7th ed. Stamford, CN: Appleton & Lange; 1999.*)

(a) Bony anatomy: the hard palate consists of the premaxilla (anteriorly) and vertical segments of the palatine bone (posteriorly) which contain the greater palatine foramina and the lesser palatine foramina
(b) Greater palatine foramen: contents include the greater palatine vessels and greater palatine nerve
(c) Lesser palatine foramen: lesser palatine nerves
(d) Muscles: are all innervated by CN X except tensor veli palatini (innervated by V3)
   ○ Levator veli palatini
   ○ Tensor veli palatini
   ○ Palatoglossus
   ○ Palatopharyngeus
   ○ Musculus uvula
(e) Primary blood supply
   ○ Hard palate: greater palatine artery
   ○ Soft palate: descending palatine branch of the facial artery, palatine branch of the ascending pharyngeal artery, and lesser palatine artery

Embryology (Figure 46-2)

- Lip
   (a) Gestational week 4: paired maxillary prominences begin to appear from the first pharyngeal arches and frontonasal prominence (only unpaired prominence) from mesenchyme ventral to forebrain
   (b) Gestational week 5: nasal placodes invaginate forming medial and lateral nasal prominences
   (c) Gestational weeks 6-7: medial growth of paired maxillary prominences meet paired medial nasal prominences and frontonasal prominence forming upper lip

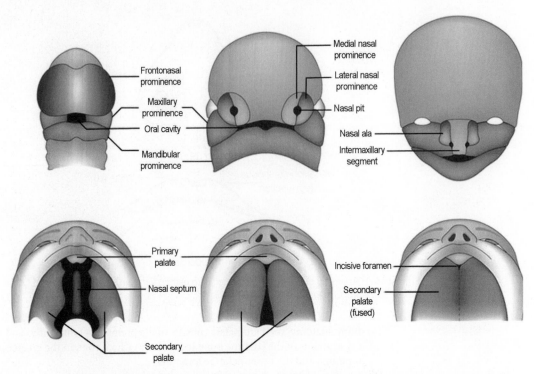

Figure 46-2 Embryologic development of the midface. The upper row is a frontal view of lip development during gestation and the lower row is an axial view of palatal development during gestation. (*Reproduced with permission from Dixon MJ, Marazita ML, Beaty TH, Murray JC. Cleft lip and palate: understanding genetic and environmental influences. Nat Rev Genet. Mar 2011;12(3):167-178.*)

- Palate
  - (a) Gestational weeks 5-12: maxillary prominences push medial nasal prominences medially and fuse by 12 weeks; intermaxillary segment (with four incisor teeth buds) is formed by fusion of the paired medial nasal prominences
  - (b) Gestational weeks 5-6: soft palate musculature migrates toward midline from both sides of the developing oropharynx
  - (c) Gestational weeks 6-7: palatal shelves grow medially from maxillary prominences
  - (d) Gestational weeks 9-10: soft palate muscles have moved into a horizontal orientation, paralleling the palatine shelves
  - (e) Gestational weeks 8-12: fusion of palatal shelves form the secondary palate, secondary palatal fusion occurs from anterior (incisive foramen) to posterior (uvula), by the 12th week the soft palate tissue and muscles fuse

Epidemiology/Incidence (Tables 46-1 and 46-2)

- Cleft incidence varies widely depending on geographic origin, racial and ethnic group, environmental exposures, and socioeconomic status
  - (a) Cleft Lip w/ or w/o cleft palate: 1 in 1000
  - (b) Cleft Palate w/o cleft lip: 1 in 2,500 live births

Table 46-1 **Epidemiology of Clefts**

(CL ± P)	*Isolated Cleft Palate (CPO)*
0.2-2.3/1000 births	0.1-1.1/1000 births
Varies across ethnicities:	Uniform across ethnicities
• American Indian 3.6:1000	
• Chinese 1.7:1000	
• European descent 1:1000	
• African descent 0.7:1000	
Up to 30% associated with syndromes	Up to 50% associated with syndromes
Male:Female 1.5-2.0:1	Male:Female 0.5-0.7:1

Table 46-2 **What Are the Next Child's Chances of a Clefting Defect?**

	Cleft Lip ± Palate (%)	*Cleft Palate (%)*
Parents normal, first child is affected		
No affected relatives	4	2
Affected relatives	4	7
Parents normal, two affected relatives	9	10
One parent affected, no affected children	4	6
One parent affected, one child affected	17	15

(c) Parent has cleft: 3% to 5% risk for each child
(d) One affected sibling: 2% to 4% risk for each child
(e) Two affected siblings: 8% to 10% risk for each child
(f) Sibling + parent: 10% risk
(g) Racial characteristics: Asian and Pacific islanders > White > African Americans

Etiology

- Genetics Factors
  (a) Twin concordance rates
    ○ Monozygotic concordance rate: 50% to 60%
    ○ Dizygotic concordance rate: 5%
  (b) Nonsyndromic
    ○ 70% of cleft lip w/ or w/o cleft palate
    ○ 50% of cleft palate
  (c) Syndromic
    ○ Van der Woude: autosomal dominant (IRF6 gene on Chromosome 1)

- Lower lip pits (90% penetrance) and cleft lip and/or cleft palate
- Pierre Robin sequence: may be syndromic (with other associated abnormalities) or nonsyndromic
  - Classic triad: micrognathia, glossoptosis, U-shaped cleft palate (micrognathia is primary cause that leads to glossoptosis and cleft palate)
- Stickler: autosomal dominant (mutations in genes involved in collagen production)
  - Flattened facial appearance, eye abnormalities (high myopia, glaucoma, cataracts, retinal detachments), cleft palate as part of Pierre Robin sequence, hearing loss, joint abnormalities (hypermobile; kyphosis/scoliosis/platyspondyly)
- 22q11.2 Deletion syndrome (Velocardiofacial syndrome, DiGeorge syndrome): autosomal dominant (deletion of Ch 22q11.2)
  - Cleft palate, cardiac anomalies, unique facial characteristics, minor learning disabilities, velopharyngeal insufficiency (can be without cleft palate), medial displacement of carotid arteries, immune deficiency/absent thymus, hypocalcemia, cardiac defects
- Others: Treacher-Collins, Down, CHARGE, Hemifacial microsomia, Apert, median facial dysplasia
  (d) Implicated genes: Msx1 gene, IRF6, TGF-alpha and TGF-beta
- Environmental risks
  (a) Teratogens: retinoids, smoking, alcohol abuse, illicit drugs, nitrate compounds, organic solvents, lead, anticonvulsants
  (b) Nutrition: inadequate folic acid (vitamin B9), vitamins B6 and B12
  (c) Amniotic band sequence
  (d) Increasing birth order has higher risk of clefting

Classification

- A variety of classification schemes have been suggested for typical and atypical clefting.
- The features used to initiate classification of a cleft lip w/ or w/o palate include laterality, completeness, severity (wide vs narrow), and presence of abnormal tissue.
- Diminutive clefts are described as microform, occult, minor or forme fruste.
- Complete cleft lip: extends through the lip and the nasal sill.
- Incomplete cleft lip: extends through the orbicularis oris and skin, but intact lip persists.
- Cleft alveolus can be considered complete or notched.
- Simonart band: web-like tissue that extends form the lips' cleft side to the noncleft side at the nasal sill that often contains orbicularis oris muscle (if present, it does not constitute an incomplete cleft).
- Unilateral cleft palate: one palatal shelf attaches to the nasal septum.
- Bilateral cleft palate: the palatal shelves do not attach to the nasal septum.
- Veau classification: group I: cleft of the soft palate, group II: cleft of the soft and hard palate to the incisive foramen (secondary palate cleft), group III: unilateral cleft extending though entire palate (secondary and primary palate) to the alveolus, group IV: complete bilateral clefts.

Management

- Multidisciplinary care
  (a) A multidisciplinary approach is recommended in assessing a child with orofacial clefting.
  (b) Initial evaluations are performed by a pediatrician, geneticist, surgeon, feeding specialist, and social worker.
  (c) The patient will also require hearing assessment to evaluate for congenital sensorineural hearing loss and conductive hearing loss (Eustachian tube dysfunction is associated with a cleft palate).
  (d) Dental and maxillofacial evaluation are crucial.
      ◦ Presurgically, orthopedics are discussed (nasoalveolar molding).
      ◦ Postsurgically, palatal expansion, dental alignment, alveolar bone grafting, and orthognathic surgery may be recommended.
  (e) When appropriate, speech and language pathology is consulted as there is a high risk of speech-language disorders.
  (f) Periodic assessment of the psychosocial needs of both the patient and the family are recommended.
- Early management
  (a) Cleft patients may present as early as the prenatal period due to the ability to make the diagnosis on a prenatal ultrasound.
  (b) After birth, initial management includes ensuring proper feeding and evaluation for other comorbidities.
  (c) Breast feeding is unlikely with a cleft palate, but in select cases may be possible.
  (d) May require bottle feeds utilizing a specialized nipple that controls the flow rate, such as a Haberman or pigeon-type nipple.
  (e) Monitor the infant for adequate weight gain.
  (f) Early airway management may be necessary (especially in the setting or Pierre Robin sequence) including positioning, nasal trumpet, and mandible distraction.
  (g) Consider genetic evaluation and counseling.
- Late management
  (a) Various procedures may be necessary during the first two decades of life (Figure 46-3).
- Surgical assessment
  (a) Cleft repair goal: restore the normal function and anatomic features of the lip and/or palate
  (b) Consider the overall width of the cleft, as a wide cleft could make the repair difficult and place undesirable tension on the closure (may lead to breakdown and scarring)
      ◦ Presurgical devices may assist in narrowing the cleft (lip taping, oral appliance, nasoalveolar molding)
      ◦ Other options included performing a two-staged repair with primary lip adhesion or delaying the repair to allow increased growth

Cleft Lip

- Timing of repair
  (a) Generally based off the rule of 10s (> 10 weeks old, > 10 lb, > 10 hemoglobin)
  (b) Usually performed during the first year of age

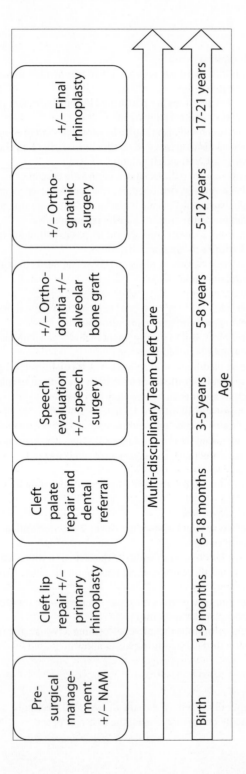

Figure 46-3 Timeline for the management of patients with cleft lip/palate. The multidisciplinary cleft team facilitates management throughout the years.

(c) Many consider waiting three months will allow safer anesthesia, improved accuracy of repair, and parental acceptance of the malformation
- Surgical goals
  (a) Restore function of the orbicularis oris muscle.
  (b) Alignment and recreation of the philtral ridges and groove, white roll, and mucocutaneous ridge.
  (c) In a bilateral lip, the goal is also to generate a balanced lip and nose with adequate columella length and proper philtral landmarks.
- Unilateral cleft lip
  (a) Relevant anatomy
    ○ Orbicularis oris muscle is disrupted and possesses abnormal attachments to the base of the nasal sill on the cleft side and the base of the columella on the non-cleft side.
    ○ Columella is shorter on the cleft side and the base is deviated to the noncleft side.
    ○ The lower lateral cartilage is displaced inferiorly, laterally, and posteriorly on the cleft side.
    ○ The nasal tip is displaced and the dome on the cleft side is obtuse.
    ○ The caudal nasal septum is deflected to the noncleft side.
    ○ The maxilla on the cleft side is hypoplastic.
    ○ The nasal floor is absent in complete cleft lips.
  (b) Surgical techniques
    ○ Multiple techniques and variations have been described (straight line closure, geometric lip repair, advancement-rotation, etc).
    ○ The principles of advancement and rotation were popularized by Millard.
    ○ Millard technique.
      – Flaps are created as illustrated (see Figure 46-4).
      – The orbicularis oris muscle is released from its abnormal attachments at the alar base and columella and the ends approximated to create a functional sphincter.
      – The alar base on the cleft side is released and realigned symmetrically with the contralateral base.
      – The philtral ridge on the cleft side is rotated to equal the philtral ridge on the non-cleft side approximated to the non-cleft upper lip.
      – The mucocutaneous border is meticulously aligned.
      – The nasal floor and sill are closed.
      – Primary rhinoplasty may be performed to improve overall nasal symmetry.
- Bilateral cleft lip
  (a) Relevant anatomy
    ○ The premaxillary segment is separated from the lateral maxillary segments and there is a tendency for the premaxilla to protrude anteriorly and superiorly (this may cause tension on a lip repair).
    ○ Muscle fibers and the white roll are absent in the prolabial segment.
    ○ The nasal floor is absent in complete bilateral cleft lips.
    ○ The columella length is shortened.
    ○ The nasal tip is widened.
  (b) Surgical techniques
    ○ Major goals of reconstruction include:
      – Reconstruction of a functional muscular sphincter
      – Symmetric alar base narrowing

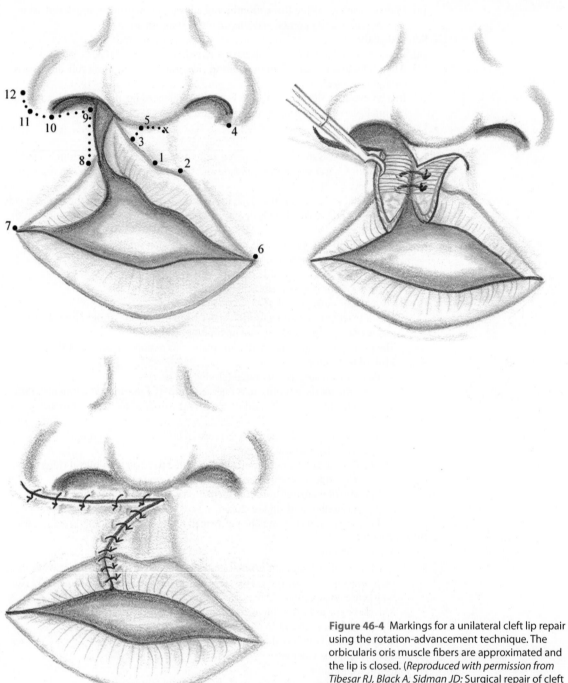

Figure 46-4 Markings for a unilateral cleft lip repair using the rotation-advancement technique. The orbicularis oris muscle fibers are approximated and the lip is closed. (*Reproduced with permission from Tibesar RJ, Black A, Sidman JD:* Surgical repair of cleft lip and palate, Otolaryngol Head Neck Surg. *2009 Dec;20(4):245-255.*)

– Creation of a philtral column that will widen with growth
– Aesthetic red lip and vermillion approximation
○ Multiple surgical techniques have been advocated, including a bilateral repair in infancy with a delayed columellar lengthening at a later date, a one stage cleft repair that may or may not include a primary rhinoplasty, and a lip adhesion early in life with a delayed repair several months later (Figure 46-5).

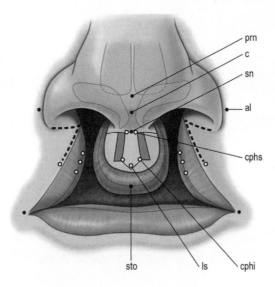

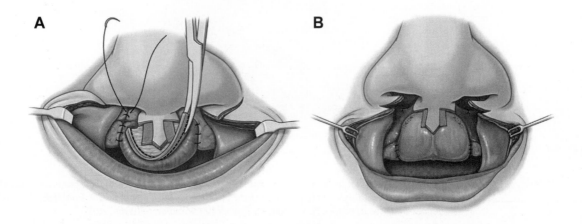

Figure 46-5 *(Continued)*

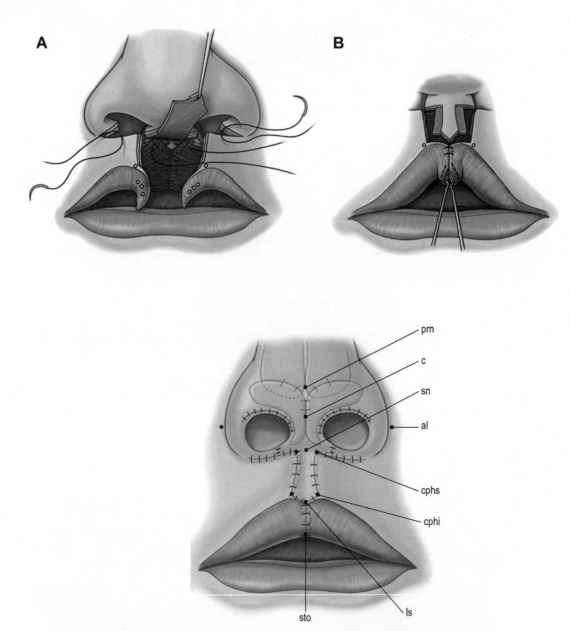

Figure 46-5 The markings for a bilateral cleft lip repair. The orbicularis oris muscle fibers are approximated and the flaps are closed to reconstruct the lip. (*Reproduced with permission from Neligan PC, Rodriguez ED, Losee JE, editors:* Plastic surgery. *Philadelphia: Saunders-Elsevier; 2012.*)

- Postsurgery care
  - (a) The primary goals include prevention of infection and wound tension, provide pain relief, and promote adequate nutrition.
- Complications
  - (a) Often associated with increased tension of the closure, infection, or in children with poor nutrition.
  - (b) Complications include lip dehiscence, vermillion notching, misalignment of the white roll, orbicularis oris muscle discontinuity.
- Primary rhinoplasty
  - (a) Performed at the time of the cleft lip repair
  - (b) Early treatment of nasal deformity minimizes nasal asymmetries and allows the nose to grow symmetrically
  - (c) Technique
    - ◦ The lower later cartilages are released from the skin soft tissue envelope.
    - ◦ The nasal dome and lower lateral cartilages are repositioned in order to improve alar symmetry and tip projection using contouring sutures.
    - ◦ Some surgeons will use tie-over bolsters and/or nasal conformers to aid proper healing.

Cleft palate

- Timing of repair
  - (a) In an appropriately developing child, the standard is to repair the palate before 18 months of age and earlier when possible (most repairs are performed between 6 and 16 months of age).
  - (b) The timing of repair is a balance between poor speech and language development related to late surgery and the potential impairment of maxillary growth related to early surgery.
- Relevant anatomy (Figure 46-6)
  - (a) Anatomical differences of the hard palate
    - ◦ The nasal mucosa joins with oral mucosa medially along the cleft margin.

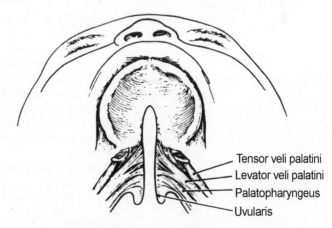

Tensor veli palatini
Levator veli palatini
Palatopharyngeus
Uvularis

Figure 46-6 Schematic diagram of clefting of the secondary palate. Note the abnormal attachment of the levator veli palatini to the posterior edge of the hard palate instead of meeting in the midline. (*Reproduced with permission from Meyers AD*: Biological Basis of Facial Plastic Surgery. *New York, NY: Thieme Medical Publishers; 1993.*)

- In a unilateral cleft palate repair, the nasal layer is formed medially from the mucosa of the vomer.
- In a bilateral cleft or an isolated cleft of the hard palate, the vomer is midline and the mucosa is not continuous with the mucosa of the palatine shelves (during repair, the vomer can be incised in the midline and each side of the nasal layer is incorporated in the repair).

(b) Anatomical differences of the soft palate
- The levator palatini muscle orients in an anterior-posterior direction, attaching to the posterior aspect of the palatine bone and the anterior half of the cleft margin (whereas the normal configuration is the extension from lateral to medial, creating a muscular sling).
- The tensor veli palatini muscle is thinner and commonly inserts as thick bundle into the anterior portion of the levator muscle (this orientation limits its ability to open the Eustachian tube and contributes to the middle ear disease of patients with cleft palates).

(c) Anatomical differences of a submucous cleft palate
- Intact mucosa with underlying dehiscence and anterior-posterior alignment of the palatal musculature
- Classic physical findings: bifid uvula, zona pellucida (hyperlucent line in the middle of the soft palate), notch at the middling of the posterior palate
- May be associated with velopharyngeal insufficiency, feeding concerns, and otologic disease

- Surgical goals
  (a) Restore the functional anatomy of the palate
  (b) Separate the oral and nasal layers in order to aid the processes of eating, swallowing, articulation, and resonance associated with speech
  (c) Produce a functional velopharyngeal mechanism
- Surgical techniques
  (a) Various techniques and modifications have been developed for cleft palate repair (two-flap, double-opposing Z-plasty, intravelar veloplasty, V-Y, pushback, von Langenbeck, etc)
  (b) The type of cleft (hard vs soft palate) and the width are evaluated in order to select an appropriate technique to accomplish the goals of repair
  (c) Submucous cleft palates can be monitored closely and repaired only if there is evidence of feeding, otologic, or speech problems
  (d) Common techniques include the two-flap palatoplasty with intravelar veloplasty and the double-opposing Z-plasty popularized by Furlow
  (e) Two-flap palatoplasty with intravelar veloplasty technique (Figure 46-7)
    - Indication: widely used for all palatal clefts.
    - Two mucoperiosteal flaps are raised on either side of the cleft based on the greater palatine vasculature.
    - The soft palatal muscles are released from the posterior aspect of the hard palate.
    - The nasal layer is approximated.
    - An intravelar veloplasty is performed, reorienting and approximating the levator sling.
    - The oral layer is approximated.
  (f) Double opposing Z-plasty (Furlow palatoplasty) (Figure 46-8)
    - Indication: commonly used for soft palate clefts and submucous cleft palates, but may be combined with other techniques for closure of all palatal clefts.

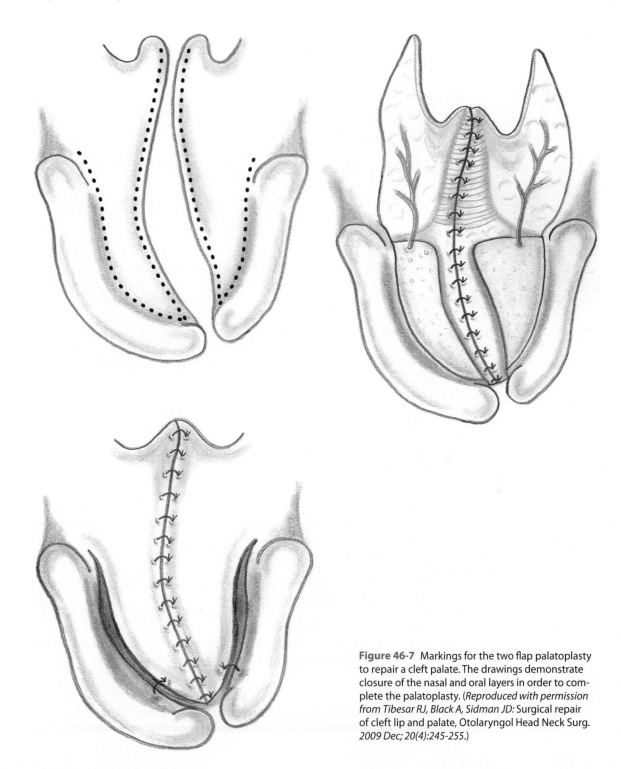

Figure 46-7 Markings for the two flap palatoplasty to repair a cleft palate. The drawings demonstrate closure of the nasal and oral layers in order to complete the palatoplasty. (*Reproduced with permission from Tibesar RJ, Black A, Sidman JD:* Surgical repair of cleft lip and palate, Otolaryngol Head Neck Surg. *2009 Dec; 20(4):245-255.*)

A   **B**

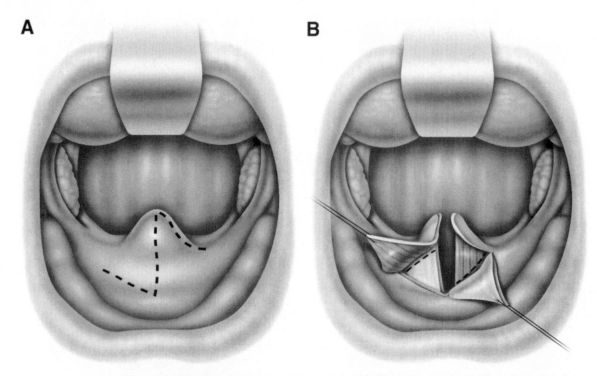

Figure 46-8 The steps involved in completing the Furlow double opposing Z-plasty. (*Reproduced with permission from Muntz HM.* Current techniques for treatment of velopharyngeal insufficiency, Otolaryngol Head Neck Surg. *2001 Dec;12(4):204-209.*)

- ○ Double opposing Z-plasty incisions are made and flaps elevated on the oral and nasal layers.
  - – Typically on the oral layer, a left posteriorly based myomucosal flap and a right anteriorly based mucosal flap are raised.
  - – Typically on the nasal layer, a left anteriorly based mucosal flap and a right posteriorly based myomucosal flap are raised.
  - ○ The Z-plasties are then transposed in an opposing fashion, thus reorienting the levator muscle and lengthening the palate.
- • Postsurgery care
  - (a) The primary goals include prevention of infection and wound tension, provide pain relief, and promote adequate nutrition.
- • Complications
  - (a) Oronasal fistula in up to 10%
  - (b) Velopharyngeal insufficiency (hypernasal speech, increased resonance, nasal regurgitation, and nasal emission during phonation) in up to 25%

Additional Associated Factors
- • Otologic disease
  - (a) A poorly functioning tensor veli palatini muscle and abnormal levator veli palatini muscle insertion contribute to poor middle ear pressure equalization in those with cleft palates.

(b) Other potential causes of Eustachian tube dysfunction in those with cleft palate include the abnormal curvature of the Eustachian tube lumen and hypoplasia of the lateral cartilage relative to normal patients.

(c) Pressure equalization tubes are often necessary early in life (often placed at the time of the lip repair).

(d) The middle ear disease frequently improves after repair of the palate and as the patient ages.

- Speech
  (a) Speech issues are noted in approximately 25% of patients with cleft palate.
  (b) All patients with clefts should undergo aggressive speech evaluations—these should occur often enough to assure adequate documentation of the patient's progress, so that interventions can be made early.
  (c) A cleft palate is a known structural cause of velopharyngeal insufficiency.
  (d) Velopharyngeal insufficiency (VPI).
    ○ Occurs when there is incomplete closure of the nasopharynx by the soft palate, allowing air to escape through the nose with speech.
    ○ Hypernasal speech with sounds other than /n/, /m/, and /ng/.
    ○ Other manifestations: increased resonance, nasal regurgitation, nasal emission with phonation.
    ○ A multispecialty team is helpful in the workup, including a speech-language pathologist, otolaryngologist, prosthodontist, and a surgeon trained in velopharyngeal surgery.
    ○ Evaluation- perceptual speech evaluation by a speech-language pathologist, video nasopharyngeal endoscopy and/or video fluoroscopy.
    ○ Treatment.
      – Initial aggressive speech therapy is indicated.
      – Surgical intervention is recommended in those with velopharyngeal insufficiency that does not improve with therapy and/or structural insufficiency is visualized demonstrating an incomplete velopharyngeal closure pattern with non-nasal words and phrases.
      – Prosthetic devices may be fashioned for poor surgical candidates.
    ○ Common surgical options.
      – Posterior pharyngeal augmentation
        ◊ Varying implants and injectables (fat, hydroxyapatite)
        ◊ Tendency for migration, extrusion, or foreign body reaction
        ◊ Used for small, central velopharyngeal gaps
      – Double opposing Z-plasty (see Figure 46-8)
        ◊ Repositions the levator muscles and lengthens the palate
        ◊ Used for small midline velopharyngeal gaps and submucous cleft palate
      – Radical intravelar veloplasty
        ◊ Repositions and reconstructs the levator muscles
        ◊ Used for submucous cleft palates
      – Pharyngeal flap (Figure 46-9)
        ◊ Recruits tissue from posterior pharyngeal wall to attach to soft palate in order to obstruct the central portion of the velopharyngeal gap
        ◊ Used for all cases of VPI, especially large velopharyngeal gaps and those with an adynamic velopharyngeal mechanisms
      – Sphincter pharyngoplasty (Figure 46-10)

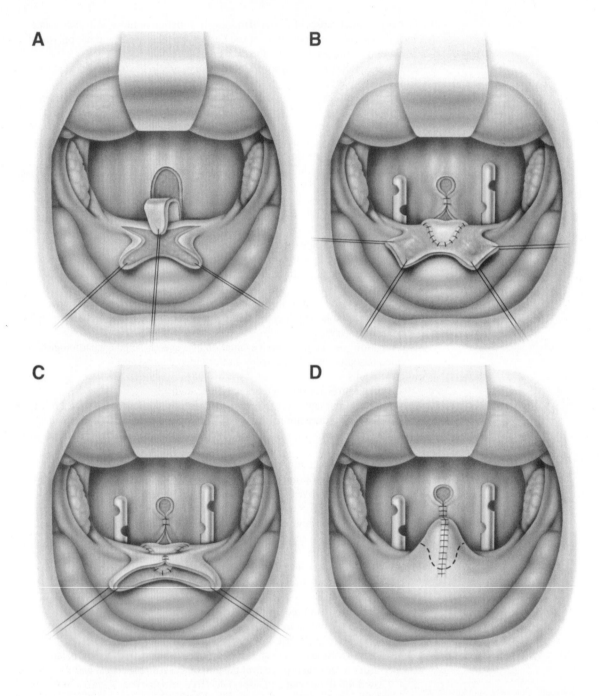

Figure 46-9 The steps involved in completing a superiorly based pharyngeal flap. (*Reproduced with permission from Muntz HM. Current techniques for treatment of velopharyngeal insufficiency, Otolaryngol Head Neck Surg. 2001 Dec;12(4):204-209.*)

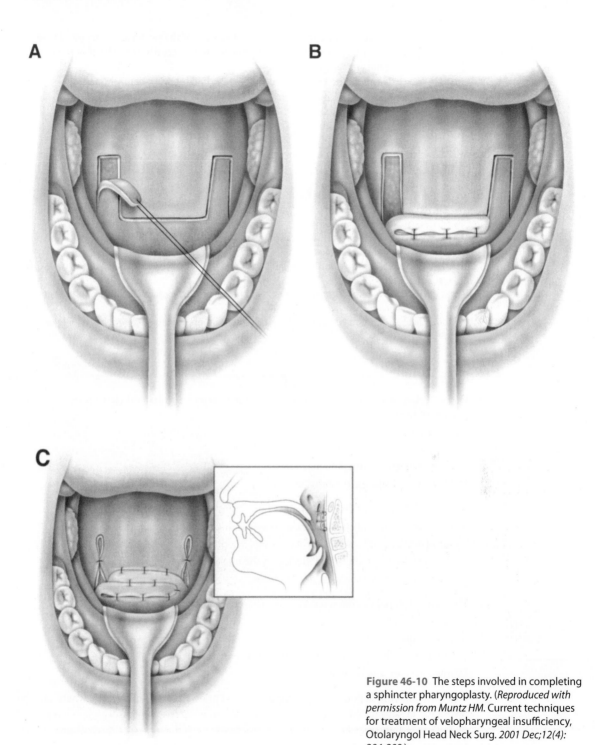

Figure 46-10 The steps involved in completing a sphincter pharyngoplasty. (*Reproduced with permission from Muntz HM.* Current techniques for treatment of velopharyngeal insufficiency, Otolaryngol Head Neck Surg. *2001 Dec;12(4): 204-209.*)

◊ Recruits tissue from both lateral aspects of the posterior pharyngeal wall in order to secure them at a recipient site posteriorly at the level of the velopharyngeal sphincter
◊ Narrows the velopharyngeal port and maintains a central opening
◊ Used for VPI with lateral velopharyngeal gaps or those with "bowtie" closure patterns
◊ Can be combined with a double opposing Z-plasty palatoplasty

Bibliography

Allori AC, Marcus JR. Modern tenets for repair of bilateral cleft lip. *Clin Plastic Surg.* 2014;41:179-188.
Cotton RT, Myer CM III. Cleft lip and palate. In: Lee KJ, ed. *Essential Otolaryngology.* 7th ed. Stamford, CN: Appleton & Lange; 1999.
Dixon MJ, Marazita ML, Beaty TH, Murray JC. Cleft lip and palate: understanding genetic and environmental influences. *Nat Rev Genet.* 2011;12(3):167-178.
Muntz HM. Current techniques for treatment of velopharyngeal insufficiency. *Operative Tech Otolaryngol.* 2001;12:204-209.
Sykes JM, Senders CW. Pathologic anatomy of cleft lip, palate and nasal deformities. In: Meyers AD, ed. *Biol Basis Facial Plast Surg.* 1993;5:57-71.
Tibesar RJ, Black A, Sidman JD. Surgical repair of cleft lip and palate. *Operative Tech Otolaryngol.* 2009;20:245-255.

Questions

1. In the Millard rotation-advancement technique to repair a unilateral cleft lip repair, which portion of the lip is rotated?
   A. The cleft side
   B. The noncleft side
   C. Both the cleft and the noncleft sides
   D. Neither the cleft nor the noncleft side

2. All of the following differences are noted in a child with a unilateral cleft lip except
   A. the lower lateral cartilage on the cleft side is displaced inferiorly and posteriorly
   B. the orbicularis oris muscle forms a complete sphincter
   C. the caudal nasal septum is deflected to the non-cleft side
   D. the nasal dome on the cleft side is obtuse

3. The following are key characteristics of a submucous cleft palate except
   A. zona pellucida
   B. bifid uvula
   C. notch in midline of the posterior hard palate
   D. intact levator muscular sling

4. When performing a double opposing Z-plasty (Furlow) palatoplasty, from where are the myomucosal flaps based?
   A. Both based posteriorly.
   B. Both based anteriorly.

    C. The oral myomucosal flap is based posteriorly and the nasal myomucosal flap is based anteriorly.

    D. The oral myomucosal flap is based anteriorly and the nasal myomucosal flap is based posteriorly.

5. All of the muscles of the soft palate are innervated by CN X except

    A. palatopharyngeus

    B. palatoglossus

    C. tensor veli palatini

    D. levator veli palatini

Chapter 47
Pediatric Otolaryngology: Head and Neck Surgery

General Information

This chapter focuses on otolaryngologic issues in children. The chapter is divided into (1) Ears and Hearing; (2) Nose, Nashopharynx, and Paranasal Sinuses; (3) Mouth and Upper Digestive Tract; (4) Airway; and (5) Head and Neck.

Ears and Hearing

Outer Ear (Pinna, External Auditory Canal [EAC], Tympanic Membrane[TM])

Developmental Anatomy

A. Prenatal development
   i. 5 weeks' gestation
      a. Auricle develops from first (mandibular) and second (hyoid) arches that give rise to six Hillocks of His.
      b. Controversial, but first Hillock gives rise to tragus, second to helical crus, third to remainder of helix, fourth to antihelix, fifth to antitragus, sixth to lobule. Lobule is last to form and some feel not derived from Hillocks.
   ii. 8 weeks' gestation
      a. Cartilaginous (outer third) of EAC derived from invagination of concha cavum (first branchial groove).
      b. Bony EAC (inner two thirds) derived from invagination of meatal plug (solid epithelial core) from primary meatus to primitive tympanic cavity to form meatal plate.
   iii. 21 weeks' gestation
      a. Epithelial cells resorb to canalize bony EAC. Incomplete resorption results in atresia or stenosis.
      b. Tympanic membrane has three layers.
         1. Outer epithelial layer from ectoderm of first branchial groove.
         2. Middle fibrous layer.
         3. Inner mucosal layer from endoderm of first pharyngeal pouch.
         4. Pars tensa composed of three layers. Pars flaccida composed of two (outer and inner) layers. Perforations in pars tensa that heal and look thin are composed of outer and inner layers (missing middle layer) and should be called dimeric membrane (rather than monomeric membrane which is a misnomer).

    B. Postnatal development
        i. Medial EAC ossifies by 2 years of age and reaches adult size by 9 years of age.
        ii. TM almost adult size at birth but horizontally oriented. Becomes more vertical as EAC lengthens.
        iii. Pinna is 80% of adult size by age 5, adult size by age 9. Lobule may continue to grow thereafter.

Signs and Symptoms

Visible lesion, drainage, infection, abnormally shaped pinna.

Clinical Assessment

Close inspection of pinna and remainder of head and neck for associated features as described below.

Pathologies

Congenital

    A. Preauricular tag
        i. Most common ear anomaly.
        ii. Due to supernumerary hillock formation.
        iii. May be associated with branchio-oto-renal (BOR) syndrome involving hearing loss, branchial cleft cyst and renal anomalies or other craniofacial syndromes.
        iv. May be removed electively.
    B. Preauricular pit
        i. Likely due to failure of fusion of hillocks.
        ii. Most commonly at helical root. Pit below tragus more likely to be first branchial cleft anomaly.
        iii. May be associated with BOR.
        iv. Acute infection warrants antibiotics and drainage if necessary.
        v. Definitive excision after resolution of inflammation. Removal of entire tract plus cartilage at base of tract is necessary to prevent postoperative infection and recurrence.
    C. Protruding ears
        i. Larger than average distance from helical rim to mastoid.
        ii. Usually bilateral.
        iii. Due to under development of antihelix and deep conchal bowl.
        iv. Elective otoplasty at 5 or 6 years of age. Leave both ears undraped and address more severely deformed ear first. Mustarde suture recreates antihelical fold. Furnas suture sets back conchal bowl. Cartilage scoring, retropositioning of the helical tail, and suture techniques without incisions have also been described.
    D. Microtia
        i. Clinical features
            a. Prevalence 1:600-12,000
            b. More often male, unilateral, right side.
            c. More common in Hispanic, Aboriginal, Asian and Andean descent.
            d. Associations.
                1. Syndromic (60%): Oculo-auriculo-vertebral spectrum (OAVS) (ie, Goldenhar/hemifacial microsomia-holoprosencephaly, facial asymmetry, macrostomia, oral cleft, microphthalmia, vertebral anomaly, limb reduction, polydactyly, renal and cardiac anomaly; Treacher Collins (bilateral condition); BOR; Townes-Brocks; Miller; Meier-Gorlin
                2. Other: Aural atresia, hearing loss (90%), facial nerve palsy
            e. Absence of lobule is unusual and more likely associated with retinoic embryopathy and CHARGE syndrome.

    ii. Assessment

        a. Clinical examination to rule out concomitant atresia or syndrome.

        b. Weerda classification selected by American J Med Genetics for reporting:

            1. First degree: All components present. Length more than 2 standard deviation (SD) below normal. Reconstruction only occasionally requires additional skin or cartilage.

            2. Second degree: Some components present. Length more than 2 SD below normal (ie, rudimentary helix). Partial reconstruction requires some additional skin and cartilage.

            3. Third degree: Structures present but not recognizable (ie, peanut ear). Also includes anotia. Total reconstruction requires skin and large amounts of cartilage.

        c. Bone conduction auditory brain stem response (ABR) prior to 4 months of age to avoid anesthetic.

   iii. Management

        a. Counselling involving parents and child.

        b. Nonsurgical

            1. Masking with longer hair.

            2. Adhesive retained prosthesis.

        c. Surgical

            1. Bone anchored auricular prosthesis (BAAP)

              • Advantages: Good for burns, auricular avulsion, failed microtia repair

              • Disadvantages: Requires removal of auricular remnant precluding future microtia repair, daily make-up application, replacement due to degradation

            2. Microtia repair

              • Reconstruction at 5 or 6 years of age so rib is large enough to match other side. Reconstructed ear should grow with child.

              • Performed 3 to 4 months prior to atresia repair.

              • Three types of implant material:

                (a) Autogenous rib graft

                    ○ Three-staged approach (Brent method)

                      – *Stage 1: harvest rib cartilage, place framework*

                      – *Stage 2: transpose lobule*

                      – *Stage 3: elevate auricle for projection using skin graft*

                    ○ Two-staged approach (Nagata method)

                      – *Stage 1: harvest rib cartilage, place framework, transpose lobule*

                      – *Stage 2: elevate auricle for projection using skin graft*

                    ○ Advantages: Maintenance free after healed.

                    ○ Disadvantages: Bleeding, infection, skin or cartilage loss, poor cosmetic result, pneumothorax.

                (b) Synthetic implant

                    ○ Medpore

                      – Advantages: can perform at age 3, fewer stages, no rib donor site morbidity

                      – Disadvantages: varied success, no long-term data, extrusion.

                (c) Irradiated rib

                    ○ Largely abandoned due to high rate of resorption.

  E. Aural atresia

    i. Clinical features

a. Incidence 1:20,000 live births.

b. More often male, unilateral, right side.

c. Associations
   1. Apert, Crouzon, Pfeiffer, Goldenhar (hemifacial microsomia), Treacher Collins, Duane, Turner, trisomies 13,14,15,18, 21,22.
   2. Renal dysgenesis

ii. Assessment

   a. Bone conduction auditory brainstem response (ABR) prior to 4 months of age to avoid anesthetic.
   b. CT imaging (high resolution, low-dose, nonenhanced) of temporal bone if canal stenosis and unable to examine EAC to rule out canal cholesteatoma or if there is drainage from canal or pit near canal. Otherwise, defer imaging until prior to surgical repair due to risk of sedation.

iii. Management

   a. Monitor hearing carefully. Early amplification where appropriate.
   b. Treat occult ear infections.
   c. Unilateral atresia
      1. Early repair only if canal cholesteatoma.
      2. Early air conduction hearing aid in side with patent EAC. Bone conduction hearing aid (adhesive or headband) on atretic side.
   d. Bilateral atresia
      1. Early bone conduction hearing aid (adhesive or headband).
   e. Surgical management
      1. Percutaneous abutment retained bone conduction aid (ie, BAHA).
         • Bone conduction threshold must be 40-45 dB in at least one ear to be effective.
         • Usually one stage but may be two stages in young children with thin calvaria (delayed placement of abutment on screw until osseointegration complete).
         • Advantages: Superior and more consistent hearing compared to atresia repair, no risk to facial nerve, not dependent on patent auditory canal, no risk of restenosis or drainage, no water precautions necessary.
         • Disadvantages: Failure to osseointegrate, soft tissue infection, cosmesis.
      2. Transcutaneous magnet retained bone conduction aid (ie, Sophono).
         • Advantages: As per percutaneous abutment retained device but with improved cosmesis.
         • Disadvantages: Skin breakdown and discomfort at magnet site.
      3. Atresia repair
         • Usually delayed until over 5 years of age.
         • Performed after microtia repair to minimize injury to skin flap.
         • Likelihood of significant improvement in hearing following surgery associated with anatomical findings on CT imaging (Jahrsdoerfer criteria). Score of 8 or better out of 10 predicts better outcomes:
            (a) Stapes present (2 points)
            (b) Oval window patent (1 point)
            (c) Round window patent (1 point)
            (d) Incus-stapes connection (1 point)
            (e) Malleus-incus complex (1 point)
            (f) Facial nerve position (1 point)
            (g) Middle ear space aerated (1 point)

    (h) Mastoid pneumatized (1 point)

    (i) External ear appearance (1 point)

- Advantages: Creates EAC to house hearing aid which is usually required.
- Disadvantages: Sensorineural hearing loss, facial nerve palsy, canal restenosis, high revision rate (up to 34%), degradation of audiological results over time, persistent otorrhea, tympanic membrane perforation.

  F. First branchial cleft cyst, Work type I (see Head and Neck section)

Infectious

A. Otitis externa

  i. Acute

    a. Change from acidic to alkaline environment predisposes to bacterial infection.

    b. Most commonly *Pseudomonas aeruginosa, Staphylococcus aureus*, mixed flora.

    c. Symptoms include moderate to severe otalgia (tender tragus), itching, aural fullness, hearing loss, otorrhea.

    d. Diagnosis based on symptoms of rapid onset ear canal inflammation (otalgia, itching, fullness) and signs (tender, diffuse canal edema or erythema).

    e. Beware malignant otitis externa (osteomyelitis) in diabetic and immunocompromised patients. Requires addition of parenteral antibiotics.

    f. Treatment includes debridement, analgesia, acidifying agents (acetic acid) and/or topical antibiotic/steroid drops +/− otowick if significant canal edema.

  ii. Chronic

    a. Same bacteria as acute otitis externa.

    b. Symptoms include itching, mild discomfort, drainage.

    c. Treatment same as acute otitis externa. Prolonged treatment can lead to otomycosis (*Aspergillus* and *Candida*) which may require topical clotrimazole.

Traumatic

A. Auricular hematoma

  i. Associated with wrestling. Left untreated, may result in "cauliflower ear."

  ii. Requires incision and drainage and sandwiching of pinna between two dental rolls for 7 to 14 days to prevent reaccumulation of blood under perichondrium.

  iii. Antibiotic prophylaxis.

  iv. Suspect abuse if identified in nonambulatory infant.

B. Auricular laceration and avulsion

  i. Laceration

    a. Copious irrigation, debridement, primary closure, antibiotics, rabies, or tetanus prophylaxis if indicated, bolster if perichondrium raised off cartilage.

  ii. Avulsion

    a. < 1.5 cm: reattach missing segment or primary closure.

    b. > 1.5 cm: composite graft from opposite ear or local flap.

    c. Complete options include: microvascular reimplantation, banking of deepithelialized cartilage under temporalis fascia for later reconstruction, reconstruction using costal cartilage, or auricular prosthesis.

C. Exostoses

  i. Overgrowth of immature lamellar bone likely due to cold water exposure.

  ii. Bilateral, broadly based lesions in medial half of external auditory canal.

  iii. Surgical removal only if symptomatic (ie, hearing loss, infection).

D. Osteoma

  i. Overgrowth of cancellous bone.

  ii. Unilateral, pedunculated lesions in outer half of external auditory canal.

      iii. Surgical removal only if symptomatic (ie, hearing loss, infection).

  E. Keratosis obturans

     i. Desquamation of hyperplastic epithelium leading to EAC obstruction.

     ii. Symptoms include otalgia and hearing loss.

     iii. Treatment includes acetic acid irrigations or surgical removal.

Neoplastic

  A. Benign

     i. Dermoid

       a. Two cell layers (mesoderm and ectoderm).

       b. May cause hearing loss and recurrent otitis externa.

       c. Surgical removal if symptomatic.

     ii. Pilomatricoma (formerly pilomatrixoma, calcifying epithelioma of Malherbe)

       a. Benign neoplasm from hair cortex cells.

       b. More common in Caucasian females.

       c. Painless, superficial, firm, bluish discoloration over skin.

       d. Diagnosis may require ultrasound to demonstrate calcification.

       e. Treatment options include observation versus surgical excision.

     iii. Fibrous dysplasia

       a. Monostotic (70%), polyostotic (24%) or Albright syndrome (6%).

       b. Symptoms include temporal bone mass, otorrhea, conductive hearing loss.

       c. CT demonstrates lesion with ground-glass appearance.

       d. Surgery only if symptomatic.

     iv. Langerhans cell histiocytosis

       a. Clonal proliferation of Langerhans cells.

       b. Symptoms include postauricular swelling, temporal bone mass, otorrhea, conductive hearing loss, aural polyp.

       c. CT demonstrates punched-out lytic lesions.

       d. Bone scan recommended to assess number of sites affected.

       e. Pathology demonstrates Birbeck granules.

         1. Treatment options

           • Monostotic disease: Surgery with possible addition of steroids

           • Polyostotic disease: Chemotherapy or radiation

  B. Malignant

     i. Rhabdomyosarcoma

       a. Aggressive tumor of striated muscle (15% have distant metastases at diagnosis).

       b. 3% occur in temporal bone.

       c. Three types:

         1. Embryonal (most common type in head and neck)

         2. Alveolar (more common in adolescents)

         3. Pleomorphic

         4. Sclerosing (rare, poor prognosis)

       d. Symptoms include mass in ear canal, polyp, discharge, bleeding, pain, hearing loss, facial nerve palsy.

       e. CT or MRI demonstrate enhancement and destruction.

       f. Diagnosis based on biopsy. Pathology shows small round blue cells with hyperchromatic nuclei, large polygonal tumor cells with abundant eosinophilic cytoplasm with cross striations. Molecular genetics of embryonal rhabdomyosarcoma shows deletion of short arm of chromosome 11 (11p15).

       g. Treatment includes chemotherapy and radiation (see Head and Neck section).

        ii. Ewing sarcoma
- a. Aggressive tumor of bone.
- b. < 6% of Ewing sarcoma involve temporal bone.
- c. Diagnosis based on biopsy. Pathology demonstrates sheets of small round blue cells with scant cytoplasm and inconspicuous nucleoli. Molecular genetic translocation t(11:22)(q24;q12) pathognomonic.
- d. Treatment includes chemotherapy, radiation +/- surgical decompression if compressive symptoms (see Head and Neck section).

       iii. Leukemia and lymphoma
- a. 20% of leukemic patients have temporal bone involvement.
- b. Infiltration of tympanic membrane, middle ear, mastoid, petrous apex.
- c. Diagnosis based on biopsy. Pathology demonstrates small round blue cells.
- d. Improves with treatment of underlying disease. Treat secondary infections.

       iv. Other
- a. Chondrosarcoma
- b. Liposarcoma
- c. Hemangiosarcoma

Middle Ear (Ossicles, Eustachian Tube [ET])

Developmental Anatomy

A. Prenatal development
- i. 3 weeks' gestation
  - a. First pharyngeal pouch forms tubotympanic recess. At 7 weeks' gestation, tubotympanic recess becomes constricted by second branchial arch to form Eustachian tube and tympanic cavity.
- ii. 4 to 6 weeks' gestation
  - a. Ossicles begin to develop. At 8 weeks' gestation malleoincudal and incudostapedial joints form. Ossicles are adult size and shape at birth.
    1. First arch (mandibular arch) gives rise to head of malleus, short process and body of incus, tensor tympani tendon.
    2. Second arch (hyoid arch) gives rise to manubrium of malleus, long process of incus, stapes suprastructure, stapedius tendon. Stapes footplate derives from otic capsule.
- iii. 21 weeks' gestation
  - a. Mastoid antrum appears.

B. Postnatal development
- i. Eustachian tube doubles in length from birth to adulthood.
- ii. Mastoid tip poorly developed at birth. Facial nerve is therefore more superficial and prone to surgical injury.
- iii. Mastoid air cells grow in first 2 to 3 years of life.

Signs and Symptoms

A. Otorrhea
B. Conductive hearing loss
C. Otalgia
D. Dysequilibrium

Clinical Assessment

A. Otoscopic examination including pneumatic otoscopy.
B. Audiological testing including tympanometry.
C. Computed tomography and/or magnetic resonance imaging.

Pathologies
Congenital
A. Ossicular anomalies
   i. Suspect when conductive hearing loss and normal otoscopic examination.
  ii. Syndromic:
     a. Apert/Crouzon (see below)
       1. Ankylosis of malleus and incus to lateral wall, deformed stapes.
     b. Beckwith-Wiedemann
       1. Overgrowth disorder (macroglossia or hemihypertrophy) with a predisposition to tumor development (Wilms tumor, hepatoblastoma).
       2. May also have hypoglycemia, abdominal wall defects, visceromegaly, adrenocortical cytomegaly, and renal anomalies.
       3. Due to mutation or deletion on chromosome 11p15.
       4. CT demonstrates anterior bony fixation of malleus and stapes fixation. Also have ear lobule crease.
     c. Branchiootorenal (BOR) syndrome (see below)
       1. Fused malleoincudal complex
     d. CHARGE syndrome (see below)
       1. Abnormally shaped incus and stapes, ossicular chain fixation, absent stapedius tendon, absent stapes footplate.
     e. Congenital stapes footplate fixation (aka x-linked stapes gusher, Phelp syndrome) (see below)
       1. Stapes fixed to oval window. Therefore manipulation may lead to dead ear.
     f. DiGeorge
       1. **C**ardiac anomalies, **A**bnormal facies, **T** cell deficit due to thymic hypoplasia, **C**left palate, **H**ypocalcemia due to hypoparathyroidism (acronym CATCH22).
       2. Due to mutations in TBX1 gene on chromosome 22q11.
       3. CT demonstrates ossicular malformations and Mondini malformation.
     g. Goldenhar (aka Oculo-Auriculo-Vertebral dysplasia)
       1. Prevalence 1/45,000.
       2. May be caused by mutation in 14q32 leading to first and second branchial arch anomalies.
       3. Clinical features (unilateral):
         • Epibulbar dermoids: benign white tumors over sclera
         • Conductive hearing loss, facial nerve deviation
         • Vertebral anomalies (hemi or fused)
         • Parotid agenesis
         • Cleft lip/palate and hypoplastic mandible
       4. Ossicles may be fused as one block which is commonly fused to wall of hypopolastic middle ear cavity. May also have absent ossicles.
       5. Treatment:
         • Ophthalmology consultation
         • Conventional or bone anchored hearing aids
         • Correction of cleft lip/palate and mandible
     h. Hurler
       1. Inherited mucopolysaccharidosis whereby lack of lysosomal enzymes leads to inability to degrade glycosaminoglycans or mucopolysaccharides which in turn accumulate in tissue.

      2. Due to mutation on chromosome 4p16 encoding alpha-L-iduronidase.

      3. Thick mucosa in middle ear due to lysosomes filled with glycosaminogly-cans (Hurler cells). Hurler cells have also been found in middle ear ossicles, spiral ganglion neurons, the organ of Corti and the vestibulocochlear nerve.

    i. Klippel-Feil (see below)

      1. Deformed head of the malleus, rudimentary head of the incus, short or absent long process of the incus or absent incus, missing parts of stapes or complete absence, fixed stapes footplate (risk of gusher at surgery).

  iii. Nonsyndromic:

    a. Congenital stapes ankylosis (accounts for 50%-70% of stapes fixation).

      1. Management initially with hearing aids

      2. Stapedectomy when older

    b. Juvenile otosclerosis (15% develop symptoms as children)

      1. Progressive hearing loss from 10 years of age.

      2. Usually bilateral (90%).

      3. Family history in one half of patients.

B. Cholesteatoma

  i. Keratinized squamous epithelium in middle ear or mastoid space.

  ii. Pressure and degradative enzymes erode soft tissue and bone.

  iii. Clinical features:

    a. Congenital

      1. Well-circumscribed pearly white mass behind intact tympanic membrane in absence of otorrhea, perforation, or prior otologic surgery.

      2. Likely results from persistent epithelial rests at the time of neural groove closure between third and fifth weeks' embryogenesis.

      3. Usually undiagnosed until 2.5 to 5 years of age.

      4. More often male (3:1), unilateral (97%).

      5. Present as hearing loss or facial nerve paralysis.

    b. Acquired

      1. Primary acquired

        • Negative middle ear pressure creates retraction pocket leading to buildup of keratinous debris.

      2. Secondary acquired

        • Due to implantation of keratin from prior surgery or trauma.

      3. Present as foul smelling ear with discharge through perforated tympanic membrane and keratin in middle ear space. Hearing loss, vertigo, or facial nerve paralysis possible if left untreated.

  iv. Diagnosis

    a. Fine cut (0.625-mm thickness) CT temporal bone without contrast.

    b. MRI shows lesion to be isointense on T1 (cholesterol granuloma is intense on T1) without enhancement from contrast and hyperintense on T2. Diffusion-weighted imaging is sensitive/specific for recurrent/persistent postsurgical disease.

  v. Management

    a. Surgical removal with goal of obtaining dry, safe ear. Hearing preservation is secondary.

    b. Small lesions removed through tympanomeatal flap. Larger lesions may require tympanomastoidectomy. Canal wall may be left up, taken down to reach diseased areas, or reconstructed to obliterate the mastoid space.

    C. Vascular anomalies
        i. Aberrant carotid artery
           a. Anteroinferior quadrant of tympanic membrane
           b. Symptoms of pulsatile tinnitus
        ii. High-riding jugular bulb
           a. Posteroinferior quadrant of tympanic membrane.
           b. Do not perform myringotomy if there is any suspicion of this finding.
        iii. Persistent stapedial artery

Infectious

    A. Acute otitis media (AOM) (AAP Clinical Practice Guideline 2013)
        i. Most common bacterial infection of childhood.
        ii. Diagnosis based on any one of the following:
           a. Rapid onset of inflammation in middle ear.
           b. Moderate to severe bulging of TM.
           c. Mild bulging of TM and recent ear pain (< 48 hours) or intense erythema.
           d. New onset otorrhea not due to otitis externa.
        iii. Most common organisms:
           a. *S Pneumonia* (35%)
           b. *H Influenza* (nontypeable: ie, not type B, etc) (25%)
           c. *M Catarrhalis* (10%)
           d. *S Aureus* and *S Pyogenes*
           e. Anaerobes (newborns)
           f. Gram-negative enteric organisms (infants)
           g. Viral
        iv. Incidence of beta-lactamase producing organism is 20% to 30%.
        v. Predisposing factors:
           a. Male
           b. First nations/Inuit
           c. Craniofacial abnormality
           d. Immunodeficiency
           e. Bottle propping
           f. Day care
           g. Smoke exposure
           h. Sibling with history of recurrent AOM.
           i. Infection in child less than 6 months of age.
        vi. Complications:
           a. Intratemporal (within temporal bone)
               1. Conductive hearing loss
               2. TM perforation
               3. Mastoiditis
               4. Facial nerve palsy
               5. Labyrinthitis
               6. Petrositis
               7. SNHL
               8. Bezold abscess (abscess in sternocleidomastoid muscle)
           b. Intracranial (within cranium)
               1. Meningitis. Recurrent meningitis due to AOM warrants evaluation using imaging for cochlear or temporal bone malformation.
               2. Sigmoid sinus thrombosis.

3. Otitic hydrocephalus.
4. Epidural abscess.
5. Subdural abscess.
6. Intracranial abscess.
 vii. Management:
  a. Exclusive breastfeeding for first 6 months of life.
  b. Avoid tobacco smoke.
  c. Influenza vaccine after 6 months of age (up to 55% reduction in AOM).
  d. Pneumococcal conjugate vaccine (29% reduction in AOM if given before 24 months of age).
  e. Assess and treat pain.
  f. Antibiotic therapy:
   1. May closely observe without antibiotics if:
- Parents reliable.
- Age 6 months to 2 years and unilateral non severe AOM. (Severe = moderate otalgia, otalgia lasting 48 hours, fever 39°C)
- Age > 2 years and nonsevere bilateral AOM.
- No head/neck anomalies, immunodeficiency, chronic cardiac or pulmonary disease.
- Give antibiotics if worsens or fails to improve after 48-72 hours.
   2. Treatment with antibiotics if fails to fulfill above criteria.
- First-line treatment if no previous antibiotics: High-dose amoxicillin (cefdinir, cefuroxime, or ceftriaxone if penicillin allergic).
- If failure of initial antibiotic treatment: Amoxcillin-clavulanate (ceftriaxone or clindamycin if penicillin allergy).
- Do not prescribe prophylactic antibiotics.
   3. Myringotomy and tubes for recurrent AOM.
- Three episodes in 6 months.
- Four episodes in 1 year with one episode in preceding 6 months.
B. Otitis media with effusion (OME) (Clinical Practice Guideline 2013)
 i. Diagnosis
  a. Middle ear fluid without signs of infection or inflammation.
  b. Conductive hearing loss.
  c. Otoscopy shows retraction, amber fluid, meniscus.
  d. Flat tympanogram.
 ii. Predisposing factors
  a. Acute otitis media.
  b. Poor Eustachian tube function (ie, cleft palate).
 iii. Management
  a. Observation with serial audiograms (90% resolve within 3 months).
  b. Tympanostomy tube indications:
   1. Chronic bilateral OME (> 3 months) with hearing loss.
   2. Chronic unilateral or bilateral OME with vestibular or behavioral problems, ear discomfort, poor school performance.
   3. Children at risk (sensory, physical, cognitive, behavioural deficits) with OME of any duration that is unlikely to resolve (flat tympanograms).

Traumatic
A. Perforation due to foreign body
 i. Most heal spontaneously.

      ii. Vertigo or SNHL warrants audiological assessment. Consider middle ear exploration.

   B. Temporal bone fracture

      i. Less common in children.

      ii. Rarely follow "classic" descriptions of oblique versus longitudinal. However, more likely to be oblique.

      iii. Less likely to be associated with facial nerve palsy or SNHL.

Neoplastic

   A. Benign

      i. Choristoma

         a. Aggregates of normal tissue (such as salivary or neural) in an abnormal location.

      ii. Paraganglioma (glomus jugulare and glomus tympanicum)

         a. Derived from chemoreceptive cells of neural crest origin along parasympathetic nerves.

         b. Usually benign. Rarely can be malignant.

         c. Slow growing, expansile, locally destructive.

         d. CT angiography shows lesion, blood supply, extent of bone destruction. MRI shows avidly-enhancing salt-pepper appearance.

         e. Pathology shows clusters of chief cells called *zellballen*.

         f. Complete surgical resection optimal with adjuvant chemo/radiation for nonresectable or malignant disease. Test for catecholamine secretion preoperatively.

      iii. Fibrous dysplasia

      iv. Langerhans cell histiocytosis (see below)

   B. Malignant

      i. Rhabdomyosarcoma

      ii. Ewing sarcoma

      iii. Leukemia and lymphoma

      iv. Chondrosarcoma

      v. Liposarcoma

      vi. Hemangiosarcoma

      vii. Adenocarcinoma

      viii. Fibrosarcoma

Inner Ear (Cochlea, Vestibule, Internal Auditory Canal [IAC])

Developmental Anatomy

   A. Prenatal development

      i. 3 weeks' gestation

         a. Otic placode appears. Later invaginates to become otocyst/otic vesicle which develops into membranous labyrinth.

      ii. 5 weeks' gestation

         a. Endolymphatic duct (first to develop), cochlear duct and vestibular precursor form on otocyst.

         b. Otocyst has two parts:

            1. Pars superior: becomes ampulla and semicircular canals. Semicircular canals develop in following order (superior, posterior, lateral).

            2. Pars inferior: becomes saccule and cochlea.

      iii. 6 weeks' gestation

   a. Cochlear duct grows from saccule. At 10 weeks' reaches full 2.5 turns. At 20 weeks' reaches full adult size. At 21 weeks' organ of Corti becomes functional.
   B. Postnatal development
      i. Endolymphatic sac and duct grow until age 3-4 years.

Signs and Symptoms
   A. Speech delay
   B. Behavioral problems
   C. Dysequilibrium

Clinical Assessment
   A. History
      i. Risk factors for childhood permanent hearing loss [Joint Committee on Infant Hearing (JCIH), 2007]. Neonates who pass the infant hearing screen but possess these risk factors should undergo audiologic monitoring every 6 months until 3 years of age.
         a. Family history of permanent childhood hearing loss.
         b. In-utero infections such as CMV and TORCH.
         c. Stigmata of syndrome known to include hearing loss or Eustachian tube dysfunction.
         d. Craniofacial anomalies.
         e. Syndromes associated with progressive hearing loss (ie, Alport, Jervell, and Lange-Nielsen, Neurofibromatosis, Osteopetrosis, Pendred, Usher, Waardenburg).
         f. Neurodegenerative disorders (ie, Charcot-Marie Tooth, Friedrich ataxia, Hunter).
         g. Postnatal infections associated with hearing loss such as bacterial and viral (herpes, varicella) meningitis.
         h. Admission of 48 hours or greater to a NICU.
         i. Hyperbilirubinemia requiring serum exchange transfusion, persistent.
         j. Pulmonary hypertension associated with mechanical ventilation, ECMO.
         k. Ototoxic medications (including chemotherapy), loop diuretics.
         l. Head trauma.
         m. Recurrent or persistent OME for at least 3 months.
         n. Caregiver concern regarding hearing, speech, language or developmental delay.
   B. Auditory function tests
      i. Physiological tests
         a. Otoacoustic emissions (OAE): Low-intensity sounds produced by outer hair cells of the cochlea as they expand and contract. Used as infant hearing screen and to test for functional hearing loss. Drawback is that OAEs can estimate hearing sensitivity only within a limited range of frequencies.
         b. Auditory brainstem response (ABR): Auditory evoked potential generated by brief click or tone pip transmitted via insert earphone. Waveform peaks denote functionality of different parts of auditory pathway.
         c. Tympanometry: Test of middle ear function. Not as useful in infants due to increased compliance of EAC.
      ii. Behavioral tests
         a. Visual reinforcement audiometry (VRA): Responses in soundfield (not ear-specific) are rewarded visually (ie, clapping clown). Used for children 8 months to 3 years of age.

      b. Conditioned play audiometry: Ear-specific responses. Used for children 3 to 5 years of age.

      c. Conventional audiometry: Ear-specific air conduction (AC) and bone conduction (BC) thresholds. Used for children greater than 5 years of age.

C. Vestibular testing (see Chapter 16)

D. Imaging the temporal bone

    i. Low dose fine cut (0.625 mm) temporal bone CT scan is the standard.

    ii. MRI may be helpful for internal auditory canal (IAC) (ie, number of nerves on sagittal section), endolymphatic sac, patency of cochlear duct, mass lesions.

Pathology/Treatment/Complications

Congenital Hearing Loss

A. Genetic: Nonsyndromic

    i. Autosomal recessive

      a. Connexins (GJB2 and GJB6 encoding connexins 26 and 30, respectively).

        1. Most common genetic nonsyndromic SNHL.

        2. 35delG mutation accounts for 80% of connexin 26 mutations.

        3. Dysfunctional gap junctions impair potassium ion recycling in stria vascularis.

      b. Enlarged vestibular aqueduct (EVA)

        1. May also have sensorineural hearing loss (mild to profound, audiogram flat or downsloping high-frequency loss), conductive hearing loss (low frequency), may be isolated or associated with Mondini malformation.

        2. May have sudden hearing loss with head trauma.

        3. Do not have SLC26A4 mutation or thyroid problems.

      c. Mitochondrial A1555G mutation

        1. Maternally inherited mutation in mitochondrial 12S RNA.

        2. 15% of patients in United States with SNHL due to aminoglycosides have this mutation. Much more common in Mongolia.

      d. Otoferlin mutation/auditory dyssynchrony

        1. Mutation in OTOF gene causes vesicle membrane fusion problem.

        2. Causes auditory dyssynchromy: present OAE, absent ABR, variable auditory thresholds.

    ii. Autosomal dominant

      a. Wolfram

        1. Most common cause of dominantly-inherited low-frequency SNHL.

        2. Progressive hearing loss.

B. Genetic: Syndromic (over 400 types in total)

    i. Autosomal recessive

      a. Pendred

        1. 2% of profound congenital SNHL.

        2. Mutations in SLC26A4 or PDS lead to defect in iodine-chloride transporter.

        3. SNHL (unilateral or bilateral, progressive), Mondini malformation.

        4. Associated with thyroid goiter (euthyroid), thyroid malignancy.

        5. Test for SLC26A4, TSH, T3, T4. Do not remove thyroid unless malignancy present.

      b. Usher

        1. 3% of deaf population, 50% of deaf/blind population.

        2. Mutations in MYO7A, USH2A and others lead to defective tip links and Usherin protein.

      3. SNHL, vestibular dysfunction, retinitis pigmentosa.

      4. Three types:

- USH1 (MYO7A mutation) (40% of cases): Profound congenital bilateral SNHL, absent vestibular function, early retinitis pigmentosa by 10 years of age.
- USH2 (USH2A mutation) (60% of cases): Moderate SNHL, normal vestibular function, later onset retinitis pigmentosa.
- USH3 (3% of cases, mostly Norwegian): Progressive SNHL, variable vestibular function.

  c. Jervell & Lange-Nielsen

      1. 1/1000 of profoundly deaf population.

      2. Mutation in KVLQT1 leads to dysregulation of potassium channel.

      3. Severe/profound SNHL, prolonged QT and large T waves on ECG.

      4. Presents as 20-30-year-old healthy person with sudden onset syncope and sudden death.

      5. Treat with beta blocker.

      6. Test first degree relatives for Ward-Romano syndrome due to similar cardiac problem without hearing loss.

  d. Biotinidase deficiency

      1. 1/60,000

      2. Lack enzyme to recycle Biotin.

      3. Leads to hair loss, hearing loss, seizures, hypotonia, coma and death.

      4. Tested as part of infant screening program because it is preventable with dietary replacement.

 ii. Autosomal dominant

  a. Waardenburg

      1. Most common inherited congenital deafness (2%).

      2. Mutation in neural crest cells leads to defective intermediate layer of stria vascularis.

      3. Clinical features

- White forelock (25% of cases, varying age of first appearance).
- Hearing loss (unilateral or bilateral, EVA in 50%).
- Synophores (eyebrows grow together).
- Dystopia canthorum (lateral displacement of inner canthi).
- Blue eyes or heterochromia iridis (different colors).
- Pinched nose.
- Hirschsprung disease (absent ganglia in distal colon).
- Limb defects.

      4. Four types:

- WS1 (most common): PAX3 mutation, dystopia canthorum, hearing loss (20%)
- WS2A (Tietz syndrome): MITF mutation, no dystopia canthorum, hearing loss (50%)
- WS3 (Klein-Waardenburg): Unilateral ptosis, eyelid and limb anomalies
- WS4 (Shah-Waardenburg): SOX10 mutation, Hirshsprung

  b. Apert/Crouzon

      1. Craniosynostosis of coronal suture leads to prominent forehead and flat occiput. Large fontanelles close at later age.

      2. Due to mutation in FGFR2 gene on chromosome 26.

      3. 70% normal intelligence, 30% delayed.

      4. Fused vertebrae (40%).

      5. Conductive hearing loss, ankylosis of malleus and incus to lateral wall and deformed fixed stapes footplate, wide cochlear aqueduct, absent internal auditory canal (prohibits cochlear implantation).

      6. Downslanting palpebral fissures.

      7. Proptosis and exposure keratitis.

      8. Apert involves syndactyly (fingers and toes 2,3,4 fused in middigital mass), whereas Crouzon does not.

      9. Treatment includes eye care for keratitis, craniofacial surgery and Tessier procedure for separating fused digits.

  c. Branchiootorenal (aka Melnick-Fraser)

      1. 2% of deaf children, 1/40,000.

      2. Autosomal dominant. Many mutations are de novo and are specific to individual families. High penetrance, variable expressivity, successive anticipation (worse with every generation).

      3. Due to mutation in EYA1 gene on chromosome 8q13.

      4. Clinical diagnosis based on 3 major, 2 major/2 minor, or 1 major and first degree relative with diagnosis:

         • Major criteria

           (a) Hearing loss (conductive, SNHL, or mixed). Often mild and goes undiagnosed therefore audiogram recommended in all patients with family history of branchial anomalies.

           (b) Prehilical pits.

           (c) Branchial cleft cyst or fistula.

           (d) Renal dysplasia/malformed calyces, aplasia, polycystic kidneys.

         • Minor criteria

           (a) External ear

           (b) Middle ear

           (c) Inner ear

           (d) Tags, facial asymmetry, palatal abnormalities

      5. Temporal bone features pathognomonic (1) fused malleoincudal complex; (2) facial nerve on medial side of cochlea; (3) hypoplastic apical turn of cochlea; (4) funnel-shaped internal auditory canal; and (4) patulous Eustachian tube; and (5) medially displaced carotid arteries.

      6. Confirmatory diagnosis by genetic testing for EYA1 mutation (only 40% have mutation in EYA1 gene).

      7. Treatment includes hearing screen, hearing aid if loss diagnosed, genetics in family members.

  d. CHARGE

      1. Stands for **C**oloboma of the eye, **H**eart defects, **A**tresia choanae, **R**etardation of growth/development, **G**enitourinary abnormalities, **E**ar anomalies and deafness.

      2. Due to sporadic microdeletions in CHD7 gene on chromosome 8 (only 50% of patients have this mutation).

      3. Clinical diagnosis based on major and minor criteria:

         • Major criteria

           (a) Coloboma of the eye (cleft of iris, retina, macula or disc, not eyelid), microphthalmos, anophthalmos.

    (b) Ear anomalies: outer (wide ear with little or no lobe, antihelix discontinuous with tragus).

    (c) Ear anomalies: middle (abnormally shaped incus and stapes, ossicular chain fixation, absent stapedius tendon and stapes footplate and conductive loss).

    (d) Ear anomalies: inner (absent oval window, Mondini malformation, hypoplastic or absent semicircular canals).

    (e) Choanal atresia.

    (f) Cranial nerve anomalies (missing olfactory nerve, abnormal facial nerve course and facial palsy, swallowing difficulties, aspiration).

- Minor criteria
  - (a) CHARGE behavior (perseverance, obsessive, compulsive).
  - (b) Growth hormone deficiency.
  - (c) CHARGE facies, prominent forehead, arched eyebrows, thick nostrils, facial asymmetry.
  - (d) Cleft lip and palate.
  - (e) Tracheoesophageal fistula.
  - (f) Heart defects such as tetralogy of Fallot.
  - (g) Renal anomalies (absent, small, misplaced).
  - (h) Genitourinary (small penis, undescended testes, small labia, small or missing uterus).

e. Neurofibromatosis Type 2 (NF2)
1. Autosomal dominant
2. Mutation in tumor suppressor gene schwannomin on chromosome 22 leads to abnormal production of protein merlin.
3. Hearing loss around age 20 years, tinnitus, imbalance, vertigo.
4. Diagnostic criteria:
   - Bilateral acoustic neuromas.
   - First degree relative with NF2 PLUS patient has unilateral acoustic neuroma OR two other tumors (neurofibroma, meningioma, glioma, schwannoma)

f. Otosclerosis (aka otospongiosus)
1. Endochondral bony sclerosis of stapes footplate to oval window.
2. Autosomal dominant, incomplete penetrance (25%).
3. 1% of Caucasian adults.
4. More common in females.
5. Conductive and sensorineural hearing loss.

g. Stickler
1. Myopia, cataracts, retinal detachment.
2. Progressive mixed hearing loss (80%).
3. Midface hypoplasia.
4. Robin sequence.
5. Hypermobile joints and arthritis.

h. Treacher-Collins (aka mandibulofacial dysostosis)
1. Mutation in chromosome 5q leads to abnormal treacle protein.
2. May be due to maternal sensitivity to vitamin A.
3. Bilateral features.
4. Diagnostic criteria:
   - Microtia (also have aural atresia, conductive hearing loss, sensorineural hearing loss and vestibular dysfunction)

- Midface hypoplasia (underdevelopment of zygomatic arch)
- Downsloping palpebral fissures
- Coloboma of outer third of lower eyelid with absence of lashes
- Micrognathia (may have cleft palate, velopharyngeal insufficiency)

   i. Klippel-Feil
  1. Failure of segmentation of cervical vertebrae leading to fused appearance.
  2. Due to mutations in GDF6 gene on chromosome 8q22, MEOX1 gene on chromosome 17q21 and GDF3 gene on chromosome 12p13.
  3. CT demonstrates narrow down-sloping external auditory canals, deformed head of the malleus, rudimentary head of the incus, short or absent long process of the incus or absent incus, missing parts of stapes or complete absence, fixed stapes footplate (risk of gusher at surgery), dehiscence of facial nerve, absence of one or all semicircular canals, cochlear malformation or absence.

C. X-linked
   i. Nonsyndromic
     a. Congenital fixation of stapes footplate with perilymphatic gusher
  1. Most common x-linked deafness.
  2. Due to mutation of POU3F4 gene on Xq21 locus.
  3. Affected males have stable hearing at birth, then progressive mixed hearing loss or sensorineural loss which is often bilateral (75%).
  4. Carrier females have mild hearing loss and less severe middle ear anomalies.
  5. Family history of hearing loss.
  6. Large internal auditory canal, absent lamina cribrosa.
  7. Entry into cochleovestibular apparatus leads to gush of perilymphatic fluid which can lead to a dead ear.

  ii. Syndromic
     a. Alport
  1. Mostly due to x-linked mutation in COL4A5. 15% autosomal recessive due to mutations in COL4A3 or COL4A4.
  2. Progressive high frequency sensorineural hearing loss.
  3. Retinal flecks, anterior lenticonus (protrusion of the lens), spherophakia (spherical lens), congenital cataracts.
  4. Glomerulonephritis, hematuria and progressive renal failure.
     b. Deafness dystonia (rare)
  1. Hearing loss, blindness, dystonia, mental deterioration
     c. Norrie (rare)
  1. Hearing loss, blindness, mental deterioration
     d. Otopalatodigital (rare)
  1. Conductive hearing loss due to ossicular malformations
  2. Cleft palate
  3. Broad fingers, large spaces between toes
     e. Wildervanck
  1. Familial
  2. Affects females only
  3. Mixed hearing loss
  4. CN6 palsy
  5. Fused cervical vertebrae

    D. Chromosomal
       i. Down syndrome
         a. Most common chromosomal anomaly.
         b. 90% are trisomy 21. 5% are due to translocations.
         c. Superior helix folded over, stenotic external auditory canal, middle ear and mastoid disease, sensorineural hearing loss, hypoplastic lateral semicircular canal bony island, superior semicircular canal dehiscence, narrow internal auditory canal, cochlear nerve stenosis, large vestibular aqueduct.
       ii. Turner syndrome
         a. Absence of one X chromosome
         b. Short stature
         c. Conductive and sensorineural hearing loss
         d. Webbed neck
         e. Shield chest
         f. Gonadal dysgenesis
    E. Environmental
       i. Fetal alcohol
         a. Microcephaly, mental retardation, seizures
         b. Narrow forehead, eyelid ptosis, midface hypoplasia, short nose
         c. Conductive and sensorineural hearing loss

Infectious Hearing Loss

    A. Congenital TORCH infections
       i. Clinical features
         a. **T**oxoplasmosis.
         b. **O**ther: syphilis, varicella, parvovirus B19 ("Fifth disease", "slapcheek").
         c. **R**ubella: Developmental delay, meningoencephalitis, SNHL, cataracts, retinopathy, glaucoma, patent ductus arteriosus, pulmonary artery stenosis.
         d. **C**ytomegalovirus: Most common infectious cause of congenital SNHL. Severe symptoms in 5%. Intrauterine growth retardation (IUGR), microcephaly, large cerebral ventricles, intracerebral calcification, SNHL, retinitis, hepatosplenomegaly, thrombocytopenia, jaundice.
         e. **H**erpes.
    B. Meningitis: any organism may cause hearing loss
    C. Mumps

Traumatic

    A. Ototoxic medications
       i. Clinical features
         a. Chemotherapeutics (cisplatin, carboplatin)
         b. Loop diuretics (furosemide). May be reversible.
         c. Aminoglycoside antibiotics. Predisposition to hearing loss if A1555G mutation in maternally inherited mitochondrial DNA.
    B. Noise
    C. Temporal bone fracture

Management

    A. Early identification is crucial (universal infant hearing screening)
    B. Amplification
    C. Cochlear implantation
    D. Sign language

Neoplastic

    A. Acoustic neuroma (see Neurofibromatosis).

Nose, Nasopharynx, and Paranasal Sinuses _____

Developmental Anatomy

A. Prenatal development
  i. 3 weeks' gestation
    a. Anterior neuropore at skull base persists medial to optic recess.
    b. Fonticulus nasofrontalis
      1. Space between inferior part of frontal bone and nasal bones.
      2. Entrapped tissue becomes extranasal encephalocele (meninges with or without brain tissue).
    c. Prenasal space
      1. Potential space posterior to nasal bones.
      2. Between 3 and 8 weeks': dura projects through foramen cecum (hole in skull base) and down through prenasal space. As foramen cecum closes, the diverticulum retracts into the cranium. Entrapped tissue becomes intranasal glioma (no meningeal connection) or intranasal encephalocele (retains meningeal connection).
  ii. 4 weeks' gestation
    a. External nasal development.
    b. Neural crest proliferation creates nasal placode. Adjacent cells give rise to medial and lateral nasal processes.
      1. Medial nasal process: joins maxillary process to form columella and philtrum. Overgrowth leads to pyriform aperture stenosis.
      2. Frontal prominence: joins medial nasal/maxillary processes to form frontonasal process which develops into frontal/nasal bones, ethmoids, cartilaginous nose.
    c. Nasal pits invaginate and nasobuccal membrane ruptures (5-6 weeks') forming nasal cavities. Failure to rupture leads to choanal atresia.
    d. Nasal septum development.
    e. Grows downward from nasofrontal process.
    f. Fuses to palatine process anteriorly (at 9 weeks') then posteriorly (at 12 weeks'). Septomaxillary ligament joining septum to anterior nasal spine pulls on maxilla.
  iii. 10 to 16 weeks' gestation
    a. Paranasal sinus development
    b. Maxillary sinus (10 weeks')
      1. First to develop
      2. Pneumatization from middle meatus into ethmoid cartilage. Extension into maxilla at 5 months.
      3. Radiologically visible at birth.
    c. Ethmoid sinus (4 months')
      1. Pneumatization from middle and superior meatus into ethmoid capsule. Secondary pneumatization between birth and 2 years of age.
      2. Basal lamella of middle turbinate separates anterior and posterior ethmoid cells.
    d. Sphenoid sinus (4 months')
      1. Sphenoethmoid recess becomes constricted.
      2. Secondary pneumatization between 6 and 7 years of age.
      3. Sphenoid and frontal sinuses commonly absent in Down syndrome.
    e. Frontal sinus (4 months')

          1. Begins with mucosal invaginations.

          2. Secondary pneumatization at 6 months to 2 years, but not radiologically visible until 6 years of age.

    B. Postnatal development

       i. Vomer and perforated portions of cribriform plate ossify by 3 years of age.

       ii. Adenoids peak in size from 3 to 5 years of age and regress by 8 years of age.

       iii. Maxillary sinus floor is superior to nasal floor at birth, same level as nasal floor at 8 years of age, and 5 mm below nasal floor by adulthood.

       iv. Ethmoid, sphenoid, and frontal sinuses continue to grow as above.

       v. External nasal dimensions mature by 13 years of age in females and 15 years of age in males.

Signs and Symptoms

    A. Infants are obligate nasal breathers for several weeks so nasal obstruction leads to respiratory distress.

    B. After they begin to breathe orally, obstruction manifests as sleep apnea and feeding difficulties.

    C. Purulent rhinorrhea.

    D. Mass effect.

Clinical Assessment

    A. Complete head and neck examination noting dysmorphic features.

    B. Examine from anteriorly to posteriorly and then superiorly to inferiorly.

    C. Anterior rhinoscopy for septum, vestibule and anterior nasal cavity.

    D. Flexible nasopharyngoscopy for nasal passage, nasopharynx, oropharynx and larynx.

    E. Physical examination may be limited for sinus pathology.

    F. X-ray, CT or MRI depending on suspected pathologies.

Pathology/Treatment/Complications

Congenital

    A. Pyriform aperture stenosis

       i. Clinical features

         a. Due to overgrowth of nasal process of maxilla.

         b. Presentation similar to choanal atresia.

         c. May be associated with single central incisor, holoprosencephaly or pituitary deficiency.

       ii. Diagnosis

         a. Based on physical examination and CT scan.

         b. MRI brain for pituitary abnormalities.

       iii. Management

         a. Conservative measures such as suction and saline (one side at a time).

         b. Airway compromise warrants sublabial incision and drillout of pyriform apertures.

    B. Nasolacrimal duct obstruction/cyst

       i. Clinical features

         a. Due to failed canalization of caudal nasolacrimal duct.

         b. 90% unilateral.

         c. Symptoms appear at 1 to 3 weeks of age. These include epiphora, medial canthal discharge, and noninjected conjunctiva.

       ii. Diagnosis

         a. Cystic lesion in inferior meatus.

   iii. Management
       a. May resolve spontaneously as cyst ruptures into nasal passage.
       b. Marsupialization.
       c. Associated duct stenosis may require dilatation.
   C. Choanal atresia/stenosis
       i. Clinical features
          a. Failure of resorption of bucconasal membrane of Hochstetter at 5 weeks.
          b. 1:5000 live births.
          c. Twice as common in females than males.
          d. Twice as likely to be unilateral than bilateral.
          e. Majority are mixed bony and membranous.
          f. 50% of patients have other congenital anomalies.
          g. Associated with CHARGE and Treacher-Collins (see above).
          h. Bilateral atresia presents in newborn as "cyclical cyanosis" with airway obstruction and cyanosis at rest that resolves with crying and agitation (due to open-mouth posture).
          i. Unilateral atresia presents later in life as unilateral nasal obstruction and thick, stringy, unilateral nasal discharge.
       ii. Diagnosis
          a. Classic consultation is for "inability to pass suction catheter through nose." However, flexible nasopharyngoscopy with direct visualization is required.
          b. CT scan of choanae confirms diagnosis and extent of atresia. The nose should be suctioned and decongested with oxymetazoline prior to imaging.
       iii. Management
          a. Oral airway or McGovern nipple (feeding nipple with end cut off) while infant is obligate nasal breather.
          b. Bilateral choanal atresia almost always requires early surgical repair.
          c. Unilateral atresia can be repaired when problematic, usually prior to starting school.
          d. Endoscopic or transpalatal repair with or without placement of stents.
          e. Syndromic choanal atresia may have poorer outcomes and require tracheotomy.
   D. Nasal encephalocele/glioma/dermoid
       i. Encephaloceles and gliomas develop due to failure of closure of foramen cecum at 3 weeks' gestation. No communication with skin.
          a. Encephalocele (no communication with skin)
             1. At root of nose, maintain communication with subarachnoid space.
             2. 1:35,000 live births.
             3. 35% have other abnormalities.
             4. 4 types:
                • Nasal
                   (a) Nasofrontal: between nose and forehead
                   (b) Nasoethmoid: between nose and ethmoid
                   (c) Nasoorbital: between nose and orbit
                • Frontal
                • Atretic/parietal
                • Occipital
          b. Glioma (no communication with skin)
             1. No communication with subarachnoid space.
             2. 15% have fibrous stalk continuous with dura.

ii. Dermoid (communication with skin/pit in nasal dorsum)
   a. Ectodermal elements.
   b. May pass through foramen cecum to cranial fossa.
iii. Diagnosis
   a. Encephalocele is soft and compressible, transilluminates, and has positive Furstenberg test (expands with crying, Valsalva maneuver, or compression of jugular vein).
   b. Gliomas are firm, noncompressible, do not transilluminate, and have negative Furstenberg test.
   c. Imaging important to assess communication with intracranial space. CT for bony skull base defect. MRI for CSF communication.
iv. Management
   a. Antibiotics for infection.
   b. Surgical excision for definitive management.
   c. Involve neurosurgery if intracranial connection.

E. Tornwald cyst
  i. Clinical features
   a. Persistence of pharyngeal bursa (first described by Mayer, then Luschka).
   b. Present as midline nasopharyngeal cyst or chronic crusting.
  ii. Diagnosis
   a. Clinical or using MRI or CT.
  iii. Management
   a. Surgical excision or marsupialization.

F. Primary ciliary dyskinesia
  i. Clinical features:
   a. Defective dynein arms lead to poor mucociliary clearance, otitis media, sinusitis and bronchiectasis.
   b. May be due to autosomal recessive mutations in DNAI1 and DNAH5 (38%).
   c. Can be associated with Kartagener syndrome (50%).
     1. Sinusitis, bronchiectasis
     2. Situs inversus
     3. Infertility
  ii. Diagnosis requires ciliary biopsy from nasal or tracheal mucosa.
  iii. Management is symptomatic at present.

G. Cystic fibrosis
  i. Clinical features
   a. Most common fatal autosomal recessive disorder (1/2000 live births).
   b. Mutations in CFTR gene (delta F508 most common) causes defect in cell membrane chloride ion transport.
   c. Increased mucus viscosity impairs clearance leading to infection.
   d. Suspect in children under 10 years of age with nasal polyps.
   e. Nasal obstruction and chronic sinusitis (30%).
     1. Most common bacteria cultured are *S aureus* (47%) and *P aeruginosa* (26%) (*P aeruginosa* more common in patients older than 8 years of age). Both of these bacteria found in same sinus in only 7% of patients, suggesting separate specimens should be obtained from several sinuses.
     2. Sinus bacteria highly predictive of pulmonary bacteria in children over 8 years of age.
   f. Persistent productive cough, bronchitis, bronchiectasis.

g. Pancreatic insufficiency, fat malabsorption, coagulopathy (due to vitamin K deficiency), meconium ileus.

h. Cirrhosis and hepatomegaly.

i. Nephrolithiasis.

j. Infertility.

k. Reduced bone density.

l. Venous thrombosis.

ii. Diagnosis

   a. Clinical symptoms of CF in one organ system.

   b. Evidence of dysfunctional cystic fibrosis transmembrane conductance regulator protein evidenced by any of the following:

      1. Elevated sweat chloride level (first line, diagnostic if greater or equal to 60 mmol/L).

      2. Genetic testing (used if sweat chloride intermediate, less than 60 mmol/L).

      3. Abnormal nasal potential difference (false negative if inflammation).

      4. Immunoreactive trypsin test (IRT) during neonatal screening (identifies 50% of cases).

   c. CT shows bilateral pansinusitis.

iii. Treatment

   a. Medical management

      1. Nasal steroid sprays.

      2. Oral macrolide antibiotics for acute exacerbations.

   b. Surgical management

      1. For alleviation of nasal obstruction after failure of maximal medical therapy.

      2. No evidence that sinonasal surgery improves pulmonary function.

      3. Check coagulation preoperatively.

Trauma

A. Septal deviation

  i. Neonatal septal deviation

   a. Relatively common.

   b. Most improve spontaneously.

   c. Severe deviations with airway compromise should be corrected early.

  ii. Acquired septal deviation

   a. Impact of early surgery on facial growth controversial. Conservative therapy with minimal removal of cartilage advocated.

B. Septal hematoma

  i. Nasal obstruction.

  ii. Diagnosed on examination.

  iii. Management

   a. Drainage and nasal packing to minimize risk of abscess, perforation and saddle nose deformity.

C. Septal abscess

  i. Nasal obstruction, pain, and fever.

  ii. Leads to cartilage loss and saddle nose deformity.

  iii. Management

   a. Drainage, packing and antibiotics (to cover *S pneumoniae* and group A beta-hemolytic *streptococci*).

   b. Suspect child abuse in children under 2 years of age.

D. Nasal fractures
    i. Most common facial fracture of childhood.
    ii. Greenstick fractures common.
    iii. Rule out septal hematoma/abscess or CSF leak.
    iv. Diagnosis
        a. Based on clinical examination.
        b. Radiographs not helpful.
    v. Management
        a. Closed reduction if obvious cosmetic deformity.
        b. Reduce immediately before swelling occurs or 5 to 7 days after trauma when swelling subsides.

E. Nasoethmoid fractures
    i. Uncommon in children.
    ii. Rule out intracranial and cervical spine injuries.
    iii. May require reconstructive surgery.

F. Orbital floor fractures
    i. Clinical features
        a. Hypoesthesia of infraorbital nerve
        b. Inferior rectus muscle entrapment
        c. Enophthalmos
        d. Globe injuries
    ii. Management
        a. May require reconstructive surgery.

G. Nasal foreign body
    i. Associated with malodorous rhinorrhea, often unilateral.
    ii. Button/disk batteries must be removed immediately due to risk of necrosis and septal perforation.

Infectious/Inflammatory

A. Rhinitis of infancy
    i. May cause airway obstruction and feeding difficulties in infants.
    ii. Onset at birth or within first month of life.
    iii. Seasonal variation, more common in fall and winter.
    iv. May be due to RSV, chlamydia, GERD, meconium aspiration.
    v. Management
        a. Bulb suction for nose. Ear suction used in nose is more slender and less traumatic.
        b. Topical vasoconstrictor for 3 days and saline drops. If no improvement in 5 days add steroid drops or spray.
        c. Culture may be helpful.
        d. CT reserved for nonresponders.

B. Allergic rhinitis
    i. Itchy nose with discharge and obstruction. Bruising under eyes "allergic shiners" and "supratip crease" (from rubbing nose upwards) common.
    ii. IgE-mediated response (type 1).
    iii. Types:
        a. Seasonal (grass, trees, pollen, ragweed)
        b. Perennial (allergens within home)
        c. Sporadic (intermittent to specific allergen)
        d. Occupational

      iv. Family history of atopy in 50% to 75% of children.

      v. Examination shows pale, boggy edematous mucosa, inferior turbinate hypertrophy, thin clear rhinorrhea, +/− polyps.

      vi. Diagnosis:

        a. Based on clinical history alone.

        b. May confirm with skin prick test, intradermal tests, radioallergosorbent assay testing (RAST) or enzyme-linked immunosorbent assay (ELISA)

          1. Management

        a. Avoidance

        b. Pharmacotherapy (nasal saline, decongestants, steroid sprays, antihistamines, leukotriene inhibitors, mast cell stabilizers, anticholinergics)

        c. Immunotherapy

C. Viral rhinitis

      i. Common in childhood.

      ii. Pathogens include rhinovirus, coronavirus, adenovirus, and respiratory syncytial virus.

D. Bacterial rhinitis

      i. Diphtheria: pseudomembrane formation on nasal septum.

      ii. Pertussis: associated with prolonged cough.

      iii. Chlamydia: red nasal mucosa in neonate with rhinorrhea. Vertical transmission from mother to child during delivery.

      iv. Syphilis—congenital infection

        a. First stage—presents in first 3 months of life with watery rhinorrhea which progresses to mucopurulent drainage.

        b. Second stage—presents later in childhood with "snuffles" and gumma formation in nasal cavity.

E. Adenoid hypertrophy

      i. Clinical features

        a. Nasal obstruction.

        b. Hyponasal speech.

        c. "Adenoid facies": Open mouth, flat midface, long lower face, high-arched palate. Open mouth posture leads to unopposed compressive action of masseter muscles on maxilla and overgrowth of molars due to lack of contact.

        d. Rhinorrhea.

        e. Sleep apnea.

        f. Eustachian tube dysfunction.

        g. Recurrent acute otitis media.

      ii. Diagnosis

        a. Flexible nasopharyngoscopy (benefits: faster, no radiation, and allows evaluation of effect of palate location on size of choanal aperture).

        b. X-ray (benefit: no scope for uncooperative children; risks: radiation, crying children elevate soft palate which makes nasal aperture look smaller thus over-estimating adenoid size.)

      iii. Management

        a. Nasal steroids.

        b. Add montelukast for mild cases.

        c. Surgery for moderate/severe cases.

        d. Recurrent obstruction following surgery responds better to nasal steroids than prior to surgery. Failure to improve warrants revision adenoidectomy.

    e. Biopsy recurrent adenoid regrowth to rule out lymphoma.

    f. Complications of surgery include velopharyngeal insufficiency, bleeding, infection, torticollis (Grisel syndrome), nasopharyngeal stenosis, Eustachian tube injury and atlantoaxial subluxation (ie, Down syndrome: avoid neck extension even if they have "normal" flexion/extension cervical spine x-rays.)

F. Rhinosinusitis

  i. Acute

    a. Clinical features

      1. Purulent rhinorrhea more than 10 days with fever.

      2. Uncomplicated infections due to:
- *S pneumoniae* (30%)
- *H influenzae* (20%)
- *M catarrhalis* (20%)
- *S pyogenes* (5%)

      3. Complicated infections due to
- Polymicrobial
- *S anginosis*
- Anaerobes
- Methicillin-resistant *S aureus* (MRSA)

      4. Communicating location of infection (Chandler classification). These are not progressive and are only descriptive.
- Preseptal cellulitis
- Orbital cellulitis (associated with chemosis)
- Subperiosteal abscess
- Orbital abscess
- Venous/cavernous sinus thrombosis

      5. Risks of spread
- Frontal bone (Pott puffy tumor)
- Meningitis
- Abscess (subdural, epidural, brain)

    b. Diagnosis

      1. Uncomplicated sinusitis based on clinical symptoms. Radiographic sinus opacification is nonspecific in young children.

      2. Complications require urgent CT scan.

    c. Treatment

      1. Uncomplicated: Oral amoxicillin 10 to 14 days. Beta-lactamase inhibitor if severe symptoms or if no improvement after 72 hours.

      2. Complications: Intravenous antibiotics that have good soft tissue and CNS penetration. Consult ophthalmology and/or neurosurgery as required. May require urgent surgical drainage.

  ii. Recurrent acute

    a. Clinical features

      1. Free of symptoms for 2 weeks between episodes.

    b. Diagnosis

      1. Rule out immunodeficiency, cystic fibrosis (CF), primary ciliary dyskinesia (PCD), and gastroesophageal reflux disease (GERD).

      2. Assess adenoid size.

    c. Treatment

      1. Adenoidectomy if adenoids obstructive.

iii. Chronic
  a. Clinical features
    1. Congestion, rhinorrhea, headache, postnasal drip, cough, halitosis.
    2. Low-grade symptoms lasting more than 12 weeks.
    3. Infections due to:
      - *S aureus*
      - Anaerobes
      - Fungi
  b. Diagnosis
    1. Cultures from middle meatus/ethmoid/maxillary sinus helpful if
      - Immunocompromised
      - Systemic illness
      - Progression despite appropriate therapy
      - Suppurative complications
  c. Treatment
    1. Antibiotic therapy 4 to 6 weeks.
    2. Adenoidectomy may be helpful in younger children.
    3. Endoscopic sinus surgery for failed medical management. Limited to involved sinuses (usually maxillary and anterior ethmoids).
G. Nasal polyps
  i. Antrochoanal polyp
    a. Clinical features
      1. Extends from maxillary sinus into nasal cavity.
      2. Most unilateral.
    b. Diagnosis
      1. Flexible nasopharyngoscopy
      2. CT or MRI
    c. Management
      1. Endoscopic removal. Send to pathology to rule out inverting papilloma.
  ii. Multiple polyps
    a. Related to allergy, chronic sinusitis or cystic fibrosis (see above)

Neoplasms
Most sinonasal tumors in children are benign.
A. Benign
  i. Juvenile nasopharyngeal angiofibroma (JNA)
    a. Clinical features
      1. Most common benign nasopharyngeal tumor.
      2. Incidence 1:5,000-1:60,000.
      3. Mostly males.
      4. Commonly 14 to 8 years of age.
      5. Originates in sphenopalatine recess. Extend laterally to pterygomaxillary space and superiorly to cavernous sinus and middle cranial fossa.
      6. Nasal mass, obstruction, epistaxis, facial deformity and proptosis.
    b. Diagnosis
      1. History and examination. Biopsy contraindicated due to risk of bleeding.
      2. CT, MRI, and magnetic resonance angiography (MRA) for extent.
    c. Treatment
      1. Preoperative embolization 48 hours prior to minimize blood loss.
      2. Surgical approach depends on extent of lesion. Approaches include:

- Endoscopic (most common)
- LeFort I osteotomy and midface degloving
- Lateral rhinotomy
- Transpalatal
- Lateral infratemporal fossa
            3. Tumors with intracranial extension require neurosurgical consultation.
            4. Radiation for unresectable lesions. Risk of malignant transformation.
            5. Use of hormonal therapy unclear.
    ii. Fibrous dysplasia
        a. Clinical features
            1. Normal bone replaced by fibrous tissue.
            2. Types:
                - Monostotic (70%)
                - Polyostotic (24%)
                - McCune-Albright syndrome (6%): multiple café au lait spots, precocious puberty
            3. Nasal mass, obstruction, sinusitis.
            4. Often incidental finding on CT or MRI performed for other reason.
        b. Diagnosis
            1. CT shows ground-glass appearance.
        c. Management
            1. Surgery only if symptomatic.
            2. Contouring of bone for cosmetic appearance where resection not possible.
    iii. Teratoma (rare)
        a. Clinical features
            1. Usually present at birth.
            2. Tissue from all three germ layers present: ectoderm, mesoderm, endoderm.
            3. Rare malignant potential.
            4. Nasal obstruction.
        b. Diagnosis
            1. CT or MRI
        c. Treatment
            1. Surgical excision
B. Malignant
    i. Rhabdomyosarcoma (see above)
    ii. Lymphoma (see above)

Idiopathic

A. Granulomatosis with polyangitis (GPA, formerly known as Wegener granulomatosis)
    i. Clinical features
        a. Autoimmune disease
        b. Rare, less than 1:100,000
        c. Teen females more common than males
    ii. Diagnostic criteria in children requires 3 of 6 features (EULAR 2010)
        a. Sinonasal (recurrent epistaxis or septal perforation) or oral inflammation
        b. Abnormal pulmonary chest x-ray or CT
        c. Abnormal urinalysis or necrotizing pauci-immune glomerulonephritis
        d. Granuloma within or around an artery on pathology
        e. Laryngotracheobronchial involvement with stenosis
        f. Positive PR3/cANCA or MPO/pANCA

       iii. Management
- a. Trimethoprim/sulfamethoxazole prevents flareups in upper respiratory tract.
- b. Cyclophosphamide + prednisone for acute life-threatening exacerbations.
- c. Methotrexate + prednisone for maintenance therapy.

Oral cavity/Oropharynx
Developmental Anatomy
A. Prenatal development
- i. 4 week's gestation
  - a. Tongue forms from mesenchymal proliferations on floor of oral cavity.
  - b. Anterior 2/3 develops from lateral lingual swellings (first arch) and median tuberculum impar.
  - c. Posterior 1/3 develops from copula (second arch) and hypobranchial eminence (third and fourth arches).
  - d. Tongue musculature develops from occipital somites.
- ii. 6 weeks' gestation
  - a. Upper lateral lip forms as maxillary prominences meet nasal prominences. Upper medial lip forms as both nasal prominences meet.
  - b. Palatal shelves grow medially from maxillary prominences.
- iii. 7 weeks' gestation
  - a. Bilateral Meckel cartilages begin intramembranous ossification on lateral aspect of mandibular symphysis. This spreads anteriorly and posteriorly. Fusion at symphysis does not occur until after birth.
- iv. 12 weeks' gestation
  - a. Medial nasal prominences fuse forming intermaxillary segment with four incisor tooth buds.
  - b. Secondary palate fuses from incisive foramen to uvula.

B. Postnatal development
- i. All structures of the oral cavity grow postnatally.
- ii. Tonsils peak in size by age 5 to 8 years.

Signs and Symptoms
A. Stertor
B. Airway obstruction
C. Visible lesion
D. Feeding difficulties
E. Sialorrhea
F. Altered speech

Clinical Assessment
Direct examination of oral cavity from anteriorly and using nasopharyngoscope from posterosuperiorly.

Pathology/Treatment/Complications
Congenital
A. Ankyloglossia (tethered lingual frenulum, "tongue-tie")
- i. Clinical features
  - a. Congenital anomaly
  - b. May interfere with feeding or speech
- ii. Diagnosis
  - a. Inability of tongue to extend past red-white junction of lower lip may be predictive of success following division.

      iii. Treatment

         a. Frenulectomy (division) or frenuloplasty (division plus suture closure of defect) for feeding or speech issues.

B. Ranula

    i. Clinical features

      a. Cystic lesion in anterolateral floor of mouth.

      b. Due to obstruction of sublingual gland.

      c. Plunging ranula: extends below mylohyoid muscle.

    ii. Diagnosis

      a. Unilateral cystic lesion in floor of mouth.

      b. Filled with thick, clear fluid.

      c. Differentiate from macrocystic lymphatic malformation.

      d. May require MRI or CT to confirm diagnosis.

    iii. Treatment

      a. Excision of sublingual gland eradicates disease.

      b. Careful preservation of submandibular duct orifice to prevent sialadenitis and lingual nerve to prevent numbness.

      c. Marsupialization of cyst not recommended due to high rate of recurrence.

C. Floor of mouth dermoid

    i. Well-circumscribed cyst filled with keratin.

    ii. Surgical excision.

D. Midline rhomboid glossitis

    i. Soft tissue mass in posterior midline tongue.

    ii. Due to defect in posterior tongue development (tuberculum impar).

    iii. No treatment necessary.

E. Lingual thyroid gland

    i. Clinical features

      a. Due to abnormal descent of thyroid from foramen cecum to lower neck.

      b. Increases in size with age, infection and other thyroid disorders.

      c. May cause airway obstruction, speech and feeding difficulties.

      d. May be the patient's only functioning thyroid tissue.

    ii. Diagnosis

      a. Thyroid scan to detect other functioning thyroid tissue lower in neck.

      b. Thyroid function studies.

    iii. Treatment

      a. Observation if minimal or no symptoms.

      b. Thyroid suppression.

      c. Surgery if fails medical management or suspicion of malignancy.

F. Lingual thyroglossal duct cyst

    i. Clinical features

      a. Due to abnormal descent of thyroid from foramen cecum to lower neck.

      b. Cystic swelling in base of tongue (intrinsic to musculature).

    ii. Diagnosis

      a. MRI (T2 sagittal) for location and to ensure there is normal thyroid gland in neck to decrease chances of removing only functioning thyroid.

    iii. Treatment

      a. Suspension microlaryngoscopy and surgical removal using laser, bipolar cautery (to minimize swelling) or microdebrider.

      b. Consider overnight intubation until swelling subsides.

      c. Consider thyroid function tests postoperatively.

G. Vallecular cyst
  i. Clinical features
    a. Retention cyst from obstructed minor salivary gland.
    b. Cystic swelling in vallecula between tongue base and epiglottis (extrinsic to tongue musculature).
  ii. Diagnosis
    a. MRI (T2 sagittal) for location.
  iii. Treatment
    a. Suspension microlaryngoscopy and surgical removal using laser, cautery or microdebrider.
    b. Consider overnight intubation until swelling subsides.
H. Macroglossia
  i. Large anterior tongue
    a. Beckwith-Wiedemann
      1. Clinical features
        • Due to mutation on chromosome 11 in imprinting control region (ICR) leading to abnormal gene methylation or paternal uniparental disomy (UPD) where both paternally expressed genes are active
        • Macrosomia (birthweight over 10 lb)
        • Hypoglycemia
        • Auricular pits
        • Omphalocele
        • Hepatosplenomegaly
        • Tumors develop in 10% (Wilms, rhabdomyosarcoma, hepatoblastoma)
      2. Treatment
        • Wedge resection of anterior tongue to allow child to close mouth
    b. Glycosaminoglycan (GAG) storage diseases
      1. Hurler syndrome (mucopolysaccharidosis I)
        • Autosomal recessive.
        • Deficient lysosomal alpha-L-iduronidase leads to GAG storage.
        • Deafness, coarse facial features, low nasal bridge, cardiac anomalies, stunted growth.
        • Treatment includes ECG, genetic testing, urine tests for mucopolysaccharides, spine x-ray, enzyme therapy with intravenous Iduronidase.
      2. Hunter syndrome (mucopolysaccharidosis II)
        • X-linked recessive.
        • Deficient enzyme iduronate-2-sulfatase leads to storage of heparan sulfate and dermatan sulfate.
        • Large head, prominent forehead, flattened nasal bridge, large tongue.
        • Treatments include testing for I2S gene and wedge resection of tongue where necessary.
    c. Congenital hypothyroidism
      1. Due to myxedema of tongue.
      2. Diagnosed as part of neonatal screening.
      3. Treatment includes early thyroid replacement to reverse symptoms.
  ii. Large tongue base
    a. Trisomy 21 (Down syndrome).
    b. Treatment includes lingual tonsillectomy, midline posterior glossectomy +/− genioglossus advancement for severe obstructive sleep apnea.

I. Glossoptosis
    i. With retrognathia
        a. Clinical features
            1. Pierre-Robin sequence
                - Retrognathia leads to severe glossoptosis. Tongue prevents fusion of palate in midline causing U-shaped cleft of secondary palate.
                - Mandible requires 4 to 6 months to grow and alleviate obstruction.
            2. Stickler syndrome
                - Most autosomal dominant mutation in collagen genes (COL)
                - Myopia before 10 years of age, retinal detachment
                - Hearing loss (mixed conductive and sensorineural)
                - Joint problems
            3. Nager syndrome (Acrofacial dysostosis)
                - Auricular anomalies including atresia
                - Malar hypoplasia
                - Downslanting palpebral fissures
                - Eyelid coloboma
                - Cleft palate
                - Thumb hypoplasia
            4. Treacher Collins syndrome (Mandibulofacial dysostosis)
                - Most autosomal dominant mutation in TCOF1 gene
                - Malar hypoplasia with deficient zygomatic arch
                - Eyelid coloboma
                - Hearing loss, bilateral microtia and atresia
                - Choanal atresia
        b. Treatment depends on degree of obstruction.
            - Positioning on side or prone
            - McGovern nipple (nipple with tip cut off, better tolerated than oral airway)
            - Nasal trumpet
            - Tongue-lip adhesion (benefits controversial)
            - Subperiosteal release of floor of mouth (SRFM; 84% effective)
            - Mandibular advancement
            - Tracheotomy
    ii. Without retrognathia
        a. Clinical features
            1. Tongue prolapses posteriorly despite mandible being in proper position.
        b. Treatment depends on degree of airway obstruction.
            - Positioning on side or prone
            - McGovern nipple
            - Nasal trumpet
            - Tongue-lip adhesion (benefits controversial)
            - Subperiosteal release of floor of mouth (SRFM; 84% effective)
            - Tongue suspension or genioglossus advancement
            - Tracheotomy
J. Velopharyngeal insufficiency
    i. Clinical features
        a. Nasal air escape on consonant sounds, hypernasality on vowel sounds.
        b. Compensatory misarticulations (m, n, ng, w do not require closure).
        c. May have nasal regurgitation of food.
        d. 25% to 40% after cleft palate repair.

      ii. Diagnosis
         a. Perceptual speech evaluation
         b. Nasometry
         c. Nasendoscopy to look for velopharyngeal closure patterns
         d. Fiberoptic endoscopic evaluation of swallowing (FEES)
      iii. Management
         a. Speech therapy: for sound-specific VPI and compensatory misarticulations.
         b. Furlow palatoplasty to lengthen palate.
         c. Sphincter pharyngoplasty: superomedial rotation of bilateral muscle flaps from posterior pharyngeal wall to recreate Passavant ridge.
         d. Pharyngeal flap: superior rotation of midline muscle flap from posterior pharyngeal wall with attachment to soft palate.
         e. Palatal lift or obturator (last resort).

Neoplastic

A. Benign
    i. Epulis (granular cell tumor)
       a. Most commonly from maxillary gingiva.
       b. Mostly female (4:1).
       c. Treat with surgical excision.
    ii. Epignathus
       a. Teratoma from palate or pharynx in basisphenoid region (Rathke pouch).
       b. Diagnosed on prenatal ultrasound, confirmed on fetal MRI.
       c. Associated with polyhydramnios, midline facial defects, airway obstruction.
       d. May require EXIT procedure to secure airway.
    iii. Hamartoma
       a. Normal tissue in normal location growing in disorganized fashion.
       b. Treat with surgical excision if problematic.
    iv. Choristoma
       a. Normal tissue in abnormal location.
       b. Treat with surgical excision if problematic.

B. Malignant
    i. Rhabdomyosarcoma: see Head and Neck section.
    ii. Lymphoma: see Head and Heck section.
    iii. Squamous cell carcinoma
       a. Rare in children
       b. Tongue most commonly involved but lip, palate or gingiva may be as well.
       c. Rapid growth.
       d. Early regional metastases.
       e. Treatment similar to that recommended for adults.

Infectious/Inflammatory

A. Tonsillitis
    i. Viral (majority of tonsillitis)
       a. Adenovirus, rhinovirus, echovirus, Coxsackie, RSV, influenza, parainfluenza.
       b. Epstein Barr virus (human herpes virus 4, infectious mononucleosis)
          1. Clinical features
             • High fever and malaise.
             • Grayish-white coating on tonsils.
             • Petechiae at hard-soft palate junction.
             • Hepatosplenomegaly.
             • Develop rash with amoxicillin.

2. Diagnosis
- CBC shows 50% lymphocytes, 10% atypical.
- ESR more likely to be elevated in EBV than bacterial infection.
- Monospot positive (85% sensitive—less in first two weeks, 100% specific). If initial test negative, repeat once per week for 6 weeks.
- EBV serology: use if monospot negative after 6 weeks.

ii. Bacterial
  a. Clinical features
    1. Group A beta-hemolytic *Streptococcus pyogenes* (most common).
    2. May be associated with rheumatic fever or glomerulonephritis.
    3. May be cause of periodic fever, aphthous ulcers, pharyngitis, cervical adenitis (PFAPA).
       - Each episode lasts 3 days
       - At least 3 episodes
       - Reccur every 3 weeks
       - Symptom-free intervals
       - Rule out cyclical neutropenia.
  b. Diagnosis
    1. Sore throat plus one of exudate, adenopathy, positive RADT or GABHS culture, temperature greater than 38.3°C.
    2. Rapid antigen detection test (RADT). If negative, perform throat culture. Antistreptolysin-O (ASO) titres not recommended as they only indicate prior infection.
  c. Treatment
    1. Antibiotics to avoid complications.
    2. Tonsillectomy if 7 episodes in 1 year, 5 episodes per year for each of 2 years, or 3 episodes per year for each of 3 years.

B. Peritonsillar abscess
  i. Purulent infection of Weber glands in potential space between tonsil and pharyngeal constrictor.
  ii. Due to mixture of anaerobic and aerobic bacteria.
  iii. Clinical features
    a. Trismus (best indicator)
    b. Antecedent pharyngitis
    c. Fever
    d. Odynophagia
    e. Airway obstruction
    f. Unilateral palatal enlargement and deviation of uvula to contralateral side
  iv. Diagnosis
    a. Clinical examination.
    b. May attempt drainage with needle if unsure whether cellulitis or abscess.
    c. CT scan of neck with contrast not routinely indicated but may help if clinical picture unclear or suspicion of spread.
  v. Treatment
    a. Intravenous antibiotics +/− steroids.
    b. Drainage is mainstay of therapy.
    c. Recurrence rate 17%. Tonsillectomy recommended after second abscess.

C. Retropharyngeal abscess
   i. Infection of lymph nodes (of Rouviere) in retropharyngeal space between visceral and alar fasciae. Usually disappear by age 5 years.
   ii. Infection may extend inferiorly to mediastinum.
   iii. Most common organisms
       a. Beta-hemolytic *Streptococcus*
       b. Anaerobic streptococci
       c. *S aureus*
   iv. Clinical features
       a. Torticollis (best indicator)
       b. Antecedent pharyngitis
       c. Fever
       d. Odynophagia
       e. Airway obstruction
       f. Sialorrhea
       g. Bulge in posterior pharyngeal wall (best appreciated with nasopharyngoscopy)
   v. Diagnosis
       a. Lateral neck x-ray shows thickening of prevertebral tissue and loss of lordosis due to spasm of prevertebral muscles. Neck must be extended to prevent false appearance of thickened tissue. Thickening greater than one half the width of the vertebral body at the same level is pathological.
       b. CT scan of neck with contrast distinguishes phlegmon (nondrainable) from abscess (drainable) and helps define level and angle of entry for drainage.
   vi. Treatment
       a. Intravenous antibiotics
       b. Incision and drainage of abscess (fluid filled with rim enhancement)
D. Tonsillar hypertrophy
   i. Clinical features
       a. May cause obstructive sleep apnea.
          1. Inspiratory effort in the absence of air flow.
          2. Signs and symptoms in children (different from adults):
             • Heroic snoring
             • Pauses
             • Gasping
             • Neck hyperextension
             • Nocturnal diaphoresis
             • Nocturnal enuresis
             • Parasomnias (tooth grinding, sleepwalking)
             • Morning headache
             • Excessive daytime sleepiness
             • Attention deficit or hyperactivity
             • Poor school performance
       b. May cause dysphagia
   ii. Diagnosis
       a. Parental observation (use clock and count number of episodes per hour).
       b. Sleep study (not oxygen saturation study) is gold standard.
          1. Differentiates obstructive from central apnea and degree of obstruction.

2. Obstructive sleep apnea defined as apnea-hypopnea index (AHI) >1 (2 apneas or hypopneas in 2 consecutive breaths per hour) or drop in oxygen saturation to less than 92%. Many consider surgery when AHI > 5/hour.

iii. Indications for treatment

    a. Obstructive sleep apnea with tonsil hypertrophy (grade 3 or 4).

       1. Tonsillectomy and adenoidectomy (many reserve surgery for AHI > 5/hour).

       2. Single intraoperative dose dexamethasone for postoperative nausea.

       3. No role for routine postoperative antibiotics.

       4. Advocate for pain control (avoid codeine).

    b. Asymmetric tonsils in children with immunosuppression and solid organ transplant to rule out posttransplant lymphoproliferative disorder (PTLD).

iv. Complications of tonsillectomy and adenoidectomy

    a. General anesthetic

    b. Loose/chipped teeth

    c. Primary bleeding (< 24 hour, 0.2%-2.2%); Secondary bleeding (> 24 hour, 0.1%-3.0%)

    d. Velopharyngeal insufficiency

    e. Aspiration pneumonia

    f. Torticollis

    g. Respiratory distress/airway obstruction

    h. Death

Traumatic

A. Penetrating trauma of the oral cavity

  i. Clinical features

    a. Impalement of oropharynx and palate usually from running while holding sharp object.

    b. Risk of carotid injury (higher risk if injury lateral to anterior tonsillar pillar).

  ii. Management

    a. Most injuries do not require surgical repair.

    b. CT neck with contrast if concerned about carotid injury.

    c. Injuries in infants who are not yet walking should alert to abuse.

Larynx/Subglottis

Developmental Anatomy

A. Prenatal development

  i. 4 weeks' gestation

    a. Ventral wall of foregut (laryngotracheal groove) develops thickening.

    b. Laryngotracheal groove divides into ventral (trachea) and dorsal (esophagus) components. Divided by tracheoesophageal septum.

  ii. 6 weeks' gestation

    a. Laryngeal lumen obliterated by mesenchyme.

  iii. 8 weeks' gestation

    a. Larynx, trachea, and esophagus are formed.

  iv. 10 weeks' gestation

    a. Recanalization of larynx and trachea. Failure to do so results in laryngeal/tracheal atresia.

  v. 12 weeks' gestation

    a. Vocal cord movement detectable.

      vi. Branchial arches contribute to each of the following structures.

        a. Second arch: hyoid upper body and lesser horn.

        b. Third arch: hyoid lower body and greater horn.

        c. Fourth arch: thyroid cartilage, cricothyroid muscle (superior laryngeal nerve).

        d. Fifth arch: cricoid, cuneiform, corniculate, arytenoid cartilages. Intrinsic muscles except cricothryoid (recurrent laryngeal nerve).

  B. Postnatal development

    i. Neonatal glottis measures 7 mm anteroposteriorly and 4 mm laterally.

    ii. Subglottis is narrowest part measuring 4 to 5 mm in diameter.

    iii. Larynx descends in neck with growth.

      a. At level of C4 at birth, C5 at 2 years, C6 at 5 years, and C6-C7 at 15 years.

Signs and Symptoms

  A. Voice change

  B. Drooling

  C. Stridor (inspiratory, expiratory, biphasic)

  D. Tachypnea

  E. Tachycardia

  F. Tracheal tug, chest wall retractions, abdominal breathing.

  G. Desaturation first, followed by bradycardia.

  H. Feeding difficulties and weight loss (burn calories breathing and preferentially breathe rather that eat).

Clinical Assessment

  A. Inspect nose for flaring, lips for cyanosis, neck for tracheal tug, chest for indrawing.

  B. Auscultation over trachea for stridor.

  C. Flexible nasopharyngoscopy for vocal cord movement and pathology.

  D. Direct laryngoscopy and bronchoscopy under anesthesia may be required.

Pathology/Treatment/Complications

Laryngomalacia

  A. Clinical features

    i. Most common cause of stridor in infants.

    ii. Inspiratory stridor within first 6 weeks of life.

    iii. Worse lying supine and when agitated.

    iv. Improves sitting up and prone.

    v. Ninety percent spontaneously resolve by 12 months.

    vi. Neurologically impaired children may have progressive laryngomalacia.

    vii. May be associated with airway compromise (stridor, retractions, desaturation, cyanosis), feeding difficulties and failure to thrive.

  B. Diagnosis

    i. Flexible nasopharyngoscopy

      a. Short aryepiglottic folds

      b. Omega-shaped epiglottis

      c. Prolapse of epiglottis into laryngeal inlet

      d. Redundant tissue over arytenoid cartilages due to inspiration against closed glottis leading to acid reflux.

    ii. 10% to 20% incidence of secondary synchronous airway lesion. More severe or atypical symptoms warrants laryngoscopy and bronchoscopy.

  C. Management

    i. Monitor growth on growth curve.

    ii. Most do not require intervention due to high rate of spontaneous improvement.

      iii. Treating gastroesophageal reflux may break the cycle and improve respiratory symptoms.

      iv. Infants with severe laryngomalacia (cyanotic episodes, failure to thrive) may benefit from supraglottoplasty.

      v. Beware of syndromes such as CHARGE whereby supraglottoplasty leads to epiglottic collapse and worsens respiratory distress.

Vocal Cord Dysfunction

A. Clinical features
    i. Second most common laryngeal anomaly of infancy.
    ii. Mostly idiopathic in infants, iatrogenic in older children.
    iii. Left vocal cord more commonly affected due to longer, more circuitous route.

B. Etiology
    i. Congenital
        a. Complex congenital heart disease.
        b. CNS anomalies
           1. Hydrocephalus
           2. Spinal cord anomalies
           3. Nucleus ambiguus dysgenesis (usually familial and bilateral)
           4. Kernicterus
        c. Other associations
           1. Moebius syndrome—associated with bilateral facial nerve palsy
           2. Trisomy 21 (Down syndrome)
           3. Mediastinal anomalies
           4. Trauma—usually improves in 4 to 6 months
           5. Diaphragmatic hernia
           6. Erb palsy
    ii. Acquired
        a. Arnold-Chiari malformation
           1. Unilateral or bilateral paresis
           2. May also have central sleep apnea
        b. Infectious
           1. Poliomyelitis
           2. Guillain-Barré
           3. Botulism
           4. Diphtheria
           5. Syphilis
         c. Iatrogenic
           1. Cardiac surgery
           2. Thyroidectomy
           3. Intubation injury

C. Diagnosis
    i. MRI brain, neck, chest (entire length of recurrent laryngeal nerves)
    ii. Palpation of arytenoid cartilages to rule out dislocation

D. Management
    i. Dependent on degree of airway compromise.
    ii. Spontaneous recovery may occur up to several years later.
    iii. Observation if no desaturations, cyanosis or respiratory distress.
    iv. Chiari malformation may require decompression.

     v. Unilateral palsy requires feeding assessment to rule out aspiration.

     vi. Bilateral palsy may require tracheotomy.

     vii. Reserve destructive procedures such as vocal cord lateralization, arytenoidectomy and posterior costal cartilage graft laryngotracheoplasty for longstanding bilateral vocal cord paralysis with respiratory distress or poor quality of life.

Laryngeal Cleft

A. Clinical features

     i. Incomplete fusion of posterior cricoid lamina and tracheoesophageal septum.

     ii. Incidence 1/10,000-1/20,000 live births.

     iii. More common in males.

     iv. Present with coughing with feeds (worse with thin liquids) and recurrent pneumonia.

     v. Associated with CHARGE, VACTERL/VATER, Opitz, Pallister Hall syndromes.

B. Diagnosis

     i. Video swallow study shows aspiration.

     ii. Rigid laryngoscopy with distraction of arytenoids is essential. Flexible nasopharyngoscopy not adequate for ruling out laryngeal cleft.

     iii. Benjamin and Inglis classification based on inferior extent of cleft

        a. Type I: Interarytenoid cleft down to but not below true vocal folds.

        b. Type II: Extension into cricoid cartilage but not through it.

        c. Type III: Extension through entire cricoid +/− into cervical trachea.

        d. Type IV: Extension into thoracic trachea.

        e. Deep interarytenoid notch

           1. A deep interarytenoid notch that does not extend to the vocal folds may still cause aspiration requiring treatment.

        f. Type IV may be subdivided to better reflect need for different approach.

           1. IVA: Extension into proximal thoracic trachea.

           2. IVB: Extension into distal thoracic trachea.

C. Treatment

     i. Types I and II: may be injected temporarily with filler to determine the effect of treatment and temporize until endoscopic suture repair can be performed.

     ii. Types I, II, and shallow type III may be amenable to endoscopic suture repair.

     iii. Long type III and shallow type IV not extending past the innominate artery require open surgical repair. This is best performed using a transtracheal approach with placement of posterior costal cartilage graft and interposing fascia.

     iv. Long type IV require open surgical repair. This is best performed using cricotracheal separation to obviate the need for bypass with placement of interposing fascia.

Subglottic Stenosis

A. Clinical features

     i. Congenital

        a. Due to cricoid malformation (ie, elliptical cricoid)

        b. Types of presentation

           1. No issues at birth, followed by recurrent croup.

           2. Stridor at birth.

           3. Failure to extubate.

        c. Types

           1. Membranous

           2. Cartilaginous

      ii. Acquired
         a. Due to trauma such as prolonged intubation.
         b. Exacerbated by GERD, eosinophilic esophagitis and infection.
         c. Congenital stenosis may predispose to acquired stenosis.
  B. Diagnosis
      i. Rigid laryngoscopy and bronchoscopy.
      ii. Sizing of airway to assess degree of stenosis (Cotton-Myer grading system).
         a. Grade 1: 0%-50% stenosis.
         b. Grade 2: 51%-70% stenosis.
         c. Grade 3: 71%-99% stenosis.
         d. Grade 4: 100% stenosis.
      iii. Rule out concomitant GERD, EE, MRSA that portend poorer outcomes.
         a. Management
      iv. Treat GERD, EE MRSA where present.
      v. Staging of procedures
         a. Single stage: patient does not have tracheotomy at end of procedure.
         b. Double stage: patient has tracheotomy removed at later date.
      vi. Endoscopic (scar division, balloon dilatation, steroid injection).
      vii. Open laryngotracheal reconstruction (LTR)
         a. Anterior cricoid split with thyroid ala or costal cartilage graft
         b. Posterior cricoid split with costal cartilage graft
         c. Anterior and posterior cricoid splits with costal cartilage grafts
         d. Cricotracheal reconstruction (CTR)
         e. Cervical slide tracheoplasty

Subglottic Cyst

  A. Acquired from intubation injury.
  B. Due to blocked mucous gland.
  C. Treatment
      i. Suspension microlaryngoscopy with excision/marsupialization of cyst.
      ii. Inhaled steroid and antibiotic to facilitate healing of denuded cartilage.

Subglottic Hemangioma

  A. Most common neoplasm of pediatric airway.
  B. Arise from hematopoietic progenitor cells from placenta or stem cells followed by genetic alterations and cytokine expression (ie, MMP-9, VEGF, b-FGF, TGF-beta).
  C. Twice as common in females.
  D. Clinical features
      i. Biphasic stridor at 6 weeks of age (85% present by 6 months of age).
      ii. Progressive symptoms as lesion grows in proliferative phase.
      iii. Plateau at 1 year of age.
      iv. Spontaneous involution by 18 months to 2 years of age.
      v. 60% of hemangiomata in "beard" distribution also have subglottic lesion.
  E. Diagnosis
      i. High kV AP neck x-ray shows unilateral subglottic mass (usually left side).
      ii. Rigid bronchoscopy
         a. Do not intubate prior to visualizing or lesion may become compressed and go unnoticed.
         b. Vascular blush on vocal cord.
         c. Rounded vascular lesion in subglottis (usually left side).
         d. Biopsy not required.

       iii. Rule out PHACES syndrome: **P**osterior fossa malformations, **H**emangioma typically involving the face, **A**rterial lesions of the head and neck, **C**ardiac abnormalities (coarctation of the aorta), **E**ye abnormalities and **S**ternal cleft or **S**upraumbilical hernia

  F. Management
     i. Minimal manipulation and awaken patient.
     ii. Secure airway via intubation only if essential.
     iii. Propranolol or Nadolol.
     iv. Intravenous or injectable steroids may be required.
     v. Historically, CO_2 laser, open surgical excision and alpha interferon were options but these are reserved for patients who fail medical management.

Granular Cell Tumor

  A. Benign tumor resembling hemangioma.
  B. Rare in children.
  C. Up to 10% found in larynx.
  D. Clinical features
     i. Hoarseness, cough, stridor, hemoptysis, dysphagia, pain.
  E. Diagnosis
     i. High kV AP neck x-ray.
     ii. Rigid bronchoscopy reveals yellow to gray-pink, firm, nonulcerated lesion.
     iii. Histology demonstrates large fusiform or polygonal cells with abundant pale cytoplasm and marked cell membrane. Eosinophilic granules in cytoplasm may induce pseudoepitheliomatous hyperplasia which can be confused with squamous cell carcinoma.
  F. Management
     i. Surgical excision with ample margins to prevent recurrence.

Neurofibroma

  A. Benign tumor of Schwann cell with low malignant potential.
  B. Located on arytenoid cartilages or aryepiglottic folds.
  C. May be associated with neurofibromatosis (see above).
  D. Management involves suspension microlaryngoscopy with surgical excision.

Malignant Laryngeal Tumors

  A. Rare in children.
  B. Clinical features:
     i. Differential diagnosis
       a. Embryonal variant of rhabdomyosarcoma (most common)
       b. Squamous cell carcinoma
       c. Choriocarcinoma
       d. Primitive neuroectodermal tumor (PNET)
       e. NUT midline carcinoma
     ii. Progressive airway obstruction, dysphonia, dysphagia
  C. Management:
     i. Flexible nasopharyngoscopy.
     ii. Rigid laryngoscopy and bronchoscopy with biopsy.
     iii. Consider tracheotomy based on current and predicted airway obstruction.
     iv. CT and MRI with metastatic workup.
     v. Chemotherapy, radiation, surgery dependent on nature of malignancy.

Infectious/Inflammatory

  A. Laryngotracheobronchitis (croup)

      i. Clinical features

         a. Viral infection, most commonly parainfluenza.

         b. Bacterial superinfection (*H influenzae* or *S aureus*) may follow.

         c. More common in children under 2 years of age.

         d. Present with barky cough and biphasic stridor.

         e. Variable degree of airway compromise.

         f. Recurrent croup (3 or more episodes) is unusual, suspect underlying subglottic stenosis.

      ii. Diagnosis

         a. High kV neck x-ray

            1. AP rather than PA, as it is easier to restrain child in this orientation and the patient is closer to the film so there is less magnification.

            2. Ensure arms are down at side (unlike chest x-ray).

            3. "Steeple sign" in subglottis.

            4. Lateral x-ray may show narrowing.

         b. Flexible nasopharyngoscopy may help rule out other etiologies.

         c. No indication for routine rigid laryngoscopy or bronchoscopy.

      iii. Treatment

         a. Humidification, hydration, oxygen.

         b. Nebulized epinephrine.

         c. Consider nebulized steroids.

         d. Oral or intravenous steroids.

         e. Recurrent croup warrants repeat high kV neck x-ray when infection resolves (minimum 6 weeks following infection) to rule out underlying subglottic pathology. Consider rigid laryngoscopy and bronchoscopy if x-ray does not resolve this question.

  B. Epiglottitis

      i. Clinical features

         a. Usually caused by *H influenzae* type B (Hib).

         b. Incidence has fallen dramatically after introduction of Hib vaccine.

         c. Must consider immunization status, other bacteria, leukemia, caustic injury.

         d. Rapid onset sore throat, fever, inspiratory stridor, respiratory distress, drooling, "tripod position" (hands on knees) due to inability to swallow secretions.

         e. After diagnosis confirmed, avoid irritating child.

      ii. Diagnosis

         a. High kV lateral neck x-ray shows "thumb sign" (widened epiglottis). Child should be accompanied in radiology suite by physician skilled at intubating.

      iii. Management

         a. Intubation in the operating room with tracheotomy tray prepared.

         b. Administer inhalational anesthetic.

         c. Blood and airway cultures can be obtained following intubation.

  C. Recurrent respiratory papillomatosis (RRP)

      i. Clinical features

         a. Most common benign neoplasm of the larynx in children.

         b. Second most common cause of hoarseness in children (nodules are first).

         c. Incidence 4/100,000 in United States, 0.24/100,000 in Canada.

         d. Usually diagnosed between 2 and 5 years of age.

         e. May involve any transition from squamous to columnar epithelium such as mucosal abrasion, tracheotomy site, etc.

1. Larynx (most common)
2. Oral cavity
3. Trachea
4. Bronchi

ii. Classification
   a. Juvenile (< 12 years of age)
      1. More aggressive.
      2. Due to vertical transmission or sexual abuse.
      3. Human papillomavirus (HPV) 6 and 11 most common (same as genital condylomata), 16 and 18 less common but higher risk malignant transformation (2%-3%).
   b. Adult (20-40 years of age)
      1. Less aggressive.
      2. Sexually acquired.
      3. Extralaryngeal involvement in 16% of patients.

iii. Diagnosis
   a. Flexible nasopharyngoscopy shows exophytic protruberances on vocal fold with multiple pinpoint dimples.
   b. Rigid laryngoscopy with biopsy confirms diagnosis.
   c. Histopathology shows pedunculated, finger-like projections with fibrovascular core, covered by stratified squamous epithelium).
   d. PCR confirms viral subtype.
   e. Chest CT if pulmonary involvement.

iv. Management
   a. Goals of treatment
      1. Maintain patent airway.
      2. Preserve lamina propria to preserve voice.
      3. Prevent injury to trachea to decrease risk of extralaryngeal spread.
   b. Multiple treatments required per year, decreases in frequency as child ages.
   c. Microdebrider or laser (CO_2 and KTP) most commonly used.
   d. Indications for adjuvant therapy
      1. More than six procedures per year
      2. Distal spread
      3. Rapid recurrence
   e. Adjuvant therapies
      1. Intralesional cidofovir
      2. Interferon-alpha
      3. Photodynamic therapy
      4. Indole-3-carbinol
   f. Annual biopsies to rule out malignant transformation.
   g. Quadrivalent vaccine for prevention of HPV types 6,11,16, and 18 has promise for decreasing the incidence of RRP. Vaccine therapy for those already affected with HPV is under study.

Iatrogenic
A. Intubation injury
   i. Acute
      a. Edema, granulation tissue, ulceration, soft scar, arytenoid dislocation.
   ii. Chronic
      a. Granulation tissue, ulceration, fibrotic scar, arytenoid fixation.

Idiopathic

A. Paradoxical vocal fold movement
   i. Clinical features
      a. Vocal cord adduction on inspiration, abduction on expiration.
      b. More common in females with social stressors (ie, athletes).
      c. Inspiratory stridor and strained voice.
      d. Associated with laryngopharyngeal reflux.
      e. Often misdiagnosed as asthma.
   ii. Diagnosis
      a. Flexible nasopharyngoscopy reveals abnormal vocal cord movement while awake and normal movement while asleep.
      b. May need to perform nasopharyngoscopy while patient on treadmill to notice episode.
   iii. Management
      a. Reassurance
      b. Panting exercises (leads to vocal cord relaxation).
      c. Topical lidocaine may have minor benefit.
      d. Proton pump inhibitor.
      e. Voice therapy, massage and biofeedback.
      f. Counselling by professional with experience treating conversion disorders.
      g. Severe respiratory distress may warrant helium-oxygen therapy (heliox) to reduce airway turbulence, botox, or anticholinergic agents such as inhaled ipratropium.
      h. Counsel family that the patient may pass out, but this will allow them to breathe again.

Tracheobronchial Tree

Developmental Anatomy

A. Prenatal development
   i. Lung bud grows at distal end of laryngotracheal tube.
   ii. Divides into two bronchial buds which form primitive primary bronchi, lower airway, and lung parenchyma.
   iii. 5 weeks' gestation:
      a. Esophagotracheal septum regresses leading to separation of laryngotracheal tube and esophagus.
      b. Incomplete separation results in tracheoesophageal fistula.
   iv. 8 weeks' gestation:
      a. Tracheal cilia appear.
   v. 20 weeks' gestation:
      a. All major microscopic features of trachea are visible.
   vi. 24 weeks' gestation:
      a. Surfactant secretion begins. Sufficient quantity to prevent lung collapse by 28 to 32 weeks'.
B. Postnatal development
   i. Trachea lengthens and descends deeper into mediastinum.
   ii. Trachea grows from 4 cm at birth to 12 cm in adult.
   iii. Trachea becomes more firm.
   iv. Division of bronchioles and alveoli continues for at least 8 years.

Signs and Symptoms
   A. Dyspnea
   B. Cough
   C. Aspiration, recurrent pneumonia
   D. Failure to thrive

Clinical Assessment
   A. Auscultation.
   B. Chest x-ray (AP and lateral).
   C. Fluoroscopy.
   D. CT.
   E. Rigid laryngoscopy and bronchoscopy (gold standard).
   F. Some advocate flexible bronchoscopy in the awake patient in clinic but this is still under investigation.

Pathology/Treatment/Complications
Congenital
   A. Tracheomalacia (intrinsic tracheal narrowing)
      i. Clinical features
         a. Trachealis muscle moves anteriorly to narrow tracheal lumen.
         b. Barking or honking stridor on forceful expiration.
         c. Not usually associated with respiratory distress.
      ii. Diagnosis
         a. Rigid bronchoscopy with spontaneous ventilation without positive pressure.
         b. Rule out extrinsic pulsatile vascular compression (vascular ring or sling).
         c. May be detected on sagittal fluoroscopy.
      iii. Management
         a. Reassurance and observation usually sufficient.
         b. Continuous positive pressure ventilation.
         c. Aortopexy to pull trachea anteriorly to decrease degree of trachealis obstruction being investigated.
         d. Suturing of trachealis muscle to prevertebral fascia being investigated.
         e. Tracheotomy as last resort, as pressure makes trachealis muscle weaker.
   B. External compression of trachea (extrinsic tracheal narrowing)
      i. Clinical features
         a. Compression of trachea (mostly anterior) narrows lumen.
         b. Stridor, respiratory distress, cyanosis, recurrent or chronic lung infections.
      ii. Diagnosis
         a. Rigid bronchoscopy with spontaneous ventilation without positive pressure.
         b. Pulsatile vascular compression of trachea.
         c. Tracheal cross section shaped like sideways "teardrop" usually with narrow point on patient's left side.
         d. CT chest with contrast and three-dimensional reconstruction of trachea and vasculature to confirm responsible vessel.
      iii. Management
         a. Continuous positive pressure ventilation with slow wean.
         b. Aortopexy or division of vascular ring as required.
         c. Shortening of trachea (using slide tracheoplasty or resection) to alter relationship of trachea and offending vessel.
         d. Tracheotomy last resort due to risk of tracheotomy tip eroding into vessel.
         e. Metallic stents only in palliative cases due to high risk of erosion into vessel.

C. Tracheoesophageal fistula (TEF or TOF)
  i. Clinical features
     a. Communication between trachea and esophagus.
     b. Incidence 1/2500 live births.
     c. More common in males.
     d. Due to incomplete separation of foregut at 4 to 5 weeks' gestation.
     e. Defective signalling in Sonic Hedgehog pathway in mice.
     f. Associated with polyhydramnios in utero.
     g. Associated with VACTERL syndrome: **V**ertebral, **A**nal atresia, **C**ardiac, **T**racheoesophageal fistula, **E**sophageal atresia, **R**adial or renal atresia, **L**imb anomalies.
     h. Coughing with feeds, cyanotic episodes, dysphagia, regurgitation, recurrent pneumonia.
  ii. Diagnosis
     a. Majority are proximal esophageal atresia with distal TEF.
        1. X-ray shows anterior bowing of trachea from distended esophageal pouch.
        2. Feeding tube passed through nose down esophageal atresia with injection of air into pouch. If esophageal atresia is present along with air in stomach, then a fistula exists.
     b. "Pullback" esophagram for H-type fistula or recurrent TEF.
        1. Nasogastric tube inserted into esophagus and pulled backward up esophagus as contrast is injected under force during fluoroscopy.
        2. Air bronchogram (white outline of tracheobronchial tree) indicates presence of fistula.
     c. Rigid bronchoscopy
        1. Primary fistulae easily detected. Rule out secondary fistula.
        2. Secondary fistulae more difficult to detect.
           • May require insertion of nasogastric tube into distal esophagus with forceful injection of large volume of air while looking for bubbles in trachea.
           • Fogarty catheter inserted to distal esophagus, followed by inflation of balloon and slow withdrawal while investigating posterior tracheal wall is an alternative.
     d. Four main types of TEF
        1. Proximal esophageal atresia with distal TEF (90%)
        2. H-type fistula (2%-4% of primary TEF, 100% of secondary TEF)
        3. Proximal TEF with distal esophageal atresia (1%)
        4. Proximal esophageal atresia with TEF and distal esophageal atresia with second TEF (1%)
  iii. Management
     a. Thoracoscopic or open surgery
        1. TEF closed at same time as esophageal atresia repair.
        2. Recurrence rate 20%. Minimized by:
           • Less extensive mobilization of esophagus
           • Absorbable sutures
           • Complete division of tract rather than ligation
           • Noncontiguous tracheal and esophageal suture lines
           • Minimal tension on anastomosis
           • Interposing tissue between layers
           • Minimal postoperative trauma

    b. Endoscopic
      1. Reserved for recurrent fistulae following open approach (20%).
      2. De-epithelialization of tract using electrical or chemical cautery with or without addition of fibrin glue.
      3. Success rates vary from 60% to 90% with average of two attempts required.
      4. Clip placed in esophagus may facilitate closure of recalcitrant TEF.
    c. Slide tracheoplasty or tracheal resection
      1. For recalcitrant TEF unable to be closed by any other method.
      2. Obliteration of TEF by shortening trachea to separate tracheal and esophageal suture lines.

D. Complete tracheal rings
  i. Clinical features
    a. Due to unequal partitioning of foregut into trachea and esophagus.
    b. Associated with congenital heart disease, lung agenesis, duodenal atresia, and Down syndrome.
  ii. Diagnosis
    a. Flexible or rigid bronchoscopy.
      1. Location: helpful to place scope at proximal end of stenosis, turn off room lights and visualize whether light is superior or inferior to clavicles. This determines whether needs to be repaired via cervical or thoracic approach.
      2. Length.
      3. Degree of narrowing.
    b. CT with contrast and 3D reconstruction of trachea and vasculature helps to delineate extent of stenosis and associated cardiac anomalies.
    c. Cardiac echocardiogram for concurrent cardiac anomalies.
  iii. Management
    a. Depends on degree of airway compromise.
    b. Observation as patient outgrows stenosis. Often require medical management for symptomatic episodes.
    c. Medical
      1. Often required for symptomatic episodes during observation period.
      2. Steroids.
      3. Inhaled epinephrine.
      4. Heliox.
      5. Bag/mask ventilation.
      6. Laryngeal mask airway. Works well for elective surgery.
      7. Intubation as last resort. Should be performed by most experienced person with placement of endotracheal tube just below vocal cords. Forcing tube distally leads to edema and loss of airway.
    d. Extra-Corporeal Membrane Oxygenation (ECMO).
      1. May be required for acute airway obstruction as bridge to surgery.
    e. Slide tracheoplasty
      1. Reserved for severely symptomatic patients in first few months of life or patients with poor exercise tolerance around age 5 years.
      2. Performed simultaneously with cardiac repair if required.
      3. Patient usually placed on cardiac bypass or ECMO.
      4. Multiple flexible bronchoscopies for bronchopulmonary lavage required following surgery.
      5. Often requires several balloon dilatations until trachea relaxes.

E. Sleeve trachea
  i. Clinical features
     a. Continuous smooth span of cartilage without tracheal rings or intercartilaginous ligaments.
     b. Associated with Pfeiffer syndrome: autosomal dominant craniosynostosis, midface hypoplasia, proptosis, syndactyly caused by mutations in chromosome 8 or FGFR2 gene.

Infectious/Inflammatory

A. Allergic bronchopulmonary aspergillosis
  i. Clinical features
     a. Wheezing, mucous production, pulmonary infiltrates, elevated IgE.
     b. Associated with reactive airway disease or cystic fibrosis.
     c. May be unilateral, therefore confused with foreign body aspiration.
  ii. Diagnosis
     a. Based on retrieval of cast from bronchial tree.
  iii. Treatment
     a. Removal of airway casts.
     b. Systemic treatment of atopy.
B. Tuberculosis (TB)
  i. Granulomas may be seen in tracheobronchial tree.
  ii. Diagnosis based on biopsy of lesion.
  iii. Treatment as per systemic tuberculosis.

Foreign Body Aspiration

A. Clinical features
  i. 1000 deaths per year in the United States.
  ii. Most common cause of accidental death in children less than 1 year of age.
  iii. 25% of airway foreign bodies have been present for over 2 weeks.
  iv. Ingestion may be observed or unobserved. Any suspected foreign body aspiration must be thoroughly investigated.
  v. Initial episode usually involves coughing, gagging or sputtering, that usually resolves as foreign body moves past vocal cords.
  vi. Chronic cough, lung infection or bronchiectasis if present for long time.
  vii. Symptoms related to level and degree of obstruction.
     a. Larynx: change in voice, cough, odynophagia, airway obstruction
     b. Trachea: palpable thud, expiratory wheeze
     c. Bronchus: cough, unilateral wheeze
  viii. Location in decreasing order:
     a. Right main bronchus (60%)
     b. Left main bronchus (30%)
     c. Hypopharynx (2%-5%)
     d. Trachea (3%-12%)
     e. Larynx (1%-7%)
B. Diagnosis
  i. History alone may prompt bronchoscopy even if no foreign body on x-ray.
  ii. Physical findings as above.
  iii. X-ray:
     a. AP and lateral
        1. Radiopaque lesion seen <25% of time.
        2. Mediastinal shift away from foreign body.

3. Elevated contralateral hemidiaphragm.
4. Postobstructive collapse if present for long time.
5. Pneumomediastinum.
6. Pneumothorax.
   b. Inspiratory and expiratory films in lateral decubitus.
   1. Dependent lung should collapse but looks hyperinflated if foreign body blocking bronchus.
   2. Only in 50% of patients with foreign body (specific but not sensitive).
   iv. CT scan:
   a. Some advocate CT for visualizing airway foreign bodies.
   b. More sensitive than x-ray, less sensitive than bronchoscopy.
   c. Risk of sending patient with airway foreign body to CT scanner.
   d. May require anaesthetic for CT and another for bronchoscopy.
   e. Suggest using only following negative bronchoscopy where symptoms persist, to look for object in subsegmental bronchi and help plan next bronchoscopy.
   v. Bronchoscopy:
   a. Gold standard for diagnosis.
   C. Management
   i. Rigid laryngoscopy and bronchoscopy with spontaneous ventilation.
   ii. Sharp edges are retrieved into bronchoscope to minimize trauma.
   iii. Rarely, tracheotomy is required for removal of large foreign bodies.

Esophagus

Developmental Anatomy
A. Prenatal development (see laryngeal development)
   i. Upper esophagus and upper esophageal sphincter.
   a. fourth, fifth, and sixth branchial arches give rise to striated muscle.
   b. Innervated by vagal nerve and recurrent laryngeal nerve.
   ii. Middle esophagus
   a. Somites and endoderm give rise to smooth and skeletal muscle.
   iii. Lower esophagus and lower esophageal sphincter.
   a. Mesenchyme of somites surrounding foregut.
   iv. 6 weeks' gestation
   a. Circular muscle and ganglion cells of myenteric plexus form.
   v. 7 weeks' gestation
   a. Blood vessels enter submucosa.
   vi. 9 to 13 weeks' gestation
   a. Myenteric plexus has cholinesterase activity and ganglion cells differentiate.
   b. Peristalsis begins in first trimester.
   vii. 16 weeks' gestation
   a. Ciliated epithelium replaced by stratified squamous epithelium.
   b. Residual islands of ciliated epithelium give rise to esophageal glands.
B. Postnatal development
   i. Peristalsis matures and regurgitation decreases.
   ii. Pressure at lower esophageal sphincter reaches maturity at 3 to 6 weeks of age.

Signs and Symptoms
A. Feeding difficulties.
B. Aspiration.
C. Regurgitation.
D. Foreign bodies in the esophagus may present as stridor and respiratory distress.

Clinical Assessment
  A. X-ray to look for air in esophagus and bowel.
  B. Passage of nasogastric tube can demonstrate patency.
  C. Gastrograffin or barium swallow:
      i. Stricture
      ii. Filling defect denotes foreign body
      iii. Tracheoesophageal stricture

Pathology/Treatment/Complications
Congenital
  A. Tracheoesophageal fistula (see above)
  B. Esophageal stenosis
      i. Usually in distal one-third.
      ii. Can occur anywhere along length of esophagus.
  C. Achalasia: rare in children
      i. Clinical features
          a. Decreased ganglion cells in enteric nervous system within smooth muscle.
          b. Chronic aspiration and chronic pulmonary disease.
          c. Failure to thrive.
      ii. Diagnosis
          a. Chest x-ray: widened mediastinum
          b. Barium swallow
              1. "Bird-beak" deformity: dilated proximal esophagus and tapering of distal esophagus.
          c. Manometry
              1. Increased tone in lower esophageal sphincter (LES)
              2. Failure of LES to relax on swallow
              3. Absence of peristalsis
      iii. Treatment
          a. Medical management to improve peristalsis and decrease LES tone
          b. Dilatation
          c. Myotomy for nonresponders

Neoplastic
Neoplastic lesions are rare in children.

Infectious/Inflammatory
  A. Eosinophilic esophagitis (EE)
      i. Clinical features
          a. Chronic inflammation of esophagus due to infiltration of eosinophils.
          b. Due to food or environmental allergies. May be post infectious.
          c. Other risk factors
              1. Male
              2. Allergies (food or seasonal), asthma
              3. Family history of EE
              4. Living in cold, dry climate
          d. Symptoms include
              1. Gastroesophageal reflux disease unreponsive to proton pump inhibitors.
              2. Vomiting (61%).
              3. Dysphagia (39%). More common if endoscopic findings or eosinophils in blood.
              4. Abdominal pain (34%).

5. Feeding disorders (14%).

6. Heartburn (14%).

7. Food impaction (7%).

8. Vague chest pain (5%).

9. Diarrhea (5%).

10. Failure to thrive.

  ii. Diagnosis

    a. Esophagoscopy may or may not raise suspicion, therefore biopsy required.

      1. Majority of children have no findings on esophagoscopy.

      2. White exudate.

      3. Esophageal rings ("trachealization" or corrugation).

      4. Linear furrows.

      5. Pallor.

      6. Congestion.

      7. Loss of vascularization.

    b. Biopsy

      1. Multiple biopsies required from proximal, mid and distal esophagus.

      2. Persistent esophageal eosinophilia > 15 eosinophils per high power field after 2 months of proton pump inhibitor therapy or with normal pH study.

      3. Degranulated eosinophils.

      4. Eosinophilic microabscesses (clusters of 4 or more eosinophils).

      5. Eosinophils in superficial layers of squamous mucosa.

      6. Patchy or diffuse distribution of eosinophils through entire length of esophageal squamous mucosa.

      7. Lamina propria fibrosis.

  iii. Management

    a. Referral to gastroenterologist and allergist.

    b. Elimination and elemental diets to decrease allergen exposure. Must be supervised by dietician due to risk of nutritional deprivation.

    c. Proton pump inhibitor +/− promotility agents for acid reflux.

      1. 1/3 have good response to proton pump inhibitor alone.

    d. Swallowed topical glucocorticoid.

      1. Decreases esophageal inflammation.

      2. Fluticasone via metered dose inhaler without spacer is sprayed into mouth and swallowed.

      3. Patients should not inhale or eat or drink for 30 minutes after.

      4. Dose in children ranges from 88 to 440 µg/day in divided doses.

      5. Responders do so within 1 week. Treatment continued for 8 weeks.

      6. Relapse rates 14% to 91% when stopped.

      7. Nonresponders should try oral viscous budesonide.

    e. Careful esophageal dilatation for strictures not responsive to medical management as may lead to perforation.

B. Juvenile dermatomyositis

  i. Clinical features

    a. Systemic autoimmune inflammatory muscle disorder and vasculopathy.

    b. Expanded diagnostic criteria (2006 international consensus survey).

      1. Heliotrope rash over eyelids, Gottron papules over metacarpophalangeal joints and proximal interphalangeal joints.

2. Calcinosis cutis (firm lump in skin).
3. Symmetrical proximal muscle weakness.
4. Elevated muscle enzymes.
5. Myopathic changes on electromyopathy.
6. Abnormal muscle biopsy findings.
7. Muscle MRI and US abnormalities.
8. Nailfold capillaroscopy abnormalities.
   - Dysphonia
   c. Vasculopathy may affect gastrointestinal tract
C. Stevens-Johnson syndrome
   i. Life-threatening skin condition whereby cell death leads to separation of epidermis from dermis.
   ii. Hypersensitivity complex reaction due to medications, infections, and cancer.

Traumatic

A. Foreign body ingestion
   i. Clinical features
      a. Dysphagia
      b. Drooling
      c. History of choking episode.
      d. May cause compression of trachea and airway obstruction.
      e. Diagnosis may be delayed.
   ii. Diagnosis
      a. X-ray
         1. AP and lateral x-rays from mouth to anus.
         2. Must rule out button battery.
            - Halo sign (visible double density ring on AP film).
            - Step sign (visible step on lateral film).
            - Batteries must be removed as soon as possible.
         3. Must rule out two or more magnets.
            - One magnet will not cause problems but two will.
            - Stick to each other through bowel wall leading to perforation.
      b. Contrast esophagram
         1. May help rule out radiolucent foreign body.
         2. Coating marshmallow in barium may detect nonobstructive object like fishbone that may be missed with liquid contrast.
   iii. Treatment
      a. Rigid esophagoscopy and removal using optical forceps.
      b. Esophageal button batteries require emergent removal due to risk of liquefaction necrosis, perforation and stricture. Batteries that have passed into the stomach can be followed radiographically until they pass the rectum.
      c. Nasogastric tube to prevent stricture if severe circumferential injury.
      d. Sucralfate may be beneficial for severe circumferential injury. Binds to exposed proteins for protection, inhibits pepsin, and binds bile salts.
      e. Two or more magnets require emergent removal. May leave one magnet behind as long as there are no other magnets to be attracted to.
      f. Coins most commonly lodge at thoracic inlet.
B. Caustic ingestion
   i. Clinical features
      a. Accidental ingestion most common in first 3 years of life.

      b. Degree of injury related to type of corrosive, amount, concentration, duration of contact.

      c. Types of corrosives

        1. Alkali (NaOH, KOH, NH$_4$OH)
- Found in drain cleaners and button batteries.
- Cause liquefaction necrosis that diffuses into deep tissue layers.

        2. Acids (HCl, H$_2$SO$_4$, HNO$_3$)
- Cause coagulation necrosis where degree of injury is more superficial.

        3. Phenol (ie, Lysol)

        4. Hypochlorous acid (HClO)
- Found in bleach.
- Forms hydrochloric acid when oxygen is released.

ii. Assessment

    a. Determine substance ingested.

    b. Intraoral signs do not correlate with esophageal exposure.

    c. Assess entire patient to rule out airway involvement and perforated viscus.

iii. Management

    a. Observation if few symptoms and benign physical examination.

    b. Clear liquid diet during observation with intravenous hydration if necessary.

    c. Steroids

      1. May minimize injury in first 8 hours.

      2. Do not give steroids if severe esophageal injury noted at time of endoscopy due to risk of perforation.

    d. Antibiotics may hasten re-epithelialization.

    e. Esophagoscopy

      1. If indicated, should be performed 24 to 72 hours after incident to delineate areas of injury. Earlier endoscopy may underestimate degree of injury.

      2. Endoscope should not be advanced beyond area of significant injury to minimize risk of esophageal rupture.

    f. Nasogastric tube passed under direct vision if severe esophageal injury.

    g. Gastrostomy tube may be required.

    h. Esophageal stricture may require dilatation or resection.

Idiopathic

A. Gastroesophageal reflux disease (GERD)

  i. Clinical features

    a. Regurgitation of stomach contents into esophagus.

    b. Very common in infants.

    c. Symptoms and signs

      1. Arching of back and discomfort

      2. Cough

      3. Hoarseness

      4. Laryngospasm

      5. Bronchospasm

      6. Apneic episodes

  ii. Diagnosis

    a. Flexible nasopharyngoscopy

      1. Redundant, erythematous tissue over arytenoid cartilages.

      2. Pooling of frothy clear secretions at esophageal inlet.

      3. Vocal cord nodules or granulomata.

      4. "Cobblestoning" of posterior pharyngeal wall (lymphatic hypertrophy).

b. Barium swallow
   1. May show reflux of contrast or hiatus hernia.
c. Impedance probe
   1. Detects frequency and level of acid and nonacid reflux up the esophagus.
d. pH probe
   1. Detects frequency of acid reflux up the esophagus.
e. Upper GI endoscopy
   1. Allows inspection of mucosa, lower esophageal sphincter and biopsies.

iii. Treatment
   a. Physical measures
      1. Elevate head of bed by placing wedge under mattress or book under bed frame. Extra pillows merely kink the neck and do not improve reflux.
      2. Allow ample time for digestion prior to going to bed.
      3. Eliminate acidic foods and caffeine (ie, spices, tomatoes, chocolate, caffeinated drinks).
      4. Thicken feeds.
      5. Small frequent feeds.
   b. Pharmacological
      1. Acid suppression
         • Antacids
         • H$_2$ blockers
         • Proton pump inhibitors: must be given on empty stomach 1 hour before meal or else do not work. Supplement with vitamin D drops to prevent decreased calcium absorption from long-term PPI use.
      2. Prokinetic agents
         • Domperidone
         • Metoclopramide
         • Cisapride: For patients with unusual, debilitating problems for whom there is no alternative therapy in the United States due to risk of cardiac arrhythmia.
   c. Surgical
      1. Nissen fundoplication: complete or partial wrap.
      2. Feeding gastrojejunostomy (GJ) tube: poorer quality of life for patient and caregiver due to need for continuous feeds and frequent loose stools.

Head and Neck

Developmental Anatomy

A. Prenatal development
   i. Embryology in first 8 weeks' determines pathway an anomaly will follow.
   ii. Six branchial arches. External clefts lined with ectoderm, internal pouches lined with endoderm. The fifth branchial arch degenerates.
   iii. Each arch has a nerve, artery, cartilaginous bar, muscle.
      a. First arch: trigeminal nerve; malleus head/neck, anterior malleolar ligament, incus body/short process, mandible, sphenomandibular ligament; tensory tympani, tensor veli palatini, muscles of mastication, digastric anterior belly, mylohoid.
      b. Second arch: facial nerve; external carotid artery; malleus manubrium, incus long process, stapes (not vestibular side of footplate), pyramidal eminence,

styloid process, hyoid lesser cornu and upper half body; stapedius tendon, muscles of facial expression, digastric posterior belly, stylohyoid.
- c. Third arch: glossopharyngeal nerve; internal and common carotid arteries; hyoid greater cornu and lower half body; stylopharyngeus.
- d. Fourth arch: superior laryngeal nerve; right subclavian artery, aortic arch; thyroid cartilage, cuneiform cartilage; cricothyroid membrane, inferior pharyngeal constrictors.
- e. Sixth arch: recurrent laryngeal nerve; right pulmonary artery, ductus arteriosus; cricoid, arytenoid, corniculate; intrinsic laryngeal muscles (except cricothyroid).
- iv. Cysts, sinuses and fistulae course deep to derivatives of their own branchial arch and superficial to derivatives of the next branchial arch. The origin of third and fourth branchial anomalies is controversial.
- v. Types of anomalies
  - a. Cyst (lined by mucosa or epithelium, no external opening, arises from embryonic rests trapped inside developing tissue).
  - b. Sinus (from incomplete closure of pouches and clefts, communicates with single body surface that may be either the skin or the pharynx).
  - c. Fistula (from incomplete closure of pouches and clefts, communicates with two body surfaces).
- B. Postnatal development
  - i. Majority of these structures continue to grow postnatally, with the exception of arytenoid cartilages that attain adult size at birth.

Signs and Symptoms
- A. Neck mass
- B. Compressive symptoms
- C. Fever, chills, night sweats, weight loss

Clinical Assessment
- A. Complete head and neck examination including cranial nerves.
- B. Flexible nasopharyngoscopy.
- C. Imaging usually necessary for determining type and extent of lesion.

Pathology/Treatment/Complications
Congenital
- A. Vascular anomalies (ISSVA classification 2014). Even though not all are congenital, the entire classification is delineated here for simplicity.
  - i. Vascular tumors
    - a. Benign
      - 1. Infantile hemangioma (IH)/hemangioma of infancy
        - • Clinical features
          - (a) Most common tumor of childhood (10% of Caucasians).
          - (b) More common in preterm infants.
          - (c) 3 times more common in females.
          - (d) Present at birth as flat discoloration with no mass.
          - (e) Three phases of growth:
            - ○ Proliferative phase begins around 4 weeks, rapid growth until 4 months, plateau around 1 year.
            - ○ Quiescent phase between proliferation and involution.
            - ○ Involution phase can last up to 10 years.
            - ○ May be associated with Kasabach-Merritt syndrome consumptive coagulopathy and systemic hemangiomata.

- Diagnosis
  - (a) Based on history and physical.
  - (b) MRI with gadolinium confirms diagnosis.
  - (c) Biopsy only if clinical picture unclear.
  - (d) Glut-1 positive on histopathology.
  - (e) Hemangioma in beard distribution more likely to also have subglottic hemangioma. Therefore stridor warrants rigid bronchoscopy.
- Treatment
  - (a) Observation for small lesions not at risk of causing functional or long-term cosmetic deformity.
  - (b) Beta blocker (propranolol or nadolol) if loss of function such as impaired vision, ulceration or bleeding.
  - (c) Short-term steroids may control growth.
  - (d) Pulsed dye laser for ulcerated lesions.
  - (e) Surgical excision for persistence following medical management. Try to resect after lesion has entered involution phase.
2. Congenital hemangioma (CH)
   - Clinical features
     - (a) Fully formed at birth. Three subtypes:
       - ○ RICH: rapidly involuting congenital hemangioma
       - ○ NICH: noninvoluting congenital hemangioma
       - ○ PICH: partially involuting congenital hemangioma
   - Diagnosis
     - (a) Glut-1 negative on histopathology.
   - Treatment
     - (a) RICH disappear within weeks to months, but may take longer. NICH should be observed to ensure they are not RICH and then may require surgical excision in absence of involution.
3. Tufted angioma
4. Spindle-cell hemangioma
5. Epithelioid hemangioma
6. Pyogenic granuloma (aka lobular capillary hemangioma)

b. Locally aggressive or borderline vascular tumors (not congenital but included here to maintain structure of ISSVA classification for completeness).
   1. Kaposiform hemangioendothelioma
   2. Retiform hemangioendothelioma
   3. Papillary intralymphatic angioendothelioma (PILA; Dabska tumor)
   4. Composite hemangioendothelioma
   5. Kaposi sarcoma

c. Malignant vascular tumors (for completeness)
   1. Angiosarcoma
   2. Epithelioid hemangioendothelioma

ii. Vascular malformations
   a. Simple
      1. Capillary malformations (CM)
         - Cutaneous or mucosal (aka "port-wine" stain)
         - Telangiectasia (ie, hereditary hemorrhagic telangiectasia)
         - Cutis marmorata telangiectatica (CMTC)
         - Nevus simplex/salmon patch/"angel kiss," "stork bite"

   2. Lymphatic malformations (LM)
- Common (cystic) LM
  - (a) Clinical features.
  - (b) Present at birth and grow in proportion to child.
  - (c) May enlarge with viral or bacterial infection.
  - (d) Classification:
    - Microcystic LM: usually above myelohyoid muscle
    - Macrocystic LM: usually below myelohyoid muscle
    - Mixed cystic LM
  - (e) Diagnosis
    - T2-MRI shows lesion well as bright anomaly, no radiation.
    - US or CT with contrast may also be used.
  - (f) Treatment
    - Antibiotics for acute infection.
    - Microcystic LM: surgical resection (often difficult due to infiltration into normal structures) or sclerotherapy.
    - Macrocystic LM: surgical resection or sclerotherapy.
- Generalized lymphatic anomaly (GLA)
- LM in Gorham-Stout disease
- Channel type LM
- Primary lymphedema

   3. Venous malformations (VM)
- Common VM
- Familial VM cutaneo-mucosal (VMCM)
- Blue rubber bleb nevus (Bean) syndrome VM
- Glomuvenous malformation (GVM)
- Cerebral cavernous malformation (CCM)

   4. Arteriovenous malformations (AVM)
- Clinical features
  - (a) Associated with palpable thrill, bruit, hypertrichosis, hyperthermia, hyperhydrosis.
  - (b) Subtypes:
    - Sporadic
    - In HHT
    - In CM-AVM
  - (c) Treatment
    - Embolization followed by surgical resection.

   5. Arteriovenous fistula
- Sporadic
- In HHT
- In CM-AVM

  b. Combined
  c. Of major named vessels
  d. Associated with other anomalies

B. Branchial cleft anomalies
  i. Clinical features
    a. Cysts are lined by mucosa or epithelium with no external opening. Present as mass that may become enlarged or infected (erythematous, warm, painful) with respiratory illness.

b. Sinuses communicate with a single body surface. Present as skin pit that discharges sticky exudate. May become infected.

c. Fistulae communicate with two body surfaces. Present as neck mass or recurrent thyroiditis (third branchial anomalies).

d. First branchial anomalies (5%-25%): Work divided these postoperatively based on histology and location, however, some use this classification preoperatively (with caution) to plan surgery.

    1. Work I (less common)
- Ectoderm-derived duplication of external auditory canal lined by squamous epithelium.
- Usually anteromedial to EAC but may be posterior to pinna.
- Course lateral to facial nerve. May course under annulus into middle ear and attach to umbo of malleus.

    2. Work II (more common)
- Ectoderm and mesoderm derived, lined by squamous epithelium and contain adnexae and cartilage.
- Open into external auditory canal or concha as fistula or cyst and also as fistula on face at angle of mandible.
- Pass superficial (57%), deep (30%) or between (13%) branches of facial nerve. Deep to facial nerve more common in females, young children, fistulae rather than sinuses, and tracts not opening into external auditory canal.

e. Second branchial anomalies (40%-95%)

    1. Present as neck mass along anterior border of sternocleidomastoid muscle.

    2. Unilateral fistula (more common on right side) may be seen along anterior border of sternocleidomastoid muscle midway between mandible and clavicle.

f. Pyriform fossa abnormalities (formerly known as third and fourth branchial anomalies) (2%-8%)

    1. Present as recurrent thyroiditis, thyroid abscess or fistula if previous incision and drainage. Most on left side of neck.

ii. Diagnosis

a. Work I anomalies: CT with contrast for relation to bony structures.

b. Work II anomalies: MRI with gadolinium to visualize parotid gland.

c. Second branchial cleft sinuses: no imaging required.

d. Second branchial cleft cysts: CT with contrast or MRI.

e. Pyriform fossa/third branchial anomalies: CT with contrast or MRI. Gas bubbles along tract are diagnostic. Confirmation of pyriform fossa fistula on laryngoscopy essential prior to surgery.

iii. Treatment

a. Antibiotics for acute infection. May require incision and drainage.

b. Surgical excision

    1. Work I anomalies: use nerve monitor. Begin with small preauricular incision and be prepared for full parotidectomy approach.

    2. Work II anomalies: use nerve monitor and begin with parotidectomy approach. Mastoid tip less developed in children thus facial nerve superficial.

    3. Second branchial cleft sinuses: place lacrimal probe in sinus, elliptical incision around sinus and dissection of tract.

    4. Second branchial cleft cysts: excise cyst and tract.

    5. Pyriform fossa/third branchial anomalies: Place probe into pyriform fossa on direct laryngoscopy, open neck, identify probe and resect tract, usually with hemithyroidectomy. Some advocate electrocautery of pyriform sinus tract alone, however, potential risk of injury to recurrent laryngeal nerve exists.

C. Thyroglossal duct cyst

  i. Clinical features

    a. Midline lesion anywhere from foramen cecum at base of tongue to pyramidal lobe of thyroid gland. Extensive branching of ductal system especially above hyoid bone.

    b. Usually presents as neck mass due to upper respiratory tract infection.

    c. Elevates with tongue protrusion.

    d. Most contain small rim of thyroid tissue.

    e. Rarely may contain the only functioning thyroid tissue or may develop into thyroid malignancy.

  ii. Diagnosis

    a. Ultrasound

      1. Ensures thyroid gland is in normal location (decreases chances that cyst is only functioning thyroid tissue).

      2. May distinguish thyroglossal duct cyst from dermoid cyst. Helps consent patient and plan extent and duration of surgery. Presence of septae, irregular wall and solid components are more indicative of thyroglossal duct cyst than dermoid cyst (SIST score).

    b. Nuclear imaging

      1. May be used when orthotopic thyroid is not evident to ensure thyroglossal duct cyst is not the only functioning thyroid tissue.

  iii. Treatment

    a. Antibotics +/− incision and drainage for acute infection.

    b. Surgical excision (Sistrunk)

      1. After resolution of infection.

      2. Recommend delineation of cyst, puncture with small needle to determine thyroglossal (mucus-filled) versus dermoid (keratin-filled) cyst. Thyroglossal warrants excision of all contents between strap muscles (not just following tract) down to and including pyramidal lobe of thyroid, plus resection of middle third of hyoid bone (Sistrunk procedure) with a cuff of tongue muscle to minimize chances of recurrence.

D. Dermoid cyst

  i. Clinical features

    a. Usually asymptomatic lesion in midline of the neck.

    b. May become acutely infected.

    c. Does not elevate with tongue protrusion.

  ii. Diagnosis

    a. See thyroglossal duct cyst.

  iii. Treatment

    a. Antibiotics for acute infection.

    b. Surgical excision (simple cystectomy)

      1. After resolution of infection.

      2. Delineation of cyst, puncture with needle. Dermoid cyst warrants simple cystectomy.

Neoplastic
A. Salivary gland tumors
    i. Clinical features
        a. Most common presentation is asymptomatic mass.
        b. Parotid neoplasms
            1. Benign (75%): Pleomorphic adenoma, hemangioma.
            2. Malignant (25%): Mucoepidermoid carcinoma, acinic cell carcinoma.
        c. Submandibular neoplasms
            1. Majority are benign (opposite to what is seen in adults).
    ii. Diagnosis
        a. US to delineate infection versus neoplasm.
        b. MRI for diagnosis and surgical planning.
    iii. Management
        a. Superficial versus deep lobe parotidectomy with negative margins.
        b. Serial surveillance MRI postoperatively to look for recurrence for malignant lesions.
B. Rhabdomyosarcoma
    i. Clinical features
        a. Most common soft tissue malignancy of childhood.
        b. Arises from mesenchymal tissue, may originate in nonstriated muscle.
        c. 40% present by 5 years of age, 70% by 12 years of age.
        d. Most common sites of origin (decreasing frequency):
            1. Orbit: best prognosis, rapid onset proptosis in children younger than 10 years.
            2. Nasopharynx: unilateral Eustachian tube dysfunction, nasal obstruction, rhinorrhea. Usually late diagnosis.
            3. Middle ear/mastoid: Unilateral otorrhea with aural polyp.
            4. Sinonasal: obstruction. Usually late diagnosis.
    ii. Diagnosis
        a. Prompt surgical biopsy.
        b. Intraoperative frozen section shows small round blue cell tumor.
        c. Pathological subtyping requires immunohistochemistry.
            1. Embryonal (includes botryoid and spindle)
                • Young children
                • Due to mutations in chromosome 11
            2. Pleomorphic
                • Older children and adults
            3. Alveolar and undifferentiated
                • Mostly outside head and neck
                • Poor prognosis
            4. Sclerosing
                • Very rare
                • Very poor prognosis
        d. Staging
            1. MRI or CT of primary site.
                • Whichever is best for primary is usually good enough for imaging lymphadenopathy. If MRI is used for the primary and the lymph nodes are not visualized well enough, CT may be added.
            2. CT chest

       3. Bone scan

       4. Bone marrow biopsy

  iii. Treatment

    a. Surgical excision if feasible with little to no mutilation.

    b. Chemotherapy (lasting approximately 1 year).

    c. Radiation (beginning at approximately week 12).

    d. Outcome

       1. Depends on site, clinical stage and pathological subtype.

       2. 5-year failure-free survival rate 81% for patients 1-9 years of age.

       3. Lower if outside this age range.

C. Lymphoma

  i. Hodgkin lymphoma

    a. Clinical features

       1. Malignancy of lymphoreticular system associated with Epstein-Barr virus.

       2. Adolescents and young adults, rarely children less than 5 years of age.

       3. More common in males.

       4. Presents as cervical and supraclavicular neck mass.

       5. Spleen is most common extranodal site (denotes disease progression).

    b. Diagnosis

       1. Lymph node excisional biopsy

         • Specimen must be sent fresh without formalin.

         • Send separate specimen for flow cytometry.

         • Avoid preoperative steroids because they degrade the specimen.

       2. Pathology

         • Diagnosis based on presence of Reed-Sternberg cells (multinucleated giant cells).

         • Two subtypes (WHO classification)

           (a) Classical Hodgkin lymphoma (CHL)

           (b) Nodular lymphocyte-predominant Hodgkin lymphoma (NLPHL)

    c. Staging

       1. CT chest, abdomen, pelvis.

       2. Whole body PET scan (detects metastases including bone lesions and gages response to therapy).

       3. Bone marrow and lumbar puncture only in select patients.

    d. Treatment

       1. Dependent on stage of disease at presentation.

       2. Surgery

         • For diagnosis and staging, not resection or cure.

       3. Chemotherapy

         • For all stages.

         • Stage determines number of courses of chemotherapy.

       4. Radiation

         • Need depends on initial stage plus initial response to chemotherapy (as determined by repeat CT PET).

    e. Outcome

       1. 90% have good initial response regardless of stage.

       2. Event free survival 85% to 90%. Overall survival 95%.

       3. Potential for significant late effects (cardiac, secondary malignancies, infertility).

ii. Non-Hodgkin lymphoma (NHL)
  a. Clinical features
    1. Comprises multiple pathological entities
      • B-cell such as Burkitt, Burkitt-like, and Burkitt leukemia.
      • Diffuse large B-cell, lymphoblastic, anaplastic large cell.
    2. Children age 2 to 12 years.
    3. Males more common.
    4. Immunosuppressed children more common.
    5. Presents as asymptomatic adenopathy.
    6. May involve Waldeyer ring
    7. Children more commonly present with advanced disease.
  b. Diagnosis
    1. Pathological diagnosis required.
    2. Each entity has own pathological appearance.
    3. Staged according to St. Jude/Murphy system
      • CT chest, abdomen, pelvis.
      • Bone marrow aspirate and biopsy.
      • Lumbar puncture.
  c. Treatment
    1. Most entities treated with aggressive chemotherapy.
    2. Limited role for radiation.
  d. Outcome
    1. Prognosis depends on stage at presentation.
    2. Patients with CNS or bone marrow involvement have worse outcomes.
    3. 70% to 95% survival depending on entity.
iii. Burkitt lymphoma (type of NHL)
  a. Clinical features
    1. A type of non-Hodgkin lymphoma.
    2. Associated with Epstein-Barr virus (EBV) infection.
    3. Almost exclusively seen in children.
    4. Males more commonly affected.
    5. Most rapidly proliferating human cancer.
    6. Endemic disease (associated with high malaria zones and EBV)
      • Affects maxilla, may affect mandible.
      • Present with loose dentition, facial distortion, proptosis, and trismus.
    7. North American disease
      • Most common presentation is abdominal mass.
      • 25% have head and neck involvement (asymptomatic adenopathy).
      • Nasopharyngeal and tonsillar involvement have been reported.
  b. Diagnosis
    1. Pathology
      • Diffuse proliferation of uniform, undifferentiated cells with small nuclei. Classically described as a "starry sky pattern" because of interspersed large macrophages.
    2. Staging—similar to NHL.
  c. Treatment
    1. Chemotherapy
    2. Surgical debulking for bowel obstruction
  d. Outcome

1. 90% have complete response to therapy initially.
2. Overall 2-year survival is 90% to 95%.
3. Children with CNS and marrow involvement do worse.

D. Histiocytosis
   i. Clinical features
      a. Three major classes:
         1. Langerhans cell histiocytosis (Histiocytosis X)
         2. Malignant histiocytosis syndrome (T-cell lymphoma)
         3. Non-Langerhans cell histiocytosis (hematophagocytic syndrome)
      b. Langerhans cell histiocytosis (Histiocytosis X)
         1. 3 overlapping states of clonal proliferation of Langerhans cells.
            • Eosinophilic granuloma
               (a) Localized, benign, monostotic. Excellent prognosis.
            • Hand-Schuller-Christian disease
               (b) Skull lesions, exophthalmos, diabetes insipidus. Chronic course.
            • Letterer-Siwe disease
               (c) Disseminated form, multiple organ involvement, presents by 3 years of age, rapidly progressive course.
         2. Incidence 1/200,000.
         3. May be genetic, oncologic or autoimmune.
         4. Mainly 5 to 10 years of age.
         5. Males more common.
   ii. Diagnosis
      a. Pathology
         1. Non neoplastic proliferation of Langerhans cells
         2. Birbeck granules (organelles within nuclear cytoplasm)
            • Skeletal survey or bone scan
            • Serum electrolytes
            • Urine specific gravity for diabetes insipidus
   iii. Treatment
      a. Debridement and curettage of focal lesions
      b. Adjuvant therapy for systemic involvement
      c. Radiation for nonresectable lesions

Infectious/Inflammatory
   A. Atypical mycobacteria
      i. Clinical
         a. Prolonged erythema over skin that eventually turns violaceous in color.
         b. May drain spontaneously.
         c. Not responsive to antibiotics that cover skin flora.
         d. Most commonly *Mycobacterium avium intracellulare* or *Mycobacterium scrofulaceum.*
      ii. Diagnosis
         a. Culture and sensitivity may be diagnostic.
         b. Avoid incision and drainage due to risk of persistent fistulous tract.
      iii. Treatment
         a. Treat empirically with clarithromycin.
         b. Surgery
            1. If fails to respond to clarithromycin.

2. Place incision 1 to 2 cm away from site of infection, elevate small skin flap and curette lesion and undersurface of skin. Continue clarithromycin postoperatively.

B. Cat scratch
   i. Clinical
      a. History of exposure to cats, usually kittens.
      b. Caused by *Bartonella henselae* (gram-negative bacillus).
      c. Rarely have systemic involvement.
   ii. Diagnosis
      a. Blood test for bacteria.
   iii. Treatment
      a. Treat empirically with clarithromycin.

C. Kawasaki disease (aka mucocutaneous lymph node syndrome)
   i. Clinical features
      a. Multisystem vasculitis of unknown etiology.
      b. Children less than 5 years of age.
      c. Most common cause of acquired heart disease in children (coronary artery aneurysm).
   ii. Diagnosis (American Heart Association) using FEBRILE acronym:
      a. Fever longer than 5 days plus 4 of the following:
      b. Exanthem: generalized polymorphous nonvesicular rash.
      c. Bulbar conjunctivitis: bilateral, nonexudative, painless.
      d. Redness: lip erythema, fissuring and crusting, strawberry tongue, diffuse erythema of oral cavity.
      e. Internal organ involvement (not part of the criteria).
      f. Lymphadenopathy: acute, nonpurulent, diameter > 1.5 cm, unilateral.
      g. Extremity changes: red or edematous palms and soles, followed by desquamation or transverse grooves across finger and toe nails (Beau lines).
   iii. Treatment (to prevent coronary complications)
      a. Aspirin and antiplatelet medications
      b. Intravenous immunoglobulin therapy (IVIG)
      c. Echocardiogram at time of diagnosis, 2 weeks later and 2 months later
      d. Corticosteroids
      e. Methotrexate
      f. Infliximab
      g. Anticoagulants if unresponsive to treatment or complications

D. Kikuchi disease (aka histiocytic necrotizing lyphadenitis)
   i. Clinical features
      a. Cervical lymphadenopathy with or without systemic signs.
      b. Generally self-limited, however, may rarely be fatal.
   ii. Diagnosis
      a. Biopsy may be mistaken for lymphoma or systemic lupus erythematous.
   iii. Treatment
      a. Self-limiting

Traumatic

A. Fibromatosis colli/pseudotumor of infancy/congenital torticollis
   i. Clinical features
      a. Lateral neck mass within sternocleidomastoid muscle.

  b. Presents in first 6 weeks of life.

  c. Associated with breech position in utero and congenital hip dysplasia.

 ii. Diagnosis

  a. Based on physical examination

  b. Confirmed with ultrasonography

  c. No need for CT or MRI

 iii. Treatment

  a. Urgent referral to physiotherapy plus home programme (> 90% success).

  b. Botox injections to weaken affected muscle (rarely required).

  c. Surgical excision of mass with reapproximation of muscle (rarely required).

B. Facial nerve palsy

 i. Clinical presentation

  a. Risk factors

   1. Primiparous mother

   2. Large birth weight

   3. Prolonged labor

   4. Assisted (forceps or vacuum) vaginal delivery

  b. Signs of trauma, ecchymosis, fractures, laceration.

 ii. Diagnosis

  a. Physical examination

 iii. Treatment

  a. 90% recover spontaneously.

Bibliography

American Academy of Pediatrics, Joint Committee on Infant Hearing. Year 2007 position statement: principles and guidelines for early hearing detection and intervention programs. *Pediatrics.* 2007;120(4):898-921.

Baugh RF, Archer SM, Mitchell RB, et al. Clinical practice guideline: tonsillectomy in children. *Otolaryngol Head Neck Surg.* 2011;144(1 Suppl): S1-S31.

Dasgupta R, Fishman SJ. ISSVA classification. *Semin Pediatr Surg.* 2014;23(4):158-161.

Lieberthal AS, Carroll AE, Chonmaitree T, et al. The diagnosis and management of acute otitis media. *Pediatrics.* 2013;131(3):e964-e999.

Rosenfeld RM, Schwartz SR, Pynnonen MA, et al. Clinical practice guideline: tympanostomy tubes in children. *Otolaryngol Head Neck Surg.* 2013;149(1 Supp.):S1-S35.

Acknowledgements

The authors acknowledge Kathleen Sie, Seattle Children's Hospital, for a previous version of this text; Paul Nathan and Sumit Gupta, Division of Hematology/Oncology, Hospital for Sick Children, for their experience regarding management of head and neck malignancies; Susan Blaser, Division of Neuroradiology , Hospital for Sick Children, for her expertise regarding temporal bone anomalies in various syndromic conditions.

Questions

1. Which of the following is **true** regarding acute otitis media.
   A. Diagnosis requires evidence of fluid but not inflammation.
   B. Most common organisms are *S Pneumoniae, H Influenza B,* and *M Catarrhalis.*
   C. The incidence of beta-lactamase producing organisms is 60% to 70%.
   D. May closely observe without antibiotics if parents are reliable and child is 6 months to 2 years of age with unilateral non severe AOM or > 2 years of age with nonsevere bilateral AOM.
   E. First-line treatment if no previous antibiotics is amoxicillin-clavulanate.

2. A 6-year-old boy presents with a chronically draining right ear. All of the following are reasonable next steps **except**:
   A. microdebridement of the ear.
   B. fine cut CT scan of the temporal bone.
   C. audiogram with myringotomy and tube if hearing loss is present.
   D. diffusion-weighted MRI with gadolinium.
   E. application of topical antibiotic/steroid suspension in ear.

3. You are consulted regarding a newborn because the nurse is not able to pass a flexible nasal suction catheter through either side of the nose. All of the following are correct next steps **except**:
   A. make a diagnosis of CHARGE syndrome and obtain consent for surgery.
   B. perform bilateral flexible nasopharyngoscopy.
   C. perform CT scan following administration of decongestant and suctioning.
   D. cut the end off the nipple from his bottle and place it in his mouth.
   E. send blood for genetic testing of CHD7 gene.

4. Obstructive sleep apnea in children may be associated with all of the following EXCEPT:
   A. nocturnal enuresis.
   B. attention deficit or hyperactivity (ADD or ADHD).
   C. two apneas or hypopneas in two consecutive breaths per hour or a drop in oxygen saturation to less than 92%.
   D. desaturation to less than 90% on oximetry.
   E. benefit from intraoperative dexamethasone during tonsillectomy and adenoidectomy but not postoperative antibiotics.

5. Which of the following are **true** regarding subglottic lesions?
   A. The gold standard for diagnosing subglottic stenosis is high kV x-ray.
   B. Eosinophilic esophagitis, defined as >25 eosinophils per high power field after 2 months of proton pump inhibitor therapy, should be treated prior to open airway reconstruction.
   C. Subglottic cysts should be treated with propranolol +/− steroids.
   D. A subglottic hemangioma is most commonly located on the right side.
   E. None of the above.

Part 7
Facial Plastic and Reconstructive Surgery

Chapter 48
Facial Plastic Surgery

Facial Analysis

General Facial Assessment
- Ideal width to length ratio of face: 3:4
- Vertical fifths: Each fifth approximates the width of one eye or the intercanthal distance
- Horizontal thirds: Demarcated by trichion, glabella, subnasale, and menton

Facial Landmarks (Figure 48-1)
A. Trichion: hairline in the midsagittal plane
B. Glabella: most prominent portion of forehead in midsagittal plane, above root of the nose
C. Nasion: deepest point in the nasofrontal angle, corresponds to nasofrontal suture
D. Radix: root of nose
E. Rhinion: junction of bony and cartilaginous nasal dorsum; thinnest skin of the nose
F. Tip defining point: most anterior projection of nasal tip, corresponds to the apex of the lobular arch of the lower lateral cartilage
G. Nasal base: includes the tip in addition to the columella, alar side walls, and nasal sill
H. Subnasale: the point at which the nasal columella merges with the upper cutaneous lip
I. Pogonion: most prominent anterior projection of chin
J. Menton: inferiormost border of chin
K. Cervical point: innermost area between the submental region and the neck

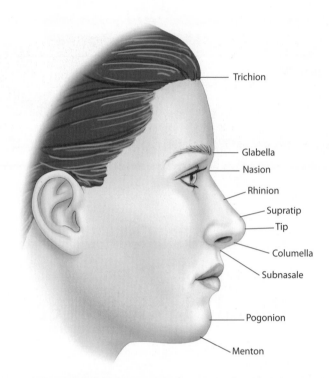

Figure 48-1 Facial anatomic landmarks. *(Adapted with permission from Taub PJ and Baker SB: Rhinoplasty. New York, NY: McGraw-Hill Education; 2011.)*

Facial Angles (Figure 48-2)

Nasofacial angle: angle between the plane of the face (glabella to pogonion) and the nasal dorsum; normally 30 to 40 degree

    A. Nasolabial angle: angle between a line from the upper lip mucocutaneous border to the subnasale and a line from the subnasale to the most anterior point on the columella; ideal range is 90 to 105 degree in men, and 95 to 120 degree in women

    B. Nasofrontal angle: angle between the nasal dorsum and a tangent passing through the nasion and the glabella; ideal range is 115 to 130 degrees

    C. Nasomental angle: angle between the nasal dorsum and the nasomental line (nasal tip to pogonion); ideal range is 120 to 132 degree

    D. Cervicomental angle: angle between a line from the glabella to the pogonion and a line from the menton to the cervical point; ideal range is 80 to 90 degree

Methods of Facial Analysis

- Cephalometrics: involves measurement of bony landmarks on x-ray (radiographic craniofacial relationships)
- Photometrics: direct consideration of soft-tissue proportion on facial photographs
  - (a) Frankfort horizontal line: reference plane used for photos and analysis
    - ◦ An imaginary line drawn from the superior portion of the cartilaginous external auditory canal through the infraorbital rim.
- Gestalt: the intuitive appreciation of the face as a whole as determined by our inborn and sociocultural influences.

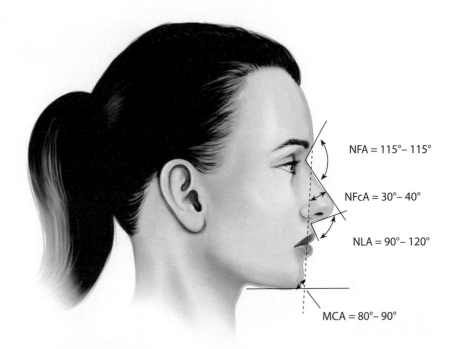

Figure 48-2 Facial Angles.

Bony Facial Skeleton Aesthetic Surgery

By altering the facial skeleton, the surgeon can create profound aesthetic changes. This involves the surgeon's understanding of basic aesthetic principles of facial forms, skeletal balance and the volumetric contours they create. There are three major promontories that determine a person's facial contours. These are the nose, the two malar zygomatic eminences and the chin-jawline. The strength and volume characteristics of each promontory affect their relative balance with each other. The surgeon can accomplish this balance by using alloplastic implants or alteration of the skeletal size, shape, and position.

Management of Chin Deficiencies (Figure 48-3)
Methods of Evaluating Chin Projection
Roughly, the anterior projection of the chin should be at a line dropped from the red-white lip junction. (In males, slightly anterior to the line; in females, slightly posterior to the line.)

- Gonzales-Ulloa: chin should approximate a line perpendicular to Frankfort horizontal line that intersects nasion
- Merrifield Z-angle: angle between Frankfort horizontal line and line connecting soft-tissue pogonion and most anterior part of lip should be 80 degrees +/- 5
- Differentiate microgenia (small chin requiring augmentation or sliding genioplasty) and retrognathia (retrodisplaced mandible requiring sagittal split osteotomies)

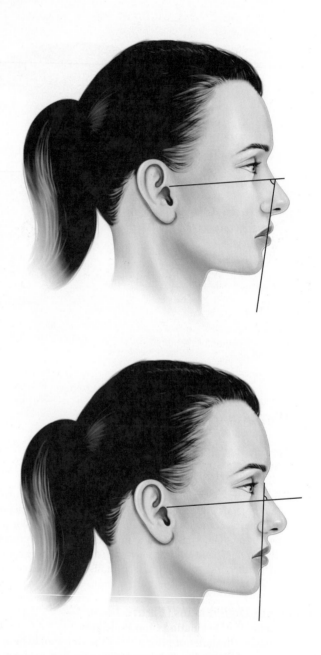

Figure 48-3 Management of chin deficiencies.

Techniques

Sliding Genioplasty

- Horizontal osteotomy of the mandibular symphysis (usually below cuspid apices and mental foramina), advancement of the mobilized inferior segments, plate or wire in new position

Indications

- More severe cases of retrognathia
- Insufficient vertical heights
- Hemifacial atrophy
- Failed implant

Advantage

- Possible to alter vertical height of the chin

Disadvantages

- Increased surgical time
- Longer healing time
- Risk of injury to teeth
- Risk of lower lip incompetence (poor reapproximation of mentalis muscle)

Complications

- Mental nerve injury
- Malposition
- Poor bony union
- Damage to tooth roots during osteotomy

Chin Implants

- Various implants are available to help augment the chin. These include but are not limited to silastic (most common), e-PTFE, porous polyethylene and acrylics.

Surgical Techniques for Chin Implant

- Subperiosteal placement of implant is desirable.
- Intraoral or extraoral (more common) approach:
  - (a) Intraoral: requires gingivobuccal incision; risk of intraoral contamination, suture irritation, inability to stabilize implant internally, anterior gingivobuccal sulcus scar contracture
  - (b) Extraoral: incision in the submental crease carried down and through the periosteum, lateral subperiosteal envelopes are created, allows implant to be suture stabilized to periosteum
- Final soft tissue augmentation represents 70% of implant width.

Complications

- Implant malplacement/displacement
- Infection
- Bony resorption
- Improper size
- Mental nerve injury
- Hypertrophic scar

Orthognathic Surgery

- Cephalometric analysis can assist in identifying inappropriate maxillomandibular relationship.
- Angle Classification System
  - (a) Class I occlusion: Mesial buccal cusp of the first maxillary molar fits in mesobuccal groove of first mandibular molar

(b) Class II malocclusion: Mesial buccal cusp of the first maxillary molar is anterior to the first mandibular molar

(c) Class III malocclusion: Mesial buccal cusp of the first maxillary molar is posterior to the first mandibular molar

- Methods to address retrognathia
  (a) Mandibular sagittal split osteotomy or vertical osteotomies and bone grafting
  (b) Distraction osteogenesis

Midfacial Augmentation

Indications

- Lack of malar prominence
- Adjunct to face-lift surgery if patient has deepened melolabial folds
- Accentuation of malar prominence
- Asymmetry of malar prominence from congenital deformity, surgical resection or incomplete reduction of malar fracture

Evaluation

- Decision based more on aesthetic appreciation than actual measurements.
- Malar region should appear full, and not fall more than 5 mm posterior to nasolabial fold (NLF) on true lateral projection.

Surgical Technique for Implant

- Intraoral or subciliary approach: former is most common approach with a canine fossa incision. Elevation of periosteum superiorly and laterally over malar eminence and zygoma. The implant is usually pre-soaked in antimicrobial solution and saline. The implant is inserted subperiosteally and secured by the confines of the pocket, or with sutures and bolster. Care is taken to avoid the infraorbital nerve.

Complications

- Malpositioned implant or displacement
- Infection
- Intraoral implant exposure

The Aging Face

Physiologic changes of the aging face:

A. Thinning of papillary dermis: approximately 1% per year in adult life
B. Decreased collagen production with shorter, more coarse bundles
C. Reduction in production of elastin and increased fragmentation of elastin chains resulting in disordered collection of fibers
D. Increased skin laxity and wrinkling (rhytidosis)
E. Photodamage
F. Dermal atrophy
G. Soft tissue ptosis
H. Loss of soft tissue volume including decreased subcutaneous fat
I. Bone resorption of facial skeleton: particularly involving maxilla (medial and pyriform region), orbital rim (superomedial, inferolateral), and mandible (pre-jowl)

Common age-related issues of the upper third of the face:

A. Brow ptosis
B. Forehead rhytids
C. Glabellar furrowing

Forehead Lifting

The primary goal of "forehead" or "brow" lifting is to restore the normal position of the ptotic brow in order to produce an attractive and youthful appearance. Secondary goals of forehead lifting can include improvement of the glabellar and forehead rhytids.

Ideal brow position
- Medial: The eyebrow should start on a plane extended vertically from the medial canthus.
- Lateral: The eyebrow should end at a point on a line that is extended from the nasal ala through the lateral canthus of the eye.
- Superior: In men, the brow should sit at the level of the superior orbital rim and have a horizontal shape. In women, the brow should sit above the superior orbital rim with an apex located between the lateral limbus and lateral canthus. The lateral brow should sit slightly higher than the medial brow on the horizontal plane.

Commonly Employed Surgical Techniques for Correction of the Ptotic Brow

Coronal Forehead Lift
- Surgical approach: A coronal incision is made 4 to 6 cm behind the anterior hairline with the incision beveled parallel to the hair follicles. The forehead tissues are elevated in a subgaleal, supraperiosteal plane to the level of the superior orbital rims. Medially, careful dissection is performed in the regions of the supraorbital and supratrochlear neurovascular bundles in order to avoid postoperative hypoesthesia. Laterally, the plane of dissection is immediately overlying the deep temporalis fascia in order to avoid trauma to the frontal branch of the facial nerve which lies in the temporoparietal fascia. The corrugator and procerus muscles can be partially resected in order to reduce glabellar rhytids and the frontalis muscle can be scored to reduce forehead rhytids as appropriate. The soft-tissue is then redraped superiorly and a 1 to 2 cm strip of skin and soft-tissue is usually excised along the length of the incision prior to closure.
- Advantages:
  (a) Scar is well hidden within the hairline (should be avoided in alopecic male)
  (b) Predictable and secure results
  (c) Unparalleled exposure
  (d) Ability to precisely address different muscle groups
- Disadvantages:
  (a) More extensive procedure
  (b) Elevates hairline
  (c) Scalp hypoesthesia posterior to incision line

Trichophytic Forehead Lift
Surgical approach: Performed similarly to the coronal forehead lift, but the incision is placed just within the first few rows of hairs of the anterior hairline, tapering into the hairline laterally. The incision is made perpendicular to the axis of the hair follicles in order to allow the hair shafts to grow through the scar and the wound is closed meticulously to reduce the visibility of the scar.
- Advantages:
  (a) Excellent exposure
  (b) Will not alter the height of the hairline and is, therefore, a good option for individuals with a pre-existing high hairline where elevation of the vertical height of the forehead would not be appropriate. It also shortens the height of a tall forehead.
- Disadvantages:
  (a) Potentially visible scar
  (b) Scalp hypoesthesia posterior to incision line

Endoscopic Forehead Lift
- Surgical approach: Several small incisions are made in the scalp posterior to the hairline. Periosteal elevators are inserted through these incisions to elevate the brow soft-tissues in a subperiosteal plane. Dissection is performed down to the supraorbital rims, and laterally over the temporalis fascia. An endoscope is introduced through an adjacent incision to allow visualization of the neurovascular bundles in order to avoid trauma to these structures. Specially designed, curved grasping forceps and cautery may be used to resect procerus and corrugator musculature. The mobilized forehead tissues are suspended in an elevated position using sutures with bone-tunnels, or bio-absorbable screws or fixation devices.
- Advantages:
  - (a) Less invasive procedure
  - (b) Absence of long scars
  - (c) Able to address brow position
  - (d) Able to address dynamic rhytids related to muscle activity
- Disadvantages:
  - (a) Occasional problems with fixation devices (infection, palpability, tissue reaction)
  - (b) May be unable to achieve same degree of lift as coronal approach, particularly for patients with more marked ptosis and heavy forehead soft tissues
- Complications
  - (a) Hematoma
  - (b) Infection
  - (c) Asymmetry
  - (d) Nerve injury (frontal branch of CN VII, supraorbital, supratrochlear nerves)
  - (e) Poor scarring
  - (f) Alopecia
- Common age-related issues of the middle-third of the face
  - (a) Lateral periorbital rhytids (crow's feet)
  - (b) Dermatochalasis of the upper eyelids, pseudoherniation of fat of the upper eyelids versus orbital hollowing
  - (c) Pseudoherniation of fat in the lower eyelids, lower eyelid laxity

Upper Eyelid Blepharoplasty
Important Terms
- Dermatochalasis—Excess upper eyelid skin laxity. (Pseudoherniation of the central and medial fat compartments can also contribute to upper eyelid fullness.)
- Blepharochalasis—Uncommon condition involving recurrent episodes or eyelid edema and inflammation. Typically occurs in the younger patient.
- Hering law of Equal Innervation: Bilateral levator palpabrae muscles receive same level of innervation for motor power, despite any asymmetries. Unilateral ptosis repair can thus result in descent of contralateral "normal" eyelid. Preoperative test to determine whether this will occur: Ptotic eye is covered, or the lid is elevated manually. Contralateral eyelid will drop 0.5 to 1 mm in seconds to minutes.

Important Anatomy
- Distance from the lash line to the upper eyelid crease is usually 8 to 10 mm.
- The upper lid may cover a small portion of the iris, but should be situated above the pupil.
- The lid crease should be at the level of the nasion.

Relevant History
- Visual acuity, field defects, history of dry eye symptoms, ocular history, glaucoma, cataracts, history of previous upper lid surgery (higher risk of lagophthalmos)

- Systemic comorbidities: hyperthyroidism, Sjogren syndrome, hypertension, use of anticoagulants

Important Physical Examination Elements

- Brow ptosis, lid ptosis, visual field testing, vision testing, dry eye testing (Schirmer test, tear break up time), pseudoherniation of medial and central fat compartments, fullness of lacrimal gland, associated skin lesions.
- Differentiate brow ptosis from upper lid dermatochalasis. A ptotic brow cannot be elevated with a blepharoplasty.
- Determine degree of lid laxity.

Surgical Technique

The patient is marked in the sitting position. The lower marking is placed precisely in the pre-existing palpebral crease which is most commonly located 8 to 10 mm from the lash line. Excess skin is assessed using Green forceps whereby excision of skin will cause a slight eversion of the lash line without causing lagophthalmos. Care is taken to mark out excess eyelid skin without excision of superior brow skin. Generally, more skin is removed laterally than medially. In women, the lateral extent of the excision may be carried past the lateral canthus, however, extension beyond the orbital rim should be avoided. For patients with lateral hooding, the incision should be extended superiorly rather than violating the thicker orbital skin. After injection of local anesthetic solution containing epinephrine, the skin ellipse is excised revealing the underlying orbicularis oculi muscle. A small strip of muscle may be excised to deepen the eyelid crease and conservative resection of excess fat of the central or medial compartment may be performed. The incision is then closed with 7-0 sutures that are removed on the fifth postoperative day.

Complications

Orbital hematoma—rare, but potentially catastrophic. Key steps in management include prompt recognition, ophthalmologic consultation, decompression by opening incision, cooling, and elevation of the head of the bed. Consideration should be given to perform lateral canthotomy and cantholysis if necessary, as well as administration of mannitol, Diamox, and steroids. Hematoma causing optic nerve compression may result in permanent vision loss.

- Poor scarring: erythema, hypertrophy, milial deposits. Milia may be treated by uncapping the lesions.
- Blepharoptosis: Undiagnosed preoperative unilateral ptosis may be unmasked by the correction of upper lid laxity. Minimal ptosis (< 2 mm) can be treated with transconjunctival Mueller muscle resection. Larger degree of ptosis is addressed best with levator resection or levator aponeurosis dehiscence repair. Ptosis can also be caused by intraoperative injury to the levator muscle, aponeurosis or tarsal plate.
- Lagophthalmos: Usually resolves with time but, if persistent, may rarely require full thickness skin grafting for correction. Results from overzealous skin excision. Always leave absolute minimum of 20 mm of distance from lash-line to lower brow.

Lower Lid Blepharoplasty

Important Terms

- Negative vector: Globe projects anterior to the infraorbital rim.
- Festoons: Redundant folds of lax skin or orbicularis muscle that hang from canthus to canthus.
- Malar bags: Areas of soft tissue fullness and edema on the lateral edge of the infraorbital ridge and zygomatic prominence. Difficult to improve with lower blepharoplasty.

Relevant History

- Dry eyes, previous ophthalmic surgery including laser vision correction, and any medical condition that may lead to eyelid problems (hyperthyroidism, Sjogren syndrome, hypertension).
- Patients with dry eyes may, seemingly paradoxically, have excessive tearing.

Important Physical Elements

- Lid retraction test: Lower lid is pulled inferiorly with finger. Medial canthus should move less than 3 mm.
- Lid distraction test (snap test)-Lower lid is pulled away from globe and released. Lid should snap back firmly against globe. Distraction greater than 1 cm is abnormal and suggests lower lid should be tightened.

Surgical Techniques

- *Skin flap*: Indicated in patients with excess skin laxity only
  - (a) Technique: Subciliary incision through skin only. Skin flap is raised to a level just below infraorbital rim. The flap is redraped, excess skin trimmed leaving 1 mm of redundancy to avoid postoperative ectropion.
- *Skin-muscle flap*: Indicated for orbicularis oculi hypertrophy, fat pseudoherniation, and excessive skin
  - (a) Surgical technique: Performed through subciliary incision 2 to 3 mm below lash line. Extends from 1 mm lateral to inferior punctum to 8 to 10 mm lateral to lateral canthus. Retention suture placed for retraction. Skin-muscle flap raised to level of orbital rim, and fat is removed if necessary just level with infraorbital rim. Skin-muscle flap redraped superotemporally. Redundancy excised with blade beveled caudally to excise 1 to 2 mm more muscle than skin to avoid bulging ridge of muscle at incision line. Canthoplasty or lid shortening procedure should be performed if there is any indication of lax lower lid in order to avoid postoperative lid retraction.
- *Transconjunctival approach*: Indicated when fat pseudoherniation is the dominant issue and minimal skin excess is present.
  - (a) Surgical technique: Transverse incision is made through the conjunctiva. The incision can be placed 2 mm below the tarsal plate to create a pre-septal plane, or 4 mm below the tarsal plate to create a postseptal plane whereby the fat compartment is directly entered. Excess fat is resected, level with the infraorbital margin. Excess eyelid skin can be resected through a "skin pinch" where excess skin is gathered and excised below the lash line externally.

Complications

- Dry eyes
- Lid rounding/retraction
- Ectropion
- Epiphora
- Hematoma
- Poor scarring
- Milia
- Inferior oblique injury

The Lower Face

Analysis of the aging face by zones allows proper management of each segment. The lower third of the face plays host to a series of age-related abnormalities which can be categorized and addressed as needed.

Issues in the lower two-thirds of the face:

A. Generalized skin laxity, rhytids

    B. Prominent melolabial and melomental folds
    C. Jowling (sagging soft-tissues along mandible)
    D. Submental laxity and fat deposition

Important Terms
- Dedo classification system for the neck
  - (a) Class I: minimal skin laxity
  - (b) Class II: skin laxity alone
  - (c) Class III: submental jowling and excess fat
  - (d) Class IV: anterior platysmal banding
  - (e) Class V: congenital or acquired micrognathia which might benefit form adjunctive chin augmentation
  - (f) Class VI: low-lying hyoid bone

Surgical Techniques

The aging middle and lower face is addressed through a variety of techniques. Rhytidectomy alone will not correct many issues of the cervicomental angle and adjunctive procedures such as submental liposuction, direct excision of submental fat, platysmaplasty, and or genioplasty may be necessary.

Types of Rhytidectomy

    A. Skin only: Rarely used

    B. Superficial musculoaponeurotic system (SMAS) plication technique

        i. Plane of Dissection—Subcutaneous Surgical technique—The standard procedure involves elevation of anterior (temporal and preauricular) and posterior (post-auricular and cervical) skin flaps. The incision courses from the temporal region (either within or just along the temporal tuft of hair), along the margin of the root of the helix, posterior to the tragus, around the lobule, and onto the postauricular surface of ear. It is commonly extended into the posterior hairline. The skin is elevated just deep to the hair follicles in the hair-bearing portion of the flap, and just deep to the subdermal plexus in the remaining portion. The skin is elevated medial enough to accommodate plication sutures within the SMAS and can be elevated to the midline in the central neck region if desired. The SMAS is then plicated under tension with heavy sutures in order to provide a deep suspension. The flaps are then redraped and tailored prior to closure while avoiding any tension on the skin.

    C. SMAS imbrication techniques

        i. Surgical technique—SMAS imbrication technique begins just as the SMAS plication technique described above. Once the SMAS is exposed on its superficial surface, the SMAS itself is elevated off the parotidomasseteric fascia. Usually, the sub-SMAS plane is elevated 1 to 2 cm beyond the anterior parotid. The SMAS is then repositioned superolaterally under tension and the overlapping SMAS is either redraped or resected. The skin flaps are then redraped and tailored without skin tension prior to closure.

        ii. Advantage:
            a. Greater mobility of SMAS flap and ability to produce greater improvement in jowls.

        iii. Disadvantage:
            a. Limited midface correction

    D. Deep plane facelift technique

        i. Plane—sub-SMAS plane laterally transitioning to a supra-SMAS plane in the superior-medial cheek directly on the anterior surface of the zygomaticus major and minor muscles. Because these nerves are innervated on their deep surfaces, the risk of facial nerve injury is limited. In the neck, a preplatysmal plane is elevated centrally, and sub-platsymal plane elevated laterally.

    ii. Advantage: allows repositioning of the cheek fat pad, and thus has a more dramatic effect on the nasolabial fold.

       a. Disadvantage: Increased risk of injury to the facial nerve

  E. Adjunct techniques

    i. Submental liposuction

    ii. Submentoplasty: midline platysma plication or imbrication +/− inferior cutback, +/− subplatysmal direct fat removal

Complications

A. Hematoma: Occurs in 3% to 15% of cases, manifests with unilateral pain or swelling. When untreated, necrosis of overlying skin flaps may occur causing permanent scarring and/or cutaneous irregularity. Timely evacuation is imperative.

B. Skin necrosis: Occurs in setting of excessive tension on skin, or poor local or systemic vascularity. The postauricular area is the most common site. Skin loss manifests with dark eschar at wound edges. Most often, complete healing occurs but scar tissue can be common.

C. Hair loss: Alopecia may occur in hair-bearing areas if hair follicles are traumatized during flap elevation. Incisions should be made parallel to hair follicles and cautery should be avoided in hair-bearing regions.

D. Nerve injury:

    i. Sensory—the most common nerve injury is to the great auricular nerve (7% incidence) which may be encountered during flap elevation over the sternocleidomastoid.

    ii. Motor—Distal branches of the facial nerve are encountered in the surgical field. Cervical and temporal branches are most commonly injured. Incidence of temporary nerve injury is 1%, and permanent nerve injury occurs in 0.1% of cases.

E. Other complications: Infection, prolonged edema/ecchymosis, hypertrophic or widened scarring, "wind-swept" or over-done look.

Aesthetic Nasal Surgery

Surgical Anatomy of the Nose

- Nasal thirds
  - (a) Upper third: nasal bone, skin
  - (b) Middle third: upper lateral cartilages, septum, skin
  - (c) Lower third: lower lateral cartilages, septum
- Nasal tip support
  - (a) Major
    - ○ Size, shape, and resilience of medial and lower lateral crura
    - ○ Medial crural footplate attachment to caudal border of quandrangular cartilage
    - ○ Attachment of upper lateral cartilage (caudal border) to alar cartilage (cephalic border)
  - (b) Minor
    - ○ Ligamentous sling spanning paired domes of alar cartilages
    - ○ Cartilaginous septal dorsum
    - ○ Sesamoid complex extending the support of the lateral crura to piriform aperture

- Attachment of alar cartilages to overlying skin and musculature
- Nasal spine
- Membranous septum

Nasal Analysis

- Nasal-facial analysis
  (a) The face is divided into equal vertical thirds by horizontal lines and vertical lines which divide the face into fifths, with nasal base width equal to intercanthal distance and width of each eye.
  (b) In profile, nose should project from face with proportion of 3-4-5 right angle triangle, or 60% of nasal length.
  (c) Nasofrontal angle begins at level of supratarsal crease.
- Nasal skin
  (a) Critical factor in determining final results. Moderate skin thickness is best.
  (b) Thick sebaceous skin: more postoperative edema, may yield poor results even when underlying structures are appropriately contoured.
  (c) Thin skin: reveals minor irregularities.
  (d) Nasal skin is generally thicker at nasion and becomes thinner over the rhinion.
  (e) From rhinion to supratip, the skin becomes thick again.
- Frontal view
  (a) Assess brow-tip aesthetic line, should be a smooth line from medial brow to ipsilateral nasal tip defining point
  (b) Width of nasal dorsum and alar base: rule of facial fifths
  (c) Nasal length: nasion to tip defining point
  (d) Nasal tip: double break, symmetry, width and size
  (e) Alar-columellar margin forms a 'gull in flight' outline
- Profile view
  (a) Nasofrontal angle: angle between line from nasion tangent to glabella and line tangent to nasal tip, 115 to 130 degree
  (b) Nasal dorsum: line drawn from nasion to desired tip projection, nasal dorsum should lie at or slightly (1-2 mm) posterior and parallel to this line
  (c) Dorsal height: rule of facial thirds, nasion to subnasale should be equivalent to middle one-third of facial length
  (d) Tip projection: distance between anterior facial plane to tip of nose
  (e) Tip rotation: degree of inclination of nasolabial angle
    - Nasolabial angle: angle between line from most anterior and posterior point of nostril to vertical line dropped along upper lip; men 90 to 95 degree, women 95 to 110 degree.
    - More rotation is acceptable in shorter individuals.
    - Increasing rotation generally increases projection but decreases nasal length.
  (f) Alar-columellar relationship: alar rim should arch 2 to 4 mm above columella on lateral view
- Base view
  (a) Should reveal an equilateral triangle
  (b) Assess size, shape, orientation and symmetry of nostril, width and length of columella, height of lobule
  (c) Columella to lobule ratio 2:1
- Intranasal examination
  (a) Adequacy of nasal airway, position of septum, internal and external nasal valve competence, condition of mucosa and inferior turbinate

- Chin
  - (a) Chin should align with a vertical line from vermilion border of lower lip (in women, chin may be slightly behind this line).

Rhinoplasty Incisions

- Marginal: follow the caudal edge of lower lateral cartilage
- Intercartilaginous: incision between lower and upper lateral cartilage
- Trans/intracartilaginous: incision through lower lateral cartilage
- Transcolumellar: used for open approach rhinoplasty, inverted V or stairstep
- Transfixion and hemitransfixion: between caudal portion of septum and medial crura through-and-through, or on one side only

Rhinoplasty Approaches

Closed (Endonasal)

- Nondelivery: intercartilaginous incisions are made between upper and lower lateral cartilages
  - (a) Advantage: no major tip support disrupted, no external scar, preserved intact caudal rim
  - (b) Disadvantage: minimal exposure of lower lateral cartilage, limited tip modification possible, potential vestibular valve scar
- Delivery: combined intercartilaginous and marginal incisions, to allow delivery of lower lateral cartilage as a bilateral pedicled chondrocutaneous flap
  - (a) Advantages: improved visualization of entire lower lateral cartilage, good access to nasal tip and dome, no external incision
  - (b) Disadvantages: compromise one major tip support mechanism (attachment of lower lateral cartilage to upper lateral cartilage), limited tip modification possible, higher revision rates than open

Open (External)

- Transcolumellar and bilateral marginal incisions
- Indications: significant tip work, revision rhinoplasty, cleft nose, non-Caucasian nose, crooked nose, teaching yourself and others
  - (a) Advantages: complete exposure of nasal tip structures, cartilaginous and bony nasal dorsum, good for teaching purposes, allow for precise graft and suture placement, lower revision rates than closed
  - (b) Disadvantages: external scar, potentially more postoperative edema

Which approach to use? If you can diagnose the deformities and correct them as well with a closed approach, do it closed. If not, use open approach.

Common Indications for Rhinoplasty

Nasal Dorsal Hump

- Can be bony or cartilaginous (more common)
- For bony hump reduction, can use Rubin osteotome and/or nasal rasp with serially smaller teeth to create a smooth surface

Correction of Crooked Nose

- Management depends on etiology, may include one or a combination of below techniques
- Goal is to create a smooth brow-nose aesthetic line

(a) Upper third: osteotomies

(b) Middle third: spreader grafts, septoplasty, onlay grafts

(c) Lower third: septoplasty, camouflage graft, nasal tip work

Osteotomies

- Indications: close an open roof defect, straighten a crooked nose, narrow a broad upper third
- Medial osteotomy: completed in absence of an open roof, between upper lateral cartilage and nasal septum and continue through the nasal bones to free it from perpendicular plate of ethmoid
- Lateral osteotomy: low to high cut along nasomaxillary groove, initiating above the level of inferior turbinate to prevent nasal obstruction
- Intermediate osteotomies: indicated for excessively wide or convex nasal bone, or asymmetry of nasal side wall

Tip Modification

- The key to modifying the nasal tip is to achieve appropriate nasal tip shape and position, without losing significant tip support.
- In general, think of retaining cartilage strength and structural support through maximal suture sculpting and minimal cartilage excision. "Preserve and conserve. Do not resect and regret."
- Nasal tip surgery and tip dynamics are best understood in the context of the Tripod Theory and M-Arch Model.
- Techniques for bulbous tip:
  (a) Cephalic trim: should maintain 8 to 10 mm of alar cartilage width for support
  (b) Suture tip contouring (preferred to aggressive cartilage excision)
  (c) Lateral crural strut grafts: cartilage grafts sewn to undersurface of lateral crura to flatten contour. (Can also be used to strengthen lateral crura to alleviate prolapse or collapse.)

Tip Projection

- Methods to increase tip projection
  (a) Transdomal or interdomal suture
  (b) Lateral crural steal
  (c) Cartilage graft: shield graft, CAP graft
  (d) Columellar strut
  (e) Septocolumellar suture
- Methods to decrease tip projection
  (a) Complete transfixion incision
  (b) Retrodisplacement and reposition of medial crura
  (c) Incise and overlap medial or lateral crura (medial crural or lateral crural overlay)

Tip Rotation

- Methods to increase tip rotation
  (a) Reduce caudal septum anteriorly
  (b) Anterior placement of medial crura along septum (tongue-in-groove)
  (c) Augment premaxilla
  (d) Shorten lateral crura (lateral crural overlay)
  (e) Removal of dorsal hump (apparent increase in tip rotation)
  (f) Note that excessive cephalic lower cartilage resection creates margin retraction, crural collapse and airway obstruction.
- Methods to decrease tip rotation
  (a) Shorten medial crural footplate or medial crural overlay

(b) Caudal septum excision near spine
(c) Dorsal augmentation (apparent decrease in tip rotation)

Revision Rhinoplasty and Complications

- 5% to 10% of open, and 10% to 15% of closed rhinoplasties require revision
- Recommended to wait for 1 year prior to revision surgery

Postoperative Complications

- Pollybeak deformity
  (a) Supratip prominence projecting beyond the nasal tip
  (b) Etiologies can be cartilaginous or soft tissue, including excess resection of nasal dorsum, inadequate removal of cartilaginous dorsum, loss of nasal tip support, soft tissue scarring in the supratip
  (c) Management: depends on etiology
    ○ Soft tissue scarring: steroid injection, or direct excision
    ○ Dorsal defect: onlay grafting or supratip cartilage resection
    ○ Reestablish nasal support, that is columellar strut
- Saddling
  (a) Etiologies: excessive reduction of nasal dorsum
  (b) Management: lateral osteotomies, dorsal onlay graft, extended height spreader grafts
- Open roof deformity
  (a) Etiology: failure to perform lateral osteotomies, leaving the medial aspect of nasal bones wide and flat
  (b) Management: lateral osteotomies, spreader/spacer grafts
- Inverted-V deformity
  (a) Visible transition between caudal border of nasal bone and cephalic border of upper lateral cartilage, medial prolapse of upper lateral cartilages
  (b) Etiology: weakening of attachment of upper lateral cartilage to nasal bones, collapse of upper lateral cartilage due to over resection of dorsum
  (c) Management: revision rhinoplasty, placement of spreader grafts, osteotomies, onlay grafts
- Alar deformity
  (a) Retracted or notched
  (b) Etiologies can be excessive lower lateral cartilage excision with retraction, vestibular skin removal or poorly closed marginal incision
  (c) Management: lower lateral cartilage graft, rim graft, composite graft
- Tip defects
  (a) Bossae: bulbous deformity in the domal region caused by irregular scarring or inadequate support, usually due to over-resection
  (b) Pinched tip: excess narrowing of nasal tip usually due to over-resection, and narrow intact rim strip
  (c) Tip ptosis: disruption of major tip support, poor healing, inadequate tip support
  (d) Management: lobule sutures, onlay or underlay cartilage grafts to recreate normal anatomy
- Persistent Nasal Obstruction
  (a) Etiologies: persistent septal deformity, intranasal scarring/synechiae, nasal valve collapse
  (b) Management: dependent on etiology-can include septoplasty, spreader grafts, lateral crural strut grafts, scar lysis, turbinate reduction, steroid injection

Otoplasty _____

Anatomy

- Auricular structure is comprised of a complex structure of fibroelastic cartilage
  - (a) Covered with skin that is closely adherent anteriorly, more loosely attached posteriorly
  - (b) Exhibits several prominences, grooves and folds

Important Landmarks

- Helix
- Superior crus
- Inferior crus
- Antihelix
- Cymba concha and cavum concha
- Fossa triangularis

Preoperative Evaluation

- Size and relation to scalp
- Auricular components and convolutions (helix, antihelix, scaphoid fossa, fossa triangularis, lobule)
- Compare to opposite ear
- Normal measurements
  - (a) Vertical height: 6 cm
  - (b) Width: 55% length
  - (c) Auriculocephalic angle: 20 to 30 degree
  - (d) Lateral helix to mastoid skin: 2 to 2.5 cm
- Preoperative photograph
  - (a) Anterior full face, posterior full head, close-up photographs of involved ears
- Most common aesthetic auricular defect: Protruding ear
  - (a) Auriculocephalic angle > 30 degree
  - (b) Poor antihelical fold
  - (c) Overdeveloped conchal cartilage
  - (d) Superior helix > 20 mm from scalp
- Timing
  - (a) Best before child starts school, age 5 to 6 years
  - (b) Ear is 85% to 90% of adult size, cartilage has adequate strength
  - (c) Reduce teasing, anxiety

Goals of Aesthetic Otoplasty

- Symmetry
  - (a) Adequate auriculomastoid separation
  - (b) Anatomical remodeling of antihelix without acute angles or edges
  - (c) Well-hidden scar
  - (d) Lasting results
  - (e) Superior poles 15 to 20 mm from scalp

Correcting the Protruding Ear: Surgical Techniques

- Overdeveloped conchal bowl

(a) Conchomastoid suture technique: Furnas
  ○ Permanent sutures through conchal cartilage and mastoid periosteum
  ○ Placement of conchomastoid suture as far posteriorly to avoid narrowing of external auditory canal
  ○ When done first, may reduce/eliminate need for Mustarde sutures
(b) Cartilage sculpting techniques: Converse, Farrior, Pitanguy
  ○ Involves variable reshaping, splitting or removal of auricular cartilage
  ○ Farrior technique includes a combination of suture and cartilage sculpting technique
  ○ Problems: cartilage irregularities, asymmetries
- Underdeveloped antihelical fold
(a) Suture technique: Mustarde
  ○ Postauricular incision followed by undermining in supraperichondrial plane, 2 to 3 horizontal mattress sutures along the scapha to create an antihelical fold. All sutures placed prior to final tightening
  ○ Problems: accuracy of suture placement, resilience of cartilage, suture exposure, does not address conchal bowl

Postoperative Care

- This is often as important as the surgical procedure
- Pressure head dressing for 1 week, followed by up to 6 weeks of head band at night

Complications

- Inadequate correction (most common)
- Suture extrusion
- Chondritis
- Hematoma
- 'Telephone ear' deformity: upper and lower pole of auricle protrude on anterior view due to undercorrection of concha, overcorrection of helix
- Cartilage irregularities (cartilage cutting techniques)

Facial Skin Rejuvenation/Resurfacing

The principles behind skin resurfacing involve removal of epidermis and creation of a controlled papillary to upper reticular dermal injury. The healing process stimulates production of new collagen and a resurfaced epidermis from deeper, less sun-damaged cells, to result in cosmetic improvement in actinically damaged, aged or scarred skin. These methods include dermabrasion which causes mechanical injury, chemical peel (chemexfoliation) and laser, which causes thermal injury.

Skin Anatomy

- Epidermis
(a) Stratum corneum
(b) Stratum granulosum
(c) Stratum lucidum

(d) Stratum spinosum
(e) Stratum basale
- Dermis
  (a) Papillary dermis: thin, loose collagen surrounding adnexal structures; abundant elastic fibers
  (b) Reticular dermis: thick, compact collagen. Damage to this layer results in permanent scar
- Subcutaneous layer

Skin Analysis

Analysis of patient's skin color, type, and degree of photoaging is important. The Fitzpatrick skin type system is one of the most commonly used classification systems. Fitzpatrick III through VI may be at higher risk for pigmentary dyschromia (particularly with medium and deep chemical peels). Glogau classification I-IV defines degree of skin rhytids. Of importance is degree of skin thickness.

Fitzpatrick Classification of Skin Types
- Class I: very white, always burns, never tans
- Class II: white, usually burns, tans minimally
- Class III: white to olive, sometimes burns, tans
- Class IV: brown, rarely burns, always tans
- Class V: dark brown, very rarely burns, tans profusely
- Class VI: black, never burns, tans profusely

Glogau Classification of Photoaging
- Class I: no wrinkles
- Class II: wrinkles in motion
- Class III: wrinkles at rest
- Class IV: only wrinkles

Dermabrasion

Dermabrasion is a mechanical method of removing the epidermis to create a papillary dermal wound. This induces new collagen and resurfaced epidermis from deeper, less damaged cells to yield cosmetic improvement. This is limited to the papillary dermis (pinpoint bleeding) or superficial reticular dermis to avoid scarring. Adjuncts include preoperative topical tretinoin treatment for 2 weeks, and freezing of skin prior to abrading to allow for rigid surface.

Indications
- Acne scarring
- Facial wrinkles
- Premalignant solar keratosis
- Rhinophyma
- Adjunct for scar revision

Advantages
- Inexpensive, portable and widely available
- Precise depth level

Complications
- Milia
- Acne flares
- Erythema beyond 2 weeks
- Herpes simplex infection
- Hyperpigmentation/hypopigmentation

Chemical Peeling

Chemical peeling involves the application of a chemical exfoliant to wound the epidermis and dermis for the removal of superficial lesions and to improve texture of skin.

Indications
- Postacne scarring
- Scar revision
- Actinic keratosis
- Seborrheic keratosis
- Photodamaged skin
- Pigment irregularities

Common Chemical Peel Agents
- Classified by depth of penetration
- *Very superficial*: exfoliate stratum corneum down to stratum granulosum
- *Superficial*: necrosis of stratus granulosum and basal cell layer
- *Medium*: necrosis of epidermis and wounding of papillary dermis
- *Deep*: necrosis and wounding from epidermis through papillary dermis and into reticular dermis

Depth of Penetrating Factors
- Chemical agent, skin thickness, use of retinoic acid or lactic acid, use of prepeel agent (enhance peels), occlusion versus nonocclusion

Contraindications
- Active herpetic lesions
- History of keloids
- Collagen vascular disease
- Pustular acne
- Prior radiation

Common Peels

Superficial Chemical Peeling
- Exfoliation of stratum corneum to basal cell layer to encourage regrowth with less photodamage and a more youthful appearance.
- Examples: glycolic acid, 10% to 20% TCA, Jessner solution (14 g resorcinol, 14 g salicylic acid, 14 mL lactic acid in 100 mL ethanol)
- Period of recovery: 1 to 5 days
- May require repetitive sessions to obtain maximum results.

Medium Depth Chemical Peeling
- Controlled damage to the papillary dermis to reticular junction
- Example: 35% TCA
- Period of recovery: 7 to 10 days

Deep Chemical Peeling
- Controlled damage to the reticular dermis
- Examples: 50% TCA, Gordon Baker phenol peel (phenol USP 88%, 2 mL tap water, 3 gtts croton oil, 8 gtts soap solution)
  - (a) Phenol peel causes liquefactory necrosis in deep dermis (washing and degreasing skin results in deeper penetration)
    - ○ Toxicity: cardiac arrhythmias, renal and hepatic toxicity
    - ○ Avoid by careful preoperative screen of patients with cardiac or renal or hepatic risk factors, intravenous hydration pre-, during, and postprocedure, application

of phenol peel one facial subunit at a time with 15 minutes wait between units, cardiac monitoring of the patients
- Period of recovery: 10 to 14 days

Complications
- Hyperpigmentation/hypopigmentation
- Scarring: keloid, sun exposure post peel, Accutane therapy, postradiation
- Cutaneous infection: bacterial, fungal, herpes simplex activation
- Renal toxicity (phenol)
- Cardiac arrhythmia (phenol)
- Areas treated with external beam radiation
- Melasma
- Ectropion
- Prolonged erythema
- Persistent rhytides

Laser Skin Resurfacing

Laser can be divided into ablative and nonablative. Laser utilizes the concept of selective thermolysis which is determined by absorbance of skin constituents (chromophore, oxyhemoglobin, and melanin), the power and spot size. Ablative lasers target and remove the epidermis and portions of the superficial dermis. This induces collagen remodeling and new collagen production in the months after the procedure. The advantage of ablative skin resurfacing relate to the ability to produce results in a precise and controlled fashion at the appropriate depth. The skin then heals over a period of time with thicker and smoother texture. Non-ablative lasers do not cause disruption or injury to the epidermis. The primary advantage is decreased downtime.

Types of Ablative Lasers
  A. CO_2 laser is the most commonly used
    i. Target chromophore: water
    ii. Wavelength: 10600 nm
    iii. Depth of penetration: 20 to 60 μm first pass (more with additional passes)
    iv. Advantages
      a. Best outcome in terms of removing severe sun damage and correction of elastosis and deeper wrinkling of skin
    v. Disadvantages
      a. Postoperative downtime: 10 to 14 days is required for reepithelialization, followed by erythema that may last 1 to 3 months
      b. Risk of pigmentary changes, scarring and infection
  B. Erb:YAG
    i. Target chromophore: water
    ii. Wavelength: 2940 nm
    iii. Depth of penetration: 3-5 μm
    iv. Produce more superficial ablation than CO_2 laser
    v. Advantages
      a. Faster healing time (5 days) with less erythema (3-4 weeks)
      b. Useful in treating more superficial rhytids
    vi. Disadvantages
      a. Less collagen remodeling and tightening
      b. Unable to manage deeper wrinkles and more severe photodamage

C. Fractionated laser

    i. Microzones of injury surrounded by normal intervening skin; allow rapid healing of injured tissue.

        a. 100 μm diameter area of injury is surrounded by 250 μm of normal tissue.

    ii. Wavelength: 1550 nm.

    iii. Depth: deep dermis, varies with millijoules used.

        a. Typical penetration is 30 μm.

    iv. Advantages:

        a. Decreased downtime : Reservoir of undamaged skin adjacent to sites of laser injury allows for rapid reepithelialization after treatment through migration of viable cells into wounded area.

    v. Typically a series of multiple treatments are performed at 7 to 30 day intervals.

    vi. MTZ (microthermal injury zone) are created over approximately 12% to 20% of entire treatment area.

Indications

- Rhytids
- Dyschromias
- Scarring conditions
  - (a) Superficial/shallow acne
  - (b) Elevated scars
- Skin lesions
  - (a) Lentigines and seborrheic keratoses
  - (b) Actinic keratoses
  - (c) Early superficial BCC

Contraindications

- Active or recent use of isotretinoin
  - (a) Skin resurfacing delayed 6 months to 2 years
- Active infection
- History of HSV
- Radiation therapy, collagen vascular disease (eg, scleroderma), hypertrophic scar or keloid

Complications

- Milia
- Infection: HSV, bacterial, fungal
- Hyperpigmentation/Hypopigmentation
- Scarring
- Ectropion
- Lack of improvement
- Persistent redness

Treatment Protocol

Preoperative preparation

- Skin may be prepared for up to 6 weeks prior to resurfacing procedure using one or a combination of retinoic acid, alpha-hydroxy acid and hydroquinone. Prophylactic oral antiviral and antibacterial medications should be prescribed.

Technique

- Local, regional or general anesthesia is administered based on patient and surgeon's preferences. Depth of tissue vaporization can be controlled by varying laser parameters, and number of passes. Depth of penetration is determined to be superficial, deep or upper reticular dermis. Avoidance of injury beyond adnexal structures in order to avoid scarring.

Postoperative care
- Application of semiocclusive dressing to promote wound healing
  (a) Open: Vaseline, Aquaphor
  (b) Closed: composite foam, hydrogel, plastic mesh, polymer film
- Laser wounds reepithelialize in 7 to 10 days
- Sun protection for 3 to 6 months

Types of Nonablative Lasers
- Infrared laser: target dermal water to induce collagen production and remodeling leading to improvements in fine lines and skin texture
  (a) ND:YAG: 1320 nm
  (b) Diode laser: 1450 nm
  (c) ND:YAG: 1064 nm
- Pigment-specific laser: lighten lentigines and ephelides
  (a) QS ND:YAG: 532 and 1064 nm
  (b) QS ruby: 694 nm
  (c) QS alexandrite: 755 nm
- Vascular-specific lasers: target erythema, flushing and telangiectasia
- Intense pulsed light: broad wavelength that can target both vascular and pigmentary alterations
- Often combination is used

Advantage
- Improve mild to moderate rhytids and acne scars with no external wounding

Disadvantage
- Not capable of achieving results seen with ablative procedures

Aesthetic Injectables

Botulinum Toxin
- Produced by *Clostridium botulinum* bacteria
- Clinical application was established for investigation of nonsurgical treatment of strabismus
- Types: Eight serotypes, with type A being the most potent and most commonly used in clinical practice
  (a) Onabotulinumtoxin A (Botox)
  (b) Abobotulinumtoxin A (Dysport)
  (c) Incobotulinumtoxin A (Xeomin)
  (d) RimabotulinumtoxinB (Myobloc)
- Botox (Allergen, Irvine, California) was initially approved by the Food and Drug Administration for the treatment of strabismus, blepharospasm, cervical dystonia

Mechanism of Action
- Blockade of presynaptic acetylcholine release, muscle fibers become functionally denervated which results in muscle fiber atrophy and flaccid paralysis

Preparation and Pharmacology
- Botox (Allergan) is typically available in 100 or 200 U vials.
- Each vial is lyophilized complex consisting of 100 U of toxin, 0.5 mg of human albumin and 0.9 mg of sodium chloride.
- Reconstitution.

(a) Desired volume of sterile unpreserved saline (most commonly 1 cc) by injection with a 1-cc tuberculin syringe and 1 ½ in 25G needle.

(b) Areas of controversy: appropriate dilution of reconstituted toxin and length of viability.

(c) Reconstituted solution should be stored at 2°C to 8°C.

Clinical Efficacy

- Onset of action: 6 to 36 hours after exposure
- Maximum effect: up to 7 to 14 days
- Duration of effect: 3 to 4 months (new neuromuscular junctions and axonal sprouts eventually replace nonfunctional junctions and restore muscle function in 3-6 months)
- Common aesthetic regions: glabellar complex, orbicularis oculi muscle, frontalis muscle, platysma muscle, other facial muscle such as orbicularis oris, mentalis, depressor anguli oris)
  (a) Others: facial nerve disorders, parotid gland fistula, headache, hyperhidrosis, gustatory sweating

Complications

- Local: pain, edema, erythema, ecchymosis, headache, short term hyperesthesia, eyelid ptosis
- Immunologic: acute type 1 reaction
- Systemic: nausea, fatigue, malaise, flulike symptoms, distant rash
- Therapeutic failure: circulating neutralizing antibodies

Contraindications

- Hypersensitivity to ingredients (albumin)
- Neuromuscular disease: myasthenia gravis, Eaton Lambert syndrome
- Patients treated with aminoglycoside, penicillamine, quinine, calcium channel blocker
- Pregnancy/lactation
- Patients on anticoagulation therapy/aspirin
- Phobia of injection
- Poor psychological adjustment

Injectable Fillers

Indications

- Soft tissue augmentation to decrease the prominence of facial grooves and creases, provide volume to atrophied tissue
- Ideal filler: Inexpensive, safe, painless to inject, hypoallergenic, long lasting, consistent and predictable results, feels natural, ready to use, little or no downtime to patient, low risk of complications

Technique

- Varies for the particular facial regions being addressed
- Immediate correction
- Intradermal: facial rhytids
- Subcutaneous: NLF, glabellar crease, marionette lines
- Intramuscular/subcutaneous: lip, cheek, temple
- Supra-periosteal: cheek, chin, prejowl

Materials

- Collagen
  (a) Major structural component of skin

   (b) Bovine collagen was the first FDA-approved dermal filler
      ○ Required pretreatment allergy testing
      ○ Taken off the market in 2010
      ○ Others: human, porcine
- Hyaluronic acid (HA)
   (a) Most prominent glycosaminoglycan in the skin
   (b) Most commonly used filler material worldwide
   (c) Binds to water when injected into skin, volumizes, softens and hydrates the skin
   (d) Since 2010, all FDA-approved HA products contain lidocaine
   (e) Last about 6 to 12 months depending on location with increased longevity in less mobile areas of the face
   (f) Advantage: no allergy testing required, predictable and lasting soft tissue augmentation, hyaluronidase available for overcorrection or undesirable migration (off-label use)
- Synthetic fillers
   (a) Poly-L-lactic acid (Sculptra): deep dermal or supraperiosteal injection, stimulates collagen synthesis, requires multiple treatment with effects lasting years. (Correction is not immediate.)
   (b) Calcium hydroxyapatite: identical to mineral portion of bone, placement in deep dermis or supraperiosteal
- Autologous fat (see section below)
- Others less commonly used
   (a) Autologous cell therapy
   (b) Micronized AlloDerm
   (c) Autologous Fibroblast
   (d) Silicone
   (e) Polymethylmethacrylate (ArteFill)

Complications
- Allergic reaction, skin necrosis, blindness (embolization)

Autologous Fat (Microlipoinjection)
- Most facial volume loss is secondary to fat tissue loss
- Autologous fat transfer involves harvest of fat and transfer with cannula injection during same procedure

Indications
- Facial rhytids, grooves and volume correction

Advantages
- Autologous
- Completely biocompatible
- Available in sufficient quantities
- Naturally integrated into host tissue
- Potentially permanent
- No allergy testing
- Inexpensive and simple to obtain

Disadvantages
- Results can be unpredictable
- Viability of transferred fat varies depending on surgical technique and patient factors

Technique

- 3 steps: (1) harvesting of fat via liposuction, (2) Refinement and isolation of fat cells, (3) fat cell transplantation
- Harvesting technique: "Nontraumatic"
  (a) Infiltrate donor site with tumescent solution.
  (b) 3-mm puncture incision, harvesting cannula with a blunt tip is attached to a 10-mL Luer-lock syringe.
  (c) Cannula is pushed through the harvest site as the surgeon uses digital manipulation to pull back on the plunger of the syringe and create gentle negative pressure.
  (d) Once syringe is filled, it is disconnected from the cannula and replaced with a plug that seals the Luer-Lock end of the syringe.
- Refine and transfer
  (a) Centrifugation can be used to separate denser components from less dense components.
  (b) Upper level: least dense-oil; middle portion-fatty tissue; lower portion-blood, water and aqueous element (lidocaine).
  (c) Recommended centrifuge speed: 3000 rpm, 3 minutes.
  (d) Decant oil layer and wick off any remaining oil using an absorbent material; remove Luer-Lock plug to release densest liquid layer.
- Transplantation and Placement
  (a) Cannula technique preferred.
  (b) Accuracy of volume, location and level of placement is critical to success.

Scar Revision

Important Terms

- Relaxed skin tension lines (RSTL)—created by the intrinsic tension of the skin at rest. These lines generally fall perpendicular to the underlying musculature, and parallel to facial rhytids except around the eye where RSTLs are parallel to the orbicularis oculi.
- Lines of maximal extensibility (LME)—usually perpendicular to the RSTLs and represent the direction in which closure can be performed with the least tension. Typically parallel to the muscle fibers.

Approaches to Scar Revision

Excision

- Excision of the scar along RSTLs, normal facial creases, and the junctions between distinct facial aesthetic units, with meticulous everted closure. Serial excision of larger scars may be performed in stages according to these principles. Usually best for scars 0 to 30 degrees from the RSTLs.

Irregularization

- **Z-plasty**: Interdigitated triangular flaps interposed to reorient a scar that does not lie in the RSTLs. This both lengthens and reorients the scar. Created by the addition of two limbs, one at either end of the existing scar, similar to the length of the scar and at 30, 45, or 60 degree angles to it. This will lengthen the scar by 25, 50, and 75 percent, respectively. Multiple Z-plasties can be employed along a single scar to lengthen the line. Z-plasty is usually best for scars that are oriented 30 to 60 degrees from the RSTLs.

- **W-plasty**: Created by a series of interdigitating triangles on either side of the scar. It distributes tension and breaks up a linear scar. Usually best for scars 60 to 90 degrees from the RSTLs.
- **Geometric broken line closure**: Involves outlining of one side of the scar to be excised with an irregular composite of rectangular, triangular, and semicircular shapes, and is creating a complimentary template for interdigitation on the other side. The new scar carries an irregularly irregular pattern that is less conspicuous. Usually best for very long scars 60 to 90 degrees from the RSTLs.

Abrasion Techniques

Mechanical dermabrasion or laser resurfacing can serve as a primary scar treatment modality or as an adjunct to surgical scar revision (6 weeks after scar revision).

Questions

1. What is junction of bony and cartilaginous nasal dorsum?
   A. Nasion
   B. Radix
   C. Rhinion
   D. Subnasale

2. What is the ideal width to length ratio of the face?
   A. 2:3
   B. 4:5
   C. 1:2
   D. 3:4

3. Which of the following describes Fitzpatrick Class IV skin?
   A. Brown, rarely burns, always tans
   B. White to olive, sometimes burns, tans
   C. White, usually burns, tans minimally
   D. Dark brown, very rarely burns, tans profusely

4. The following are all methods to increase tip rotation except for?
   A. Augment premaxilla
   B. Shorten medial crural footplate or medial crural overlay
   C. Shorten lateral crura (lateral crural overlay)
   D. Reduce caudal septum anteriorly

5. All of the following are major tip support except for
   A. size, shape and resilience of medial and lower lateral crura
   B. attachment of upper lateral cartilage to alar cartilage
   C. cartilaginous septal dorsum
   D. medial crural footplate attachment to caudal border of quandrangular cartilage

Chapter 49
Reconstructive Head and Neck Surgery

In the past, ablative surgery for head and neck cancer, osteoradionecrosis, or major facial trauma resulted in significant cosmetic and functional deficits that severely impacted patients' quality of life, and often led to social isolation. Our faces form much of our personal identities, and it is through the head and neck region that we communicate with others via speech and facial expression. Moreover, our abilities to taste, swallow, and enjoy food are essential to our sense of wellness and community. Today, the head and neck surgeon has a number of tools in his or her armamentarium to address most reconstructive problems in this region. Reconstructive plans that took months and several operative procedures four decades ago can now be accomplished at the time of resection with the advent of microvascular free tissue transfer. Following a brief description of defect analysis, this chapter will describe various reconstructive techniques ranging from simple to complex.

Defect Considerations

- Composition (which tissues need to be replaced)
  - (a) Skin
  - (b) Mucosa
  - (c) Muscle
  - (d) Bone
  - (e) Cartilage
  - (f) Nerve(s)
- Functional considerations
  - (a) Bone stock for skeletal framework and/or osseointegration
  - (b) Soft tissue coverage of vital structures (eg, carotid artery, intracranial contents)
  - (c) Muscle strength (eg, oral competence in lip reconstruction)
  - (d) Pliability
  - (e) Volume
  - (f) Secretory mucosal surface
  - (g) Provision of sensibility
  - (h) Vascularized tissue for support of free grafts, and/or treatment of fistulae, osteomyelitis and/or osteoradionecrosis
- Location
- Patient's health status

    (a) Previous irradiation
    (b) Infection
    (c) Fistulae
    (d) Comorbidities

The Reconstructive Ladder

The traditional concept of the reconstructive ladder allows the surgeon to analyze various approaches to defect repair, using a hierarchical system that emphasizes simplicity. The surgeon is to choose the technique(s) that is most expedient for addressing the reconstructive problem with contingency plans in case of flap/graft failure or recurrence.

- Microneurovascular free tissue transfer
- Prosthetic reconstruction
- Regional flaps
- Local flaps
- Skin, cartilage, bone, nerve, and composite grafting
- Primary closure
- Healing by secondary intention

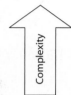

Healing by Secondary Intention

Concave surfaces that heal well by secondary intention	Surfaces that heal fairly well by secondary intention
Lateral forehead	Nasal sidewall
Glabella	Lateral canthal area
Medial canthal area	
Depressed areas of ear	
Perinasal melolabial fold	

Skin Grafts

- Completely dependent on recipient bed for survival via neovascularization
- Contraindicated in irradiated and infected sites
- Generally heal well over the fat, muscle, perichondrium, and fascia
- Requirements for success include
  - (a) Effective immobilization and avoidance of shearing by use of bolsters, quilting stitches, intraoral prosthodontic devices, and/or staples
  - (b) Avoidance of hematoma
  - (c) Avoidance of infection including timely removal of bolsters to prevent bacterial colonization

Split-Thickness Skin Grafts (STSGs)

- Harvested from thigh or buttocks using powered dermatome.
- Thickness varies from 0.012 to 0.016 in. Thinner grafts exhibit more reliable neovascularization, but more contracture than thicker grafts.
- Donor site is covered with a porous dressing or occlusive semipermeable dressing for 1 week.
- Disadvantages include poor color match, texture, and possible contracture.
- Applications:
  (a) Small defects of oral cavity.
  (b) Maxillectomy cheek flap defect (internal lining).
  (c) Temporalis fascia flap cover for auricular and periorbital reconstruction.
  (d) Auricular reconstruction.
  (e) Coverage of free flap donor sites.
  (f) Meshed grafts may be used to cover large defects in the scalp, but are cosmetically unacceptable in other facial areas.

Full-Thickness Skin Grafts (FTSGs)

- Donor sites include postauricular, upper eyelid, supraclavicular, preauricular, and nasolabial areas.
- Graft is defatted, and donor site is closed primarily.
- Appropriate for small (1-5 cm), externally visible facial defects.

Cartilage Grafts

Reconstruction of the cartilaginous skeleton of the ear and upper aerodigestive tract frequently require grafting with like tissues. Grafts taken from curved portions of cartilage are prone to warping due to cartilage memory.

Septal Cartilage Grafts

- Care must be taken to leave 1.5 cm caudal and dorsal struts when harvesting septal cartilage in order to maintain support of the nasal dorsum and tip.
- Applications:
  (a) Used primarily for nasal dorsal and tip minor support and augmentation in the form of onlay grafts, alar batten grafts, columellar strut grafts, spreader grafts, and tip grafts
  (b) Reconstruction of small orbital floor defects
  (c) Reconstruction of eyelid lacerations involving the lid margin and tarsal plate

Auricular Cartilage Grafts

- Typically harvested from the conchal bowl with no cosmetic deficit.
- Indications are similar to those for septal cartilage grafts.
- Also used for reconstruction of large nasal alar and septal cartilage defects.

Costal Cartilage Grafts

- Straight segments of the sixth to the eighth ribs are used for large nasal dorsal reconstruction defects (eg, saddle nose deformities).
- Curved and straight segments of the sixth through the eighth ribs are used for auricular reconstruction.
- Rib cartilage is also used for laryngotracheal reconstruction.

Bone Grafts

Free bone grafts are easily sculpted to donor defects. However, all free bone grafts are nonliving scaffolds that are replaced by mesenchymal cells that differentiate into osteoblasts. This limits the size and thickness of free bone grafts due to need for vascular invasion. Resorption is a common problem, and cortical bone grafts must be rigidly immobilized to reduce the incidence of this complication.

Cortical Free Bone Grafts

- Harvest sites
  - (a) Split calvarium
  - (b) Split rib
  - (c) Iliac crest
- Applications
  - (a) Nasal dorsal augmentation
  - (b) Malar and chin augmentation
  - (c) Posttraumatic reconstruction of facial buttresses
  - (d) Prevention of relapse in orthognathic surgery
  - (e) Prevention of relapse and filling of defects in correction of craniosynostoses

Cancellous Bone Grafts

- More quickly vascularized than cortical bone
- Have no structural integrity, so cannot be used for load bearing
- Harvest sites
  - (a) Iliac crest
  - (b) Tibia
- Applications
  - (a) Repair of mandibular nonunion and small segmental mandibular defects up to 5 cm with a bone cage
  - (b) Alveolar bone grafting in cleft lip and palate
  - (c) Sinus obliteration
  - (d) Repair of small cranial contour defects

Nerve Grafts

Nerve interposition grafts in head and neck reconstruction are primarily used for facial reanimation. Common donor sites include

- Greater auricular nerve, which is often in the operative field and therefore easy to harvest
- Medial antebrachial cutaneous nerve
- Radial nerve
- Sural nerve

Composite Grafts

Composite skin and cartilage grafts are routinely harvested from the conchal bowl, and are used to reconstruct defects of the nasal ala and columella. As with skin grafts, composite grafts are dependent on the recipient bed for neovascularization, and therefore are contraindicated in irradiated and infected beds. Composite grafts up to 1.5 cm may be used, but grafts 1 cm or less in diameter are more apt to take. Epidermolysis and skin slough may occur during the first week.

Local Flaps

- Also termed random pattern flaps because they are based upon subdermal plexuses and do not have a dominant vascular supply.
- Superior color match and texture to skin grafts.
- Flap design considerations:
  (a) Mechanical properties of skin.
    ○ Skin is anisotropic meaning that it's mechanical properties vary with direction.
    ○ Relaxed skin tension lines (RSTLs) are lines of minimal tension, whereas lines of maximal tension are perpendicular to the RSTLs. Flap design should minimize tension.
    ○ Aging skin has less tension, and therefore more creep than younger skin.
  (b) A traditional length-to-width ratio of 3:1 or less is used to ensure adequate flap perfusion.
- Commonly used designs include advancement, rotation, bilobed, island transposition, and rhomboid transposition flaps (Figure 49-1).

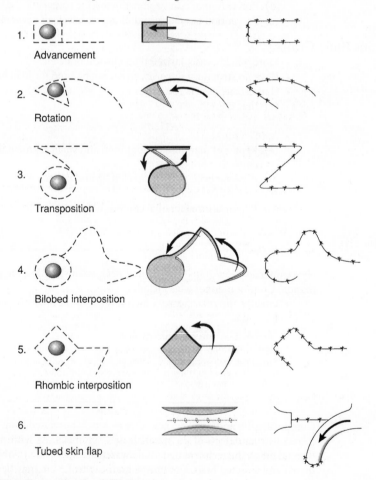

1. Advancement

2. Rotation

3. Transposition

4. Bilobed interposition

5. Rhombic interposition

6. Tubed skin flap

Figure 49-1 Six common local skin flaps.

- Tension and smoking have a negative impact on the success of these flaps.
- Applications:
  (a) Defects of the facial skin and scalp.
  (b) Nasolabial interpolation flaps may be used for small defects of the buccal mucosa and floor of mouth.
  (c) Nasolabial flaps, nasal dorsal flaps, septal mucosal flaps, and inferior turbinate mucosal flaps may be used for internal lining of nasal defects.
  (d) Buccal mucosal flaps may be used for repair of intranasal defects.

Regional Flaps

- These flaps have an axial pattern based on one or more dominant vessels.
- Flap design is based on the concept of angiosomes.
  (a) An angiosome is the tissue volume supplied by a single source artery and vein.
  (b) "Choke" or oscillating arteries connect adjacent angiosomes.
  (c) An adjacent angiosome may be captured in flap design by interrupting the adjacent source artery due to reversal of physiologic flow (flap training).
  (d) The risk of partial flap necrosis is significantly greater when the design extends beyond the adjacent angiosome.

Fascial, Fasciocutaneous, and Mucosal Flaps
Paramedian Forehead Flap
- Based on supratrochlear artery
- Applications include reconstruction of nasal, upper lip, and medial cheek skin defects
Temporal Fascia Flaps
- The temporal fascias (superficial, temporoparietal and deep) may be transferred as single or bilobed flaps based on branches of the superficial temporal artery.
- Primarily used as vascularized tissue bed for STSGs used in auricular, forehead, and periorbital reconstruction.
- May also be used for skull base reconstruction.
Deltopectoral Flap
- Largely of historic interest
- Based on perforators of the internal mammary artery in the first two intercostal spaces
- Applications include central neck cutaneous reconstruction, staged pharyngoesophageal reconstruction, and cheek reconstruction
Palatal Island Flap
- Based on greater palatine artery
- Use for defects of the central palate, or defects of the central palate including the maxillary alveolus posterior to but not including the canine teeth

Muscular and Myocutaneous Flaps
- Regional muscle flaps may be transferred or transposed with or without overlying skin.
- Myocutaneous flaps consist of defined territories of the skin overlying the muscles that are perfused by perpendicularly oriented perforators. This vascular orientation allows circumferential suturing around the transferred skin islands without compromising vascularity.

Temporalis Flap
- Muscular flap based on the deep temporal artery
- Historically used for facial reanimation, primarily in the lower face

Pectoralis Major Flap
- Ease of dissection and versatility make this a workhorse flap with many applications.
- Based on the pectoral branch of the thoracoacromial artery.
- Simultaneous harvest without patient repositioning and primary closure of donor site are advantages.
- A segment of rib may be harvested with this flap for mandibular reconstruction, but the blood supply to this bony segment is tenuous.
- Transposition of the flap is limited by the arc of rotation of the flap pedicle over the clavicle. With superiorly located defects, removal of a segment of the clavicle may increase the reach of the flap.
- Applications:
  (a) This flap can reach as superiorly as the hard palate and superior helix. It is suitable for reconstruction of facial, oral, and pharyngeal defects below this level.
  (b) To avoid transfer of hair-bearing tissue into the mouth, the muscle with its overlying fascia may be transferred into an oral defect and then skin-grafted.
  (c) The muscle with its overlying fascia may be transferred into the neck without the skin paddle to provide coverage of the ipsilateral carotid artery.
  (d) The flap may be tubed on itself for pharyngoesophageal reconstruction.
- Disadvantages:
  (a) Inferiorly pedicled flaps exhibit a tendency toward dehiscence the superior defect due to gravity and the bulk of the flap, which is greater in women.
  (b) The most distal aspect of the skin paddle, which is the most poorly perfused, is necessarily inset into the most superior aspect of the defect.

Trapezius System of Flaps
- Disadvantages to use of these flaps include variable vascular anatomy and the need to skin graft the donor site.
- The *lateral island* flap is used to reconstruct defects of the lateral scalp, neck, and cheek.
  (a) Dependent on identification of a transverse cervical artery and vein that are coursing under the anterior border of the trapezius muscle and not intertwined in the branches of the brachial plexus
- The *lower island* flap is used for delivery of skin to the lateral scalp, neck, and cheek.
  (a) It has the widest arc of rotation of the trapezius flaps.
  (b) Its two major pedicles include the transverse cervical artery and the dorsal scapular artery.
  (c) The transverse cervical artery may be compromised if there has been a previous neck dissection.
- The *superior trapezius* flap is used for reconstruction of the lateral neck and lower cheek.
  (a) It is based on paraspinous perforating branches of the intercostal vessels.
  (b) This flap is less inclined to pull away from the defect, but results in an unfavorable cosmetic deformity.

Latissimus Dorsi Flap
- Broad, thin muscle that may be transposed into the head and neck either subcutaneously or via a transaxillary approach
- Based on the thoracodorsal artery
- Used to reconstruct the lateral neck and scalp

- Disadvantages
  - (a) Need for decubitus positioning
  - (b) Unreliability
  - (c) Frequent donor site wound dehiscence

Sternocleidomastoid Flap

- Superiorly based flap used to buttress oral and pharyngeal suture lines
- Based on occipital artery
- Rotation limited by spinal accessory nerve's entry into anterior border of muscle
- Contraindicated in high-stage neck dissections

Other Muscle Flaps

- Superiorly based levator scapulae and posterior scalene flaps may be used as the sterno-cleidomastoid flap is used.
- Bipedicled or inferiorly pedicled strap muscle flaps survive via microvascular blood supply transmitted through their bony origins, and are used for reconstruction of partial laryngectomy defects.

Free Microneurovascular Tissue Transfer

Microneurovascular free tissue transfer is the reconstructive method that most closely replaces missing tissue with nearly identical tissues. The "free flap" is also to some extent free of the geometric limitations imposed by pedicles. The use of microneurovascular free tissue transfer in the past three decades has decreased the incidences of partial flap loss and dehiscences.

Characteristics of the Ideal Donor Site

- Long, large-caliber, anatomically consistent vascular pedicle
- Minimal donor site functional and aesthetic morbidity
- Simultaneous two-team approach
- Where applicable
  - (a) Provision for functional motor or sensate capability
  - (b) Secretory mucosa
  - (c) Bone stock capable of accepting osseointegrated implants

Preoperative Assessment

- A history of ischemic heart disease may preclude a prolonged operative time, and patients in need of cardiac revascularization should be considered candidates for shorter procedures.
- Previous treatment may affect the availability of recipient vessels, and these patients should be considered for preoperative head and neck angiography.
- Patients who do not have recipient vessels within the reach of the defect should be consented for vein grafts, or alternatively, an arteriovenous fistula may be formed in the neck using a saphenous or cephalic vein graft before the planned microvascular reconstruction.

Points of Technique

- The external jugular vein should be preserved when possible as a potential recipient vein or vein graft.
- Major arteries and veins that are to be sacrificed should be handled with care, and transected some distance from their takeoffs in order to leave a stump for anastomosis.
- Enteric, muscle, and bone-containing free flaps are the most sensitive to ischemia time.
- Complete dissection of the flap in situ, as well as preparation of the recipient vessels should be performed prior to pedicle transection in order to decrease ischemia time.

- Flap cooling with iced saline during the ischemia time reduces metabolic demand and extends available time prior to irreversible changes.
- Attention to detail in flap design and insetting (pedicle geometry, tension, and kinking) should minimize the risk of vascular compromise.

Avoiding Complications

- Most failures occur within 72 hours of revascularization, hence the need for vigilant monitoring.
- Vessel wall dissection, disruption, and suture puncture result in endothelial discontinuity and exposure of thrombogenic subendothelial collagen.
- This forms the basis for use of postoperative aspirin, low-molecular-weight dextran-40, and even heparin after revascularization.
- Restoration of endothelial continuity occurs over the ensuing 2 weeks.
- Perfusion is maintained through maintenance of normal blood pressures and euvolemia.
- Maintenance of normothermia will minimize peripheral vasoconstriction and sympathetic outflow which are deleterious to microvascular blood flow.

Fascial and Fasciocutaneous Flaps

Temporoparietal Fascia Free Flap

- The temporoparietal fascia, with or without overlying skin, may be transferred as a free flap based on the superficial temporal vessels.
- Harvest dimension of 17 × 14 cm can be achieved.
- Split calvarial bone may be harvested with this flap to create a composite flap.
- Applications:
  - (a) Reconstruction of oral mucosal defects, usually with a skin graft
  - (b) Reconstruction of facial contour defects
  - (c) Reconstruction of difficult orbital and temporal bone defects
  - (d) Reconstruction of hemilaryngectomy defects
- Disadvantages:
  - (a) Small-caliber donor vessels.
  - (b) Vein is superficial to the fascia, making it vulnerable during flap harvest.
  - (c) Risk of injury to the frontal branch of the facial nerve.
  - (d) Risk of alopecia.

Radial Forearm Free Flap

- Fascial or fasciocutaneous design based on the long, large-caliber radial vessels.
- Fasciocutaneous vessels are transmitted to the skin paddle via the lateral intermuscular (brachioradialis - flexor carpi ulnaris) septum.
- Sensate capabilities are provided by the lateral and medial antebrachial cutaneous nerves.
- Versatility, pliability, and dependability make this a workhorse flap with multiple applications.
- Simultaneous harvest without patient repositioning allows for two-team approach.
- Absence of a complete palmar arch precludes use of this flap, so a preoperative Allen's test must be performed to ascertain palmar arch integrity.
- Applications:
  - (a) Tongue reconstruction
  - (b) Floor of mouth reconstruction
  - (c) Palatal reconstruction
  - (d) Total lower lip reconstruction with suspension using palmaris longus tendon

      (e) Pharyngoesophageal reconstruction

      (f) Reconstruction of the cheek

      (g) Nasal reconstruction

      (h) Reconstruction of the skull base

- Disadvantage includes cosmetic deformity at donor site with fasciocutaneous flap harvest.

Lateral Arm Free Flap

- Fascial or fasciocutaneous design based on the posterior branches of the radial collateral vessels.
- Fasciocutaneous perforators are transferred to the skin through the lateral intermuscular (brachialis-brachioradialis-triceps) septum.
- Sensate capabilities are provided by the posterior cutaneous nerve of the forearm and the posterior cutaneous nerve of the arm.
- Transfer of a portion of the humerus (1×10 cm) has been described with this flap.
- Donor site may be closed primarily.
- Skin and subcutaneous tissues of the arm in this area are thicker and less pliable than the forearm.
- Skin in this area is the best color match for facial skin of all the free flaps.
- Pedicle entry in the center of this flap limits its applications.
- Applications:

      (a) Tongue reconstruction

      (b) Pharyngoesophageal reconstruction

      (c) Cheek reconstruction

- Disadvantages:

      (a) Cosmetic deformity at donor site.

      (b) Pedicle dissection is more difficult than that of the forearm flap.

      (c) Pedicle is shorter than that of the forearm flap.

      (d) Lateral arm numbness.

      (e) Elbow pain due to release of the triceps from the humerus.

Anterolateral Thigh Free Flap

- May be harvested as a fasciocutaneous, or musculofasciocutaneous flap including the vastus lateralis and based on the lateral circumflex femoral artery.
- Sensate capability provided by lateral femoral cutaneous nerve.
- Versatility allows for multiple skin and/or muscle paddles to be harvested for complex defects.
- Subcutaneous tissues may be trimmed to make the skin paddle(s) more pliable.
- Simultaneous harvest without patient repositioning allows for two-team approach.
- A large skin surface (the entire lateral thigh) may be harvested and then skin grafted.
- Relatively inconspicuous donor site.
- Applications:

      (a) Cheek reconstruction

      (b) Lower lip/chin complex reconstruction

      (c) Tongue reconstruction

      (d) Pharyngoesophageal reconstruction

- Disadvantage is variable pedicle anatomy.

Lateral Thigh Free Flap

- Fasciocutaneous design based on the septocutaneous perforators of the profunda femoris vessels.
- Sensate capability provided by lateral femoral cutaneous nerve.

- Simultaneous harvest without patient repositioning allows for two-team approach.
- Large surface area can be harvested (up to 25 × 14 cm or more).
- Relatively inconspicuous donor site can be closed primarily, but may be skin grafted.
- Flap is less pliable than forearm flap due to thicker subcutaneous tissue, but may be tubed.
- Applications are the same as those for the anterolateral thigh free flap.
- Disadvantages:
  - (a) Difficult pedicle dissection
  - (b) Variable pedicle anatomy
  - (c) Thickness of flap correlates with patient's body habitus
  - (d) Risk to nutrient artery of the femur, which is a branch of the second perforator of the profunda femoris

Muscular and Myocutaneous Flaps

Latissimus Dorsi Free Flap

- May be harvested as a muscle only or myocutaneous flap based on the thoracodorsal artery.
- The muscle component of this flap is broad and thin, making it a pliable flap that is easy to contour to defects.
- The thoracodorsal artery is a branch of the subscapular artery, so the latissimus dorsi may be harvested as part of a "superflap" based on the subscapular artery and incorporating the scapular and parascapular free flaps.
- Applications:
  - (a) Reconstruction of large scalp defects
  - (b) Reconstruction of cranio-orbital defects
  - (c) Cheek and maxillectomy reconstruction
  - (d) Lower lip/chin complex reconstruction
  - (e) Tongue reconstruction
  - (f) Pharyngoesophageal reconstruction
- Disadvantages:
  - (a) Need for decubitus positioning
  - (b) Frequent donor site wound dehiscence

Rectus Abdominus Free Flap

- May be harvested as a muscle only or myocutaneous flap based on the inferior epigastric vascular pedicle.
- May be designed in various orientations.
- Simultaneous harvest without patient repositioning allows for two-team approach.
- Relatively inconspicuous donor site.
- Flap is less pliable than forearm flap due to thicker subcutaneous tissue, but may be tubed.
- Applications:
  - (a) Skull base reconstruction
  - (b) Reconstruction of cranio-orbital defects
  - (c) Cheek and maxillary reconstruction
  - (d) Lower lip/chin complex reconstruction
  - (e) Tongue reconstruction
  - (f) Pharyngoesophageal reconstruction
- Disadvantages:
  - (a) Abdominal wall weakness resulting from muscle harvest is possible.
  - (b) Thickness of flap correlates with the patient's body habitus.

Gracilis free flap

- Muscle flap based on the terminal branch of the adductor artery, a branch of the profunda femoris.
- Motor capability provided by the anterior branch of the obturator nerve.
- Relatively inconspicuous donor site is closed primarily with minimal functional deficit.
- A skin paddle up to 10 x 25 cm can be transferred with this muscle, but the musculocutaneous perforators are variable and sometimes absent.
- Applications:
  - (a) Primary application is facial reanimation due to capacity for motor innervation.
  - (b) Folded flap may also be used for tongue reconstruction.
- Disadvantage is bulk of the flap.

Bone-Containing Free Flaps

Radial Forearm Free Flap

- This flap may include a monocortical segment of the radius up to 10 cm in length by incorporating a cuff of the flexor pollicis longus muscle.
- Immediate plating (load sharing) of the radial defect is required to allow faster return to function and decrease risk of pathologic fracture.
- The segment of bone that may be harvested with this flap is inadequate for osseointegrated implants.

Fibular Free Flap

- May be transferred as a bone-only or osseocutaneous flap based on the peroneal vessels.
- Skin component perfused by septocutaneous vessels transmitted via the posterior crural septum.
- Sensate capability provided by lateral sural cutaneous nerve.
- Considered a workhorse flap, it may be contoured without compromising vascularity.
- Simultaneous harvest without patient repositioning allows for two-team approach.
- Relatively inconspicuous donor site.
- Absence of anterior tibial vessels (peroneal arteria magna) or involvement of the anterior tibial vessels with severe atherosclerotic disease precludes the use of this flap, so preoperative angiography is necessary.
- Applications:
  - (a) Osseous component may be used to reconstruct an entire mandible.
  - (b) Maxillary and palatal reconstruction.
- Disadvantages:
  - (a) While placement of osseointegrated implants may be possible with this free flap, the small diameter of the fibula often warrants "double barreling" of the osseous component of the flap in order to achieve adequate bone height for implants. This shortens the pedicle and may compromise the skin perforators.
  - (b) The anatomy of the skin perforators is variable, and they are often not present.
  - (c) A STSG is occasionally needed to resurface the donor site in larger reconstructions.
  - (d) Transient ankle stiffness frequently occurs after flap harvest.

Iliac Crest Free Flap

- Composite flap consisting of skin, subcutaneous tissue, internal oblique muscle, and iliac crest is based on the deep circumflex iliac artery.
- Simultaneous harvest without patient repositioning allows for two-team approach.
- Relatively inconspicuous donor site.

- Applications:
  - (a) Oromandibular reconstruction
  - (b) Mandible/chin reconstruction
  - (c) Palatomaxillary reconstruction
- Disadvantages:
  - (a) Volume of tissue and lack of rotation of soft tissue component with respect to osseous component can make inset of this flap difficult.
  - (b) Significant donor site morbidities can include chronic pain and gait disturbance
  - (c) Risk of hernia.

Scapular Free Flaps

- The subscapular system of flaps is the most versatile donor site for composite tissue transfer and is based on the circumflex scapular artery, which is a branch of the subscapular artery.
- Separation of the soft tissue and bone flaps is possible, allowing the most freedom of rotation for three-dimensional insetting of any composite free flap.
- The latissimus dorsi and serratus anterior muscles with overlying skin and adjacent rib may be harvested with the subscapular flaps as one large "superflap" based on the subscapular artery for reconstruction of large, complex defects.
- The transversely oriented *scapular free flap* is based on the transverse cutaneous branch of the circumflex scapular artery.
- The vertically oriented *parascapular free flap* incorporates the lateral border of the scapula.
  - (a) Based on the descending branches of the circumflex scapular artery.
  - (b) A straight segment of bone 3 cm in width and up to 14 cm in length may be harvested.
- The tip of the scapula has a separate blood supply from the lateral border (angular branch of the thoracodorsal artery), and may be harvested as a separate bone-containing segment of the same flap to reconstruct bone defects that are separated in space.
- Relatively inconspicuous donor site.
- Applications:
  - (a) Oromandibular reconstruction
  - (b) Zygomaticofacial reconstruction
  - (c) Orbital reconstruction
  - (d) Palatomaxillary reconstruction
  - (e) Lower lip/chin complex reconstruction
- Disadvantages:
  - (a) Need for decubitus positioning
  - (b) Bone stock is thin and not adequate for osseointegrated implants
  - (c) Variable vascular anatomy
  - (d) Division of the teres major is necessary for pedicle dissection, and this may weaken the shoulder girdle
  - (e) Potential for brachial plexus injury

Visceral Free Flaps

Jejunal Free Flap

- May be transferred as a tubed interposition graft for segmental pharyngoesophageal reconstruction, or an open "patch graft" based on mesenteric arcade vessels.
- Transfers a secretary mucosal surface, which is useful in cases of previous irradiation.
- Flap must be inset isoperistaltically.

- A "sentinel loop" of "test intestine" may be developed and brought out through the neck incision for monitoring.
- Limited by the level at which it is safe to perform an anastomosis to the remaining esophagus (thoracic inlet) without a thoracotomy.
- Disadvantages:
  - (a) Need for laparotomy and enteric anastomosis.
  - (b) Two enteric anastomoses are needed in the neck.
  - (c) The risk of anastomotic stricture is high.
  - (d) Risk of intrathoracic anastomotic leak.
  - (e) A feeding jejunostomy is required.
  - (f) The mesenteric vessels are known for their friability and tendency toward intimal separation.
  - (g) Postoperative dysphagia caused by peristalsis that is not coordinated with native pharyngeal swallowing mechanism.
  - (h) Poor vocal result with tracheoesophageal puncture.
  - (i) Significant possible donor site morbidity (prolonged ileus, abdominal adhesions).

Omental Free Flap

- Based on the right gastroepiploic vessels, the omental free flap provides vascularized tissue that is ideal for infected or irradiated sites.
- This flap may be compartmentalized based on vascular arcades.
- Applications:
  - (a) Resurfacing of large scalp defects with an STSG
  - (b) Closure of pharyngocutaneous fistulae
  - (c) Treatment of osteoradionecrosis and osteomyelitis of the craniofacial skeleton
  - (d) Augmentation of facial soft tissue defects
- Disadvantages:
  - (a) Need for laparotomy
  - (b) Variation in length and width of the omentum
  - (c) Prior abdominal surgery or peritonitis causes significant scarring and contraction of the omentum, which usually makes it unsuitable for reconstructive use

Facial Reanimation

- Determining the best approach to management of facial reanimation is based on the following:
  - (a) An understanding of the cause of paralysis
  - (b) Site of lesion and
  - (c) Duration of paralysis
- With potentially reversible causes of facial nerve paralysis, such as Bell palsy, no procedure that interrupts continuity of the nerve should be done while a chance of recovery exists.
- If uncertainty as to the integrity of the nerve exists, for example in the case of temporal bone trauma, exploration is necessary.
- Traumatic and iatrogenic transections of the facial nerve should be repaired by neurorrhaphy, with or without interposition grafting, at the time of injury to optimize the chances of recovery (physiologic nerve repair).
  - (a) Interposition grafting is indicated when the distance between healthy cut ends of the nerve is 1 cm or more because excessive mobilization of the nerve leads to devascularization.

(b) In general, peripheral nerve injuries distal (medial) to the pupillary line are not repaired due to sufficient neural anastomoses in the midface.

- When planned resection of the nerve is necessary, strategies for reanimation should be anticipated and implemented at the time of resection, if possible.
- Long-standing cases of facial paralysis are characterized by collagenization and fibrosis of nerve tubules, which hampers axon regeneration. This process begins 3 months after denervation.
- Muscle atrophy occurs due to denervation, and is irreversible after 2-3 years.

Synergistic Nerve Crossover

- Indications:
  (a) Sufficient proximal motor input is lacking
  (b) Muscle atrophy has not yet occurred
  (c) One or more peripheral branches of the facial nerve is intact on the affected side
- Important to transect preexisting innervation, even if it does not produce movement, as innervated muscle fibers will not accept new innervation, even if existing axons are too dilute to produce movement.
- Connects nonessential buccal branches of contralateral nerve to paralyzed side with sural nerve graft.
- The more distal the branches used on the normal side, the less the fire power provided.
- The more proximal the branches used, the greater the donor deficit.
- Controversy exists as to the value of crossfacial grafting because of the limited number of axons available for reinnervation.
- This is commonly used as the first step in microsurgical reconstruction of facial paralysis (neuromuscular pedicle transfer).

Nerve Substitutions

- Indications are the same as those for synergistic nerve crossover.
- The most common substitution is the hypoglossal-facial substitution.
  (a) Contraindicated in patients with lower cranial nerve deficits due to negative impact on swallowing.
  (b) The XII nerve is transected just before it enters the tongue, transposed under the digastric, and sutured to the VIIth nerve main trunk.
  (c) Alternatively, the XIIth nerve is partially transected, and an interposition graft connects the transected portion of the XII nerve to the VIIth nerve, avoiding complete hemitongue denervation and atrophy (hypoglossal-facial jump graft).
  (d) Results:
    ○ Movement seen after 4 to 6 months.
    ○ Mass synkinesis occurs in 80% of patients.
    ○ Spontaneous, reflexive facial function rarely achieved.
    ○ 10% of patients develop animation with speech.
    ○ Excessive facial tone, hyperactivity, and/or spasm complicate 15% of cases.
- Masseteric nerve substitution:
  (a) Similar to the hypoglossal-facial substitution
    ○ Closer to ipsilateral facial nerve branches and can be sutured without need for interposition graft
    ○ Less morbidity than the hypoglossal-facial substitution

(a) May be used with an interposition graft for crossfacial nerve grafting as the first step in microsurgical reconstruction of facial paralysis (neuromuscular pedicle transfer)

(b) Used for reinnervation of neuromuscular transplants in patient with Moebius syndrome

- Other historic nerve substitutions:
  (a) Spinal accessory-facial substitution
  (b) Ansa hypoglossi-facial substitution

Neuromuscular Pedicle Transfer

- Indicated in cases where muscle atrophy may be present and/or extratemporal facial nerve is not intact.
- First step is crossfacial nerve grafting.
- After clinical evidence of arrival of nerve fibers to contralateral side (usually 1 year), the microsurgical transfer of a muscle with its motor nerve is performed with microvascular and microneural anastomoses.
- The muscle is inset from the zygomatic arch to the oral commissure on the affected side to reanimate the lower face.
- Possible muscle transfers.
  (a) Gracilis muscle with anterior branch of the obturator nerve
  (b) Serratus or latissimus dorsi muscle with the subscapular, long thoracic nerve
  (c) Pectoralis major muscle with the medial and lateral pectoral nerves
  (d) Pectoralis minor muscle with the medial and lateral pectoral nerves
  (e) Abductor hallucis with a branch of the medial plantar nerve
  (f) Internal oblique with intercostal and infracostal neurovascular pedicles
  (g) Adductor magnus muscle with posterior branch of the obturator nerve
  (h) Trapezius muscle with its branch of the spinal accessory nerve
  (i) Inferior rectus abdominus
  (j) Short head of the biceps femoris
  (k) Extensor digitorum brevis
- Volitional movement and symmetric emotive firing of the reanimated hemiface can be achieved.
- Disadvantages:
  (a) Need for multiple stages.
  (b) Ancillary procedures are needed for upper facial reanimation.

Muscle Transposition

- Indications are the same as those for neuromuscular pedicle transfer.
- Also indicated in patients who cannot or choose not to undergo neuromuscular pedicle transfer.
- The central third of the temporalis muscle is inset to the oral commissure to reanimate the lower face.
- Results:
  (a) Elevation of the oral commissure occurs in most patients.
  (b) Emotional movement occurs in only 10%.
  (c) Results may be enhanced by motor-sensory reeducation techniques.
  (d) As with neuromuscular pedicle transfer, ancillary procedures are needed for upper facial reanimation.

Static Procedures

Although considered ancillary, static procedures are useful adjuncts in the management of facial paralysis, particularly in the upper face.

Static Slings
- Indications are the same as those for muscle transposition.
- Provide elevation of the oral commissure without volitional movement.
- Common materials used:
  (a) Temporalis fascia
  (b) Fascia lata
  (c) Acellular dermal allograft

Eyelid Procedures
- *Browlifting* may be indicated to correct obstruction of visual field deficits and restore resting symmetry of the upper face.
- *Upper eyelid implants* use gravity to effect eye closure.
- *Canthoplasty* procedures elevate lax lower eyelids to improve eye closure.
- *Tarsorrhaphy* may be indicated in severe cases of eyelid denervation when more conservative approaches are inadequate in preventing drying of the cornea.

Lip Reconstruction

- The goals of perioral reconstruction are the following:
  (a) Oral competency
  (b) Adequate oral access
  (c) Mobility
  (d) Normal anatomical proportions
- When all goals cannot be achieved, the first two take precedent.
- Because most lip cancers start in the mucosa, early cutaneous malignancies can usually be managed with excision and local mucosal advancement flaps.
- Partial-thickness skin defects can be managed with primary closure, skin grafts, or a number of local flaps as previously described.
- The remainder of the section will concern itself with management of full-thickness defects of the lips.

Upper Lip

Defects not Involving the Philtrum
- *Defects of less than ¼ of the lip width* can be closed primarily.
- *Defects of ¼-⅓ of the lip width* can be closed with unilateral perialar crescenteric advancement.
- *Defects involving the entire lateral subunit, but not the oral commissure,* can be corrected using an Abbe flap.
- *Defects involving the entire lateral subunit and the oral commissure* can be corrected with an Estlander flap.

Defects Involving the Philtrum
- *Central defects involving the philtrum only* can be repaired with primary closure, or more aesthetically appropriate, an Abbe flap.
- *Defects of less than ¾ of the lip width.*

(a) Bilateral perialar crescentic advancement flaps with an Abbe flap for central subunit reconstruction

(b) Bilateral Karapandzic flaps with or without an Abbe flap for central subunit reconstruction

- *Defects ⅔ to total lip width.*

(a) Bilateral full-thickness melolabial flaps with or without an Abbe flap for central subunit reconstruction if there is adequate cheek skin laxity

(b) If cheek skin laxity is inadequate,
  ○ Bilateral Karapandzic flaps with or without an Abbe flap for central subunit reconstruction
  ○ Microvascular free tissue transfer

Lower Lip

- *Defects ¼-⅓ of the lip width* can be closed primarily.
- *Defects ⅓-½ of the lip width.*
  (a) Bilateral full-thickness advancement flaps
  (b) If not involving the oral commissure, an Abbe flap can be used
  (c) If involving the oral commissure, an Estlander flap is indicated
- *Defects ½-⅔ of lip width* can be addressed with bilateral Karapandzic flaps.
- *Defects ⅔ to total lip width.*
  (a) Bernard—von Burow or Giles fan flaps
  (b) Microvascular free tissue transfer

Prosthetic Reconstruction

Prosthetic reconstruction complements surgical techniques in cases of amputation (eg, traumatic auricular avulsion), or in major facial defects resulting from ballistic and other injuries, or from major facial resections for neoplasms or invasive infections. Osseointegrated implants typically form the anchor for facial prostheses including those used for dental rehabilitation. Because these implants require good bone stock for stability, the importance of providing a platform for osseointegrated implants, even by free tissue transfer if necessary, cannot be overstated. Other requirements include healthy soft tissue around the implant posts, and therefore an implant site with soft tissue that is thin enough that the posts do not become buried, but robust enough to prevent exposure of the abutments. This may require thinning of subcutaneous tissues over the abutments. Patient compliance with care of the implants is necessary to prevent infection. In addition to auricular prostheses, craniofacial implants are used to improve cosmesis in patients with orbital and nasal defects, often using eyeglasses as a camouflage.

Composite Facial Allotransplantation

Composite facial allotransplantation offers an opportunity for restoration of appearance and function for patients with severe disfigurement when other reconstructive options have failed or are limited. Cosmetic results are immediate, but there is a paucity of data on functional outcomes. Facial transplants have been well-accepted by most patients despite ethical concerns regarding issues of identity. Early acute rejection has been reported in several cases of facial transplantation, though it is too early to determine if chronic rejection and graft-versus-host disease will be significant problems with this method of facial reconstruction. Opportunistic infections and lymphoproliferative disorders resulting from immunosuppression have been reported following facial allotransplantation with some fatalities. Reluctance to consent to donation by patient families has limited the availability of facial allotransplants. Contingency plans for autologous coverage or repeat transplantation in cases of facial allotransplantation failure may be difficult or impossible. Facial allotransplantation is still considered experimental, and the issues surrounding this method of facial reconstruction include the need for lifelong immunosuppression, patient selection, donor and recipient confidentiality, and cost to society. Functional outcome studies on facial allotransplantation will inform the risk to benefit ratio of these procedures.

Future Trends

Prefabrication of a vascularized mandibular segment using regenerative medicine approaches has been demonstrated, and is a logical extension of current microsurgical techniques. Ongoing advances in tissue engineering of osseous, adipose, cartilaginous, and neural tissues hold promise for development of customized replacement tissues that can be transferred with little to no donor site morbidity. These developments, along with the recent successes of facial and laryngeal allotransplantation, forecast an exciting new era in head and neck reconstructive surgery.

Bibliography

Bascom DA, Schaitkin BM, May M, Klein S. Facial nerve repair: a retrospective review. *Facial Plast Surg.* 2000;16(4):309-313.

Coffman KL, Siemionow MZ. Ethics of facial transplantation revisited. *Curr Opin Organ Transplant.* 2014;19:181-187.

Delacure MD. Reconstructive head and neck surgery. In: Lee KJ, ed. *Essential Otolaryngology.* 9th ed. New York, NY: McGraw-Hill; 2008:740-754:chap. 29.

Jiang H, Pan B, Lin L, Zhao Y, Guo D, Zhuang H. Fabrication of three-dimensional cartilaginous framework in auricular reconstruction. *J Plast Reconstr Aesthet Surg.* 2008;61(Suppl 1):S77-S85.

Sherris DA, Larrabee WA, Jr. *Principles of Facial Reconstruction.* New York, NY: Thieme; 2010.

Shindo M. Facial reanimation with microneurovascular free flaps. *Facial Plast Surg.* 2000;16(4):357-359.

Urken ML. *Multidisciplinary Head and Neck Reconstruction: A Defect-Oriented Approach.* New York, NY: Lippincott, Williams and Wilkins; 2010.

Urken ML, Cheney ML, Sullivan MJ, Biller HJ. *Atlas of Regional and Free Flaps for Head and Neck Reconstruction.* New York, NY: Raven Press; 1995.

Warnke PH, Springer IN, Wiltfang J, et al. Growth and transplantation of a custom vascularised bone graft in a man. *Lancet.* 2004;364(9463):766-770.

Windfuhr JP, Chen YS, Güldner C, Neukirch D. Rib cartilage harvest in rhinoplasty procedures based on CT radiological data. *Acta Otolaryngol.* 2011;131(1):67-71.

Yoleri L, Mavioğlu H. Total tongue reconstruction with free functional gracilis muscle transplantation: a technical note and review of the literature. *Ann Plast Surg.* 2000;45(2):181-186.

Questions

1. All of the following are true regarding the pectoralis major myocutaneous flap except
    A. it is based on a branch of the thoracoacromial artery
    B. transposition of the flap is limited by the arc of rotation of the pedicle over the clavicle
    C. it can be used to reconstruct scalp defects
    D. the most distal aspect of the skin paddle is the most poorly perfused
    E. gravity may cause superior dehiscence of the flap

2. Synergistic nerve crossover
    A. is the first step in microsurgical reconstruction of facial paralysis
    B. is performed before transection of pre-existing innervation
    C. is used when there is sufficient proximal motor input
    D. connects the marginal mandibular branches of the contralateral nerve to the paralyzed side with a sural nerve graft
    E. cannot be used if there are other lower cranial nerve deficits

3. Which of the following statements about skin grafts is incorrect?
    A. They heal well over the fat, muscle, perichondrium, and fascia.
    B. They depend on formation of a hematoma for survival.
    C. They require immobilization and avoidance of shear to take.
    D. The thinner the graft, the greater the risk of contracture.
    E. Meshed grafts can be used to cover large scalp defects.

4. The scapular system of free flaps
    A. provides good bone stock for osseointegrated implants
    B. may be harvested with two separate bone-containing segments to reconstruct bone defects that are separated in space
    C. has the least freedom of rotation of the soft tissue component with respect to the osseous component of all the bone-containing free flaps
    D. does not require decubitus positioning for harvest through a transaxillary approach
    E. is based on the thoracodorsal artery

5. A full-thickness defect of the upper lip not involving the philtrum, and measuring <¼ of the lip width should be closed
    A. with a perialar crescenteric flap
    B. with perialar crescentic flaps combined with an Abbe flap
    C. with an Estlander flap
    D. with a Karapandzic flap
    E. primarily

Chapter 50
Craniomaxillofacial Trauma

Causes

- Facial injuries can vary from the most minor laceration to the most severe disruption of the face, as seen in shotgun blasts.
- Often described as blunt or penetrating and by the amount of energy.
- Low-impact (so-called "low energy") injuries are often due to falls and fights.
- Moderate-energy injuries are often due to low-velocity vehicular trauma, falls from moderate height, and interpersonal trauma that involves a blunt weapon.
- High-energy injuries are often due to high-speed vehicular trauma and recreational vehicles, industrial accidents, and falls from height.
- Penetrating injuries are often due to gunshots and can vary from small holes and limited damage to areas of destruction and major tissue loss.
- Management depends on the nature of the injury.

Anatomy

- The face includes an underlying bony skeletal support structure with a very complicated three-dimensional (3D) structure.
- Skeleton provides facial shape (important for both function and cosmesis).
- Skeleton also provides support and protection for viscera (eyes, brain, etc).
- The paranasal sinuses are mucosal-lined cavities within the facial skeleton. These may lighten the face/head, and also serve as a protective "crumple zone" for the nearby viscera.
- The upper and lower jaws contain teeth, which are important for chopping food for both swallowing and digestion.
- The lower jaw is mobile and is suspended from the cranium by the two temporomandibular joints.
- The bony skeleton is covered by soft tissues of various thicknesses, including the periosteum, muscles, fat, and skin.
- Viscera of the facial area include the brain, eyes, oral structures, major and minor salivary glands, as well as nerves, blood vessels, and lymphatics.
- Facial injuries may affect any of the aforementioned structures. Familiarity with normal anatomy is the key to being able to reestablish it after it has been disrupted by an injury.
- Visceral injuries are managed to reestablish function.

- Soft tissue repair is done to reestablish covering and to minimize the visibility of any scars. Acute repair may require the use of local or other flaps or grafts.
- Facial nerve injuries should be identified early, and if there is a peripheral nerve injury, exploration and repair at the earliest opportunity should be considered.
- Similarly, injuries to main salivary ducts should be explored and repaired.
- The focus is on the craniomaxillofacial (CMF) skeleton.
- For purposes of this chapter, the CMF skeleton is divided into three areas: upper third, middle third, lower third.
  - (a) Upper third includes the forehead, including the frontal bones, supraorbital rims, and glabella.
  - (b) Middle third includes the zygomas, maxillae, nasal bones, and orbits, and it can include the vertical rami of the mandible.
  - (c) Lower third is composed of the mandible, generally anterior to the vertical rami.
  - (d) The nasal septum is a midline structure in both the middle and lower thirds.

Diagnosis

- In any trauma setting, we must assess ABCs first.
- Always consider cervical spine injury.
- Always assess neurological status and obtain consultation as indicated.
  - (a) Clinical
  - (b) Observation
    - Soft tissue tears, loss.
    - Swelling.
    - Bleeding.
    - Look for and account for missing teeth (may have been aspirated or swallowed).
    - Look for evidence of ocular injury.
    - Assess occlusion (the relationship between the maxillary and mandibular dentition).
  - (c) Palpation
    - Bony step-offs
    - Mobility of bony fragments
    - Midface mobility (indicates disarticulation of the tooth-bearing segment of the maxillae from the more solid bone above)
  - (d) Information from patient (when possible)
    - Assess sensory nerve function (trigeminal: V1, V2, V3).
    - Assess motor nerve function (extraocular movement: cranial nerves [CN] III, IV, VI; facial movement: CN VII; tongue movement: CN XII).
    - Assess special senses including vision and hearing (smell may be affected by swelling and bleeding so more difficult to assess, and taste is not generally assessed in the setting of acute trauma).
  - (e) Radiological
    - Plain x-rays are rarely used today (unless CT is not available).
    - Computed tomography (CT) scanning should be performed and viewed in three planes (axial, coronal, sagittal). (3D reconstructions help the clinician form a conception of the injuries, but they are less precise and therefore are not a replacement.)
    - Axial CT is best for vertical structures, for example, the medial orbital walls, pterygoid plates.

- Coronal CT is best for horizontal structures, for example, the orbital floors and anterior and posterior walls of the frontal sinuses.
- Sagittal CT is best for viewing the orbital floor; note that if done at the angle of the orbital plane, it may better demonstrate the status of the optic canal.
- For mandible fractures, orthopantomograms (note that the term "Panorex" refers to a company name) are frequently used. These are 2D panoramic tomograms of the entire mandible that are generally inexpensive and easily accessible.

Fracture Classification

- Upper third
  - (a) Frontal sinus
    - Anterior wall
    - Posterior wall
    - Floor (includes the sinus outflow tract)
  - (b) Superior orbital rims
- Middle third
  - (a) Includes separation of the maxillary alveoli containing the teeth from the more solid bone above
    - Le Fort I extends across the maxillae and nasal septum and pterygoid plates at a level just above the maxillary alveoli.
    - Le Fort II or pyramidal fracture extends from the lateral maxillae above the alveoli more superiorly toward the orbit, then crosses the inferior and medial orbit and crosses the midline at or below the frontonasal junction, still crossing the nasal septum and pterygoid plates.
    - Le Fort III traverses the orbits from medial to lateral and completes the separation laterally by crossing the zygomatic arches. Like the Le Fort II, it separates the nose from the skull at the frontonasal junction. It also crosses the nasal septum and pterygoid plates, thereby creating a complete craniofacial dysjunction.
  - (b) Naso-orbital-ethmoid (NOE) (also known as the nasoethmoid complex [NEC])
    - Direct trauma to the nasal root which separates from the frontal bone and is telescoped posteriorly between the orbits. The maxillary, lacrimal, and ethmoid portions of the medial orbits are typically involved.
    - Loss of medial attachment of medial canthal ligament(s) allows lateral displacement.
    - Causes telecanthus, that is, telescoping laterally of the medial canthus.
    - Appearance of hypertelorism—called pseudohypertelorism.
  - (c) Orbital fractures
    - Orbital floor most common.
      - Entrapment of inferior rectus leads to limitation of extraocular movement (mainly up gaze, though can be both up and down and even all directions).
      - White-eyed fracture in children often associated with vagal reflex symptoms of nausea and vomiting.
      - May be due to direct globe trauma and/or trauma to the inferior orbital rim.
    - Medial wall also common, but easily missed.
    - Superior and lateral walls less frequent.
    - Enlargement of orbital volume can lead to enophthalmos—sinking in of the globe.
    - Loss of floor support can create hypophthalmos (inferior displacement of the globe).
    - Also associated with zygomatic fractures (see the following text).

    (d) Zygomatic fractures
- Zygoma typically separates from attachments to the frontal bone, temporal bone, maxilla, and sphenoid bone.
- Can be pushed in, rotated laterally or rotated medially.
- Less frequently rotated inferiorly.
- Involves medial and inferior walls of the orbit.
- Can rotate into the orbit and compress the orbital structures, typically causing proptosis (exophthalmos), or more rarely, compression of the orbital apex.
- Compression of the orbital apex can cause superior orbital fissure syndrome (involving CN III, IV, V_1, VI, and the sympathetics) or orbital apex syndrome (which adds compression of the optic nerve)—these are surgical emergencies.

    (e) Nasal and septal fractures
- Can be displaced or nondisplaced.
- Must assess for septal hematoma and manage if present—untreated may lead to loss of septal support and saddle nose deformity.
- Loss of support of the upper lateral cartilages is common and may lead to internal valve stenosis and nasal obstruction.

- Lower third

    (a) Mandible fractures
- Symphyseal fractures involve the body of the mandible between the mental foramina (some people call the midline the symphysis and anything off the midline parasymphyseal).
- Body fractures involve the mandible between the mental foramina and the angle.
- Angle fractures typically extend from the region of the posterior body posterior to or through the region of the third molar, so that they occur behind the dentition.
  - Dentition is therefore not available to assist with stabilization of the fracture.
- If the posterior edge of the fracture is behind the angle of the mandible, it is in the ramus.
- Fractures that traverse the sigmoid notch (between the coronoid and condylar segments) and exit the posterior mandible behind the angle are subcondylar fractures.
- If they exit anterior to the angle, they are vertical ramus fractures.
- If they extend anteriorly from the notch, they are coronoid fractures.
- If they traverse the ramus horizontally, they are horizontal ramus fractures.
- Patients with teeth are dentulous; those without teeth are edentulous. The presence or absence of teeth (as well as their quality) has significant implications for fracture repair.
- Over time, the edentulous mandible atrophies from the top down, leaving the bone thin and atrophic and both vulnerable to fracture and difficult to repair.
- Alveolar fractures involve the tooth bearing segments and separate them from the remainder of the mandible.

Management

- Upper third
  (a) Frontal fractures involve the frontal bones.
  (b) Fractures that do not traverse the frontal sinus(es) are cranial vault fractures.

(c) Fractures involving only the anterior wall of the frontal sinus(es) do not affect sinus function and therefore are cosmetic concerns only.

- Not all displaced anterior wall fractures will lead to a deformity.
- Fracture may be repaired to avoid deformity or if deformity is present, or a depression may be covered with an implant to correct any deformity (camouflage).
- Major fractures are generally opened and repaired.
- If camouflage is chosen, the surgeon and patient can wait to see if a significant deformity is going to develop before deciding if repair is indicated.
- Small fractures with overlying lacerations can be repaired using the laceration (uncommon).
- Larger fractures or if no laceration is present, a coronal approach is generally utilized to avoid scarring on the forehead (the brow or gull wing incision is rarely used today due to the likelihood of unsightly scarring as well as injury to the supraorbital and supratrochlear nerves).
- Repair involves the use of small plates or mesh screwed in place so as to hold the bones in position and reestablish the proper contour of the forehead.

(d) Fractures involving the posterior wall of the frontal sinus(es) indicate a risk of dural tear and/or intracranial injury.

- If the fracture is nondisplaced and the sinus is fully aerated and clear on CT, exploration is not required.
- If the fracture is displaced and/or there is density in the sinus, cerebrospinal fluid (CSF) leak cannot be ruled out, or worse, plugging of the defect with brain similarly cannot be ruled out, and some form of exploration is necessary.
  - Exploration may include open procedure (by osteoplastic bone flap or other means) or an endoscopic procedure.
- When the posterior wall of the frontal sinus(es) is disrupted, some form of obliteration of the sinus should be considered. This requires complete removal of all mucosa followed by obliteration of the frontal sinus outflow tracts.
  - If the back wall remains, the sinus is generally filled with some obliteration material, typically cancellous bone or abdominal fat.
  - If the back wall is shattered, cranialization of the sinus (complete removal of the back wall) may be considered.
  - Obliteration is supposed to create a "safe sinus"; however, this is not guaranteed, and meningitis and brain abscess have been reported after frontal sinus obliteration.
- Damage to the floor of the frontal sinus implies injury to the frontal sinus outflow tract.
  - If the back wall is disrupted, obliteration is the current standard of care.
  - If the back wall is in position, if the patient is likely to cooperate with careful follow-up, observation, and management of the frontal sinus expectantly may be considered. Note that this approach requires careful follow-up and a low threshold for intervention if the sinus remains cloudy or sinusitis develops. Otherwise, obliteration should be carried out.
- Supraorbital rim fractures will often create step-offs that require reduction.
  - The sensory nerves of V_1 may be compressed and may therefore require decompression.
  - These may extend along the orbital roof.

- Middle third
  - (a) Orbital fractures may involve any of the four orbital walls.
    - ○ Orbital roof fractures rarely require repair, and these may require intracranial repair.
    - ○ Medial wall, lateral wall, and floor fractures are repaired to restore the correct orbital volume and correct/prevent enophthalmos or exophthalmos as well as to relieve any entrapment of the extraocular muscles and correct diplopia and/or limitation of eye movement.
    - ○ Entrapment requires release of any tissue trapped in the fracture—if it is a crack in the bone, a small implant or even a piece of fascia or cartilage or Gelfilm may adequately resolve the problem and prevent recurrence.
    - ○ Defects must be repaired with implants or grafts to restore both orbital contour and volume.
    - ○ The medial wall may be approached via transcutaneous ortranscaruncular (through orbital mucosa) approach or transnasally using an endoscopic approach.
      - – A transnasal approach allows repair with an implant or through stenting of the medial wall.
    - ○ The orbital floor may be approached via a transcutaneous approach through the lower lid or a transconjunctival approach through the lower lid. It may also be approached through the maxillary sinus or the nose using endoscopes, though this is more controversial.
      - – A transcutaneous or transconjunctival approach allows for a wider variety of implants, including implants with titanium which shows up on a post-op CT.
      - – A transconjunctival incision may be made preseptal or postseptal. Both are used.
      - – When an orbital fracture occurs along with other midfacial fractures (eg, zygomatic, Le Fort), it is generally best to repair other fractures before attending to the orbital walls.
  - (b) Zygomatic fractures:
    - ○ The key to reduction in zygomatic fractures is to remember that it has complex 3D anatomy and must be repositioned properly in all three dimensions.
      - – Align the zygomaticomaxillary area when possible (sometimes this is impossible due to comminution) via a gingivobuccal sulcus exposure.
        - ◊ For simple fractures, rigid fixation with plates in this area after proper reduction may be adequate.
        - ◊ Use small (mini, not micro) plates and screws and ensure at least two or three screws in each side of the fracture, taking care to avoid injury to the infraorbital nerve.
      - – If necessary, reduction and fixation may be carried out along the infraorbital rim and the frontozygomatic region.
        - ◊ Infraorbital rim may be reached via the gingivobuccal sulcus incision, but this puts the infraorbital nerve at risk. Generally reached via a lower lid incision.
        - ◊ Infraorbital rim should be repaired using microplates or wires, since fixation of the skin to the plate may lead to lid malposition.
        - ◊ Frontozygomatic fracture may be reached via an upper lid crease incision or an infra or supra brow incision (incision generally should not violate the brow, as the scar may separate the hair and be more visible).
        - ◊ When coronal incision has been used, the frontozygomatic region is reached via this approach.

- When 3D repositioning of the zygoma in space is difficult due to comminution, the zygomaticosphenoid suture is exposed inside the lateral orbit and used to assist with reduction. Generally exposure is enough to ensure position, though, occasionally, this suture may be plated inside the orbit.
- When comminution is severe, exposure of the zygomatic arch via a coronal incision will allow direct repositioning and repair of the arch.
  ◊ Generally done with wires or microplates
  ◊ Critical to ensure proper reconstruction of the arch—note that it is usually not a true arch, but rather has a straight portion anteriorly and becomes an arch posteriorly

(c) Zygomatic arch fractures:
  ○ Generally repaired percutaneously.
  ○ Rarely require fixation.
  ○ An instrument is advanced under the arch and is used to lift the arch into position, where it typically stays.
    - Gillies' approach is performed from above.
      ◊ Incision within the temporal hair.
      ◊ Taken through the temporalis fascia.
      ◊ Elevation between the fascia and muscle allows access to the arch medially since the fascia inserts on the arch and the muscle continues to the coronoid process of the mandible.
    - Keen approach is performed via an intraoral incision in the gingivobuccal sulcus elevated up to and under the zygoma and then advanced posteriorly along the medial zygomatic arch.
    - For severe comminution requiring open repair, a coronal approach is typically used (quite uncommon in the absence of more complex fractures).

(d) Le Fort fractures:
  ○ For all fractures involving the bone that supports dentition, a means of ensuring reestablishment of proper occlusion is key and, in fact, supersedes precise repositioning of all bone fragments.
    - Various means of fixing occlusion are used.
    - Most common technique employs Erich arch bars, which are stainless steel bars with hooks for attaching wires or rubber bands.
      ◊ These are fixed to the teeth using wires.
    - Modern arch bars may be screwed to the bone of the maxillae and mandible.
    - Teeth may be wired directly (Ernst ligatures, Ivy loops).
    - Screws with eyes or slots may be screwed into the bone of the maxillae and mandible.
  ○ Le Fort I.
    - After occlusion is established, the bones may be in proper anatomic position.
      ◊ If not, they are reduced and rigid fixation may be applied using small (1.5-2.0 mm) plates and screws.
      ◊ Once rigid fixation has been properly applied, the surgeon may decide to remove the appliance used to establish occlusion.
  ○ Le Fort II.
    - Similar to Le Fort I, except that fixation is performed at a higher level due to the more superior position of the fractures.
    - Since the fracture crosses the orbital floors, decision needs to be made as to whether or not orbital exploration is indicated.

- There is a tendency for the fracture to rotate superiorly at the nasofrontal junction, which can lead to an open bite deformity of the occlusion.
  - ◊ Maxilla-mandibular fixation (MMF) may appear to compensate for this, but the mandible may be pulled forward and superiorly at the joints, thereby giving the false appearance of proper reduction—great care must be exercised to ensure that the maxillae have been properly reduced.
  - ◊ If the maxillae are impacted, Rowe disimpaction forceps or a wire through the nasal root may be necessary to ensure that proper reduction is accomplished prior to placing any rigid fixation appliances.
- Like Le Fort I, MMF is applied prior to fixation.
- Fixation of the fractures with small (1.5-2.0 mm, not micro) plates ensuring at least two to three screws on each side of each fracture is performed.
- Fixation along the infraorbital rim may be used if needed—again, micro plates are best in this area to avoid visibility and palpability in the lower lid region.
- Fixation may be applied if needed and if exposure has been performed at the nasofrontal junction.

- Le Fort III.
  - Pure Le Fort III fractures are rare, and these often represent a mixture of Le Fort II level fractures with zygomatic fractures, as well as other fractures that may be present; some consider the nomenclature confusing.
  - This is a more complex series of fractures and typically requires multiple surgical exposures for repair.
  - Coronal approach to the frontozygomatic and nasofrontal areas commonly utilized.
  - Also provides access to the zygomatic arches if needed.
  - Allows access to the NOE region if needed.
  - Exposure of the orbital floors and/or medial orbits may be needed as well.
  - Since pure Le Fort III fractures are uncommon, it is likely that a gingivobuccal sulcus incision will be required to repair any lower maxillary fractures present along with the Le Fort III craniofacial separation which will be present superiorly.
  - In a true classic Le Fort III, the zygomas remain attached to the maxillae, so that repair of the frontozygomatic areas, the nasofrontal area, and the zygomatic arches (as needed) will result in complete stability.
  - Occlusion is established first.
  - Disimpaction is performed if needed.
  - In the more common mixed fractures, repair is generally recommended going from the stable to the unstable. Thus repair of all areas where the mobile facial skeleton is separated from the nonmobile cranial skeleton should be performed first. Fixation is then continued from the top down, completing the repair at the Le Fort I level. If facial symmetry and occlusion have been established and there is a minor bony discrepancy persisting at the Le Fort I level, this may be disregarded. Ellis has even recommended fracturing at the Le Fort I level if symmetry has been established above and there is occlusal discrepancy present at this final point of the procedure.

- NOE/NEC fractures.
  - Can be easily missed since telecanthus may be absent or minor initially, but may progress later to a significant facial deformity.

- Important to recognize and repair, since delayed repair is much more difficult and frequently leads to unsatisfactory outcomes.
- In addition to telecanthus, there is often a loss of nasal dorsal height.
- If loss of nasal dorsal height occurs, this must be repaired or a bone graft should be placed.
- In addition to telecanthus, an epicanthal fold may develop—the risk of this is lessened by reestablishing proper nasal dorsal height.
- NOE fractures have been classified as types 1, 2, and 3, depending on the status of the medial canthal ligament and its bony attachment.
    ◊ Type 1
        * The ligament is fixed to a moderately large fragment.
        * This can be repaired by properly stabilizing this fragment to solid surrounding bone.
    ◊ Type 2
        * The ligament remains attached to bone, but the fragment is too small to be stabilized with rigid fixation techniques.
        * Repair requires transcanthal (transnasal) fixation with either wire or permanent suture.
        * The bone fragment(s) may be included, or the ligament may be freed converting it into a type 3 and fixed directly transnasally.
    ◊ Type 3
        * The ligament is completely disrupted and no longer attached to the bone.
        * Requires repair by fixing the ligament across the nose to the opposite side.
    ◊ For both types 2 and 3, it is critical to properly reposition the ligament posteriorly, medially, and superiorly, as the natural tendency of the ligament is to move anteriorly, laterally, and inferiorly when left unattached. This is the key to proper repair.
    ◊ When the medal anterior orbit is deficient, repair is best performed by first bone grafting the medial orbital wall defect.
    ◊ A drill hole in the graft will allow proper placement of the transcanthal/transnasal repair.
  ○ Nasal fractures.
    - Nasal fractures may be repaired using open reduction (essentially an acute rhinoplasty), closed reduction and delayed repair (delayed rhinoplasty).
    - Septal hematomas must be drained acutely to avoid abscess and loss of the cartilaginous septum with resultant development of a saddle nose deformity.
        ◊ Closed reduction is done by analyzing the deformity and attempting to correct it by manipulating the bones into their native position manually using instruments.
            * If the entire dorsum is shifted, it is important to lift the nasal bones prior to moving them laterally.
        ◊ Open reduction is essentially an acute (septo)rhinoplasty.
            * Some surgeons advocate this, while others suggest that it may lead to unplanned fractures if osteotomies are attempted.
        ◊ In the absence of septal hematoma, delayed intervention may be considered.
            * Most surgeons recommend waiting at least 6 months for healing of the bones to proceed before osteotomies are attempted.
            * A formal (septo)rhinoplasty is then carried out.

- Lower third
  - (a) The lower third is essentially the mandible.
    - ○ In the dentate patient, most, if not all, fractures through the tooth-bearing bone will be compound (open into the mouth) and therefore contaminated—the use of prophylactic antibiotics is therefore advocated by most surgeons from the time of the fracture until the time of repair.
    - ○ Fractures behind the dentition in dentate patients, and most fractures in edentulous patients will be closed.
  - (b) Mandible fracture repair is different from repair of fractures of the middle and upper thirds of the face in that the mandible is a weight-bearing bone. The forces of mastication are such that there are large forces of compression and distraction acting on the bone during function.
    - ○ Like the maxillae, the mandible has the teeth.
    - ○ Occlusion must be reestablished.
    - ○ Arch bars are the most common means of establishing and maintaining the correct occlusal relationships (though other means may be used; see the preceding text).
    - ○ Once occlusion has been established, the key to stabilization of mandible fractures is to apply fixation so that the forces of distraction during function are overcome and may even be converted into compressive forces.
      - – Since teeth are only in the superior border of the mandible, the forces of mastication are transmitted downward along the teeth where chewing is taking place.
      - – When the bolus being chewed is at a distance from a fracture, it tends to distract the alveolar portion of the fracture and compress the inferior border.
      - – When the bolus is chewed in the area of the fracture, it would likely lead to compression of the alveolar border and distraction of the inferior border.
        - ◊ This is much less likely due to pain and splinting that tend to occur at the fracture site.
      - – Therefore, most distracting forces in function will be at the alveolar (superior or dental) border, and the compressive forces will generally be inferior.
      - – Therefore, overcoming the distracting forces along the alveolar border will generally lead to healing.
      - – Means of accomplishing this:
        - ◊ A well-applied arch bar can control the distracting forces along the alveolar border.
        - ◊ A mini-plate (1.5-2.0 mm, locking or nonlocking) below the dental roots will generally prevent distraction along the alveolar border and distribute the inferior border compressive forces along the length of the fracture.
          - * Since this is close to the tooth roots and the inferior alveolar nerve, only monocortical screws can be used.
        - ◊ A mandibular reconstruction plate (MRP) (typically ≥ 2.0 mm) placed bicortically along the inferior border with at least three or preferably four screws in each side will generally stabilize the bones and overcome all distraction forces.
        - ◊ For fractures of the mandibular body from angle to angle, monocortical mini-plates may be used along the so-called "ideal line of osteosynthesis."
          - * This sits below the tooth roots from third molar to third molar, with two plates required in the symphyseal region.

* At the angle, the plate is placed along the oblique line from the lingual side of the proximal (ramus) fragment to the buccal side of the distal (body) fragment.
◊ Fractures of the ramus are generally bridged with one or two mini-plates.
◊ Subcondylar fractures may be treated closed with elastic MMF to train the occlusion, which is preferred to rigid MMF.
  * Note that this is a form of "forced adaptation" of the occlusion, since this does not reduce the fracture.
◊ Open reduction of subcondylar fractures may be performed transorally or from an external approach.
  * The transoral approach is often done using endoscopic assistance.
  * The external approach may be done from below using a submandibular (Risdon) incision, retromandibular (transparotid) approach, or using a preauricular approach which requires facial nerve dissection.
  * The amount of fixation required remains controversial, though two mini-plates or as single larger plate seem to be preferred.
◊ For overlapping fragments, the use of lag screws is important to fix the fragments together without distracting them.
  * Lag screws may also be used across the midline due to its curvature to stabilize symphyseal fractures.
◊ Note that for managing mandible fractures, familiarity with the locations of the tooth roots and the inferior alveolar nerves is important.
◊ Most American surgeons do not open fractures of the condylar head at this time, so this will not be addressed.
◊ For areas of bone loss, the most dependable means of repair involves the placement of a long, strong plate that is strong enough to replace the mandible.
  * An MRP will usually do this successfully as long as at least three or preferably four screws are placed into solid bone on either side of the defect area.
  * Note that since an MRP is strong enough to replace a segment of missing bone, it is also an excellent "fall-back" tool for managing any fracture of the mandible where there is doubt about the ability to utilize any other form of fixation.
◊ For the edentulous mandible:
  * If there is no atrophy, it can be treated in a manner similar to the dentate mandible.
  * When atrophy is present, the bone to bone contact is usually inadequate to take advantage of the compressive forces of function; therefore, an MRP should be used, since the very weak bone tends to function for all intents and purposes like a defect area.
◊ For areas of comminution:
  * Note that comminuted fragments of bone do not support force well and tend to behave like a defect area; therefore, an MRP should be utilized to bridge areas of comminution.
  * Note that fragments may be pieced together with wires and/or mini or even micro plates before application of the MRP to bridge the weakened area.

- A note about pediatric fractures:
  ◊ The presence of mixed dentition makes the use of arch bars more difficult, and dental splints may be very helpful
  ◊ Note the presence of the tooth buds in the bone during the period of deciduous dentition.
    * This provides limited access for placement of plates and screws without injuring the developing teeth.
    * Great care must be utilized in placing any appliances.
- Do not forget that when the dentition is adequate and the patient will cooperate, there is always the option of managing mandible fractures using arch bars and MMF and avoiding open reduction altogether.
  ◊ Though this approach has fallen out of vogue in recent years, it should be in the surgical armamentarium.
  ◊ External fixation may be used to stabilize fractures in the unstable patient.
- Complications
  (a) Infection
    ○ Common with dirty wounds.
      - May require drainage
    ○ With bone repair, the stability of the repair needs to be assessed.
      - If stable, wound should be cleansed and cultured and antibiotics used.
      - If bone fixation remains stable, it will generally go on to successful healing.
      - Rarely, will develop posttraumatic osteitis.
        ◊ Best treated by removing hardware, debriding bone, replacing a longer, stronger repair, with or without a cancellous bone graft
  (b) Malposition
    ○ A malposition may be significant or minimal
      - If significant, early reoperation and repositioning and restabilization can rescue an inadequate repair.
      - If minimal, unless it is in an area that causes a functional problem (such as a malocclusion or diplopia), it can usually be ignored or camouflaged later.
      - Note that a malpositioned bone in a tooth-bearing region will generally cause a malocclusion.
        ◊ Minimal may be manageable using occlusal grinding.
        ◊ Moderate may respond to orthodontia.
        ◊ Severe will usually require secondary surgery.
      - Also note that proper healing in the wrong position is called a "malunion."
      - This must be distinguished from a "nonunion" which is a failure of a fracture to heal.
      - A significant malposition that has no effect on function may still create a significant cosmetic deformity and therefore necessitate some form of repair.
  (c) Other complications
    ○ Scars
      - Hypertrophic, unsightly; may revise
    ○ Eyelid malpositions
      - Particular risk from repair of orbital floor fractures.
      - Some may be prevented by using a Frost stitch to stretch the lower lid during the immediate postoperative period.
      - Mild cases may respond to massage.
      - More significant may require surgical repair.

- ○ Lacrimal injuries
  - – May be due to the trauma
  - – May be iatrogenic
- ○ Nerve injuries
  - – Traumatic from the injury
    - ◊ Best to identify pre-op to avoid it being attributed to surgery
  - – Iatrogenic
    - ◊ Trigeminal injuries not uncommon.
      - * Supraorbital doing frontal repairs
      - * Infraorbital doing orbital and maxillary repairs
      - * Inferior alveolar doing mandibular repairs
    - ◊ Facial nerve injuries should be repaired if possible.
- ○ Dental injuries
  - – Inadvertent extractions
  - – Tooth root injuries
    - ◊ Particularly common using MMF screws and similar risk with screw-in arch bars
- ○ Missed fractures
  - – NOE is most common.
    - ◊ Intervene as soon as the problem is identified.
- ○ Sinus problems
  - – Should be managed using rhinological techniques
- ○ CSF leaks/meningitis
  - – Must be managed aggressively to minimize risk of significant neurologic morbidity

Questions

1. Since atrophic, edentulous mandibles are very small in height, when the body of such a mandible is fractured, it is best repaired using which of the following techniques?
   A. Wire fixation to minimize damage to the small bone
   B. Mini-plates to match the plates to the size of the bone
   C. Mandibular reconstruction plates to replace the strength of the bone
   D. Compression plates to maximize the force across the fracture and promote healing

2. When the orbit is fractured along with a zygomatic fracture, and there is clinical evidence of enophthalmos, which of the following represents the best approach to repair?
   A. Stabilize the zygoma and then repair the orbital floor with an implant.
   B. Stabilize the zygoma and don't worry about the orbit; you can repair it later if the problem persists.
   C. First attend to the defect in the orbital floor, and once this is repaired, the zygoma can be fixed.
   D. Don't worry about the zygoma; repair the orbit and the zygoma can be repaired later if it presents a problem.

3. When managing subcondylar fractures of the mandible, which of the following is most correct?

    A. These do not require attention, since the patient will get better on his/her own.

    B. Open reduction and placement of a mandibular reconstruction plate is the best approach today.

    C. Placing the patient in rigid MMF will reduce the fracture and result in the best outcome for most patients.

    D. Transoral open reduction and placement of mini-plates is a reasonable approach to these fractures.

4. NOE fractures are best managed using which of the following approaches?

    A. Closed reduction

    B. Percutaneous transnasal wiring

    C. Open reduction with transnasal wiring

    D. Delayed repair to see if such a difficult surgery is actually necessary

5. When the anterior wall of the frontal sinus is fractured, which of the following is most likely to be true?

    A. The patient will require a coronal incision if he/she wants to have the fracture reduced and plated in position.

    B. The patient will require a gull wing incision to best access the fracture and perform reduction and plate fixation.

    C. The patient will need a frontal sinus obliteration using abdominal fat to obliterate the sinus and make it safe.

    D. The best repair will involve cranialization of the frontal sinus.

Chapter 51
Orbital Fractures

Orbital fractures are injuries frequently encountered both acutely in the emergency room as well as in the office as chronic conditions. They are seen in isolation or in association with other head and neck injuries. This chapter covers the clinical presentation, evaluation, examination findings, and management of orbital fractures organized from an anatomical perspective. The bulk of the discussion focuses on floor fractures, as these are the most frequent orbital fractures encountered. Other orbital fractures are then discussed in a more succinct fashion to highlight the unique features based on their anatomic location. Basic orbital anatomy is not discussed; for a review of orbital anatomy, refer to Chapter 6.

Orbital Floor Fractures

Background

A. Orbital floor fractures are the most common orbital fracture encountered.
   i. Most common location is posteromedial floor (maxillary bone), medial to infra-orbital neurovascular bundle.
B. *Blow-out fracture*: floor fracture with intact orbital rim.
C. Floor is shortest orbital wall, in shape of equilateral triangle.
D. Mechanism:
   i. *Smith and Converse*: cadaveric study (1956).
      a. Blunt trauma (usually object smaller in diameter than orbit) pushes orbital contents posteriorly.
      b. Resultant increase in intraorbital pressure causes fracture at weakest point: posteromedial orbital floor (hydraulic theory).
   ii. *Buckling theory*: direct blow to orbital rim causes buckling at weakest point of orbital floor.
E. *Blow-in fracture*: direct trauma to orbital rim causing bone fragment to be displaced into orbit (rather than into maxillary sinus); presents with exophthalmos, not enophthalmos.

Clinical Presentation

A. *Symptoms*: pain, blurred vision, binocular vertical/oblique diplopia
B. Signs of periocular injury
   i. Eyelid edema

  ii. Ecchymosis

  iii. Subcutaneous or orbital emphysema

  iv. Subconjunctival hemorrhage

  v. Enophthalmos (volume expansion) or exophthalmos (soft tissue swelling/edema)

  vi. Globe ptosis

C. Ocular injuries

  i. *Corneal abrasion*: foreign-body sensation, photophobia, blurred vision

  ii. *Traumatic iritis*: photophobia, blurred vision, brow ache

  iii. *Hyphema*: layer of blood in anterior chamber

   a. May have associated problems with intraocular pressure

  iv. *Lens dislocation*: blurred vision; may occlude pupil causing angle closure glaucoma

  v. *Retinal detachment*: acute, painless loss of vision. Associated with flashes of light and visual field defect

  vi. *Commotio retinae*: injury to outer retinal layers caused by shockwave from blunt trauma with resultant edema; may cause blurred vision if macula involved

  vii. Open globe injury

D. Motility defects

  i. Trapdoor fracture:

   a. Small floor fracture.

   b. Orbital pressure causes orbital soft tissue to protrude through defect.

   c. Orbital bone recoils faster than soft tissue, trapping soft tissue in defect.

   d. Resultant motility restriction with greatest limitation in upgaze.

   e. *Vagal symptoms*: nausea, vomiting, bradycardia.

   f. May cause ischemia to extraocular muscles (EOMs) and later fibrosis and restrictive strabismus.

   g. Most common in children due to more flexible bones (greenstick fracture—"white eyed" blow-out fracture).

  ii. Contusive injury to EOM may cause generalized restriction in motility.

  iii. *Retrobulbar hemorrhage* may cause orbital compartment syndrome: proptosis, pain, loss of vision, and frozen globe (complete restriction of EOM).

Evaluation

A. Basic examination

  i. *Visual acuity*: vision assessed with one eye at a time, using near card with full spectacle correction. If no near card available, ask patient to read hospital badge.

  ii. *Pupillary examination*: assess for afferent pupillary defect, anisocoria, and peaked/irregular pupil.

  iii. *Intraocular pressure*: most emergency rooms have a Tono-Pen available these days.

  iv. *Motility*: particular attention to limitation in upgaze suggestive of entrapment.

   a. *Diplopia fields*: Have patient follow your finger in horizontal and vertical directions.

   b. Increase in intraocular pressure (1-15 mm Hg) on upgaze compared to primary position suggests entrapment of inferior rectus.

  v. Cranial nerve assessment, particularly III, IV, V, VI, and VII.

  vi. *Ophthalmic examination*: slit lamp biomicroscopy and dilated funduscopic examination.

  vii. Exophthalmometry.

B. *External photography*: to document facial injury, EOM restriction, and other associated findings

       i. Worm's eye view good angle to show enophthalmos
      ii. Helpful in postoperative period to assess success of surgical intervention
  C. *Forced ductions*: used to distinguish paretic muscle from entrapped (restricted) muscle
       i. Fine-toothed forceps (eg, 0.5 forceps) are used to grab tissue at limbus after topical anesthetic administered.
         a. *Note*: for assessment of horizontal motility, the limbus is grasped at 12 and 6 o' clock to prevent corneal abrasion if forceps slip. Conversely, for vertical ductions, the limbus is grasped at 3 and 9 o' clock.
      ii. Patient is asked to look in direction being examined and globe is then rotated in the same direction.
     iii. Degree of restriction is noted.
     iv. In acute setting this test may not be helpful as edema and hemorrhage of muscle capsule may cause restriction and simulate an entrapped muscle.
      v. This test may be most helpful intraoperatively, done both at the beginning of surgery and then after orbital contents have been reposited and fracture has been reduced to ensure that all soft tissue has been freed.
  D. *CT scan*: allows for evaluation of orbital fracture extent, size, and configuration; also orbital soft tissue, entrapment, orbital volume, and hemorrhage

Management

Surgical intervention versus conservative management of orbital floor fractures is a somewhat controversial topic.
  A. Smith and Converse advocated early surgical intervention, within 2 to 3 weeks of injury, to minimize late enophthalmos and diplopia.
  B. Putterman (1974) argued that all cases may be followed for 4 to 6 months or longer prior to surgical intervention.
       i. Found that patients with diplopia had resolution in functional positions of gaze without surgical intervention.
      ii. One-quarter of patients had persistent diplopia, but in extremes of gaze, and were without functional limitations.
  C. Dutton proposed the following recommendations that are generally accepted as guidelines for surgical intervention:
       i. Symptomatic persistent diplopia with positive forced ductions, computed tomography (CT) evidence of orbital tissue or muscle entrapment, and no clinical improvement over 1 to 2 weeks
      ii. Early enophthalmos of 3 mm or more
     iii. Significant globe ptosis
     iv. Floor defect of greater than 50% likely to result in late enophthalmos
      v. Associated rim and facial fractures
  D. Other indications:
       i. *Blow-in fracture*: position of bone fragments may compromise vision.
      ii. *Persistent diplopia interfering with occupational demands*: pilots, painters, mechanics or professional athletes.
     iii. Vagal signs (*oculocardiac reflex*) such as intractable nausea and vomiting and bradycardia are signs of EOM entrapment and suggest a more emergent indication for decompression.
     iv. Herniation of globe into maxillary sinus is also an indication for emergent repair.
      v. Progressive.

Treatment and Repair

A. *Nasal precautions*: avoid nose blowing, sneezing with a closed mouth, sucking through a straw.

B. *Timing of fracture repair*: fractures are general observed for 7 to 10 days to allow edema and hemorrhage to decrease.

   i. Preferably repaired within 2 weeks of injury; injuries greater than 6 weeks become increasingly difficult to repair.

   ii. Delayed repair of floor fracture may result in persistent enophthalmos, secondary to fibrosis and contracture of traumatized orbital soft tissue.

C. *Surgical technique*: subciliary incision may be used for surgical approach; however, the authors' preference is transconjunctival incision which is described in the following text.

   i. General anesthesia.

   ii. Forced ductions performed at beginning of case as described previously.

   iii. Traction suture placed in lower lid (eg, 4-0 silk).

   iv. Jaeger plate is used to protect globe and provide gentle retraction, as lower lid is retracted by traction suture.

   v. Monopolar cautery with Colorado needle is used to make conjunctival incision below tarsus from the punctum to the lateral canthus.

      a. Canthotomy and cantholysis may also be performed to increase visibility/exposure.

   vi. Second traction suture is placed through conjunctiva and retractors (that have now been disinserted from tarsus) and a heavy hemostat is used to provide upward traction on the flap, which is pulled over the cornea.

   vii. Desmarres retractor then placed in the lower lid to retract downward.

   viii. Dissection is continued in the preseptal plane to the orbital floor.

   ix. The periorbita is incised with monopolar cautery and the periorbita is elevated with a periosteal elevator.

   x. Periorbital elevation is continued posteriorly.

   xi. Malleable retractors are used to retract orbital contents as the surgeon uses freer in one hand and suction in other hand to continue periosteal elevation to anterior edge of fracture.

   xii. All edges of fracture are identified and prolapsed orbital content is reposited into orbit.

   xiii. Various implant materials are available for floor fracture repair; the authors' preference is the thinnest Supramid available (0.1-0.4 mm).

   xiv. The implant is cut in the shape of a guitar pick and placed in the orbit to cover floor defect. The implant may need to be trimmed.

   xv. Some surgeons fixate their implant; we have found this is unnecessary.

   xvi. Alternatively screws may be used to fixate the implant, or two small parallel incisions may be placed in the central anterior edge of the implant and the central portion may be depressed and then wedged into the anterior edge of the defect for stability.

   xvii. Forced ductions are repeated to ensure no additional restriction is present.

   xviii. The periosteum is closed with 4-0 Vicryl sutures in an interrupted fashion.

   xix. If lateral canthotomy/cantholysis is performed, the lateral canthal tendon is then reattached with the same 4-0 Vicryl suture. Skin closure is with 5-0 or 6-0 fast-absorbing gut suture.

       xx. The conjunctival traction suture is removed. However, it is the authors' preference to leave the eyelid traction suture and secure it above the brow with Steri-Strips for 2 to 5 days to provide gentle upward traction and prevent lower eyelid retraction.

D. Postoperative care
    i. Routine postoperative care is recommended as with other orbital procedures including limitation of activity as well as nasal precautions.
    ii. Prophylactic antibiotics are prescribed for 7 to 10 days.
    iii. Narcotic/acetaminophen combination analgesics are prescribed.
    iv. The patient is seen at 2 to 5 days for Frost suture removal and then again 2 weeks postoperatively.

Complications

A. Related to trauma
    i. Vision loss
        a. Direct and indirect traumatic optic neuropathy
        b. Retrobulbar hemorrhage
        c. *Ocular injury*: open globe, retinal detachment, etc (as described previously)
    ii. *Enophthalmos*: caused by volume expansion, or by atrophy of traumatized orbital contents
    iii. *Superior sulcus deformity*: hollowing of superior sulcus secondary to downward displacement of orbital fat
    iv. *Strabismus/persistent diplopia*: restrictive secondary to EOM trauma and fibrosis
    v. Persistent V2 hypoesthesia/paresthesia
    vi. Hypoglobus
B. Related to repair
    i. Lower eyelid retraction
    ii. Cicatricial ectropion (subciliary incision) or entropion (transconjunctival incision)
    iii. Hematic cyst formation (depending on implant material used)

Medial Wall Fractures

Background

A. The medial wall is the thinnest of all orbital walls (lamina papyracea).
B. May be associated with nasal bone fractures (naso-orbito-ethmoidal [NOE] fracture or NOE).
C. In addition to previously described mechanisms of injury, it was proposed by Pfeiffer and later supported by Erling that isolated medial wall fractures may be a result of direct contact of the globe with the medial wall.
D. Classification:
    i. *Type I*: isolated medial wall fracture
    ii. *Type II*: combined medial wall and floor fracture (most common)
    iii. *Type III*: combined medial wall and floor fracture continuous with orbital rim and malar fracture
    iv. *Type IV*: medial wall fracture associated with complex midfacial fractures (eg, NOE)

Clinical Presentation

A. *Symptoms and signs*: similar to floor fracture; isolated medial wall fractures may go unnoticed
B. *Epistaxis*: secondary to sheering of sinus mucosa
C. *Orbital hemorrhage*: caused by damage to the anterior or posterior ethmoidal arteries; may be subperiosteal or extend into orbital soft tissue if periosteum is disrupted
D. Less commonly associated with EOM entrapment; orbital fat or intermuscular septum, however, may be incarcerated
   i. May cause various forms of horizontal dysmotility depending on where the medial rectus is restricted in respect to the globe (anteriorly, at equator, or posteriorly)
E. Enophthalmos more likely in types II-IV given significant volume expansion of orbit compared to floor or medial wall fracture alone

Evaluation

A. Again, similar to above. Special attention should be given to the medial canthus to evaluate for traumatic telecanthus, as well as nasal examination to assess for telescoping.

Management

A. Conservative management is similar to floor fracture; prophylactic antibiotics, nasal precautions, etc.
B. Indications for repair:
   i. Horizontal or vertical duction deficits that persist in absence of significant orbital edema and with CT findings suggestive of entrapment.
   ii. Early enophthalmos.
   iii. CT findings suggesting significant orbital volume expansion.
   iv. Telecanthus and other deformities associated with types III and IV fractures.

Treatment and Repair

A. Timing of surgical repair is described previously.
B. *Surgical technique*: the same subciliary or transconjunctival approach is used as above. Differences are listed in the following text.
   i. Again, "swinging lower eyelid" may aid in exposure; however, for medial wall fractures, this can be combined with a transcaruncular incision to increase visualization of the medial wall fracture.
   ii. When placing implant, inferior oblique may need to be disinserted at its origin; there is no need to directly reattach the inferior oblique.
   iii. Various implant material can be used; however, in contrast to isolated floor fractures, medial wall fractures will likely require fixation of the implant. The authors prefer to use porous polyethylene with titanium implants for combined floor and medial wall fractures.
      a. *Note*: These implants should not be fixated to the anterior orbital rim; they are meant to be fixated posterior to the orbital rim.

Complications

A. Complications are similar to those described previously with addition of
   i. *CSF rhinorrhea*: may occur as result of injury or as surgical complication
   ii. Epistaxis

      iii. *Telecanthus*: as result of injury or neglecting to address/inadequately addressing medial canthal tendon

      iv. Nasal deformity

Lateral Wall/Orbitozygomatic Fractures

Background

A. *Early 1900s*: simple reduction without fixation.
B. *Adams (1942)*: first described using wires for internal fixation.
C. Swiss AO group and other investigators began using miniplates for fixation.
D. May involve zygomatic arch in isolation or "tripod" fracture:
    i. Zygomatic arch
    ii. Inferior orbital rim
    iii. Frontozygomatic buttress
    iv. Zygomaticomaxillary buttress
E. *Biomechanics*: multiple vectors of force act on zygoma, making immobilization of fracture difficult.
    i. Masseter and temporalis exert dominant dynamic forces; these must be overcome at fracture site for stabilization.
    ii. Two types of bony union can form at fracture site:
      a. *Callous bone formation*: movement at fracture site, fibroblastic response which then differentiates into bone
      b. *Primary healing*: immobilization of bone allows alignment of haversian canals, allowing direct ossification at fracture site; this is stronger bony union.
    iii. Bony resorption occurs with inadequate reduction and stabilization of fracture.
      a. Contributes to enophthalmos

Clinical Presentation

Signs and symptoms are as described earlier, with addition of malar flattening.

Evaluation

A. *History*: obtain mechanism of injury to distinguish low-velocity injury from high-velocity injury.
B. *Physical examination*: in addition to aforementioned standard examination:
    i. *Trismus*: suggests impingement of displaced arch fracture on coronoid process
    ii. *Dental occlusion*: to assess for associated mandibular or maxillary fractures
C. Classification:
    i. *Type I*: no significant displacement of bony fragments and remains attached at zygomaticomaxillary, zygomaticofrontal sutures, and the zygomatic arch
    ii. *Type II*: incomplete downward and laterally displaced fragment (zygomaticomaxillary suture) with attachment remained at zygomaticofrontal suture
      a. Associated with blunt force trauma from laterally to inferior orbital rim
    iii. *Type IIIa*: incomplete downward and laterally displaced fragment hinged on zygomaticomaxillary suture with detachment at zygomaticofrontal suture
      a. Associated with blunt injury directed inferiorly from above

iv. *Type IIIb*: incomplete superiorly and posteriorly displaced fragment, again hinged at zygomaticomaxillary suture with detachment at zygomaticofrontal suture
  a. Associated with blunt force injury directed superiorly from below
v. *Type IV*: complete fracture displaced inferiorly with internal rotation of the inferior orbital rim and medial displacement of zygoma
  a. Associated with blunt force trauma directed directly to zygomatic arch

Management

A. General considerations regarding repair of orbitozygomatic fractures
  i. Can these fractures be classified according to severity and then managed accordingly?
  ii. If so, which of these fractures can be reduced only? Which require reduction and fixation?
  iii. Does the method of fixation affect long-term results?
A. Summary of clinical data
  i. A small subset of orbitozygomatic fractures can be treated with reduction only: low-velocity injury that is stable after reduction.
  ii. High-velocity fractures comminution and displacement require open reduction and rigid fixation.
  iii. Combination of microplate and miniplate fixation is the best tolerated fixation method and provides optimal rigid stabilization.
    a. Miniplate applied to zygomaticomaxillary buttress to counteract action of masseter.
    b. Microplate used for infraorbital rim and zygomaticofrontal areas, except for high-energy fractures, which require miniplate.

Treatment and Repair

A. *Isolated arch fracture*: Gillies procedure
  i. 2- to 3-cm incision made in temporal hairline.
  ii. Dissection continued deep to temporalis fascia.
  iii. Dingman elevator used to elevate arch.
  iv. If fracture is stable, no further intervention necessary.
  v. If fracture is unstable, there are two options.
    a. ORIF through transcoronal incision
    b. Stenting unstable fracture with spinal needle passed transcutaneously beneath the arch and back out through the skin. This is left in place for 10 days.
B. Orbitozygomatic fractures
  i. Nondisplaced: conservative management with soft diet, malar protection, and close follow-up
  ii. Displaced: classified as low or high velocity
    a. As previously mentioned, low-velocity fractures may be fixated with a combination of miniplates and microplates. High-velocity fractures require miniplates only.
C. Surgical approach for orbitozygomatic fractures
  i. Three separate incisions used:
    a. Lateral upper lid crease incision
    b. Gingivobuccal sulcus incision
    c. Lower eyelid incision (transconjunctival with "swinging" eyelid vs subciliary)
  ii. Zygomatic arch is key to repair.

D. Surgical technique
   i. *Fracture reduction*: Carol Gerard screw placed in the zygomatic body through lower eyelid incision (after periosteum has been elevated). Alternatively, Dingman elevator can be placed below the zygomatic arch through upper lid crease incision.
      a. Must directly visualize reduction at all fracture sites prior to fixation; anatomical reduction at one site may be accompanied by malalignment of other fracture location
   ii. After adequate reduction confirmed at all sites, rigid plate fixation of the fragments is performed from superior to inferior and from lateral to medial working from a stable structure to an unstable one.
      a. Zygomaticofrontal fracture is fixated first.
   iii. Care taken in zygomaticomaxillary buttress to prevent injury to roots of teeth in area of alveolar ridge.
   iv. Infraorbital rim fixated with microplate or miniplate.
   v. Reduction and fixation of associated orbital floor fracture performed at this point.
   vi. For comminuted zygomatic fractures with loss of projection, zygomatic arch will need to be plated; approached through transcoronal approach.
   vii. After fixation is completed, periosteum is closed as described previously.
   viii. Skin is closed with fast-absorbing gut suture.

Naso-orbito-ethmoidal Fractures

Background

A. Naso-orbito-ethmoidal (NOE) fractures were partly discussed previously with medial wall fractures. This segment will serve as a supplement to previous discussion.
B. It is worth mentioning that while many patients present acutely, other patients present for revisional surgery after already having one or more procedures performed already.

Clinical Presentation

As described previously.

Evaluation

A. Patient history
   i. Mechanism of injury
   ii. Previous procedures, if any
   iii. Patient concerns, symptoms (enophthalmos, epiphora, breathing difficulty, sinus issues)
B. Clinical examination
   i. Assess degree of facial asymmetry, telecanthus, and enophthalmos (exophthalmometry).
   ii. Evaluation of external nose, nasal septum, airway.
   iii. Examine lacrimal drainage system if symptomatic or radiologic evidence of compromise.
C. *Review studies*: CT orbits or maxillofacial

Management

As described previously.

Treatment and Repair

A. Surgical techniques
   i. Transnasal wiring
   ii. Microplate fixation
B. Description of techniques
   i. Transnasal wiring
      a. *Surgical access*: bicoronal, gingivobuccal sulcus, and/or transconjunctival/caruncular incisions.
         1. May also use previous scars/incisions
      b. Three anatomic subgroups must be address:
         1. Medial canthus
            - Bone fragment with attached medial canthal tendon identified.
            - Bone freed with osteotomies and repositioned medially.
            - Two drill holes placed posteriorly to insertion of medial canthal tendon and 28-gauge wire passed from temporal to nasal through both holes,
            - Wires passed transnasally with awl and fixated to plate in supratrochlear region of contralateral orbit.
            - If the bone fragment is too small or if the tendon has been stripped from the bone (class II and III injury, respectively), the posterior crus of the medial canthal tendon itself can be purchased with a figure-of-eight 28-gauge wire and passed as above.
            - Compression plates may be placed at the conclusion of repair to maintain medial canthal position and prevent hematoma formation.
            - Medial canthus is last anatomic subunit to be addressed.
         2. Nose
            - Nasal width corrected by infracturing nasal pyramid with or without osteotomy and repositioning central maxillary buttress
            - Nasal dorsum height and length restored with bone grafts
         3. Medial wall/orbital floor
            - Subperiosteal dissection to identify fracture, reposit prolapsed soft tissue, and placement of orbital implant of choice (based on surgeon preference, size of defect, available support)
   ii. *Cantilevered miniplate fixation*: Y-shaped titanium miniplate cantilevered from lateral nose, and directed posteriorly into orbit, and bone fragment with medial canthal tendon fixated to plate

Complications

A. Persistent telecanthus
B. Epiphora/damage to nasolacrimal system
   i. Must handle medial canthal tissue carefully
   ii. Low threshold for silicone stent placement

Orbital Roof Fractures

Background

A. Although all the previously described fractures may require an interdisciplinary approach, fractures of the orbital roof will almost always require multiple specialty intervention.

B. Fractures of the upper face are less commonly encountered.
   i. In a patient presenting with any facial fracture, 3% to 9.3% will involve the orbital roof.
   ii. More common in children, with incidence of 18% to 35% of all pediatric facial fractures.
C. Adult bone of forehead/supraorbital ridge is thicker compared to pediatric bone; also the cranium is proportionately larger in children.
D. *"Pure" fracture*: only the orbital roof is fractured without involving orbital rim.
E. *"Impure" fracture*: involves the orbital roof and rim.
   i. Impure blow-in fracture is the most commonly encountered type of roof fracture.

Clinical Presentation

A. Signs and symptoms as above with the following additions:
   i. Upper eyelid hematoma that may show delayed expansion
      a. May be result of intracranial or intraorbital hemorrhage decompressing into the superior anterior orbit and upper eyelid
   ii. Forehead hypoesthesia
   iii. Contour deformity of forehead and supraorbital ridge
   iv. Cerebrospinal fluid (CSF) rhinorrhea
   v. Neurologic deficits
   vi. Proptosis secondary to prolapsed intracranial contents

Evaluation

As described previously, though more extensive neurologic evaluation may be required.

Management

A. As previously mentioned, these cases will certainly involve an interdisciplinary approach, including ENT (ear, nose, and throat), neurosurgery, and ophthalmology at a minimum.
B. Intracranial injury takes precedence, followed by globe injury.
C. Minimal displaced or nondisplaced fractures of supraorbital region or roof, not involving frontal sinus (*lateral injury*), may be observed.
   i. Displaced roof fracture in this setting may also be observed in asymptomatic patient; however, the patient must be monitored for the development of pulsatile proptosis.
   ii. Visible bony contour deformities require reduction and fixation.
D. Isolated CSF leak may be observed for 1 week for spontaneous resolution; persistent CSF leak may require dural repair.
E. Fractures involving frontal sinus (*medial injury*) with minimally or nondisplaced anterior frontal sinus wall may be observed; displaced anterior table fractures, however, must be repaired.
   i. Nasofrontal duct should be investigated; if compromised, sinus obliteration should be performed.
F. Medial injuries involving posterior wall of frontal sinus are more complicated and are associated with high-velocity injuries.
   i. In setting of minimally displaced fracture with no CSF leak, posterior wall fracture is observed and anterior wall fracture is managed, as described previously.
   ii. In setting of minimally displaced or nondisplaced posterior wall fracture with CSF leak can be cautiously observed for spontaneous resolution as described above; lumbar drain may help promote resolution.

      iii. Persistent CSF leak must be treated by cranialization of the sinus.

      iv. Displaced posterior wall without CSF leak and intact nasofrontal duct may be observed (and anterior wall may be addressed as needed).

      v. Displaced posterior wall without CSF leak and compromised nasofrontal duct may be treated either by obliteration of frontal sinus or cranialization of sinus.

G. Proptosis, persistent diplopia, or signs of muscular impingement may also be indications for surgery.

H. Optic canal injury with bony fragment impingement on optic nerve and signs of optic neuropathy remains a controversial indication for optic canal decompression; at a minimum a skilled and experienced team of surgeons are required to attempt such an intervention.

Treatment and Repair

A. The surgical approach often may utilize preexisting lacerations; otherwise, a coronal incision may be used.

    i. Care should be taken to identify supraorbital and supratrochlear neurovascular bundle.

B. Adjunctive incisions:

    i. Upper lid crease

    ii. Lynch

    iii. Infrabrow

    iv. Suprabrow/gull wing

C. Reconstruction of orbital roof is generally preferred to reduction in setting of comminution.

    i. Bone graft

      a. Outer table cranial bone graft or inner table cranial bone graft harvested from full-thickness craniotomy (with outer table then replaced)

      b. Rib

      c. Iliac crest

    ii. Titanium mesh

Complications

A. Diplopia/strabismus secondary to cranial nerve injury or direct trauma to EOM

B. Loss of vision due to globe or optic nerve injury

C. Vertical globe dystopia, enophthalmos, proptosis (also pulsatile proptosis)

D. Mucocele or mucopyocele

Bibliography

Burnstine MA. Clinical recommendations for repair of isolated orbital floor fractures: an evidence-based analysis. *Ophthalmology.* 2002;109(7):1207-1210.

Dutton JJ. Management of blow-out fractures of the orbital floor. *Surv Ophthalmol.* 1991;35:279.

Holck DE, Ng JD. *Evaluation and Treatment of Orbital Fractures: A Multidisciplinary Approach.* Philadelphia, PA: Elsevier; 2006.

Jordan DR Allen LH, White J, Harvey J, Pashby R, Esmaeli B. Intervention within days for some orbital floor fractures: the white-eyed blowout. *Ophth Plast Reconstr Surg.* 1998;14(6): 379-390.

Smith B, Regan WF. Blowout fracture of the orbit. *Am J Ophthalmol.* 1957;44:733.

Questions:

1. Which of the following indicates a need for urgent repair of orbital floor fractures?
   A. Persistent symptomatic diplopia with evidence of entrapment
   B. Early enophthalmos of 3 mm or more
   C. Nausea, vomiting, and bradycardia
   D. Floor defect of greater than 50%
   E. Associated rim and facial fractures

2. Which of the following are causes of blurred vision acutely following orbital trauma?
   A. Corneal abrasion
   B. Traumatic iritis
   C. Retinal detachment
   D. Commotio retinae
   E. All of the above

3. Enophthalmos is most likely following which type of medial wall fractures?
   A. Type I
   B. Type II
   C. Type III
   D. Type IV
   E. B, C, and D
   F. None of the above

4. Which of the following incisions may be used when approaching orbitozygomatic fractures?
   A. Temporal hairline
   B. Upper lid crease
   C. Transconjunctival
   D. Gingivobuccal
   E. Gull wing
   F. All of the above
   G. A,B, C, and D

5. All of the following are signs of an orbital roof fracture except
   A. delayed upper eyelid hematoma
   B. V2 hypoesthesia
   C. contour deformity of forehead and supraorbital ridge
   D. CSF rhinorrhea
   E. neurologic deficits

Chapter 52
Related Ophthalmology

Anatomy

    A. The orbit forms a quadrilateral pyramid: floor, roof, medial wall, and lateral wall.
- i. *Roof*: orbital process of the frontal bone, lesser wing of the sphenoid
- ii. *Floor*: orbital plate of maxilla, orbital surface of zygoma, orbital process of the palatine bone
- iii. *Medial wall*: frontal process of maxilla, lacrimal bone, sphenoid bone, lamina papyracea of the ethmoid bone
- iv. *Lateral wall*: lesser and greater wings of the sphenoid, zygoma

    B. The trochlea, a pulley through which runs the tendon of the superior oblique (SO) muscle, is located between the roof and the medial wall. A displaced trochlea causes diplopia on downward gaze.

    C. The inferior orbital fissure is in the floor of the orbit. It is bound by the greater wing of the sphenoid, orbital surface of the maxilla, and orbital process of the palatine bone. It transmits the infraorbital nerve, infraorbital vessels, zygomatic nerve, fine branches from the sphenopalatine ganglion to the lacrimal gland, and ophthalmic vein branch.

    D. The anterior and posterior ethmoid foramina are situated at the junction between the frontal and ethmoid bones, in the frontal side of the suture line.

    E. The superior orbital fissure lies between the roof and the lateral wall of the nose. It is a gap between the lesser and the greater wings of the sphenoid. It transmits cranial nerves III, IV, V1, VI, the superior orbital vein, ophthalmic vein, orbital branch of the middle meningeal artery, and recurrent branch of the lacrimal artery.

    F. The optic canal runs from the middle cranial fossa into the apex of the orbit. It is formed by a curvilinear portion of the lesser wing of the sphenoid bone, and through it courses the optic nerve and ophthalmic artery.

    G. The upper lid contains the following:
- i. Orbicularis oculi
- ii. Levator palpebrae superioris
- iii. Müller muscle
- iv. Sweat glands
- v. Meibomian glands
- vi. Wolfring glands
- vii. Tarsal plate

    H. The lower lid contains the following:
- i. Tarsal plate

     ii. Lower lid retractors
    iii. Orbicularis oculi
    iv. Sweat glands
     v. Meibomian glands
    vi. Wolfring glands

I. The lateral ends of the tarsi unite to form the lateral palpebral ligament, which fixes onto the orbital surface of the zygomatic bone. A displaced lateral canthal ligament may give rise to an inferiorly displaced canthus or slight ptosis. Also, with loss of the inferior fornix, prosthesis will not stay in place, if such is necessary.

J. The medial ends divide into deep and superficial heads. The superficial heads unite and form the medial canthal tendon, which anchors the eyelids medially. If this support is lost, a rounding of the medial aspect of the eyelid will occur, resulting in pseudohypertelorism. The deep heads form the muscular diaphragm over the lacrimal fossa, envelope the punctae, and swing back to attach to the posterior lacrimal crest, establishing the "lacrimal pump" mechanism. Disruption of this muscle attachment may result in epiphora.

K. The septum orbitale is the orbital periosteum, which extends into the lid to attach to the tarsal plates. The orbital septum separates the eyelid from the orbital contents. If fat is exposed, the orbit has been entered, as there is no subcutaneous fat in the eyelids. The superior orbital septum attaches to the levator apparatus with subsequent attachment to the tarsal plate, whereas the inferior septum attaches directly into the tarsal plate. Medially, it is fused with the palpebral ligament leading toward the posterior lacrimal crest.

L. The suspensory ligament of Lockwood is a continuous band of fibrous tissue slung beneath the eyeball from side to side. The ends of the suspensory ligament blend with the cheek ligaments and with the medial and lateral horns of the aponeurosis of the levator palpebrae superioris.

M. The lower lid retractors are the capsulopalpebral heads of the inferior rectus/inferior oblique complex, and cause a slight retraction of the lower lid with forced openings. Fibers can be separated supplied by the sympathetic nerves as well as the third cranial nerve.

Control of Eye Movement

A. The upper lid is opened by the levator palpebrae superior (nerve III) and Müller muscle (sympathetic fibers). It is closed by the orbicularis oculi (nerve VII). The ophthalmic division of nerve V is responsible for the sensory innervation to the upper lid, and the lower lid is innervated by the first two divisions of nerve V.

B. *Entropion*: turning in of the lid margin. *Ectropion*: turning out of the lid margin.

C. *Horner syndrome*: paralysis of the sympathetic nerve, especially the superior cervical sympathetics, giving rise to ptosis, miosis, and anhidrosis. The ptosis is caused by weakness or paralysis of Müller muscle, which can account for 3 to 6 mm of upper lid retraction.

Muscles

A. The six extraocular muscles and their functions are as follows:
    i. Lateral rectus (LR), to adduct
    ii. Medial rectus, to abduct

      iii. Superior rectus, to elevate (and intort)

      iv. Inferior rectus, to depress (and extort)

      v. SO, to intort (and depress)

      vi. Inferior oblique, to extort (and elevate)

B. The LR is innervated by nerve VI. The SO is innervated by nerve IV. The rest of the extraocular muscles are innervated by nerve III.

C. The inferior rectus muscle is the most commonly trapped muscle in a blowout fracture, the second being the inferior oblique. When these muscles are trapped, the patient may experience difficulty looking upward. This condition is not due to paralysis but rather due to the trapping of the two muscles mentioned previously. To differentiate paralysis of the elevators from trapping of the inferior rectus and the inferior oblique muscles, the "forced duction test" is performed under local or general anesthesia. The forced duction test consists of grasping the globe adjacent to the limbus with small forceps and rotating it up, down, in, and out. If the globe moves freely, there is no entrapment of these muscles. The degree of movement should be compared to that of the unaffected opposite globe.

D. There are six cardinal directions of gaze, each controlled by a set of two muscles:

      i. Eyes to right, right LR and left medial rectus

      ii. Eyes to left, right medial rectus and left LR

      iii. Eyes up and right, right superior rectus and left inferior oblique

      iv. Eyes down and right, right inferior rectus and left SO

      v. Eyes up and left, right inferior oblique and left superior rectus

      vi. Eyes down and left, right SO and inferior rectus

E. When diplopia occurs, it may exist in more than one direction. The muscles suspected of being involved are those controlling the direction of gaze in which the images of the diplopia are farthest apart. It is usually obvious as to which eye is involved. However, when such is not the case, each eye should be covered in turn and tested. The eye that sees the peripheral image is the one that is injured.

F. The evaluation of diplopia is very difficult and requires a detailed ophthalmologic examination. It should be ascertained whether the diplopia is vertical, horizontal, or rotational and whether it occurs in at a distance or near, up, or down gaze positions.

G. Injury to the trochlea can occur during frontal sinus floor trephine or external ethmoidectomy, causing SO dysfunction and subsequent diplopia.

Lacrimal System

A. The lacrimal gland (a serous gland predominantly) is located in a fossa within the zygomatic process of the frontal bone. The lacrimal sac lies in a fossa bound by the lacrimal bone, the frontal process of the maxilla, and the nasal process of the frontal bone.

B. The lacrimal gland secretes tears through 17-20 openings. Although the gland is developed, secretion of tears does not take place until 2 weeks after birth. The tears are composed of watery, oily, and mucoid components, which are present in both basic and reflex tearing.

C. When cannulating the inferior and superior canaliculi, it is important to remember that each canaliculus has a vertical portion (~2 mm) and a longer horizontal portion (~8 mm). The canaliculi join into a common canaliculus of variable length. A laceration of one or both canaliculi requires insertion of a silicone tube, which is looped between the inferior and superior puncti in the medial corner of the eye, brought through the nasolacrimal duct, and tied together within the nasal cavity. The laceration can be sutured over the tube, which is left in place for 6 weeks to 3 months. The lacrimal sac is about 12 mm long and the duct about 17 mm long. The nasolacrimal duct empties into the anterior portion of the inferior meatus. The most common site of congenital obstruction in the lacrimal system is a stricture of the valve of Hasner, of the nasolacrimal duct, at the inferior meatus. Acquired causes of the blockage, primarily in the upper collecting system, include infection (dacryocystitis)—often with the formation of dacryoliths—trauma, and idiopathic causes. The idiopathic conditions are commonly seen in postmenopausal women.

Graves Orbitopathy

A. Malignant exophthalmos is caused by an endocrine disorder. One of the causes is an oversecretion of "exophthalmos factor" by the anterior pituitary. This factor is possibly linked to thyroid-stimulating hormone (TSH). The more severe form of exophthalmos is caused by excessive orbital edema, giving rise to an increase in bulk of the extraocular muscles and adipose tissues. These adipose tissues are found at such time to contain a greater amount of mucopolysaccharides than normal. The extraocular muscles are particularly affected by this inflammatory process, which eventually leads to deposition of collagen and fibrosis. Imaging studies with computed tomography (CT) or A-scan ultrasound often demonstrate significant thickening of the middle and posterior aspects of the extraocular muscles. The globe decompresses itself through the anterior orbit, creating the observed proptosis. Upper eyelid retraction with upper scleral show may be evident. Ocular symptoms include mild burning, foreign-body sensation, and tearing from corneal exposure, progressing to severe loss of vision from compressive optic neuropathy. Management of Graves orbitopathy is based on the severity of the disease and should be coordinated by a team consisting of the endocrinologist, ophthalmologist, and otorhinolaryngologist. Medical management for more severe symptoms has included the use of anti-inflammatory medications, corticosteroids, and radiation.

B. The exophthalmos is not only esthetically undesirable but can also lead to the following:
   i. Corneal exposure and desiccation due to failure to close lids over cornea.
   ii. Chemosis secondary to venous stasis.
   iii. Fixation of the extraocular muscles, causing ophthalmoplegia. The earliest limitation noted is in upward gaze.
   iv. Retinal venous congestion leading to blindness.
   v. Conjunctivitis due to exposure, desiccation, and inflammation.

C. Because the consequences of malignant exophthalmos are grave, many surgical corrections have been devised.
   i. Krönlein procedure removes the lateral orbital wall to allow the orbital contents to expand into the zygomatic area.
   ii. Naffziger procedure removes the roof of the orbital cavity to allow expansion of the orbital contents into the anterior cranial fossa. It does not expose any of the paranasal sinuses, and it preserves the superior orbital rim. Postoperatively, the cerebral pulsations may be noted in the orbit.
   iii. Sewell procedure consists of an ethmoidectomy and removal of the floor of the frontal sinus for expansion.

Table 52-1 **Werner's Detailed Classification**	
Class	*Description*
0	No physical signs or symptoms
1	Only signs (upper lid retraction, stare, and eyelid lag)
2	Symptoms (irritation, etc) along with class 1 signs
3	Proptosis
4	Extraocular muscle involvement
5	Corneal involvement
6	Visual loss with optic neuropathy

  iv. Hirsch procedure removes the orbital floor to allow decompression into the maxillary sinus. A ridge of bone around the infraorbital nerve is preserved to support the nerve.

  v. Historically, the Ogura procedure combined the floor and medial wall resections for maximal decompression.

  vi. Scleral grafts to lengthen the upper lids may be required when scarring has shortened the lids through retraction.

  vii. Currently, the treatment of choice is the endoscopic decompression of the medial orbit via an ethmoidectomy with removal of the lamina papyracea and a partial resection of the floor of the orbit.

  viii. Classification of thyroid ophthalmopathy has been based on Werner's detailed degree of orbital involvement (Table 52-1), with classes 5 and 6 most often requiring decompression surgery.

  ix. Thyroid orbitopathy is primarily managed through medical control of the hyperthyroidism. Decompression is generally indicated in euthyroid patients who continue to have persistent corneal exposure, motility disturbances, and/or progressive visual loss.

Exophthalmos and Proptosis

 A. Causes of exophthalmos and orbital proptosis include the following:
  i. Pseudotumor
  ii. Lymphoma
  iii. Hemangioma
  iv. Thyroid orbitopathy (Graves)
  v. Orbital cellulitis/abscess
  vi. Metastatic tumor
  vii. Paranasal sinus mass
  viii. Carotid-cavernous fistula

 B. Pseudotumor of the orbit is usually seen in young adults and is quite responsive to high-dose parenteral steroids. It is idiopathic in origin.

 C. Lymphedema of the orbit can often be diagnosed by CT or magnetic resonance imaging (MRI), with a confirmatory biopsy or needle aspiration. Open biopsy may require using a medial or lateral orbitotomy approach.

D. Vascular tumors of the orbit can usually be diagnosed by orbital ultrasound with confirmation by magnetic resonance angiography (MRA) or arteriogram. Surgical approach is required to prevent impending blindness, while radiation therapy may be indicated to retard the growth of the tumor.

E. Orbital cellulitis often causes proptosis without ophthalmoplegia. When globe movement is reduced, presence of an orbital abscess must be suspected, and a CT or MRI scan obtained. Most inflammatory conditions of the orbit originate from paranasal sinus disease, with surgical drainage via an anterior orbitotomy required. Fungal orbital infection is a surgical emergency. Inflammation of the lid anterior to the orbital septum generally remains localized to the lid (preseptal cellulitis), while if posterior to the septum, it is by definition, an orbital infection.

F. Metastatic tumors of the orbit are usually of breast origin. A complete physical examination will reveal the breast tumor, although a mammogram may be indicated if not obvious. Orbital exenteration is usually not performed, in favor of chemotherapy and radiation therapy.

G. Tumors of the paranasal sinuses may encroach upon the orbit—adenocarcinoma or squamous cell carcinoma. En bloc resection of the sinus tumor with orbital exenteration is usually indicated. Polypoid disease of the sinuses, as well as a frontal sinus osteoma, may push into the orbit, causing proptosis.

H. A carotid artery–cavernous sinus fistula can occur after head or facial trauma and presents with pulsatile exophthalmos. An enhanced CT or MRA will demonstrate the fistula, and an orbital bruit can be auscultated. This condition requires intracranial closure of the fistula.

Questions

1. The roof of the orbit consists of the orbital process of the frontal bone and the lesser wing of the sphenoid.
   A. True
   B. False

2. A displaced trochlea causes diplopia on upward gaze.
   A. True
   B. False

3. The meibomian glands are located in the upper lid only.
   A. True
   B. False

4. Horner syndrome includes ptosis, miosis, and anhidrosis.
   A. True
   B. False

5. The nasolacrimal duct drains into the anterior aspect of the middle meatus.
   A. True
   B. False

Part 8
Allergy

Chapter 53
Immunology and Allergy

Introduction

- Immune system:
  - (a) Composed of a complex set of elements that is designed to distinguish "self" from "nonself."
  - (b) Protects against foreign pathogens while preserving components of self.
  - (c) Expresses and controls a specific recognition system utilizing cellular and humoral mediators.
  - (d) *The primary physiologic function of the immune system is defense against infectious microbes.*
- Innate and adaptive immunity
  - (a) Immune system defense mechanisms are mediated through two interactive processes:
    - ○ Innate immunity (also called natural or *native immunity*)
      - – Consists of genetically based mechanisms in place prior to exposure
      - – Capable of rapid responses to exposure to microbes
      - – Involves physical, chemical, and cellular barriers
    - ○ Adaptive immunity (also called *specific immunity*)
      - – More highly evolved mechanism of responding to host attack
      - – Coordinated response, with memory for prior antigen exposure and amplification in magnitude with successive antigen stimulation
      - – Involves lymphocytes and their products

- Characteristics of the innate immune system:
  (a) Specificity
    ○ Responses are specific to groups of recognized microbial antigens.
    ○ Immune responses are mediated through toll-like receptors (TLR) that coordinate various cytokine-generated, complement-mediated, and phagocytic responses.
  (b) Diversity
    ○ Limited to small range of microbial groups
  (c) Memory
- None
  (a) Nonreactivity to self
    ○ Host antigens do not under normal or healthy conditions promote an immune response.
- Characteristics of the adaptive immune system:
  (a) Specificity
    ○ Immune responses are specific for distinct antigens, microbial and nonmicrobial.
      – Structural components of single complex proteins, polysaccharides, or other macromolecules.
    ○ Portions of molecules that are recognized by lymphocytes are known as *antigenic determinants* or *epitopes*.
    ○ Mediated through antigen-specific receptors on the surfaces of T and B lymphocytes and antibodies.
  (b) Diversity
    ○ The total number of antigenic specificities recognized by lymphocytes is known as the *lymphocyte reservoir*.
    ○ Mammalian immune system can discriminate 10^9-10^{11} distinct antigenic determinants.
  (c) Memory
    ○ Exposure of the immune system to an antigen enhances its responses when again presented with that antigen.
    ○ Responses to subsequent exposures are more rapid and pronounced than initial responses.
  (d) Self-regulation
    ○ Normal immune responses decrease over time after antigen stimulation.
    ○ Immune system returns to basal resting state (homeostasis).
    ○ Antigens and immune responses stimulate self-regulatory mechanisms through ongoing, interactive feedback control.
  (e) Nonreactivity to self
    ○ Normal immune system is able to recognize and eliminate foreign materials while avoiding harmful responses to host tissues.
    ○ Immunologic unresponsiveness is known as *tolerance*.
    ○ Abnormalities in the induction or maintenance of tolerance to self leads to autoimmunity and the induction of a range of diseases.

Adaptive Immune System

- Principal cells of the immune system are (Figure 53-1).
  (a) Lymphocytes
    ○ T lymphocytes
    ○ B lymphocytes

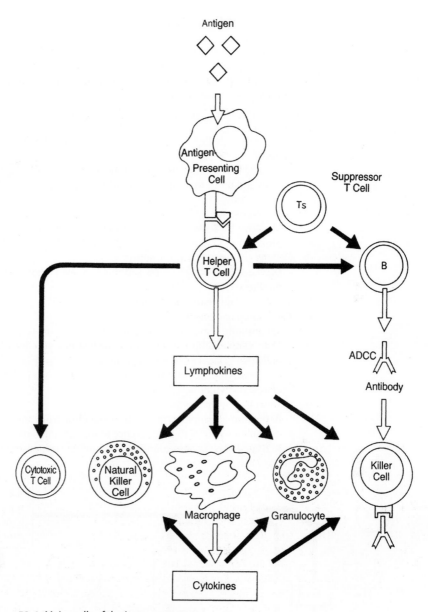

Figure 53-1 Major cells of the immune system.

    (b) Accessory cells
        ◦ Mononuclear phagocytes
        ◦ Dendritic cells (antigen-presenting cells [APCs])
    (c) Effector cells
        ◦ Activated (effector) T lymphocytes
        ◦ Mononuclear phagocytes
        ◦ Other leukocytes

- - Neutrophils
    - Eosinophils
    - Basophils
    - Mast cells
- Immunity is mediated through antigen-specific receptors on the surfaces of T and B lymphocytes and through specific antibodies.
- Immune response is triggered by exposure to antigen.
  - (a) Antigen
    - Any molecule that can be specifically recognized by the adaptive immune system
  - (b) Antibody
    - Specific immunoglobulin (Ig) produced by a specific B lymphocyte that recognizes and binds to antigens recognized as nonself
- Types of immunity
  - (a) Humoral immunity
    - Mediated by B lymphocytes and their secreted antibodies and related soluble products
  - (b) Cellular (cell-mediated) immunity
    - Mediated by T lymphocytes and their secreted cytokines and other related products
- Phases of the adaptive immune response (Figure 53-2)
  - (a) *Recognition of antigen*
    - All immune responses are initiated by the specific recognition of antigens.
    - Every individual possesses numerous lymphocytes derived from a single clonal precursor (clonal selection hypothesis).
      - These lymphocytes respond to a distinct antigenic determinant and activate a specific lymphocyte clone.
  - (b) *Activation of lymphocytes*
    - Activation of lymphocytes requires signaling from antigen exposure and innate immune responses to the presence of foreign antigens.
    - Activated lymphocytes coordinate an immune response consisting of the following:

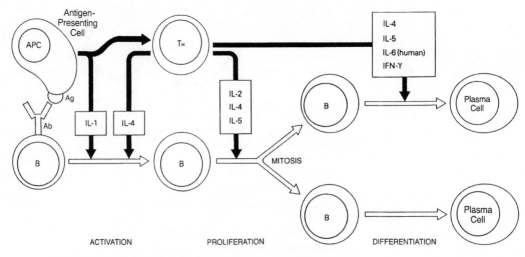

Figure 53-2 Sequence of cellular response to sensitization.

- Synthesis of new proteins
  ◊ Cytokines
  ◊ Cytokine receptors
  ◊ Proteins involved in cell division and gene transcription
- Cellular proliferation
  ◊ Expansion of specific clonal lymphocytes
- Cellular differentiation
  ◊ Effector cells
  ◊ Memory cells

(c) *Clearance of antigen*
  ○ Activated lymphocytes coordinate an effector response designed to clear foreign antigens
    - Antibodies, T lymphocytes, and other effector cells, in coordination with innate immune system defenses, clear the offending antigens

Organs and Tissues of the Immune System

- Adaptive immune responses in peripheral organs that make up the primary lymphoid system
  (a) Thymus
  (b) Bone marrow
  (c) Lymph nodes
  (d) Spleen
  (e) Cutaneous immune system
  (f) Mucosal immune system
- Thymus
  (a) Site of T-cell maturation.
  (b) Contains *thymocytes*, or T cells at various stages of maturation.
  (c) Highly vascularized with efferent lymphatics to mediastinal lymph nodes.
  (d) Only mature T cells exit the thymus and enter the peripheral circulation.
- Bone marrow
  (a) Site of generation of all circulating blood cells in the adult.
  (b) Site of B-cell maturation.
  (c) All blood cells originate from a common *stem cell* that differentiates into various cells with unique functionality.
  (d) Proliferation and maturation of cells in the bone marrow is stimulated and controlled by cytokines.
  (e) Contains numerous *plasma cells*, responsible for secretion of antibodies.
- Lymph nodes (Figure 53-3)
  (a) Site of adaptive immune responses to antigens delivered through lymphatic mechanisms.
  (b) Afferent lymphatics enter the node in multiple sites through the cortex of the node.
  (c) Efferent lymphatics exit the node through a single efferent lymphatic vessel in the hilum of the node.
  (d) Histologic anatomy of the lymph node:
    ○ Cortex
      - Outer region of node, inside capsule
      - Location of the *lymphoid follicles*
      - Rich population of B cells

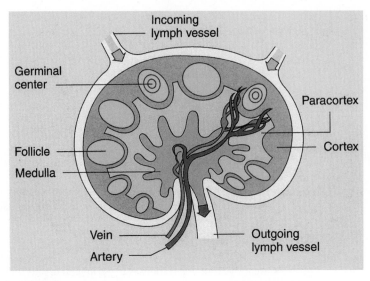

Figure 53-3 Lymph node.

- Paracortex
  - Primarily populated with T cells and antigen-processing cells
- Medulla
  - More centrally located in the lymph node
  - Presence of T cells, B cells, and plasma cells
  - Presence of macrophages
- Spleen
  - (a) Site of immune responses to blood-borne antigens
  - (b) Lymphoid follicles surround small arterioles in *periarteriolar lymphoid sheaths* (PALS)
    - Follicles contain germinal centers.
  - (c) Arterioles end in vascular sinusoids
    - Interface with large numbers of macrophages, dendritic cells, lymphocytes, and plasma cells.
  - (d) Acts as a filter for clearing the blood of microbes and other antigenic particles
    - Important in the immune response to encapsulated organisms, for example, pneumococci
- Cutaneous immune system
  - (a) Specialized network of immune cells and accessory cells that is centered in the skin.
    - Responsible for detection and surveillance of environmental antigens
  - (b) Principal cell populations include the following:
    - Keratinocytes
    - Melanocytes
    - Langerhans cells
    - T cells
  - (c) Langerhans cells are immature dendritic cells found in the skin and are active in the processing of antigen detected by the cutaneous immune system.
    - As antigens are captured by Langerhans cells, under the influence of proinflammatory cytokines, these cells migrate into the dermis and then to the regional lymph nodes for stimulation of a specific immune response.
- Mucosal immune system (Figure 53-4)

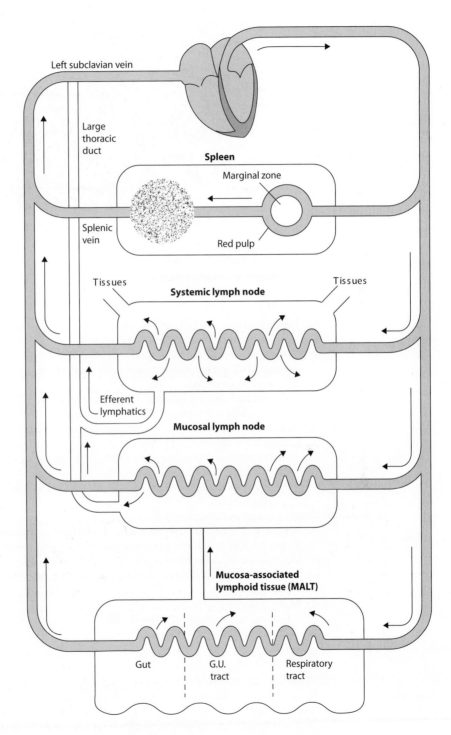

Figure 53-4 Recirculation. Mucosa-associated lymphoid tissue (MALT).

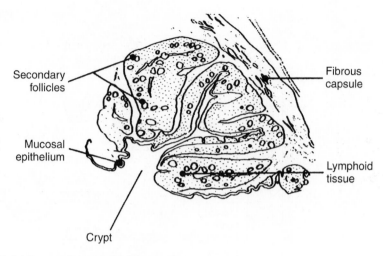

Secondary follicles

Fibrous capsule

Mucosal epithelium

Lymphoid tissue

Crypt

Figure 53-5 Microscopic structure of the tonsil.

    (a) Network of immune cells and supporting cells found in mucosal surfaces of the gastrointestinal (GI) and respiratory tracts.
- Responsible for immune response to inhaled and ingested antigens

    (b) Mucosa of GI tract demonstrates scattered collections of lymphocytes in clusters known as *Peyer patches*.
- Cells at each site have distinct functional properties.
- The majority of lymphocytes in these locations are T cells.

    (c) Tonsils/adenoids are mucosal lymphoid follicles analogous to Peyer patches and located in the upper aerodigestive tract.

    (d) Immune response to oral antigens differs from the response noted at other sites.
- High levels of IgA antibody production
- Tendency of antigens processed orally to induce T-cell tolerance rather than T-cell activation

- Tonsils and adenoids (Figure 53-5)

    (a) System of channels or clefts covered by specialized epithelium that permits contact between antigens in the upper aerodigestive tract and immune competent cells

    (b) Contain specialized epithelial cells, M (membranous) cells
- Actively transport macromolecules from surface into germinal centers through pinocytosis

    (c) Major immune function
- Generation of antigen-specific B cells in the tonsillar follicles
- Production of secretory IgA

Cells of the Immune System (Figure 53-6)

- Lymphocytes

    (a) The only cells capable of specifically recognizing and distinguishing different antigenic determinants

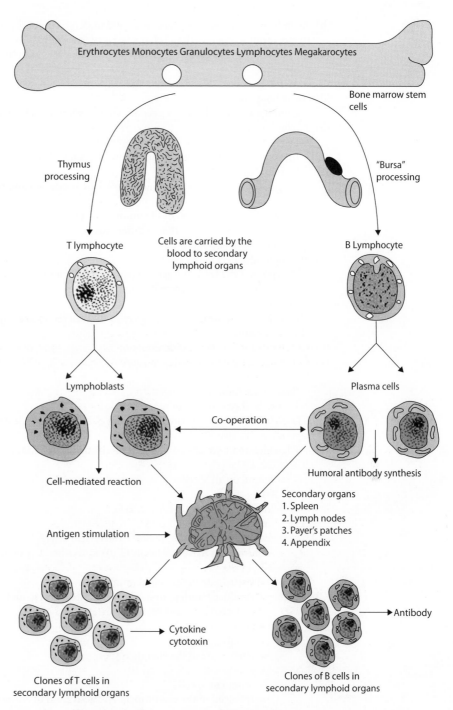

Figure 53-6 Humoral and cellular responses of the immune system.

(b) Arise from bone marrow progenitors and undergo complex patterns of maturation that determine the functional characteristics of specific cells

(c) Responsible for two primary functions of the adaptive immune system
  ◦ Specificity
  ◦ Memory

(d) Naïve lymphocytes
  ◦ Lymphocytes that have not been previously stimulated by antigen

(e) B lymphocytes
  ◦ Derived from bone marrow in mammals
  ◦ Involved in antibody production (humoral immunity)

(f) T lymphocytes
  ◦ Precursors arise in the bone marrow and are processed and mature in the thymus
  ◦ Involved in coordination of the immune response (cell-mediated immunity)
    – Stimulate B-cell growth and differentiation
    – Activate macrophages

(g) NK (natural killer) lymphocytes
  ◦ Receptors differ from those found on B and T lymphocytes
  ◦ Primarily involved in innate immunity

- Cluster of differentiation (CD) system
  (a) Molecules on the surface of lymphocytes that are recognized by a cluster of mono-clonal antibodies
  (b) CD stands for "cluster of differentiation"
  (c) CD status of lymphocytes depends on
    ◦ Cell lineage
    ◦ Stage of maturation
    ◦ Degree and type of immune activation
  (d) CD surface molecules distinguish among classes of lymphocytes

- T lymphocytes (Figure 53-7)
  ◦ Classification into subsets depends on the pattern of CD antigens
    – CD2, CD3
      ◊ Found on all T cells
    – CD4
      ◊ Identify category of T *helper cells*
        * 60% of peripheral T cells
      ◊ Induce cytotoxic/suppressor T cells (CD8 cells)
      ◊ Mature from naïve CD4 cells (T_H0) into either T_H1 or T_H2 cells
        * T_H1 cells
          ▪ Participate in microbial immunity
          ▪ Produce interleukin-2 (IL-2) and interferon gamma (IFN-γ) when activated
          ▪ Inhibit B cells
        * T_H2 cells
          ▪ Participate in the allergic response
          ▪ Produce IL-4, 5, 6, and 10
          ▪ Stimulate B cells
          ▪ Involved in the recruitment and activation of eosinophils
    – CD4 + CD25
      ◊ Recently characterized third subset of T helper cells, known as TH17 cells.

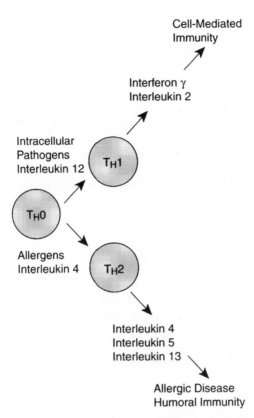

Cell-Mediated
Immunity

Interferon γ
Interleukin 2

Intracellular
Pathogens
Interleukin 12

T_H1

T_H0

Allergens
Interleukin 4

T_H2

Interleukin 4
Interleukin 5
Interleukin 13

Allergic Disease
Humoral Immunity

Figure 53-7 T_H1 and T_H2 effector cells.

* T_H17 cells
    ▪ Respond to host infections with specific bacterial and fungal species
    ▪ Involved in the recruitment and activation of neutrophils
    ▪ Create profound local inflammatory changes
    ▪ Appear to be involved in autoimmune diseases such as multiple
      sclerosis
◊ Another T-cell subset has also been identified, known as T regulatory (T_{reg})
   cells.
    * T_{reg} cells
        ▪ Regulate immune responses in vivo
        ▪ Exert suppressor effects on effector T cells and APCs
        ▪ Involved in prevention of autoimmunity
        ▪ Involved in induction of immune tolerance
            • Play a central role in therapeutic effects noted with allergy
              immunotherapy
– CD8
    ◊ Identify category of *T suppressor (cytotoxic) cells*
        * 20% to 30% of peripheral T cells
        * Specifically kill target cells
            ▪ Lysis of virus-infected cells

- Lysis of tumor cells
  * Inhibit the response of B cells and other T cells
  * Important in immune tolerance
- B lymphocytes
  (a) Produce antibodies
  (b) Carry endogenously produced immunoglobulins (Ig) on surface
    ○ Act as antigen receptors
  (c) Maturation occurs in the bone marrow
  (d) Differentiate into plasma cells
    ○ Produce genetically programmed specific Ig
    ○ Stimulated by contact with antigen
      – Act collaboratively with T cells and macrophages
  (e) Account for 10% to 15% of circulating lymphocytes
  (f) Positive for CD19, CD21
- Natural killer (NK) cells
  (a) Also referred to as *null cells*
  (b) Large, granular lymphocytes that are neither T nor B cells
  (c) Major function is innate immunity
    ○ Able to lyse and eliminate virus-infected cells and tumor cells
    ○ Involved in autoimmunity (antibody-dependent cellular cytotoxicity)
  (d) Account for 10% of circulating lymphocytes
  (e) Rarely found in lymph nodes
  (f) Positive for CD16
- Myeloid cells
  (a) Macrophages
  (b) Antigen-presenting (processing) cells (APCs)
  (c) Dendritic cells
  (d) Polymorphonuclear granulocytes
    ○ Neutrophils
    ○ Basophils
    ○ Eosinophils
    ○ Mast cells
    ○ Other granulocytes

Accessory Factors Involved in Immune System Function

- Major histocompatibility complex (MHC) proteins (Figure 53-8)
  (a) Central to the function of the immune system
  (b) Specialized proteins responsible for displaying antigens for recognition of antigens by and presentation of peptides to T cells
    ○ Antigen receptors of T cells are specific for complexes of foreign peptides and self-MHC molecules.
    ○ MHC proteins are involved in both external immunity and autoimmunity.
  (c) Coded by a broad locus of highly polymorphic genes
  (d) MHC molecules
    ○ Contain cell surface glycoprotein that is encoded in each species by the MHC gene complex.
    ○ Principal function is to bind fragments of foreign protein, thereby forming complexes that are recognized by T cells.

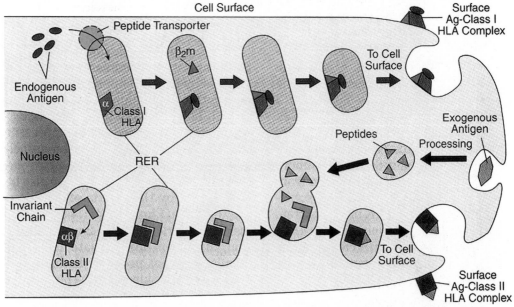

Figure 53-8 Antigen processing.

- ○ Two types of polymorphic MHC genes:
  - – *Class I*: membrane associated glycoproteins present on nearly all nucleated cells
  - – *Class II*: normally expressed only on B lymphocytes, macrophages or dendritic cells, endothelial cells, and a few other cell lines
  - ○ Each MHC molecule contains an extracellular peptide-binding region and a pair of Ig-like domains, and attaches to the cell by transmembrane and cytoplasmic components (Figure 53-9).
    - – Ig-like domains act as binding sites for CD4 and CD8.
- Cytokines
  - (a) Proteins secreted by cells of the innate and adaptive immune system in response to stimulation with antigen and that mediate the function of these immune cells.
  - (b) Produced in response to antigens and stimulate diverse cellular responses.
    - ○ Stimulate growth and differentiation of lymphocytes
    - ○ Activate effector cells to eliminate microbial and other antigens
    - ○ Stimulate the development of hematopoietic cells
  - (c) Cytokines are often classified by their cellular sources or by their action on immune cells.
    - ○ *Lymphokines*: cytokines produced by lymphocytes
    - ○ *Interferons*: potent antiviral agents
    - ○ *Colony-stimulating factors*: involved in maturation and systemic release of bone marrow precursor cells
    - ○ *Tumor necrosis factors*: principal mediators of acute inflammatory response to gram-negative bacteria

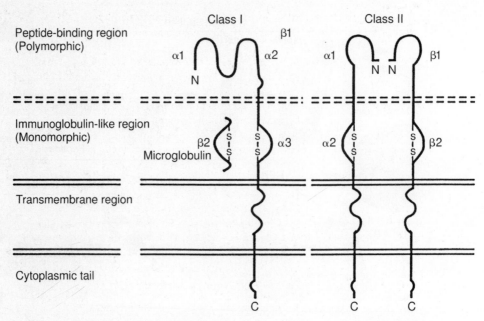

Figure 53-9 Structure of major histocompatibility complex (MHC) classes I and II molecules.

- o *Interleukins*: cytokines produced by leukocytes that act on other leukocytes
  - – Individual interleukins are assigned an IL number that is used to classify their function (eg, IL-1, IL-5).
- (d) Properties of cytokines:
  - o Cytokine secretion is brief and self-limited.
  - o The actions of cytokines are often redundant.
  - o Cytokines often influence the synthesis and action of other cytokines.
  - o Cytokine actions may be local and/or systemic.
  - o Cytokines initiate their actions by binding to specific membrane receptors on target cells.
  - o Cytokines act through regulation of gene expression in target cells.
- • Principal cytokines involved in the allergic response
  - (a) IL-2
    - o Growth factor for antigen-stimulated T cells and responsible for T-cell clonal expansion
    - o Derived from T cells
    - o Promotes the proliferation and differentiation of other immune cells
  - (b) IL-3
    - o Promotes development and expansion of immature bone marrow elements
      - – Promotes mast cell proliferation
      - – Promotes eosinophil activation
      - – Derived from CD4+ T cells
  - (c) IL-4
    - o Principal cytokine that stimulates B-cell isotype switching to the IgE isotype
      - – IgE is the primary immunoglobulin involved in the allergic response.

- Stimulates the development of T_H2 cells from naïve CD4+ cells
- Derived from CD4+ T cells and mast cells

(d) IL-5
  - Activates eosinophils and links T-cell activation and eosinophilic inflammation
  - Stimulates the growth and differentiation of eosinophils and the activation of mature eosinophils
  - Involved in stimulating eosinophil chemotaxis to areas of inflammation
  - Derived from CD4+ T cells

(e) IL-10
  - Inhibits activated macrophages
  - Inhibits cytokine synthesis in various cells
  - Maintains homeostatic control of innate and cell-mediated immune reactions
  - Derived from activated macrophages and CD4+ T cells
  - Suppresses antigen-presenting capacities of APCs
  - Acts as an important regulator of the immune system

(f) IL-13
  - Functions in a similar manner to IL-4
  - Induces adhesion molecules at sites of allergic inflammation contributing to increased populations of eosinophils and lymphocytes

Overview of the Cell-Mediated Immune System

- Cell-mediated immunity
  (a) The adaptive immune response to antigens is mediated by T lymphocytes, which recognize specific antigens and produce cytokines that stimulate inflammation.
  (b) Induction of cell-mediated immunity involves antigen recognition by T cells in peripheral lymphoid organs, proliferation of these T cells, and their differentiation into effector lymphocytes.
  (c) The specificity of the immune response is due to T cells.
  (d) Antigen-presenting cells (APCs) (Figure 53-10).

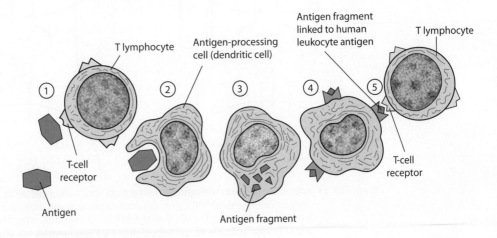

Figure 53-10 T-cell activation.

- ○ T cells respond to antigens presented by other cells in the context of MHC proteins.
  - – Proteins may be presented by macrophages (dendritic cells), endothelial, or glial cells
  - – Dendritic cells
    - ◊ Specialized macrophages found in the skin, mucosa, lymph nodes, spleen, and thymus
- ○ APCs ingest and process the antigen.
- ○ APCs present the antigen to T cells in association with Class II MHC molecules (Figure 53-11).
- ○ In the spleen and thymus, these APCs may be important in the recognition of self-antigens.
- (e) T-cell activation.
  - ○ Resting T cells are activated by cellular signaling.
  - ○ When activated, these T cells
    - – Proliferate
    - – Differentiate
    - – Produce cytokines and various effector functions
- (f) Migration of activated T cells and other leukocytes.
  - ○ Migration of leukocytes to sites of inflammation is stimulated by cytokines.
    - – Cytokines induce the expression of adhesion molecules on endothelial cells and the chemotaxis of leukocytes.
  - ○ Previously activated effector and memory T cells migrate to the site of inflammation.

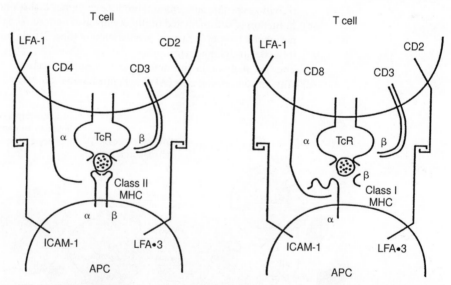

Figure 53-11 Interaction of T cells with antigen and antigen-presenting cell (APC). Left: CD4 T (helper) cell where the TcR interacts with antigen (stippled area) and major histocompatibility complex (MHC) class II on the APC. Accessory molecules LFA-1, ICAM-1, CD2, and LFA-3 facilitate the interaction. Right: CD8 T (suppressor) cell where the TcR interacts with antigen and MHC class I on the APC.

Overview of the Humoral Immune Response

- Humoral immunity
  - (a) Humoral immunity is mediated by secreted antibodies.
  - (b) The primary function of humoral immunity is the defense against extracellular microbes and microbial toxins.
  - (c) Antibodies are produced by B cells and plasma cells in the lymphoid organs and bone marrow, but antibodies perform their effector functions at sites distant from their production.
  - (d) Antibodies may be derived from cells produced at the time of primary exposure and activated again through a secondary immune response mediated by memory B cells.
  - (e) Features of an antibody (Figure 53-12).
    - ○ Four polypeptide chains connected with disulfide bonds
    - ○ Two identical light polypeptide chains (25,000 MW)
      - – The light chain determines light chain class.
        - ◊ Kappa
        - ◊ Lambda
    - ○ Two identical heavy polypeptide chains (50,000-77,000 MW)
      - – The heavy chain binds to host tissues and complement and determines Ig class.
    - ○ Constant region (C-terminal end of the Ig molecule) or Fc fragment
    - ○ Variable region (N-terminal end) of F_{ab} fragment
  - (f) Classes of immunoglobulins (Figure 53-13)
    - ○ IgG
      - – Major antibody involved in secondary immune responses
      - – Important activity against viruses, bacteria, parasites, and some fungi
      - – Only Ig class that crosses the placenta
        - ◊ Provides 3 to 6 months of immunity after birth
      - – Fixes complement through the classic pathway
    - ○ IgM
      - – Primary antibody associated with the early immune response
      - – Pentamer associated with a J chain
      - – Fixes complement through the classic pathway

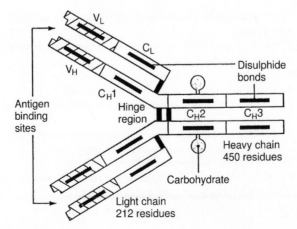

Figure 53-12 Structure of Ig molecule.

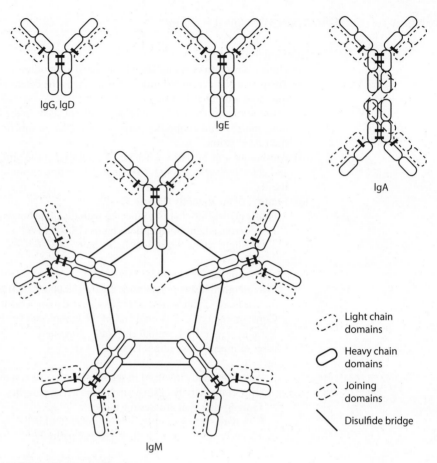

Figure 53-13 Structure of Ig classes.

- ○ IgA
  - – Predominant Ig in seromucinous secretions (saliva, tracheobronchial secretions)
  - – Dimer associated with "secretory component" (prevents proteolysis by digestive enzymes) and J chain
- ○ IgD
  - – Found in large quantities on circulating B cells
  - – May be involved in antigen-induced lymphocyte proliferation
- ○ IgE
  - – Involved in type I immediate hypersensitivity reactions
  - – Classic Ig involved in anaphylaxis and atopy
  - – Unique biologic properties
    - ◊ Cell-associated IgE molecules of a particular antigenic specificity can be cross-linked by their appropriate antigen.
  - – Present in smallest amount of all of the five Ig classes

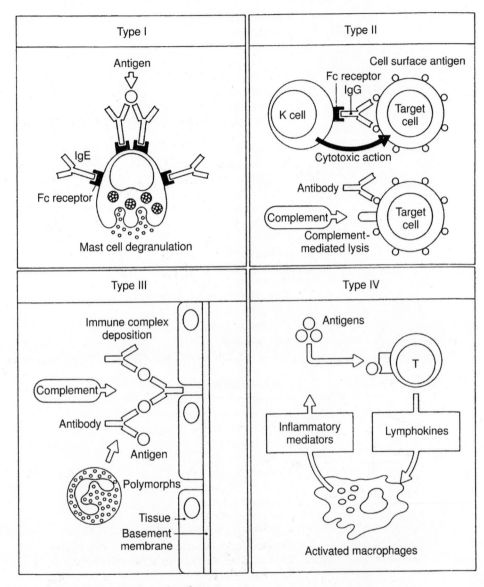

Figure 53-14 Gell and Coombs classification.

(g) Hypersensitivity reactions (also known as the "Gell and Coombs" classes" [Figure 53-14])
- *Type I: anaphylactic*
  - Immediate hypersensitivity reaction
  - Symptoms apparent within minutes of exposure
  - Upper respiratory symptoms
    ◊ Sneezing

    ◊ Itching

    ◊ Rhinorrhea

    ◊ Congestion

  – Lower respiratory symptoms

    ◊ Cough

    ◊ Bronchospasm

    ◊ Wheezing

      * Shortness of breath

  – Skin symptoms

    ◊ Urticaria

    ◊ Angioedema

    ◊ Itching

    ◊ Whealing

  – Inciting agents

    ◊ Inhalants

    ◊ Foods

    ◊ Drugs

    ◊ Insect stings

  – Mechanism

    ◊ Crosslinking of IgE molecules on mast cells

    ◊ Degranulation of mast cells

    ◊ Release of histamine

 ○ *Type II: cytotoxic*

  – Involved in various systemic hypersensitivities

    ◊ Hemolytic anemia

    ◊ Transfusion reactions

    ◊ Hyperacute graft rejection

    ◊ Goodpasture syndrome

    ◊ Myasthenia gravis

  – Inciting agents

    ◊ Unknown

  – Mechanism

    ◊ IgG or IgM mediated

    ◊ Antibodies react with antigens on cell surface

    ◊ Activation of complement

 ○ *Type III: immune complex-mediated*

  – Onset of symptoms may be delayed for up to days.

  – Involved in various system hypersensitivities.

    ◊ Serum sickness

    ◊ Poststreptococcal glomerulonephritis

    ◊ Arthus reaction

    ◊ Angioedema

    ◊ GI intolerance

  – Inciting agents:

    ◊ Drugs

    ◊ Bacterial products

    ◊ Often unknown

  – Mechanism:

    ◊ Immune complexes are formed, usually with IgG antibodies.

◊ Complexes deposited in tissues.
◊ Activation of complement.
◊ Initiation of acute inflammatory response.
○ *Type IV: delayed (cell-mediated) hypersensitivity*
 – Involved in acute and chronic dermatitis
 – Involved in granulomatous diseases
 ◊ Tuberculosis
 ◊ Sarcoidosis
 – Involved in some fungal diseases
 ◊ Candidiasis
 – Inciting agents
 ◊ Poison ivy, sumac, oak
 ◊ Cosmetics
 ◊ Various metals and chemicals
- Nickel
 – Mechanism
 ◊ Mediated by direct T-cell activation
 ◊ Cell-mediated inflammation

The Allergic Response

- Allergy overview
 (a) Allergy is the most common disorder of immunity and affects 20% to 25% of all individuals in the United States.
 (b) Allergic reactions occur with exposure to normally harmless antigens among susceptible individuals.
 (c) The susceptibility to develop an allergic response is known as *atopy*, which implies a genetic predisposition toward the expression of allergic diseases.
 ○ Atopic individuals demonstrate a skewing of T helper responses to the T_H2 pattern.
 ○ The overproduction of IgE antibodies in this setting creates a milieu in which allergic symptoms can be expressed.
 (d) In genetically predisposed individuals, an environmental protein antigen, commonly referred to as an *allergen*, stimulates CD4+ T cells to differentiate into T_H2 effector cells.
 (e) A cascade of events occurs in which allergic symptoms occur through this immediate hypersensitivity response.
- Sequence of events in immediate hypersensitivity responses
 (a) Initial exposure to an antigen among susceptible individuals stimulates naïve T cells to differentiate into T_H2 effector cells.
 (b) Activated T cells secrete IL-4 and contact-mediated signals promote differentiation of B cells specific for that antigen into IgE-producing cells.
 (c) IgE produced by these cells circulates throughout the body and binds to high-affinity F_c receptors on the surfaces of circulating basophils and on tissue mast cells.
 (d) Subsequent reexposure to the antigen results in binding of the antigen to IgE molecules on the surface of mast cells and basophils.
 (e) Crosslinking of adjacent IgE molecules initiates signal transduction in mast cells and basophils, resulting in the release of preformed mediators stored in cytoplasmic granules in these cells, as well as the rapid synthesis and release of other, newly formed mediators.

(f) Clinical and pathological manifestations of the allergic response are due to the effects of these mediators on target cells.
- ○ "Wheal and flare" response
  - – Vascular leakage of plasma
  - – Vasodilation
- ○ Smooth muscle stimulation
- ○ Bronchoconstriction
- ○ Acute and chronic inflammation
- • Specifics of the allergic response
  - (a) Production of IgE
    - ○ Type I immediate hypersensitivity reactions are primarily mediated by IgE antibodies.
    - ○ The presence of a factor in the serum that was capable of transferring the allergic wheal and flare reaction was first demonstrated by Prausnitz and Kustner (1921).
      - – This serum factor was termed regain.
    - ○ IgE was first isolated and characterized by Ishizaka (1967).
      - – Noted to be a new class of Ig, and termed IgE
  - (b) Production of antigen-specific IgE antibodies
    - ○ Requires active collaboration between macrophages (APCs), T cells, and B cells.
    - ○ Allergen exposure
      - – Introduced through the respiratory tract, GI tract, or skin.
      - – Reacts with APCs that process the antigen.
      - – Presented to appropriately sensitized T cells with interaction at the T-cell receptor.
      - – B cells, in the presence of the APC, antigen, and sensitized T cells are stimulated to develop into plasma cells.
      - – Plasma cells synthesize and secrete antigen-specific IgE.
        - ◊ IgE-producing plasma cells are primarily located in the lamina propria of the skin, respiratory tract, and GI tract.
  - (c) Binding of the IgE to mast cells
    - ○ IgE antibodies bind to mast cells.
      - – Receptors on mast cells specific for the Fc region of the epsilon heavy chain.
      - – IgE-laden mast cells are distributed throughout the body through passive transfer into the serum.
    - ○ Mast cells:
      - – Located in perivascular connective tissue
      - – Circulate in the serum as similar cells, *basophils*
      - – Contain 5000-500,000 antigen-specific IgE antibodies on their surfaces
      - – Contain potent mediators of immediate hypersensitivity
  - (d) Reexposure to antigen
    - ○ The binding of IgE antibody to mediator cell receptors is directly related to serum IgE concentration.
      - – The higher the serum IgE level, the greater the binding of IgE to mast cells and basophils.
    - ○ The greater the patient sensitivity, the lesser antigen is required to initiate an allergic response.
    - ○ Antigen interaction with antigen-specific IgE bound to the surface of mast cells (Figure 53-15).

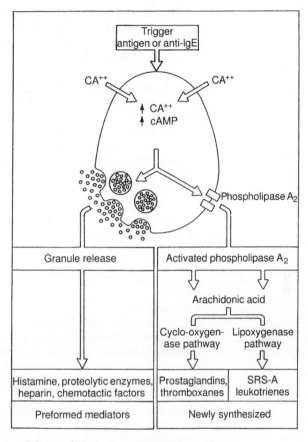

Figure 53-15 Mast cell degranulation.

- Repeat allergen stimulation by the same specific allergen initiates the cross-linking of two or more mast cell bound IgE molecules.
- Signal is transmitted to the cell interior that initiates a specific molecular response.
  ◊ Increased ratio of cyclic guanosine monophosphate (cGMP) to cyclic adenosine monophosphate (cAMP).
  ◊ F_c receptors are linked to a transmembrane coupling protein and adenylate cyclase.
  ◊ Coupling protein activates adenylate cyclase when cross-linking of antigen to two IgE antibodies occurs.
  ◊ Adenylate cyclase reduces adenosine triphosphate (ATP) to AMP.
  ◊ AMP decreased by kinase enhances mediator release.
- Preformed cytoplasmic granules.
  ◊ Migrate to the cell surface membrane
  ◊ Fuse with each other and with the cell membrane
  ◊ Extrude through the membrane and released into the external microenvironment

       – Enhances the influx of Ca2+ from the extracellular space.
         ◊ Release of mediators of type I anaphylaxis
         ◊ Production of newly formed mediators, leukotrienes and prostaglandins, via the activation of arachidonic acid metabolism

(e) Mast cell degranulation
   ○ When triggered by an antigen, the mast cell membrane allows Ca2+ influx, which triggers degranulation and the release of granule-associated preformed mediators.
     – Histamine
       ◊ Main mediator of the allergic reaction
       ◊ Tissue effects include
         * Vasodilation
         * Increased capillary permeability
         * Bronchoconstriction
         * Tissue edema
       ◊ Exerts effects through various receptor subtypes
         * H_1-H_3
     – Tryptase
       ◊ Proteolytic enzymes
     – Heparin
       ◊ Anticoagulant
       ◊ Suppresses histamine production
       ◊ Enhances phagocytosis
     – Chemotactic factors
       ◊ Involved in chemotaxis of both eosinophils and neutrophils
     – Kininogenase
       ◊ Promotes vasoactive mucosal edema
   ○ Newly generated inflammatory mediators are also released through metabolism of arachidonic acid.
     – Leukotrienes
       ◊ Formed through the lipoxygenase pathway
       ◊ Potent mediators of inflammation
       ◊ Vasoactive
       ◊ Chemotactic
       ◊ Involved in bronchoconstriction
     – Prostaglandins
       ◊ Formed through the cyclooxygenase pathway
       ◊ Involved in bronchoconstriction
       ◊ Encourage platelet aggregation
       ◊ Promote vasodilation
     – Platelet-activating factor (PAF)
       ◊ Chemotactic for eosinophils
       ◊ Stimulates other cells to release mediators

(f) Promotion of allergic signs and symptoms
   ○ Eyes
     – Allergic shiners
       ◊ Darkening under the eyes from chronic deposition of hemosiderin in tissues
     – Long, silky eyelashes

- Periorbital edema and puffiness
- Dennie's lines
  ◊ Fine horizontal lines in the lower lids
  ◊ Occur through spasms of Mueller muscles in the lids
- Conjunctival lymphoid aggregates
- Injection of the bulbar conjunctiva
○ Nose
  - Itching
  - Supratip horizontal crease
    ◊ Develops through chronic rubbing of the nose
  - Facial grimacing
  - "Allergic salute"
    ◊ Characteristic rubbing of the nose with the heel of the hand
  - Nasal obstruction
    ◊ Mucosal edema
    ◊ Turbinate hypertrophy
    ◊ Increased mucus secretion
  - Sneezing
  - Rhinorrhea
○ Mouth
  - Chronic mouth breathing
    ◊ Secondary to nasal obstruction
  - Palatal itching
  - Nocturnal bruxism
○ Pharynx
  - Dry, irritated, inflamed mucosa
    ◊ Related to direct allergen exposure
    ◊ Related to chronic mouth breathing
  - Repeated throat clearing
    ◊ Also associated with laryngopharyngeal reflux
  - "Cobblestoning" of the posterior pharyngeal wall
    ◊ Presence of lymphoid aggregates or patches on the posterior pharyngeal wall
○ Larynx
  - Intermittent dysphonia
  - Increased tenacious mucus
  - Throat clearing
  - Cough
○ Lungs
  - Cough
  - Wheezing
  - Dyspnea
  - Interference with sleep
(g) Phases of the allergic response (Figure 53-16)
○ Early phase
  - Primarily histamine mediated.
  - Occurs rapidly after exposure to a previously sensitized antigen.
    ◊ Usually occur within 5 to 10 minutes.
    ◊ Immediate symptoms can last for several hours.

Early phase reaction (epr) occurs within minutes of allergen exposure in sensitized subjects

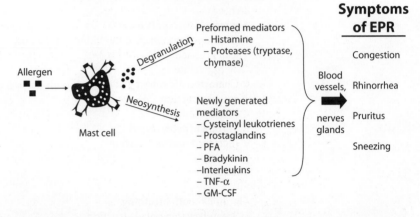

Late phase reaction (lpr) occurs 3 to 12 hours post allergen exposure

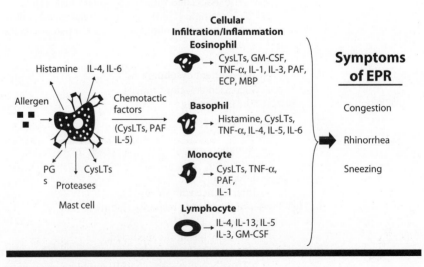

Figure 53-16 Early- and late-phase allergic responses.

  - Symptoms primarily include itching, sneezing, tearing, wheezing, mild congestion, and rhinorrhea.
  ○ Late phase (delayed)
  - Primarily mediated by newly generated mediators of inflammation and cellular infiltration.
    ◊ Leukotrienes, eosinophils
  - Occur after a delay.
    ◊ Generally begin in 4 to 8 hours after exposure
    ◊ May occur after initial resolution of acute symptoms
    ◊ Can last for 24 hours or more
  - Symptoms include increasing congestion, increased rhinorrhea, wheezing.

Overview of Inhalant Allergens

- Four broad categories of allergic triggers
  (a) Inhalants
    ○ Pollens, animal danders, molds
  (b) Ingestants
    ○ Foods, medications
  (c) Injectables
    ○ Medications, insect venom
  (d) Contactants
    ○ Nickel, poison ivy, medications
- Inhalant allergy
  (a) US classification divides inhalant allergy into two categories:
    ○ Seasonal allergy
      - Occurs in relation to outdoor allergens
      - Discrete identifiable seasons with onset, peak, and decline
        ◊ Spring, tree pollen
        ◊ Summer, grass pollen
        ◊ Fall, weed pollen
    ○ Perennial allergy
      - Occurs primarily in relation to indoor allergens
        ◊ Dust mites, cockroach, indoor molds, animal danders
      - Present throughout the year with little or no seasonality
  (b) International (World Health Organization) classifies allergy according to the ARIA (Allergic Rhinitis and its Impact on Asthma) guidelines.
    ○ Use categories based on persistence and severity of symptoms (Figure 53-17)
      - Intermittent allergic rhinitis
        ◊ Less than 4 days a week or less then 4 weeks yearly
      - Persistent allergic rhinitis
        ◊ Greater than 4 days a week and greater than 4 weeks yearly
      - Grades severity as mild or moderate/severe
        ◊ *Mild*: no impact on quality of life or function
        ◊ *Moderate/severe*: symptoms impact quality of life or function, for example, sleep, work, school performance

Intermittent • <4 days per week OR • <4 weeks	**Persistent** • 4 days per week AND • >4 weeks

Mild
Normal sleep AND
• No impairment of daily
  activities, sport, leisure
• Normal work and school
• No troublesome symptoms
	Moderate-severe
	One or more:
	• Abnormal sleep
	• Impairment of daily
	  activities, sport, leisure
	• Abnormal work or school
	• Troublesome symptoms

Figure 53-17 Allergic Rhinitis and Its Impact on Asthma (ARIA) classification of allergy severity and chronicity.

(c) Seasonal allergic rhinitis.
  ◦ Pollens from outdoor plants are released into the air at discrete times during the year.
  ◦ Pollens need to be disbursed in the atmosphere in such a way as to come into contact with human populations and create symptoms.
  ◦ Antigenicity of a pollen is determined by *Thommen's postulates*:
    – In order for a pollen to be an effective allergen, it must be
      ◊ Windborne
      ◊ Light enough to be carried large distances in the air
      ◊ Produced in large quantities
      ◊ Abundantly distributed in the environment
      ◊ Able to be allergenic to sensitive individuals
  ◦ Distribution of allergens varies based on climate, elevation, and other local agricultural characteristics.
  ◦ Effective management of seasonal allergy requires an awareness of the locally significant pollens in a specific geographic area.
  ◦ Seasons for various classes of pollens can be broadly grouped as the following:
    – *Trees*: winter and spring allergens, generally February to May
      ◊ Birch
      ◊ Oak
      ◊ Maple
      ◊ Sycamore
      ◊ Cedar
    – *Grasses*: later spring and summer allergens, generally April to August
      ◊ Timothy
      ◊ Johnson
      ◊ Bermuda
    – *Weeds*: later summer and fall allergens, generally July to first frost
      ◊ Ragweed
      ◊ Sage
      ◊ Lamb's quarter
(d) Perennial allergic rhinitis
  ◦ Allergens are present in the environment year-round and are difficult to avoid.

- Classes of perennial allergens include dust, dust mite, cockroach, animal dander, and indoor molds.
- Dust:
  - Composite of various antigens rather than a discrete antigen.
  - Composed of dust mite and cockroach elements, human skin, fibers, paints, animal danders.
  - Dust is not generally tested or treated as a discrete antigen currently, but rather assessed and treated by its important component elements.
- Dust mites:
  - Small arachnids present in large quantities around human habitation.
  - Two primary species important in US allergic disease.
    ◊ *Dermatophagoides pteronyssinus*
    ◊ *Dermatophagoides farinae*
  - Primary antigenic proteins.
    ◊ DerP1
    ◊ DerF1
  - Found primarily in humid environments at or near sea level.
  - Prefer 70° to 80°F and 35% to 70% relative humidity.
  - Most allergenic element of the dust mite is its feces.
    ◊ Highly allergenic and easily distributed
  - Feed on human skin scales.
  - Found in large quantities in bedrooms.
- Animal danders
  - Cat
    ◊ Primary antigen is FelD1.
    ◊ Found in cat pelt, cat saliva, and cat urine.
    ◊ Highly allergenic and persistent in environment.
  - Dog
    ◊ Primary antigen is CanD1.
    ◊ Often less allergenic than cat.
    ◊ Allergen is not well understood.
  - Mouse, rat, guinea pig, horse, etc
    ◊ Other animal danders may be significant in situations where individuals come into regular contact with these antigens.
      * Rodent allergy appears to be increasing in frequency in the inner city.
      * Lab workers may develop allergy to the lab animals in their care.
- Molds
  - Molds that demonstrate significance in perennial allergy are generally found in or near the home.
    ◊ Indoor plants, moist areas indoors, basements, refrigerators, air-conditioning units
    ◊ Associated with plants or decaying matter near the home outdoors
  - Mold antigens vary widely in their size and their antigenicity.
    ◊ May promote both types I and IV responses
  - Leading offenders
    ◊ *Alternaria, Aspergillus, Curvularia, Hormodendrum, Cladosporium, Pullaria, Penicillium*
- Cockroach
  - Important allergen in inner-city environments.

      – Very potent allergen, involved in both allergic rhinitis and asthma.
      – Allergen appears to involve decaying whole-body antigens.
        ◊ May be secreted by the insect
      – Difficult avoid.

Diagnosis of Allergy

- Diagnosis of allergy involves three elements
  (a) History
  (b) Physical examination
  (c) Diagnostic testing
- History of the allergic patient
  (a) Types of symptoms
    ○ Nasal
      – Sneezing
      – Itching
      – Rhinorrhea
      – Congestion
    ○ Ocular
      – Tearing
      – Itching
      – Redness
    ○ Lower respiratory
      – Wheezing
      – Cough
      – Dyspnea
    ○ Skin
      – Itching
      – Redness
      – Swelling
  (b) Magnitude of symptoms
  (c) Duration of symptoms
    ○ Transient versus persistent
  (d) Triggers to symptoms
    ○ Inhalants
    ○ Foods
    ○ Contact irritants
    ○ Medications
  (e) Seasonality of symptoms
    ○ Seasonal versus perennial
  (f) Family history of allergy
    ○ First-degree relatives versus more distant
    ○ History of allergic rhinitis, conjunctivitis, asthma
  (g) Present environments
    ○ Home
    ○ School
    ○ Work
    ○ Time spent indoor versus outdoor

(h) Past medical history
(i) Past and current treatment
- ○ Medications
- ○ Immunotherapy
- Physical examination of the allergy patient
  - (a) Overall appearance
    - ○ Presence of cough, sniffling, sneezing, etc
  - (b) Facial appearance
    - ○ Dennie's lines, allergic shiners, periorbital edema, nasal crease
    - ○ Nasal rubbing, grimacing, or wiping
    - ○ Mouth breathing
  - (c) Eyes
    - ○ Conjunctival redness or injection
    - ○ Conjunctival edema or tearing
  - (d) Nose
    - ○ Size of inferior turbinates
    - ○ Color of nasal mucosa
    - ○ Presence of mucoid or mucopurulent secretion
    - ○ Position of nasal septum
  - (e) Oral cavity/oropharynx
    - ○ Size of tonsils
    - ○ Presence of cobblestoning on posterior pharyngeal wall
  - (f) Lungs
    - ○ Presence of wheezing
- Diagnostic testing of the allergic patient
  - (a) Nasal cytology
    - ○ Designed to evaluate for the presence of eosinophils versus neutrophils in the nasal mucus.
    - ○ Has been done historically to differentiate allergic rhinitis from other types of rhinitis.
    - ○ Test is poorly sensitive and specific, and can frequently be inaccurate.
      - – Nasal polyps
      - – NARES (nonallergic rhinitis and eosinophilia syndrome)
      - – Local allergic rhinitis
        - ◊ Production of local IgE and immune mediators in the nose itself, without systemic presence of IgE
        - ◊ Controversial topic, with increasing evidence that it may be operational in some patients
        - ◊ Increased interest in developing diagnostic methods to detect local allergic rhinitis
  - (b) Specific allergen testing
    - ○ Designed to assess the presence of discrete allergens to which the patient shows hypersensitivity.
    - ○ Can be done through either in vivo (skin testing) or in vitro (serum testing) methods.
    - ○ Goal is to identify:
      - – Whether the patient is allergic
      - – The antigens to which the patient is allergic
      - – The degree of sensitization

- ○ Testing for inhalant allergens has been conducted for over 100 years and has been demonstrated to be safe and useful.
- ○ *Proviso*: A patient may have positive allergy tests without any allergic symptoms.
  - – Suggests that the patient is atopic, but may not have sufficient sensitization to be symptomatic.
  - – Presence of symptoms is necessary to classify the patient as "allergic."
- ○ In vivo allergy tests:
  - – Can be classified as *epicutaneous* or *percutaneous*
  - – Epicutaneous techniques
    - ◊ Introduction of antigen into epidermis only
    - ◊ Include scratch, prick, and puncture tests
  - – Percutaneous techniques
    - ◊ Introduction of antigen into the superficial dermis
    - ◊ Include various intradermal techniques
  - – Scratch testing
    - ◊ Epicutaneous method
    - ◊ First describe by Blackley in 1873
    - ◊ Technique
      - * 2-mm superficial lacerations are made in the patient's skin.
      - * A drop of concentrated antigen is applied to the scratch.
      - * Usually conducted on the patient's back.
    - ◊ Advantages
      - * Generally safe
        - ▪ Systemic reactions are uncommon.
      - * Rare delayed skin reactions
      - * Large surface area for testing
    - ◊ Disadvantages
      - * False-positive reactions are common.
        - ▪ Related to traumatic reactions of the skin rather than immune-mediated allergic reactions
      - * More painful than other types of testing.
      - * Tests are poorly reproducible.
    - ◊ Because of variable sensitivity, poor specificity, and lack of reproducibility, scratch testing is not currently recommended as a diagnostic procedure for assessment of inhalant allergy.
  - – Prick/puncture testing
    - ◊ Epicutaneous metody
    - ◊ First described by Lewis and Grant in 1926
    - ◊ Most widely used allergy testing method worldwide
    - ◊ Technique
      - * Various methods are used for prick/puncture testing.
        - ▪ A drop of antigen is placed on the skin and a small needle or lancet is used to penetrate into the epidermis through this drop.
        - ▪ As an alternate, single- and multiple-prick devices can be used that hold the antigen in small tines for introduction into the epidermis.
      - * 10-20 minutes is allotted for the skin to react.
      - * Measurement of the reaction can be done through a subjective system (eg, 0 to 4+) or through direct measurement of wheal diameters.
    - ◊ Advantages

* Rapid and easily performed.
* Inter-rater consistency is good.
* High degree of safety.
  * Rare systemic reactions
* Excellent screening test for the presence or absence of allergy
◊ Disadvantages
* Allows only a qualitative assessment of allergen sensitization.
* May by less sensitive to low degrees of allergy sensitization.
  * Can result in false negative responses
* Grading of skin response is less objective than with intradermal techniques.
◊ Summary
* Prick/puncture testing is an excellent screening method for the presence or absence of allergy to individual antigens.
* Testing can be done rapidly and safely, with little intertester variability.
* May be less sensitive to presence of low degrees of allergic sensitization for individual antigens.
– Intradermal testing
◊ Percutaneous method
◊ First described by Cooke in 1915
◊ Can involve single- or multiple-dilutional techniques
◊ Technique (single-dilutional)
* Use a small gauge (eg, # 26) needle to inject intradermally a small amount of antigen, ranging from 0.01 to 0.05 mL.
* Concentrations of injected antigens can vary, but are generally prepared as 1:500 to 1:1000 weight/volume.
* 10 to 20 minutes are allotted for the skin to react.
* Erythema and induration (whealing) are measured using either a subjective (eg, 0 to 4+) method or through measurement of the diameter of the response.
◊ Advantages (single-dilutional)
* Highly sensitive
  * Very low degrees of allergy can be detected.
* Moderately reproducible
◊ Disadvantages (single-dilutional)
* Can be poorly specific.
  * Higher likelihood of false-positive responses
* Standardization of response is poor.
* Can elicit significant systemic reactions if used without prior prick/puncture screening or testing with dilute concentrations of antigen intradermally.
  * Danger of anaphylaxis with single intradermal tests alone
◊ Summary (single-dilutional)
* Single-dilutional intradermal tests can be highly sensitive yet less specific than prick/puncture testing, and can be associated with increased systemic morbidity.
– Intradermal dilutional testing (IDT)
◊ Formerly referred to as *skin endpoint titration* (SET)
◊ First developed by Hansel and refined by Rinkel in 1962

◊ Frequently used by otolaryngologists in testing for inhalant allergy
◊ Involves the sequential administration of fivefold diluted antigens, beginning with very dilute concentrations and progressively administering more concentrated antigens until a specific response is obtained on the skin
◊ Technique
  * Fivefold dilutions of each antigen are prepared and labeled from # 1 through # 6.
    ▪ 1 cc of antigenic concentrate (1:20 w/v) is mixed with 4 cc of inert diluent.
    ▪ First diluted preparation is referred to as the # 1 dilution.
    ▪ Each dilution is subsequently diluted further, through the sixth dilution (# 6).
  * The test material, starting with the # 6 dilution, is injected intradermally.
    ▪ About 0.01 mL of extract is injected, with the goal of creating a precise 4 mm round wheal in the skin.
  * The injection is observed for 10 minutes for any skin reaction.
    ▪ 4-mm wheal will generally enlarge to 5 mm in 10 minutes simply through physical diffusion of material in the skin.
    ▪ A wheal size of 7 mm or greater (2 mm larger than that expected from physical diffusion alone) would be considered a positive whealing response.
  * If there is no significant growth of the wheal after 10 minutes, the next stronger dilution (# 5) is similarly injected.
    ▪ In the absence of allergy, no whealing will be observed with any concentration
    ▪ In the presence of allergy, a progression of the whealing response will be observed.
    ▪ The *endpoint* is defined as the dilution that initiates progressive positive whealing.
  * Positive whealing and determination of the endpoint:
    ▪ After the demonstration of a first positive wheal (reaction at least 2 mm > negative wheal), the next stronger concentration is applied to assess the continuation of progressive whealing.
    ▪ With an additional growth of at least 2 mm in diameter, this second wheal is considered positive.
      ◆ This positive second wheal is referred to as the "confirming wheal," and verifies the prior wheal as the endpoint.
  * Examples of positive IDT responses (endpoint underlined).
    ▪ 5-5-<u>7</u>-9
    ▪ 5-5-7-<u>7</u>-9
    ▪ 5-<u>8</u>-11
◊ Advantages
  * Quantitative as well as qualitative determination of allergic sensitization
  * Highly reproducible results with little intertester variability
  * Very sensitive to low-level allergy
  * Very safe
    ▪ Very low incidence of systemic responses
◊ Disadvantages
  * Specificity can be poor with high concentrations of antigen.

- May be an increase in false-positive test responses
- Should never test with or determine a # 1 endpoint, as many of these responses are likely irritant responses
  * Test is time-consuming and tester-dependent.
  * More supplies are necessary to complete a full IDT battery.
  * Cost of testing materials is greater than with other techniques.
  ◊ Summary
    * IDT has been shown to have excellent utility in the diagnosis of allergy, and in guiding the preparation of sera for safe immunotherapy.
– Modified quantitative testing (MQT)
  ◊ Blended epicutaneous/percutaneous technique
  ◊ First described by Krouse in 2003
  ◊ Involves the use of prick/puncture testing as the initial testing modality to determine an approximation of the degree of allergic sensitization
    * Select intradermal tests are used to refine the initial prick/puncture results and to estimate an endpoint for calculation of initial immunotherapy dose.
  ◊ Utilizes fivefold dilutions and terminology standard and accepted by practicing otolaryngologists
  ◊ Technique
    * Prick/puncture tests are first applied to the patient's forearm using a multiple-pronged testing device.
    * Responses are read at 20 minutes to determine the presence or absence of whealing.
      - Wheal diameters are measured and recorded in mm.
      - If wheals are noted at least 9 mm in diameter to a specific antigen, intradermal testing is not conducted on that antigen, and its sensitivity is assigned an endpoint of # 6.
    * Select intradermal tests are then placed based upon the response to initial prick/puncture testing.
      - If initial whealing to prick/puncture testing is 3 mm or less, a single # 2 intradermal test is placed on the upper arm.
      - If initial whealing is between 3 and 8 mm in diameter, a single # 5 intradermal test is placed.
    * Following the pattern of whealing of both prick/puncture and intradermal tests, an algorithm is used to estimate an endpoint for each antigen (Figure 53-18).
      - The endpoint is determined conservatively in order to decrease the likelihood of any adverse systemic reaction with initiation of immunotherapy.
  ◊ Advantages
    * Provides quantitative information regarding degree of allergic sensitization without the need to complete a full IDT battery
    * Has excellent sensitivity and very good specificity for determination of allergy
    * Rapid, reproducible, and not tester-dependent
    * Requires fewer supplies as lesser cost than IDT
    * Shown to be highly correlated with full IDT test batteries
  ◊ Disadvantages

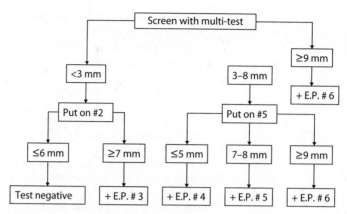

Figure 53-18 Modified quantitative testing (MQT) algorithm.

- * Endpoint determination is conservative and does involve initiation of immunotherapy with slightly weaker antigens than IDT.
- * Can have large local skin reactions with intradermal testing.
- ◊ Summary
  - * MQT provides an excellent alternative to full IDT.
  - * Results of MQT correlate highly with those determined with IDT batteries, but at lower cost and with lesser time involved for testing.
  - * MQT allows use of endpoints and preparation of immunotherapy in a standard manner employed by otolaryngologists practicing allergy.
- – Concurrent medications and skin testing
  - ◊ Antihistamines
    - * Suppress the wheal and flare response.
    - * Persistence of wheal and flare suppression varies with specific antihistamine.
      - ▪ First-generation antihistamines (eg, diphenhydramine, chlorpheniramine).
        - ♦ Wheal suppression can persist for 48 to 72 hours.
        - ♦ Should not test during this period.
      - ▪ Second-generation antihistamines (eg, loratadine, cetirizine, fexofenadine).
        - ♦ Wheal suppression can persist for 7 days.
        - ♦ Should not test during this period.
        - ♦ Desloratadine can suppress whealing for 10 to 14 days.
      - ▪ First-generation antihistamines are often found in other over-the-counter (OTC) products, including cold remedies, sleep medications, and vestibular suppressants.
    - * Tricyclic antidepressants (eg, amitriptyline, imipramine)
      - ▪ Have antihistaminic properties
      - ▪ Can suppress the wheal and flare response for up to 7 days
      - ▪ Should not test during this time period
    - * Leukotriene receptor antagonists (eg, montelukast)
      - ▪ Have not been shown to suppress wheal and flare in several trials.
      - ▪ Isolated clinical anecdotes of wheal suppression have been reported.

- If suspected to have suppressed wheal and flare in a specific patient, stop drug for 7 days and retest.
  * Oral and topical nasal corticosteroids
    - No effect on wheal and flare
  * Other medications generally do not suppress wheal and flare.
    - Include decongestants, cromolyn sodium, and inhaled bronchodilators
  * Beta blockers
    - Both topical and oral beta blockers can increase resistance to epinephrine, and as such should be avoided in patients undergoing testing or treatment for allergy.
    - Epinephrine is used as a rescue medication in episodes of suspected anaphylaxis, and patients on beta-blocking medications, including topical eye drops, are resistant to standard doses.
      - Unopposed alpha stimulation in this setting can lead to critical hypertension and arrhythmia.
  ○ In vitro allergy testing
    − Original in vitro assay was the *RAST* (radioallergosorbent test).
      ◊ Developed in the 1970s as a method of assessing quantities of specific IgE in the serum.
      ◊ Original technique was poorly sensitive, and the scoring and interpretation system was recalculated.
      ◊ Updated system has been known as the *modified RAST* (mRAST).
    − Classic RAST technique (Figure 53-19):

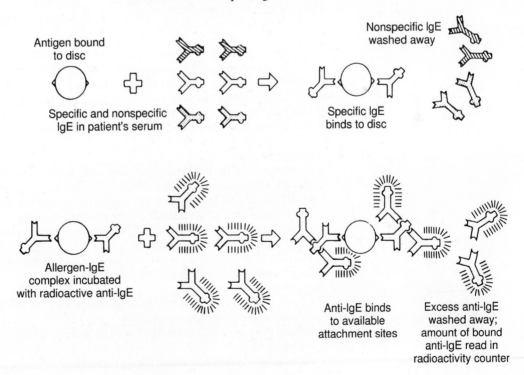

Figure 53-19 Radioallergosorbent test (RAST): basic mechanism.

◊ RAST measures the serum level of allergen-specific IgE.
◊ Technique:
  * Antigen-bound paper disc is used for assessment.
  * Disc is placed in a test tube, to which patient's serum is added.
  * Allergen-specific IgE present in the serum binds to antigen on the disc.
  * Excess nonspecific IgE is washed away.
  * Radiolabeled anti-IgE antibody is added and binds to the patient's IgE bound to the antigen on the disc.
  * Excess anti-IgE is washed away.
  * The amount of bound radiolabel is then measured with a gamma counter.
  * Proper controls must be used for best sensitivity and specificity of the test.
– Modifications of classic RAST technique:
  ◊ Specific IgE antigens can be presented in other formats.
    * Solid-phase, three-dimensional units, etc
  ◊ Labels other than radioactive labels can be used.
    * Fluorescent labels, enzyme-lined assays, etc
  ◊ Length of time for antigen to interact with serum can be varied.
    * Increased time generally improves accuracy of test.
  ◊ Scoring/measurement systems can vary.
    * Counts, units, etc
– Advantages of in vitro assays:
  ◊ Eliminate variability of the skin response.
  ◊ Eliminate drug effects on the skin.
  ◊ Permit safe testing in patients on beta-blockers.
  ◊ Allow testing for numerous antigens to be conducted on a single serum sample.
  ◊ Provide a quantitative assessment that can be used to estimate degree of allergic sensitization and for preparation of allergy sera for immunotherapy.
  ◊ Demonstrate greater specificity than skin testing.
– Disadvantages of in vitro assays:
  ◊ Generally more expensive than skin testing
  ◊ May demonstrate lesser sensitivity than skin testing, especially with older assay techniques
– Total IgE measurement:
  ◊ Measurement of the total amount of nonspecific IgE in the serum has been suggested as a screening tool for allergy.
  ◊ High levels of total IgE (eg, >200 IU) suggest the presence of allergy.
  ◊ Low levels of total IgE do not rule out the presence of allergy.
    * Patients with low total IgE may still have one or more allergens that demonstrate significant levels of specific IgE.
  ◊ Total IgE can be useful as a screen, but low levels do not necessary eliminate the presence of clinically significant allergy.
– Indications for in vitro testing:
  ◊ Patients requiring allergy testing to determine presence of allergy and to estimate degree of allergic sensitization
  ◊ Patients not responding to environmental control and conservative medical management
  ◊ Apprehensive children in whom allergy seems likely

◊ Symptomatic patients with conditions in which in vivo skin testing is contraindicated (eg, dermatographism, eczema)
◊ Patients on beta-blocking medications
◊ Patients on antihistamines who are unwilling or unable to discontinue medications
◊ Patients doing poorly on immunotherapy
◊ Venom sensitivity
◊ Diagnosis of IgE-mediated food sensitivity
– Contraindication for in vitro testing:
  ◊ Primary contraindication is for the diagnosis of non–IgE-mediated disorders.

Treatment of Allergy

- All patients with allergy need to be actively involved in their treatment.
  ○ Education regarding allergic sensitivities and their management is essential for all allergy patients.
- The treatment of allergy generally relies on a three-pronged strategy, with the combination of these approaches individualized for each patient.
  ○ Environmental control/avoidance
  ○ Pharmacotherapy
  ○ Immunotherapy
- Environmental control:
  ○ Involves decreasing the allergen load to which the patient is exposed by altering the environment of the patient.
  ○ While conceptually attractive, avoidance can be difficult to do and is of questionable efficacy in routine use.
    – Pollens
      ◊ Difficult to avoid due to wide airborne distribution
      ◊ Avoidance of outdoor activities in the morning
        * Pollen released in greater amounts in the morning
      ◊ Use of air-conditioners in the home
        * Keeping windows closed to prevent pollens from entering the indoor environment
      ◊ Limit presence of offending plants in the immediate vicinity
    – Molds
      ◊ Avoid damp environments
      ◊ Avoid dense landscaping with decaying organic material near the house
      ◊ Prevent moisture accumulation indoors around pipes, air conditioners, refrigerators, bathroom fixtures
    – Dust/dust mites
      ◊ Use of synthetic carpets or elimination of carpets
      ◊ Regular and frequent vacuuming
        * HEPA vacuums distribute lesser levels of dust into the air and decrease symptoms in susceptible individuals.
      ◊ Regular changing of filters in the heating and air-conditioning systems
      ◊ Use of impervious pillow and mattress covers on bedding
      ◊ Regular washing of bedding in hot (>140°F) water

◊ HEPA filters in the bedroom and other frequently occupied areas of the home
    * Filter must be of adequate capacity for size of room.
– Animal danders
    ◊ Removal or avoidance of the pet
        * If impractical, removing the pet from the bedroom or confining the pet to a space not regularly occupied
    ◊ Weekly washing of pets
- Pharmacotherapy:
    (a) Primary treatment for majority of symptomatic allergic patients
    (b) Indicated in all patients with inhalant allergy
    (c) Antihistamines
        ○ H1-receptor antagonists (also considered *reverse agonists*) that act mainly be dose-dependent competitive binding of H1 receptors on target cells in the eyes, nose, skin, lungs.
        ○ Work best on the immediate, early-phase allergic response.
        ○ Have little effect on congestion.
            – Congestion driven significantly by late-phase mediators.
            – *Exception*: topically applied antihistamines have been shown to have clinically significant effects on reduction in nasal congestion.
        ○ Classified by generation:
            – First-generation oral antihistamines
                ◊ Developed in the 1940s
                ◊ Include agents such as diphenhydramine, chlorpheniramine, triprolidine, azatadine
                ◊ Highly lipophilic
                    * Cross the blood-brain barrier readily
                    * Result in high incidence of sedation and central nervous system (CNS) suppressive effects
                ◊ Highly anticholinergic
                    * Drying of mucous membranes
                    * Increase in mucus tenacity
                    * Blurring of vision
                    * Constipation
                    * Urinary retention
                ◊ May be accompanied with tachyphylaxis
                    * Efficacy decreases with continued use.
            – Second-generation oral antihistamines
                ◊ Developed in the 1980s through engineering of previous agents
                ◊ Include medications such as loratadine, fexofenadine, cetirizine, desloratadine, levocetirizine
                ◊ Lipophobic
                    * Do not cross the blood-brain barrier as readily
                    * Less likely to result in sedation or CNS effects
                        ▪ Can be dose related
                ◊ Little or no anticholinergic activity
                    * Safe to use in patients with asthma
                ◊ Little if any tachyphylaxis

- Topical antihistamines
  ◊ Work directly through application at the target organ (eg, eye, nose)
  ◊ Medications include azelastine, olopatadine
  ◊ Demonstrate usual antihistaminic effects, but with increased efficacy in congestion and more rapid onset of action
  ○ Antihistamines demonstrate effects on other receptors, which can lead to both useful and unwanted effects.
  ○ Sedation is a major concern, primarily with first-generation antihistamines.
  - Patients can exhibit cognitive and psychomotor impairment without subjective sense of sedation.
  - First-generation antihistamines should be used judiciously due to their significant adverse impact on performance and quality of life.

(d) Decongestants
  ○ Administered either orally or topically to decrease nasal obstruction
  ○ Have minimal effect on rhinorrhea, itching, or sneezing
  ○ Work as alpha-2 agonists
  - Bind to alpha-2 receptors on target organs
  - Decrease vascular engorgement through vasoconstrictive mechanism
  ○ Systemic decongestants
  - Include pseudoephedrine and phenylephrine
    ◊ Pseudoephedrine available only behind the pharmacy counter due to its ability to be converted chemically to methamphetamine
  - Often combined with antihistamines to provide decongestant effect.
  - Can be accompanied with significant alpha-adrenergic side effects.
    ◊ Increased blood pressure in hypertensive patients
    ◊ Increased appetite
    ◊ Increased cardiac symptoms
      * Tachycardia
      * Arrhythmia
  - Vasoconstrictive effect decreases hyperemia, congestion, and edema.
  - Can infrequently be accompanied with significant tachyphylaxis (rebound rhinitis).
  ○ Topical decongestants
  - Include oxymetazoline, phenylephrine, naphazoline, tetrahydrozoline.
  - Work rapidly to decrease nasal congestion with excellent efficacy.
  - Rapid rebound congestion can develop with use for as few as 3 days.
    ◊ Rapid tachyphylaxis develops, leading to increased frequency of use.
    ◊ Mucosal hypoxia and neurotransmitter depletion occur.
    ◊ Leads to *rhinitis medicamentosa*, a severe representation of nasal congestion.
  - Use should be limited to no more than 3 days at a time.

(e) Corticosteroids
  ○ Can be used systemically or topically.
  ○ Block the generation and release of mediators and the influx of inflammatory cells.
  ○ Work on genetic transcription and protein synthesis in the nucleus of cells.
  ○ Wide range of effects are noted.
  - Cellular (mast cells, eosinophils, macrophages, lymphocytes, neutrophils)
  - Humoral mediators (histamine, eicosanoids, leukotrienes, cytokines)

○ Parenteral corticosteroids:
  – Have been administered through IM injections seasonally
    ◊ Anecdotally noted to have benefit for 2 to 3 months with single depot injection.
    ◊ Depot injections of corticosteroids are discouraged by current guidelines due to potentially significant prolonged adverse effects.
      * Psychiatric (eg, psychosis, mood swings).
      * Musculoskeletal (eg, joint and soft tissue abnormalities.
      * Cataract formation.
      * Once a depot preparation is injected, it cannot be removed if adverse events occur.
      * Oral preparations are therefore recommended preferentially to depot injections of steroids.
○ Oral corticosteroids:
  – Preferential to parenteral corticosteroids for the management of allergic rhinitis
  – Can be used for short courses in serious allergic inflammation
  – Often notice effects within 12 to 24 hours
  – Commonly used oral corticosteroids
    ◊ Prednisone
    ◊ Methylprednisolone
    ◊ Dexamethasone
○ Topical corticosteroids
  – Used commonly in the treatment of allergic rhinitis
  – Increase local concentrations of effective agent with concurrent limitation of systemic absorption and adverse effects
  – Newer agents generally free of hypothalamic-pituitary-adrenal (HPA) axis suppression
  – Demonstrate broad local anti-inflammatory benefits and significant reduction in nasal symptoms
  – Agents
    ◊ Beclomethasone dipropionate
      * Higher systemic bioavailability than other, more recent preparations
      * Has been demonstrated to cause growth suppression in prepubescent children
    ◊ Flunisolide
      * Does have significant systemic bioavailability
      * Often poorly tolerated due to propylene glycol base
      * Use has largely been supplanted by newer agents
    ◊ Budesonide
      * Aqueous-based spray
      * Scent-free, taste-free
      * Only topical nasal corticosteroid with a pregnancy class B
    ◊ Triamcinolone acetate
      * Aqueous-based spray
      * Scent-free, taste-free
      * Available "over-the-counter" in the United States

◊ Fluticasone propionate
* Aqueous-based spray.
* Low systemic bioavailability.
* Onset of action within 12 hours.
* Indication for both allergic rhinitis and nonallergic rhinitis.
* Floral scent and taste often limit patient tolerability.
  ▪ Secondary to phenylethyl alcohol
* Widely available as a generic preparation.
◊ Mometasone furoate
* Aqueous-based spray
* Scent-free, taste-free
* Low systemic bioavailability
* Onset of action within 12 hours
* Indication for both allergic rhinitis and nasal polyps
* Approved for use down to age 2
◊ Fluticasone furoate
* Aqueous-based spray
* Scent-free, taste-free
* Low systemic bioavailability
* Onset of action within 12 hours
* Indication for allergic rhinitis and labeled effectiveness for eye symptoms
* Approved for use down to age 2
◊ Ciclesonide
* Aqueous-based spray
* Scent-free, taste-free
* Low systemic bioavailability
  ▪ Administered as a prodrug and activated by tissue esterases
* Indication for allergic rhinitis
– Topical agents have very similar demonstrated efficacy in treatment of allergic rhinitis.
  ◊ Individual preferences and formulary availability are large driving factors in use.
  ◊ Variability in labeled indications often directs prescribing practices.
(f) Cromolyn sodium
  ○ Mechanism of action
  – Stabilizes mast cell membranes and inhibits degranulation and release of histamine
  ○ Lipophobic without systemic absorption
  – Free of systemic adverse effects
  ○ Available in topical form for both ocular and nasal symptoms
  – Must be administered three to four times daily due to very short half-life
  – Will not treat symptoms once exposure has occurred and mast cells have degranulated
  – Needs to be used prophylactically
  ○ Efficacy is mild to moderate at best

(g) Leukotriene receptor antagonists
- Block the binding of leukotrienes to target cells.
- Efficacy demonstrated in the treatment of allergic rhinitis.
- Systemic use also has therapeutic effect with lower airway disease.
- Agent:
  - Montelukast
    ◊ Only agent approved for use in allergic rhinitis
      * Also indicated for asthma and exercise-induced bronchospasm
    ◊ Indicated for use down to 6 months of age
    ◊ Safe and well tolerated
- Immunotherapy
  (a) Process of administering allergen either subcutaneously or sublingually over time to induce allergic tolerance and reduction of allergic symptoms
  (b) Effects
    - Change in balance of T helper cell populations
      - Shift in skewing of T cells from the T_H1 phenotype to the T_H2 phenotype
      - Induction in maturation and distribution of T regulatory (T_{reg}) cells
      - Concurrent shift in T-cell–induced cytokines
        ◊ Increase in IL-10 and IL-12
        ◊ Reduction in IL-4 and IL-5
    - Reduction in
      - Mediator release (eg, histamine, kinins, prostaglandins)
      - Trafficking of inflammatory cells (eg, lymphocytes, eosinophils)
      - Clinical symptoms, both early and late phase
    - Other observed immunologic effects (Figure 53-20)
      - Initial rise in specific IgE levels, with suppression in specific IgE levels over time with treatment
      - Increase in specific IgG4 levels for treated allergens
        ◊ Formerly thought to induce immune tolerance as "blocking antibodies"
        ◊ Probably more a marker of T helper regulation than a true mediator of effect

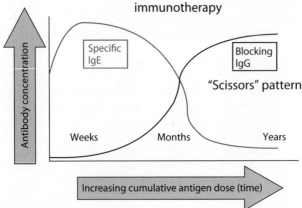

Figure 53-20 Scissors effect.

    (c) Satisfactory response to immunotherapy requires
- Identifying the offending allergens responsible for symptoms
- Correlating positive skin or in vitro testing results with generation of clinical symptoms
- Providing an adequate therapeutic dose for treatment
  - Aggregate dose over time correlates with persistence of immunotherapy effect.
- Treating for an adequate period of time
  - Immunotherapy generally is felt to require at least 3 to 5 years of regular administration to permit persistence of benefits after discontinuation.

    (d) Subcutaneous immunotherapy (SCIT)
- Involves the injections of sequentially greater concentrations of allergens over time to induce hyposensitization and immune tolerance
- Has been practiced for nearly 100 years with excellent profile of safety, efficacy, and tolerability
- Begins with very dilute concentrations of allergenic sera, injected once or twice weekly, and advanced until maximal tolerability and delivery of adequate dosage of antigen is achieved
  - Starting doses should be
    - ◊ High enough to rapidly induce an immune response
    - ◊ Low enough to avoid any significant local or systemic adverse reactions
- Theoretical advantages of quantitative testing
  - Safely able to begin immunotherapy with greater concentrations of antigen, as safety has been established through testing
  - Able to achieve maintenance dosage levels more rapidly due to initially stronger starting doses
  - Able to adjust the concentrations of each antigen based on its degree of skin reactivity
- Dose escalation
  - Purpose of escalation is to achieve the *maintenance dose*, which is the target dose where maximal antigen is delivered with each dose, yet without systemic or large local reactions.
  - Maintenance dose should deliver a targeted cumulative level of antigen when given over a period of 3 to 5 years.
  - Some degree of local skin reactivity is expected and tolerated at maintenance.
  - After starting immunotherapy, the dose should be increased as quickly as possible, up to twice weekly.
    - ◊ Generally, increasing by 0.05 cc weekly is very safe.
    - ◊ Increasing by 0.10 cc weekly is often safe and well tolerated.
    - ◊ Increasing by 0.05-0.10 cc twice weekly can often be tolerated and safe in patients without significant asthma or history of anaphylaxis.
  - In large local reactions or significant systemic reactions suddenly occur, look for the following:
    - ◊ Concurrent exposure to large allergenic load (eg, coseasonal administration of allergen)
    - ◊ Presence of upper or lower respiratory infection
    - ◊ Poorly controlled asthma
    - ◊ Error in dosing, wrong patient, other error

- Maintenance dose:
  ◊ No specific level is appropriate for all patients.
  ◊ Goal is to administer highest tolerated concentration of antigen per injection.
  ◊ Should control symptoms for at least 1 week.
  ◊ Local reaction of 3 to 4 cm would suggest that maintenance dose is achieved.
    * Systemic reactions are more likely after large local reactions.
- Dosing intervals can be increased from weekly to every 2 to 3 weeks after 6 to 12 months of injections and if symptoms are adequately controlled between injections.
  ◊ Breakthrough symptoms are not uncommon with large antigen exposures.
  ◊ Even with successful immunotherapy, some medications may be necessary for complete control of symptoms.
○ Stopping immunotherapy
  - Many patients are able to discontinue SCIT in 3 to 5 years after achieving maintenance dose.
  - Should be monitored after discontinuation for recurrence of symptoms.
○ Indications and contraindications for SCIT
  - Indications
    ◊ Symptoms demonstrated to be initiated by IgE antibodies
    ◊ Presence of respiratory allergy (eg, nasal allergy or atopic asthma)
    ◊ Severe symptoms
      * Poorly controlled by avoidance and pharmacotherapy
    ◊ Perennial allergy or long, overlapping allergy seasons
  - Contraindications
    ◊ Nonimmune mechanism responsible for symptoms
    ◊ Absence of demonstrated IgE on skin or in vitro testing
    ◊ Mild symptoms easily controlled with other methods
    ◊ Atopic dermatitis or food allergies
    ◊ Very short seasons with transient pollenosis
    ◊ Poorly adherent patients
    ◊ Concurrent use of beta blockers
    ◊ Uncontrolled asthma
  - Complications of SCIT
    ◊ Usually related to
      * Inadvertent use of the wrong antigen
      * Giving a treatment dose from the wrong SCIT vial
      * Too rapid escalation of dose
      * Concurrent respiratory infection
      * Poorly controlled asthma or current asthma exacerbation
    ◊ Local reactions
      * Local induration is expected as higher concentrations of antigen are delivered.
      * Reactions of greater than 3 to 4 cm would suggest a mild adverse reactions.
    ◊ Systemic reactions
      * May include symptoms of cough, throat tightening, wheezing, and shortness of breath
      * Urticaria and/or angioedema
        ▪ Can suggest early anaphylaxis

* In severe cases can result in true anaphylaxis
  - Laryngeal edema
  - Bronchospasm
  - Hypotension
  - Cardiovascular collapse
◊ Anaphylaxis
* Usually apparent within seconds to minutes after SCIT injection
* Patient complains of
  - Nasal congestion
  - Flushing and warmth
  - Heaviness in chest
  - Shortness of breath
  - Throat closing
  - Itching
  - Nausea, vomiting
  - Sense of "impending doom"
* Treatment
  - Lay patient down.
  - Take vital signs.
  - Early use of epinephrine:
    • 0.3 cc SC (adults)
    • 0.1–0.2 cc SC (children)
  - Oxygen.
  - Tourniquet proximal to injection site.
  - Intravenous access for fluid administration.
  - Diphenhydramine 50 mg IV.
  - Dexamethasone 8 mg IV.
  - Establish airway if necessary.
  - Transfer to intensive care unit (ICU) setting for further treatment.
    • Pressor support
  - Remember that late reactions do occur even with successful reversal of immediate symptoms.

(e) Sublingual immunotherapy (SLIT)
  ○ Involves the administration of allergens orally or as drops or tablets under the tongue to achieve hyposensitization and induce immune tolerance.
    – Dosages may be given in fixed or escalating schedules.
  ○ Developed in Europe over the past 50 years in response to perceived risks of SCIT and several episodes of death with immunotherapy.
  ○ Efficacy in Europe well established using single-dose antigen studies.
    – Numerous randomized trials with various antigens have demonstrated benefit.
    – Multiple-antigen SLIT has not been well studied to date.
  ○ Has increased in popularity in the United States due to excellent safety and patient ease of use.
  ○ Currently available as (1) commercially manufactured sublingual tablets, with the Food and Drug Administration (FDA) approval for use; (2) physician-prepared sera made with allergen extracts designed for SCIT.
    – Physician-prepared SLIT drops vary widely in composition and concentration due to individual philosophies and practices of allergy professionals.
    – Efficacy with these physician-prepared SLIT sera in the United States has not been well established through scientific trials.

○ Several commercial tablets were approved by the FDA for use in the United States in 2014 and are now marketed.
  – Sublingual tablets are currently available in the United States for timothy grass and ragweed, with others (eg, dust mite) under clinical trial.
○ In order for SLIT to be widely accepted and well established in United States allergy practice, certain questions are going to need to be addressed.
  – Safety and efficacy in polysensitized individuals, especially those with asthma and other concurrent medical illnesses
  – Necessary dosage levels to achieve both subjective symptomatic relief and immune modulation
    ◊ Many preparations have traditionally underdosed with antigen concentration, and are of questionable efficacy.
  – Cost of therapy
    ◊ Physician-prepared SLIT treatments have traditionally been considered noncovered expenses by most third-party insurers.
    ◊ Care must be taken in using appropriate codes and descriptions of therapy in billing insurers.
○ Recent report from the Cochrane Collaboration has shown excellent efficacy in adults with single-antigen therapy.
  – Safety in multiple clinical trials has been excellent.

Food Allergy

- Definition
  (a) Food allergy is an *immune-mediated pathological reaction to ingested food antigens*.
    ○ Food allergy must be distinguished from other adverse reactions to food and to food intolerance.
  (b) Adverse reactions to food include both toxic and nontoxic reactions.
    ○ Toxic reactions
      – Occur in response to food contaminants, such as bacterial toxins and chemicals
      – Will occur in any exposed individual with sufficient dose
    ○ Nontoxic reactions
      – Immune-mediated reactions
        ◊ Food allergy
          * IgE-mediated reactions to known allergenic foods
          * Non–IgE-mediated reactions
            ▪ These reactions are poorly understood and poorly characterized.
      – Non–immune-mediated reactions
        ◊ Food intolerance
          * Lactose intolerance
          * Vasoactive amines in certain foods produce a pharmacologic effect
      – Undefined food intolerances
        ◊ Can involve poorly characterized immune and nonimmune mechanisms
          * Reactions to foods that induce endogenous histamine release
          * Reactions to food additives (eg, dyes, tartrazine, sulfites, glutamate, etc)
- Common symptoms of food allergy

    (a) Pharynx
- Lip swelling
- Pharyngeal itching and edema
  - Oral allergy syndrome

    (b) Stomach
- Reflux gastroenteritis and laryngopharyngitis
- Nausea
- Vomiting

    (c) Intestine
- Abdominal pain
- Malabsorption syndromes
- Diarrhea
- Constipation
- Fecal blood loss

- Pathophysiology of food allergy

    (a) Studies suggest that both IgE-mediated and non–IgE-mediated mechanisms may be involved in hypersensitivity reactions to foods.
- While it is tempting to speculate that cytotoxic delayed reactions may occur secondary to food exposure, tissue damage of this sort (eg, immune-complex–mediated pathophysiology) has not been confirmed in vivo.

    (b) Food allergy involves the breakdown of natural oral tolerance to foods.
- Barrier disruption to macromolecules early in life appears to be a factor in early IgE sensitization to foods.
- Increased amounts of protein antigens may be able to circulate in an undegraded state, leading to development of IgE antibodies to certain types and classes of foods.

    (c) There appears to be a genetic predisposition to the development of food allergy.
- Susceptible individuals appear to have
  - Predominance of T_H2 lymphocytes
  - Increased production of IL-4 and IL-5
  - Enhanced mast-cell releasability
- Lack of immune-protective factors
- Increased antigen resorption
  - Loss of mucosal integrity

    (d) Food allergic reactions can be seen in patients without evidence of specific IgE to those foods either in skin testing or in in vitro assays.
- This absence of IgE documentation has been used as an argument for other mechanisms of food allergy.
  - Speculation of IgG-mediated allergy or "cyclic food allergy"
- Recent studies imply that local IgE production in the gut, in the absence of significant levels of circulating IgE, may be responsible for many of these cases of food allergy.
- Diagnosis and treatment of these non–IgE-mediated food sensitivities is controversial.
  - No good evidence base to support the use of these approaches.

    (e) Diagnosis of food allergy:
- History
  - Symptoms
  - Presence of other atopic diseases

- Presence of other GI complaints or systemic diseases
- Potential triggers for induction of symptoms
  ◊ Most common food allergens
    * Peanut
    * Tree nuts
    * Milk proteins (casein)
    * Egg whites (albumin)
    * Wheat products (gluten)
  ◊ Other foods involved in food intolerance
    * Corn and corn products
    * Soy and soy products
    * Yeasts and yeast-containing products
○ GI examinations
  - Endoscopy, colonoscopy
    ◊ Can be useful in examining for other potential diseases
      * Eosinophilic esophagitis
      * Crohn disease
      * Ulcerative colitis
○ Laboratory studies
  - Total and specific IgE levels
    ◊ In vivo assays demonstrating elevated IgG levels to specific foods *does not* imply allergy, only exposure to those foods in the diet.
    ◊ Elevated IgG levels to foods are not suggestive or diagnostic of food allergy.
○ Provocation tests
  - Skin-prick testing
  - Elimination diet and challenge
  - Double-blind placebo-controlled food challenge (DBPCFC)
    ◊ Proposed as the "gold standard" for the diagnosis of food allergy
    ◊ Risk of anaphylaxis in true IgE-mediated food allergy
    ◊ Poorly sensitive and poorly specific
    ◊ High incidence of inaccuracy due to patient self-reported symptoms and placebo effect
○ Empiric treatment
  - Food elimination
  - Food avoidance
  - Oral cromolyn therapy
○ Desensitization
  - Highly controversial
  - High risk of systemic reactions an anaphylaxis
  - Currently under investigation in controlled clinical trials in major academic medical centers
    ◊ Early results are encouraging, but more study is clearly necessary.

Bibliography

Brozek JL, Bousquet J, Baena-Cagnani CE, et al. Allergic rhinitis and its impact on asthma (ARIA) guidelines: 2010 revision. *J Allergy Clin Immunol.* 2010;126:466-476.

Burton MJ, Krouse JH, Rosenfeld RM. Extracts from the Cochrane Library: sublingual immunotherapy for allergic rhinitis. *Otolaryngol-Head Neck Surg.* 2011;144:149-153.

Krouse JH, Chadwick SJ, Gordon BR, Derebery MJ. *Allergy and Immunology: An Otolaryngic Approach.* Philadelphia, PA: Lippincott, Williams and Wilkins; 2002.

Krouse JH, Mabry RL. Skin testing for inhalant allergy 2003: current strategies. *Otolaryngol-Head Neck Surg.* 2003;129:33-49.

Marple BF, Mabry RL. *Quantitative Skin Testing for Allergy: IDT and MQT.* New York, NY: Thieme; 2006.

Questions

1. Histamine is released from which cell on allergic exposure?
   A. Mast cell
   B. Eosinophil
   C. Plasma cell
   D. Neutrophil
   E. NK cell

2. Which statement is *not true* concerning prick testing for inhalant allergy?
   A. Prick testing may underestimate the degree of low-level allergy.
   B. Prick testing should not be done in a patient on beta blockers.
   C. Prick testing is effective as a screen for the presence of allergy.
   D. Prick testing is more sensitive than intradermal testing.
   E. Prick testing has been conducted for over 50 years.

3. Which class of immunoglobulin is responsible for the allergic response?
   A. IgG
   B. IgM
   C. IgA
   D. IgD
   E. IgE

4. Which whealing pattern to IDT would not suggest a positive response?
   A. 5-5-5-7-9
   B. 5-5-8-11
   C. 5-6-7-9-11
   D. 5-5-5-5-6
   E. 5-7-9

5. Which statement is *not true* concerning sublingual immunotherapy (SLIT)?
   A. SLIT has been demonstrated to have good efficacy.
   B. Allergen extracts are not FDA-licensed for sublingual use.
   C. Dosing of SLIT extracts has not been precisely determined.
   D. SLIT is less safe than SCIT.
   E. Multiple-antigen SLIT has not been well studied.

Chapter 54
Highlights and Pearls

Embryology

A. *Branchial arch derivatives*: nerve, muscles, cartilage, artery
  i. First arch (mandibular)
    a. *Nerve*: trigeminal (V)
    b. *Muscle*: muscles of mastication, tensor veli palatini, mylohyoid, anterior digastrics, tensor tympani
    c. *Skeletal structure*: sphenomandibular ligament, anterior malleal ligament, mandible, malleus, incus
    d. *Artery*: maxillary
    e. *Pouch and derivative*: eustachian tube, middle ear
  ii. Second arch (hyoid)
    a. *Nerve*: facial (VII)
    b. *Muscle*: stapedius, posterior digastric, stylohyoid, muscles of facial expression
    c. *Skeletal structure*: stapes, styloid process, stylohyoid ligament, lesser cornu/upper portion of hyoid
    d. *Artery*: stapedial
    e. *Pouch and derivative*: palatine tonsil
  iii. Third arch
    a. *Nerve*: glossopharyngeal (IX)
    b. *Muscle*: stylopharyngeus

   c. *Skeletal structure*: greater cornu of the hyoid, lower body of hyoid
   d. *Artery*: common and internal carotid
   e. *Pouch and derivative*: thymus and inferior parathyroid
   iv. Fourth arch
   a. *Nerve*: superior laryngeal (X)
   b. *Muscle*: constrictors of the pharynx, cricothyroid
   c. *Skeletal structure*: laryngeal cartilages
   d. *Artery*: subclavian on right, arch of aorta on left
   e. *Pouch and derivative*: superior parathyroid, parafollicular cells of thyroid
   v. Sixth Arch
   a. *Nerve*: recurrent laryngeal (X)
   b. *Muscle*: intrinsic laryngeal muscles
   c. *Skeletal structure*: laryngeal cartilages
   d. *Artery*: pulmonary artery on right, ductus arteriosus on left
B. Hillocks of His
   i. Fifth week of gestation
   a. External ear develops from six small buds of mesenchyme.
   b. Hillocks of His fuse during the 12th week.
   c. 1 to 3 (from first arch) develop into tragus, helical crus, helix.
   d. 4 to 6 (from second arch) develop into antihelix, antitragus, and lobule.
C. Tongue
   i. Anterior two-thirds of tongue form from:
   a. Tuberculum impar in midline
   b. Two lateral lingual prominences
   ii. Posterior one-third of tongue form from copula.
D. Thyroid
   i. At 3 to 4 weeks gestation, starts as epithelial proliferation at the base of tongue (foramen cecum) between tuberculum impar and cupola.
   ii. Connected to foregut by thyroglossal duct as it descends into neck.
   iii. Thyroglossal duct obliterates.
   iv. Ultimobranchial body contributes parafollicular cells of thyroid.
E. Nasal dermal sinus
   i. *Foramen cecum*: anterior neuropore at anterior floor of cranial vault.
   ii. *Prenasal space*: potential space beneath nasal bone running from anterior aspect of nasal bone to frontal bone/foramen cecum area.
   iii. *Fonticulus frontalis*: embryologic gap between nasal and frontal bones.
   iv. Dura and nasal skin lie in close proximity and become separated with foramen cecum closure. Persistent dural-dermal connection via foramen cecum and pre-nasal space (or less frequently via fonticulus frontalis) produces gliomas, meningoceles, or encephaloceles projecting from above. Projecting from below may be dermal sinuses or dermoids.

Anatomy

A. Skin
   i. *Epidermis*: stratum corneum, stratum granulosum, stratum lucidum, stratum spinosum, stratum basale
   ii. Dermis
   iii. Subcutis

B. Contents of skull base foramina (Figures 54-1 through 54-8)
  i. Cribriform plate—olfactory nerves
  ii. Optic canal
    a. Optic nerve
    b. Ophthalmic artery
    c. Central retinal artery
  iii. Superior orbital fissure
    a. Cranial nerve (CN) III
    b. CN IV
    c. CN V1 branches (frontal nerve, lacrimal nerve, nasociliary nerve)

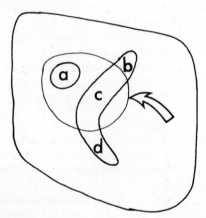

Figure 54-1 Left orbit. Arrow points to tendon of Zinn, which divides the orbital fissures into three compartments. Structures passing through (a) are the optic nerve and the ophthalmic artery. Structures passing through (b) are the trochlear nerve and the lacrimal and frontal divisions of V₁ as well as the supraorbital vein. Structures passing through (c) are the oculomotor and abducens nerves and the nasociliary division of V_1. Structures passing through (d) are the zygomaticofacial and zygomaticotemporal divisions of V_2 and the inferior ophthalmic vein.

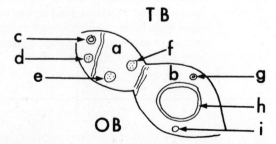

Figure 54-2 Right jugular foramen. (TB, temporal bone; OB, occipital bone; a, pars nervosa; b, pars vasculara; c, inferior petrosal sinus; d, glossopharyngeal nerve; e, vagus nerve; f, accessory nerve; g, posterior meningeal artery; h, internal jugular vein; i, nodes of Krause.)

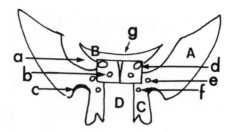

Figure 54-3 Sphenoid bone. (A, greater wing; B, lesser wing; C, pterygoid process; D, nasal cavity; a, foramen rotundum; b, pterygoid canal; c, jugum. Note: Pterygoid processes have medial and lateral plates [the lateral plate is the origin for both pterygoid muscles] and the hamulus [for tensor palati]).

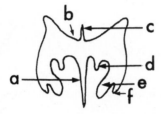

Figure 54-4 Ethmoid bone. (a, perpendicular plate; b, cribriform plate; c, crista galli, d, superior turbinate; e, middle turbinate; f, uncinate process.)

  d. CN VI
  e. Superior ophthalmic vein
  f. Inferior ophthalmic vein branch
  g. Middle meningeal artery (orbital branch)
 iv. Inferior orbital fissure: CN V2 branches (zygomatic nerves, sphenopalatine branch)
 v. Foramen rotundum: CN V2
 vi. Foramen ovale: CN V3
  a. Accessory meningeal artery
  b. Lesser petrosal nerve
  c. Emissary vein
 vii. Foramen spinosum
  a. Middle meningeal artery

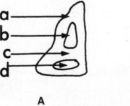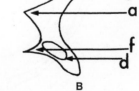

Figure 54-5 Right arytenoid. A. anterior view; B. lateral view. (a, colliculus; b, triangular pit; c, arcuate crest; d, oblong pit; e, corniculate; f, vocal process.)

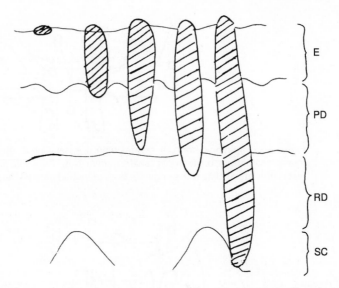

Figure 54-6 Clinicopathologic staging of melanoma. (E, epidermis; PD, papillary dermis; RD, reticular dermis; SC, subcutaneous tissue; BANS, back, upper arm, posterolateral neck, posterior scalp.)

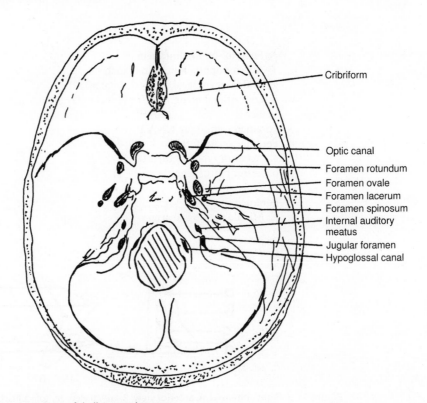

Figure 54-7 Base of skull, internal aspect.

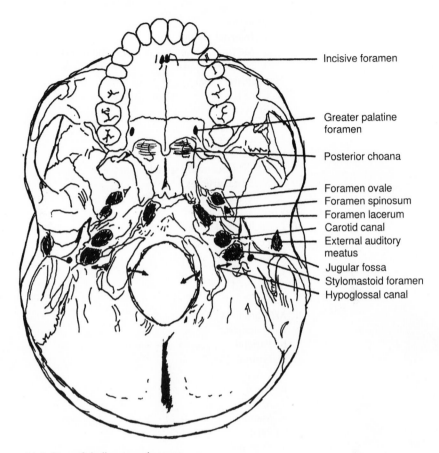

Figure 54-8 Base of skull, external aspect.

  viii. Foramen lacerum
    a. Cartilage
    b. Internal carotid artery (traverses)
    c. Deep petrosal nerve
    d. Greater petrosal nerve
    e. Terminal branch of ascending pharyngeal artery
    f. Emissary vein
  ix. Internal auditory canal (IAC)
    a. CN VII (including nervus intermedius)
    b. CN VIII
    c. Labyrinthine artery
  x. Jugular foramen
    a. Anterior—inferior petrosal sinus
    b. Middle
      1. CN IX
      2. CN X
      3. CN XI

        c. Posterior
           1. Internal jugular vein
           2. Meningeal branches from occipital and ascending pharyngeal arteries
           3. Nodes of Krause
     xi. Hypoglossal canal
        a. CN XII
        b. Emissary vein
        c. Lymphatics
    xii. Foramen magnum
        a. Medulla oblongata
        b. CN XI (ascending spinal rootlets)
        c. Vertebral arteries
        d. Anterior and posterior spinal arteries
  C. Skull bones
     i. Endochondral bones
        a. Petrous
        b. Occipital
        c. Ethmoid
        d. Mastoid
        e. Sphenoid
    ii. Membranous bones
        a. Sphenoid
        b. Parietal
        c. Frontal
        d. Lacrimal
        e. Nasal
        f. Maxillae
        g. Mandible
        h. Palate
        i. Zygoma
        j. Premaxilla
        k. Tympanic ring
        l. Squamosa
       m. Vomer
       n. Bony modiolus
  D. Cranial nerves
     i. CN I (olfactory nerve)
        a. Sensory nerve
        b. Located in olfactory foramina in cribriform plate
        c. *Afferent pathway*: olfactory epithelium → olfactory nerve → olfactory bulb → primary olfactory cortex (prepyriform and entorhinal areas)
    ii. CN II (optic nerve)
        a. Sensory nerve
        b. *Visual pathway*: optic nerve → optic chiasm → optic tract → lateral geniculate nucleus → optic radiation → primary visual cortex
    iii. CN III
        a. *Mainly motor*: innervates levator palpebrae superioris, superior rectus, medial rectus, inferior rectus, and inferior oblique
        b. *Autonomic*: lateral nucleus of Edinger-Westphal: preganglionic parasympathetic fibers to ciliary muscles and sphincter pupillae

iv. CN IV: motor fibers for superior oblique muscle

v. CN V

   a. *Somatic* sensory

     1. Sensory for pain, thermal, tactile sense from skin of face and forehead, mucous membranes of nose and mouth, teeth, and dura

     2. Proprioceptive inputs from teeth, periodontal ligaments, hard palate, and temporomandibular joint

     3. Stretch receptors for muscles of mastication

   b. *Motor* fibers

     1. Motor to muscles of mastication (temporalis, masseter, and lateral and medial pterygoid), mylohyoid, anterior digastrics, tensor tympani, and tensor veli palatini muscles

   c. Branches of mandibular nerve (V3)

     1. Trunk

- Tensor tympani
- Tensor veli palatini
- Meningeal
- Medial pterygoid

     2. Anterior divisions

- Long buccal
- Lateral pterygoid
- Temporalis branches
- Masseteric

     3. Posterior divisions

- Auriculotemporal
- Lingual
- Inferior alveolar

vi. CN VI: motor fibers for lateral rectus muscle; longest intracranial course of the cranial nerves

vii. CN VII:

   a. Nervus intermedius

     1. *Somatic* sensory for the external auditory canal (EAC)

     2. *Visceral* afferent

- Sensation from nose, palate, and pharynx
- Taste from anterior two-thirds of tongue

     3. *Visceral efferent*: parasympathetic fibers traveling from the superior salivary nucleus via the nervus intermedius:

- To chorda tympani to submandibular and sublingual glands
- To greater superficial petrosal nerve (GSPN) to the pterygopalatine ganglion and then to the lacrimal gland and minor salivary glands to the palate and nasal cavity

   b. *Motor*

     1. Motor to stapedius, posterior belly of digastric, and muscles of facial expression.

     2. Lower facial muscles receives only cross fibers, whereas upper facial muscles receives both crossed and uncrossed fibers.

viii. CN VIII

   a. *Auditory afferent*: spiral ganglion fibers ascend to dorsal and ventral cochlear nuclei → to ipsilateral superior olivary nucleus (or may cross via the reticular formation and the trapezoid body to opposite olivary nucleus) → ascend via

lateral lemniscus → to inferior colliculus or the medial geniculate body → terminate in cortex of the superior temporal gyrus
- b. *Vestibular afferent*: ascend to vestibular nuclei or descend via medial longitudinal fasciculus to vestibulospinal tract

ix. CN IX
- a. *Visceral* afferent
  1. Taste from posterior one-third of tongue to inferior (petrosal) ganglion and tractus solitarius to its nucleus
  2. Sensation from oral cavity, oropharynx, and hypopharynx via the tractus solitarius
- b. *Visceral* efferent
  1. From the inferior salivatory nucleus via Jacobson nerve to the otic ganglion to the auriculotemporal nerve to the parotid gland
- c. Motor
  1. Motor to stylopharyngeus muscle
    - CN X
- d. *Somatic sensory* via Arnold nerve for EAC and posterior auricle
- e. *Motor* to striated muscles of the velum, pharynx, and larynx
- f. *Visceral* afferent
  1. For receptors of respiration, cardiac activity, gastric secretions, and biliary function
- g. Visceral efferent
  1. From dorsal nucleus to smooth muscle of the esophagus, stomach, small intestine, upper colon, gallbladder, pancreas, lungs, and inhibitory fibers to the heart

x. CN XI
- a. *Cranial portion*: arises in nucleus ambiguous
  1. Contains special and general visceral efferent fibers that join the vagus and are distributed with it
- b. *Spinal portion*: arises from motor cells in the first five segments of cervical spinal cord
  1. Travels upward via the foramen magnum, across the occipital bone to the jugular fossa, where it pierces the dura and enters the neck via the jugular foramen to innervate the sternocleidomastoid and trapezius muscles

xi. *CN XII*: motor to the muscles of the tongue

xii. Ganglia
- a. Ciliary ganglion (CN III): parasympathetic ganglion and receives:
  1. Preganglionic, parasympathetic fibers from the Edinger-Westphal nucleus
  2. Postganglionic fibers go to ciliary muscles and sphincter papillae muscles
- b. Sphenopalatine ganglion (CN VII) receives:
  1. Preganglionic, parasympathetic fibers via the greater superficial petrosal nerve from the superior salivary nucleus
  2. Postganglionic fibers innervate the lacrimal and minor salivary glands
- c. Submandibular ganglion (CN VII) receives:
  1. Preganglionic, parasympathetic fibers from the superior salivary nucleus via the chorda tympani
  2. Postganglionic fibers innervate the submandibular and sublingual glands

      d. Otic ganglion (CN IX) receives:
        1. Preganglionic, parasympathetic fibers from the inferior salivary nucleus via Jacobson nerve
        2. Postganglionic fibers innervate the parotid gland.
E. Branches of the external carotid artery
   i. Superior thyroid artery
     a. Infrahyoid artery
     b. Superior laryngeal artery
     c. Sternomastoid artery
     d. Cricothyroid artery
   ii. Lingual artery
     a. Suprahyoid artery
     b. Dorsalis linguae artery
     c. Sublingual artery
   iii. Facial artery
     a. Cervical branches
       1. Ascending palatine artery
       2. Tonsillar artery
       3. Submaxillary artery
       4. Submental artery
       5. Muscular branches
     b. Facial branches
       1. Muscular branches
       2. Inferior labial artery
       3. Superior labial artery
       4. Lateral nasal artery
       5. Angular artery
   iv. Occipital artery
     a. Muscular branches
     b. Sternomastoid artery
     c. Auricular artery
     d. Meningeal branches
   v. Posterior auricular artery
     a. Stylomastoid branch
     b. Stapedial branch
     c. Auricular branch
     d. Occipital branch
   vi. Ascending pharyngeal artery
     a. Prevertebral branches
     b. Pharyngeal branches
     c. Inferior tympanic branch
   vii. Superficial temporal artery
     a. Transverse facial artery
     b. Middle temporal artery
     c. Anterior auricular branches
   viii. Internal maxillary artery
     a. Maxillary portion
       1. Anterior tympanic branch

        2. Deep auricular branch
        3. Middle meningeal artery
        4. Accessory meningeal artery
        5. Inferior dental artery
     b. Pterygoid portion
        1. Deep temporal branch
        2. Pterygoid branch
        3. Masseteric artery
        4. Buccal artery
     c. Sphenomaxillary portion
        1. Posterior superior alveolar artery
        2. Infraorbital artery
        3. Descending palatine artery
        4. Vidian artery
        5. Pterygopalatine artery
        6. Sphenopalatine artery
        7. Posterior nasal artery
F. Blood supply to tonsil
    i. Facial artery
      a. Tonsillar artery
      b. Ascending palatine artery
   ii. Lingual artery
      a. Dorsal lingual branch
  iii. Internal maxillary artery
      a. Descending palatine artery
      b. Greater palatine artery
   iv. Ascending pharyngeal artery
G. Blood supply to adenoids
    i. Ascending palatine branch of facial artery
   ii. Ascending pharyngeal artery
  iii. Pharyngeal branch of internal maxillary artery
   iv. Ascending cervical branch of thyrocervical trunk
H. Ethmoid arteries
    i. Branches of ophthalmic artery.
   ii. Anterior ethmoid artery is approximately 24 mm posterior to the anterior lacrimal crest.
  iii. Posterior ethmoid artery is approximately 12 mm posterior to the anterior ethmoid artery.
   iv. Optic nerve is approximately 6 mm posterior to the posterior ethmoid artery.
I. Orbit
    i. *Seven bones*: maxillary, frontal, ethmoid, zygomatic, sphenoid, palatal, and lacrimal
   ii. Communicates with:
      a. Infratemporal fossa via inferior orbital fissure
      b. Pterygopalatine fossa via inferior orbital fissure
      c. Middle cranial fossa via optic canal and superior orbital fissure
      d. Nose via nasolacrimal duct
  iii. Upper eyelid anatomy
      a. Skin
      b. Orbicularis oculi

  c. Orbital septum

  d. Prelevator fat (medial compartment with two fat pads and lateral compartment)

  e. Levator palpebrae superioris

  f. Müller muscle (superior tarsal muscle)

  g. Conjunctiva

 iv. Lower eyelid anatomy

  a. Skin

  b. Orbicularis oculi

  c. Orbital septum

  d. Orbital fat (medial, central, and lateral compartments with inferior oblique muscle between the central and medial compartments)

  e. Inferior tarsal muscle

  f. Conjunctiva

J. Ear

 i. External auditory canal

  a. Lateral half is cartilage and medial half is bone.

  b. *Fissures of Santorini*: small fenestrations within the anterior inferior cartilaginous EAC, which allow spread of infection to the parotid region and skull base.

  c. *Foramen of Huschke*: embryologic remnant that may persist as a communication from the anterior inferior aspect of the medial EAC, allows spread of tumors and infection to or from preauricular area/parotid.

 ii. Tympanic membrane

  a. *Three layers*: squamous epithelium, fibrous layer, and cuboidal mucosal epithelium

  b. Pars flaccida (Shrapnell membrane)

  c. Blood supply to tympanic membrane (TM)

   1. *External*: deep auricular artery

   2. *Internal*: anterior tympanic artery

 iii. Middle ear

  a. Regions

   1. Epitympanum

    • Portion of middle ear superior to TM

    • Contains head of malleus, body, and short process of incus

    • Bounded superiorly by tegmen tympani

   2. Mesotympanum

    • Portion which can be visualized through TM

    • Contains manubrium of malleus, long process of incus, and stapes

   3. Hypotympanum

    • Portion inferior to TM

    • *Hyrtl fissure*: an embryologic remnant that normally obliterates but may persist as a hypotympanic connection to the subarachnoid space

   4. Retrotympanum

    • Contains facial recess and sinus tympani

   5. Protympanum

    • Portion anterior to TM

  b. Ossicular chain

   1. *Malleus*: tensor tympani tendon originates from cochleariform process and connects to malleus neck

2. *Incus*: lenticular process connects to stapes
3. *Stapes*: stapedius tendon originates from pyramidal process and is innervated by the facial nerve
    iv. Prussak space
        a. *Anterior*: lateral malleal fold
        b. *Posterior*: lateral malleal fold
        c. *Superior*: lateral malleal fold
        d. *Inferior*: lateral process of malleus
        e. *Medial*: neck of malleus
        f. *Lateral*: Shrapnell membrane
    v. Muscles of eustachian tube
        a. Levator veli palatini
        b. Tensor veli palatini
        c. Salpingopharyngeus
        d. Dilator tubae
    vi. Facial nerve course:
        a. Facial motor nucleus → loops dorsomedially around abducens nucleus → exits at pontomedullary junction → joins nervus intermedius (nuclei are superior salivatory and nucleus solitarius) to become facial nerve proper → intracranial (23-24 mm) → enters porus acusticus in anterior superior quadrant → intrameatal (8-10 mm) → angles 120 degree anterior superior laterally → exits meatal foramen → labyrinthine (3-4 mm) → geniculate ganglion at processus cochleariformis → angles 75-90 degree posteriorly → tympanic (10-11 mm) → gentle arc posterior laterally → at pyramidal eminence, it becomes the mastoid portion (13-15 mm) → dives toward stylomastoid foramen → extracranial segment → first major division at pes
        b. Blood supply to facial nerve:
            1. *Intracranial*: anterior inferior cerebellar artery (AICA)
            2. *Intrameatal*: labyrinthine artery
            3. *Labyrinthine*: no defined (watershed of labyrinthine and superior petrosal arteries)
            4. *Tympanic*: superior petrosal and stylomastoid arteries
            5. *Mastoid*: stylomastoid artery
    vii. Contents of internal auditory canal
        a. Facial motor nerve
        b. Nervus intermedius
        c. Cochlear nerve
        d. Superior division of vestibular nerve
        e. Inferior division of vestibular nerve
        f. Labyrinthine artery
        g. Labyrinthine vein
    viii. *Jacobson nerve*: branch of IX that traverses the promontory and carries parasympathetics to the parotid gland
    ix. *Arnold nerve*: branch of X that supplies innervation to EAC
    x. *Facial recess*: bounded by facial nerve posteriorly, chorda tympani anteriorly, and incudal buttress superiorly
    xi. *Sinus tympani*: space medial to facial nerve, bounded anteriorly by promontory, superiorly by facial canal, laterally by pyramidal eminence (subiculum beneath, ponticulus above)

K. Nose and paranasal sinuses
   i. *External nasal valve*: area in the vestibule, under the nasal ala, formed by the caudal septum, medial crura of the alar cartilages, alar rim, and nasal sill
   ii. *Internal nasal valve*: nasal septum, caudal margin of upper lateral cartilage, anterior end of inferior turbinate, floor of nose
   iii. *Septum*: composed of quadrangular cartilage, perpendicular plate of the ethmoid, vomer
   iv. Ethmoid labyrinth is divided by four parallel bony lamellae
     a. Uncinate process
     b. Ethmoid bulla
     c. Ground lamella of middle turbinate
     d. Ground lamella of superior turbinate
   v. Three attachments of the middle turbinate
     a. *Anterior*: parasagittal into cribriform plate
     b. *Middle*: coronal into lamina papyracea
     c. *Posterior*: axial into lamina papyracea
   vi. Boundaries of infratemporal fossa
     a. *Superior*: greater wing of sphenoid, infratemporal crest
     b. *Anterior*: posterior curvature of maxillary bone
     c. *Medial*: lateral surface of lateral pterygoid plate
     d. *Lateral*: medial surface of mandibular ramus
     e. *Posterior*: spine of sphenoid, mandibular fossa
     f. *Inferior*: alveolar border of maxilla

L. Oral cavity
   i. Tongue
     a. Musculature
       1. Genioglossus, styloglossus, hyoglossus, palatoglossus
       2. All innervated by CN XII, except palatoglossus (CN X)
     b. Innervation
       1. *Motor*: CN XII
       2. *Taste*: anterior two-thirds by CN VII (via chorda tympani), posterior one-third by CN IX
       3. *Sensation*: anterior two-thirds by CN V3, posterior one-third by CN IX
     c. Papillae
       1. *Fungiform*: most numerous
       2. *Circumvallate*: immediately anterior to foramen cecum and sulcus terminalis
       3. *Foliate*: laterally on the tongue
     d. Sulcus terminalis
       1. Inverted V-shape groove (posterior to circumvallate papillae) on tongue dividing anterior two-thirds and posterior one-third of tongue.
       2. Foramen cecum lies at posterior aspect of the sulcus terminalis.
   ii. Palatal muscles
     a. Palatoglossus, palatopharyngeus, levator veli palatine, musculus uvulae, tensor veli palatini
     b. Innervated by CN X except for tensor veli palatini (CN V)

M. Pharynx
   i. *Muscles*: palatopharyngeus, stylopharyngeus, salpingopharyngeus, superior constrictor, middle constrictor, inferior constrictor.

      ii. Inner musculature is longitudinal (palatopharyngeus, stylopharyngeus, salpingopharyngeus).

      iii. Outer musculature is circular (constrictors).

      iv. Passavant ridge is a constriction of the superior margin of the superior constrictor muscle.

      v. All muscles are innervated by CN X except for stylopharyngeus (CN IX).

      vi. Pharyngeal constrictors

         a. *Superior*: spans from pharyngeal raphe and occipital bone to medial pterygoid, pterygomandibular ligament, and mandible

         b. *Middle*: spans from pharyngeal raphe to the hyoid bone

         c. *Inferior*: spans from pharyngeal raphe to the thyroid and cricoids cartilages

      vii. Killian triangle

         a. Site of least resistance between inferior constrictor and cricopharyngeus.

         b. Zenker diverticulum tends to develop here, usually emanate from left posterior esophagus.

      viii. Parapharyngeal space

         a. Boundaries

            1. *Superior*: skull base

            2. *Lateral*: mandible, medial pterygoid, parotid

            3. *Medial*: superior constrictor, buccopharyngeal fascia

            4. *Anterior*: pterygomandibular raphe, pterygoid fascia

            5. *Posterior*: carotid sheath, vertebral fascia

            6. *Interior*: lesser cornu of hyoid

         b. Compartments

            1. *Prestyloid*: internal maxillary artery, inferior alveolar nerve, lingual nerve, auriculotemporal nerve

            2. *Poststyloid*: carotid artery, internal jugular vein, CN IX-XII, cervical sympathetic chain

N. Salivary glands

    i. *Parotid duct*: along a line from the tragus to the midportion of the upper lip

    ii. Parasympathetic innervation

       a. Parotid gland

          1. Inferior salivary nucleus → CN IX (Jacobson nerve) enters middle ear via tympanic canaliculus → lesser superficial petrosal nerve (LSPN) via foramen ovale (otic ganglion → auriculotemporal branch of V3) → parotid gland

       b. Submandibular and sublingual gland

          1. Superior salivary nucleus → facial nerve (nervus intermedius) → chorda tympani → leaves ear via petrotympanic fissure → lingual branch of V3 (in infratemporal fossa) → submandibular ganglion → submandibular and sublingual glands

    iii. Sympathetic innervation

       a. Thoracic spinal cord → sympathetic trunk → superior cervical ganglion → external carotid artery → salivary glands

O. Neck

    i. Triangles

       a. Anterior

          1. *Submental*: anterior digastrics, midline of neck, hyoid

          2. *Digastric*: mandible, anterior and posterior bellies of digastric

          3. *Carotid*: Sternocleidomastoid muscle (SCM), posterior digastrics, anterior omohyoid

        4. *Muscular*: SCM, anterior omohyoid, midline of neck

     b. Posterior

        1. *Occipital*: trapezius, SCM, posterior omohyoid

        2. *Supraclavicular*: clavicle, SCM, posterior omohyoid

    ii. Blood supply to the SCM

     a. Occipital artery

     b. Branches of superior thyroid artery

     c. Branches of thyrocervical trunk

P. Larynx

    i. Supraglottis

     a. Extends from epiglottis to the level of the laryngeal ventricles, includes the epiglottis, aryepiglottic folds, arytenoids, false vocal folds, preepiglottic space, and the paraglottic space

     b. *Preepiglottic space*: fat-filled space limited superiorly by the hyoid and posteriorly by the epiglottis

     c. *Paraglottic space*: fat-filled space lateral to false and true vocal folds

     d. *Quadrangular membrane*: poorly developed ligamentous membrane bounded by aryepiglottic fold, anterior surface of arytenoids, vestibular fold, and lateral epiglottis

    ii. *Glottis*: true vocal folds and anterior and posterior commissures

    iii. Subglottis

     a. Extends from inferior aspect of the true vocal folds to the cricoids cartilage.

     b. Lateral margin is conus elasticus.

     c. *Conus elasticus*: arises from anterosuperior cricoids, sweeps up and medially to join anteriorly and attach to thyroid cartilage, and posteriorly to the vocal process of arytenoids, in between is the vocal ligament.

    iv. Superior laryngeal nerve (SLN)

     a. Originate in the nodose ganglion of CN X, which is just inferior to the skull base

     b. *External branch*: motor to cricothyroid

     c. *Internal branch*: sensory to distal pharynx and larynx cephalad to true vocal cords

    v. Recurrent laryngeal nerve (RLN)

     a. Motor to laryngeal musculature except for cricothyroid and sensation for area below the level of true vocal cords.

     b. The most important laryngeal muscle of respiration and airway protection is posterior cricoarytenoid muscle (the only abductor).

Radiology

A. Computed tomography (CT)

    i. Contrast used to evaluate neck to highlight malignancy or infection

    ii. Contrast not needed for bony anatomy (sinus or temporal bone)

B. Magnetic resonance imaging (MRI)

    i. *T1*: fat is bright, muscles are intermediate, fluid is dark. Fat saturation is often applied on postgadolinium T1-weighted images.

    ii. *T2*: fluid is bright.

    iii. Gadolinium contrast agent to highlight pathology.

C. Positron emission tomography (PET)
   i. Uses radioactive sugar (^{18}F-florodeoxyglucose or FDG) to highlight areas of increased metabolic activity. It has high negative predictive value.
   ii. Asymmetry can suggest malignancy.
   iii. Used to assess for unknown primaries, posttreatment evaluation, and in searching for metastases.
D. MRI is study of choice to assess malignancy; CT is helpful for assessing infectious and inflammatory processes.
E. Inner ear and temporal bone
   i. Cochlear malformations
      a. *Mondini*: bony and membranous cochlear dysplasia with 1.5 turns or less of cochlea, associated with perilymph fistula
      b. *Michel*: complete aplasia of bony and membranous labyrinth, looks like solid bone
   ii. Petrous apex
      a. Arachnoid cyst
         1. *CT*: fluid-filled mass without aggressive features
         2. *MRI*: low on T1, bright on T2, no enhancement
      b. Cholesteatoma
         1. *CT*: soft tissue mass with bony erosion
         2. *MRI*: intermediate on T1, bright on T2, no enhancement
      c. Cholesterol granuloma
         1. *CT*: expansile lesion
         2. *MRI*: bright on T1 and T2, no enhancement
      d. Chondrosarcoma
         1. *CT*: bony erosion and soft tissue mass with calcifications
         2. *MRI*: intermediate to low on T1, bright on T2, shows contrast enhancement
      e. Mucocele
         1. Similar to cholesterol granuloma
      f. Petrous apicitis
         1. *CT*: fluid-filled air cells +/− bony erosion
         2. *MRI*: low on T1, bright on T2, may show contrast enhancement
   iii. Otosclerosis
      a. CT reveals decreased density of bone anterior to oval window (fissula ante fenestram).
      b. Cochlear otosclerosis may reveal ring of lucency around the cochlea (Halo sign).
F. Cerebellopontine angle (CPA)
   i. Acoustic neuroma
      a. *CT*: widening of IAC
      b. *MRI*: intermediate on T1 and T2 (unless tumor is cystic), shows postgadolinium enhancement; filling defect on high resolution T2 images
   ii. Arachnoid cyst
      a. *CT*: fluid-filled mass without aggressive features
      b. *MRI*: low on T1, bright on T2, no enhancement
   iii. Epidermoid cyst
      a. Similar to arachnoid cyst
   iv. Meningioma
      a. *CT*: intermediate intensity mass
      b. *MRI*: intermediate on T1 and T2 with increased postgadolinium enhancement, "dural tail" seen on T1 postcontrast images

G. External ear
  i. *Malignant otitis externa (OE)*: diagnosed with MRI or Technetium[99] radioisotope scan
  ii. Follow treatment course with Gallium scan
H. Nose and paranasal sinuses
  i. Esthesioneuroblastoma
    a. *CT*: homogeneous soft tissue mass with contrast enhancement and bony erosion and molding
    b. *MRI*: locally invasive soft tissue mass that is hypointense on T1, bright on T2, and enhances with gadolinium
  ii. Fungal sinusitis
    a. Invasive
      1. *Acute*: aggressive soft tissue mass with bone and soft tissue destruction, contrast enhancement is often absent secondary to angioinvasion
      2. *Chronic*: similar to allergic fungal sinusitis but with less fulminant course
    b. Noninvasive
      1. Allergic fungal sinusitis
        • *CT*: soft tissue masses of multiple sinuses with mucosal thickening, sinus opacification, and bone remodeling
        • Heterogeneous density is often seen as a result of inspissated secretions and increased iron content
      2. *Mycetoma*: increased density and calcifications on CT
  iii. Inverting papilloma
    a. *CT*: mass extending from middle meatus into maxillary sinus and nasal cavity
    b. *MRI*: intermediate T1 and T2 signal intensity with postcontrast enhancement
  iv. Juvenile nasal angiofibroma
    a. *CT*: contrast enhancing mass with Holman-Miller sign (anterior displacement of the posterior maxillary sinus wall)
    b. *MRI*: prominent flow voids and postgadolinium enhancement
  v. Mucus retention cyst
    a. *CT*: low-intermediate density soft tissue mass
    b. *MRI*: intermediate on T1, bright on T2, variable contrast enhancement
I. Nasopharynx
  i. Rhabdomyosarcoma
    a. *MRI*: aggressive process with isointense T1, intermediate T2, and postgadolinium enhancement
  ii. Nasopharyngeal carcinoma
    a. *MRI*: soft tissue mass (often centered around fossa of Rosenmüller) with isointense T1, intermediate T2, and postgadolinium enhancement
  iii. Thornwaldt cyst
    a. *CT*: hypodense
    b. *MRI*: bright on T1 and T2, with no enhancement
J. Oral cavity
  i. *Sialadenitis*: CT may reveal calculi.
  ii. *Venous malformations*: bright on T1 (postcontrast) and T2 MRI.
K. Neck
  i. Abscess
    a. *CT*: low-density mass with ring enhancement

      ii. Branchial cleft cyst
         a. *CT*: unilocular, cystic mass displacing the submandibular gland anteriorly and the SCM posteriorly
      iii. Cystic hygroma
         a. *CT*: low density
         b. *MRI*: heterogeneous T1 and T2 without postgadolinium enhancement
      iv. Paraganglioma
         a. *CT*: postcontrast enhancement
         b. *MRI*: mild enhancement on T2, intense T1 postcontrast enhancement with "salt and pepper" appearance secondary to flow voids
         c. Types
            1. *Carotid body tumor*: Lyre sign
            2. Glomus jugulare
            3. Glomus tympanicum
            4. *Glomus vagale*: displaces carotid anteromedially

Dermatology

  A. Fitzpatrick scale
     i. Type I—very white—always burns, never tans
     ii. Type II—white—burns easily, tans minimally
     iii. Type III—white to olive—sometimes burns, slowly tans to light brown
     iv. Type IV—brown—burns minimally, always tans to dark brown
     v. Type V—dark brown—rarely burns, tans well
     vi. Type VI—black—never burns, deeply pigmented
  B. Benign neoplasms
     i. *Actinic keratosis*: small lesions of epidermal proliferation. May evolve (1%) into squamous cell carcinoma (SCCA).
     ii. *Chondrodermatitis nodularis helicis/antihelices*: ulcerative lesion of helix or antihelix. Results from pressure and may be treated with surgical excision.
     iii. *Keratoacanthoma*: fast-growing tumors that are difficult to distinguish from SCCA. Distinguished from SCCA by absence of epithelial membrane antigen.
     iv. Nevi:
        a. *Intraepithelial*: benign
        b. *Junctional*: premalignant
        c. *Intradermal*: benign
        d. *Blue (Spitz)*: benign
     v. Seborrheic Keratosis: originate in keratinocytes and tend to increase with age. May have various colors (tan, brown, black) and often have a "pasted on" appearance. Easily treated with curettage.
  C. Malignant neoplasms
     i. Systemic diseases associated with skin cancers include albinism, xeroderma pigmentosum (SCCA), Gorlin syndrome (basal cell carcinoma [BCCA]), dysplastic nevus syndrome (melanoma), Bowen disease (SCCA)
     ii. Mohs surgery
        a. Maximum control rates for nonmelanoma skin cancer and maximum preservation of normal tissue.

    b. Indications:
        1. Recurrent BCCA
        2. Sclerosing BCCA
        3. Poorly differentiated SCCA
        4. Need to preserve soft tissue (ie, eyelid)
    c. The preauricular region has the highest rate of recurrence following Mohs surgery for BCCA of the face.

iii. Basal cell carcinoma
    a. Most common cutaneous malignancy in adults
    b. High association with ultraviolet (UV) exposure
    c. Potential for "skip" lesions secondary to neurotropism
    d. Low risk for metastases but may become locally aggressive
    e. Subtypes
        1. Superficial
           • Slow-growing, nonaggressive, scaly, erythematous plaques
           • Topical agents (ie, 5% fluorouracil), cryotherapy, photodynamic therapy, curettage, or Mohs
        2. Nodular
           • Histology shows groups of cells with decreased cytoplasm and "palisading" nuclei.
           • Pearly papules with telangiectatic borders.
           • Local excision (0.5-cm margins) or Mohs excision.
        3. Sclerosing/morpheaform
           • Small stands of tumor extend out from central lesion (skip lesions) resulting in high recurrence rates and large surgical defects
           • Mohs surgery
        4. Basosquamous
           • Characterized by squamous differentiation and keratinization
           • Can be confused with SCCA
           • Mohs or wide local excision

iv. SCCA
    a. Second most common cutaneous malignancy in adults
    b. High association with UV exposure and radiation burn scars
        1. *Marjolin ulcer*: aggressive, ulcerating SCCA in area of previous trauma, inflammation, or scar
    c. Precursors include actinic keratosis or Bowen disease
    d. May result in nodal disease and distant metastases
    e. Types
        1. *Bowen disease*: SCCA in situ (5% progress to invasive SCCA). Cryotherapy and photodynamic therapy
        2. Well differentiated
           • Squamous cells in cords with "intercellular bridges" and "keratin pearls"
           • Stain for cytokeratins
           • Mohs or wide local excision
        3. Poorly differentiated
           • Less intercellular bridges and keratin pearls
           • Mohs or wide local excision with 1-cm margins

   v. Melanoma
      a. Third most common cutaneous malignancy in adults.
      b. Incidence is growing at 5% annually.
      c. Associated with UV exposure, large congenital nevi, and those with more than 50 benign nevi.
      d. *Histological markers*: S-100, Melan-A, HMB-45 ("Human Melanoma Black"— antibody against melanoma antigen) is most specific.
      e. Types:
         1. Atypical junctional melanocytic hyperplasia, lesion between nevus and lentigo maligna.
         2. Lentigo maligna (melanoma in situ or Hutchinson freckle) (4%-15%):
            • Lesions confined to the epidermis
         3. *Lentigo maligna melanoma*: lesions with dermal violation.
         4. Superficial spreading (70%):
            • Most common
            • Usually develop from preexisting nevi
            • Radial growth
         5. Nodular (15%-30%):
            • Early invasion and vertical growth
         6. Desmoplastic (2%):
            • Neurotropic
         7. *Mucosal*: very rare (2%) and carries a 5-year survival rate of 10% and recurrence rate of 50%. The major failure is local recurrence, not regional lymph node metastases. Elective neck dissection is *not* beneficial.
   D. *ABCDEs*: *A*symmetry, irregular *B*orders, *C*olor variation, *D*iameter (> 6 mm), *E*volving lesion
   E. *Prognostic factors*: thickness, ulceration, satellite lesions, and lymph node involvement
   F. 5-year survival
      i. Clark I, 100% (epidermis)
      ii. Clark II, 93% (papillary dermis)
      iii. Clark III, 74% (junction of papillary and reticular dermis)
      iv. Clark IV, 39% (reticular dermis)
   G. Biopsy—Do not do shave biopsy. Need to assess depth, so perform excisional biopsy with 1- to 2-mm margins
   H. Treatment
      i. *Lentigo maligna*: square technique, Mohs, Woods light with 5-mm margins
      ii. Wide surgical excision with sentinel lymph node biopsy if lesion is greater than 1.0-mm Breslow depth
         a. Sentinel node dissection should be offered to all patients with a clinically negative nodal basin and a primary melanoma greater than 1 mm in depth. It may be considered in melanoma 0.76 to 1 mm in thickness with adverse features including lymphovascular invasion, age <40, significant vertical growth phase, increased mitotic rate.
         b. *Lesions under 2-mm Breslow depth*: 1-cm margins
         c. *Lesions over 2-mm Breslow depth*: 2-cm margins
      iii. Radiation
      iv. Interferon (IFN alpha-2b)

Ophthalmology

    A. *Pupillary reflex*: direct and consensual components:
       i. Optic nerve → optic tract → superior colliculus → pretectal area → visceral nuclei of oculomotor complex → preganglionic fibers via CN III to ciliary ganglion → postganglionic fibers from ciliary ganglion to sphincter of the iris
    B. Corneal reflex:
       i. Ophthalmic branch of the trigeminal nerve → motor nuclei of CN VII → orbicularis oculi
    C. *Argyle-Robertson pupil*: miotic pupils. Does not contract to light but does to accommodation (suggests syphilis).
    D. *Marcus-Gunn pupil*: pupil dilation in response to direct light (afferent pupillary defect). Results from optic nerve injury with decreased afferent input to brain.
    E. Optic chiasm lesions may result in bitemporal hemianopsia, whereas optic tract lesions result in a contralateral hemianopsia.

Pharmacology

    A. Amide local anesthetic
       i. Lidocaine, bupivacaine, mepivacaine, prilocaine, ropivacaine, etidocaine
       ii. Metabolized by liver dealkylation
    B. Ester local anesthetic
       i. Cocaine, procaine, chloroprocaine, tetracaine, benzocaine
       ii. Metabolized by plasma and liver cholinesterases
    C. Local anesthetic toxicity
       i. Central nervous system (CNS) effects
         a. *Excitatory*: blurred vision, tingling, tinnitus, numbness, disorientation, sweating, seizures, sweating, vomiting
         b. *Inhibitory*: decreased level of consciousness, coma
       ii. Cardiovascular system (CVS) effects
         a. Bradycardia, hypotension, cardiorespiratory arrest
       iii. Management
         a. Airway, breathing, circulation
         b. Stop procedure/stop injection
         c. Oxygen, IV, fluids
    D. Side effects of corticosteroids
       i. Fluid imbalance
       ii. Electrolyte disturbance
       iii. Glycosuria
       iv. Susceptibility to infection
       v. Hypertension
       vi. Hyperglycemia
       vii. Peptic ulcer disease
       viii. Osteoporosis
       ix. Cataracts
       x. Behavioral disturbances

        xi. Cushingoid habitus

        xii. Central obesity

        xiii. Acne

        xiv. Hirsutism

        xv. Avascular necrosis

E. Antiemetics

    i. Emetic center in medulla (reticular formation), acetylcholine and histamine receptors present

    ii. Chemoreceptor trigger zone in fourth ventricle, dopamine receptors present

        a. Phenothiazines work well, antidopaminergic and anticholinergic.

        b. Metoclopramide is antidopaminergic.

        c. *Odansetron and granisetron*: 5HT3 receptor antagonist.

F. Expectorants

    i. Stimulates secretions in respiratory tract via vagus nerve

    ii. Ammonium salts, iodide salts, guaifenesin

Otology

A. Audiology

    i. Range of human hearing is 20 to 20,000 Hz.

    ii. Speech sounds are concentrated between 250 and 6000 Hz.

    iii. *Decibel*: 10 log 10.

    iv. Interaural attenuation is 0 dB for bone conduction and 40 to 60 dB for earphones.

    v. Masking required for

        a. Air conduction when test tone is 40 to 60 dB louder than bone thresholds of nontest ear

        b. Bone conduction when there is any difference between air conduction and bone conduction thresholds

        c. Masking dilemma occurs when there is bilateral 50 dB air-bone gap and requires special audiometric techniques

    vi. *Threshold*: softest intensity level for a pure tone to be detected 50% of the time

    vii. *Speech reception threshold (SRT)*: lowest intensity level required for patient to recognize 50% of bisyllabic words (spondee)

        a. Should be within 10 dB of the pure tone average (PTA)

    viii. Word recognition—patient's ability to recognize monosyllabic words presented 40 dB above SRT

    ix. Conductive hearing loss (CHL)

        a. *50-60 dB*: ossicular discontinuity with intact TM

        b. *Less than 50 dB*: otosclerosis

        c. *30-50 dB*: ossicular discontinuity and TM perforation

        d. *10-30 dB*: TM perforation

    x. Stenger test

        a. Used to detect pseudohypacusis, "functional" hearing loss, nonorganic loss and malingering

        b. Based on the principle that a listener will only hear the louder of two tones when identical tones of different intensity levels are presented to the two ears

        c. Tester presents subthreshold tone in "bad" ear and suprathreshold tone in "good" ear

    d. If the patient has a functional loss, they will state that they cannot hear any-thing despite the fact that they should hear the tone presented in the "good" ear

  xi. *Recruitment*: abnormal growth in loudness that indicates a cochlear lesion. When an acoustic neuroma is present, the finding of recruitment probably overrides the finding of auditory fatigue

  xii. *Fatigue*: Change of auditory threshold resulting from continued acoustic stimulation that indicates retrocochlear lesion

 xiii. *Rollover*: a decrease of word recognition at high intensities (from cochlear distortion of eighth nerve adaptation) and is a classic finding for retrocochlear lesions

 xiv. Tympanometry

    a. *Type A*: normal

      1. *Type A$_s$*: "S"hallow. Seen in otosclerosis, tympanosclerosis

      2. *Type AD*: "D"eep. Seen in ossicular discontinuity

    b. *Type B*: flat. Seen in middle ear effusion or TM perforation

    c. *Type C*: represents negative pressure as seen in eustachian tube dysfunction (ETD)

  xv. Acoustic reflex

    a. Cochlea → CN VIII → cochlear nuclei and contralateral olivary complex via the trapezoid body → motor nucleus of CN VII → stapedius.

    b. A unilateral stimulus results in bilateral contraction.

    c. Abnormal result is decay to less than 50% of the original amplitude within 10 seconds.

      1. Indicative of eighth nerve or brain stem lesion

    d. Factors that can affect the acoustic reflex

      1. Conductive losses of 40 dB for the ear receiving the reflex-eliciting tone or as little as 10 dB for the probe ear

      2. Sensorineural hearing losses (SNHLs) of greater than 70 dB

      3. Eighth nerve lesions

      4. Seventh nerve lesion proximal to stapedius (ie, Ramsay Hunt syndrome)

      5. Multiple sclerosis

      6. Brain stem lesions

    e. Eighth nerve or CNS lesions may have the following acoustic reflex responses:

      1. Normal reflexes

      2. Elevated reflex thresholds without decay

      3. Normal or elevated reflex thresholds with decay

      4. Absent reflexes

  xvi. Auditory brain stem response (ABR)

    a. Brain stem function can be identified on ABR testing at approximately 28 weeks' gestational age with the appearance of waves I, III, and V. "Maturity" is not reached until approximately 18 months after birth.

    b. Waves I-V represented by the mnemonic "EECOL":

      1. *Wave I*: distal *E*ighth nerve

      2. *Wave II*: proximal *E*ighth nerve

      3. *Wave III*: *C*ochlear nucleus

      4. *Wave IV*: *O*livary complex

      5. *Wave V*: lateral *L*emniscus

    c. Normal waveform latencies:

      1. I-III is 2.3 ms

      2. III-V is 2.1 ms

      3. I-V is 4.4 ms

        d. Retrocochlear lesions should be suspected if ABR results show the following:

           1. Interpeak latency difference greater than 4.4 ms

           2. Interaural latency difference of wave V greater than 0.2 ms

           3. V_3-V_5 latency of greater than 2.1 ms

xvii. *Electrocochleography (ECOG)*: diagnostic for Ménière disease if the ratio of the summating potential to the compound action potential is elevated (> 0.4)

xviii. Otoacoustic emissions

A. Distortion product otoacoustic emissions (DPOAEs) have the most clinical applications

    1. Used to monitor newborn hearing, aminoglycoside-induced hearing loss, and to help differentiate between cochlear and retrocochlear causes of SNH

    2. Auditory neuropathy—normal OAEs, abnormal CN VIII

    3. Produced by outer hair cells (OHCs)

B. Vestibular testing

    i. History may suggest disorder

      a. *Drop attacks*: crisis of Tumarkin (Ménière disease)

      b. *Vertigo with pressure changes*: Hennebert sign (Ménière disease, perilymph fistula [PLF], superior canal dehiscence syndrome, syphilis)

      c. *Noise-induced vertigo*: Tullio phenomenon (Ménière disease, PLF, superior canal dehiscence syndrome, syphilis)

      d. *Positional vertigo*: benign paroxysmal positional vertigo (BPPV)

    ii. Components of vestibular testing

      a. Nystagmus evaluation

        1. Slow phase is driven by vestibulo-ocular reflex (VOR), and is measured in degree/second.

        2. Fast phase (saccade) is driven by the paramedian pontine reticular formation.

          • Direction of nystagmus is determined by the direction of the fast phase.

        3. Testing:

          • Spontaneous

            (a) Evaluate with Frenzel goggles

            (b) Peripheral nystagmus

               ◦ Usually horizontal ± torsional component

               ◦ Decrease with visual fixation

            (c) Central nystagmus

               ◦ Vertical or purely torsional

               ◦ Does not decrease with visual fixation

          • Gaze

            (a) Peripheral nystagmus

               ◦ Fixed direction in varying gaze positions

            (b) Central nystagmus

               ◦ May change directions in different gaze positions

            (c) Degrees

               ◦ *First degree*: Nystagmus is present when looking laterally in the direction of the fast component.

               ◦ *Second degree*: Nystagmus is present when looking laterally in the direction of the fast component and in neutral position.

               ◦ *Third degree*: Nystagmus is present in all three positions.

- Positioning
  - (a) Head shaking nystagmus (HSN)
    - ○ Horizontal HSN can be seen in unilateral vestibular lesions.
- Positional
  - (a) Dix-Hallpike maneuver
    - ○ Vertical and torsional nystagmus toward downward ear (geotropic) indicates BPPV.

b. VOR/horizontal semicircular canal evaluation
  1. Calorics
     - Evaluates horizontal semicircular canal
     - Supine position with head tilted 30 degree up from horizontal (to place horizontal canal in vertical position)
     - Bithermal stimulus (water or air)
     - Most likely test to lateralize a peripheral lesion
     - Warm stimulus causes endolymph to rise and stimulate horizontal canal
  2. COWS: *Cold Opposite, Warm Same*
     - Uses peak slow-phase eye velocities (degree/second) for calculations
     - Can determine:
       - (a) Unilateral weakness (right vs left ear)
         - ○ (RW + RC) – (LW + LC)/total
         - ○ Twenty-five percent or less is normal.
         - ○ Used to evaluate symmetry.
         - ○ Negative value indicates right weakness, positive value indicates left weakness.
       - (b) Directional preponderance (right vs left movement)
         - ○ (RW + LC) – (RC + LW)/total
         - ○ Thirty-five percent or less is normal
         - ○ Present if patient has spontaneous nystagmus
  3. Rotational chair
     - Evaluates VOR (see Anatomy section for VOR description)
       - (a) Uses peak slow-phase eye velocities for calculations
       - (b) Tests across 0.01-1.28 Hz in octave steps
       - (c) Determines
         - ○ *Phase*: describes the *timing relationship* between head movement and the reflexive eye response
       - (d) If eyes and head move at the exact same velocity in opposite directions, they are *out of phase* (or 180 degree)
       - (e) *Phase lead*: Eye velocity is greater than head velocity
       - (f) Normal to have phase lead at low frequencies
       - (g) Abnormal phase leads at low frequencies—peripheral lesion
       - (h) Abnormal phase leads at all frequencies—central lesion
       - (i) *Phase lag*: Head velocity is greater than eye velocity
       - (j) Occurs in peripheral lesions or in presence of poor gains
         - ○ Gain
       - (k) *Ratio* of the peak amplitude of slow-phase eye velocity to the amplitude of the head velocity
       - (l) Should be 1 (except at low frequencies)
       - (m) Insufficient gain suggests ototoxic process or central lesion
         - ○ Symmetry

      (n) Comparison of the slow-phase eye velocities when the head is rotated to the right compared with rotation to the left

      (o) Corresponds to directional preponderance

  c. Oculomotor evaluation

    1. Evaluates eye movement function for various stimuli in the absence of vestibular stimulation

- *Saccades*: Evaluate velocity, accuracy, and latency of fast-phase eye movements.
- *Smooth pursuit*: Results should show smooth, sinusoidal tracking. Abrupt, jerky eye movements may indicate central pathology.
- Opticokinetic nystagmus: Tracks multiple stimuli. Results in nystagmus-like eye movements. Evaluate for symmetry between eyes.

  d. Posturography

    1. Evaluates:

- Balance
- Visual, proprioceptive, and vestibular signal processing

    2. Conditions tested:

- 1: Eyes open, support stable, visual field fixed
- 2: *Eyes closed*, support stable, visual field fixed
- 3: Eyes open, support stable, *visual field sway referenced*
- 4: Eyes open, *support tilted*, visual field fixed
- 5: *Eyes closed, support tilted*, visual field fixed
- 6: Eyes open, *support tilted, visual field sway referenced*

    3. Vestibular dysfunction can be determined by abnormal values in 5 or 6.

 iii. Electronystagmography (ENG) incorporates nystagmus, VOR/HSCC (horizontal semicircular canal), and oculomotor testing

  a. Helps determine site of lesion

  b. Supports the diagnosis of

    1. BPPV

    2. Labyrinthitis

    3. Ménière disease

    4. Ototoxicity

    5. Vestibular neuritis

C. External ear

  i. Aural atresia

  a. Clinical findings include absent ear canal and 40 to 65 dB air-bone gap.

  b. Often sporadic but may be associated with:

    1. Treacher-Collins syndrome

    2. Goldenhar syndrome (Hemifacial microsomia)

  c. Treatment options:

    1. Bone anchored hearing aid (BAHA) placement

    2. Atresiaplasty

    3. Amplification (Bone conduction aids)

  d. Jahrsdoerfer criteria for surgical repair:

    1. 10 excellent, 9 very good, 8 good, 7 fair, 6 marginal, 5 or less poor

- *Stapes*: 2
- *Oval window open*: 1
- *Round window open*: 1

- *Middle ear space*: 1
- *Pneumatized mastoid*: 1
- *Normal CN VII*: 1
- *Malleus and incus*: (minus) −1
- *Incus and stapes*: 1
- *External ear*: 1

   e. Only 50% of aural atresia patients are surgical candidates.

ii. Microtia

   a. RUM:

     1. *Right* > left

     2. *Unilateral* > bilateral (4:1)

     3. *Males* > females (2.5:1)

   b. Classification:

     1. Type I—mild deformity (ie, lop ear, cup ear, etc)

     2. Type II—all structures are present to some degree, but there is a tissue deficiency

     3. Type III—"Classic" microtia, significant deformity with few recognizable landmarks, lobule often present and anteriorly displaced, and canal atresia

   c. Best time to reconstruct is between 6 and 10 years.

   d. Ear reaches 85% of adult size by 5 years of age.

iii. Frostbite

   a. Rapidly rewarm with gauze soaked in saline, that is, 38°C-42°C/100.4°F-107.6°F

   b. Tissue should not be debrided upon rewarming as demarcation may take several weeks.

   c. Treat with topical antibiotic, ointment, and oral analgesics.

iv. Otitis externa

   a. Most common organisms

     1. Bacterial
- *Staphylococcus aureus*
- *Pseudomonas aeruginosa*

     2. Fungal
- *Aspergillus niger*

   b. Agents for bacterial otitis externa—neomycin, polymyxin, ciprofloxacin, ofloxacin compounds ± steroids

   c. Agents for otomycosis

     1. Merthiolate (Thimerosal)

     2. Acetic acid

     3. Isopropyl alcohol

     4. Gentian violet

     5. Nystatin suspension, cream, ointment, or powder

     6. Azole cream, lotion, or solution

v. Malignant Otitis Externa

   a. Seen in diabetic, elderly and immunocompromised patients

   b. *P aeruginosa*

   c. Infection disseminates to skull base via fissures of Santorini.

   d. Diagnosed with MRI or Technetium[99] radioisotope scan and followed with gallium scan

e. CT may be used for confirmation of osteomyelitis, although 30% to 50% of the trabecular bone of the mastoid must be destroyed before the CT becomes obviously positive

f. Antipseudomonal antibiotics for 3 to 4 months and surgical debridement.

vi. *Exostoses*: broad-based, bony lesions (multiple) of EAC secondary to cold water exposure. Surgery required for CHL or cerumen impaction

vii. *Osteoma*: benign, pedunculated bony neoplasm (usually single) of the anterior EAC. Surgery required for CHL or cerumen impaction

viii. Referred otalgia

    a. *CN V*: oral cavity, mandible, temporomandibular joint (TMJ), palate, preauricular region

    b. *CN VII*: EAC, postauricular region

    c. *CN IX*: tonsil, tongue base, nasopharynx, eustachian tube, pharynx (transmitted via Jacobson nerve)

    d. *CN X*: hypopharynx, larynx, trachea (transmitted via Arnold nerve)

D. Middle ear

i. Cerebrospinal fluid (CSF) otorrhea

    a. Associated with 6% of basilar skull fractures

    b. Most common source in adults is mastoid tegmen secondary to meningoencephalocele

    c. Ninety percent seal spontaneously

        1. Middle fossa leaks heal rapidly due to the extensive fibrosis promoted by the rich arachnoid mesh in this area

        2. Posterior fossa leaks close more slowly, as little arachnoid is present in this area

    d. Indications for repair

        1. Persistent leak for longer than 2 weeks despite bed rest with head elevation

        2. Recurrent meningitis

        3. Brain or meningeal herniation

        4. Penetration of brain by bony spicule

ii. Cholesteatoma

    a. Congenital cholesteatoma

        1. Appears as a "pearl" in the middle ear space

        2. Usually develop from embryonic rest of epithelium in anterior-superior quadrant

        3. Often asymptomatic

    b. Acquired cholesteatoma

        1. Usually develops from retraction of pars flaccida into Prussak space (between pars flaccida and malleus neck).

        2. Epithelial migration or retraction pocket formation with internal desquamation, enzymatic erosion, and osteitis allow formation and progression of cholesteatoma.

        3. Most common location for cholesteatoma in middle ear is around long process of the incus and stapes suprastructure.

        4. Common areas for residual disease following surgery include the sinus tympani, facial recess, and anterior epitympanum.

    c. Complications of cholesteatoma

        1. Most common complication is erosion of horizontal semicircular canal.

        2. Most common ossicle eroded is the long process of the incus.

        3. Tympanic portion of facial nerve (FN) is most commonly injured during surgery secondary to confusing anatomy and frequent nerve dehiscence.

    4. Oval or round window fistulas should be patched with fascia and packed.

    5. Others:
- Extradural or perisinus abscess
- Serous or suppurative labyrinthitis
- Meningitis secondary to tegmental erosion
- Epidural, subdural, or parenchymal brain abscess
- Sigmoid sinus thrombosis/phlebitis
- Subperiosteal abscess/Bezold abscess due to erosion of the mastoid cortex
- Recurrence

d. Treatment

    1. Canal-wall-up tympanomastoid
- Higher risk of persistent or recurrent cholesteatoma
- Often requires second look surgery within 1 year and possible delay of ossicular reconstruction

    2. Canal-wall-down tympanomastoid
- Highest rate of success on initial surgery
- Requires meatoplasty
- Indications: Only hearing ear, contracted mastoid, labyrinthine fistula, EAC erosion

    3. Reasons for a persistently draining mastoid cavity are:
- Inadequate meatoplasty
- Dependent tip cell
- High facial ridge
- Exposed eustachian tube

    4. The cholesteatoma matrix is completely removed except for the following situations:
- Matrix is adherent to the dura.
- Matrix is adherent to the superior semicircular canal.
- Matrix is firmly adherent to the FN.
- Extends into the mesotympanum covering the footplate.
- Performing canal-wall-down mastoid and will be using some residual matrix to line mastoid cavity.

iii. Eustachian tube dysfunction

a. The dilator tubae portion of the tensor veli palatini muscle is primarily responsible for eustachian tube opening.

b. Tubal closure is passive.

c. Chronic ETD can generate negative pressures to 600 cm H_2O with resultant retraction pocket formation and middle ear effusion.

iv. Ossicular abnormalities

a. Teunissen classification

    1. *Class I*: congenital stapes ankylosis (fixation)

    2. *Class II*: stapes ankylosis with ossicular abnormality
- Class I and II are *good surgical candidates.*

    3. *Class III*: ossicular abnormality with mobile footplate, ossicular discontinuity, or epitympanic fixation

    4. *Class IV*: aplasia or dysplasia of round or oval window ± crossing FN or persistent stapedial artery
- Class III and IV are *poor candidates.*

     v. Otosclerosis
       a. Most common cause of conductive hearing loss between the ages of 15 and 50.
       b. Prevalence
         1. Caucasian > Asian > African American
         2. Female > male (2:1)
       c. Elevated antimeasles virus IgG in perilymph.
       d. Autosomal dominant with 40% penetrance.
       e. Hastened by pregnancy and menopause.
       f. Eighty-five percent are bilateral.
       g. Disease usually begins in region anterior to oval window niche (fissula ante fenestram) resulting in stapes fixation and CHL.
       h. Involvement of the cochlea may result in SNHL.
       i. Increased osteoblastic and osteoclastic activity resulting in "spongiosis" and eventually resulting in bone with increased mineralization.
       j. *Blue Mantles of Manasse*: finger-like projections of blue otosclerotic bone around normal vasculature.
       k. *Schwartze sign*: pinkish hue over promontory and oval window niche (represents region of thickened mucosa).
       l. Acoustic reflex testing
         1. Early in disease process—increased compliance at beginning and end of stimulus
         2. Late in disease process—decreased or absent reflex
       m. *Audiometry*: Air-bone gap (unusual to find air-bone gaps > 50 dB) with Carhart notch (elevation of bone thresholds centered around 2000 Hz). The Carhart notch is not a true indication of cochlear reserve.
       n. CT may reveal "double ring" or "halo" sign.
       o. Treatment
         1. Consider hearing aid first
         2. Stapedectomy
     vi. Tuberculosis
       a. Grey TM with multiple, small perforations
       b. Mucoid, clear drainage
       c. Incus resorption and denuded malleus head
       d. SNHL
     vii. Vascular anomalies
       a. Dehiscent carotid—pulsatile red mass in anteroinferior quadrant
       b. High-riding jugular bulb—bluish mass in posteroinferior quadrant
       c. Persistent stapedial artery
         1. Branch of the petrous internal carotid artery.
         2. Passes through obturator foramen of the stapes.
         3. Gives off the middle meningeal artery (foramen spinosum is absent).
         4. Consider terminating surgery if encountered during stapedectomy.
         5. CT may show absent foramen spinosum and widened fallopian canal.
       d. Glomus tympanicum—see Other Neck Disorders section
   E. SNHL
     i. Prevalence
       a. Less than 1% of children are born with hearing loss.
       b. Ten percent of adults have SNHL.
         1. Thirty-five percent of adults over 65 and 40% of adults over 70 have SNHL.

  ii. Asymmetric—obtain MRI to rule out CPA angle mass

  iii. Hereditary—see Pediatrics section

  iv. Noise induced

   a. Results in elevated thresholds centered around 4000 Hz

   b. Outer hair cell death

   c. OSHA (Occupational Safety and Health Administration) noise exposure limits

    1. 90 dB for 8 hours

    2. 95 dB for 4 hours

    3. 100 dB for 2 hours

    4. 105 dB for 1 hour

    5. 110 dB for 1/2 hour

   d. US Air Force and Army have chosen a more stringent exposure limit of 85 dB for 8 hours

  v. Ototoxicity

   a. Aminoglycosides, cisplatin, loop diuretics, quinine, and salicylates

   b. Outer hair cell death

  vi. Presbycusis—symmetric, high-frequency sensorineural hearing loss (HFSNHL) *and* often have diminished speech discrimination (suggesting neural involvement as well)

 vii. Sudden SNHL

   a. Obtain MRI.

   b. Autoimmune:

    1. *Cogan syndrome*: interstitial keratitis and Ménière-like attacks of vertigo, ataxia, tinnitus, nausea, vomiting, and hearing loss

    2. *Others*: Wegener granulomatosis, polyarteritis nodosa, temporal arteritis, Buerger disease (thromboangiitis obliterans), and systemic lupus erythematosus (SLE)

    3. Prednisone 1 mg/kg/d for 4 weeks followed by a slow taper if the patient responds

   c. *Idiopathic sudden SNHL (ISSNHL)*: treat with steroids; may include intratympanic steroid treatment.

   d. *Traumatic*: transverse temporal bone fractures often cause SNHL and vertigo.

   e. *Viral*: believed to be the cause of the majority of cases of ISSNHL. Researchers have shown a statistically significant increase in viral seroconversion in patients with ISSNHL compared with controls for cytomegalovirus (CMV) as well as influenza B, mumps, rubeola, and varicella zoster viruses.

   f. Between 40% and 70% of patients recover some hearing without treatment.

   g. Prognostic factors:

    1. Good

     • Minimal hearing loss

     • Low-frequency loss

     • Absence of vestibular symptoms

     • Early treatment (within 3 days)

    2. Poor

     • Advanced age

     • Total deafness

     • Vestibular symptoms

     • Vascular risk factors

     • Delayed treatment

       viii. Viruses associated with SNHL
- a. Rubella
- b. Herpes simplex 1 and 2
- c. Varicella (chickenpox or zoster oticus)
- d. Variola (smallpox)
- e. Epstein-Barr virus (EBV)
- f. Polio
- g. Influenza
- h. Adenovirus
- i. CMV (most common viral cause of SNHL)
- j. Measles
- k. Mumps (most common viral cause of unilateral SNHL)
- l. Hepatitis

F. Auditory neuropathy
- i. SNHL with poor word recognition scores
- ii. Normal outer hair cell function
- iii. Abnormal CN VIII function
- iv. HAs and cochlear implants may be of little help

G. Superior semicircular canal dehiscence syndrome
- i. Dehiscence of bone overlying the superior semicircular canal
- ii. Vertigo and oscillopsia generated by sound (Tullio phenomenon) or Valsalva
- iii. Sensitivity to bone conduction (lower bone thresholds at lower frequencies)
- iv. CHL due to dissipation of sound energy because of presence of "third" window
  - a. Intact acoustic reflexes can help differentiate from otosclerosis
- v. Diagnosed by temporal bone CT; cervical VEMP also useful (reduced threshold)
- vi. Treatment
  - a. Avoidance measures
  - b. Plugging or resurfacing of superior semicircular canal
    1. Middle fossa approach
    2. Transmastoid approach

H. Vestibular disorders
- i. *Vertigo*: sense of movement
- ii. Importance of history
  - a. Always ask patient about their first vertiginous episode
  - b. Clear understanding of duration, circumstance, and associated otologic symptoms can help narrow the differential diagnosis
  - c. Differential diagnosis can be partially tailored based on history
    1. *BPPV: seconds*, no hearing loss, provoked by head movement
    2. *Perilymphatic fistula: seconds*, hearing loss, provoked by trauma, barotrauma, or stapes surgery
    3. *Migraine: minutes to hours*, can precede headache, similar to Ménière disease but without otologic symptoms
    4. *Vertebrobasilar insufficiency: minutes*, accompany arterial hypotension (cardiac arrhythmia, orthostatic hypotension), patients with diabetes mellitus (DM), and atherosclerosis
    5. *Ménière disease*: recurrent, *hours*, hearing loss, tinnitus, aural fullness
    6. *Delayed-onset vertigo (delayed endolymphatic hydrops)*: similar to Ménière disease but develops months or years after developing SNHL

7. *Serous (toxic) labyrinthitis*: acute vertigo crisis in presence of otitis media (OM), no hearing loss
8. *Suppurative labyrinthitis*: acute vertigo crisis and hearing loss in presence of OM and fever
9. *Labyrinthine fistula*: dizziness in patient with cholesteatoma
10. *Vestibular neuronitis*: acute crisis, *hours to days*, gradual improvement over days, present with no movement, no associated otologic symptoms
11. *Viral labyrinthitis*: *similar to vestibular neuronitis* but with sudden hearing loss
12. *Ototoxic*: vertigo and hearing loss following aminoglycoside use
13. *Acoustic neuroma*: hearing loss, tinnitus, and *mild if any* vestibular symptoms
14. *Multiple sclerosis*: vertigo frequently seen, common other findings: vertical nystagmus and internuclear ophthalmoplegia (INO)

I. Auditory aids
   i. Conventional hearing aids (HAs)
      a. In general, a patient with a dynamic range of more than 45 dB is a good HA candidate, whereas a patient with a dynamic range of 25 to 45 dB is a fair candidate.
      b. Parameters for fitting HAs:
         1. Most comfortable loudness (MCL)—the level at which listening to words or speech is most comfortable (usually between 40 and 60 dB)
         2. Uncomfortable loudness (UCL)—the level at which listening to *words* or speech is uncomfortably loud
         3. Loudness discomfort level (LDL)—the level at which specific *tones* are painfully loud
      c. Dynamic range of HA:
         1. UCL—SRT
      d. Gain:
         1. Difference between the level of the input signal and the level of the output signal at a given frequency
         2. To decrease the amount of gain in the low frequencies in patients with high-frequency neural loss, consider:
            • Open venting of the earmold—allows low-frequency sounds to escape (low-frequency attenuation), thus selectively amplifying high frequencies
            • Shorten the canal of the earmold
            • Enlarge the sound bore
      e. May need to be vented to prevent the occlusion effect (hearing your own voice while speaking).
      f. A closed mold provides a more uniform amplification.
   ii. *CROS*: contralateral routing of sound. For patients with one good ear and one deaf ear
   iii. *BICROS*: bilateral contralateral routing of sound. For patients with one impaired ear and one deaf ear
   iv. *BAHA*: bone-anchored hearing aid. For patients with unilateral conductive or mixed hearing loss who cannot otherwise wear traditional HAs (ie, chronic suppurative otitis media [CSOM], atresia)
   v. Cochlear implants
      a. Severe to profound SNHL with hearing in noise test (AZ Bio) scores of 50% in the implanted ear and 60% in the contralateral ear.

      b. Worst candidate is prelingually-deafened adult.

      c. FDA approval as early as 12 months old.

      d. *Transmission pathway:* microphone → external processor → receiver-stimulator → electrodes → spiral ganglion cells and eighth nerve → cochlear nucleus

      e. Round window insertion or cochleostomy (placed anterior and inferior to the round window niche).

      f. Electrode is ideally placed in scala tympani.

J. FN injury and disorders

  i. Immediate paralysis concerning for transection

  ii. Delayed-onset palsy most likely secondary to edema

  iii. House-Brackmann (HB) classification

      a. Grade I—*normal*

      b. Grade II—slight weakness/asymmetry with movement

      c. Grade III—obvious asymmetry with movement, possible synkinesis. *Complete eye closure*

      d. Grade IV—*incomplete eye closure*, no forehead movement, asymmetry with movement

      e. Grade V—*asymmetric at rest*, minimal movement with effort

      f. Grade VI—*no movement*

  iv. Sunderland classification

      a. First degree

        1. *Neuropraxia*: pressure on nerve trunk. Blockage of axoplasm flow at site of injury

      b. Second degree

        1. *Axonotmesis*: axonal and myelin injury. Axon degenerates distal to the site of injury and proximally to the next node of Ranvier. May develop wallerian degeneration

      c. *Third degree: Neurotmesis*: injury to axon, myelin, and endoneurium. Poor prognosis

      d. *Fourth degree: Neurotmesis*: injury to axon, myelin, endoneurium, and perineurium. Poor prognosis

      e. *Fifth degree: Neurotmesis*: injury to axon, myelin, endoneurium, perineurium, and epineurium (all layers of nerve sheath). Poor prognosis

  v. Nerve testing

      a. Only done on patients with HB Grade VI.

      b. Wallerian degeneration takes 48 to 72 hours to progress to extratemporal segments of FN. Therefore, *electrophysiologic testing (nerve excitability test [NET] and electroneuronography [ENOG]) should not be done in first 3 days.*

      c. *NET*: 2.0-3.5 mA difference between sides suggests unfavorable prognosis.

      d. ENOG:

        1. Measures *compound muscle action potential* (CMAP).

        2. Greater than and equal to 90% degeneration of CMAP suggests poor recovery and is an indication for surgical exploration and decompression.

        3. Should be performed daily until nadir is reached.

      e. Electromyography (EMG):

        1. Measures *motor unit potentials* (MUP)

        2. May be useful in first 3 days following injury

          • MUP in four of five groups in first 3 days associated with satisfactory return of function in more than 90% of patients

3. Important for assessing reinnervation potential of the muscle *2 to 3 weeks after onset*
   - Fibrillation potentials suggest loss of neural supply
   - Polyphasic potentials seen in cases of reinnervation

vi. *Indications for imaging*: Progression of palsy over 3 weeks, recurrent palsy, facial hyperkinesis, development of associated cranial neuropathies. These symptoms may also suggest neoplastic involvement.

vii. Acute facial palsy

a. Bell (70%)
   1. Diagnosis of exclusion
   2. Rapid onset (< 48 hours)
   3. May affect CN V-XII
   4. Believed to be viral (herpes simples virus [HSV])

b. Herpes zoster (Ramsay Hunt syndrome) (15%)
   1. Differentiated from Bell by the presence of:
      - Cutaneous vesicles of EAC and conchal bowl
      - Otalgia
      - Higher incidence of cochlear and vestibular disturbances

c. Other symptoms related to FN paralysis
   1. Dysgeusia (chorda tympani)
   2. Hyperacusis (stapedius dysfunction)
   3. Decreased lacrimation (GSPN)

d. Site of injury is believed to be the *meatal foramen*, which is just proximal to the labyrinthine portion of FN.

e. Prednisone (1 mg/kg) divided tid for 10 days with a 10-day taper.

f. Acyclovir 800 mg five times daily for 10 days.

g. Valacyclovir may be more effective for Ramsay Hunt syndrome.

viii. Other notable causes of FN palsy

a. DM

b. *Guillain-Barré syndrome*: most common cause of *bilateral* FN paralysis

c. Hyperthyroidism

d. Lyme disease
   1. *Borrelia burgdorferi*
   2. Unilateral or bilateral facial palsy (3:1)
   3. "Bull eye" rash
   4. Tetracycline for adults, penicillin for children

e. *Melkersson-Rosenthal syndrome*: unilateral facial palsy, facial edema, and fissured tongue (lingua plicata)

f. *Mobius syndrome*: bilateral facial and abducens nerve palsies

g. Mononucleosis

h. Multiple sclerosis

i. Mumps

j. Myasthenia gravis

k. Neoplasia

l. OM
   1. *AOM*: amoxicillin and myringotomy
   2. *CSOM*: surgical removal of disease and nerve decompression
   3. *MOE*: see External Ear section

    m. Perinatal
      1. FN at risk due to lack of mastoid tip
      2. Compression by mother's sacrum or delivery forceps
      3. Excellent spontaneous recovery
    n. Sarcoidosis
      1. Heerfordt disease (uveoparotid fever) consists of uveitis, mild fever, non-suppurative parotitis, and CN paralysis
      2. FN is most commonly involved (may be *bilateral*)
      3. Elevated serum angiotensin-converting enzyme (ACE) generally confirms the diagnosis
    o. *Trauma*: penetrating wounds or temporal bone fracture
    p. Wegener granulomatosis
  i. Complications
    a. "Crocodile tears"—cross-innervation from LSPN to GSPN
  ii. Repair of transected nerve
    a. Best result will be HB III
    b. Types
      1. Before 18 months
        • End to end
      2. Best option
      3. FN can be mobilized 2 cm
        • Cable graft
      4. Used if greater than 2 cm is needed
        • CN XII-VII
      5. After 18 months
        • Dynamic muscle sling (ie, temporalis)
      6. Make sure V_3 is intact prior to performing temporalis sling

Rhinology

  A. Chandler classification of orbital cellulitis:
    i. Periorbital edema
    ii. Periorbital cellulitis
    iii. Subperiosteal abscess
    iv. Orbital abscess
    v. Cavernous sinus thrombosis
  B. *Samter triad*: aspirin sensitivity, asthma, nasal polyposis.
  C. Allergic fungal sinusitis:
    i. Benign, noninvasive fungal disease resulting in a hypersensitivity reaction within the paranasal sinuses
    ii. Immunocompetent adults
    iii. Type I hypersensitivity response to fungi
    iv. Microbiology
      a. Dematiaceous molds, that is, *Pseudallescheria boydii*
    v. Diagnosis (Bent and Kuhn criteria)
      a. Eosinophilic mucin (Charcot-Leyden crystals)
      b. Noninvasive fungal hyphae
      c. Nasal polyposis

      d. Type 1 hypersensitivity by history, skin tests, or serology

      e. Characteristic radiologic findings

         1. *CT*: Rim of hypointensity with hyperdense central material (allergic mucin)

         2. *CT*: speckled areas of increased attenuation due to ferromagnetic fungal elements

         3. *MRI*: peripheral hyperintensity with central hypointensity on both T1 and T2

         4. *MRI*: central void on T2

D. Differential diagnosis of nasal mass:

    i. *Congenital*: glioma, encephalocele, dermoid, teratoma

    ii. *Infectious*: tuberculosis, rhinoscleroma, rhinosporidiosis

    iii. *Inflammatory/granulomatous*: allergic polyp, sarcoid

    iv. *Benign tumors*: squamous and schneiderian papilloma, juvenile angiofibroma, paraganglioma, leiomyoma, schwannoma, adenoma

    v. *Malignant tumors*: SCCA, adenocarcinoma, adenoid cystic carcinoma, lymphoma, rhabdomyosarcoma, melanoma, esthesioneuroblastoma, chordoma, plasmacytoma, histiocytosis X

E. Paranasal malignancy:

    i. Paranasal sinus cancers account for 3% of aerodigestive and 1% of all malignancies.

    ii. Maxillary > ethmoid > sphenoid > frontal sinuses.

    iii. Risk factors:

      a. Wood dust

      b. Nickel

      c. Chromium

      d. Volatile hydrocarbons

      e. Organic fibers found in the wood, shoe, and textile industries

      f. At least one study has found smoking to be a significant risk factor

      g. Human papilloma virus (HPV) may be involved in the malignant degeneration of inverting papillomas

      h. At least one study suggests that chronic sinusitis is a risk factor for paranasal sinus cancer with a 2.3-fold increase in risk compared with the general population

    iv. Diagnosis:

      a. CT—identifies bony involvement and erosion

      b. MRI

         1. Identifies neural involvement

         2. Superior to CT with 94% to 98% correlation with surgical findings

    v. Most patients have advanced disease at the time of diagnosis.

      a. One exception to this is tumors of the maxillary sinus (tumors inferior to Ohngren line).

F. Anosmia:

    i. Associated with

      a. Alzheimer disease

      b. Chronic rhinitis

      c. Chronic sinusitis

      d. Nasal polyps

      e. Nasal allergy

      f. Head trauma with or without cribriform fracture

      g. Postviral

    h. Malignancy of the nasal cavity/nasopharynx/ethmoid sinus/frontal sinus

    i. Psychiatric disorders

    j. Medications

    k. Nasal surgery

    l. Hypogonadism (Kallmann syndrome)

G. *Hutchinson rule*: Herpes zoster involvement of the nasal tip is associated with a high incidence of herpes zoster ophthalmicus due to retrograde spread via the nasociliary nerve. Early ophthalmology consultation advised.

H. Nasal obstruction:

    i. Septal deviation, septal hematoma, turbinate hypertrophy, nasal narrowing, nasal valve collapse, tip ptosis, choanal atresia, nasopharyngeal obstruction/mass, trauma

    ii. Nasal tumor, foreign body

    iii. Inflammation due to nasal/sinus infection, allergy, granulomatous process, atrophic rhinitis (AR), septal abscess

    iv. Medication, hypothyroidism, pregnancy

    v. Psychogenic, hyperpatency

I. Septal perforation etiologies:

    i. Iatrogenic

    ii. Cocaine use

    iii. Septal abscess

    iv. Nose picking

    v. Infections such as syphilis, tuberculosis, leprosy, and rhinoscleroma

    vi. Inflammatory etiologies include Wegener granulomatosis, sarcoidosis, lupus, and other collagen vascular disease

    vii. Neoplasms include nasal lymphoma and other malignancies

Head and Neck

A. Angioedema

    i. Causes

        a. Allergy (treat with Benadryl and epinephrine)

        b. ACE inhibitor use

        c. Familial—C1 esterase deficiency

    ii. Treatment

        a. Airway protection

        b. Steroids, H_1 and H_2 blockers, subcutaneous epinephrine

B. Benign pigmentation changes

    i. Melanosis—physiologic pigmentation (dark patches) on mucosa

    ii. Amalgam tattoo—tattoo of gingival from dental amalgam

C. Bitter sensation is better appreciated through the glossopharyngeal nerve.

D. Sensation for ammonia and hot chilli peppers is mediated by the trigeminal nerve.

E. Craniopharyngioma:

    i. Epithelial tumors derived from the Rathke cleft (embryonal precursor to the adenohypophysis)

        a. Craniopharyngeal duct is the structure along which the eventual adenohypophysis and infundibulum migrate.

      b. Tumors can occur anywhere along the course of this duct (pharynx, sella turcica, third ventricle).

    ii. Clinical presentation

      a. Headaches

      b. Visual loss (possible bitemporal hemianopsia)

      c. Optic atrophy

      d. Hypopituitarism

      e. Enlargement of sella turcica

      f. Parasellar calcifications

    iii. Differential diagnosis

      a. Optic glioma

      b. Primary pituitary tumors

      c. Parasellar metastases

F. Dental pathology:

    i. Enamel discoloration—antibiotic (tetracycline) exposure prior to eruption

    ii. Treatment for dislodged tooth is immediate replacement

    iii. Odontogenic cysts and tumors

      a. Dentigerous (follicular) cyst—defect in enamel formation. Results in unerupted tooth crown. Ameloblastoma formation occurs in cyst wall.

      b. Lateral periodontal cyst—small lucent cysts (usually at mandibular premolars).

      c. Primordial cyst—rare cyst that develops instead of a tooth.

      d. Periapical/radicular cyst—most common. Burned out tooth infection

      e. Odontogenic keratocyst—can arise from any cyst. Distinguished by keratinizing lining. Aggressive and difficult to remove. Need larger resection. Part of basal cell nevus syndrome (BCNS)/Gorlin syndrome.

      f. Nonodontogenic cysts—bone cysts, aneurysmal bone cyst (ABC), gingival cysts.

      g. Ameloblastoma—most common odontogenic tumor. Benign but locally aggressive. Wide excision (eg, segmental mandibulectomy).

G. Granular cell tumor:

    i. Nonulcerated, painless nodules with insidious onset and slow growth

    ii. Involves tongue in 25% of cases

    iii. Histology shows pseudoepitheliomatous hyperplasia

    iv. Three percent become malignant

    v. Conservative excision

H. Immunosuppression (acquired/iatrogenic) results in an increase in lymphoproliferative disorders and should be kept in mind when evaluating lesions of Waldeyer ring, salivary glands, or cervical nodes.

I. Infections:

    i. Adenotonsillitis

    ii. Candidiasis

      a. Predisposing factors

        1. Antibiotics, steroids

        2. Infants, elderly

        3. Diabetes, malnutrition, immunosuppression

      b. Clinical features

        1. Patches of creamy white pseudomembrane

        2. Odynophagia

        3. Dysphagia

        4. Angular cheilitis

        5. Laryngitis

    c. Diagnosis—Sabouraud medium

    d. Treatment—nystatin, amphotericin B

        1. Herpangina
- Minute vesicles on the anterior tonsillar pillars and soft palate
- Coxsackie A virus (hand, foot, and mouth disease)

        2. Histoplasmosis
- Etiology

        3. *Histoplasma capsulatum*

        4. Endemic in Missouri and Ohio River valleys
- Clinical features

        5. Lung involvement

        6. Rhinitis, pharyngitis, epiglottitis

        7. Nodular lesions of tongue, lip, and oral mucosa (oral lesions much more common than in *Blastomyces* and *Coccidioides*)

        8. Dirty white mucosa or true cords
- Pathology—epithelioid granulomas
- Diagnosis

        9. Skin test

      10. Complement fixation

      11. Latex agglutination

      12. Laryngeal lesions require direct laryngoscopy (DL) and biopsy with fungal stains
- Treatment—amphotericin B

      13. Pharyngitis
- Symptoms—throat pain, fever, pharyngeal erythema/exudates, cervical lymphadenopathy in the absence of coryza, cough, and hoarseness
- Pathogens

      14. *Streptococcus pyogenes* (most important pathogen)

      15. *S aureus*

      16. *Streptococcus pneumoniae*

      17. *Moraxella catarrhalis*

      18. *Haemophilus influenzae*

      19. *Mycoplasma pneumoniae* (may account for 30% of adult pharyngitis)

      20. *Corynebacterium diphtheriae*

      21. Gonococcal
- Treatment—erythromycin, amoxicillin

J. Malignant lesions:
- i. Risk factors
  - a. Tobacco and alcohol use
  - b. Poor oral hygiene
  - c. HPV 16 and 18
  - d. Betel nut
- ii. Types
  - a. SCCA
  - b. Minor salivary gland malignancies
    1. Adenocarcinoma
    2. Adenoid cystic carcinoma

　　　　3. Mucoepidermoid carcinoma
　　　c. Lymphoma—commonly seen in tonsillar fossa
　　iii. Staging
　　　　a. T1 less than and equal to 2 cm
　　　　b. T2 greater than 2 cm, less than and equal to 4 cm
　　　　c. T3 greater than 4 cm
　　　　d. T4 invades surrounding structures
　　iv. Lymph node disease
　　　　a. Tumors of the tongue and floor of mouth have a high rate of nodal metastases
　　　　　1. Lateral tumors drain to ipsilateral submandibular and jugulodigastric nodes
　　　　　2. Midline tumors may have bilateral drainage
　　　　b. Presence of lymph node disease halves the survival for any given T stage
　　v. Treatment
　　　　a. Oral cavity
　　　　　1. Surgery or (XRT) for early lesions (Stage I and II)
　　　　　2. Surgery and XRT for advanced lesions (Stage III and IV)
　　　　b. Oropharynx
　　　　　1. Surgery or XRT for early lesions
　　　　　2. Surgery and XRT or chemoradiation (organ preservation) for advanced lesions
　　　　c. Neck dissection
　　　　　1. Advanced tumors.
　　　　　2. Tumors approaching midline often require bilateral neck dissection.
　　　　　3. Tumors with 2 mm or greater tongue invasion.
　　　　　4. Tumors of the soft palate.
　　　　　5. Tumors of the pharyngeal wall require bilateral neck dissection.
　　　　　6. Tumors with bony involvement of mandible.
K. Nasopharyngeal carcinoma:
　　i. Presenting symptoms
　　　　a. Cervical lymphadenopathy
　　　　b. Epistaxis
　　　　c. Serous effusion
　　　　d. CN VI paralysis
　　ii. Commonly arises at the fossa of Rosenmüller
　　iii. Male:female: 2.5:1
　　iv. Increased incidence in people from southern China
　　v. Associated with EBV infection
　　　　a. Can follow treatment success with serial measurements of EBV viral capsid antigen in WHO II and III tumors
　　vi. Treatment—radiation therapy
　　vii. No neck dissection unless for persistent disease
L. Nutritional deficiencies:
　　i. Vitamin B_2 (riboflavin)—atrophic glossitis, angular cheilitis, gingivostomatitis
　　ii. Vitamin B_6 (pyridoxine)—angular cheilitis
　　iii. Vitamin B_{12}—pernicious anemia, tongue with lobulations and possible shiny, smooth, and red appearance
　　iv. Vitamin C—scurvy, gingivitis, and bleeding gums
　　v. Iron deficiency—oral mucosa is gray and tongue is smooth and devoid of papillae
　　vi. Nicotinic acid—angular cheilitis

M. Obstructive sleep apnea (OSA):
  i. One in five American adults has at least mild OSA.
  ii. Minimal diagnostic criteria for OSA are at least 10 apneic events per hour. Events include:
     a. Complete cessation of airflow for at least 10 seconds
     b. Hypopnea in which airflow decreases by 50% for 10 seconds or decreases by 30% if there is an associated decrease in the oxygen saturation or an arousal from sleep
  iii. Apnea-hypopnea index (AHI) grades severity of OSA. AHI is also sometimes referred to as the respiratory disturbance index (RDI).
     a. 5 is normal
     b. 5-15 is mild
     c. 15-30 is moderate
     d. Greater than 30 is severe
  iv. Symptoms
     a. Morning headaches
     b. Daytime hypersomnolence
     c. Decreased productivity
     d. Lethargy
     e. Depression
  v. Long-term sequelae
     a. Intellectual deterioration
     b. Impotence
     c. Cardiac arrhythmias
     d. Pulmonary hypertension (HTN)
  vi. Diagnosis
     a. Polysomnogram
     b. Determining the site of obstruction is essential
        1. Fiberoptic endoscopy in the supine position with Müeller maneuver
        2. Cephalometric measurements are required in many cases
  vii. Medical evaluation and treatment
     a. Treatment of allergies and sinusitis.
     b. Weight loss.
     c. Several devices are available and have found some use in selected patients.
        1. Nasal airways, nasal valve supports, tongue-advancement devices, and bite prostheses to maintain an open bite.
        2. Nasal continuous positive airway pressure (CPAP) is available, but patient tolerance is often a limiting factor.
     d. Surgical treatment *must address site of obstruction.*
        1. Septoplasty.
        2. Adenoidectomy and tonsillectomy.
        3. Partial midline or posterior glossectomy or radiofrequency ablation.
        4. Uvulopalatopharyngoplasty—When excising any portion of the soft palate, remember that the middle one-third of the palate is the most important from a functional standpoint. Therefore, remove more laterally rather than centrally.
        5. Hyoid suspension.
        6. Genioglossal advancement ± hyoid myotomy.
        7. Maxillomandibular advancement.
        8. Tracheotomy—gold standard.

N. Papillomas of the oral cavity are most frequently seen on the tonsillar pillars and soft palate. May be premalignant.

O. Pemphigus:
  i. Types:
    a. Vulgaris—rapid acute form
    b. Vegetans—indolent chronic form
  ii. Affects the oral cavity in approximately two-thirds.
  iii. In those with oral cavity involvement, about half subsequently develop skin lesions.
  iv. Suprabasal *intraepidermal* bullae:
    a. Autoantibodies are present to the epithelial intercellular substance.
  v. Acantholysis is seen on biopsy, and there is a positive Nikolsky sign.
  vi. All areas of the gastrointestinal (GI) tract can become involved and are the usual source of sepsis and death.
  vii. Treatment—steroids.

P. Pemphigoid:
  i. Types
    a. Bullous
      1. Oral lesions are seen in one-third of patients.
    b. Benign mucous membrane
      1. Lesions are usually limited to the oral cavity and conjunctiva.
      2. *Subepidermal* bullae are present and tend to be smaller than pemphigus and more tense.
      3. No acantholysis is present and Nikolsky sign is negative.
      4. Autoantibodies are present to the basement membrane.
      5. Both forms are more successfully treated with intermittent systemic steroids.
      6. Penicillamine may allow healing in resistant cases.

Q. Premalignant lesions:
  i. Leukoplakia
    a. Hyperkeratotic lesion
    b. 5% to 10% will progress to SCCA
  ii. Erythroplakia
    a. Granular, erythematous region
    b. Often seen in association with leukoplakia
    c. 50% will show dysplasia or carcinoma in situ (CIS) on biopsy

R. Thornwaldt cyst:
  i. Most common congenital nasopharyngeal lesion
  ii. Develops in the midline as the notochord ascends through the clivus to create the neural plate

S. TMJ syndrome
  i. Associated with:
    a. Bruxism
    b. Dental trauma or dental surgery
    c. Mandibular trauma/abnormalities/asymmetry
    d. Myofascial or cervical tension
  ii. Treatment begins with soft diet, warm compresses, and nonsteroidal anti-inflammatory drugs (NSAIDs). A thorough dental/maxillofacial evaluation is advised.

Salivary Glands

   A. Salivary duct—acinus (surrounded by myoepithelial cells) $\Rightarrow$ intercalated duct $\Rightarrow$ striated duct $\Rightarrow$ excretory duct

   B. Saliva

      i. Made in the acinus and modified in the duct

      ii. High in potassium and low in sodium

     iii. Parotid secretions are watery (due to increased serous cells), low in mucin, and high in enzymes

     iv. Submandibular and sublingual secretions are thicker due to increased levels of mucin

     v. Important in dental hygiene

     vi. Antibacterial activity—IgA, lysozymes, leukotaxins, opsonins

   C. Nonneoplastic disease

      i. Infectious

        a. Mumps (viral parotitis)

          1. Paramyxovirus

          2. Affects children 4-6 years of age

          3. Bilateral parotid swelling

          4. Other symptoms

- Encephalitis
- Meningitis
- Nephritis
- Pancreatitis
- Orchitis

          5. Self-limited disease

          6. MMR (measles, mumps, and rubella) vaccine has significantly decreased incidence

        b. Sialadenitis

          1. Acute

- Seen in debilitated and dehydrated patients
- S *aureus*
- Treatment

          2. Anti-*Staphylococcus* antibiotics

          3. Warm compresses

          4. Hydration

          5. Sialogogues

          6. Chronic

- Recurrent, painful enlargement of gland
- Caused by decreased salivary flow (sialolith, stasis)
- Treatment

          7. Hydration

          8. Sialogogues

          9. Salivary duct dilation

         10. Occasional sialoadenectomy

         11. Granulomatous

- Chronic unilateral or bilateral swelling with minimal pain
- Frequently seen in patients with HIV
- Causes

(a) Actinomycosis
- Acute illness—inflammation and trismus.
- Chronic illness—firm, progressively enlarging, painless facial mass with increasing trismus, often confused with a parotid tumor
- Draining sinus tracts are common
- *Etiology: Actinomyces israelii*
- *Culture*: branching, anaerobic, or microaerophilic gram-positive rods (must be grown on blood agar in anaerobic conditions), sulfur granules
- Associations
  (a) Mucous membrane trauma
  (b) Poor oral hygiene
  (c) Dental abscess
  (d) Diabetes
  (e) Immunosuppression
- Treatment
- Penicillin (4-6 weeks)
- Incision and drainage required in some cases
- Cat scratch disease
- Sarcoid—Heerfordt disease (uveoparotid fever) consists of uveitis, mild fever, nonsuppurative parotitis, and CN paralysis
- Tuberculosis
- Wegener granulomatosis

    ii. Noninfectious

      a. Sialolithiasis

1. Most commonly affects the submandibular glands (80%)
2. Sixty-five percent of parotid sialoliths are radiolucent and 65% of submandibular sialoliths are radiopaque
3. Pain and swelling of affected gland
4. Treatment
   - Sialolithotripsy (ultrasonic, pulsed dye laser)
   - Endoscopic removal
   - Sialodochoplasty (open removal)

      b. Sjögren disease

1. See Connective Tissue Disorders section
2. Medications
   - Pilocarpine (Salagen)—cholinergic agonist for post-XRT and Sjögren disease
   - Cevimeline (Evoxac)—cholinergic agonist for Sjögren disease

      c. Xerostomia

1. Commonly seen with aging, radiation therapy, Sjögren disease, dehydration, diabetes, and medications
2. Medications
   - Chemoprotectants such as Amifostine can help prevent radiation-induced xerostomia.
   - Pilocarpine (Salagen)
   - Cevimeline (Evoxac)—approved for Sjögren disease but sometimes used as second-line therapy for post-XRT xerostomia.

      d. Neoplastic disease

1. One percent of all head and neck tumors
2. Eighty percent of tumors occur in parotid and 75% to 80% of these are benign

3. Fifteen percent of tumors occur in submandibular gland and 50% to 60% of these are malignant
4. Benign tumors
   - Pleomorphic adenoma
     (a) Most common salivary gland neoplasm
     (b) Most common location is the parotid (85%); 90% occur in the tail of the superficial lobe
     (c) Slow-growing, painless, and firm mass
     (d) Histology shows epithelial, myoepithelial, and stromal elements—benign mixed tumor
     (e) Treatment is excision with a cuff of normal tissue
     (f) Risk of conversion to carcinoma ex-pleomorphic adenoma
   - Warthin tumor
     (a) Second most common benign parotid neoplasm
     (b) Rarely seen outside of parotid gland
     (c) Seen in older white males
     (d) Slow-growing, painless, and firm mass
     (e) Exhibit uptake on Technetium[99] scans
     (f) Histology—papillary cystadenoma lymphomatosum
     (g) Treatment is excision with a cuff of normal tissue
   - Oncocytoma
     (a) Two percent of benign epithelial salivary
     (b) Seen in older individuals
     (c) Slow-growing, painless, and firm mass
     (d) Exhibit uptake on Technetium[99] scans
     (e) Histology shows sheets, nests, or cords of oncocytes (granular-appearing cells)
     (f) Treatment is excision with a cuff of normal tissue
     (g) Malignant tumors
   - Most commonly seen in fifth to sixth decade
   - Pain, CN VII involvement, and fixation imply poor prognosis
   - Types
     (a) Mucoepidermoid
     (b) Thirty-four percent of salivary gland malignancies
     (c) Most common parotid malignancy (85%)
     (d) Second most common submandibular and minor salivary gland malignancy
     (e) Grades
       ○ Low
       ○ Higher ratio of mucous to epidermoid cells
       ○ Presence of cystic spaces
       ○ Smaller, partially encapsulated, with long history
       ○ High
       ○ Higher ratio of epidermoid to mucous cells
       ○ May resemble SCCA on histology
       ○ More aggressive with a shorter history
       ○ 25% present with facial paralysis
     (f) Treatment
       ○ Low grade—wide excision

- High grade—wide excision and postoperative XRT
- Adenoid cystic
  - (a) Twenty-two percent of salivary gland malignancies
  - (b) Second most common parotid malignancy
  - (c) Most common submandibular and minor salivary gland malignancy
  - (d) *Perineural invasion* with "skip lesions"
  - (e) Three histologic subtypes: cribriform, tubular, and solid
  - (f) Prognosis depends on cell type: tubular (best) > cribriform > solid (worst)
  - (g) Treatment—wide excision with postoperative XRT
  - (h) Metastases occur most commonly in first 5 years but will continue to occur over 20 years; lung is most common site of metastasis
- Adenocarcinoma
  - (a) Eighteen percent of salivary gland malignancies
  - (b) High or low grade
  - (c) Treatment is wide excision with postoperative XRT
- Malignant mixed tumor
  - (a) Thirteen percent of salivary gland malignancies
  - (b) Seventy-five percent originate in parotid gland
  - (c) Types
    - Primary malignant mixed tumor
    - De novo metastasizing neoplasm
      - Contains myoepithelial and epithelial cells
      - Highly lethal (0% 5-year survival)
      - Carcinoma ex-pleomorphic adenoma
      - Malignant transformation within preexisting pleomorphic adenoma
      - Slow-growing mass which suddenly increases in size
      - Only contains epithelial cells
      - Local and distant metastases (lung) common
      - Treatment wide excision with postoperative radiation
      - Poor prognosis
    - Acinic cell carcinoma
  - (d) Seven percent of salivary gland malignancies
  - (e) 80% to 90% occur in parotid
  - (f) Low-grade to intermediate-grade malignancy
  - (g) Histology—serous acinar cells and cells with clear cytoplasm
  - (h) Well circumscribed and surrounded by fibrous capsules
  - (i) Calcification may be prominent
  - (j) Treatment is wide surgical excision
  - (k) Radiation is ineffective
  - (l) Metastases are rare, but tend to be hematogenous to bone and lungs
    - SCCA
  - (m) Very rare
  - (n) Must exclude
    - Metastatic SCCA
    - Invasive SCCA
    - High-grade mucoepidermoid carcinoma
  - (o) Treatment is wide excision and postoperative XRT

- Histologic derivation of salivary malignancies
  - (a) Acinic cell carcinoma—acinar and intercalated duct cells
  - (b) Malignant mixed—myoepithelial and acinar cells
  - (c) Mucoepidermoid—excretory duct cells
  - (d) SCCA—excretory duct cells
- Frey syndrome
  - (a) Preauricular gustatory sweating
  - (b) Parasympathetic salivary nerves from the auriculotemporal nerve innervate the sweat glands of the skin flap
  - (c) Diagnosed by Minor starch-iodide test
  - (d) Treat with topical antiperspirant, topical glycopyrrolate, or topical atropine
- The accuracy of fine-needle aspiration (FNA) biopsies and frozen section specimens in salivary gland lesions varies with the experience of the pathologist

Laryngology

A. True vocal fold
  i. Superior edge of cricothyroid ligament
  ii. 1.7 mm in thickness
  iii. Layers
      a. Stratified squamous epithelium
      b. Superficial layer of lamina propria (corresponds to Reinke space)
      c. Vocal ligament
         1. Intermediate layer of lamina propria
         2. Deep layer of lamina propria
      d. Vocalis muscle
  iv. Phonation
      a. Air from the lungs causes Bernoulli effect and vocal fold vibration.
      b. Mucosal wave produces a fundamental tone accompanied by several nonharmonic overtones.
      c. Sound is modified by the volume of airflow, movements of the vocal tract, and the degree of vocal cord tension.
      d. Voice fundamental frequency increases in aging men but decreases in aging women.
B. Benign lesions
  i. Amyloidosis
      a. Larynx is the most common site of airway involvement.
      b. Submucosal mass of the true or false fold.
      c. Histology shows apple-green birefringence after staining with Congo red dye.
      d. Treatment is surgical excision.
  ii. Chondroma
      a. Firm, smooth lesion usually involving posterior cricoid cartilage.
      b. Treatment is surgical excision.
  iii. Cysts
      a. Mixed group of benign lesions that may involve any laryngeal structure with the exception of the free edge of the true vocal cords (TVCs)

b. Lined with ciliated pseudostratified columnar (respiratory) epithelium, columnar epithelium, squamous epithelium, or a combination of all three

c. Types
1. *Ductal cysts (75%)*: develop from an obstructed mucous duct, which subsequently leads to cystic dilation of the mucous gland
2. Saccular cysts (24%)
   - Disorders of the saccule represent a spectrum from enlarged saccule to laryngocele, to saccular cyst.
   - Mucous-filled dilations of the laryngeal saccule.
   - Anterior saccular cysts protrude anteromedially between the true and false vocal folds.
   - Lateral saccular cysts extend superolaterally to involve the false vocal cord, aryepiglottic fold, and vallecula and may extend to the extralaryngeal tissues via the thyrohyoid membrane.
3. Thyroid cartilage foraminal cysts are extremely rare, herniation of subglottic mucosa through a persistent thyroid ala foramen

iv. Gastroesophageal reflux
a. Erythema and edema
b. Pachydermia
c. Pseudosulcus

v. Granuloma
a. Develop from extrinsic trauma (ie, intubation, gastroesophageal reflux disease [GERD])
b. Arise posteriorly in the region of the vocal process of the arytenoids
c. Treat with speech therapy, proton pump inhibitor (PPI), and removal of source of trauma

vi. Granular cell tumor
a. Yellow lesion on posterior one-third of vocal fold
b. Also found on the tongue, skin, breast, subcutaneous tissues, and respiratory tract
c. Histology shows pseudoepitheliomatous hyperplasia
d. Three percent become malignant
e. Conservative excision

vii. Nodules
a. Develop from vocal trauma
b. Bilateral white lesions often found at the junction of the anterior one-third and posterior two-thirds of the vocal fold
c. Treat with speech therapy

viii. Polyps
a. Associated with vocal trauma and smoking
b. Unilateral, pedunculated lesion commonly found between anterior one-third and posterior two-thirds of the vocal fold
c. Treat with micro DL and excision

ix. Recurrent respiratory papillomatosis (RRP)
a. Onset is usually between 2 and 4 years
b. Self-limited disease
c. Associated with HPVs 6 and 11
d. Papilloma virus resides in the superficial epithelial layer.

e. Two occult sites for RRP
  1. Nasopharynx
  2. Undersurface of the true vocal folds
f. Treatment
  1. Micro DL with stripping and/or CO2 laser ablation
  2. Intralesional injection of cidofovir (5 mg/mL)
g. Avoid jet ventilation, since this can potentially seed lower respiratory airways

x. Reinke edema
  a. Associated with smoking
  b. Accumulation of fluid in superficial layer of lamina propria
  c. Bilateral, edematous changes of vocal fold
  d. Treat with smoking cessation and surgery in severe cases

xi. Sarcoid
  a. Epiglottis is the most common site of involvement.
    1. Pale pink, turban-like epiglottis

xii. Tuberculosis
  a. Most commonly seen in the interarytenoid area and the laryngeal surface of the epiglottis.

C. Malignant lesions
  i. Risk factors
    a. Tobacco and alcohol use
    b. HPVs 16 and 18
    c. GERD
    d. Radiation exposure
  ii. Types
    a. SCCA (> 90%)
    b. Minor salivary gland malignancies
      1. Adenoid cystic carcinoma
      2. Mucoepidermoid carcinoma
    c. Chondrosarcoma—posterior cricoid cartilage
  iii. Fixed cords are usually the result of involvement of the thyroarytenoid muscle
  iv. Staging
    a. Different schemas for supraglottis, glottis, and subglottis.
    b. T1 lesions involve one subsite.
    c. T2 lesions extend to adjacent subsite ± impaired vocal fold mobility.
    d. T3 lesions are all characterized by true vocal fold fixation (supraglottic tumors may be T3 if there is preepiglottic or postcricoid involvement).
    e. T4 lesions have extralaryngeal spread.
    f. Nodal staging is the same as oral cavity and oropharynx.
  v. Treatment
    a. Glottic CIS—serial micro DL and stripping until eradication of the malignancy. Current trends include laser excision after biopsy documentation.
    b. Chondrosarcoma should be narrowly excised without postoperative radiation.
    c. Stage I and II SCCA may be treated with surgery or XRT.
    d. Stage III and IV SCCA may be treated with concomitant chemoradiation (organ preservation) or surgery ± XRT.

     e. Hemilaryngectomy—for unilateral T1 and T2 disease. Tumor can have less than 1-cm subglottic extension and can involve the anterior commissure or anterior aspect of contralateral true fold.

     f. Supraglottic laryngectomy—voice-preserving approach for T1, T2, or T3 (pre-epiglottic space involvement only) supraglottic lesions without anterior commissure involvement, tongue involvement past the circumvallate papillae, or apical involvement of the pyriform sinus. True cords, arytenoid, and thyroid cartilages are preserved. Patients must have good pulmonary status. Try to preserve SLN to prevent postoperative aspiration.

     g. Supracricoid laryngectomy—voice-preserving approach for tumors of the anterior glottis. Preserves cricoid and at least one arytenoid cartilage. Fifty percent of patients remain tracheostomy dependent.

     h. Total laryngectomy—for T3 and T4 tumors with cartilaginous invasion and extralaryngeal/neck involvement.

     i. Neck dissection:

       1. Bilateral selective neck dissection (II-IV) should be performed on clinically normal necks for all supraglottic and advanced (T3-T4) laryngeal tumors.

       2. Extended neck dissections should be performed for confirmed neck disease.

  vi. Tracheoesophageal speech

     a. Prosthesis directs air into pharynx when tracheostoma is occluded

     b. Prosthesis prone to candidal infections

     c. Requires cricopharyngeus myotomy for optimal results

       1. Inadequate cricopharyngeus myotomy can be tested for with Botox.

D. Vocal cord paralysis

  i. Vocal cord position

     a. RLN—*Paramedian*

     b. Vagal—*Lateral/intermediate* and patient will have *hypernasal* speech

  ii. Vocal cord medialization

     a. Permanent paralysis

       1. Medialization laryngoplasty

       2. Injection laryngoplasty with Teflon or autologous collagen/fat, requires injection lateral to vocalis muscle

     b. Temporary paralysis, Gelfoam

E. Other

  i. Airway lengthening techniques:

     a. Mobilization after blunt dissection of the larynx and trachea (3 cm)

     b. Incision of the annular ligaments on one side of the trachea proximal to the anastomosis and on the opposite side distally (1.5 cm)

     c. Laryngeal release

       1. Suprahyoid (5 cm)

       2. Infrahyoid (often results in dysphagia)

  ii. Autoimmune airway obstruction.

  iii. Gutman sign is associated with SLN paralysis. In the normal individual, lateral pressure over the thyroid cartilage causes an increased voice pitch, whereas anterior pressure causes a decrease. In SLN paralysis, the reverse is true.

  iv. Myasthenia gravis—vocal fatigue, which improves with rest. Test with edrophonium (Tensilon test).

     v. Passy-Muir valve aids in swallowing and helps prevent aspiration by increasing subglottic pressure.

     vi. Supraglottitis—Most common bacteria in adults is *S aureus*.

     vii. Venturi jet ventilation:

       a. Used in pediatric endoscopic procedures, excision of laryngeal papillomata, and endolaryngeal laser procedures.

       b. Complications of this technique include hypoventilation, pneumothorax, pneumomediastinum, subcutaneous emphysema, abdominal distention, mucosal dehydration, and distal seeding of malignant cells or papillomavirus particles.

Other Neck Disorders

A. Necrotizing fasciitis

  i. Progressive, rapidly spreading, inflammatory infection located in the deep fascia, with secondary necrosis of the subcutaneous tissues.

  ii. Seen in patients with trauma, recent surgery, or medical compromise (immunocompromised).

  iii. Bacteria:

    a. *S pyogenes* (group A hemolytic streptococci) and *S aureus* are the most common inciting bacteria

    b. Others include:

      1. *Bacteroides*

      2. *Clostridium perfringens* (classic gas-producing organism)

      3. *Peptostreptococcus*

      4. *Enterobacteriaceae*

      5. *Proteus*

      6. *Pseudomonas*

      7. *Klebsiella*

  iv. Clinical examination reveals rapidly spreading, erythematous skin changes with skin discoloration and subcutaneous emphysema.

  v. CT reveals necrosis, fascial thickening, and subcutaneous gas.

  vi. Treatment:

    a. Blood sugar control

    b. Surgical debridement

    c. Broad-spectrum antibiotics with anaerobic and aerobic coverage

    d. Hyperbaric oxygen

B. Paragangliomas

  i. Arise from neuroendocrine cells (paraganglia) of the autonomic nervous system

    a. Carotid paraganglia—located in the adventitia of the posteromedial aspect of the bifurcation of the common carotid artery

    b. Temporal bone paraganglia—accompanying Jacobson nerve (from CN IX) or Arnold nerve (from CN X), or in the adventitia of the jugular bulb

    c. Vagal paraganglia—located within the perineurium of the vagus nerve

  ii. Capable of producing vasoactive substances

    a. Catecholamines, norepinephrine, dopamine, somatostatin, vasoactive intestinal polypeptide (VIP), calcitonin

b. If patient has headache, palpitations, flushing, diarrhea, or HTN
1. Obtain 24-hour urine vanillylmandelic acid (VMA) and serum catecholamine levels
   - If catecholamines are elevated
2. Obtain abdominal CT to rule out pheochromocytoma
   - Treat adrenergic symptoms
iii. May be familial (autosomal dominant)—family members should have screening MRIs every 2 years
iv. Ten percent are multicentric, about 10% malignant, and about 10% hormonally active
v. Radiology
   a. Arteriography is the gold standard.
   b. CT shows postcontrast enhancement and MRI shows mild enhancement on T2 image, intense postcontrast enhancement, and "salt and pepper" appearance secondary to flow voids.
vi. Histology shows
   a. Chief cells (amine precursor and uptake decarboxylase cells) and sustentacular cells (modified Schwann cells) organized in clusters known as Zellballen
vii. Types
   a. Carotid body tumors
      1. Sixty percent of paragangliomas
      2. Slow-growing, painless neck mass that has often been present for years
      3. Mass is often pulsatile and mobile in a horizontal axis
      4. May have hoarseness, vocal cord paralysis, or dysphagia
      5. Arteriography reveals characteristic splaying of the internal and external carotid arteries (*Lyre sign*)
      6. Treatment
         - Surgery ± preoperative embolization
         - In certain situations (recurrent tumor, incomplete resection, and elderly patients), XRT may be used as primary therapy
   b. Glomus jugulare and tympanicum
      1. Tympanicum is the most common tumor of the middle ear.
      2. Female to male ratio of 4:1.
      3. May present with *pulsatile tinnitus*, aural fullness, hearing loss, and cranial neuropathies.
      4. Examination may show vascular middle ear mass, which exhibits Brown sign (blanching of mass with positive pneumatoscopic pressure).
      5. Gold standard of diagnosis is arteriography.
      6. Treatment
         - Surgery ± preoperative embolization
         - XRT
   c. Glomus vagale
      1. Account for 3% of paragangliomas
      2. More common in females
      3. Commonly arise from the nodose ganglion (inferior ganglion of vagus nerve)
      4. Often present with a painless neck mass with tongue weakness, hoarseness, dysphagia, and a Horner syndrome
      5. Radiography reveals vascular lesion that displaces the internal carotid artery anteromedially

6. Gold standard of diagnosis is arteriography
7. Treatment
   - Surgery ± preoperative embolization
   - In certain situations (recurrent tumor, incomplete resection, and elderly patients), stereotactic radiation may be used as primary therapy.

C. Peripheral nerve sheath tumors
   i. Schwannomas
      a. Encapsulated, round tumor derived from Schwann cells
      b. Adherent or partially displacing involved nerve
      c. Histology shows Antoni A and Antoni B tissue
      d. Treatment—surgery (can often preserve nerve function)
   ii. Neurofibroma
      a. More common than schwannomas
      b. Nonencapsulated, fusiform tumor
      c. Intertwined with involved nerve
      d. Associated with von Recklinghausen disease (neurofibromatosis type 1 [NF-1])
      e. Treatment—surgery (often lose nerve function)

Head and Neck Oncology Considerations

A. Cervical metastases from occult primary tumors:
   i. Five percent of cases present with adenopathy
   ii. Squamous is predominant histologic type
   iii. Ninety percent of primaries eventually found with repeated examination, biopsies, and scanning
   iv. Frequent sites of primary
      a. Nasopharynx
      b. Tonsil
      c. Vallecula/base of tongue
      d. Pyriform sinus
      e. Metastatic disease
   v. Panendoscopy and directed biopsies
B. Chyle fistula:
   i. Can result from dissection in the supraclavicular fossa
   ii. Volumes of less than 500 to 700 mL/d can be treated with
      a. Pressure and a low-fat diet.
      b. If using hyperalimentation, medium-chain triglycerides (MCT) can be used as a caloric source.
      c. Octreotide has been shown to help resolve chyle fistulas.
   iii. For volumes greater than 500 to 700 mL/d
      a. Exploration and ligation
C. C-myc—most commonly mutated proto-oncogene in head and neck cancer.
D. p53—most commonly mutated tumor suppressor gene in head and neck cancer.
E. Flaps:
   i. Regional skin and fascial
      a. Deltopectoral—first to fourth perforators from internal mammary artery
      b. Paramedian forehead—supratrochlear artery

    c. Pericranial
      1. Supraorbital and supratrochlear
      2. Provides watertight barrier
    d. Temporoparietal—superficial temporal

ii. Myocutaneous
    a. Latissimus dorsi—thoracodorsal artery
    b. Pectoralis major—thoracoacromial artery and internal mammary artery perforators
    c. Platysma—occipital, postauricular, facial, superior thyroid, and transverse cervical
    d. Sternocleidomastoid—occipital artery (loops around 12th CN) superior thyroid artery, transverse cervical artery
    e. Trapezius—occipital, dorsal scapular, and transverse cervical arteries

iii. Osteomyocutaneous
    a. Pectoralis major with rib (see above)
    b. Sternocleidomastoid with clavicle (see above)
    c. Trapezius with scapular spine (see above)

iv. Free flaps
    a. Fibula
      1. Peroneal artery
      2. Mandibular defects
      3. Evaluate preoperative blood supply with magnetic resonance angiogram (MRA)
    b. Iliac crest
      1. Deep circumflex iliac artery
      2. Mandibular defects
    c. Jejunum
      1. Superior mesenteric arterial arcade
      2. Esophageal defects above thoracic inlet
    d. Lateral arm—posterior radial collateral artery
    e. Lateral thigh
      1. Profunda femoris artery
      2. Hypopharynx and esophageal defects above thoracic inlet
    f. Latissimus dorsi
      1. Thoracodorsal artery
      2. Total glossectomy defect
    g. Radial forearm
      1. Radial artery
      2. Oral cavity defects requiring skin
      3. Tongue defects (anterior two-thirds)
      4. Hypopharynx and esophageal defects above thoracic inlet
    h. Rectus
      1. Deep inferior epigastric artery
      2. Total glossectomy defect
    i. Scapula
      1. Circumflex scapular artery
      2. May harvest with two skin paddles
      3. Oral cavity defects requiring skin ± mandible
      4. Mandibular defects
      5. Hypopharynx and esophageal defects above thoracic inlet

F. HPVs 16 and 18 are associated with head and neck SCCA.
G. Hyperfractionated radiation techniques permit a higher cumulative dose per treatment.
H. Lip carcinoma:
    i. BCCA—often seen on upper lip
    ii. Squamous carcinoma
        a. Often seen on lower lip
        b. Upper lip SCCA metastasizes early
    iii. Oral commissure has worst prognosis
I. Lymph node staging:
    i. N1—less than and equal to 3 cm
    ii. N2a—single ipsilateral lymph node greater than 3 cm, less than and equal to 6 cm
    iii. N2b—multiple ipsilateral nodes, none greater than and equal to 6 cm
    iv. N2c—bilateral or contralateral lymph nodes, none greater than and equal to 6 cm
    v. N3—greater than 6 cm
J. Postlaryngectomy patients have a high likelihood of recurrence when a Delphian node is involved.
K. Postoperative radiation therapy
    i. Advanced stage
    ii. Close or positive margins
    iii. Lymph node involvement
    iv. Extracapsular spread
    v. Perineural invasion
L. Postoperative radiation therapy should be started by 6 weeks after resection even if there is a healing wound.
M. Retinoids appear to reduce the likelihood of developing second primaries in patients with head and neck squamous carcinomas.
N. Syndrome of inappropriate antidiuretic hormone (SIADH)—can result increased intracranial pressure from bilateral neck dissection.

Endocrine

A. Thyroid follicle
    i. Spheroidal, cyst-like compartment with follicular epithelium, colloid center, para-follicular cells, capillaries, connective tissue, and lymphatics
    ii. Principal component of colloid is large iodinated glycoprotein called thyroglobulin
B. Thyroid hormone
    i. Thyroid peroxidase is responsible for iodination of thyroglobulin molecules.
    ii. Iodinated thyroglobulin molecules are coupled to form T3 and T4.
    iii. T3 and T4 are mostly bound to carrier proteins (> 99%).
    iv. T3 is most biologically active.
C. Calcitonin
    i. Produced in thyroid C cells
    ii. Reduces blood calcium levels
    iii. Used as a marker in medullary thyroid cancer

D. Laboratory tests
   i. T3 and T4—used in conjunction with thyroid-stimulating hormone (TSH)
   ii. TSH
      a. Elevated reflects hypothyroidism
      b. Decreased levels should be studied in conjunction with T4 levels
         1. Low TSH and high T4—*hyperthyroidism*
         2. Low TSH and low T4—*secondary hypothyroidism* (possible nonthyroidal illness)
         3. Low TSH and normal T4
            • Order T3
               (a) Normal T3—*subclinical hyperthyroidism*
               (b) High T3—*T3 toxicosis*
   iii. Thyroglobulin—useful marker in thyroid cancer. Values above 10 mg/dL indicate persistent disease
   iv. Calcitonin—useful marker in monitoring medullary thyroid cancer. Not used as a screening test (estimated cost of detecting one case of medullary cancer with calcitonin is $12,500)
   v. Antithyroid peroxidase antibodies—elevated in Hashimoto thyroiditis
   vi. Thyroid-stimulating antibody—elevated in Graves' disease
E. Thyroid nodules
   i. Clinically apparent in 4% to 7% of the population (W > M 5:1).
   ii. Ninety-five percent are either adenomas, colloid nodules, cysts, thyroiditis, or carcinoma.
   iii. Most are benign with carcinoma being detected in 5% of all lesions.
   iv. Findings of concern:
      a. Age less than 20, greater than 60 years
      b. Male
      c. Size greater than 4 cm
      d. History of radiation exposure
      e. Vocal fold fixation
      f. Rapid growth
   v. FNA:
      a. Nodules greater than or equal to 1 cm.
      b. Most accurate tool for selecting patients requiring surgery, has increased the percentage of malignant nodules excised by 60% to 100% and reduced percentage of benign nodules excised by 34% to 70%.
      c. Overall accuracy exceeds 95%.
      d. Four cytopathologic categories:
         1. Malignant
         2. Suspicious (microfollicular, Hürthle cell predominant)
         3. Benign (macrofollicular)
         4. Nondiagnostic
      e. Microfollicular may be follicular adenoma or follicular carcinoma:
         1. Needs surgical biopsy to evaluate for vascular or capsular invasion (carcinoma)
      f. Hürthle cell predominant may represent adenoma or carcinoma:
         1. Needs surgical biopsy.
         2. Hashimoto and multinodular goiter may have Hürthle cells, so FNA of these lesions may result in unnecessary surgery.

    vi. Thyroid scintigraphy:
- a. Utilizes radioisotopes of iodine or Technetium[99]
- b. Less cost-effective and more controversial than FNA
- c. Considered primary test in two scenarios
  1. Low TSH (autonomous nodule)
  2. Suspicion for Hashimoto thyroiditis
- d. Sometimes used after FNA reveals microfollicular pattern to further distinguish between autonomous adenomas and cold lesions, which may represent follicular carcinoma

    vii. Ultrasound (US):
- a. More detail than scintigraphy
- b. Most cost-effective way of screening for thyroid adenoma
- c. Reveals additional nodules in 20% to 48% of patients referred for solitary nodule
- d. Helpful in
  1. Assisting FNA of cystic and nonpalpable nodules
  2. Following cystic nodules after aspiration

F. Adenomas
- i. Monoclonal neoplasms arising from follicular epithelium or Hürthle cells
- ii. May be autonomous
- iii. May be macrofollicular or microfollicular on FNA
  - a. Macrofollicular adenomas are benign
  - b. Microfollicular adenomas that do not exhibit vascular or capsular invasion are considered benign
- iv. Treatment
  - a. Nontoxic
    1. Macrofollicular
       - May be watched
       - Twenty percent or less of patients will have a decrease in nodule size with T4 therapy
    2. Microfollicular
       - Surgical excision to evaluate for capsular or vascular invasion
       - Toxic adenomas
         (a) Beta blockers
         (b) Thionamide therapy (methimazole and propylthiouracil)
            ○ Inhibits thyroperoxidase, blocks T3 and T4 synthesis
            ○ Propylthiouracil blocks the peripheral conversion of T4 to T3, causes liver failure, and is no longer first line
    3. I[131] ameliorates hyperthyroidism and reduces total thyroid volume by 45% in 2 years
    4. Surgery

G. Colloid nodules
- i. Develop within multinodular goiters
- ii. Focus of hyperplasia within the thyroid architecture
- iii. Macrofollicular on FNA and benign
- iv. Treatment
  - a. I[131] (hyperthyroidism)
  - b. Surgery (hyperthyroidism or aerodigestive compromise)
  - c. T4 has been shown to interfere with goitrogenesis and prevent new nodule formation but does not reduce the size of solitary thyroid nodules

H. Cysts
    i. Primarily develop from degenerating adenomas
    ii. Suddenly appearing or painful neck mass may represent a hemorrhagic cyst
    iii. Zero percent to 3% contain malignant cells (often papillary)
    iv. Treatment
        a. Benign cysts may be treated with FNA (25%-50% disappear after aspiration)
        b. Surgery
I. Thyroiditis
    i. Hashimoto thyroiditis
        a. Lymphocytic infiltration, germinal center formation, Hürthle cells, and follicular atrophy
        b. Elevated antithyroid peroxidase antibodies
        c. Thyroid lymphoma usually arises from Hashimoto thyroiditis
        d. Treat resultant hypothyroidism with T4
    ii. Lymphocytic thyroiditis
        a. Painless, postpartum thyroiditis
        b. Hyperthyroidism followed by hypothyroidism
        c. Self-limited
    iii. Riedel struma
        a. Inflammatory process of unknown etiology
        b. Woody goiter fixed to surrounding structures and progressive aerodigestive symptoms
    iv. Subacute granulomatous thyroiditis (SGT)
        a. Most common cause of *painful* thyroid
        b. Viral etiology
        c. Hyperthyroidism followed by hypothyroidism
        d. Self-limited
J. Top causes of hyperthyroidism
    i. Graves' disease
        a. Females 20-40
        b. Immunoglobulins that bind with the TSH receptor
        c. Accumulation of glycosaminoglycans in tissues leading to
            1. Exophthalmos
            2. Dermopathy (pretibial myxedema)
            3. Osteopathy
        d. Treatment
            1. Beta blockers
            2. Thionamides
            3. Radioactive iodine
            4. Subtotal thyroidectomy
    ii. Toxic multinodular goiter
    iii. Autogenous adenoma
    iv. SGT
K. Top causes of hypothyroidism
    i. Hashimoto thyroiditis
    ii. Iatrogenic
    iii. Excessive iodine intake
    iv. SGT

L. Carcinoma
  i. Patients are frequently euthyroid
  ii. Well differentiated
    a. Associated with Gardner syndrome (familial colonic polyposis) and Cowden disease (familial goiter and skin hamartomata)
    b. Cady AMES staging (there is also Hay AGES)
      1. *Age, Metastases, Extent* of primary tumor, size
      2. Low risk
        • Men less than 41 and women less than 51 without distant metastases
        • Men greater than 41 and women greater than 51, with no metastases, tumor confined to the thyroid gland and less than 5 cm in diameter
      3. High risk
        • All patients with distant metastases
        • Men greater than 41 and women greater than 51 with extrathyroidal tumor (or major capsular involvement for follicular) and greater than or equal to 5 cm in diameter
    c. Papillary (80% of thyroid malignancies)
      1. Spontaneous
      2. Cystic
      3. Lymphotropic with high rate of nodal metastasis
      4. Histology—papillae, lack of follicles, *psammoma bodies*, large nuclei, and prominent nucleoli (*Orphan Annie eye*)
    d. Follicular (10% of thyroid malignancies)
      1. Unifocal.
      2. Hematogenous spread with higher rate of distant metastasis.
      3. Hürthle cell carcinoma is a more aggressive subtype of follicular carcinoma.
      4. Differentiated from follicular adenoma by pericapsular vascular invasion.
    e. Treatment
      1. Surgery is primary therapy
        • Ten-year survivals of 98% (papillary) and 92% (follicular)
        • Total thyroidectomy allows physicians to follow postoperative patients with thyroglobulin and I^{131} scans
        • Subtotal thyroidectomy requires postablation with I^{131}
        • Palpable lymph nodes should be excised as part of a level 2-6 neck dissection
      2. T3 may be given during first 2 weeks to minimize symptoms of hypothyroidism
      3. I^{131} imaging (and ablation with 30-50 mCi for subtotal thyroidectomy patients) should be performed 4 to 6 weeks after surgery. Postoperative I^{131} ablation reduces local and regional recurrence and disease-specific mortality in high-risk patients
      4. Following treatment, patients should receive T4 to minimize potential TSH stimulation of tumor growth
      5. Repeat thyroid scintigraphy when thyroglobulin is greater than 5 mg/mL
  iii. Medullary (5% of thyroid malignancies)
    a. Seventy-five percent sporadic
    b. Twenty-five percent familial
      1. Multiple endocrine neoplasia (MEN) 2a (Sipple)—medullary thyroid carcinoma, pheochromocytoma, hyperparathyroidism

      2. MEN 2b—medullary thyroid carcinoma, pheochromocytoma, mucosal neuromas

      3. Familial non-MEN medullary thyroid carcinoma (FMTC)

    c. *RET* proto-oncogene is associated with MEN 2a and 2b.

      1. *REarranged* during transfection.

      2. *RET* is a tyrosine kinase

    d. Arises from parafollicular C cells and secretes calcitonin

    e. Tendency for paratracheal and lateral node involvement

    f. Histology shows sheets of amyloid-rich cells

    g. Main treatment is surgery

      1. Total thyroidectomy with neck dissection for cervical disease

      2. Recommend thyroidectomy at age 6 years in MEN 2a and at 2 years in MEN 2b

    h. T4 therapy should be started after surgery to maintain euthyroidism

    i. Follow with serum calcitonin

  iv. Anaplastic (1%-5% of thyroid malignancies)

    a. Extremely aggressive and uniformly fatal

    b. Twenty percent of patients have history of differentiated thyroid cancer

    c. Ninety percent have regional or distant spread at presentation

    d. Treatment is often palliative with chemoradiation/XRT

      1. Doxorubicin and XRT may increase the local response rate to 80% with subsequent median survival of 1 year (Kim et al, 1987, Cancer)

  v. Lymphoma (1%-5% of thyroid malignancies)

    a. Non-Hodgkin lymphoma

    b. Strong association with Hashimoto thyroiditis

    c. Treatment

      1. XRT for local disease

      2. Chemotherapy for metastatic disease

M. Hyperparathyroidism

  i. Primary

    a. Frequently seen in 30- to 50-year old, postmenopausal women

    b. Usually caused by isolated parathyroid adenoma (85%)

    c. Associated with MEN 1 (Werner) and MEN 2a

    d. Symptoms

      1. Hypercalcemia with elevated 24-hour urine calcium

        • Other causes of hypercalcemia—CHIMPs

          (a) *Cancer*

          (b) *Hyperthyroid*

          (c) *Iatrogenic*

          (d) *Multiple* myeloma

          (e) *Primary* hyperparathyroidism

          (f) Painful bones (arthralgia), kidney stones (nephrolithiasis), abdominal groans (constipation, N/V, pancreatitis), psychic moans (depression), and fatigue overtones

      2. Cardiovascular—HTN and arrhythmias

    e. Localization

      1. Ultrasound—60% to 90% sensitivity for localizing a single adenoma.

      2. Sestamibi scan—uses Technetium[99], initially taken up in thyroid and parathyroids. Over time, sestamibi washes out of thyroid and remains in parathyroids. Scan has 70% to 100% sensitivity.

- Limitations
  - (a) Adenomas less than 5 mm
  - (b) Multigland disease (ie, four-gland hyperplasia)
  - (c) Coexisting thyroid pathology
  - (d) Previous surgery
- f. Treatment
  1. Parathyroidectomy.
  2. Reimplantation may be used in setting of four-gland hyperplasia.
  3. Intraoperative parathyroid hormone (PTH) monitoring may be helpful. Half-life of PTH is 3 to 5 minutes. Decrease in PTH of 50% at 10 minutes indicates likely success.
- g. Hypocalcemia after uneventful removal of solitary parathyroid adenoma may indicate "hungry bone syndrome, caused by adenoma's prior suppression of other parathyroids
- ii. Secondary—results from hypocalcemia secondary to renal disease
- iii. Tertiary—autonomous secretion of PTH following prolonged period of secondary hyperparathyroidism

Esophagus and Trachea

- A. Esophagus
  - i. Upper one-third—skeletal muscle
  - ii. Lower two-thirds—smooth muscle
  - iii. Physiology of swallowing
    - a. Oral phase—bolus preparation
    - b. Pharyngeal phase
      1. Nasopharyngeal closure—constriction of superior constrictor and tensor and levator veli palatini
      2. Breathing stopped and glottis closed
      3. Bolus propulsion—base of tongue elevation and contraction of pharyngeal constrictors
      4. Laryngeal elevation—stylopharyngeus, stylohyoid, and salpingopharyngeus
      5. Epiglottic rotation
      6. Dilation of cleft palate (CP)
    - c. Esophageal phase
  - iv. Benign disease
    - a. Achalasia
      1. Lack of peristalsis
      2. Failure of esophageal sphincter (LES) relaxation
      3. Caused by degeneration of Auerbach plexus
      4. "Birds beak" esophagus on esophagram
      5. Treatment
        - Medical
          - (a) Calcium channel blockers
          - (b) Botox of the LES
        - Surgical
          - (a) Dilation
          - (b) Heller myotomy—gold standard

    b. LES myotomy and partial fundoplication
    c. GERD
       1. Most common esophageal disorder in the US
       2. Results from LES relaxation and abnormalities in esophageal peristalsis
       3. May lead to Barrett esophagitis
       4. Classic symptoms
         • Heartburn
         • Regurgitation
       5. Atypical symptoms
         • Laryngospasm
         • Cough
         • Hoarseness
         • Globus
         • Wheezing
       6. Diagnosis
         • History
         • Response to over-the-counter (OTC) antacids or trial PPI is the presently considered gold standard
         • Esophageal manometry—normal in 40% of people with GERD
         • pH monitoring—greater than 90% sensitivity and specificity
       7. Treatment
         • Behavioral—weight loss, smoking cessation, dietary modification (abstain from fatty foods, spicy foods, chocolate, caffeine, dairy-rich products, nuts, and eating close to bedtime), elevate head of bed
         • Medical
           (a) H_2 blockers
           (b) PPIs
              ◦ Irreversibly block the hydrogen/potassium adenosine-5'-triphosphate (ATP) enzyme system (gastric proton pump) of the parietal cell
         • Surgery—Nissen fundoplication
    d. Leiomyoma—most common benign tumor of the esophagus
    e. Polymyositis—see Connective Tissue Disorders section
    f. Scleroderma—see Connective Tissue Disorders section
    g. Zenker diverticulum
       1. Occurs in posterior wall of Killian triangle
       2. Symptoms
         • Dysphagia
         • Regurgitation of undigested food
         • Bad breath
       3. Diagnosis—esophagram
       4. Treatment—surgery
         • Transcervical approach
         • Endoscopic stapling of cricopharyngeal bar
    h. Webs
       1. Dysphagia develops slowly.
       2. Commonly develop on anterior wall.
       3. Associated with Plummer-Vinson syndrome.
         • Esophageal web
         • Iron deficiency anemia

- Hypothyroidism
- Gastritis
- Cheilitis
- Glossitis

v. Malignant lesions
- a. Barrett esophagitis
  1. Metaplasia of esophageal mucosa
     - Squamous epithelium ⇒ columnar epithelium
       (a) May progress to carcinoma in 10% to 15% of cases
       (b) Treatment—PPI ± fundoplication
- b. Esophageal carcinoma
  1. Associations
     - Barrett esophagitis
     - Alcohol
     - Tobacco
     - Achalasia
     - Oculopharyngeal syndrome
     - Caustic burns
     - Plummer-Vinson syndrome
     - Pernicious anemia
  2. Male:female—5:1
  3. Symptoms
     - Dysphagia is the most common symptom
     - Odynophagia
     - Weight loss
     - Hoarseness
  4. Cancers arising in upper third are SCCA
  5. Cancers arising in lower two-thirds are usually adenocarcinoma
  6. Treatment
     - Esophagectomy (transhiatal vs transthoracic)
     - No benefits have been seen with neoadjuvant or adjuvant chemoradiation/XRT

B. Trachea
- i. Bacterial tracheitis—see Pediatric section
- ii. Differential diagnosis of hemoptysis
  - a. Acute
    1. Pneumonia
       - Primary
       - Secondary
    2. Tumor
    3. Foreign body
    4. Aspiration
    5. Pulmonary infarct
    6. Acute bronchitis
    7. Infection—bronchitis, abscess, tuberculosis
    8. Iatrogenic—tracheotomy, intubation, bronchoscopy, needle biopsy
    9. Cancer
  - b. Chronic
    1. Tuberculosis
    2. Bronchial carcinoma

    c. Recurrent
      1. Chronic bronchitis
      2. Neoplasm
      3. Bronchiectasis
      4. Cystic fibrosis
      5. Pulmonary HTN
      6. Osler-Weber-Rendu syndrome
      7. Arteriovenous fistula
    d. Cardiovascular disease
      1. Mitral valve disease
      2. Left ventricular failure
      3. Pulmonary embolus
    e. Investigations
      1. Chest x-ray (CXR) film
      2. Endoscopy with or without laser coagulation
      3. Cytology
      4. Culture and sensitivity tests
      5. Occasional bronchogram, angiogram, lung scan
iii. Stenosis
    a. Congenital, extrinsic, idiopathic, or posttraumatic
    b. Commonly seen in patients requiring ventilatory support
      1. Overinflated balloon cuffs (> 25 mm Hg) result in mucosal ischemia and loss, inflammation, and scarring
      2. May result in
        • Granulation tissue at cuff or tracheostomy site
        • Circumferential scars at level of cuff and cricoid cartilage
    c. Treatment
      1. Antireflux measures
      2. Incision (laser or cold) and dilation, ± mitomycin C application
      3. Cricotracheal resection (CTR)
iv. Neoplasms
    a. Benign
      1. Chondroma—see Laryngology section
      2. Hemangioma—see Pediatrics section
      3. Papilloma—see Laryngology section
    b. Malignant
      1. SCCA
      2. Adenoid cystic carcinoma

Pediatrics

A. Audiometry
  i. Less than 6 months—ABR, DPOAE, *behavior observation audiometry* (warble tones)
  ii. 6 months to 3 years—ABR, DPOAE, *visual response audiometry* (child localizes to a object, ie, Teddy bear)
  iii. 3-6 years—conventional *play audiometry* (child performs an activity each time sound is heard)
  iv. Greater than 6 years—standard audiometry

B. Adenotonsillar disease
  i. Tonsillitis
    a. Common pathogens
      1. *S pyogenes* (most important treatable pathogen)
      2. *Streptococcus viridans*
      3. *S aureus*
      4. *H influenzae*
    b. Adult tonsils show mixed infections, and three-fourths of patients have beta-lactamase-producing organisms
    c. Classic finding in *S pyogenes* infection is a tonsillar exudate
    d. EBV (mononucleosis) causes abundant exudates
    e. Complications
      1. Peritonsillar abscess with potential spread to the deep neck spaces
    f. Treatment
      1. Keflex ± Flagyl
      2. Augmentin (if mononucleosis has been ruled out)
      3. Clindamycin
  ii. Indications for adenoidectomy and tonsillectomy
    a. 6-7 episodes of acute tonsillitis in 1 year, five episodes per year for 2 years, three episodes per year for 3 years (tonsillectomy)
    b. Peritonsillar abscess (tonsillectomy)
    c. Chronic tonsillitis (tonsillectomy)
    d. OSA (adenotonsillectomy)
    e. Adenotonsillar hypertrophy with dysphagia, speech abnormalities, and occlusive abnormalities (adenotonsillectomy)
  iii. Studies suggest that adenoidectomy, regardless of adenoidal size, is helpful in children with chronic OM with effusion requiring multiple sets of tubes
C. Caustic ingestion
  i. Bases cause most esophageal injuries (60%-80%)
    a. Sodium, potassium, and ammonium hydroxide
    b. *Liquefactive necrosis* with full-thickness burns
  ii. Acids are less harmful than bases
    a. Bleach, lysol.
    b. *Coagulative necrosis*
    c. Coagulum limits penetration of acid and prevents full-thickness burns
  iii. Diagnosis
    a. Evaluate chin, lips, tongue, and palate for evidence of burns
      1. Severity of oral cavity burns do not correlate with esophageal symptoms but can help in diagnosis
    b. CXR to rule out free air
    c. Esophagoscopy within the first 24 to 48 hours
      1. Do not advance esophagoscope past ulcers or circumferential burns
    d. Children presenting after 48 hours should have esophagram
  iv. Treatment
    a. Steroids
    b. Antibiotics
    c. Varying opinions exist regarding the placement of a nasogastric (NG) tube at the time of esophagoscopy
    d. Strictures can often be treated with esophageal dilation

D. Ciliary dysmotility
   i. Numerous forms
   ii. Clinical tests of ciliary function using methylene blue and saccharin
   iii. Electron microscope study of cilia biopsy in glutaraldehyde
   iv. Kartagener syndrome
      a. Lacks dynein side arms on A-tubules
      b. Triad of recurrent sinusitis, bronchiectasis, and situs inversus
E. Cleft lip (CL) and cleft palate (CP)
   i. Syndromic versus nonsyndromic
   ii. Multifactorial inheritance and etiology
   iii. Consider syndromic until proven otherwise
   iv. Risk factors for CL/CP
      a. Single gene transmission
         1. Highest risk is seen when one child and one parent has cleft (18%)
      b. Chromosome aberrations
      c. Teratogens—alcohol, thalidomide, vitamin A
      d. Environmental—amniotic band syndrome, maternal diabetes
   v. CL anatomical relationships
      a. Nasal ala on the affected side is displaced inferolaterally
      b. Caudal septum displaced to contralateral side
   vi. CP anatomical relationships
      a. Levator veli palatini, which normally forms a sling across the palate, is oriented parallel to the cleft
      b. Tensor veli palatini runs in a more anterior-posterior direction resulting in ETD and the need for tympanostomy tubes
   vii. When to repair CL (rule of 10s)—10 weeks, 10 lb, hemoglobin of 10; Millard rotation advancement flap
   viii. When to repair CP—10-18 months (when deciduous molars arrive). Cleft palate flaps are designed to reconstruct muscular sling and are based on the descending palatine, which is located in the greater palatine foramen
      a. Lengthening—V to Y and Furlow Z-plasty
      b. Posterior flaps—pharyngeal flap and sphincter pharyngoplasty
F. Congenital otologic abnormalities—see Otology section
G. Cystic fibrosis
   i. AR disease (CFTR gene) of children and young adults
   ii. Generalized dysfunction of exocrine glands
   iii. Features
      a. Pancreatic insufficiency
      b. Chronic obstructive pulmonary disease (COPD)/bronchiectasis/pneumonia
      c. Malabsorption
      d. Cirrhosis of the liver
      e. Nasal polyps/chronic sinusitis
      f. High sweat chloride/salt wasting
      g. Dehydration
   iv. Diagnosis—sweat chloride values greater than 60 mEq/L
   v. Aggressive management of polyps and sinusitis with steroids, regular sinus irrigations with tobramycin, and endoscopic sinus surgery
   vi. Children who undergo polypectomy alone will experience a 90% recurrence

H. Down syndrome
    i. Frequent upper respiratory infections (URIs)
    ii. Frequent OM secondary to ETD
    iii. Abnormal nasopharynx shape
    iv. Poor tone of tensor veli palatini
I. Enlarged vestibular aqueduct (EVA)
    i. Most common inner ear abnormality in children with congenital hearing loss
    ii. Associated with Mondini malformation, Pendred syndrome, and branchio-otore-nal syndrome.
    iii. Upper limit of normal is less than or equal to 1.5 mm at the midpoint of the aqueduct
    iv. Progressive SNHL (or mixed hearing loss) that may worsen in a stepwise fashion
    v. Hearing loss may worsen after minor trauma—avoid contact sports.
    vi. Treatment
        a. HAs
        b. Cochlear implantation
J. Esophageal atresia and tracheoesophageal fistula (TEF)
    i. Associated with VACTERL
        a. *V*ertebral
        b. *A*nal
        c. *C*ardiac
        d. *T*racheo*E*sophageal
        e. *R*enal
        f. *L*imb abnormalities
    i. Also associated with VATER syndrome
    ii. Types
        a. Esophageal atresia with distal TEF—most common (85%)
        b. Esophageal atresia without TEF—second most common (7%)
        c. TEF without atresia
        d. Esophageal atresia with proximal and distal TEF
        e. Esophageal atresia with proximal TEF
K. Foreign bodies
    i. Children less than 6 years of age do not possess molars to grind nuts and raw vegetables
    ii. A foreign body should be ruled out if a child has unilateral wheezing
    iii. Tracheal/bronchial
        a. Stridor/wheezing
        b. Cough without associated illness
        c. Recurrent or migratory pneumonia
        d. Acute aphonia
    iv. Esophageal
        a. Odynophagia
        b. Drooling
        c. Vomiting/spitting
        d. Airway compromise due to impingement of posterior trachea
    v. Radiograph
        a. CXR
            1. Visualize foreign body
            2. Evaluate for atelectasis on the side affected
            3. Overinflation due to air trapping

b. Lateral decubitus
1. Evaluates for mediastinal shift
2. Uninvolved side down results in shift of mediastinum down secondary to gravity
3. Involved side down results in no shift due to air trapping
vi. Anesthesia
a. Deep inhalational
b. Allows patient to spontaneously ventilate
c. Neuromuscular paralysis
1. Must determine whether patient can ventilate if paralyzed
2. This will prevent laryngospasm (also consider topical lidocaine on vocal cords)
3. Prevents patient movement during retrieval
vii. Five levels at which a foreign body is likely to lodge in the esophagus
a. Cricopharyngeus muscle
b. Thoracic inlet
c. Level of aortic arch
d. Tracheal bifurcation
e. Gastroesophageal junction
viii. Ingestion of disc battery
a. Contains lithium, NaOH, KOH, mercury
b. One hour—mucosal damage
c. 2-4 hours—damage to muscular layer
d. 8-12 hours—potential perforation
e. If battery passed into stomach, demonstrated by x-ray
1. Send home and monitor stool for battery
2. Repeat x-ray if not passed in 4 to 7 days
3. With larger batteries (23 mm), repeat x-ray in 48 hours following observation of battery in stomach
4. If still in stomach, remove endoscopically
L. Hereditary hearing loss
i. Less than 1% of children are born with hearing loss
ii. Greater than 90% of deaf children have normal hearing parents
iii. Diagnosis is usually delayed until approximately 2.5 years of age
iv. Seventy percent are nonsyndromic
a. Eighty percent are recessive transmission (DFNB)
1. Most common cause is abnormalities of the connexin 26 (or GJB2) gene
2. Commonly have "cookie bite" audiogram
b. Twenty percent dominant transmission (DFNA)
c. Less than 2% X-linked or mitochondrial transmission
v. 15% to 30% are syndromic
a. Autosomal recessive "JUP"
1. *Jerville-Lange-Nielsen*—SNHL, prolonged QT with syncopal events and sudden death
2. *Usher*—SNHL, retinitis pigmentosa ± vestibular symptoms. Most common syndrome to affect the eyes and ears. Diagnosed with electroretinogram
3. *Pendred*—SNHL, euthyroid goiter. Patients have abnormal perchlorate uptake test (reduced thyroid radioactivity over time). Associated with Mondini malformation and EVA

    b. Autosomal dominant
      1. Achondroplasia—most common skeletal dysplasia. Disorder of endochondral bone formation. Associated abnormalities include a narrow foramen magnum with potential for brain stem compression, hydrocephalus, spinal canal stenosis, respiratory infections, apnea, otitis, and CHL
      2. Branchio-otorenal syndrome—branchial apparatus abnormalities (clefts, cysts, or fistulas), preauricular pits, hearing loss (SNHL, CHL, or mixed), and renal malformations
      3. Crouzon syndrome—CHL, craniosynostosis, maxillary hypoplasia, ocular hypertelorism with exophthalmos, mandibular prognathism
      4. NF-2—bilateral acoustic neuromas. Candidates for auditory brain stem implants
      5. Stickler—SNHL or mixed, flattened facial appearance with Pierre Robin sequence, myopia
      6. Treacher–Collins syndrome (mandibulofacial dysostosis)—CHL, SNHL, or mixed, midface hypoplasia, micrognathia, malformed ears, lower lid coloboma, downward slanting eyes
      7. Waardenburg syndrome—SNHL, vestibular abnormalities, dystopia canthorum, pigmentary changes of the eyes, skin, and hair (ie, white forelock)
    c. X-linked
      1. Alport (may also rarely be recessive)—SNHL, renal failure with hematuria, and ocular abnormalities

M. Infant hearing loss is associated with certain high-risk groups who should have early ABR or OAE testing.
    i. Bacterial meningitis, especially *H influenzae* Type B (HIB) (Although streptococci are the most common cause of childhood meningitis, a greater percentage of those children with *H influenzae* develop hearing loss)
    ii. Congenital perinatal infections (TORCH)
      a. *Toxoplasmosis*
      b. *Other* (ie, syphilis)
      c. *Rubella*—"Cookie bite" audiogram, cataracts, cardiac malformations
      d. *Cytomegalovirus*
      e. *Herpes*
    iii. Family history of congenital hearing loss
    iv. Concomitant head and neck anomalies
    v. Birth weight less than 1500 g
    vi. Hyperbilirubinemia
    vii. Initial Apgar score less than 4 at birth, no spontaneous respirations at birth, or prolonged hypotonia persisting to 2 hours of age
    viii. Prolonged neonatal intensive care unit (NICU) stay (5%-10% of post-NICU infants have some degree of measurable hearing loss)

N. Nasal anomalies
    i. Midline nasal masses
    a. Dermoid
      1. Ectodermal and mesodermal tissues (hair follicles, sweat glands, sebaceous glands, etc)
      2. Commonly on the lower third of nasal bridge ± overlying tuft of hair
      3. CT scan may reveal skull base defect and intracranial involvement via foramen cecum
      4. External surgical excision

    b. Glioma

      1. Males:females—3:1

      2. Glial cells in a connective tissue matrix with or without a fibrous connection to the dura via fonticulus frontalis

      3. No fluid-filled space connected to the subarachnoid space

      4. Firm and noncompressible

      5. Intranasal gliomas most often arise from the lateral wall and are more often associated with dural attachment (35%)

      6. External excision unless dural connection

    c. Encephalocele

      1. Herniation of meninges ± brain through fonticulus frontalis

      2. Connected to subarachnoid space (contains CSF)

      3. Nasofrontal, nasoethmoid, naso-orbital, or skull base

      4. Soft, compressible intranasal lesions (may be confused for polyps)

      5. *Positive Furstenberg sign*: mass expands with crying

      6. CT and MRI to evaluate for skull base defect and neural tissue

      7. Intracranial then extracranial excision

  ii. Choanal atresia

    a. Neonates are obligate nasal breathers until approximately 6 weeks of age

    b. Failure to pass a 5 or 6 Fr catheter at least 3 cm into the nasal cavity

    c. "FURB"

      1. *Female predominance.*

      2. *Unilateral atresia is more common and presents later in childhood.* Initial approaches are usually transnasally, although transpalatal approaches have less recurrence

      3. Two-thirds are unilateral, more commonly on the *R*ight side

      4. Ten percent of atresia plates are mucosal only, while 90% have a *B*ony and/or cartilaginous component

    d. Fifty percent are associated with congenital anomaly

      1. CHARGE association

        • *C*oloboma

        • *H*eart defects

        • Choanal *A*tresia

        • *R*etarded growth

        • *G*enital hypoplasia

        • *E*ar abnormality

      2. Apert syndrome

      3. Crouzon disease

      4. Treacher-Collins syndrome

      5. Trisomy 18 syndrome

      6. Velocardiofacial syndrome

    e. Bilateral atresia presents at birth with cyclical apnea and crying, and urgently requires an oral airway and surgical correction before hospital discharge

    f. CT scan with bone cuts to evaluate for bony component

O. Neck masses

  i. Congenital

    a. Branchial cleft abnormalities

      1. May exist as either cysts, sinuses, or fistulae

      2. Often present after URI

3. In general, abnormality passes deep to the structures of its branchial arch but superficial to the contents of the next highest branchial arch
4. First branchial cleft cyst
   - Type I is an ectodermal duplication anomaly of the EAC
   - Type II passes through parotid gland, below the angle of the mandible and open in the anterior neck above the level of the hyoid bone. Relation to FN is variable (may pass medial to or bifurcate around nerve)
   - Surgical excision
1. Second branchial cyst
   - *Most common* type (90%)
   - *Pathway*: anterior border of SCM ⇒ deep to platysma, stylohyoid, and posterior digastric ⇒ superficial to CN IX and XII ⇒ between external and internal carotid artery ⇒ tonsillar fossa
2. Third branchial cyst
   - *Pathway*: anterior border of SCM ⇒ deep to CN IX ⇒ deep to internal carotid artery ⇒ penetrates thyrohyoid membrane (superior to SLN) ⇒ pyriform sinus
   b. Dermoid cyst
   1. Midline mass composed of mesoderm and ectoderm (hair follicles, sebaceous glands, and sweat glands)
   2. Frequently misdiagnosed as thyroglossal duct cysts
   3. Do not elevate with tongue protrusion
   c. Laryngocele
   1. Enlargement of the laryngeal saccule
   2. Internal causes distention of false vocal cord and aryepiglottic fold
   3. External presents as compressible, lateral neck masses that penetrate the thyrohyoid membrane
   d. Plunging ranula
   1. May pierce the mylohyoid and present as a paramedian or lateral neck mass
   2. Fluid with high levels of protein and salivary amylase
   3. Excision in continuity with the sublingual gland of origin
   e. Sternocleidomastoid tumor of infancy
   1. Similar presentation as torticollis (chin pointed toward opposite side)
   2. May result from hematoma during delivery
   3. Physical therapy
   f. Teratoma
   1. Midline neck mass composed of all three germ cell layers
   2. Often larger than dermoids and may result in aerodigestive compromise
   g. Thyroglossal duct cyst
   1. Most common midline mass
   2. Results from failure of involution of thyroglossal duct
   3. Asymptomatic midline mass at or below the hyoid bone that elevates with tongue protrusion
   4. Confirm normal thyroid tissue with US prior to surgical excision with Sistrunk procedure
   h. Vascular lesions—see vascular lesions in this section
ii. Inflammatory
   a. Viral—most common cause of pediatric lymphadenitis
   1. Rhinovirus, adenovirus, and enterovirus

2. EBV—patients may develop pink, measles-like rash if given amoxicillin
b. Bacterial
   1. Most common bacterial cause of cervical adenitis is *S aureus* and group A streptococci.
   2. Parapharyngeal and retropharyngeal spaces are the most common neck spaces to be involved in pediatric neck abscesses.
   3. Lemierre syndrome—septic thrombophlebitis of the internal jugular vein resulting in spiking fevers and neck fullness.
   4. FNA if mass persists past 4 to 6 weeks
   5. Cat scratch disease:
      • Most common cause of chronic cervical adenopathy in children
      • History of contact with cats
      • *Bartonella henselae*
      • Warthin-Starry stain shows small pleomorphic gram-negative rods
   6. Tuberculosis
      • "Scrofula"
      • Single large cervical lymph node
      • Skin may turn violaceous color
      • Purified protein derivative (PPD) is usually reactive
      • Isoniazid, ethambutol, streptomycin, and rifampin
   7. Atypical mycobacteria
      • Rarely exhibit fever or systemic symptoms
      • CXR is usually normal, and PPD reactions are normal or only intermediate in reactivity
      • Notoriously resistant to traditional antituberculous agents
      • Chronic draining sinuses often develop
c. Noninfectious
   1. Rosai-Dorfman disease—self-limited, nontender cervical lymphadenopathy
   2. Kawasaki disease
      • Cervical lymphadenopathy
      • Erythema of lips and tongue ("Strawberry tongue")
      • Erythema and peeling of hands and feet
      • Rash
      • Treat with aspirin and gamma-globulin to prevent coronary artery aneurysms

P. Neoplasms
   i. Juvenile nasopharyngeal angiofibroma (JNA)
      a. Occurs in young boys
      b. Originates near sphenopalatine foramen
      c. Highly vascular tumor that results in nasal obstruction and epistaxis
      d. CT classically shows Holman-Miller sign (anterior bowing of posterior maxillary sinus wall)
      e. Treatment
         1. Preoperative angioembolization
         2. Surgical resection ± XRT
   ii. Lymphoma
      a. Most common pediatric malignancy
      b. FNA (under sedation if necessary) with appropriate staining techniques to determine the cell of origin

     c. Posteroanterior (PA) and lateral chest films
     d. Intravenous pyelogram (IVP)
     e. Bone marrow aspirate, and scans as indicated
     f. Overall mortality 30%
     g. Stages
        1. 1—localized
        2. 2—limited above diaphragm with systemic symptoms
        3. 3—diffuse disease
  iii. Rhabdomyosarcoma
     a. Most common soft tissue malignancy of the head and neck in children
     b. Sites of involvement
        1. Orbit
        2. Neck
        3. Face
        4. Temporal bone
        5. Tongue
        6. Palate
        7. Larynx
     c. Often presents before age 10
     d. Rapid growth
     e. Usually embryonal subtype
     f. Orbital tumors are unique in that they tend toward locally aggressive behavior, but metastasize rarely (the converse is true of other sites)
     g. Chemotherapy and radiation are the main modalities of treatment after biopsy-proven diagnosis
        1. Intergroup Rhabdomyosarcoma Study I reported increased survival (81% vs 51%) in patients with nonorbital, parameningeal disease who were treated with chemoradiation/XRT
     h. Surgery is reserved for unresponsive lesions and residual disease following chemoradiation
     i. 3-year survivals up to 80%
Q. Ophthalmology
  i. Causes of unilateral proptosis in decreasing order of occurrence: infection ⇒ pseudotumor ⇒ dermoid ⇒ hemangioma/lymphangioma ⇒ rhabdomyosarcoma ⇒ leukemia ⇒ neurofibroma ⇒ optic nerve glioma ⇒ metastasis ⇒ paranasal tumor
R. Pharyngitis—see Oral Cavity, Oropharynx, and Nasopharynx section
S. Stridor
  i. Inspiratory—supraglottis and glottis
  ii. Biphasic—subglottis
  iii. Expiratory—trachea
  iv. Breakdown
     a. Laryngeal, 60%
        1. Laryngomalacia, 60%
        2. Subglottic stenosis, 20%
        3. Vocal cord palsy, 13%
        4. Others, 7%
     b. Tracheal, 15%
        1. Tracheomalacia, 45%
        2. Vascular compression (most commonly aberrant subclavian artery), 45%

           3. Stenosis, 5%

    c. Bronchial, 5%

    d. Infection, 5%

       1. Croup
- Parainfluenzae virus
- "Barking" cough

       2. Epiglottitis
- Historically with HIB
- HIB vaccine has significantly decreased incidence

       3. Bacterial tracheitis
- *S aureus*
- Obstructive tracheal casts
- Intubation, pulmonary toilet, suctioning, and possible bronchoscopy

    e. Miscellaneous, 15%

  v. Laryngomalacia

    a. Most common cause of stridor in children

    b. Most common congenital laryngeal abnormality

    c. Often seen in association with other findings resulting from delay in development of neuromuscular control (ie, gastroesophageal reflux, central or obstructive apnea, hypotonia, failure to thrive, and pneumonia)

    d. Self-limited

  vi. Subglottic stenosis

    a. Third most common congenital laryngeal abnormality

    b. Newborn infants have a subglottic lumen that averages 6 mm in diameter; 5 mm is regarded as borderline normal, and 4 mm is stenotic

    c. Formula for pediatric endotracheal (ET) tube selection—(age in years + 16)/4

    d. In an emergency, choose the ET tube closest to the size of the patient's pinky finger

    e. High association of subglottic stenosis in Down syndrome patients.

    f. Myer-Cotton grading

       1. Grade I—0%-50% obstruction

       2. Grade II—51%-70% obstruction

       3. Grade III—71%-99% obstruction

       4. Grade IV—complete obstruction

    g. Treatment

       1. Grade I and mild Grade II may be observed or treated with incision/dilation

       2. Grade III and IV will require trach and open repair with
- Anterior cricoid split (neonates)
- Laryngotracheal reconstruction (LTR)
- Cricotracheal resection

  vii. Tracheal rings are associated with pulmonary slings in 30% of cases.

  viii. Vocal cord paralysis

    a. Second most common congenital laryngeal abnormality

    b. Most commonly idiopathic

    c. Most common congenital CNS abnormality—Arnold-Chiari malformation

    d. The best treatment for unilateral pediatric vocal cord paralysis is speech therapy

T. Vascular lesions

  i. Hemangiomas

    a. Lesion is small at birth and has a 6- to 12-month proliferative phase

    b. Strawberry or bruised appearance

    c. Most common benign pediatric parotid tumor

    d. Suspect visceral involvement in patients with three or more cutaneous lesions

    e. Suspect glottic or subglottic involvement in neonates with progressive stridor and cutaneous hemangiomas of the face

       1. Occurs more commonly in the left posterolateral quadrant

    f. PHACE syndrome

       1. *P*osterior fossa malformations

       2. *H*emangiomas (usually of the face)

       3. *A*rterial abnormalities

       4. *C*oarctation of the aorta

       5. *E*ye abnormalities

    g. Spontaneous involution occurs over 2- to 10-year period at a rate of 10% per year (ie, 50% by 5 years, 70% by 7 years, etc)

    h. Treatment

       1. Observation

       2. Medical/surgical therapy

         • Often reserved for symptomatic infants

         • Steroids

           (a) Prednisone (2 mg/kg/d) for 4 to 6 weeks

           (b) Intralesional injection for periorbital, nasal, or lip lesions

              ◦ Periorbital injections can result in blindness

         • Laser

           (a) CO_2 laser (10,600 nm) and pulsed dye laser (585 nm) are currently favored for:

              ◦ Debulking symptomatic mucosal lesions (ie, subglottic)

              ◦ Hemangiomas with ulceration

         • Excision

           (a) Early lesions—to avoid systemic medical therapy and social trauma

           (b) Stable lesions following involution

  ii. Vascular malformations

    a. Arteriovenous malformations (AVMs)

       1. Usually present at birth and grows with patient

       2. Eventually develop pulsations secondary to arterial blood flow

       3. Differentiated from hemangioma or capillary malformation by MRI/A or US

       4. Eventually may lead to heart failure

       5. Surgical excision is the gold standard, but selective arterial embolization may be used as an adjunct or for palliation

    b. Capillary malformations

       1. "Port wine stain"

       2. Present at birth and distribution remains constant (grows with patient)

       3. Syndromes

         • Sturge-Weber

       4. Capillary malformation of V_1 distribution with calcification and loss of meninges and cortex

       5. Results in glaucoma and seizures

         • Osler-Weber-Rendu

1. Hereditary hemorrhagic telangiectasia
2. Capillary malformations of skin, mucous membranes, brain, liver, and lungs
3. Commonly have severe and recurrent epistaxis
   - Venous malformations
     (a) Usually not detected at birth
     (b) Lesion enlarges in dependent position and has a blue hue
     (c) Treatment
        ○ Compression
        ○ Sclerotherapy—alcohol-based agents frequently used for craniofacial lesions
        ○ Surgery—usually performed after sclerotherapy
  iii. Lymphatic malformations (cystic hygroma)
   a. Usually present at birth and primarily involve the head and neck.
   b. Lesions are progressive
   c. MRI is gold standard for radiologic evaluation
   d. Macrocystic and microcystic lesions
   e. Treatment
      1. Surgical excision—gold standard but has high recurrence rate.
      2. Sclerotherapy—OK-432 (*Streptococcus* that has been killed by penicillin).
      3. CO_2 laser used for glottic involvement.
      4. Diffuse disease may require tracheostomy and gastrostomy tube.
U. Velopharyngeal dysfunction
   i. Intelligibility of speech is affected more by articulation rather than resonance
   ii. "M," "n," and "ng" are normal nasal consonants, and their production is associated with an open velopharyngeal port
   iii. The hypernasal child nasalizes nonnasal phonemes /d/, /b/, /t/
   iv. Diagnosis
      a. Endoscopic evaluation of Passavant ridge
      b. Videofluoroscopy
   v. Treatment
      a. Speech therapy directed toward articulation and increasing resonance
      b. Prosthetics
         1. Indicated in children whose gap is large because of little to no motion of the velopharyngeal sphincter
      c. Palatal lift—not indicated in a child with a short palate
      d. Surgery
         1. Pharyngeal flap
            - Success depends on lateral wall motion
            - Caution must be taken to create ports less than 20 mm2 to prevent continued nasal escape; ports that are of insufficient size may result in chronic nasopharyngitis, anterior rhinorrhea, and otitis
         2. Posterior wall augmentation
            - Increase anteroposterior (AP) projection of the posterior pharyngeal wall to contact velum
            - Injectables (ie, Gelfoam, Teflon, collagen)
         3. Sphincter pharyngoplasty
            - Designed to create a dynamic pharyngeal sphincter using posterior tonsillar pillar flaps

V. Other
   i. Pediatric blood volume (mL) is approximately 7.5% of body weight (g).
   ii. Tube obstruction is the most common complication in infant tracheotomy.
   iii. Purulent rhinorrhea is the most common presenting sign for sinusitis in children.
   iv. Consider immunologic deficiency in children with chronic sinusitis.
   v. Facial trauma in children most commonly results in dental injuries.
   vi. Facial paralysis:
      a. Approximately 90% of congenital facial paralysis resolves spontaneously.
      b. Frequently caused by traumatic delivery (cephalopelvic disproportion, dystocia, high forceps delivery, intrauterine trauma).
      c. If no resolution after a period of observation, ENOG can be used to determine excitability.
      d. CT and MRI may be required for adequate evaluation.
   vii. Reflux may cause endolaryngeal granulation tissue.

Facial Plastics

A. General
   i. Dermis made of Type I and III collagen
   ii. Best measure of nutritional status—albumin
   iii. Relaxed skin tension lines (RSTLs) are perpendicular to underlying muscles
   iv. Skin grafts survive for first 48 hours by plasmatic imbibition
B. Aging
   i. Sun exposure is the most significant factor in premature aging
   ii. Decrease in overall collagen and decrease in the ratio of Type I to Type III
C. Injectables
   i. Botox
      a. Binds to cholinergic nerve terminals
      b. Translocated into the neuronal cytosol
      c. Conformational change in presence of low pH
      d. Cleaves SNARE protein, which prevents Ach vesicle docking, fusion, and subsequent release
D. Skin resurfacing
   i. General
      a. Endpoint is determined by punctate bleeding and shammy cloth appearance of the papillary dermis
      b. Accutane causes sebaceous gland atrophy and must be discontinued 6 months prior to dermabrasion or laser resurfacing
      c. Treat resurfacing patients with antiviral prophylaxis
   ii. Chemical peels
      a. Indications—fine rhytids and solar damage
      b. Agents
         1. Glycolic acid
            • Penetration is time dependent
            • Mildest results, but least complications
         2. Trichloroacetic acid
            • Intermediate-to-deep peel
            • 10% to 25%—intraepidermal

- 30% to 40%—papillary dermis
- 45% to 50%—reticular dermis
3. Phenol (with croton oil)—keratolysis and keratocoagulation
  c. Precautions
    1. Pigmented areas may lose pigmentation temporarily or permanently
    2. Peel regions rich in adnexal structures
    3. Peels for pigmentation must be superficial
  d. Complications
    1. Hypopigmentation
    2. Irregular hyperpigmentation
    3. Perioral scarring
    4. Prominent skin pores
    5. Phenol toxicity—headache, nausea, HTN, hyperreflexia, CNS depression, and *cardiotoxicity* (arrhythmias); prevents with aggressive hydration
iii. Dermabrasion
  a. Surgical procedure requires dermabrader and carries infectious transmission risk.
  b. Complications
    1. Transient postinflammatory hyperpigmentation
    2. Hypopigmentation
    3. Milia
iv. Laser
  a. Types
    1. CO_2 (10,600 nm)
    2. Erbium:YAG (2940 nm)
  b. Following laser resurfacing, bio-occlusive dressings provide a pathway of proper moisture and humidity, decreasing epithelial closure time by up to 50%
  c. Complications
    1. Transient postinflammatory hyperpigmentation
    2. Long-term hypopigmentation
    3. Infection (bacterial, viral, fungal)
v. Healing timetable
  a. 5 days—epidermis regenerates
  b. 7 days—epidermis loosely attached to dermis
  c. 2 weeks—new collagen deposited, fills out dermis, giving youthful appearance
  d. 1 month—pigmentation returns, milia possible, and requires opening
  e. 6 months—epidermis normal thickness
  f. 10 months—dermis normalizes
E. Brow lift
  i. Consider brow position before performing blepharoplasty
    a. Endoscopic and coronal approaches result in posterior displacement of hair line
    b. Pretrichial or direct do not change position of hair line
    c. Direct brow lift is most useful in patients with unilateral facial paralysis
  ii. Ideal brow position
    a. Woman—arc above the orbital rim with its apex above the lateral limbus
    b. Male—rest on superior orbital rim
  iii. Endoscopic brow lift
    a. Plane of dissection is subperosteal in the forehead and supraperiosteal over temporalis muscle

   b. Temporal branch of FN is lateral to plane of dissection. The sentinel vein indicates its location
   c. Corrugator and procerus muscles are often partially resected at the time of surgery
F. Blepharoplasty
   i. Goals—treat dermatochalasis (redundant and lax eyelid skin and muscle)
   ii. Anatomy
      a. The thickness of the eyelid skin is on average 1/100 in.
      b. Levator aponeurosis inserts into the orbicularis and dermis to form the upper eyelid crease
         1. This is usually 10 mm from the lid margin in Caucasians and absent in the Asian eyelid
      c. See Anatomy section
   iii. Preoperative assessment
      a. Ophthalmologic history.
      b. Schirmer test (> 10 mm in 5 minutes is normal).
      c. Snap test of lower lid. If abnormal (> 1 second), consider lower lid-pexy to prevent ectropion.
      d. Evaluate for negative vector. If present, consider fat repositioning of lower lid fat to prevent hollowed-out appearance.
   iv. Medical contraindications
      a. Hypothyroid myxedema
      b. Allergic dermatitis
      c. Dry eye syndrome
   v. Technique
      a. Upper lid
         1. Preserves 1 cm of skin
            • Inferior to lid crease
            • Between brow and superior incision
         2. Some orbicularis oculi muscle should be removed to enhance lid crease (preserve some of the palpebral portion of the muscle)
         3. Avoid overresection of fat to prevent hollowed-out appearance
      b. Lower lid
         1. Skin flap—allows for skin and fat excision
         2. Skin-muscle flap—allows for skin, muscle, and fat excision; higher risk for ectropion
         3. Transconjunctival—addresses fat herniation rather than skin and muscle laxity, decreased risk of ectropion
   vi. Complications
      a. Upper lid—lagophthalmos (overresection of soft tissue), ptosis (injury to levator muscle)
      b. Lower lid—ectropion, inferior oblique injury
      c. Pain, proptosis, and ecchymosis suggest hematoma
G. Rhinoplasty
   i. Anatomy
      a. Nasion—nasofrontal suture
      b. Rhinion—junction of nasal bones and upper lateral cartilages
      c. Supratip break—transition between cartilaginous dorsum and apex of lower lateral cartilages (ideal is 6 mm)

    d. Tip—apex of lower lateral cartilages

    e. Infratip break (double break)—junction between medial lower lateral crura and intermediate lower lateral crura

    f. Subnasale—nasal base

    g. Pogonion—most anterior portion of chin

    h. Menton—most inferior point of chin

    i. External valve—opening of the nostrils

    j. Internal valve—nasal septum, caudal margin of upper lateral cartilage, inferior turbinate, and floor of nose

    k. Procerus muscle—horizontal glabellar wrinkles

    l. Corrugator supercilii—vertical glabellar wrinkles

ii. Considerations

    a. Retrognathic chin may make nose appear overprojected

        1. Chin should align with vertical line dropped from nasion through Frankfort horizontal line (line between highest point of EAC and lowest portion of orbital rim)

    b. Dorsal hump may make chin appear underprojected

    c. Nasal length should be two-thirds of the midfacial height (glabella to subnasale)

    d. Nasal projection should be 50% to 60% of nasal length (3 cm-4 cm-5 cm right triangle) or the same as the width of the alar base

    e. 50% to 60% of nasal projection should be anterior to upper lip

    f. Base of nose should equal intercanthal distance

    g. Nasofrontal angle—115-130 degree

    h. Nasolabial angle—90-115 degree

    i. 2 to 4 mm of columella should be visible on profile

iii. Approaches

    a. Endonasal—marginal and intercartilaginous incisions to deliver lateral crura

        1. Technically difficult

        2. Faster healing

        3. Ideal for minimal tip work (ie, cephalic trim)

    b. Open—marginal and transcolumellar incisions

        1. Ideal approach for tip work

        2. May result in decreased tip projection (requires placement of caudal strut)

        3. Longer healing times

iv. Techniques

    a. Underprojected tip

        1. Caudal strut and alar advancement

        2. Cartilage grafts and tip suturing

    b. Underrotated tip

        1. Caudal strut

        2. Tongue and groove technique

        3. Lateral crural overlay

        4. Tip suturing

    c. Bulbous tip

        1. Tip suturing

        2. Cephalic trim

    d. Blunted nasolabial angle

        1. Trimming of posterior septal angle

        2. Removal of soft tissue

e. Compromised internal valve/narrow middle third of nasal dorsum, spreader or butterfly grafts

f. Dorsal hump
1. Resection of cartilaginous and bony dorsum
2. Osteotomies are often required to address open-roof deformity

g. Wide nasal base
1. Weir excisions

v. Complications
a. Alar notching may result from overresection of lower lateral cartilages.
b. Epistaxis.
c. Inverted V—collapse of upper lateral cartilages.
d. Open-roof deformity—inadequate osteotomies (usually lateral osteotomies) following resection of dorsal hump.
e. Pollybeak deformity—excessive bony dorsum resection with underresection of cartilaginous septum, loss of tip projection, or scar formation at supratip.
f. Rocker deformity—medial osteotomy, which results in fracture of frontal bone cephalad to radix.
g. Saddle nose deformity—overresection of dorsum.

H. Rhytidectomy
i. Goals
a. Reduce jowling
b. Decrease laxity of skin and platysma
c. Submental lipectomy

ii. Ideal candidate
a. Nonsmoker
b. Good skin tone
c. Strong facial bones and chin
d. Sharp cervicomental angle (high and posterior hyoid bone)

iii. Anatomy
a. Superficial musculoaponeurotic system (SMAS)
1. Continuous with temporoparietal fascia, lower orbicularis oculi, zygomaticus muscle, dermis of upper lip and platysma
2. Overlies parotid fascia posteriorly and masseteric fascia anteriorly

b. Facial nerve
1. Temporal branch
• Within temporoparietal fascia
• Can be found between 0.8 and 3.5 cm anterior to the EAC
• Most commonly injured nerve in rhytidectomy
2. Zygomatic and buccal
• Lay deep to the SMAS
• Buccal branch may be commonly injured during rhytidectomy as well, but is often not appreciated on examination
• Greater auricular nerve—most injured nerve during rhytidectomy

iv. Types
a. Subcutaneous
b. Sub-SMAS
1. Better long-term results than subcutaneous
2. Higher risk to FNs

    c. Composite
1. Attempts to address malar region and melolabial crease
2. Includes orbicularis oculi muscle in flap
3. Investing fascia of zygomaticus major is released
4. Higher risk to FNs than sub-SMAS technique
5. Most common area for skin loss is in postauricular region
6. Most common complication is hematoma (1%-8%)

I. Microtia—see Otology section

J. Otoplasty
    i. Most common abnormality is conchal protrusion. Treat with conchal setback with sutures (Furnas procedure)
    ii. Lack of antihelical fold. Treat with Mustardé technique—creation of antihelical fold
    iii. Perform around 6 years of age
    iv. Telephone ear can result from overresection of conchal cartilage
    v. Auriculomastoid angle—30 degree
    vi. Distance from helical rim to skull is 1 to 2 cm

K. Lip reconstruction
    i. Wedge excision with primary closure, defects up to 30% of lip length
    ii. Abbe-Estlander
      a. Defects between 30% and 60% of lip length
      b. Flap has a width of 50% of the defect
    iii. Karapandzic
      a. Total lip reconstruction
      b. Preserves neurovascular bundles
      c. Results in microstomia

L. Cleft lip and cleft palate—see Pediatrics section

M. Scar management
    i. Good time for revision is 1 year
    ii. Skin elasticity is greatest during infancy (children are more likely to form hypertrophic scars)
    iii. Keloids are more common in patients with Fitzpatrick Type III skin and above
    iv. Keloids have high recurrence rate (45%-100%) following excision
    v. Scar is Type I collagen
    vi. Tensile strength of scar at 4 weeks is 30% of original
    vii. Maximum tensile strength of a scar is 80% of original
    viii. Peak collagen production occurs at 1 week and lasts for 2 to 3 weeks
    ix. Massage
    x. Silicone sheeting/gel—unknown mechanism (hydration)
    xi. Steroids
      a. Kenalog 10 mg/mL for routine hypertrophic scars
      b. Kenalog 40 mg/mL for keloids
    xii. Dermabrasion
    xiii. Surgery
      a. Simple excision
        1. Used for shorts scars (< 2 cm) and those that fall in RSTLs
        2. Maintain 3:1 ratio to avoid standing cutaneous deformity
      b. Geometric broken line—helps camouflage long scars opposed to RSTLs
      c. Z-plasty

1. Lengthen and reorient scar
   - 30 degree $\Rightarrow$ lengthens 25% $\Rightarrow$ rotates 45 degree
   - 45 degree $\Rightarrow$ lengthens 50% $\Rightarrow$ rotates 60 degree
   - 60 degree $\Rightarrow$ lengthens 75% $\Rightarrow$ rotates 90 degree

N. Local flaps
   - i. Types
     - a. Advancement
       1. Single—cheek, forehead
       2. Bipedicle—cheek forehead
       3. V to Y—medial cheek, anterior ala, upper lip near alar base
     - b. Pivot
       1. Rotation—cheek, neck, scalp
       2. Transposition
          - Bilobe
       1. Double transposition of 45 degree (total 90 degree)
       2. One-centimeter defects of nasal tip
       3. Interpolated
          - Paramedian forehead
       4. Nasal tip, dorsum, or sidewall
       5. Based on supratrochlear vessels, which are 1.7 to 2.2 cm lateral to midline
          - Melolabial cheek—ala
          - Hinged

O. Hair replacement
   - i. Hair loss is mediated by dihydrotestosterone (DHT). (testosterone is converted to this by 5 alpha reductase)
   - ii. Medications
     - a. Minoxidil—has vasodilatory effects
     - b. Finasteride
       1. Inhibits 5 alpha reductase
       2. Also beneficial for benign prostatic hyperplasia (BPH) (Proscar)
       3. Surgery
          - Micrografts—one to two hairs
          - Minigrafts—three to six hairs
          - Follicular grafts—hair in its natural grouping of one to four hairs surrounded by adventitial sheath
       4. Takes 10-16 weeks for hair to start growing
       5. Consider pattern of hair loss and expected future loss when implanting
       6. Best transposition flap to restore frontal hair line—Juri flap

P. Lasers
   - i. Work by selective thermolysis
   - ii. Hair removal
     - a. Ruby (694 nm)
     - b. Alexandrite (755 nm)
     - c. Diode laser (800 nm)
     - d. Nd:YAG laser (1064 nm)
   - iii. Tattoo—Ruby (694 nm)
   - iv. Skin resurfacing
     - a. Erbium:YAG (2940 nm)
     - b. CO_2 (10,600 nm)

        v. Vascular lesions

          a. Potassium titanyl phosphate (KTP) (532 nm)

          b. Pulsed dye laser (585 nm)

      vi. Cutting bone

          a. Ho:YAG (2070 nm)

          b. Erbium:YAG (2940 nm)

Trauma

A. Temporal bone fracture

   i. Management

      a. First priority is airway/head injury/c-spine management.

      b. Symptoms include FN injury, hearing loss, vertigo, CSF otorrhea, TM perforation, hemotympanum, canal laceration.

   ii. Fracture patterns

      a. In 1926, Ulrich categorized as longitudinal versus transverse (most common system)

      b. Most are oblique and/or mixed

      c. May be otic capsule sparing versus otic capsule involving

   iii. Longitudinal fractures (pars squamosa to posterosuperior bony EAC to roof of middle ear anterior to labyrinth to close proximity to foramen lacerum or foramen ovale

      a. Most common type (70%-90%), hemotympanum, EAC lacerations

      b. May result in FN injury (20%) and ossicular discontinuity (CHL)

         1. The most common cause of a persistent CHL associated with temporal bone fractures is incudostapedial joint dislocation

   iv. Transverse fractures (foramen lacerum across petrous pyramid to foramen magnum)

      a. Less common (10%-30%)

      b. Frequently results in FN injury and may result in severe SNHL ± vertigo if otic capsule is destroyed

   v. FN injury occurs more often (as a percentage) with transverse fractures, but is seen more commonly with longitudinal fractures because these occur more frequently

   vi. The most common cause of posttraumatic vertigo is concussive injury to the membranous labyrinth

   vii. CSF leaks have 20% association with temporal bone fractures (usually temporary and resolve without surgery)

B. Orbital floor fractures

   i. Indication for surgical repair of orbital floor blowout fractures

      a. Rapid onset of intraorbital bleeding and decreased visual acuity

      b. Diplopia lasting more than 7 days

      c. Entrapment

      d. Enophthalmos greater than 2 mm or involvement of one-third to one-half of the orbital floor

   ii. The most common error in orbital floor reconstruction is failure to repair the posterior orbital floor

      iii. Ideal time for surgical repair is 10 to 14 days (only urgent is entrapment with oculocardiac reflex activation)

      iv. After repair is completed, forced duction test must be performed

      v. Inappropriate repair may result in enophthalmos and hypo-ophthalmos

C. Nasal

      i. 40% to 45% of all facial fractures

      ii. Evaluate for external defects, septal deviation, septal hematoma, epistaxis, and CSF rhinorrhea

      iii. Untreated septal hematoma may result in saddle nose deformity

      iv. Closed reduction should be ideally performed within hours of the accident or maybe delayed from 5 to 10 days

D. Naso-orbital-ethmoid (NOE) fractures

      i. Orbital swelling and telecanthus

      ii. Often results in skull base fracture with CSF leak

      iii. Types

         a. Type I—single, noncomminuted fragment of bone without medial canthal tendon disruption

         b. Type II—comminution of bone, but medial canthal tendon is still attached to segment of bone

         c. Type III—comminution of bone with disruption of medial canthal tendon

      iv. Goal of surgery is to accurately reconstruct the nasal root, into which the medial canthal tendon inserts.

         a. Normal intercanthal distance is 3 to 3.5 cm

         b. Medial canthal tendons may need to be reapproximated with wire

E. Maxillary fractures

      i. LeFort fractures (midface separation with mobile palate, may have different types for each half of the face)

         a. Type I—palate separated from midface. Involves the pterygoid plates

         b. Type II—involves pterygoid plates, frontonasal maxillary buttress, and skull base. Often results in CSF leak

         c. Type III—involves pterygoid plates, frontonasal maxillary buttress, and frontozygomatic buttress. Results in craniofacial separation

      ii. Occlusion (Angle classification)

         a. Class I—normal. First maxillary molar has four cusps (mesiobuccal, mesiolingual, distobuccal, and distolingual). Mesiobuccal cusp of the first maxillary molar fits in mesiobuccal groove of first mandibular molar

         b. Class II—retrognathic (mesiobuccal cusp of first maxillary molar is in between first mandibular molar and the second premolar)

         c. Class III—prognathic

F. Mandibular trauma

      i. Second most commonly fractured bone in facial trauma

      ii. Condyle, angle, and body are most common fracture locations

      iii. Bilateral fractures occur 50% of the time (ie, parasymphysial and contralateral subcondylar)

      iv. Compressive forces occur along the inferior rim and areas of tension develop along the superior rim

         a. When a fracture occurs, forces tend to distract superiorly and compress inferiorly

            1. Unfavorable fractures—displaced and distracted by pterygoid and masseter muscles

        2. Favorable fractures—reduced and aligned by pterygoid and masseter muscles

    v. Determines preinjury occlusion

    vi. Open fractures requires prophylactic antibiotics

        a. Mandibular osteomyelitis after fracture is associated with a fracture through a tooth root.

    vii. Ideal time for surgical repair is immediately following injury

    viii. Treatment

        a. Maxillomandibular fixation (MMF)

           1. Reestablishes preinjury occlusion

           2. Classically used for uncomplicated subcondylar fractures and fractures with gross comminution or soft tissue loss

           3. Contraindications closed reduction with MMF include

              • Multiple comminuted fractures

              • Elderly patients

              • Severe pulmonary disease

              • Children

              • Mentally handicapped/seizures

              • Alcoholic

              • Pregnant

        b. Open reduction internal fixation

           1. Rapid and dependable bony union with limited morbidity and complication rates

           2. Placement of plates to overcome distracting forces and take advantage of compressive forces

           3. Properly positioned miniplates can take advantage of dynamic compressive forces

              • Champy defined areas for fixation of miniplates along the ideal osteosynthesis lines

G. Laryngeal

    i. Primary objective is securing airway

    ii. Evaluate with fiberoptic examination and CT

H. Cervical injuries

    i. Zones

        a. Zone 1—sternal notch to cricoid cartilage

        b. Zone 2—cricoid cartilage to angle of mandible

        c. Zone 3—angle of mandible to skull base

    ii. There has been a trend away from mandatory exploration of all penetrating neck wounds; Immediate surgery always prudent for immediately life-threatening injuries

        a. Angiography and esophagram are often used to obtain further information in nonimmediately emergent cases

    iii. Angiography is usually the first-line treatment for Zones 1 and 3

    iv. For Zone 2, Surgical exploration (angiography is generally not needed) is frequently the first-line treatment especially with any of the following symptoms:

        a. Subcutaneous emphysema

        b. Hemoptysis

        c. Hematemesis

        d. Hematoma

        e. Significant bleeding

        f. Dysphagia

        g. Dysphonia

        h. Neurologic injury

I. Contrast studies of the aortic arch are necessary following cardiomediastinal injuries that result in the following:

    i. Widened mediastinum

    ii. Pulse rate deficit

    iii. Supraclavicular hematoma

    iv. Brachial plexus injury

    v. Cervical bruit

J. Cardiac tamponade symptoms include the following:

    i. Low cardiac output manifests as low blood pressure and increased heart rate

    ii. Muffled cardiac sounds

    iii. Increased central venous pressure

    iv. Decreased amplitude on electrocardiography (ECG)

    v. Diagnosis/treatment by pericardiocentesis

K. Air embolism

    i. Associated with head and neck trauma or venous perforation during routine head and neck procedures

    ii. "To-and-fro" murmur and decreased cardiac output can be seen with ultrasound (echocardiogram)

    iii. Place patient in Trendelenburg (head down) and left lateral decubitus position (this traps air in the ventricle and prevents ejection into pulmonary system)

    iv. Cardiac puncture may be required for aspiration of air (also possible with a Swan-Ganz catheter)

Connective Tissue Disorders

A. Characterized histologically by connective tissue and blood vessel inflammation

B. Common head and neck manifestations include skin rash, mucosal lesions, xerostomia, CN neuropathy, and hearing loss

C. Dermatomyositis and polymyositis

    i. Idiopathic inflammatory myopathies characterized by symmetric proximal muscle weakness

    ii. Difficulties phonating, dysphagia, aspiration, nasal regurgitation, and DM rashes

        a. Affects upper one-third of esophagus (striated)

        b. *Heliotrope rash*: reddish-violaceous eruption on the upper eyelids with accompanying eyelid swelling

    iii. Elevated plasma muscle enzymes (alanine aminotransferase [ALT], aspartate aminotransferase [AST], creatinkinase [CK], CK-MB, lactate dehydrogenase [LDH])

D. Relapsing polychondritis

    i. Recurring inflammation of cartilaginous structures

    ii. Ninety percent of patients develop auricular chondritis and nonerosive inflammatory polyarthritis

    iii. Chondritis develops rapidly and resolves in 1 to 2 weeks

    iv. Recurrent episodes produce cartilaginous deformity

        a. Airway collapse may lead to death

      v. The sedimentation rate is elevated

     vi.   Steroids are used in severe cases

  E. Rheumatoid arthritis

      i. Affects specific juvenile population and people in their 40s to 60s

     ii. Morning stiffness and subcutaneous rheumatoid nodules

    iii. Articular involvement

       a. Cricoarytenoid joints

         1. Best treatment for arytenoids involvement is steroids and NSAIDs

       b. Middle ear ossicles

       c. TMJ

       d. Cervical spine

     iv. Rheumatoid factor (RF) and anticitrullinated protein/peptide antibodies (ACPA) blood tests may aid in diagnosis

  F. Scleroderma

      i. Heterogeneous group of disorders characterized by thickened, sclerotic/fibrotic lesions

     ii. Eighty percent of people have esophageal dysmotility

       a. Affects lower two-thirds (smooth muscle) of esophagus and is usually the initial complaint

       b. Associated with decreased lower LES pressure

    iii. Thirty-five percent develop facial tightness

     iv. Twenty-five percent report sicca symptoms

     v. Associated with CREST

       a. *Calcinosis*

       b. *Raynaud phenomenon*

       c. *Esophageal dysfunction*

       d. *Sclerodactyly*

       e. *Telangiectasia*

  G. Sjögren disease

      i. Second most common connective tissue disease after RA

     ii. Peak incidence 40 to 60 years of age

    iii. Females to males (9:1)

     iv. Keratoconjunctivitis sicca and xerostomia (the sicca complex)

     v. Extraglandular symptoms may be seen in addition to primary exocrine gland pathology (ie, bronchiectasis)

     vi. Primary disease

       a. Not associated with connective tissue disorder

       b. Positive SS-A, SS-B, antinuclear antibodies (ANA), and erythrocyte sedimentation rate (ESR)

    vii. Secondary disease

       a. Associated with connective tissue disorders (rheumatoid arthritis, lupus erythematosus)

       b. Positive SS-A, ANA, and ESR

   viii. Patients with primary Sjögren disease have a risk for non-Hodgkin lymphoma

       a. Three percent of patients developed lymphoma during 9 years of observation.

     ix. Abnormal minor salivary gland biopsy (gold standard)

       a. Biopsy reveals lymphocytic and histiocytic infiltrate with glandular atrophy

       b. Myoepithelial cells are present in biopsy specimens of Sjögren syndrome but not in lymphoma (may be done of lip, sputum, palate)

      x. Must be distinguished from sicca-like syndromes, which have xerostomia and/or xerophthalmia, negative tests, and normal biopsy

         a. Aging

         b. Medications (diuretics, anticholinergics, antihistamines, antidepressants)

         c. Other diseases (hepatitis, autoimmune disorders)

         d. Chronic dehydration

      xi. Medications

         a. Pilocarpine (Salagen)—cholinergic agonist for post-XRT and Sjögren

         b. Cevimeline (Evoxac)—cholinergic agonist for Sjögren

H. SLE

    i. Malar and discoid rash, oral ulcerations, ulcers/perforation of nasal septum, inflammatory changes of larynx, dysphagia, sicca complex, and CN III, IV, V, VI, VII, and VIII neuropathy

    ii. ANA test—highly sensitive

    iii. Anti-dsDNA and anti-Sm antibodies—highly specific

I. Wegener granulomatosis

    i. Classic triad of respiratory granulomas, vasculitis, and glomerulonephritis

    ii. Ninety percent have head and neck symptoms at presentation

       a. Nasal obstruction and discharge

       b. Mucosal ulcerations

       c. Epistaxis

       d. Saddle nose deformity

       e. Sinusitis

       f. Gingival hyperplasia

       g. Otologic disease (serous OM) occur 20% to 25%

       h. Laryngeal edema and ulceration

       i. Subglottic stenosis

    iii. Laboratory findings include elevated ESR, C-reactive protein, and c-ANCA (cytoplasmic antineutrophil cytoplasmic antibody)

       a. C-ANCA (65%-90% sensitive). Wegener is usually associated with diffuse antibodies to cytoplasmic antigens within neutrophils (c-ANCA) against PR3 (serine proteinase 3 antigen); other autoimmune vasculitides have perinuclear antibodies to cytoplasmic antigens within neutrophils (p-ANCA) against myeloperoxidase (MPO)

       b. Nasal carriage of *Staphylococcus* is likely inciting agent. All patients should be on mupirocin nasal irrigations or bactrim prophylaxis

    iv. Biopsy confirms diagnosis

       a. Angiocentric, epithelial-type necrotizing granulomas with the presence of giant cells and histiocytes

    v. Treatment

       a. Steroids and cyclophosphamide.

       b. Mild cases can be treated with trimethoprim/sulfamethoxazole (TMP/SMX) and methotrexate instead of cyclophosphamide; plasma exchange also has been used for severe renal diseases

Other

A. Airway obstruction patients may develop

    i. Apnea after tracheotomy because respiration is driven by hypoxia in these patients. Resolution of hypoxia results in CO_2 narcosis.

    ii. Postobstructive pulmonary edema after tracheostomy or tonsillectomy due to the sudden elimination of high intraluminal pressures. Positive end-expiratory pressure (PEEP) can prevent and treat this accumulation.

B. Anesthetic agents

    i. Lidocaine

       a. Maximum dose

         1. 4.5 mg/kg for plain

         2. Seven mg/kg with epinephrine

       b. One percent lidocaine = 1 g per 100 mL or 10 mg per cc. Ten cc of 1% lidocaine contains 100 mg

    ii. Cocaine (many lawsuits settled solely due to association of cocaine use and poor cardiac outcome during case)

       a. Maximum dose

         1. 200-300 mg

       b. Forty percent are absorbed from cotton pledgets

       c. Four cc of 4% cocaine contains 160 mg

       d. Blocks uptake of epinephrine and norepinephrine

    iii. Amides have two i's in their names (ie, lidocaine)

    iv. Esters such as cocaine frequently cause more allergies

C. Invasive Aspergillosis

    i. *Aspergillus fumigatus*

    ii. Clinical features

       a. Unilateral painless proptosis

       b. Laryngeal involvement

       c. Bone erosion

    iii. Associated with immunosuppression or malignancy (prefers alkaline blood)

    iv. Biopsy shows 45 degree, branching, septate hyphae when grown on Sabouraud agar

    v. Treatment—reversal of immunosuppression and surgical removal

    vi. Causes cavitary lesions after immune function returns which can cause life-threatening hemoptysis or hemorrhage

D. Coccidiomycosis

    i. *Coccidioides immitis*

    ii. San Joaquin Valley fever

    iii. Involvement of skin, mucous membranes, thyroid, eyes, trachea, salivary glands, severe erosions of epiglottis

    iv. Diagnosis

       a. Skin test

       b. Complement fixation

       c. CXR—"coin lesions"

    v. Treatment—amphotericin B

E. Cryptococcosis

    i. *Cryptococcus neoformans*

    ii. Predisposing factors—immunosuppression, lymphoma

    iii. Membranous nasopharyngitis, meningitis, hearing loss

    iv. Diagnosis—fluorescent antibody test

    v. Treatment—amphotericin B

F. Exogenous corticosteroids

    i. The body produces 20 mg of cortisol per day, which is equivalent to 5 mg of prednisone, 4 mg of methylprednisolone, or 0.75 mg of Decadron

G. Fibro-osseous lesions
    i. Unrelated group of lesions sharing the same histologic features as their common denominator (benign cellular fibrous tissue containing variable amounts of mineralized material)
    ii. Diagnosis is often impossible by microscopy alone and requires clinical and radiographic information
    iii. Types
        a. Osseous dysplasia cementoma
            1. Asymptomatic, reactive lesion
            2. Occurs predominantly in African American women over age 20
            3. Most common location is anterior mandibular periapical alveolar bone
            4. X-ray findings
                • Early lesion periapical lucency or multiple lucencies resembling periapical granuloma or cyst, but tooth is always vital
        b. Fibrous dysplasia
            1. Develops in first to second decade of life
            2. Diffuse, painless bony swelling with facial deformity
            3. Does not cross midline
            4. Radiologic findings
                • Ground glass, multilocular, radiolucent, or irregularly mottled opaque and lucent
                • Fusiform tapered expansion
                • Diffuse margins
                • Involves and incorporates lamina dura and cortical bone
            5. Types
                • Monostotic—only one bone affected (75%)
                • Polyostotic
            6. More than one bone affected (20%)
                • Associated with Albright syndrome (5%) (precocious puberty and café au lait spots)
                • Juvenile aggressive—rapidly growing, markedly deforming lesion of maxilla that destroys tooth buds and is refractory to treatment.
        c. Ossifying fibroma (cementifying fibroma)
            1. Benign, locally aggressive neoplasm
            2. The most common site in adults is the mandible
            3. Causes painless bulge in cortical bone
            4. Radiologic findings
                • Well-demarcated lucency
                • Causes divergence of tooth roots
            5. Treatment—conservative curettage
H. Headache
    i. Intracranial pathology
        a. Traction headache
            1. Space-occupying lesion
                • Papilledema
                • Early morning headache
                • Nausea and vomiting
        b. Vascular
            1. Widespread vasodilation of cerebral vessels

   2. Aneurysm
   3. Subarachnoid hemorrhage
  c. Inflammatory
   1. Meningitis
   2. Cerebritis/encephalitis
 ii. Tension Headache
 iii. Vascular Headache
  a. Distention of scalp arteries
  b. Triggered by menses, alcohol, stress
 iv. Cluster headache
  a. Older age
  b. Bouts of episodes
  c. Hyperlacrimation, rhinorrhea
  d. Hemicranial
  e. Treatment
   1. Abortive therapy
    • Triptans (sumatriptan, zolmitriptan)
    • Ergotamine
   2. Preventive
    • Beta blockers
    • Calcium channel blockers
 v. Migraine headache
  a. Family history
  b. Vasoconstriction followed by vasodilation
  c. Aura (sensory, motor, behavioral)
  d. Hemicranial
  e. Epiphenomena (photophobia, diarrhea)
  f. Treatment
   1. Abortive therapy
    • Triptans (sumatriptan, zolmitriptan)
    • Ergotamine
   2. Preventive
    • Beta blockers
    • Calcium channel blockers
 vi. Inflammatory (sinusitis, dental) headache
 vii. Ocular headache
  a. Oculomotor imbalance
  b. Increased intraocular pressure
 viii. Tic douloureux
  a. Excruciating paroxysms of lancinating pain lasting seconds
  b. Usually V_2 and V_3
  c. Treatment
   1. Tegretol
   2. Dilantin
   3. Percutaneous radio frequency destruction
   4. Alcohol injection
 ix. TMJ dysfunction
I. Hemangiopericytoma
 i. Often involves masseter muscle

  ii. Facial mass with calcifications anterior to parotid

  iii. Histology shows Zimmerman cells

 J. Histiocytosis X (Langerhans cell histiocytosis)

  i. Family of granulomatous diseases of unknown etiology, manifest by a proliferation of mature histiocytes

  ii. Histology—Birbeck granules (tennis racket-shaped structures) found in Langerhans cells

  iii. Types

   a. Eosinophilic granuloma

    1. Children and adults

    2. Chronic course with osteolytic bone lesions (often frontal or temporal)

    3. Proptosis is seen with frontal or sphenoid involvement

    4. Acute mastoiditis, middle ear granulations, and TM perforations are common

    5. Facial paralysis is possible

    6. Surgical excision/debridement is the recommended treatment for single lesions

    7. Chemotherapy and radiotherapy have been used for recurrences and inaccessible lesions

   b. Hand-Schüller-Christian disease

    1. Children and younger adults.

    2. Subacute course with lytic skull lesions.

    3. Associated with proptosis, diabetes insipidus, and pituitary insufficiency secondary to erosion of the sphenoid roof into the sella (this constellation occurs in about 10%)

    4. Mastoid and middle ear lesions are common and can cause ossicular erosion, acute mastoiditis, and facial paralysis

    5. EAC polyps

    6. Mandibular involvement with loss of teeth

    7. Chemotherapy and/or radiotherapy are recommended

   c. Letterer-Siwe disease

    1. Infants less than 2 years of age.

    2. Acute, rapidly progressive diseases characterized by fever, proptosis, splenomegaly, hepatomegaly, adenopathy, multiple bony lesions, anemia, thrombocytopenia, and exfoliative dermatitis

    3. Chemotherapy is the treatment of choice, but the response is poor. Radiotherapy can be used for localized or unresponsive lesions

 K. Lupus anticoagulant

  i. Actually it is a procoagulant.

  ii. No special preoperative workup is required other than assuring the patient has sequential compression devices (SCDs) or subcutaneous heparin

 L. Malignant hyperthermia

  i. Associated with halogenated inhalational anesthetic agents and depolarizing muscle relaxants

  ii. Sudden increase in the calcium concentration in the muscle sarcoplasm due to either decreased uptake or excessive release of calcium from the sarcoplasmic reticulum

       iii. Hyperkalemia

       iv. Treat with dantrolene, cooling, and supplemental oxygen

M. Necrotizing sialometaplasia

       i. Benign, self-healing, inflammatory process of salivary gland tissue

       ii. Most commonly seen in nasal cavity, parotid gland, sublingual gland, palate, retromolar trigone, lip, and tongue

       iii. Histology shows lobular necrosis and pseudoepitheliomatous hyperplasia

       iv. *Treatment*: observation with expectant recovery in 6 to 12 weeks

N. Osteomas

       i. Benign, slow growing, osteogenic

       ii. Usually affect the bones of the face and skull

       iii. Usually painless, but may cause pain, headache, or facial pressure

       iv. Sites of predilection

          a. Mandible

          b. Temporal bone

          c. Frontal sinus

          d. Ethmoid sinus

          e. Maxillary sinus

          f. Sphenoid sinus

       v. Treat with surgical excision

       vi. Associated with Gardner syndrome

          a. Autosomal dominant

          b. Osteomata, soft tissue tumors, and colon polyps

             1. Polyps have 40% rate of malignant degeneration.

O. Osteosarcoma

       i. Malignant osteoid-producing tumor of bone

       ii. Twenty percent of all bone malignancies

          a. Seven percent occur in jaws, mandible, maxilla

       iii. Etiology

          a. Paget disease

          b. Fibrous dysplasia

          c. Radiotherapy

          d. Trauma

          e. Osteochondroma

       iv. Clinical features

          a. Mass (body of mandible, alveolar ridge of maxilla)

          b. Paresthesias

          c. Pain

          d. Loose dentition

       v. Radiologic findings

          a. "Sunburst" appearance (found in 25% of cases)

          b. Osteolysis and osteoblastosis

       vi. Treatment—surgery and chemoradiation

       vii. Prognosis—40% 5-year survival

P. Sarcoidosis

       i. Autoimmune disorder characterized by noncaseating granulomas involving many different organs

      ii. Lungs and lymph nodes are most commonly involved

          a. Cervical adenopathy is the most common head and neck manifestation

     iii. *Heerfordt disease (uveoparotid fever)*: seen in sarcoid patients with uveitis, mild fever, nonsuppurative parotitis, and CN paralysis

     iv. Airway obstruction in sarcoidosis involves the supraglottis

      v. Elevated ACE levels are seen in around 70% of patients with sarcoid

     vi. *Histology*: Schaumann bodies and asteroids within giant cells

    vii. Treatment

          a. Steroids ± methotrexate

Q. Teratomas

      i. Tumors of pluripotent embryonal cells

     ii. Majority recognized by 1 year

    iii. Ten percent occur in the head and neck

          a. Orbital

          b. Nasal

          c. Nasopharynx

          d. Oral cavity

          e. Neck

     iv. Types

          a. Dermoid cyst

              1. Most common

              2. Contains epidermal and mesodermal remnants

              3. Polypoid masses covered with skin and epidermal appendages

                 • In neck, occur in submental region deep to or superficial to mylohyoid membrane

                 • Superficial lesions may be confused with ranulae

              4. May cause obstruction of breathing or deglutition

              5. Excision is the treatment of choice

          b. Teratoid cyst

              1. Composed of all three germ layers

              2. Cystic with an epithelial lining

              3. Differentiation of tissues is minimal

          c. Teratoma

              1. Composed of all three germ layers

              2. Usually solid

              3. Cellular differentiation allows recognition of organ structure

              4. Often fatal

          d. Epignathi

              1. Composed of all three germ layers

              2. Most differentiated of all forms. Complete organs and body parts identifiable

              3. Often arise from midline or lateral basisphenoid and protrude through mouth

              4. Often fatal

R. Giant cells within the tunica media characterize temporal arteritis

S. Eagle syndrome is dysphagia associated with a calcified stylohyoid ligament or an elongated styloid process

      i. Calcified stylohyoid ligament is an incidental finding in about 4% of the normal population

Immunology and Allergy_____

    A. Antibodies
       i. IgA
         a. Found on mucus membranes
         b. Secreted as dimer and circulate as monomer
         c. Many bacteria contain IgA proteases
       ii. IgD: antigen receptor on B cells
       iii. IgE: Type I hypersensitivity, mediates TH-2 responses (allergic reactions)
       iv. IgG
         a. Majority of antibody-based immunity
         b. Placental transmission
         c. Has function both extracellularly and intracellularly
       v. IgM
         a. First antibody seen in response to pathogen
         b. On the surface of B cells
         c. Pentamer
         d. Largest antibody
    B. Hypersensitivities (Gel and Coombs classification)
       i. Type I (atopic)
         a. Results from exposure to a particular antigen
         b. Mediated by IgE
         c. Results in mast cell degranulation and rapid inflammation
         d. *Rhinitis, asthma, angioedema, anaphylaxis*
       ii. Type II (antibody dependent)
         a. Mediated by IgG and IgM antibodies
         b. Antibodies bind antigen and
           1. Form complexes that activate classical pathway, the complement cascade, and membrane attack complex
           2. Act as markers for natural killer cells, which cause cell death
         c. *Hashimoto thyroiditis, pemphigus*
       iii. Type III (immune complex)
         a. Immune complexes of IgG and IgM form in the blood and are deposited in tissues
         b. Activation of classical pathway, complement cascade, and membrane attack complex
         c. *Rheumatoid arthritis, serum sickness*, and *lupus*
       iv. Type IV (cell-mediated/delayed type)
         a. T-cell mediated
         b. Takes 3 days to develop
         c. *Contact dermatitis, temporal arteritis*
    C. Categories of allergic triggers
       i. Inhalants (Pollen, animal dander, molds)
       ii. Ingestants (Foods, medications)
       iii. Injectables (Medications, Insect venom)
       iv. Contactants (Nickel, poison ivy, medications)
    D. Seasons for various classes or pollens:
       i. Trees- Winter and spring, generally February to May
       ii. Grasses- Late spring and summer, generally April to August
       iii. Weeds- Late Summer and fall allergens, generally July to frost

E. Types of specific allergen testing
 i. In vivo (serum testing)
   a. Epicutaneous
     1. Introduction of the antigen into the epidermis only
     2. Include scratch, prick, and puncture tests
     3. Scratch testing has a highest false positive rate
     4. Puncture and prick testing are excellent for screening for presence or absence of allergy to individual allergens
   b. Percutaneous
     1. Introduction of antigen into superficial dermis
     2. Include various intradermal techniques
       • Single dilutional
         (a) Highly sensitive but less specific than prick or puncture testing
       • Intradermal dilutional testing (IDT)
         (a) Formerly known as skin end point titration (SET)
         (b) Is the method most commonly used by otolaryngologist
         (c) Involves the sequential administration of fivefold diluted antigens, beginning with very dilute concentrations and progressively administrating more concentrated antigens until specific response obtained on the skin
         (d) It is highly sensitive, with very low level systemic response
 ii. In vitro testing (RAST technique)
   a. RAST measures the serum level of allergen-specific IgE
     1. It is safe in patients on beta blockers
     2. Provides quantitative assessment of the degree of allergic sensitization
     3. It is more specific than skin testing
   b. Immunotherapy
     1. Process of administrating allergen either subcutaneously or sublingually overtime to induce allergic tolerance and reduction of allergic symptoms.
     2. The goal of immunotherapy shift the T-cell response from a TH1 phenotype to a TH2 phenotype.
     3. It increases specific IgG4 levels for the treated allergen.
     4. It requires at least 3 to 5 years of regular administration for continued benefits.

Genetics

A. Autosomal dominant
 i. One parent is affected.
 ii. Vertical transmission.
 iii. Each offspring has 50% chance of being affected.
 iv. Dominant genes may lack complete penetrance.
B. Autosomal recessive
 i. Each parent is at least a carrier
 ii. Each offspring has 25% chance of being affected
C. X-linked
 i. Never passed from father to son
 ii. Usually affects males, while women are usually carriers

D. Mitochondrial
   i. Inherited through mitochondrial genes, which are transmitted in the cytoplasm of the maternal oocyte
   ii. Can only be transmitted from mother

Antibiotics

A. Classes
   i. *Aminoglycosides*: gentamicin, tobramycin, amikacin, and neomycin
      a. Highly effective against *Pseudomonas*
      b. Ototoxic
   ii. *Carbapenem*: meropenem, imipenem
      a. Broad-spectrum coverage
      b. Used for serious hospital-acquired or mixed infections
   iii. Cephalosporins
      a. *First generation*: cephalexin, cephradine, and cefadroxil
         1. Primarily targeted toward gram-positive (*Streptococcus* and *Staphylococcus*) species
         2. Includes some gram-negatives like *Escherichia coli, Proteus mirabilis*, and *Klebsiella*
      b. *Second generation*: cefuroxime, cefaclor, cefprozil, cefpodoxime, and loracarbef
         1. Good gram-positive coverage and increased coverage for *H influenzae* and *M catarrhalis*
      c. *Third generation*: cefixime, ceftriaxone, ceftazidime, cefotaxime, and cefoperazone
         1. More active against gram-negatives: *H influenzae, M catarrhalis, Neisseria gonorrhoeae, Neisseria meningitidis*
         2. Less active against gram positive and anaerobes
         3. Good CNS penetration
      d. *Fourth generation*: cefepime
         1. Provides the best cephalosporin coverage against *P aeruginosa*
   iv. Clindamycin
      a. Highly effective against gram-positive and anaerobic organisms (ie, *Bacteroides fragilis*)
      b. High concentrations in respiratory tissues, mucus, saliva, and bone
      c. Increases risk for *Clostridium difficile* (treat with oral vancomycin or Flagyl)
   v. Linezolid
      a. Alternative to vancomycin for methicillin-resistant *S aureus* (MRSA)
      b. Can be given orally
   vi. Macrolides (concentrate in phagocytes), poorly effective for mucosal biofilm-mediated infections such as otitis media and sinusitis
      a. Erythromycin
         1. Primarily effective against streptococci, pneumococci, *M catarrhalis*
         2. Also effective against *Mycoplasma, Chlamydia, Legionella*, diphtheria, and pertussis
         3. In combination with sulfa (Pediazole), effective against *H influenzae*
      b. Azithromycin and clarithromycin longer acting and effective for alveolar lung disease

   vii. Metronidazole
      a. Highly effective for obligate anaerobes, protozoa, and oral spirochetes
      b. First-line agent for pseudomembranous colitis
  viii. *Monobactam*: aztreonam
      a. *Aerobic gram-negative coverage: H influenzae, N gonorrhoeae, E coli, Klebsiella, Serratia, Proteus, Pseudomonas*
      b. Increases risk for gram-positive infection unless gram-positive coverage (ie, clindamycin) is added
   ix. Penicillins (beta-lactam family)
      a. Penicillin G and V
         1. *S pyogenes, S pneumoniae*, and actinomycosis
         2. Inactivated by penicillinase
      b. *Antistaphylococcal (penicillinase resistant)*: methicillin, oxacillin, cloxacillin, dicloxacillin, and nafcillin
         1. *S aureus*
         2. MRSA is resistant
      c. Aminopenicillins—ampicillin and amoxicillin
         1. More active against streptococci and pneumococci than penicillin G and V
         2. Includes gram-negatives: *E coli, Proteus*, and *H influenzae*
      d. *Augmented penicillins*: Augmentin and Unasyn
         1. Contain beta-lactamase inhibiting compounds
         2. Restore aminopenicillin activity against *Staphylococcus, H influenzae, M catarrhalis*, and anaerobes
      e. *Antipseudomonal*: ticarcillin with clavulanate (Timentin), piperacillin with tazobactam (Zosyn)
         1. *Pseudomonas, Proteus, E coli, Klebsiella, Enterobacter, Serratia, B fragilis*
         2. Contain beta-lactamase inhibiting compounds
         3. Less effective than aminopenicillins against gram-positive upper respiratory bacteria
    x. *Quinolones*: ciprofloxacin, levofloxacin, ofloxacin, gatifloxacin, moxifloxacin
      a. Active against *Pseudomonas*, significant incidence of tendinopathy, especially when combined with steroids
      b. Respiratory quinolones (levofloxacin, gatifloxacin, and moxifloxacin) add coverage against *Streptococcus, Staphylococcus, H influenzae*, and *M catarrhalis*
      c. Moxifloxacin adds anaerobic coverage
   xi. Tetracyclines
      a. Effective against *Mycoplasma, Chlamydia*, and *Legionella*
      b. Used for acne, traveler's diarrhea, and nonspecific "flu" or atypical pneumonia
      c. Stains tooth-forming enamel and should not be used under age 10 years or in pregnancy
      d. Photosensitivity
   xii. TMP/SMX
      a. Effective adjuvant to immunosuppressive drugs for Wegener granulomatosis
      b. *Pneumocystis carinii*
  xiii. Vancomycin
      a. Good gram-positive coverage including methicillin-resistant *Staphylococcus*.
      b. Ototoxic intravenously (not ototoxic orally).
      c. Oral formulation is second-line agent for pseudomembranous colitis.

B. Antibiotic choices
   i. Otology
      a. *Acute otitis externa*: neomycin, polymyxin, ciprofloxacin, ofloxacin compounds ± steroids
      b. *AOM*: amoxicillin (high dose: 60-80 mg/kg/d)
      c. *Acute coalescent mastoiditis*: vancomycin and ceftriaxone
      d. *CSOM*: quinolone gtts and quinolone (adults), antipseudomonal penicillin or cephalosporin (children)
   ii. Rhinology
      a. *Acute sinusitis*: amoxicillin
      b. *Orbital extension of acute sinusitis*: ceftriaxone or moxifloxacin
   iii. Pharynx, head, neck
      a. Thrush-nystatin or topical azole
      b. *Tonsillitis*: keflex ± flagyl, augmentin (if mononucleosis has been ruled out), clindamycin
      c. *Pharyngitis*: erythromycin, amoxicillin
      d. *Sialadenitis*: augmentin, clindamycin
      e. *Tracheobronchitis*: erythromycin, quinolone
      f. *Epiglottitis*: Unasyn, ceftriaxone
      g. *Croup*: Unasyn, ceftriaxone
      h. *Neck abscess*: clindamycin, Unasyn
      i. *Necrotizing fasciitis*: broad-spectrum antibiotics with anaerobic and aerobic coverage. Penicillin G is one of the classic first-line agents
   iv. Other
      a. *Lyme disease*: tetracycline (adults), penicillin (children)
      b. *Pseudomembranous colitis associated with C difficile*: Flagyl (first line), oral vancomycin (second line)
   v. Preoperative
      a. *Skin*: Kefzol, clindamycin
      b. *Oral/pharyngeal*: Unasyn, clindamycin
      c. *Head and neck procedures*: clindamycin, Unasyn
      d. *Sinus surgery*: clindamycin, Unasyn
      e. *Myringotomy and tube insertion*: ciprofloxacin or ofloxacin gtts

Histology

A. Pathologic findings
   i. *Actinomycosis*: sulfur granules
   ii. Adenoid cystic carcinoma
      a. Cribriform—"Swiss cheese"
      b. Tubular
      c. Solid
   iii. *Allergic fungal sinusitis (AFS)*: Charcot-Leyden crystals
   iv. *Amyloidosis*: apple-green birefringence after staining with Congo red dye
   v. *Aspergillus*: 45 degree branching, septate hyphae when grown on Sabouraud agar
   vi. BCCA
      a. *Nodular*: palisading nuclei

      vii. *Blastomycosis*: pseudoepitheliomatous hyperplasia

     viii. *Cat scratch disease*: Warthin-Starry stain showing pleomorphic gram-negative rods

      ix. *Chordoma*: physaliferous cells

       x. Esthesioneuroblastoma

         a. Homer-Wright rosette

         b. Flexner-Wintersteiner rosette

      xi. *Fungal sinusitis*: stain with methenamine silver

     xii. Granular cell tumor-pseudoepitheliomatous hyperplasia

    xiii. *Hashimoto thyroiditis*: lymphocytic infiltrate, germinal centers, Hürthle cells, follicular atrophy

    xiv. *Hemangiopericytoma*: Zimmerman cells

     xv. *Histiocytosis X*: Birbeck granules (tennis racket-shaped structures) found in Langerhans cells

    xvi. *Histoplasmosis*: epithelioid granulomas, pseudoepitheliomatous hyperplasia

   xvii. *Hodgkin disease*: Reed-Sternberg cells

  xviii. *Ménière disease*: endolymphatic hydrops (bowing of Reissner membrane)

    xix. *Melanoma*: S100, Melan A, HMB 45

     xx. *Meningioma*: psammoma bodies

    xxi. *Necrotizing sialometaplasia*: pseudoepitheliomatous hyperplasia

   xxii. *Pemphigus*: acantholysis and positive Nikolsky sign

  xxiii. *Pleomorphic adenoma*: epithelial, myoepithelial, and stromal elements—"benign mixed tumor"

  xxiv. *P. carinii*: cysts and trophozoites

   xxv. *Rhinoscleroma*: granulation, pseudoepitheliomatous hyperplasia, Russell bodies, and Mikulicz cells

  xxvi. *Sarcoidosis*: Schaumann bodies and asteroids within giant cells

 xxvii. SCCA

         a. *Well differentiated*: squamous cells in cords with intercellular bridges (desmosomes at the electron microscopic level) and keratin pearls

         b. Cytokeratins

         c. *Verrucous carcinoma*: church-spire keratosis and broad rete pegs with pushing margins

xxviii. *Smooth muscle tumors*: vimentin

  xxix. *Syphilis*: endolymphatic hydrops (bowing of Reissner membrane) with mononuclear leukocyte infiltration and osteolytic lesions of the otic capsule

   xxx. Thyroid cancer

         a. *Papillary*: papillae, lack of follicles, large nuclei with prominent nucleoli (Orphan Annie eye), psammoma bodies

         b. *Medullary*: sheets of amyloid-rich cells

  xxxi. *Warthin tumor*: papillary cystadenoma lymphomatosum

 xxxii. *Wegener granulomatosis*: angiocentric, epithelial-type necrotizing granulomas with giant cells and histiocytes

Syndromes/Sequences

   A. *Albright syndrome*: polyostotic fibrous dysplasia, precocious puberty, and café au lait spots

   B. *Alport*: SNHL, renal failure with hematuria, and ocular abnormalities

C. *Arnold-Chiari syndrome*: cerebellar crowding at foramen magnum with cranial neuropathies and hydrocephalus

D. *BCNS*: BCCA, cysts of maxilla and mandible, ocular abnormalities

E. *Branchio-otorenal syndrome*: branchial apparatus abnormalities (clefts, cysts, or fistulas), hearing loss (SNHL, CHL, or mixed) and renal malformations

F. *Cogan syndrome*: interstitial keratitis and Ménière-like attacks of vertigo, ataxia, tinnitus, nausea, vomiting, and hearing loss

G. *Cowden disease*: familial goiter, skin hamartomata, and well-differentiated thyroid carcinoma

H. *Dandy syndrome*: oscillopsia

I. *Gardner syndrome*: familial colonic polyposis, osteomata, soft tissue tumors, and well-differentiated thyroid carcinoma

J. *Gradenigo syndrome*: otorrhea, retro-orbital pain, and lateral rectus palsy

K. *Heerfordt disease (uveoparotid fever)*: seen in sarcoid patients with uveitis, mild fever, nonsuppurative parotitis, and CN paralysis

L. *Jerville-Lange-Nielsen*: SNHL, prolonged QT with syncopal events, and sudden death

M. *Kawasaki disease*: cervical lymphadenopathy, erythema of lips and tongue ("strawberry tongue"), erythema and peeling of hands and feet, rash. Treat with aspirin and gamma-globulin to prevent cardiac complications

N. *Lemierre syndrome*: septic thrombophlebitis of the internal jugular vein resulting in spiking fevers and neck fullness

O. *NF-2*: bilateral acoustic neuromas

P. *Osler-Weber-Rendu syndrome*: hereditary hemorrhagic telangiectasia. Capillary malformations of skin, mucous membranes, brain, liver, and lungs. Commonly have severe and recurrent epistaxis. Check lung and brain MRI

Q. *Pendred*: SNHL, euthyroid goiter. Patients have abnormal perchlorate uptake test

R. *Pierre Robin sequence*: retrognathia, retrodisplacement of the tongue and respiratory compromise. Patients also often have CP

S. *Plummer-Vinson syndrome*: iron deficiency anemia, dysphagia secondary to esophageal webs, hypothyroidism, gastritis, cheilitis, glossitis

T. *Rosai-Dorfman disease*: self-limited, nontender cervical lymphadenopathy

U. *Stickler*: SNHL, flattened facial appearance with Pierre Robin sequence, myopia

V. *Sturge-Weber*: capillary malformation of V_1 distribution with calcification and loss of meninges and cortex. Results in glaucoma and seizures

W. *Treacher-Collins syndrome (mandibulofacial dysostosis)*: CHL, midface hypoplasia, micrognathia, malformed ears, lower lid coloboma, down-slanting eyes

X. *Usher*: SNHL, retinitis pigmentosa ± vestibular symptoms. Most common syndrome to affect the eyes and ears

Y. *Von-Hippel-Lindau disease*: bilateral endolymphatic sac tumors, cavernous hemangiomas (cerebellum, brain stem, retina), renal cell carcinoma

Z. *Von Recklinghausen disease (NF-1)* : Café au lait spots and neurofibromas

AA. *Waardenburg syndrome*: SNHL, vestibular abnormalities, dystopia canthorum, pigmentary changes of the eyes, skin, and hair (ie, white forelock)

Eponyms

A. *Argyle-Robertson pupil*: miotic pupils. Does not contract to light but does to accommodation (suggests syphilis)

B. *Battle sign*: postauricular ecchymosis in the setting of posterior skull base fracture

C. *Bezold abscess*: abscess in digastric groove of SCM

D. *Brown sign*: blanching of glomus tympanicum with positive pneumatoscopic pressure

E. *Crisis of Tumarkin*: drop attacks

F. *Eagle syndrome*: dysphagia associated with a calcified stylohyoid ligament or an elongated styloid process

G. *Furstenberg sign*: encephaloceles expand with crying

H. *Gradenigo syndrome*: otorrhea, retro-orbital pain, and lateral rectus palsy secondary to irritation of CN VI within Dorello canal

I. *Griesinger sign*: edema and tenderness over the mastoid cortex associated with thrombosis of the mastoid emissary vein as a result of lateral sinus thrombosis

J. *Gutman sign*: In the normal individual, lateral pressure over the thyroid cartilage causes an increased voice pitch, whereas anterior pressure causes a decrease. In SLN paralysis, the reverse is true

K. *Hennebert sign*: vertigo with pressure changes

L. *Hitzelberger sign*: numbness of ear canal in response to CN VII injury from acoustic neuroma

M. *Marcus-Gunn pupil*: pupil dilation in response to direct light (afferent pupillary defect). Results from optic nerve injury with decreased afferent input to brain

N. *Marjolin ulcer*: a skin ulceration at the site of an old scar, often from burns, with propensity for malignant degeneration

O. *Meleney ulcer*: associated with *S aureus* and nonhemolytic streptococci

P. *Schwartze sign*: pinkish hue over promontory and oval window niche (represents region of thickened mucosa) in otosclerosis

Q. *Tullio phenomenon*: noise-induced vertigo

Questions

1. The Holman- Miller sign is characteristic of which of the following?

   A. Sinonasal papilloma

   B. Juvenile nasopharyngeal angiofibroma

   C. Cystic fibrosis

   D. Olfactory neuroblastoma

   E. None of the above

2. What is the most common indication for postoperative radiation in patients with tonsil cancer?

   A. T stage

   B. Extracapsular extension

   C. Differentiation

   D. Positive margins

3. An absolute contraindication to cochlear implantation is

   A. Mondini malformation

   B. history of meningitis

   C. Michele aplasia

   D. middle ear cholesteatoma

   E. high jugular bulb

4. The artery of the second branchial arch becomes
   A. posterior inferior cerebellar artery
   B. stapedial artery
   C. superficial temporal vein
   D. superficial temporal artery

5. Which syndrome has X-linked dominant inheritance and frequent glomerulonephritis?
   A. Pendred
   B. Goldenhar
   C. Alport
   D. Apert

Answers to Chapter Questions

CHAPTER 1
1. C
2. B
3. D
4. C
5. B

CHAPTER 2
1. B
2. D
3. D
4. B
5. A

CHAPTER 3
1. B
2. E
3. C
4. C
5. A

CHAPTER 5
1. E
2. C
3. B
4. C
5. B

CHAPTER 6
1. D
2. B

3. D
4. C
5. A

CHAPTER 7
1. C
2. D
3. A
4. A
5. A

CHAPTER 8
1. C
2. C
3. D
4. E
5. C

CHAPTER 9
1. D
2. C
3. C
4. D
5. E

CHAPTER 10
1. E
2. C
3. B
4. C
5. B

CHAPTER 11
1. D
2. A
3. D
4. D
5. C

CHAPTER 12
1. C
2. D
3. E
4. C
5. C

CHAPTER 13
1. B
2. D
3. C
4. B
5. E

CHAPTER 14
1. E
2. D
3. C
4. D
5. B

CHAPTER 15
1. B
2. D
3. D
4. C
5. B

CHAPTER 16
1. A
2. B
3. D
4. D
5. B

CHAPTER 17
1. C
2. C

3. A
4. B
5. B

CHAPTER 18
1. E
2. A
3. C
4. B
5. D

CHAPTER 19
1. D
2. B, D
3. E
4. A
5. C

CHAPTER 20
1. A
2. B
3. E
4. B
5. E

CHAPTER 21
1. C
2. A
3. B
4. C
5. A

CHAPTER 22
1. B
2. D
3. C
4. A
5. B

CHAPTER 23
1. C
2. B
3. B
4. C
5. B

CHAPTER 24
1. B
2. C
3. A
4. C
5. C

CHAPTER 25
1. B
2. A
3. C
4. E
5. D

CHAPTER 26
1. D
2. E
3. C
4. A
5. E

CHAPTER 27
1. C
2. D
3. D
4. B
5. E

CHAPTER 28
1. D
2. D
3. D
4. C
5. E

CHAPTER 29
1. C
2. B
3. B
4. D
5. B

CHAPTER 30
1. C
2. A
3. A
4. E
5. C

CHAPTER 31
1. A
2. B
3. B
4. C
5. D

CHAPTER 32
1. C
2. D
3. B
4. D
5. E

CHAPTER 33
1. A
2. C
3. B
4. A
5. B

CHAPTER 34
1. C
2. D
3. C
4. E
5. D

CHAPTER 35
1. B
2. A
3. C
4. C
5. A

CHAPTER 36

1. A
2. C
3. B
4. C
5. C

CHAPTER 37

1. C
2. A
3. B
4. C
5. D

CHAPTER 38

1. C
2. B
3. E
4. E
5. B

CHAPTER 39

1. E
2. E
3. A
4. C
5. E

CHAPTER 40

1. C
2. D
3. E
4. B
5. D

CHAPTER 41

1. A
2. C
3. C
4. D
5. B

CHAPTER 42

1. D
2. A
3. B
4. C
5. A

CHAPTER 43

1. F
2. D
3. B
4. A
5. B

CHAPTER 44

1. B
2. B
3. C
4. D
5. D

CHAPTER 45

1. C
2. C
3. B
4. D
5. C

CHAPTER 46

1. B
2. B
3. D
4. A
5. C

CHAPTER 47

1. D
2. C
3. A
4. D
5. E

CHAPTER 48
1. C
2. D
3. A
4. B
5. C

CHAPTER 49
1. C
2. A
3. B
4. B
5. E

CHAPTER 50
1. C
2. A
3. D
4. C
5. A

CHAPTER 51
1. C
2. E

3. E
4. G
5. B

CHAPTER 52
1. A
2. B
3. B
4. A
5. B

CHAPTER 53
1. A
2. D
3. E
4. D
5. D

CHAPTER 54
1. B
2. B
3. C
4. B
5. C

Index

Note: Page numbers followed by *f* or *t* represent figures or tables, respectively.